Janeway's immuno biology

10TH EDITION

Kenneth Murphy
Washington University School of Medicine, Saint Louis

Casey Weaver
University of Alabama at Birmingham Heersink School of Medicine

Leslie Berg
University of Colorado Anschutz School of Medicine

With contribution by:
Gregory Barton
University of California, Berkeley

W. W. NORTON & COMPANY
Independent Publishers Since 1923

W. W. Norton & Company
Independent Publishers Since 1923

W. W. Norton & Company has been independent since its founding in 1923, when William Warder Norton and Mary D. Herter Norton first published lectures delivered at the People's Institute, the adult education division of New York City's Cooper Union. The firm soon expanded its program beyond the Institute, publishing books by celebrated academics from America and abroad. By midcentury, the two major pillars of Norton's publishing program—trade books and college texts—were firmly established. In the 1950s, the Norton family transferred control of the company to its employees, and today—with a staff of five hundred and hundreds of trade, college, and professional titles published each year—W. W. Norton & Company stands as the largest and oldest publishing house owned wholly by its employees.

Editors: Betsy Twitchell and Cailin Barrett Bressack
Editorial Advisor: Denise Schanck
Developmental Editor: Judith Kromm
Content Development Specialist: Todd Pearson
Copyeditor: Christopher Curioli
Project Editor: David Bradley
Editorial Assistant: Maggie Stephens
Managing Editor, College: Marian Johnson
Senior Production Manager: Benjamin Reynolds
Media Editor: Kate Brayton
Associate Media Editors: Jasmine Ribeaux and Lexi Malakhoff
Production Manager: Richard Bretan
Media Project Editor: Jesse Newkirk
Media Assistant Editor: Kara Zaborowsky
Managing Editor, College Digital Media: Kim Yi
Ebook Production Manager: Emily Schwoyer
Marketing Manager, Biology: Ruth Bolster
Design Director: Rubina Yeh
Design: Juan Paolo Francisco
Director of College Permissions: Megan Schindel
Permissions Editor: Patricia Wong
Photo Editor: Stephanie Romeo
Composition: Graphic World/Project Manager: Sunil Kumar
Illustrations: Blink Studios/Matthew McClements
Manufacturing: Transcontinental—Beauceville, QC

Permission to use copyrighted material is included on page C-1.

ISBN: 978-0-393-68093-5

W. W. Norton & Company, Inc., 500 Fifth Avenue, New York, NY 10110
wwnorton.com
W. W. Norton & Company Ltd., 15 Carlisle Street, London W1D 3BS

2 3 4 5 6 7 8 9 0

Preface

Since early 2020, the field of immunology has moved to an unexpectedly prominent place in daily life. As SARS-CoV-2 spread around the globe, basic questions about how the immune system combats viruses moved into the forefront of public attention. Why were individual responses to the virus so variable? Why were outcomes in older patients so much more dire than in younger infected individuals? And, most important, how quickly would a vaccine be available, would it provide adequate protection, and for how long? While some questions have been answered, notably observing the most rapid vaccine development in human history, many other questions remain outstanding. Clearly, the need for continued research into basic mechanisms controlling human immunity is undeniable.

Though somewhat overshadowed during the COVID-19 pandemic, there has been a dramatic rise in the use of various other immunotherapies in the years since the last edition of *Janeway's Immunobiology*. Multiple methods for manipulating immune responses have significantly altered the practice of clinical medicine, benefiting patients who present with a diagnosis of cancer, autoimmune disease, or chronic inflammatory disorder. In large part, these clinical advances arose from decades of basic research aimed at uncovering the molecules and pathways that regulate immune cells at steady-state conditions or during infection, inflammation, or autoimmunity.

This Tenth Edition of *Janeway's Immunobiology* strives to carry on Charlie Janeway's legacy of providing a comprehensive, up-to-date textbook focused on the mechanisms underlying the responses to infection. In keeping with this mission, this edition's text and figures have been updated throughout. The immune response to SARS-CoV-2 and the multiple vaccine strategies utilized against this infection are introduced in Chapter 1 and further discussed in Chapters 12, 16, and Appendix I. Chapter 3 now includes a detailed explanation of the mechanism by which mutations in innate sensors of infection can lead to autoimmunity. New developments in the identification of ligands for γδ T cells are highlighted in Chapter 4, and the new cryo-electron microscopy (cryo-EM) structure of the RAG-1:RAG-2 complex bound to DNA is described in Chapter 5. Recently discovered structural features of the peptide-loading machinery for antigen presentation to T cells are included in Chapter 6. The treatment of antigen receptor signaling in Chapter 7 now includes discussion of lymphocyte metabolism, a topic also revisited in the revised Chapters 9 and 11. Additionally, new information in Chapter 7 highlights the pathways targeted by checkpoint blockade immunotherapy and describes the signaling modules used to engineer chimeric antigen receptors (CARs) for cell-based therapies, a topic also elaborated in Chapter 16. The latest findings on T-cell localization and dynamics during priming interactions with dendritic cells are covered in Chapter 9, while Chapter 11 describes new insights into the development and functions of tissue-resident memory T cells. Chapter 12, which focuses on immunity at the barrier surfaces, has undergone a major overhaul and includes an expanded discussion of immune interactions with commensal microorganisms and a detailed discussion of the roles of diverse epithelial cell types in the intestine, respiratory tract, and the skin. Chapter 12 also includes a new section on respiratory virus infections, including influenza and SARS-CoV-2. Chapter 16 brings vaccines to the forefront and includes a detailed discussion of the new vaccine approaches used for SARS-CoV-2 and poliovirus vaccines. The Immunologist's Toolbox (Appendix I) has been updated with new sections on single-cell technologies such as single-cell RNA-seq and lineage-tracing approaches, antigen tetramers for identifying antigen-specific B cells, and parabiosis used to determine lymphocyte tissue residency. Also included in Appendix I is a new description of an analytic technique used to measure antibody responses to SARS-CoV-2 in infected or vaccinated individuals. End-of-chapter study questions have been reworked in the Tenth Edition, and an online learning platform for student self-assessment, InQuizitive, has been created.

We have benefited greatly from the major contribution of Gregory Barton, an expert in innate immune signaling, who has revised and updated Chapter 3. Many additional people deserve special thanks, including our thoughtful colleagues who reviewed the Ninth Edition and provided insights that helped direct revisions in this new edition. We benefited from the eagle-eyed accuracy reviewers who provided feedback on Tenth Edition chapters. All of these individuals are cited in the Acknowledgments section, and we express our gratitude for their efforts.

We have the good fortune to work with an outstanding editorial group at W. W. Norton. We thank Denise Schanck, our editorial advisor, who coordinated the entire project, guiding us gently but firmly back on track throughout the process. We thank Betsy Twitchell, our editor, who contributed her guidance, support, and wisdom. Sincere thanks also go to Judith Kromm, our developmental editor, and Christopher Curioli, our copyeditor, for their insights and attention to detail. As in all previous editions, Matt McClements has contributed his genius—and patience—reinterpreting the authors' sketches into elegant illustrations. Our editing, production, and permissions teams provided their expertise throughout; they are Maggie Stephens, David Bradley, Ben Reynolds, Stephanie Romeo, and Patricia Wong. Our media experts, Kate Brayton, Jasmine Ribeaux, Alexandra Malakhoff, and Kara Zaborowsky, created our excellent supplements package. The authors wish to thank their most important partners—Theresa, Cindy Lou, and Charles—colleagues in life who have supported this effort with their generosity of time, their own editorial insights, and their infinite patience.

We hope this Tenth Edition will continue to inspire students to appreciate immunology's beautiful subtlety—just as Charlie did. We encourage all readers to share with us their views on where we have come up short, so the next edition will further approach the asymptote. Happy reading and learning!

Kenneth Murphy
Casey Weaver
Leslie Berg

What's New in the Tenth Edition

New Coauthor

Janeway's Immunobiology is the premier text for immunology, giving students at all levels a current and authoritative understanding of immunology research. Leslie Berg joins Ken Murphy and Casey Weaver in comprehensively updating the textbook.

New Online Assessment in InQuizitive

InQuizitive for *Janeway's Immunobiology* is an award-winning, adaptive learning tool that gives students personalized learning pathways as they work through the material. Through a variety of question types and answer-specific feedback, students learn the necessary vocabulary to succeed in the immunology course and practice applying that vocabulary to core concepts.

New Norton Teaching Tools Support Classroom Instruction

The Norton Teaching Tools site for *Janeway's Immunobiology* gives instructors ready access to primary literature suggestions for each chapter, active learning activities, lecture PowerPoint files, descriptions of all the animations and videos, and much more.

New Coverage of the COVID-19 Pandemic

COVID-19 coverage has been incorporated in Chapters 1, 12, 16, and Appendix I and is highlighted on the front cover with a new illustration of the novel mRNA vaccination strategy.

Highlights of New Research

Chapter 1:
- Brief introduction to coronavirus, which is then elaborated in later chapters.

Chapter 3:
- Latest research on the Toll-like receptors and cGAS–STING pathway.
- Discussion of mutations in RIG-I, MDA-5, and cGAS–STING pathways that lead to autoimmune disorders.
- Latest information on inflammasome activation and gasdermin pore formation in secretion of inflammatory cytokines.

Chapter 5:
- New cryo-EM structure of the RAG-1:RAG-2 tetrameric complex bound to recombination signal sequences in the DNA.
- Discussion of the latest research on the evolutionary origins of RAG-dependent V(D)J recombination.

Chapter 6:
- Newly discovered structural features of the peptide-loading machinery for TAP and the peptide-loading complex (PLC).

Chapter 7:
- Latest findings on the metabolic impact of antigen receptor stimulation.

- Up-to-date research on immune checkpoint therapy with CTLA-4 and PD-1 blockade.
- New section on chimeric antigen receptors for CAR T-cell cancer immunotherapy (CAR-T therapy).

Chapter 8:
- New discussion of development of ILCs and nonconventional T cells, including regulatory T cells, iNKT cells, and CD8αα intraepithelial lymphocytes.

Chapter 9:
- Addition of new information on dendritic-cell subsets.
- New section on metabolic control of T-cell activation and differentiation.
- Latest developments in spatiotemporal control of T-cell priming by dendritic cells.
- New insights into how IL-2 signaling regulates T-cell differentiation.

Chapter 11:
- New emphasis on the relationship between antibody isotypes and immune effector modules.
- Updates on T_{FH} cells and tissue-resident memory T cells.
- New research on T-cell metabolic reprograming in formation and maintenance of T-cell memory.

Chapter 12:
- Major revision that includes more than 25 new or revised illustrations.
- Detailed discussion of the emergence of the COVID-19 pandemic and basis for viral tropism for host cells.
- Major expansion of discussion of mucosal immunity in the intestines, lungs, and skin.
- Expanded consideration of the interplay of barrier tissues with the commensal microbiota.
- Enhanced treatment of specialized epithelial cell types in barrier tissues, including tuft cells, goblet cells, Paneth cells, enteroendocrine cells, and others.
- Extended treatment of intraepithelial lymphocytes (IELs).
- New section introducing the latest findings in neuroimmune regulation.

Chapter 13:
- Expanded treatment and new figures on HIV/AIDS, including the latest findings on CCR5- and CXCR4-tropic HIV variants and use of combination antiretroviral therapy (cART).
- Latest structural information on broadly neutralizing antibodies against HIV envelope protein.
- Expanded and updated coverage of immune evasion by pathogens, including targeting of complement and interferon pathways.
- New section on viral mechanisms promoting exhaustion of T cells and NK cells.
- Updated research on mechanisms used by viral pathogens to subvert host cytokine and chemokine responses.

Chapter 16:

- Vaccines are brought to the forefront, illustrating new vaccine approaches to COVID-19 and modern vaccine technologies for poliovirus eradication.
- New discussion of checkpoint blockade and CAR T-cell technology for cancer immunotherapy.

Appendix I:

- Multiplex bead assay for flow cytometric analysis of antibody responses and its use to measure serum antibodies to SARS-CoV-2.
- Description of antigen tetramers for identification of antigen-specific B cells.

- New description of parabiosis for analysis of lymphocyte tissue residency.
- New discussion of cell lineage tracing techniques.
- Description of techniques for single-cell molecular analyses.

Resources for Instructors and Students

Instructor Resources

Instructor resources for *Janeway's Immunobiology* are available at wwnorton.com

Art of *Janeway's Immunobiology*, Tenth Edition

All the images from the book are available in both labeled and unlabeled versions in PowerPoint and JPEG formats.

PowerPoint Lecture Slides

The section headings, concept headings, and figures from the text have been integrated into customizable PowerPoint presentations.

InQuizitive

InQuizitive is Norton's award-winning, easy-to-use adaptive learning tool that personalizes the learning experience for students, helping them to master—and retain—key learning objectives. The InQuizitive course for *Janeway's Immunobiology*, Tenth Edition, includes dynamic question types focused on vocabulary and critical thinking, with clickable glossary definitions throughout. Through a variety of question types, answer-specific feedback, and pedagogical elements that promote metacognition, students are motivated to keep working until they've mastered both the concepts and the tough terminology critical to success in the immunology course. As a result, students arrive better prepared for class, giving instructors more time for discussion and activities. Because InQuizitive motivates students to keep working on a chapter until they've mastered the content, assigning it consistently can help improve course performance. A robust activity report makes it easy to identify challenging concepts, and the convenience of learning management system (LMS) integration saves time by allowing InQuizitive scores to report directly to an LMS gradebook.

Norton Teaching Tools

Searchable by chapter, phrase, or topic, the Norton Teaching Tools site is focused on resources for active learning. Each chapter offers primary literature papers with questions for classroom discussion, concept map activities to help students connect and understand complex immunological processes, relevant animations with suggestions on how to integrate them into a course, and more. For instructors looking to seamlessly weave case studies into their course, there are case study companion PowerPoints with integrated clicker questions, which will also be included in *Squarecap*, a next-generation classroom response system that promotes a high level of student engagement in the classroom through quality assessment.

Test Bank

Written by Debby Walser-Kuntz, Samira Aghlara-Fotovat, Omid Veiseh, and Cynthia Leifer, the revised and expanded Test Bank includes more than 900 questions in a variety of question formats. Questions are classified by section and difficulty, making it easy to construct tests and quizzes that are meaningful and diagnostic. Norton Testmaker brings Norton's high-quality testing materials online. Create assessments for a course from anywhere with an Internet connection, without downloading files or installing specialized software. Search and filter Test Bank questions by chapter, question type, difficulty, learning objective, and Bloom's Taxonomy. Instructors can also edit questions or create their own. Then, easily export tests to Microsoft Word or Common Cartridge files for import into an LMS.

Resources for an LMS

Easily add high-quality Norton digital resources to an online, hybrid, or lecture course. Get started building a course with our easy-to-use integrated resources; all activities can be accessed right within an existing learning management system.

Student Resources

Student resources for *Janeway's Immunobiology* are available at digital.wwnorton.com/janeway10

Ebook for *Janeway's Immunobiology*

Norton Ebooks offer an enhanced reading experience at a fraction of the cost of a print textbook. They provide an active reading experience, enabling students to take notes, bookmark, search, highlight, and even read offline. Students can access the animations directly from the ebook, and clickable key terms are linked to their definitions. Instructors can even add notes that students see as they read the text. Norton Ebooks can be viewed on—and synced across—all computers and mobile devices and can be made available for offline reading.

Case Studies in Immunology, Seventh Edition Ebook 📋

by Raif Geha and Luigi Notarangelo

Case Studies in Immunology: A Clinical Companion presents major topics of immunology through a selection of clinical cases that reinforce and extend the basic science. Each case history is preceded by essential scientific facts about the immunological mechanisms of that specific disorder. The cases themselves demonstrate how immunological problems are deconstructed in the clinic, and each one is followed by a concise summary of the clinical finding with questions that serve as discussion points. Cases are color coded to correspond to *Janeway's Immunobiology*, allowing instructors to easily find cases that complement the material in the main text. In *Janeway's Immunobiology*, diseases covered in *Case Studies* are indicated by an icon in the margin. Access to the *Case Studies in Immunology* ebook is free with every purchase of *Janeway's Immunobiology*, Tenth Edition. It is also available for purchase separately.

Animations

A set of more than three dozen animations covers some of the most important immunology concepts, such as innate recognition of pathogens, V(D)J recombination, TCR signaling, and many more. Animation-based questions in InQuizitive allow students to practice their understanding of the information presented in the animations, while links to animations in the ebook help bring these topics to life as the student reads.

Acknowledgments

We thank our spouses, families, friends, and colleagues for their continuing patience and support, without which the writing of this new edition of our textbook would not be possible. As always, we are also indebted to a large number of scientists whose generous help has been essential for making the text as clear, up to date, and accurate as possible.

Deserving special credit is Gregory Barton (University of California, Berkeley), who accepted the task of drafting Chapter 3.

In what follows, we aim to acknowledge and thank the scientists whose suggestions for the text have helped us to prepare this edition.

Chapter 1: Kenneth Frauwirth (University of Maryland), Stephen Jameson (University of Minnesota), Michael Roner (University of Texas at Arlington).

Chapter 2: Kenneth Frauwirth (University of Maryland), Teizo Fujita (Fukushima Medical University), Lora Hooper (University of Texas, Southwestern), John Hourcade (Washington University at Saint Louis), Stephen Jameson (University of Minnesota), Thomas Langmann (University of Cologne), Jenna Macciochi (University of Sussex), Rodney Newberry (University of Washington at Saint Louis), Shanna Nifoussi (University of Wisconsin–Superior), Michael Roner (University of Texas at Arlington), Frederick Sheedy (Trinity College Dublin), Kiyoshi Takeda (Osaka University Medical School), Andrea Tenner (University of California, Irvine).

Chapter 3: Mary Dinauer (Washington University at Saint Louis), Shanna Nifoussi (University of Wisconsin–Superior), David Raulet (University of California, Berkeley), Caetano Reis e Sousa (Cancer Research UK), Michael Roner (University of Texas at Arlington), Frederick Sheedy (Trinity College Dublin), Joseph Sun (Memorial Sloan Kettering Cancer Center), Tada Taniguchi (University of Tokyo), Eric Vivier (Centre d'Immunologie de Marseille–Luminy).

Chapter 4: Bob Brennan (University of Central Oklahoma), Kenneth Frauwirth (University of Maryland), K. Christopher Garcia (Stanford University School of Medicine), Paul Klenerman (Nuffield Department of Medicine, University of Oxford), Ellis Reinherz (Dana Farber Cancer Institute, Boston), Michael Roner (University of Texas at Arlington), Robyn Stanfield (The Scripps Research Institute).

Chapter 5: Bob Brennan (University of Central Oklahoma), Martin Flajnik (University of Maryland School of Medicine), Kenneth Frauwirth (University of Maryland), Paul Klenerman (Nuffield Department of Medicine, University of Oxford), Michael Krangel (Duke University School of Medicine), Michael Lieber (Keck School of Medicine, University of Southern California), Eugene Oltz (The Ohio State University), Michael Roner (University of Texas at Arlington), David Schatz (Yale School of Medicine).

Chapter 6: Peter Cresswell (Yale School of Medicine), Kenneth Frauwirth (University of Maryland), Dale Godfrey (University of Melbourne), Mitchell Kronenberg (La Jolla Institute for Immunology), Jacques Neefjes (Leiden University), Hans-Georg Rammansee (University of Tübingen), Kenneth Rock (University of Massachusetts Medical School), Michael Roner (University of Texas at Arlington), Natalie C. Steinel (University of Massachusetts Lowell), Jose Villadangos (University of Melbourne), Kai Wucherpfennig (Dana Farber Cancer Center).

Chapter 7: Michael Dustin (University of Oxford), Kenneth Frauwirth (University of Maryland), Lawrence Kane (University of Pittsburgh), Susan Pierce (National Institutes of Health), Hans-Georg Rammansee (University of Tübingen), Michael Roner (University of Texas at Arlington), Lawrence Samelson (National Cancer Institute), Andrey Shaw (Genentech), Natalie C. Steinel (University of Massachusetts Lowell), Arthur Weiss (University of California, San Francisco), Kai Wucherpfennig (Dana Farber Cancer Center), Rose Zamoyska (The University of Edinburgh).

Chapter 8: Michael Cancro (University of Pennsylvania School of Medicine), Kenneth Frauwirth (University of Maryland), Fotini Gounari (University of Chicago), Eric Huseby (University of Massachusetts Medical School), Kristin Hogquist (University of Minnesota Medical School), Joonsoo Kang (University of Massachusetts Medical School), Barbara Kee (University of Chicago), Bernard Malissen (Centre d' Immunologie de Marseille–Luminy), Diane Mathis (Harvard University), Kees Murre (University of California, San Diego), Hans-Georg Rammansee (University of Tübingen), Ellen Robey (University of California, Berkeley), Michael Roner (University of Texas at Arlington), Ellen Rothenberg (California Institute of Technology), Natalie C. Steinel (University of Massachusetts Lowell).

Chapter 9: Francis Carbone (University of Melbourne), Kenneth Frauwirth (University of Maryland), Laurie Harrington (University of Alabama at Birmingham Heersink School of Medicine), Bill Heath (University of Melbourne), Marc Jenkins (University of Minnesota Medical School), Stephanie Justice-Bitner (King's College), David Masopust (University of Minnesota Medical School), K. Kai McKinstry (University of Central Florida), James Moon (Massachusetts General Hospital), John O'Shea (National Institutes of Health), Esperanza Perucha (King's College London), Tania Watts (University of Toronto).

Chapter 10: Deepta Battacharya (The University of Arizona), John Cambier (University of Colorado School of Medicine), Michael Cancro (University of Pennsylvania School of Medicine), Marcus Clark (University of Chicago Medicine), Kenneth Frauwirth (University of Maryland), Christopher Goodnow (Garvan Institute of Medical Research), Ann Haberman (Yale University), John Kearney (University of Alabama at Birmingham Heersink School of Medicine), Stephanie Justice-Bitner (King's College), K. Kai McKinstry (University of Central Florida), David Tarlinton (Monash University), Gabriel Victora (The Rockefeller University).

Chapter 11: Kenneth Frauwirth (University of Maryland), Michael Gerner (University of Washington), Stephanie Justice-Bitner (King's College), Susan Kaech (Yale School of Medicine), David Masopust (University of Minnesota Medical School), Matthew Pipkin (The Scripps Research, Florida), Stephen McSorley (University of California, Davis, Veterinary Medicine), Dean T. Nardelli (University of Wisconsin–Milwaukee), John O'Shea (National Institutes of Health),

Gregory Sonnenberg (Weill Cornell Medicine), Sing Sing Way (Cincinnati Children's Hospital), Allan Zajac (University of Alabama at Birmingham Heersink School of Medicine).

Chapter 12: Richard Blumberg (Brigham and Women's Hospital, Harvard University), Kenneth Frauwirth (University of Maryland), Gunjan Gakhar (Washington State University Vancouver), Gunnar Hansson (University of Gothenburg), Lora Hooper (UT Southwestern Medical Center), Alessio Iannetti (Newcastle University), Stephen Jameson (University of Minnesota), Tom MacDonald (Blizard Institute–Barts and The London), Daniel Mucida (The Rockefeller University), Rodney Newberry (Washington University at Saint Louis), Dana Philpott (University of Toronto), Maria Rescigno (Humanitas University), Michael Roner (University of Texas at Arlington), Michael Russell (State University of New York, Buffalo), Phillip Smith (University of Alabama at Birmingham Heersink School of Medicine), Ramnik Xavier (Broad Institute).

Chapter 13: Shizuo Akira (Osaka University), Mary Collins (Okinawa Institute of Science and Technology), Kenneth Frauwirth (University of Maryland), Paul Goepfert (University of Alabama at Birmingham Heersink School of Medicine), Stephanie Justice-Bitner (King's College), Paul Klenerman (Nuffield Department of Medicine, University of Oxford), Scott Laster (North Carolina State University), Jordan Orange (Columbia University College of Physicians and Surgeons), Sarah L. Rowland-Jones (Nuffield Department of Medicine, University of Oxford), Tara Strutt (University of Central Florida).

Chapter 14: Cezmi Akdis (Swiss Institute of Allergy and Asthma Research), Larry Borish (University of Virginia Health), Joseph Dolence (University of Nebraska at Kearney), Kenneth Frauwirth (University of Maryland), Stephanie Justice-Bitner (King's College), Daniel Kaplan (University of Pittsburgh), Barry Kay (Deceased, Imperial College London), Brian Kim (Washington University at Saint Louis), Cathryn Nagler (University of Chicago), Steven Van Dyken (Washington University at Saint Louis), Marsha Wills-Karp (Johns Hopkins University).

Chapter 15: Robert Fairchild (Cleveland Clinic), Kenneth Frauwirth (University of Maryland), Rikard Holmdahl (Karolinska Institute), Stephanie Justice-Bitner (King's College).

Chapter 16: Tanya R. DaSylva (York University), Kenneth Frauwirth (University of Maryland), Stephanie Justice-Bitner (King's College), Joseph Larkin (University of Florida), Ken Nally (School of Biochemistry and Cell Biology, University College Cork).

Appendix I: Kenneth Frauwirth (University of Maryland), Stephanie Justice-Bitner (King's College), Lawrence Stern (University of Massachusetts Medical School), Ross Kedl (University of Colorado Anschutz School of Medicine).

We thank those scientists who were instrumental in writing and reviewing the media supplements accompanying this edition:

Samira Aghlara-Fotovat (Rice University), Paul Allen (Washington University School of Medicine), Nancy Bigley (Wright State University), William Carr (Medgar Evers College), Liliana Clemenza (University of Toronto), Maurizio Costabile (University of South Australia), Tanya R. DaSylva (York University), Mark Drew (The Ohio State University), Kenneth Frauwirth (University of Maryland), Rachel Gerstein (University of Massachusetts Medical School), Deanna Gibson (University of British Columbia), Demelza Ireland (University of Western Australia), Nuran Kumbaraci (Stevens Institute of Technology), Cynthia Leifer (Cornell University), Alan Levine (Case Western Reserve University), Adam Matthews (Wellesley College), Yanice Mendez (University of New Haven), Esperanza Perucha (King's College London), Nicholas Pullen (University of Northern Colorado), Stuart Ray (Johns Hopkins University School of Medicine), Amy Stone (Touro University Nevada), Courtney Sulentic (Wright State University), Alexander Tsygankov (Lewis Katz School of Medicine, Temple University), Omid Veiseh (Rice University), Debby Walser-Kuntz (Carleton College).

About the Authors

Kenneth Murphy is the Eugene Opie First Centennial Professor in the Department of Pathology & Immunology, Washington University School of Medicine in St. Louis. His research focuses on how the immune system selects the correct type of response appropriate for eliminating different kinds of pathogens.

Casey Weaver is the Wyatt and Susan Haskell Chair of Medical Excellence in the Department of Pathology at the University of Alabama at Birmingham Heersink School of Medicine. His research is focused on mechanisms by which CD4 T cells diverge along different developmental paths and how these cells contribute to host defense or are dysregulated in immune-mediated disease.

Leslie Berg is Professor and Chair of the Department of Immunology & Microbiology at the University of Colorado Anschutz School of Medicine. Her research focuses on understanding T-cell receptor signaling and how variations in T-cell receptor signal strength regulate T-cell development, activation, and effector-cell differentiation.

Contents in Brief

Detailed Contents

PART V THE IMMUNE SYSTEM IN HEALTH AND DISEASE

Chapter 13   Failures of Host Defense Mechanisms   587

APPENDICES

Note: Appendices II–IV are available on digital.wwnorton
.com/janeway10 and in the ebook.

Basic Concepts in Immunology

1

Immunology is the study of the body's defense against infection. We are continually exposed to microorganisms, many of which cause disease, and yet become ill only rarely. How does the body defend itself? When infection does occur, how does the body eliminate the invader and cure itself? And why do we develop long-lasting immunity to many infectious diseases encountered once and overcome? These are the questions addressed by immunology, which we study to understand our body's defenses against infection at the cellular and molecular levels.

The beginning of immunology as a science is usually attributed to Edward Jenner for his work in the late 18th century (**Fig. 1.1**). The notion of immunity—that surviving a disease confers greater protection against it later—was known since ancient Greece. **Variolation**—the inhalation or transfer into superficial skin wounds of material from smallpox pustules—had been practiced since at least the 1400s in the Middle East and China as a form of protection against that disease and was known to Jenner. Jenner had observed that the relatively mild disease of cowpox seemed to confer protection against the often fatal disease of smallpox, and in 1796, he demonstrated that inoculation with cowpox protected the recipient against smallpox. His scientific proof relied on the deliberate exposure of the inoculated individual to infectious smallpox material 2 months after inoculation. This scientific test was his original contribution.

Jenner called the procedure **vaccination**. This term is still used to describe the inoculation of healthy individuals with weakened or attenuated strains of disease-causing agents in order to provide protection from disease. Although Jenner's bold experiment was successful, it took almost two centuries for smallpox vaccination to become universal. This advance enabled the World Health Organization to announce in 1980 that smallpox had been eradicated (**Fig. 1.2**), arguably the greatest triumph of modern medicine.

Jenner's strategy of vaccination was extended in the late 19th century by the discoveries of many great microbiologists. Robert Koch proved that infectious diseases are caused by specific microorganisms. In the 1880s, Louis Pasteur

IN THIS CHAPTER

The origins of vertebrate immune cells.

Principles of innate immunity.

Principles of adaptive immunity.

The effector mechanisms of immunity.

Fig. 1.1 Edward Jenner. Portrait by John Raphael Smith.

Fig. 1.2 The eradication of smallpox by vaccination. After a period of 3 years in which no cases of smallpox were recorded, the World Health Organization was able to announce in 1980 that smallpox had been eradicated, and vaccination stopped (upper panel). A few laboratory stocks have been retained, however, and some fear that these are a source from which the virus might reemerge. Ali Maow Maalin (lower panel) contracted and survived the last case of smallpox in Somalia in 1977.

devised a vaccine against cholera in chickens and also developed a rabies vaccine that proved to be a spectacular success upon its first trial in a boy bitten by a rabid dog.

These practical triumphs led to a search for vaccination's mechanism of protection and to the development of the science of immunology. In the early 1890s, Emil von Behring and Shibasaburo Kitasato discovered that the serum of animals immune to diphtheria or tetanus contained a specific 'antitoxic activity' that could confer short-lived protection against the effects of diphtheria or tetanus toxins in unimmunized animals and people. This activity was later determined to be due to the proteins we now call **antibodies**, which bind specifically to the toxins and neutralize their activity. That these antibodies might have a crucial role in immunity was reinforced by Jules Bordet's discovery in 1899 of **complement**, a component of serum that acts in conjunction with antibodies to destroy pathogenic bacteria.

A specific response against infection by potential pathogens, such as the production of antibodies against a particular pathogen, is known as **adaptive immunity**, because it develops during the lifetime of an individual as an adaptation to infection with that pathogen. Adaptive immunity is distinguished from **innate immunity**, which—at the time von Behring was developing serum therapy for diphtheria—was already known chiefly through the work of the great Russian immunologist Élie Metchnikoff, who discovered that many microorganisms could be engulfed and digested by phagocytic cells, which thus provide defenses against infection that are nonspecific. Whereas these cells—which Metchnikoff called 'macrophages'—are always present and ready to act, adaptive immunity requires time to develop but is highly specific.

It was soon clear that specific antibodies could be induced against a vast range of substances called **antigens** because they could stimulate *anti*body *gen*eration. Paul Ehrlich advanced the development of an **antiserum** as a treatment for diphtheria and developed methods to standardize therapeutic serums. Today the term 'antigen' refers to any substance recognized by the adaptive immune system. Typically antigens are common proteins, glycoproteins, and polysaccharides of pathogens, but they can include a much wider range of chemical structures; for example, metals such as nickel, drugs such as penicillin, and organic chemicals such as the urushiol (a mix of pentadecyl-catechols) in the leaves of poison ivy. Metchnikoff and Ehrlich shared the 1908 Nobel Prize for their respective work on immunity.

This chapter introduces the principles of innate immunity and adaptive immunity, the cells of the immune system, the tissues in which they develop, and the tissues through which they circulate. We then outline the specialized functions of the different types of cells by which they eliminate infection.

The origins of vertebrate immune cells.

The body is protected from infectious agents, their toxins, and the damage they cause by a variety of effector cells and molecules that together make up the **immune system**. Both innate and adaptive immune responses depend on the activities of white blood cells, or **leukocytes**. Most cells of the immune system arise from the **bone marrow**, where many of them develop and mature. But some, particularly certain tissue-resident macrophage and lymphocyte populations (for example, the microglia of the central nervous system), originate from the yolk sac or fetal liver during embryonic development. They seed tissues before birth and are maintained throughout life as independent, self-renewing populations.

After birth, all the cellular elements of blood, including the red blood cells that transport oxygen, the platelets that trigger blood clotting in damaged tissues, and the white blood cells of the immune system, ultimately derive from the **hematopoietic stem cells (HSCs)** of the bone marrow. Because these can give rise to all the different types of blood cells, they are often known as **pluripotent** (or multipotent) hematopoietic stem cells. The hematopoietic stem cells give immediate rise to cells of more limited developmental potential, which are the progenitors of red blood cells, platelets, and the two main categories of white blood cells, the **lymphoid** and **myeloid** lineages. Once mature, immune cells reside within peripheral tissues, circulate in the bloodstream, or circulate in a specialized system of vessels called the **lymphatic system**. The lymphatic system drains extracellular fluid and immune cells from tissues and transports them as **lymph**, which is eventually emptied back into the blood system. The different types of blood cells and their lineage relationships are summarized in **Fig. 1.3**.

Principles of innate immunity.

In this part of the chapter we will outline the principles of innate immunity and describe the molecules and cells that provide continuous defense against invasion by pathogens. Although a subset of white blood cells, known as **lymphocytes**, possesses the most powerful ability to recognize and target pathogenic microorganisms, these cells need the participation of the innate immune system to initiate and mount their offensive. Indeed, the adaptive immune response and the innate immune response use many of the same destructive mechanisms to eliminate invading microorganisms.

1-1 Commensal organisms cause little host damage while pathogens damage host tissues by a variety of mechanisms.

We recognize four broad categories of disease-causing microorganisms, or **pathogens: viruses, bacteria** and archaea, **fungi**, and the unicellular and multicellular eukaryotic organisms collectively termed **parasites** (Fig. 1.4). These microorganisms vary tremendously in size and in how they damage host tissues. The smallest are viruses, which range from five to a few hundred nanometers in size and are obligate intracellular pathogens. Viruses can kill cells directly by inducing lysis during viral replication. Somewhat larger are intracellular bacteria and mycobacteria. These can kill cells directly or damage cells by producing toxins. Many single-celled intracellular parasites, such as members of the *Plasmodium* genus that cause malaria, also directly kill infected cells. Pathogenic bacteria and fungi growing in extracellular spaces can induce shock and sepsis by releasing toxins into the blood or tissues. The largest pathogens—parasitic worms, or helminths—are too large to infect host cells but can injure tissues by forming cysts that induce damaging cellular responses in the tissues into which the worms migrate.

Not all microbes are pathogens. Many tissues, especially those at the barriers of the body, such as the skin, oral mucosa, conjunctiva, and gastrointestinal tract, are constantly colonized by microbial communities—called the **microbiome**—that consist of archaea, bacteria, and fungi but cause no damage to the host. These are also called **commensal microorganisms**, because they can have a **symbiotic** relationship with the host. Indeed, some commensal organisms perform important functions, as in the case of the bacteria that aid in cellulose digestion in the stomachs of ruminants. The difference between commensal organisms and pathogens lies in whether they induce damage. Even enormous numbers of microbes in the intestinal microbiome normally cause no damage and are confined within the intestinal lumen by a protective

Fig. 1.3 All the cellular elements of the blood, including the cells of the immune system, arise from multipotent hematopoietic stem cells in the bone marrow. These multipotent cells divide to produce two types of stem cells. A common lymphoid progenitor gives rise to the lymphoid lineage (blue background) of white blood cells, or leukocytes—the innate lymphoid cells (ILCs) and natural killer (NK) cells and the T and B lymphocytes. A common myeloid progenitor gives rise to the myeloid lineage (pink and yellow backgrounds), which comprises the rest of the leukocytes, the erythrocytes (red blood cells), and the megakaryocytes that produce platelets important in blood clotting. T and B lymphocytes are distinguished from the other leukocytes by having antigen receptors and from each other by their sites of differentiation—the thymus and bone marrow, respectively. After encounter with antigen, B cells differentiate into antibody-secreting plasma cells, while

T cells differentiate into effector T cells with a variety of functions. Unlike T and B cells, ILCs and NK cells lack antigen specificity. The remaining leukocytes are the monocytes, the dendritic cells, and the neutrophils, eosinophils, and basophils. The last three of these circulate in the blood and are termed granulocytes, because of the cytoplasmic granules whose staining gives these cells a distinctive appearance in blood smears, or polymorphonuclear leukocytes, because of their irregularly shaped nuclei. Immature dendritic cells (yellow background) are phagocytic cells that enter the tissues; they mature after they have encountered a potential pathogen. The majority of dendritic cells are derived from the common myeloid progenitor cells, but some may also arise from the common lymphoid progenitor. Monocytes enter tissues, where they differentiate into phagocytic macrophages or dendritic cells. Mast cells also enter tissues and complete their maturation there.

Fig. 1.4 Pathogens vary greatly in size and lifestyle. Intracellular pathogens include viruses, such as herpes simplex (first panel), and various bacteria, such as *Listeria monocytogenes* (second panel). Many bacteria, such as *Staphylococcus aureus* (third panel), or fungi, such as *Aspergillus fumigatus* (fourth panel), can grow in the extracellular spaces and directly invade tissues, as do some archaea and protozoa (third panel). Many parasites, such as the nematode *Strongyloides stercoralis* (fifth panel), are large multicellular organisms that can move throughout the body in a complex life cycle.

layer of mucus, whereas pathogenic bacteria can penetrate this barrier, injure intestinal epithelial cells, and spread into the underlying tissues.

1-2 Anatomic and chemical barriers are the first defense against pathogens.

The host can adopt three strategies to deal with the threat posed by microbes: **avoidance**, **resistance**, and **tolerance**. Avoidance mechanisms prevent exposure to microbes and include both anatomic barriers and behavior modifications. If an infection is established, resistance is aimed at reducing or eliminating pathogens. To defend against the great variety of microbes, the immune system has numerous molecular and cellular functions, collectively called mediators, or **effector mechanisms**, suited to resist different categories of pathogens. Their description is a major aspect of this book. Finally, tolerance involves responses that enhance a tissue's capacity to resist damage induced by microbes. This meaning of the term 'tolerance' has been used extensively in the context of disease susceptibility in plants rather than animal immunity. For example, increasing growth by activating dormant meristems, the undifferentiated cells that generate new parts of the plant, is a common tolerance mechanism in response to damage. This should be distinguished from the term **immunological tolerance**, which refers to mechanisms that prevent an immune response from being mounted against the host's own tissues.

Anatomic and chemical barriers are the initial defenses against infection (**Fig. 1.5**). The skin and mucosal surfaces represent a kind of avoidance strategy that prevents exposure of internal tissues to microbes. At most anatomic barriers, additional resistance mechanisms further strengthen host defenses. For example, mucosal surfaces produce a variety of **antimicrobial proteins** that act as natural antibiotics to prevent microbes from entering the body.

If these barriers are breached or evaded, other components of the innate immune system can immediately come into play. We mentioned earlier the discovery by Jules Bordet of complement, which acts with antibodies to lyse bacteria. Complement is a group of around 30 different plasma proteins that act together and are one of the most important effector mechanisms in serum and interstitial tissues. Complement not only acts in conjunction with antibodies but can also target foreign organisms in the absence of a specific antibody; thus it contributes to both innate and adaptive responses. We will examine anatomic barriers, the antimicrobial proteins, and complement in greater detail in Chapter 2.

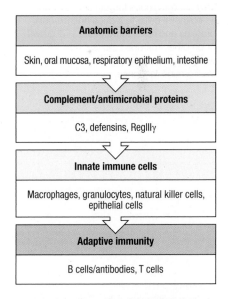

Fig. 1.5 Protection against pathogens relies on several levels of defense. The first is the anatomic barrier provided by the body's epithelial surfaces. Second, various chemical and enzymatic systems, including complement, act as an immediate antimicrobial barrier near these epithelia. If epithelia are breached, various nearby innate lymphoid and myeloid cells can coordinate a rapid cell-mediated defense. If the pathogen overcomes these barriers, the slower-acting defenses of the adaptive immune system are brought to bear.

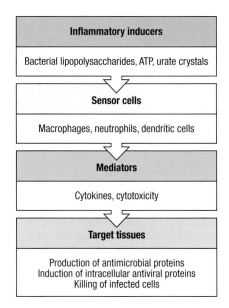

Fig. 1.6 Cell-mediated immunity proceeds in a series of steps. Inflammatory inducers are chemical structures that indicate the presence of invading microbes or the cellular damage produced by them. Sensor cells detect these inducers by their various innate recognition receptors and in response produce a variety of inflammatory mediators that act directly in defense or that further propagate the immune response. The mediators include many cytokines, and they act on various target tissues (such as epithelial cells) to induce antimicrobial proteins and resist intracellular viral growth or on other immune cells (such as ILCs), which produce other cytokines that amplify the immune response.

1-3 The immune system is activated by inflammatory inducers that indicate the presence of pathogens or tissue damage.

A pathogen that breaches the host's anatomic and chemical barriers will encounter the cellular defenses of innate immunity. Cellular immune responses are initiated when various types of **sensor cells** detect **inflammatory inducers** (Fig. 1.6) through their many **innate recognition receptors**, which are encoded by a relatively small number of genes that remain constant over an individual's lifetime. Inflammatory inducers that trigger these receptors include molecular components unique to bacteria or viruses, such as bacterial lipopolysaccharides, or molecules such as ATP, which is not normally found in the extracellular space. Triggering these receptors can activate the innate immune sensor cells to produce various **inflammatory mediators** that either act directly to destroy invading microbes or act on other cells to propagate the immune response. For example, macrophages can ingest microbes and produce toxic chemical mediators, such as degradative enzymes or reactive oxygen intermediates, to kill them. Dendritic cells may produce cytokine mediators, including many cytokines that activate target tissues, such as epithelial or other immune cells, to resist or kill invading microbes more efficiently. We will discuss these receptors and mediators briefly below and in much greater detail in Chapter 3.

Innate immune responses occur rapidly on exposure to an infectious organism (Fig. 1.7). In contrast, responses by the adaptive immune system take days rather than hours to develop. However, the adaptive immune system is capable of eliminating infections more efficiently because of the exquisite specificity of antigen recognition by its lymphocytes. In contrast to a limited repertoire

Phases of the immune response			
Response		**Typical time after infection to start of response**	**Duration of response**
Innate immune response	Inflammation, complement activation, phagocytosis, and destruction of pathogen	Minutes	Days
Adaptive immune response	Interaction between antigen-presenting dendritic cells and antigen-specific T cells: recognition of antigen, adhesion, co-stimulation, T-cell proliferation and differentiation	Hours	Days
	Activation of antigen-specific B cells	Hours	Days
	Formation of effector and memory T cells	Days	Weeks
	Interaction of T cells with B cells, formation of germinal centers. Formation of effector B cells (plasma cells) and memory B cells. Production of antibody	Days	Weeks
	Emigration of effector lymphocytes from peripheral lymphoid organs	A few days	Weeks
	Elimination of pathogen by effector cells and antibody	A few days	Weeks
Immunological memory	Maintenance of memory B cells and T cells and high serum or mucosal antibody levels. Protection against reinfection	Days to weeks	Can be lifelong

Fig. 1.7 Phases of the immune response.

of receptors expressed by innate immune cells, lymphocytes express highly specialized **antigen receptors** that collectively possess a vast repertoire of specificity. This enables the adaptive immune system to respond to virtually any pathogen and effectively focus resources to eliminate pathogens that have evaded or overwhelmed innate immunity. But the adaptive immune system interacts with, and relies on, cells of the innate immune system for many of its functions. The next several sections will introduce the major components of the innate immune system and prepare us to consider adaptive immunity later in the chapter.

1-4 The myeloid lineage comprises most of the cells of the innate immune system.

The **common myeloid progenitor (CMP)** is the precursor of the macrophages, granulocytes (the collective term for the white blood cells called neutrophils, eosinophils, and basophils), mast cells, and dendritic cells of the innate immune system. Macrophages, granulocytes, and dendritic cells make up the three classes of phagocytes in the immune system. The CMP also generates megakaryocytes and red blood cells, which will not concern us here. The cells of the myeloid lineage are shown in **Fig. 1.8**.

Macrophages are resident in almost all tissues. Many tissue-resident macrophages arise during embryonic development, but some macrophages that arise from the bone marrow in the adult animal are the mature form of **monocytes**, which circulate in the blood and continually migrate into tissues, where they differentiate. Macrophages are relatively long-lived cells and perform several different functions throughout the innate immune response and the subsequent adaptive immune response. One is to engulf and kill invading microorganisms. This phagocytic function provides a first defense in innate immunity. Macrophages also dispose of pathogens and infected cells targeted by an adaptive immune response. Both monocytes and macrophages are phagocytic, but most infections occur in the tissues, and so it is primarily macrophages that perform this important protective function. An additional and crucial role of macrophages is to orchestrate immune responses: they help induce inflammation, which, as we shall see, is a prerequisite to a successful immune response, and they produce many inflammatory mediators that activate other immune-system cells and recruit them into an immune response.

Local inflammation and the phagocytosis of invading bacteria can also be triggered by the activation of complement. Bacterial surfaces can activate the complement system, inducing a cascade of proteolytic reactions that coat the microbes with fragments of specific proteins of the complement system. Microbes coated in this way are recognized by specific **complement receptors** on macrophages and neutrophils, taken up by phagocytosis, and destroyed.

Fig. 1.8 Myeloid cells in innate and adaptive immunity. In the rest of the book, these cells will be represented in the schematic form shown on the left. A photomicrograph of each cell type is shown on the right. Macrophages and neutrophils are primarily phagocytic cells that engulf pathogens and destroy them in intracellular vesicles, a function they perform in both innate and adaptive immune responses. Dendritic cells are phagocytic when they are immature and can take up pathogens; after maturing, they function as specialized cells that present pathogen antigens to T lymphocytes in a form they can recognize, thus activating T lymphocytes and initiating adaptive immune responses. Macrophages can also present antigens to T lymphocytes and can activate them. The other myeloid cells are primarily secretory cells that release the contents of their prominent granules upon activation via antibody during an adaptive immune response. Eosinophils are thought to be involved in attacking large antibody-coated parasites such as worms; basophils are also thought to be involved in anti-parasite immunity. Mast cells are tissue cells that trigger a local inflammatory response to antigen by releasing substances that act on local blood vessels. Mast cells, eosinophils, and basophils are also important in allergic responses. Original magnification ×15,000.

Macrophage

Phagocytosis and activation of bactericidal mechanisms
Antigen presentation and cytokine production

Dendritic cell

Antigen uptake in peripheral sites
Antigen presentation and cytokine production

Neutrophil

Phagocytosis and activation of bactericidal mechanisms

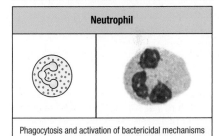

Eosinophil

Killing of antibody-coated parasites

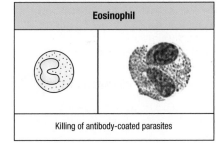

Basophil

Promotion of allergic responses and augmentation of anti-parasitic immunity

Mast cell

Release of granules containing histamine and active agents

In addition to their specialized role in the immune system, macrophages act as general scavenger cells in the body, clearing it of dead cells and cell debris.

The **granulocytes** are named for the densely staining granules in their cytoplasm; they are also called **polymorphonuclear leukocytes** because of their oddly shaped nuclei. The three types of granulocytes—neutrophils, eosinophils, and basophils—are distinguished by the different staining properties of their granules, which serve distinct functions. Granulocytes are generally relatively short-lived, surviving for only a few days. They mature in the bone marrow, and their production increases during immune responses, when they migrate to sites of infection or inflammation. The phagocytic **neutrophils** are the most numerous and important cells in innate immune responses: they take up a variety of microorganisms by phagocytosis and efficiently destroy them in intracellular vesicles by using degradative enzymes and other antimicrobial substances stored in their cytoplasmic granules. Hereditary deficiencies in neutrophil function open the way to overwhelming bacterial infection, which is fatal if untreated. Their role is discussed further in Chapter 3.

Eosinophils and **basophils** are less abundant than neutrophils, but like neutrophils, they have granules containing a variety of enzymes and toxic proteins, which are released when these cells are activated. Eosinophils and basophils are thought to be important chiefly in defense against parasites, which are too large to be ingested by macrophages or neutrophils. They can also contribute to allergic inflammatory reactions, in which their effects are damaging rather than protective.

Mast cells begin development in the bone marrow but migrate as immature precursors that mature in peripheral tissues, especially skin, intestines, and airway mucosa. Their granules contain many inflammatory mediators, such as histamine and various proteases, which play a role in protecting the internal surfaces from pathogens, including parasitic worms. Because of their localization in barrier tissues, mast cells also function as early sensors of infection or injury and, in this role, contribute to the initiation of inflammation. We cover eosinophils, basophils, and mast cells and their role in allergic inflammation further in Chapters 10 and 14.

ANIMATION 1.1

Dendritic cells were discovered in the 1970s by Ralph Steinman, a finding for which he shared the 2011 Nobel Prize. These cells form the third class of phagocytic cells of the immune system and include several related lineages whose distinct functions are still being clarified. Most dendritic cells have elaborate membranous processes, like the dendrites of nerve cells. Immature dendritic cells migrate through the bloodstream from the bone marrow to enter tissues. They take up particulate matter by phagocytosis and also continually ingest large amounts of the extracellular fluid and its contents by a process known as **macropinocytosis**. They degrade the pathogens that they take up, but their main role in the immune system is not the clearance of microorganisms. Instead, dendritic cells are a major class of sensor cells whose encounter with pathogens triggers them to produce mediators that activate other immune cells. Dendritic cells were discovered because of their role in activating a particular class of lymphocytes—T lymphocytes—of the adaptive immune system, and we will return to this activity when we discuss T-cell activation in Section 1-15. But dendritic cells and the mediators they produce also play a critical role in controlling responses of cells of the innate immune system.

1-5   Sensor cells express pattern-recognition receptors that provide an initial discrimination between self and nonself.

Long before the mechanisms of innate recognition were discovered, it was recognized that purified antigens such as proteins often did not evoke an immune response in an experimental immunization; that is, they were not

immunogenic. Rather, the induction of strong immune responses against purified proteins required the inclusion of microbial constituents, such as killed bacteria or bacterial extracts, famously called the immunologist's 'dirty little secret' by Charles Janeway (see Appendix I, Section A-1). This additional material was termed an **adjuvant**, because it helped intensify the response to the immunizing antigen (*adjuvare* is Latin for 'to help'). We know now that adjuvants are needed, at least in part, to activate innate receptors on various types of sensor cells to help activate T cells in the absence of an infection.

Macrophages, neutrophils, and dendritic cells are important classes of sensor cells that detect infection and initiate immune responses by producing inflammatory mediators, although other cells, even cells of the adaptive immune system, can serve this function. As mentioned in Section 1-3, these cells express a limited number of invariant innate recognition receptors as a means of detecting pathogens or the damage induced by them. Also called **pattern-recognition receptors (PRRs)**, they recognize simple molecules and regular patterns of molecular structure known as **pathogen-associated molecular patterns (PAMPs)** that are part of many microorganisms but not of the host body's own cells. Such structures include mannose-rich oligosaccharides, peptidoglycans, and lipopolysaccharides of the bacterial cell wall, as well as unmethylated CpG DNA (unmethylated cytosine–guanine dinucleotide in DNA), which is common to many pathogens. All of these microbial elements have been conserved during evolution, making them excellent targets for recognition because they do not change (**Fig. 1.9**).

Some PRRs are transmembrane proteins, such as the **Toll-like receptors (TLRs)** that detect PAMPs derived from extracellular bacteria or bacteria taken into vesicular pathways by phagocytosis. The role of the Toll receptor in immunity was discovered first in *Drosophila melanogaster* by Jules Hoffmann and later extended to homologous TLRs in mice by Charles Janeway and Bruce Beutler. (Hoffmann and Beutler shared the 2011 Nobel Prize along with Ralph Steinman—see Section 1-4—for their work in the activation of innate immunity.) Other PRRs are cytoplasmic proteins, such as the **NOD-like receptors (NLRs)** that sense intracellular bacterial invasion. Yet other cytoplasmic receptors detect viral infection on the basis of differences in the structures and locations of the host mRNA and virally derived RNA species and the differences between host and microbial DNA. Some receptors expressed by sensor cells detect cellular damage induced by pathogens, rather than the pathogens themselves. Much of our knowledge of innate recognition has emerged only within the past two decades and is still an active area of discovery. We describe these innate recognition systems further in Chapter 3 and discuss how adjuvants are used as a component of vaccines in Chapter 16.

Macrophages express receptors for many microbial constituents

mannose receptor

TLR-1–TLR-2 dimer

NOD1

TLR-4

glucan receptor

scavenger receptor

Fig. 1.9 **Macrophages express a number of receptors that allow them to recognize different pathogens.** Macrophages express a variety of receptors, each of which is able to recognize specific components of microbes. Some, like the mannose and glucan receptors and the scavenger receptor, bind cell-wall carbohydrates of bacteria, yeast, and fungi. The Toll-like receptors (TLRs) are an important family of pattern-recognition receptors present on macrophages, dendritic cells, and other immune cells. TLRs recognize different microbial components; for example, a heterodimer of TLR-1 and TLR-2 binds certain lipopeptides from pathogens such as Gram-positive bacteria, while TLR-4 binds both lipopolysaccharides from Gram-negative and lipoteichoic acids from Gram-positive bacteria. Other pattern-recognition receptors are intracellular, such as the nucleotide-binding and oligomerization domain (NOD)-like receptors. NOD1, for example, binds to diaminopimelic acid, a component of the cell wall of most Gram-negative bacteria.

1-6 Sensor cells induce an inflammatory response by producing mediators such as chemokines and cytokines.

Activation of PRRs on sensor cells such as macrophages and neutrophils can directly induce effector functions in these cells, such as the phagocytosis and degradation of bacteria they encounter. But sensor cells serve to amplify the immune response by the production of inflammatory mediators. Two important categories of inflammatory mediators are the secreted proteins called **cytokines** and **chemokines**, which act in a manner similar to hormones to convey important signals to other immune cells.

'Cytokine' is a term for any protein secreted by immune cells that affects the behavior of nearby cells bearing appropriate receptors. There are more than 60 different cytokines; some are produced by many different cell types, and others are produced by only a few specific cell types. Some cytokines influence many types of cells, while others influence only a few, this through the expression

 ANIMATION 3.5

Fig. 1.10 Infection triggers an inflammatory response. Macrophages encountering bacteria or other types of microorganisms in tissues are triggered to release cytokines (left panel) that increase the permeability of blood vessels, allowing fluid and proteins to pass into the tissues (center panel). Macrophages also produce chemokines, which direct the migration of neutrophils to the site of infection. The stickiness of the endothelial cells of the blood vessel wall is also changed, so that circulating cells of the immune system adhere to the wall and are able to crawl through it; first neutrophils and then monocytes are shown entering the tissue from a blood vessel (right panel). The accumulation of fluid and cells at the site of infection causes the redness, swelling, heat, and pain known collectively as inflammation. Neutrophils and macrophages are the principal inflammatory cells. Later in an immune response, activated lymphocytes can also contribute to inflammation.

pattern of each cytokine's specific receptor. The response that a cytokine induces in a target cell is typically related to amplification of an effector mechanism of the target cell, as illustrated in the remaining sections of this chapter.

Instead of presenting all the cytokines together all at once, we introduce each cytokine as it arises during our description of cellular and functional responses. We list the cytokines, their producer and target cells, and their general functions in eAppendix III, found in the ebook and on the Digital Landing Page for this book.

Chemokines are a specialized subgroup of secreted proteins that act as chemoattractants, attracting cells bearing chemokine receptors, such as neutrophils and monocytes, out of the bloodstream and into infected tissue (**Fig. 1.10**). Beyond this role, chemokines also help organize the various cells in lymphoid tissues into discrete regions where specialized responses can take place. There are about 50 different chemokines. eAppendix IV, found in the ebook and on the Digital Landing Page for this book, lists the chemokines, their target cells, and their general functions. We will discuss chemokines as the need arises during our descriptions of particular cellular immune processes.

The cytokines and chemokines released by activated macrophages act to recruit cells from the blood into infected tissues, a process known as **inflammation**, which helps to destroy the pathogen. Inflammation increases the flow of lymph, which carries microbes or cells bearing their antigens from the infected tissue to nearby lymphoid tissues, where the adaptive immune response is initiated. Once adaptive immunity has been generated, inflammation also recruits these effector components to the site of infection.

Inflammation is described clinically by the Latin words *calor, dolor, rubor,* and *tumor,* meaning heat, pain, redness, and swelling. Each of these features reflects an effect of cytokines or other inflammatory mediators on the local blood vessels. Heat, redness, and swelling result from the dilation and increased permeability of blood vessels during inflammation, leading to increased local blood flow and leakage of fluid and blood proteins into the tissues. Cytokines and complement fragments have important effects on the **endothelium** that lines blood vessels; the **endothelial cells** themselves also produce cytokines in response to infection. These alter the adhesive properties of the endothelial cells and cause circulating leukocytes to stick to the endothelial cells and migrate between them into the site of infection, to which they are attracted by chemokines. The migration of cells into the tissue and their local actions account for the pain.

The main cell types seen in the initial phase of an inflammatory response are macrophages and neutrophils, the latter being recruited into the inflamed, infected tissue in large numbers. Macrophages and neutrophils are thus also known as **inflammatory cells**. The influx of neutrophils is followed a short time later by the increased entry of monocytes, which rapidly differentiate into macrophages, thus reinforcing and sustaining the innate immune response. Later, if the inflammation continues, eosinophils also migrate into inflamed tissues and contribute to the destruction of the invading microorganisms.

1-7 Innate lymphoid cells and natural killer cells are effector cells that share similarities with lymphoid lineages of the adaptive immune system.

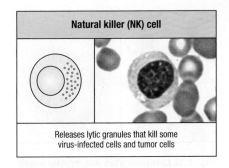

Natural killer (NK) cell

Releases lytic granules that kill some virus-infected cells and tumor cells

Fig. 1.11 Natural killer (NK) cells. These are large, granular, lymphoid-like cells with important functions in innate immunity (especially against intracellular infections), being able to kill other cells. Unlike lymphocytes, they lack antigen-specific receptors.

The **common lymphoid progenitor (CLP)** in the bone marrow gives rise both to antigen-specific lymphocytes of the adaptive immune system and to several innate lineages that lack antigen-specific receptors. Although the B and T lymphocytes of the adaptive immune system were recognized in the 1960s, the **natural killer (NK) cells (Fig. 1.11)** of the innate immune system were not discovered until the 1970s. NK cells are large lymphocyte-like cells with a distinctive granular cytoplasm that were identified because of their ability to recognize and kill certain tumor cells and cells infected with herpesviruses. Initially, the distinction between these cells and T lymphocytes was unclear, but we now recognize that NK cells are a distinct lineage of cells that arise from the CLP in the bone marrow. They lack the antigen-specific receptors of the adaptive immune system cells but express members of various families of innate receptors that can respond to cellular stress and to infections by very specific viruses. NK cells play an important role in the early innate response to viral infections, before the adaptive immune response has developed.

More recently, additional lineages of cells related to NK cells have been identified. Collectively, these cells are called **innate lymphoid cells (ILCs)**. Arising from the CLP, ILCs reside in peripheral tissues, such as the intestine, where they function as the sources of mediators of inflammatory responses. The functions of NK cells and ILCs are discussed in Chapter 3.

Summary.

Strategies of avoidance, resistance, and tolerance represent different ways to deal with pathogens. Anatomic barriers and various chemical barriers, such as complement and antimicrobial proteins, may be considered a primitive form of avoidance, and they are the first line of defense against entry of both commensal organisms and pathogens into host tissues. If these barriers are breached, the vertebrate immune response becomes largely focused on resistance. Inflammatory inducers, which may be either chemical structures unique to microbes (PAMPs) or the chemical signals of tissue damage, act on receptors expressed by sensor cells to inform the immune system of infection. Sensor cells are typically innate immune cells such as macrophages or dendritic cells. Sensor cells can either directly respond with effector activity or produce inflammatory mediators, typically cytokines and chemokines that act on other immune cells, such as the innate NK cells and ILCs. These cells then are recruited into target tissues to provide specific types of immune-response effector activities, such as cell killing or production of cytokines that have direct antiviral activity, all aimed to reduce or eliminate infection by pathogens. Inflammatory mediators released in target tissues can recruit and activate several types of inflammatory cells that are specially suited for eliminating viruses, intracellular bacteria, extracellular pathogens, or parasites.

Principles of adaptive immunity.

We come now to the components of adaptive immunity, the antigen-specific lymphocytes. Unless indicated otherwise, we shall use the term 'lymphocyte' in the remainder of this chapter to refer only to the antigen-specific lymphocytes.

Fig. 1.12 Lymphocytes are mostly small and inactive cells. The left panel shows a light micrograph of a small lymphocyte—in which the nucleus has been stained purple by hematoxylin and eosin dye—surrounded by red blood cells (which have no nuclei). Note the darker purple patches of condensed chromatin of the lymphocyte nucleus, indicating little transcriptional activity and the relative absence of cytoplasm. The right panel shows a transmission electron micrograph of a small lymphocyte. Again, note the evidence of functional inactivity: the condensed chromatin, the scanty cytoplasm, and the absence of rough endoplasmic reticulum.

Lymphocytes allow responses against a vast array of antigens from various pathogens encountered during a person's lifetime and confer the important feature of immunological memory. Lymphocytes make this possible through the highly variable antigen receptors on their surface, by which they recognize and bind antigens. Each lymphocyte matures bearing a unique variant of a prototype antigen receptor, so that the population of lymphocytes expresses a huge repertoire of receptors that are highly diverse in their antigen-binding sites. Among the billion or so lymphocytes circulating in the body at any one time there will always be some that can recognize a given foreign antigen.

A unique feature of the adaptive immune system is that it is capable of generating **immunological memory**, so that having been exposed once to an infectious agent, a person will make an immediate and stronger response against any subsequent exposure to it; that is, the individual will have protective immunity against it. Finding ways of generating long-lasting immunity to pathogens that do not naturally provoke it is one of the greatest challenges facing immunologists today.

1-8 The interaction of antigens with antigen receptors induces lymphocytes to acquire effector and memory activity.

There are two major types of lymphocytes in the vertebrate immune system, the **B lymphocytes (B cells)** and **T lymphocytes (T cells)**. These express distinct types of antigen receptors and have quite different roles in the immune system, as was discovered in the 1960s. Most lymphocytes circulating in the body appear as rather unimpressive small cells with few cytoplasmic organelles and a condensed, inactive-appearing nuclear chromatin (**Fig. 1.12**). Lymphocytes manifest little functional activity until they encounter a specific antigen that interacts with an antigen receptor on their cell surface. Lymphocytes that have not yet been activated by antigen are known as **naive lymphocytes**; those that have met their antigen, become activated, and have differentiated further into fully functional lymphocytes are known as **effector lymphocytes**.

B cells and T cells are distinguished by the structure of the antigen receptor that they express. The **B-cell antigen receptor**, or **B-cell receptor (BCR)**, is formed by the same genes that encode antibodies, therefore B-cell receptors and antibodies compose the class of proteins known as **immunoglobulin (Ig)** (**Fig. 1.13**). Thus, the antigen receptor of B lymphocytes is also known as **membrane immunoglobulin (mIg)** or **surface immunoglobulin (sIg)**. The **T-cell antigen receptor**, or **T-cell receptor (TCR)**, is related to the immunoglobulins but is quite distinct in its structure and recognition properties.

After antigen binds to a B-cell receptor, the B cell will proliferate and differentiate into **plasma cells**. These are the effector form of B lymphocytes, and they secrete antibodies that have the same antigen specificity as the plasma cell's B-cell receptor. Thus the antigen that activates a given B cell becomes the target of the antibodies produced by that B cell's progeny.

Fig. 1.13 Schematic structure of antigen receptors. Upper panel: an antibody molecule, which is secreted by activated B cells as an antigen-binding effector molecule. A membrane-bound version of this molecule acts as the B-cell antigen receptor (not shown). An antibody is composed of two identical heavy chains (green) and two identical light chains (yellow). Each chain has a constant part (shaded blue) and a variable part (shaded red). Each arm of the antibody molecule is formed by a light chain and a heavy chain, with the variable parts of the two chains coming together to create a variable region that contains the antigen-binding site. The stem is formed from the constant parts of the heavy chains and takes a limited number of forms. This constant region is involved in the elimination of the bound antigen. Lower panel: a T-cell antigen receptor. This is also composed of two chains, an α chain (yellow) and a β chain (green), each of which has a variable and a constant part. As with the antibody molecule, the variable parts of the two chains create a variable region, which forms the antigen-binding site. The T-cell receptor is not produced in a secreted form.

When a T cell first encounters an antigen that its receptor can bind, it proliferates and differentiates into one of several different functional types of **effector T lymphocytes**. When effector T cells subsequently detect antigen, they can manifest three broad classes of activity. **Cytotoxic T cells** kill other cells that are infected with viruses or other intracellular pathogens bearing the antigen. **Helper T cells** provide signals, often in the form of specific cytokines that activate the functions of other cells, such as B-cell production of antibody and macrophage killing of engulfed pathogens. **Regulatory T cells** suppress the activity of other lymphocytes and help to limit the possible damage of immune responses. We discuss the detailed functions of cytotoxic, helper, and regulatory T cells in Chapters 9, 11, 12, and 15.

Some of the B cells and T cells activated by antigen will differentiate into **memory cells**, the lymphocytes that are responsible for the long-lasting immunity that can follow exposure to disease or vaccination. Memory cells will readily differentiate into effector cells on a second exposure to their specific antigen. Immunological memory is described in Chapter 11.

1-9 Antibodies and T-cell receptors are composed of constant and variable regions that provide distinct functions.

Antibodies were studied by traditional biochemical techniques long before recombinant DNA technology allowed the study of the membrane-bound forms of the antigen receptors on B and T cells. These early studies found that antibody molecules are composed of two distinct regions. One is a **constant region**, also called the **fragment crystallizable region**, or **Fc region**, which takes one of only five biochemically distinguishable forms (see Fig. 1.13). The **variable region** of different antibody molecules, by contrast, can be composed of a vast number of different amino acid sequences that allow antibodies to recognize an equally vast variety of antigens. The basic structure of antibody molecules was determined by Gerald Edelman and Rodney Porter, who shared the 1972 Nobel Prize for their work. These biochemical studies led to subsequent X-ray crystallographic determination of the structure of the antibody Fc region.

The antibody molecule is composed of two identical **heavy chain** and two identical **light chain** polypeptides. Heavy and light chains each have variable and constant regions. The variable regions of a heavy chain and a light chain combine to form an **antigen-binding site** that determines the antigen-binding specificity of the antibody. Thus, both heavy and light chains contribute to the antigen-binding specificity of the antibody molecule. Also, each antibody has two identical variable regions, and so has two identical antigen-binding sites. The constant region determines the effector function of the antibody; that is, how the antibody will interact with various immune cells to dispose of antigen once it is bound.

The T-cell receptor shows many similarities to the B-cell receptor and antibody (see Fig. 1.13). It is composed of two chains, the TCR α and β chains, that are roughly equal in size and which span the T-cell membrane. Like antibody, each TCR chain has a variable region and a constant region, and the combination of the α- and β-chain variable regions creates a single site for binding antigen. The structures of both antibodies and T-cell receptors are described in detail in Chapter 4, and functional properties of antibody constant regions are discussed in Chapters 4 and 10.

1-10 Antibodies and T-cell receptors recognize antigens by fundamentally different mechanisms.

In principle, almost any chemical structure can be recognized as an antigen by the adaptive immune system, but the usual antigens encountered in an infection are the proteins, glycoproteins, and polysaccharides of pathogens.

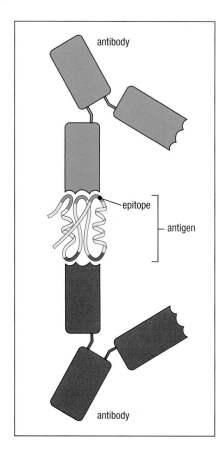

Fig. 1.14 Antigens are the molecules recognized by the immune response, while epitopes are sites within antigens to which antigen receptors bind. Antigens can be complex macromolecules such as proteins, as shown in yellow. Most antigens are larger than the sites on the antibody or antigen receptor to which they bind, and the actual portion of the antigen that is bound is known as the antigenic determinant, or epitope, for that receptor. Large antigens such as proteins can contain more than one epitope (indicated in red and blue) and thus may bind different antibodies (shown here in the same color as the epitopes they bind). Antibodies generally recognize epitopes on the surface of the antigen.

Fig. 1.15 T-cell receptors bind a complex of an antigen fragment and a self molecule. Unlike most antibodies, T-cell receptors can recognize epitopes that are buried within antigens (first panel). These antigens must first be degraded by proteases (second panel) and the epitope peptide delivered to a self molecule, called an MHC molecule (third panel). It is in this form, as a complex of peptide and MHC molecule, that antigens are recognized by T-cell receptors (TCRs; fourth panel).

An individual antigen receptor or antibody recognizes a small portion of the antigen's molecular structure, and the part recognized is known as an **antigenic determinant**, or **epitope** (**Fig. 1.14**). Typically, proteins and glycoproteins have many different epitopes that can be recognized by different antigen receptors.

Antibodies and B-cell receptors directly recognize the epitopes of native antigen in the serum or the extracellular spaces. It is possible for different antibodies to simultaneously recognize an antigen by its different epitopes; such simultaneous recognition increases the efficiency of clearing or neutralizing the antigen.

Whereas antibodies can recognize nearly any type of chemical structure, T-cell receptors usually recognize protein antigens and do so very differently from antibodies. The T-cell receptor recognizes a peptide epitope derived from a partially degraded protein, but only if the peptide is bound to specialized cell-surface glycoproteins called **MHC molecules** (**Fig. 1.15**). The members of this large family of cell-surface glycoproteins are encoded in a cluster of genes called the **major histocompatibility complex (MHC)**. The antigens recognized by T cells can be derived from proteins arising from intracellular pathogens, such as a virus, or from extracellular pathogens. A further difference from the antibody molecule is that there is no secreted form of the T-cell receptor; the T-cell receptor functions solely to signal to the T cell that it has bound its antigen, and the subsequent immunological effects depend on the actions of the T cells themselves. We will further describe how epitopes from antigens are placed on MHC proteins in Chapter 6 and how T cells carry out their subsequent functions in Chapter 9.

1-11 Antigen-receptor genes are assembled by somatic gene rearrangements of incomplete receptor gene segments.

The innate immune system detects inflammatory stimuli by means of a relatively limited number of sensors, such as the TLR and NOD proteins, numbering fewer than 100 different types of proteins. Antigen-specific receptors of adaptive immunity provide a seemingly infinite range of specificities and yet are encoded by a finite number of genes. The basis for this extraordinary range of specificity was discovered in 1976 by Susumu Tonegawa, for which he was awarded the 1987 Nobel Prize. Immunoglobulin variable regions are inherited as sets of **gene segments**, each encoding a part of the variable region of one of the immunoglobulin polypeptide chains. During B-cell development in the bone marrow, these gene segments are irreversibly joined by a process of DNA recombination to form a stretch of DNA encoding a complete variable region. A similar process of antigen-receptor gene rearrangement takes place for the T-cell receptor genes during development of T cells in the thymus.

| The epitopes recognized by T-cell receptors are often buried | The antigen must first be broken down into peptide fragments | The epitope peptide binds to a self molecule, an MHC molecule | The T-cell receptor binds to a complex of MHC molecule and epitope peptide |

Just a few hundred different gene segments can combine in different ways to generate thousands of different receptor chains. This **combinatorial diversity** allows a small amount of genetic material to encode a truly staggering diversity of receptors. During this recombination process, the random addition or subtraction of nucleotides at the junctions of the gene segments creates additional diversity known as **junctional diversity**. Diversity is amplified further by the fact that each antigen receptor has two different variable chains, each encoded by distinct sets of gene segments. In Chapter 5 we will describe the gene-rearrangement process that assembles complete antigen receptors from gene segments.

1-12 Lymphocytes activated by antigen give rise to clones of antigen-specific effector cells that mediate adaptive immunity.

There are two critical features of lymphocyte development that distinguish adaptive immunity from innate immunity. First, the process that assembles antigen receptors from incomplete gene segments, described earlier, is carried out in a manner ensuring that each developing lymphocyte expresses only one receptor specificity. Whereas the cells of the innate immune system express many different pattern-recognition receptors and recognize features shared by many pathogens, the antigen-receptor expression of lymphocytes is 'clonal,' so that each mature lymphocyte differs from others in the specificity of its antigen receptor. Second, because the gene-rearrangement process irreversibly changes the lymphocyte's DNA, all its progeny inherit the same receptor specificity. Because this specificity is inherited by a cell's progeny, the proliferation of an individual lymphocyte forms a **clone** of cells with identical antigen receptors.

There are lymphocytes of at least 10^8 different specificities in an individual human at any one time, composing the **lymphocyte receptor repertoire** of the individual. These lymphocytes are continually undergoing a process similar to natural selection: only those lymphocytes that encounter an antigen to which their receptor binds will be activated to proliferate and differentiate into effector cells. This selective mechanism was first proposed in the 1950s by Frank Macfarlane Burnet, who postulated the preexistence in the body of many different potential antibody-producing cells, each displaying on its surface a membrane-bound version of the antibody that served as a receptor for the antigen. On binding antigen, the cell is activated to divide and to produce many identical progeny, a process known as **clonal expansion**; this clone of identical cells can now secrete **clonotypic** antibodies with a specificity identical to that of the surface receptor that first triggered activation and clonal expansion (**Fig. 1.16**). Burnet called this the **clonal selection theory** of antibody production; its four basic postulates are listed in **Fig. 1.17**. Clonal selection of lymphocytes is the single most important principle in adaptive immunity.

Fig. 1.16 Clonal selection. Each lymphoid progenitor gives rise to a large number of lymphocytes, each bearing a distinct antigen receptor. Lymphocytes with receptors that bind ubiquitous self antigens are eliminated before they become fully mature, ensuring tolerance to such self antigens. When a foreign antigen (red dot) interacts with the receptor on a mature naive lymphocyte, that cell is activated and starts to divide. It gives rise to a clone of identical progeny, all of whose receptors bind the same antigen. Antigen specificity is thus maintained as the progeny proliferate and differentiate into effector cells. Once antigen has been eliminated by these effector cells, the immune response ceases, although some lymphocytes are retained to mediate immunological memory.

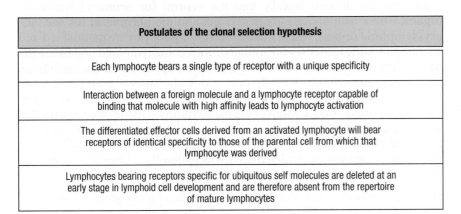

Postulates of the clonal selection hypothesis
Each lymphocyte bears a single type of receptor with a unique specificity
Interaction between a foreign molecule and a lymphocyte receptor capable of binding that molecule with high affinity leads to lymphocyte activation
The differentiated effector cells derived from an activated lymphocyte will bear receptors of identical specificity to those of the parental cell from which that lymphocyte was derived
Lymphocytes bearing receptors specific for ubiquitous self molecules are deleted at an early stage in lymphoid cell development and are therefore absent from the repertoire of mature lymphocytes

Fig. 1.17 The four basic principles of clonal selection.

1-13 Lymphocytes with self-reactive receptors are normally eliminated during development or are functionally inactivated.

When Burnet formulated his theory, nothing was known of the antigen receptors or indeed the function of lymphocytes themselves. In the early 1960s, James Gowans discovered that removal of the small lymphocytes from rats resulted in the loss of all known adaptive immune responses, which were restored when the small lymphocytes were replaced. This led to the realization that lymphocytes must be the units of clonal selection, and their biology became the focus of the new field of **cellular immunology**.

Clonal selection of lymphocytes with diverse receptors elegantly explained adaptive immunity, but it raised one significant conceptual problem. With so many different antigen receptors being generated randomly during the lifetime of an individual, there is a possibility that some receptors might react against an individual's own **self antigens**. How are lymphocytes prevented from recognizing native antigens on the tissues of the body and attacking them? Ray Owen had shown in the late 1940s that genetically different twin calves with a common placenta, and thus a shared placental blood circulation, were immunologically unresponsive, or **tolerant**, to one another's tissues. Peter Medawar then showed in 1953 that exposure to foreign tissues during embryonic development caused mice to become immunologically tolerant to these tissues. Burnet proposed that developing lymphocytes that are potentially self-reactive are removed before they can mature, a process known as **clonal deletion**. Medawar and Burnet shared the 1960 Nobel Prize for their work on tolerance. This process was demonstrated experimentally in the late 1980s. Some lymphocytes that receive either too much or too little signal through their antigen receptor during development are eliminated by a form of cell suicide called **apoptosis**—derived from a Greek word meaning the falling of leaves from trees—or **programmed cell death**. Other types of mechanisms of immunological tolerance have been identified since then that rely on the induction of an inactive state, called **anergy**, as well as mechanisms of active suppression of self-reactive lymphocytes. Chapter 8 will describe lymphocyte development and tolerance mechanisms that shape the lymphocyte receptor repertoire. Chapters 14 and 15 will discuss how immune-tolerance mechanisms can sometimes fail.

1-14 Lymphocytes mature in the bone marrow or the thymus and then congregate in lymphoid tissues throughout the body.

Lymphocytes circulate in the blood and the lymph and are also found in large numbers in **lymphoid tissues** or **lymphoid organs**, the latter being organized aggregates of lymphocytes in a framework of nonlymphoid cells. Lymphoid organs can be divided broadly into the **central (or primary) lymphoid organs**, where lymphocytes are generated, and the **peripheral (or secondary) lymphoid organs**, where mature naive lymphocytes are maintained and adaptive immune responses are initiated. The central lymphoid organs are the bone marrow and the **thymus**, an organ in the upper chest. The peripheral lymphoid organs comprise the **lymph nodes**, the **spleen**, and the mucosal lymphoid tissues of the gut, the nasal and respiratory tract, the urogenital tract, and other mucosa. The locations of the main lymphoid tissues are shown schematically in **Fig. 1.18**; we describe the individual peripheral lymphoid organs in more detail later in the chapter. Lymph nodes are interconnected by a system of lymphatic vessels, which drain extracellular fluid from tissues, carry it through the lymph nodes, and deposit it back into the blood.

The progenitors that give rise to B and T lymphocytes originate in the bone marrow. B cells complete their development within the bone marrow.

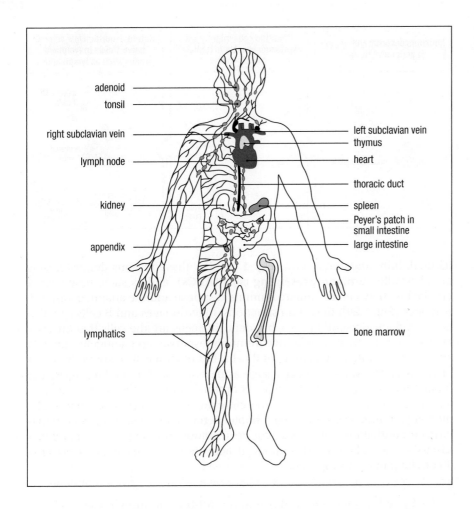

Fig. 1.18 The distribution of lymphoid tissues in the body. Lymphocytes arise from stem cells in bone marrow and differentiate in the central lymphoid organs (yellow)—B cells in the bone marrow and T cells in the thymus. They migrate from these tissues and are carried in the bloodstream to the peripheral lymphoid organs (blue). These include lymph nodes, spleen, and lymphoid tissues associated with mucosa, such as the gut-associated tonsils, Peyer's patches, and appendix. The peripheral lymphoid organs are the sites of lymphocyte activation by antigen, and lymphocytes recirculate between the blood and these organs until they encounter their specific antigen. Lymphatics drain extracellular fluid from the peripheral tissues, through the lymph nodes, and into the thoracic duct, which empties into the left subclavian vein. This fluid, known as lymph, carries antigen taken up by dendritic cells and macrophages to the lymph nodes, and it recirculates lymphocytes from the lymph nodes back into the blood. Lymphoid tissue is also associated with other mucosa such as the bronchial linings (not shown).

Although the 'B' in B lymphocytes originally stood for the **bursa of Fabricius**, a lymphoid organ in young chicks in which lymphocytes mature, it is a useful mnemonic for bone marrow. The immature precursors of T lymphocytes migrate to the thymus, from which they get their name, and complete their development there. Once they have completed maturation, both types of lymphocytes enter the bloodstream as mature naive lymphocytes and continually circulate through the peripheral lymphoid tissues.

1-15 Adaptive immune responses are initiated by antigen and antigen-presenting cells in peripheral lymphoid tissues.

Adaptive immune responses are initiated when B or T lymphocytes encounter antigens for which their receptors have specific reactivity, provided that there are appropriate inflammatory signals to support activation. For T cells, this activation occurs via encounters with dendritic cells that have picked up antigens at sites of infection and migrated to peripheral (also called secondary) lymphoid organs. Activation of the dendritic cells' PRRs by PAMPs at the site of infection stimulates the dendritic cells in the tissues to engulf the pathogen and degrade it intracellularly. They also take up extracellular material, including virus particles and bacteria, by receptor-independent macropinocytosis. These processes lead to the display of peptide antigens on the MHC molecules of the dendritic cells, a display that activates the antigen receptors of lymphocytes. Activation of PRRs also triggers the dendritic cells to express cell-surface proteins called **co-stimulatory molecules**, which support the ability of the T lymphocyte to proliferate and differentiate into

 ANIMATION 1.1

Fig. 1.19 Dendritic cells initiate adaptive immune responses. Immature dendritic cells residing in a tissue take up pathogens and their antigens by macropinocytosis and by receptor-mediated endocytosis. They are stimulated by recognition of the presence of pathogens to migrate through the lymphatics to regional lymph nodes, where they arrive as fully mature nonphagocytic dendritic cells that express both antigen and the co-stimulatory molecules necessary to activate a naive T cell that recognizes the antigen. Thus the dendritic cells stimulate lymphocyte proliferation and differentiation.

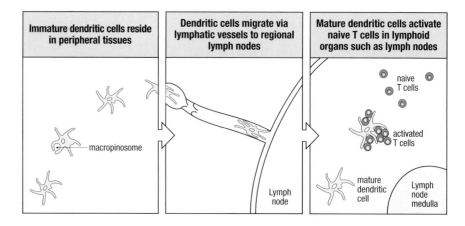

| Immature dendritic cells reside in peripheral tissues | Dendritic cells migrate via lymphatic vessels to regional lymph nodes | Mature dendritic cells activate naive T cells in lymphoid organs such as lymph nodes |

its final, fully functional form (**Fig. 1.19**). For these reasons dendritic cells are also called **antigen-presenting cells (APCs)**, and as such, they form a crucial link between the innate immune response and the adaptive immune response (**Fig. 1.20**). In certain situations, macrophages and B cells can also act as antigen-presenting cells, but dendritic cells are the cells that are specialized in initiating the adaptive immune response. Free antigens can also stimulate the antigen receptors of B cells, but most B cells respond better to antigens on the surface of cells, such as pathogens, and in addition require 'help' from activated helper T cells for optimal antibody responses. The activation of naive T lymphocytes is therefore an essential first stage in virtually all adaptive immune responses. Chapter 6 returns to dendritic cells to discuss how antigens are processed for presentation to T cells. Chapters 7 and 9 discuss co-stimulation and lymphocyte activation. Chapter 10 describes how T cells help in activating B cells.

1-16 Lymphocytes encounter and respond to antigen in the peripheral lymphoid organs.

Antigen and lymphocytes eventually encounter each other in the peripheral lymphoid organs—the lymph nodes, spleen, and mucosal lymphoid tissues (see Fig. 1.18). Mature naive lymphocytes are continually recirculating through these tissues, to which pathogen antigens are carried from sites of infection, primarily by dendritic cells. The peripheral lymphoid organs are specialized to trap antigen-bearing dendritic cells and to facilitate the initiation of adaptive immune responses. Peripheral lymphoid organs are composed of aggregations of lymphocytes in a framework of nonleukocyte stromal cells. The stromal cells provide both the basic structural organization of the tissue and survival signals to help sustain the life of the lymphocytes. Besides lymphocytes, peripheral lymphoid organs also contain resident macrophages and dendritic cells.

Fig. 1.20 Dendritic cells form a key link between the innate immune system and the adaptive immune system. Like the other cells of innate immunity, dendritic cells recognize pathogens via invariant cell-surface receptors for pathogen molecules and are activated by these stimuli early in an infection. Dendritic cells in tissues are phagocytic; they are specialized to ingest a wide range of pathogens and to display their antigens at the dendritic cell surface in a form that can be recognized by T cells.

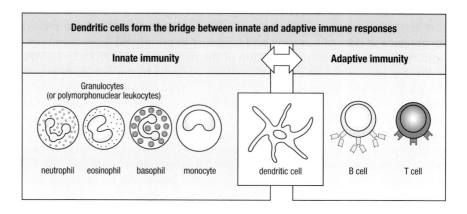

Dendritic cells form the bridge between innate and adaptive immune responses

When an infection occurs in a tissue such as the skin, free antigen and antigen-bearing dendritic cells travel from the site of infection through the afferent lymphatic vessels into the **draining lymph nodes** (**Fig. 1.21**)—peripheral lymphoid organs in which the free antigen and antigen-bearing dendritic cells activate antigen-specific lymphocytes. The activated lymphocytes then undergo a period of proliferation and differentiation, after which most leave the lymph nodes as effector cells via the efferent lymphatic vessel. This eventually returns them to the bloodstream (see Fig. 1.18), which then carries them to the tissues where they will act. This whole process takes about 4–6 days from the time that the antigen is recognized, which means that an adaptive immune response to an antigen that has not been encountered before does not become effective until about a week after infection (see Fig. 1.7). Naive lymphocytes that do not recognize their antigen also leave through the efferent lymphatic vessel and are returned to the blood, from which they continue to recirculate through lymphoid tissues until they recognize antigen or die.

The lymph nodes are highly organized lymphoid organs located at the points of convergence of vessels of the lymphatic system, which is the extensive system that collects extracellular fluid from the tissues and returns it to the blood (see Fig. 1.18). This extracellular fluid is produced continually by filtration from the blood and is called lymph. Lymph flows away from the peripheral tissues under the pressure exerted by its continual production and is carried by **lymphatic vessels**, or **lymphatics**. One-way valves in the lymphatic vessels prevent a reverse flow, and the movements of one part of the body in relation to another are important in driving the lymph along.

As noted above, **afferent lymphatic vessels** drain fluid from the tissues and carry pathogens and antigen-bearing cells from infected tissues to the lymph nodes (**Fig. 1.22**). Free antigens simply diffuse through the extracellular fluid to the lymph node, while the dendritic cells actively migrate into the lymph node, attracted by chemokines. The same chemokines also attract lymphocytes from the blood, and these enter lymph nodes by squeezing through the walls of specialized blood vessels called **high endothelial venules (HEVs)**, named for their thicker, more rounded appearance relative to flatter endothelial cells in other locations. In the lymph nodes, B lymphocytes are localized in **follicles**, which make up the outer **cortex** of the lymph node, with T cells more diffusely distributed in the surrounding **paracortical areas**, also referred to as the deep cortex or **T-cell zones** (see Fig. 1.22). Lymphocytes migrating from the blood into lymph nodes enter the paracortical areas first, and because they are attracted by the same chemokines, antigen-presenting dendritic cells and macrophages also become localized there. Free antigen diffusing through the lymph node can become trapped on these dendritic cells and macrophages. This juxtaposition of antigen, antigen-presenting cells, and naive T cells in the T-cell zone creates an ideal environment in which naive T cells can bind their specific antigen and thus become activated.

As noted earlier, activation of B cells usually requires not only antigen, which binds to the B-cell receptor, but also the cooperation of activated helper T cells, a type of effector T cell. The location of B cells and T cells within the lymph node is dynamically regulated by their state of activation. When they become activated, T cells and B cells both move to the border of the follicle and T-cell zone, where T cells can first provide their helper function to B cells. Some of the B-cell follicles include **germinal centers**, where activated B cells are undergoing intense proliferation and differentiation into plasma cells. These mechanisms are described in detail in Chapter 10.

In humans, the spleen is a fist-sized organ situated just behind the stomach (see Fig. 1.18). It has no direct connection with the lymphatic system; instead, it collects antigen from the blood and is involved in immune responses to blood-borne pathogens. Lymphocytes enter and leave the spleen via blood vessels. The spleen also collects and disposes of senescent red blood cells.

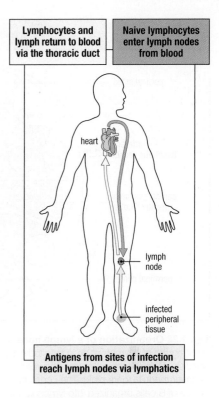

Fig. 1.21 Circulating lymphocytes encounter antigen in peripheral lymphoid organs. Naive lymphocytes recirculate constantly through peripheral lymphoid organs, here illustrated as a popliteal lymph node—a lymph node situated behind the knee. In the case of an infection in the foot, this will be the draining lymph node, where lymphocytes may encounter their specific antigens and become activated. Both activated and nonactivated lymphocytes are returned to the bloodstream via the lymphatic system.

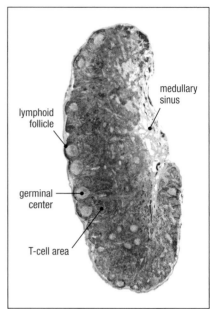

Fig. 1.22 Organization of a lymph node. As shown at left in the diagram of a lymph node in longitudinal section, a lymph node consists of an outermost cortex (the yellow and blue areas) and an inner medulla (dark pink). The cortex is composed of an outer cortex of B cells organized into lymphoid follicles and of adjacent, or paracortical, areas made up mainly of T cells and dendritic cells. When an immune response is under way, some of the follicles contain central areas of intense B-cell proliferation called germinal centers. Lymph draining from the extracellular spaces of the body carries antigens in phagocytic dendritic cells and phagocytic macrophages from the tissues to the lymph node via the afferent lymphatics. These migrate directly from the sinuses into the cellular parts of the node. Lymph leaves via the efferent lymphatic in the medulla. The medulla consists of strings of macrophages and antibody-secreting plasma cells known as the medullary cords. Naive lymphocytes enter the node from the bloodstream through specialized postcapillary venules (not shown) and leave with the lymph through the efferent lymphatic. The light micrograph at right shows a longitudinal section through a lymph node that has follicles containing germinal centers. Original magnification ×40.

Its organization is shown schematically in **Fig. 1.23**. The bulk of the spleen is composed of **red pulp**, which is the site of red blood cell disposal. The lymphocytes surround the arterioles running through the spleen, forming isolated areas of **white pulp**. The sheath of lymphocytes around an arteriole is called the **periarteriolar lymphoid sheath (PALS)** and contains mainly T cells. Lymphoid follicles occur at intervals along it, and these contain mainly B cells. An area called the **marginal zone** surrounds the follicle; it has few T cells, is rich in macrophages, and has a resident, noncirculating population of B cells known as **marginal zone B cells**. These B cells are poised to rapidly produce antibodies that have low affinity to bacterial capsular polysaccharides. These antibodies, which are discussed in Chapter 8, provide some degree of protection before the adaptive immune response is fully activated. Blood-borne microbes, soluble antigens, and antigen:antibody complexes are filtered from the blood by macrophages and immature dendritic cells within the marginal zone. Like the migration of immature dendritic cells from peripheral tissues to the T-cell areas of lymph nodes, dendritic cells in the marginal zones in the spleen migrate to the T-cell areas after taking up antigen and becoming activated; here they are able to present the antigens they carry to T cells.

1-17 Mucosal surfaces have specialized immune structures that orchestrate responses to environmental microbial encounters.

Most pathogens enter the body through mucosal surfaces, which are also exposed to a vast load of other potential antigens from the air, food, and the natural microbial flora of the body. Mucosal surfaces are protected by an extensive system of lymphoid tissues known generally as the **mucosal immune system** or **mucosa-associated lymphoid tissue (MALT)**. Collectively, the

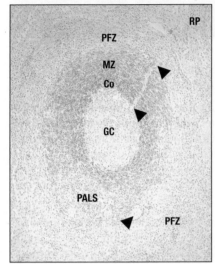

Fig. 1.23 Organization of the lymphoid tissues of the spleen.
The schematic at top left shows that the spleen consists of red pulp (pink areas), which is a site of red blood cell destruction, interspersed with the lymphoid white pulp. An enlargement of a small section of a human spleen (top right) shows the arrangement of discrete areas of white pulp (yellow and blue) around central arterioles. Most of the white pulp is shown in transverse section, with two portions in longitudinal section. The two schematics below this diagram show enlargements of a transverse section (bottom center) and longitudinal section (bottom right) of white pulp. Surrounding the central arteriole is the periarteriolar lymphoid sheath (PALS), made up of T cells. Lymphocytes and antigen-loaded dendritic cells come together here. The follicles consist mainly of B cells; in secondary follicles, a germinal center is surrounded by a B-cell corona. The follicles are surrounded by a so-called marginal zone of lymphocytes. In each area of white pulp, blood carrying both lymphocytes and antigen flows from a trabecular artery into a central arteriole. From this arteriole smaller blood vessels fan out, eventually terminating in a specialized zone in the human spleen called the perifollicular zone (PFZ), which surrounds each marginal zone. Cells and antigen then pass into the white pulp through open blood-filled spaces in the perifollicular zone. The light micrograph at bottom left shows a transverse section of white pulp of human spleen immunostained for mature B cells. Both follicle and PALS are surrounded by the perifollicular zone. The follicular arteriole emerges in the PALS (arrowhead at bottom), traverses the follicle, goes through the marginal zone, and opens into the perifollicular zone (upper arrowheads). Co, follicular B-cell corona; GC, germinal center; MZ, marginal zone; RP, red pulp; arrowheads, central arteriole.

mucosal immune system is estimated to contain as many lymphocytes as all the rest of the body, and these lymphocytes form a specialized set of cells obeying somewhat different rules of recirculation from those of lymphocytes in the other peripheral lymphoid organs. The **gut-associated lymphoid tissue (GALT)** includes the **tonsils, adenoids, appendix,** and specialized structures in the small intestine called **Peyer's patches,** and they collect antigen from the epithelial surfaces of the gastrointestinal tract. In Peyer's patches, which are the most important and highly organized of these tissues, the antigen is collected by specialized epithelial cells called **microfold cells,** or **M cells** (**Fig. 1.24**). The lymphocytes form a follicle consisting of a large central dome of B lymphocytes surrounded by smaller numbers of T lymphocytes. Dendritic cells resident within the Peyer's patch present the antigen to T lymphocytes. Lymphocytes enter Peyer's patches from the blood and leave through efferent lymphatics. Effector lymphocytes generated in Peyer's patches travel through

Peyer's patches are covered by an epithelial layer containing specialized cells called M cells, which have characteristic membrane ruffles

Fig. 1.24 Organization of a Peyer's patch in the gut mucosa. As the diagram on the left shows, a Peyer's patch contains numerous B-cell follicles with germinal centers. The areas between follicles are occupied by T cells and are therefore called the T cell–dependent areas. The layer between the surface epithelium and the follicles is known as the subepithelial dome and is rich in dendritic cells, T cells, and B cells. Peyer's patches have no afferent lymphatics, and the antigen enters directly from the gut across a specialized epithelium made up of so-called microfold (M) cells. Although this tissue looks very different from other lymphoid organs, the basic divisions are maintained. As in the lymph nodes, lymphocytes enter Peyer's patches from the blood across the walls of high endothelial venules (not shown), and leave via the efferent lymphatic. Panel a: The light micrograph shows a section through a Peyer's patch in the gut wall of a mouse. The Peyer's patch can be seen lying beneath the epithelial tissues. GC, germinal center; TDA, T cell–dependent area. Panel b: A scanning electron micrograph of the follicle-associated epithelium boxed in panel a shows the M cells, which lack the microvilli and the mucus layer present on normal epithelial cells. Each M cell appears as a sunken area on the epithelial surface. Panel c: A higher-magnification view of the boxed area in panel b shows the characteristic ruffled surface of an M cell. M cells are the portal of entry for many pathogens and other particles. Panel a, hematoxylin and eosin stain, magnification ×100; panel b, magnification ×5000; panel c, magnification ×23,000.

the lymphatic system and into the bloodstream, from where they are disseminated back into mucosal tissues to carry out their effector actions.

Similar but more diffuse aggregates of lymphocytes are present in the respiratory tract and other mucosa: **nasal-associated lymphoid tissue (NALT)** and **bronchus-associated lymphoid tissue (BALT)** are present in the respiratory tract. Like the Peyer's patches, these mucosal lymphoid tissues are also overlaid by M cells, through which inhaled microbes and antigens that become trapped in the mucous covering of the respiratory tract can pass. The mucosal immune system is discussed in Chapter 12.

Although very different in appearance, the lymph nodes, spleen, and mucosa-associated lymphoid tissue all share the same basic architecture. They all operate on the same principle, trapping antigens and antigen-presenting cells from sites of infection in order to present antigen to migratory small lymphocytes, thus inducing adaptive immune responses. The peripheral lymphoid organs also provide sustaining signals to lymphocytes that do not encounter their specific antigen immediately, so that they survive and continue to recirculate.

Because they are involved in initiating adaptive immune responses, the peripheral lymphoid organs are not static structures but vary quite markedly, depending on whether or not infection is present. The diffuse mucosal lymphoid tissues may appear in response to infection and then disappear, whereas the architecture of the organized tissues changes in a more defined way during an infection. For example, the B-cell follicles of the lymph nodes expand as B lymphocytes proliferate to form germinal centers (see Fig. 1.22), and the entire lymph node enlarges, a phenomenon familiarly known as swollen glands.

Finally, specialized populations of lymphocytes and innate lymphoid cells can be found distributed throughout particular sites in the body rather than being found in organized lymphoid tissues. Such sites include the liver and the **lamina propria** of the gut, as well as the base of the epithelial lining of the gut, reproductive epithelia, and, in mice but not in humans, the epidermis. These lymphocyte populations seem to have an important role in protecting these tissues from infection and are described further in Chapters 8 and 12.

1-18 Lymphocytes activated by antigen proliferate in the peripheral lymphoid organs, generating effector cells and immunological memory.

The great diversity of the lymphocyte receptor repertoire means that there will usually be some lymphocytes bearing a receptor for any given foreign antigen. Recent experiments suggest this number to be perhaps a few hundred per mouse, certainly not enough to mount a response against a pathogen. To generate sufficient antigen-specific effector lymphocytes to fight an infection, a lymphocyte with an appropriate receptor specificity is activated first to proliferate. Only when a large clone of identical cells has been produced do these finally differentiate into effector cells, a process that requires 4–6 days. This means the adaptive immune response to a pathogen occurs nearly a week after the initial infection has occurred and been detected by the innate immune system.

On recognizing its specific antigen on an activated antigen-presenting cell, a naive lymphocyte stops migrating, the volume of its nucleus and cytoplasm increases, and new mRNA molecules and new proteins are synthesized. Within a few hours, the cell looks completely different and is known as a **lymphoblast**. Dividing lymphoblasts are able to duplicate themselves two to four times every 24 hours over the course of 3–5 days, so that a single naive lymphocyte can produce a clone of around 1000 daughter cells of identical specificity. These then differentiate into effector cells. In the case of B cells, the differentiated effector cells are the plasma cells, which secrete antibody. In the case of T cells, the effector cells are either cytotoxic T cells, which are able to destroy infected cells, or helper T cells, which activate other cells of the immune system (see Section 1-8).

Effector lymphocytes do not recirculate like naive lymphocytes. Some effector T cells detect sites of infection and migrate into them from the blood; others stay in the lymphoid tissues to activate B cells. Some antibody-secreting plasma cells remain in the peripheral lymphoid organs, but most plasma cells generated in the lymph nodes and spleen will migrate to the bone marrow and take up residence there, secreting large amounts of antibodies into the blood system. Effector cells generated in the mucosal immune system generally stay within the mucosal tissues. Most lymphocytes generated by clonal expansion in an immune response will eventually die. However, a significant number of activated antigen-specific B cells and T cells persist after antigen has been eliminated. These cells are known as **memory cells** and form the basis of immunological memory. They can be reactivated much more quickly than naive lymphocytes, which ensures a more rapid and effective response on a second encounter with a pathogen and thereby usually provides lasting protective immunity.

The characteristics of immunological memory are readily observed by comparing an individual's antibody response to a first or **primary immunization** with the response to a **secondary (or booster) immunization** with the same antigen. As shown in **Fig. 1.25**, the secondary antibody response occurs after

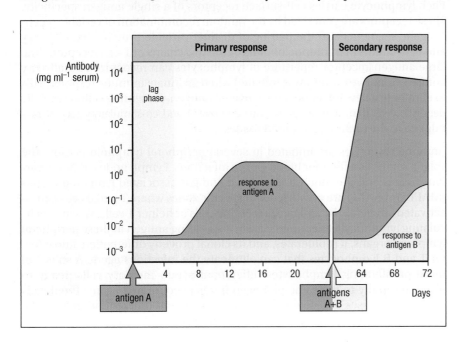

Fig. 1.25 The course of a typical antibody response. The first encounter with an antigen produces a primary response. Antigen A introduced at time zero encounters little specific antibody in the serum. After a lag phase (light blue), antibody against antigen A (dark blue) appears; its concentration rises to a plateau and then gradually declines, as is typical of a primary response. When the serum is tested for antibody against another antigen, B (yellow), there is little preset. When the animal is later challenged with a mixture of antigens A and B, a very rapid and intense antibody secondary response to A occurs, illustrating immunological memory. This is the main reason for giving booster injections after an initial vaccination. Note that the response to B resembles the primary response to A, as this is the first encounter with antigen B.

a shorter lag phase and achieves a markedly higher level than in the primary response. During the secondary response, antibodies can also acquire higher affinity, or strength of binding, for the antigen because of a process called **affinity maturation**, which takes place in the specialized germinal centers within B-cell follicles (see Section 1-16). Importantly, helper T cells are required for the process of affinity maturation, but T-cell receptors do not undergo affinity maturation. Compared with naive T cells, memory T cells show a lower threshold for activation, but as a result of changes in the responsiveness of the cell and not because of changes in the receptor. We describe the mechanisms of antibody affinity maturation in Chapter 10.

The cellular basis of immunological memory is the clonal expansion and clonal differentiation of cells that have a specific attraction for the eliciting antigen, and the memory is therefore entirely antigen-specific. It is immunological memory that enables successful vaccination and prevents reinfection with pathogens that have been repelled successfully by an adaptive immune response. In Chapter 11, we will return to immunological memory, which is perhaps the most important biological consequence of adaptive immunity.

Summary.

While the innate immune system relies on invariant pattern-recognition receptors to detect common microbial structures or the damage they cause, the adaptive immune system relies on a repertoire of antigen receptors to recognize structures that are specific to individual pathogens. This feature provides adaptive immunity with greater sensitivity and specificity. The clonal expansion of antigen-reactive lymphocytes also confers the property of immunological memory, which enhances protection against reinfection by the same pathogen.

Adaptive immunity relies on two major types of lymphocytes. B cells mature in the bone marrow and are the source of circulating antibodies. T cells mature in the thymus and recognize peptides from pathogens presented by MHC molecules on infected cells or antigen-presenting cells. An adaptive response involves the selection and amplification of clones of lymphocytes bearing receptors that recognize the foreign antigen. This clonal selection provides the theoretical framework for understanding all the key features of an adaptive immune response.

Each lymphocyte carries cell-surface receptors of a single antigen specificity. These receptors are generated by the random recombination of variable receptor gene segments and the pairing of distinct variable protein chains: heavy and light chains in immunoglobulins or the two chains of T-cell receptors. The large antigen-receptor repertoire of lymphocytes can recognize virtually any antigen. Adaptive immunity is initiated when an innate immune response fails to eliminate a new infection, and activated antigen-presenting cells—typically dendritic cells that bear antigens from pathogens and co-stimulatory receptors—migrate to the draining lymphoid tissues.

Immune responses are initiated in several peripheral lymphoid organs. The spleen serves as a filter for blood-borne infections. Lymph nodes draining various tissues and the mucosa-associated and gut-associated lymphoid tissues (MALT and GALT) are organized into specific zones where T and B cells can be activated efficiently by antigen-presenting cells or helper T cells. When a recirculating lymphocyte encounters its corresponding antigen in these peripheral lymphoid organs, it proliferates, and its clonal progeny differentiate into effector T and B lymphocytes that can eliminate the infectious agent. A subset of these proliferating lymphocytes differentiates into memory cells, ready to respond rapidly to the same pathogen if it is encountered again. The details of these processes of recognition, development, and differentiation form the main material of the central three parts of this book.

The effector mechanisms of immunity.

For activated innate and adaptive immune cells to destroy pathogens, they must employ an appropriate effector mechanism suited to each infecting agent. The different types of pathogens noted in **Fig. 1.26** have different lifestyles and require different responses for both their recognition and their destruction. Perhaps it is not surprising, then, that defenses against different pathogen types are organized into **effector modules** suited for these different lifestyles. For example, defense against extracellular pathogens can involve both phago-cytic cells and B cells, which recognize extracellular antigens and become plasma cells that secrete antibody into the extracellular environment. Defense against intracellular pathogens involves T cells that can detect peptides gen-erated inside the infected cell. Some effector T cells directly kill cells infected with intracellular pathogens such as viruses. These examples illustrate compo-nents of two distinct effector modules, one specialized for elimination of extra-cellular pathogens, and a second specialized for elimination of intracellular pathogens. In general, an effector module is a collection of cell-mediated and humoral mechanisms that involve components of both the innate and adap-tive immune systems; these mechanisms act together to achieve elimination of a particular category of pathogen. One important component of each effector module is the effector T cell response. Depending on the nature of the path-ogen, activated T cells differentiate into three major subsets of helper T cells, each of which produces different patterns of cytokines. These three subsets, discussed later, generally specialize in promoting defenses against pathogens having three major lifestyles: they can defend against intracellular infection, destroy extracellular bacteria and fungi, or provide barrier immunity directed at parasites. T cells also promote defense against extracellular pathogens by helping B cells make antibody.

Most of the other effector mechanisms used by an adaptive immune response to dispose of pathogens are the same as those of innate immunity and involve cells such as macrophages and neutrophils and proteins such as complement. Indeed, it seems likely that the vertebrate adaptive immune response evolved by the addition of specific recognition properties to innate defense mecha-nisms already existing in invertebrates. This is supported by recent findings that the innate lymphoid cells—the ILCs—show similar patterns of differenti-ation into different cytokine-producing subsets as those of T cells.

We begin this section by outlining the effector actions of antibodies, which depend almost entirely on recruiting cells and molecules of the innate immune system.

The immune system protects against four classes of pathogens		
Type of pathogen	**Examples**	**Diseases**
Viruses (intracellular)	Variola Influenza Varicella	Smallpox Flu Chickenpox
Intracellular bacteria, protozoa, parasites	*Mycobacterium leprae* *Leishmania donovani* *Plasmodium falciparum* *Toxoplasma gondii*	Leprosy Leishmaniasis Malaria Toxoplasmosis
Extracellular bacteria, parasites, fungi	*Streptococcus pneumoniae* *Clostridium tetani* *Trypanosoma brucei* *Pneumocystis jirovecii*	Pneumonia Tetanus Sleeping sickness *Pneumocystis* pneumonia
Parasitic worms (extracellular)	*Ascaris* *Schistosoma*	Ascariasis Schistosomiasis

Fig. 1.26 The major types of pathogens confronting the immune system, and some of the diseases they cause.

1-19 Innate immune responses can select from several effector modules to protect against different types of pathogens.

As we mentioned in Section 1-7, the innate immune system contains several types of cells—NK cells and ILCs—that have similarities to lymphocytes, particularly T cells. NK cells lack the antigen-specific receptors of T cells but can exhibit the cytotoxic capacity of T cells and produce some of the cytokines that effector T cells produce. ILCs develop from the same progenitor cells in the bone marrow as NK cells, and they also lack antigen-specific receptors. Very recent discoveries indicate that ILCs actually comprise several closely related lineages that differ in the specific cytokines that they will produce when activated. Remarkably, there is a striking similarity between the patterns of cytokines produced by ILC subsets and by helper T-cell subsets, as mentioned above. It appears that subsets of ILCs are the innate homologs of their helper T-cell counterparts, and NK cells are the innate homolog of cytotoxic T cells.

As mentioned in Section 1-6, there are a large number of cytokines with different functions (see eAppendix III, found in the ebook and on the Digital Landing Page for this book). A convenient way to organize the effects of cytokines is by the effector module that each cytokine promotes. Some cytokines tend to promote immunity to intracellular pathogens. One such cytokine is **interferon-γ (IFN-γ)**, which acts both by activating phagocytes to more efficiently kill intracellular pathogens and by inducing target tissues to resist intracellular pathogens. This effector module is called **type 1 immunity**. IFN-γ is produced by some but not all subsets of innate and adaptive lymphocytes, and the ILC subset making IFN-γ is called **ILC1**. Other ILC subsets produce cytokines favoring effector modules called **type 2 immunity** and **type 3 immunity**, which coordinate defense against parasitic and extracellular pathogens, respectively. The modular nature of immune effector functions will be encountered frequently throughout this book. One principle seems to be that activated sensor cells from either the innate or the adaptive immune system can activate different subsets of innate or adaptive lymphocytes that are specialized for amplifying particular effector modules that are directed against different categories of pathogens (**Fig. 1.27**).

Effector module	Cell types, functions, and mechanisms
Cytotoxicity	NK cells, CD8 T cells
	Elimination of virally infected and metabolically stressed cells
Intracellular immunity (Type 1)	ILC1, T_H1 cells
	Elimination of intracellular pathogens; activation of macrophages
Mucosal and barrier immunity (Type 2)	ILC2, T_H2 cells
	Elimination and expulsion of parasites; recruitment of eosinophils, basophils, and mast cells
Extracellular immunity (Type 3)	ILC3, T_H17 cells
	Elimination of extracellular bacteria and fungi; recruitment and activation of neutrophils

Fig. 1.27 Innate and adaptive lymphocytes share a variety of functions. The different effector modules are served by both innate and adaptive immune mechanisms. For each of the four major types of innate lymphocytes, there is a corresponding type of T cell with generally similar functional characteristics. Each set of innate lymphocyte and T cell exerts an effector activity that is broadly directed at a distinct category of pathogen.

1-20 Antibodies protect against extracellular pathogens and their toxic products.

Antibodies are found in plasma—the fluid component of blood—and in extracellular fluids. Because body fluids were once known as humors, immunity mediated by antibodies and other proteins in the plasma is known as **humoral immunity**.

Antibodies are Y-shaped molecules with two identical antigen-binding sites and one constant, or Fc, region. As mentioned in Section 1-9, there are five forms of the constant region of an antibody, known as the antibody **classes** or **isotypes**. The constant region determines an antibody's functional properties—how it will engage with the effector mechanisms that dispose of antigen once it is recognized. Each class carries out its particular function by engaging a distinct set of effector mechanisms. We describe the antibody classes and their actions in Chapters 4 and 10.

The first and most direct way in which antibodies can protect against pathogens or their products is by binding to them and thereby blocking their access to cells that they might infect or destroy (**Fig. 1.28**, left panels). This function is known as **neutralization** and is important for protection against viruses, which are prevented from entering cells and replicating, and against bacterial toxins. Neutralization is the form of immunity elicited by most vaccines against bacterial toxins.

For bacteria, however, binding by antibodies is not sufficient to stop their replication. In this case, a second function of antibodies is to enable a phagocytic cell such as a macrophage or a neutrophil to ingest and destroy the bacterium. Many bacteria evade the innate immune system because they have an outer coat that is not recognized by the pattern-recognition receptors of phagocytes. However, antigens in the coat can be recognized by antibodies, and phagocytes have receptors, called **Fc receptors**, that bind the constant region and facilitate phagocytosis of the bacterium (see Fig. 1.28, center panels). The coating of pathogens and foreign particles in this way is known as **opsonization**.

The third function of antibodies is **complement activation**. In Section 1-2 we briefly mentioned Bordet's discovery of complement as a serum factor that 'complements' the activities of antibodies. Complement can be activated by microbial surfaces even without the help of antibodies, which leads to the covalent deposition of certain complement proteins onto the bacterial surface. But when an antibody binds first to the bacterial surface, its constant region provides a platform that is much more efficient in complement activation than microbial activation of complement alone. Thus, once antibodies are produced, complement activation against a pathogen can be substantially increased.

Certain complement components that are deposited on the bacterial surface can directly lyse the membranes of some bacteria, and this is important in a few bacterial infections (see Fig. 1.28, right panels). The major function of complement, however, is to enable phagocytes to engulf and destroy bacteria that the phagocytes would not otherwise recognize. Most phagocytes express receptors that bind certain complement proteins; called complement receptors, these receptors bind to the complement proteins deposited onto the bacterial surface and thus facilitate bacterial phagocytosis. Certain other complement proteins also enhance the phagocytes' bactericidal capacity. The end result is that all pathogens and free molecules bound by antibody are eventually delivered to phagocytes for ingestion, degradation, and removal from the body (see Fig. 1.28, bottom panels). The complement system and the phagocytes that antibodies recruit are not themselves antigen-specific; they depend on antibody molecules to mark the particles as foreign.

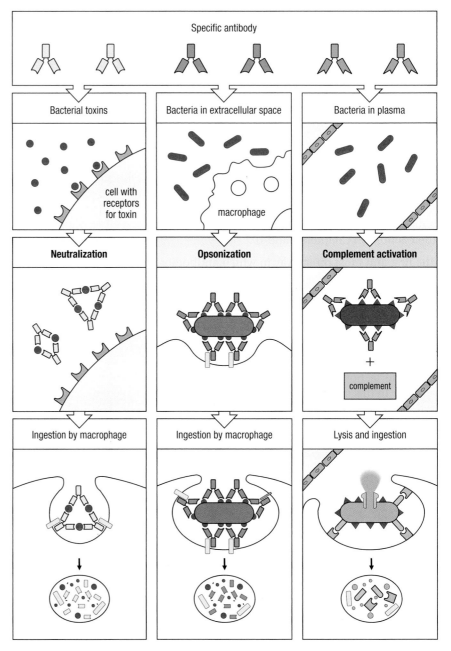

Fig. 1.28 Antibodies can participate in host defense in three main ways. The left panels show antibodies binding to and neutralizing a bacterial toxin, thus preventing it from interacting with host cells and causing pathology. Unbound toxin can react with receptors on the host cell, whereas the toxin:antibody complex cannot. Antibodies also neutralize complete virus particles and bacterial cells by binding to them and, as for toxins, preventing these microbes from interacting with host cells. For these intact microbes, neutralization by bound antibodies prevents host-cell infection and/or damage by the microbes. The antigen:antibody complex is eventually scavenged and degraded by macrophages.

Antibodies coating an antigen render it recognizable as foreign by phagocytes (macrophages and neutrophils), which then ingest and destroy it; this is called opsonization. The center panels show opsonization and phagocytosis of a bacterial cell. Antibody first binds to antigens (red) on the bacterial cell through the variable regions. Then the antibody's Fc region binds to Fc receptors (yellow) expressed by macrophages and other phagocytes, facilitating phagocytosis.

The right panels show activation of the complement system by antibodies coating a bacterial cell. Bound antibodies form a platform that activates the first protein in the complement system, which deposits complement proteins (blue) on the surface of the bacterium. This can lead in some cases to formation of a pore that lyses the bacterium directly. More generally, complement proteins on the bacterium can be recognized by complement receptors on phagocytes; this stimulates the phagocytes to ingest and destroy the bacterium. Thus, antibodies target pathogens and their toxic products for disposal by phagocytes.

1-21 T cells orchestrate cell-mediated immunity and regulate B-cell responses to most antigens.

Some bacteria and parasites, and all viruses, replicate inside cells, where they cannot be detected by antibodies, which access only the blood and extracellular space. The destruction of intracellular invaders is the function of the T lymphocytes, which are responsible for the **cell-mediated immune responses** of adaptive immunity. But T lymphocytes participate in responses to a wide variety of pathogens, including extracellular organisms, and so must exert a wide variety of effector activities.

T lymphocytes, of which there are several types, develop in the thymus. They are characterized by the type of T-cell receptors they express and by the expression of certain markers. The two main classes of T cells express either a cell-surface protein called **CD8** or another called **CD4**. These are not just random markers, but are important for a T cell's function, because they help to determine the interactions between the T cell and other cells. Recall from Section 1-10 that T cells detect peptides derived from foreign antigens that are displayed by MHC molecules on a cell's surface. CD8 and CD4 function in antigen recognition by recognizing different regions of MHC molecules and by being involved in the signaling of the T-cell receptor that is engaged with its antigen. Thus, CD4 and CD8 are known as **co-receptors** and they provide a functional difference between CD8 and CD4 T cells.

Importantly, there are two main types of MHC molecules, called **MHC class I** and **MHC class II**. These have slightly different structures, but both have an elongated groove on the outer surface that can bind a peptide (**Fig. 1.29**). The peptide becomes trapped in this groove during the synthesis and assembly of the MHC molecule inside the cell, and the peptide:MHC complex is then transported to the cell surface and displayed to T cells (**Fig. 1.30**). Because CD8 recognizes a region of the MHC class I protein while CD4 recognizes a region of the MHC class II protein, the two co-receptors functionally distinguish T cells. Therefore, CD8 T cells selectively recognize peptides that are presented by MHC class I molecules, while CD4 T cells selectively recognize peptides that are presented by MHC class II molecules.

The most direct action of T cells is cytotoxicity. Cytotoxic T cells are effector T cells that act against cells infected with viruses. Antigens derived from the virus multiplying inside the infected cell are displayed on the cell's surface, where they are recognized by the antigen receptors of cytotoxic T cells. These T cells can then control the infection by directly killing the infected cell before viral replication is complete and new viruses are released (**Fig. 1.31**). Cytotoxic T cells carry CD8, and so recognize antigen presented by MHC class I molecules. Because MHC class I molecules are expressed on most cells of the body, they serve as an important mechanism to defend against viral infections.

Fig. 1.29 MHC molecules on the cell surface display peptide fragments of antigens. MHC molecules are membrane proteins whose outer extracellular domains form a cleft in which a peptide fragment is bound. These fragments are derived from proteins degraded inside the cell and include both self and foreign protein antigens. The peptides are bound by the newly synthesized MHC molecule before it reaches the cell surface. There are two kinds of MHC molecules, MHC class I and MHC class II; they have related but distinct structures and functions. Although not shown here for simplicity, both MHC class I and MHC class II molecules are trimers of two protein chains and the bound self or nonself peptide.

Fig. 1.30 MHC class I molecules present antigen derived from proteins in the cytosol. In cells infected with viruses, viral proteins are synthesized in the cytosol. Peptide fragments of viral proteins are transported into the endoplasmic reticulum (ER), where they are bound by MHC class I molecules, which then deliver the peptides to the cell surface.

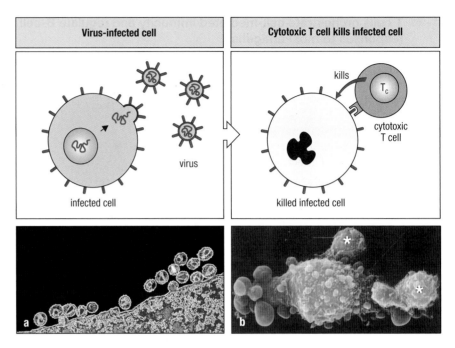

Fig. 1.31 Mechanism of host defense against intracellular infection by viruses. Cells infected by viruses are recognized by specialized T cells called cytotoxic T cells, which kill the infected cells directly. The killing mechanism involves the activation of enzymes known as caspases, which contain cysteine in their active site and cleave target proteins at aspartic acid. The caspases in turn activate a cytosolic nuclease that cleaves host and viral DNA in the infected cell. Panel a is a colored transmission electron micrograph of human immunodeficiency viruses (HIV) budding from the surface of an infected T-cell. Panel b is a scanning electron micrograph of a target cell being killed by two cytotoxic T lymphocytes (asterisks).

MHC class I molecules bearing viral peptides are recognized by CD8-bearing cytotoxic T cells, which then kill the infected cell (**Fig. 1.32**).

CD4 T cells recognize antigen presented by MHC class II molecules, which are expressed by the predominant antigen-presenting cells of the immune system: dendritic cells, macrophages, and B cells (**Fig. 1.33**). Thus CD4 T cells tend to recognize antigens taken up by phagocytosis from the extracellular environment. CD4 T cells are the helper T cells mentioned earlier in the chapter. They develop into a variety of different effector subsets, called T_H1 (for T helper type 1), T_H2, T_H17, and so on, and they produce cytokines in patterns similar to those of the subsets of ILCs mentioned earlier that activate effector modules protective against different pathogens. These subsets act primarily at sites of infection or injury in peripheral tissues. In the lymphoid tissues, a subset of CD4 T cells, called the **T follicular helper (T_{FH})** cell, interacts with B cells to regulate antibody production during the immune response. The various T helper subsets are described in Chapter 9.

For example, the T_H1 subset of CD4 T cells helps to control certain bacteria that take up residence in membrane-enclosed vesicles inside macrophages. They produce the same cytokine as ILC1 cells, IFN-γ, which activates macrophages to increase their intracellular killing power and destroy these bacteria. Important infections that are controlled by this function are tuberculosis and leprosy, which are caused by the bacteria *Mycobacterium tuberculosis* and *M. leprae*, respectively. Mycobacteria survive intracellularly because they prevent the vesicles they occupy from fusing with lysosomes, which contain a variety of degradative enzymes and antimicrobial substances (**Fig. 1.34**). However, on its surface, the infected macrophage presents mycobacteria-derived antigens that can be recognized by activated

Fig. 1.32 Cytotoxic CD8 T cells recognize antigen presented by MHC class I molecules and kill the cell. The peptide:MHC class I complex on virus-infected cells is detected by antigen-specific cytotoxic T cells. Cytotoxic T cells are preprogrammed to kill the cells they recognize.

antigen-specific T_H1 cells, which in turn secrete particular cytokines that induce the macrophage to overcome the block on vesicle fusion. T_H2 and T_H17 subsets produce cytokines that are specialized for promoting responses against parasites or extracellular bacteria and fungi, respectively. CD4 T cells, and their specialized subsets, play a pervasive role in adaptive immunity, and we will be returning to them many times in this book, including in Chapters 8, 9, 11, and 12.

1-22 Inherited and acquired defects in the immune system result in increased susceptibility to infection.

We tend to take for granted the ability of our immune systems to free our bodies of infection and prevent its recurrence. In some people, however, parts of the immune system fail. In the most severe of these **immunodeficiency diseases**, adaptive immunity is completely absent, and death occurs in infancy from overwhelming infection unless heroic measures are taken. Other less catastrophic failures lead to recurrent infections with particular types of pathogens, depending on the particular deficiency. Much has been learned about the functions of the different components of the human immune system through the study of these immunodeficiencies, many of which are caused by inherited genetic defects. Because understanding the features of immunodeficiencies requires a detailed knowledge of normal immune mechanisms, we have postponed discussion of most of these diseases until Chapter 13, where they can be considered together.

In the 1980s, a devastating form of immunodeficiency appeared, the **acquired immune deficiency syndrome**, or **AIDS**, which is caused by an infectious agent, the human immunodeficiency viruses HIV-1 and HIV-2. This disease destroys T cells, dendritic cells, and macrophages bearing CD4, leading to infections caused by intracellular bacteria and other pathogens normally controlled by such cells. These infections are the major cause of death from this increasingly prevalent immunodeficiency disease, which is discussed fully in Chapter 13 together with the inherited immunodeficiencies.

Fig. 1.33 CD4 T cells recognize antigen presented by MHC class II molecules. On recognition of their specific antigen on infected macrophages, T_H1 cells activate the macrophage, leading to the destruction of the intracellular bacteria (top panel). When T follicular helper (T_{FH}) cells recognize antigen on B cells (bottom panel), they activate these cells to proliferate and differentiate into antibody-producing plasma cells (not shown).

Acquired Immune Deficiency Syndrome (AIDS)

Fig. 1.34 Mechanism of host defense against intracellular infection by mycobacteria. Mycobacteria are engulfed by macrophages but resist being destroyed by preventing the intracellular vesicles in which they reside from fusing with lysosomes containing bactericidal agents. Thus the bacteria are protected from being killed. In resting macrophages, mycobacteria persist and replicate in these vesicles. When the phagocyte is recognized and activated by a T_H1 cell, however, the phagocytic vesicles fuse with lysosomes, and the bacteria can be killed. Macrophage activation is controlled by T_H1 cells, both to avoid tissue damage and to save energy.

1-23 Understanding adaptive immune responses is important for the control of allergies, autoimmune disease, and the rejection of transplanted organs.

The main function of our immune system is to protect the human host from infectious agents. However, many medically important diseases are associated with a normal immune response directed against an inappropriate antigen, often in the absence of infectious disease. Immune responses directed at noninfectious antigens occur in **allergy**, in which the antigen is an innocuous foreign substance; in **autoimmune disease**, in which the response is to a self antigen; and in **graft rejection**, in which the antigen is borne by a transplanted foreign cell (discussed in Chapter 15). The major antigens provoking graft rejection are, in fact, the MHC molecules, as each of these is present in many different versions in the human population—that is, they are highly **polymorphic**—and most unrelated people differ in the set of MHC molecules they express, a property commonly known as their 'tissue type.' The MHC was originally recognized by the work of Peter Gorer in the 1930s as a gene locus in mice, the **H-2 locus**, that controlled the acceptance or rejection of transplanted tumors. Genes in this locus were later studied by George Snell, who examined their role in tissue transplantation by developing mouse strains differing only at these histocompatibility loci. The human MHC molecules were first discovered during the Second World War, when attempts were made to use skin grafts from donors to repair badly burned pilots and bomb victims. The patients rejected the grafts, which were recognized by their immune systems as being 'foreign.' What we call a successful immune response or a failure, and whether the response is considered harmful or beneficial to the host, depends not on the response itself but rather on the nature of the antigen and the circumstances in which the response occurs (**Fig. 1.35**). Snell was awarded the 1980 Nobel Prize (together with Baruj Benacerraf and Jean Dausset) for his work on the MHC.

Allergic diseases, which include asthma, are an increasingly common cause of disability in the developed world. Autoimmunity is also now recognized as the cause of many important diseases. An autoimmune response directed against pancreatic β cells is the leading cause of diabetes in the young. In allergies and autoimmune diseases, the powerful protective mechanisms of the adaptive immune response cause serious damage to the individual.

Immune responses to harmless antigens, to body tissues, or to organ grafts are, like all other immune responses, highly specific. At present, the usual way to treat these responses is with immunosuppressive drugs, which inhibit all immune responses, desirable and undesirable alike. If it were possible

Antigen	Effect of response to antigen	
	Normal response	**Deficient response**
Infectious agent	Protective immunity	Recurrent infection
Innocuous substance	Allergy	No response
Grafted organ	Rejection	Acceptance
Self organ	Autoimmunity	Self tolerance
Tumor	Tumor immunity	Cancer

Fig. 1.35 Immune responses can be beneficial or harmful, depending on the nature of the antigen. Beneficial responses are shown in white boxes, harmful responses in red-shaded boxes. Where the response is beneficial, its absence is harmful.

to suppress only those lymphocyte clones responsible for the unwanted response, the disease could be cured or the grafted organ protected without impeding protective immune responses. At present, antigen-specific immunoregulation is outside the reach of clinical treatment. But as we shall see in Chapter 16, many new drugs have been developed recently that offer more selective immune suppression to control autoimmune and other unwanted immune responses. Among these, therapies using highly specific **monoclonal antibodies** were made possible by Georges Köhler and César Milstein, who shared the 1984 Nobel Prize along with Niels K. Jerne. Köhler and Milstein received the prize for their "discovery of the principle for production of monoclonal antibodies." We shall discuss the current state of understanding of allergies, autoimmune disease, graft rejection, and immunosuppressive drugs and monoclonal antibodies in Chapters 14–16, and we shall see in Chapter 15 how the mechanisms of immune regulation are beginning to emerge from a better understanding of the functional subsets of lymphocytes and the cytokines that control them.

1-24 Vaccination is the most effective means of controlling infectious diseases.

The deliberate stimulation of an immune response by immunization, or vaccination, has achieved many successes in the two centuries since Jenner's pioneering experiment. Mass immunization programs have led to the virtual eradication of several diseases that used to be associated with significant morbidity (illness) and mortality (**Fig. 1.36**). Immunization is considered so safe and so important that most states in the United States require children to be immunized against up to seven common childhood diseases. Impressive as these accomplishments are, there are still many diseases for which we lack effective vaccines. And even though vaccines for diseases such as measles can be used effectively in developed countries, technical and economic problems can prevent their widespread use in developing countries, where mortality from these diseases is still high.

The tools of modern immunology and molecular biology are being applied to develop new vaccines and improve old ones, and we discuss these advances in Chapter 16. The prospect of controlling these important diseases is tremendously exciting. The guarantee of good health is a critical step toward population control and economic development. At a cost of pennies per person, great hardship and suffering can be alleviated.

Many serious pathogens have resisted efforts to develop vaccines against them, often because they can evade or subvert the protective mechanisms of an adaptive immune response. We examine some of the evasive strategies used by successful pathogens in Chapter 13. The conquest of many of the world's leading diseases, including malaria and diarrheal diseases (the leading killers of children) as well as the more recent threat from AIDS, depends on a better understanding of the pathogens that cause them and their interactions with the cells of the immune system.

1-25 Emerging pathogens present new challenges for the immune system.

Pathogenic microbes have been besieging humans for centuries, if not millennia. Reports of the bubonic plague, caused by the bacterium *Yersinia pestis*, date back to the Philistines in 1320 BCE. Influenza virus has been causing human disease for centuries, with the earliest report of an influenza-like illness by Hippocrates, the Greek physician, in ~410 BCE. Current estimates indicate that *Mycobacterium tuberculosis*, the causative agent of tuberculosis,

Fig. 1.36 Successful vaccination campaigns. Diphtheria, polio, and measles and their consequences have been virtually eliminated in the United States, as shown in these three graphs. SSPE stands for subacute sclerosing panencephalitis, a brain disease that is a late consequence of measles infection in few individuals. When measles was prevented, SSPE disappeared 15–20 years later. However, because these diseases have not been eradicated worldwide, immunization must be maintained in a very high percentage of the population to prevent their reappearance.

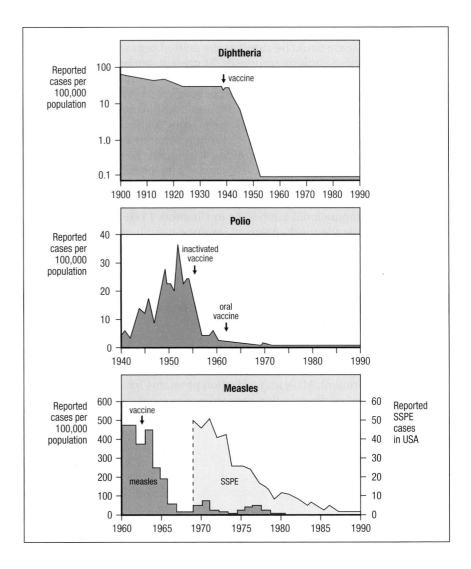

has existed for more than 70,000 years. However, as recent history has shown us, new pathogenic organisms occasionally arise and wreak devastation on the human population. Frequently, these emerging pathogens are viruses with relatively small genomes and high mutation rates, ideal conditions for the development of human-to-human transmission capabilities.

The early 21st century witnessed the emergence of several novel coronaviruses that cause respiratory infections with a high rate of transmission. These viruses are believed to have crossed into humans from bats, their natural reservoir. Two of these viruses caused epidemics with a high fatality rate, SARS-CoV in 2002–2003 and MERS-CoV in 2012, but ultimately were responsible for fewer than 1000 deaths each. A third coronavirus, SARS-CoV-2, emerged in late 2019 and rapidly spread across the globe, causing a worldwide pandemic that disrupted societies and economies and by June 2020 was responsible for more than 4000 deaths a day. Studies of the immune response to SARS-CoV-2 are proceeding at a remarkable pace, and by early 2021 multiple effective vaccines had been developed and introduced to the public.

Summary.

The responses to infection can be organized into several effector modules that target the various types of pathogen lifestyles. Innate sensor cells that detect infection generate mediators that activate innate lymphoid cells (ILCs) and T cells, which amplify the immune response and also activate various effector modules. ILCs include subsets that produce different cytokines and activate distinct effector modules. T cells fall into two major classes that are based on the expression of the co-receptors CD8 and CD4. CD8 and CD4 T cells recognize antigen presented by MHC class I or MHC class II proteins, respectively. These subsets of T cells, like their ILC counterparts, also promote the actions of distinct effector modules. NK cells and CD8 T cells can exert cytotoxic activity to target intracellular infections such as viruses. Other subsets of innate lymphoid and helper T cells can secrete mediators that activate other effector functions, ones that target intracellular bacteria, extracellular bacteria and fungi, and parasites. T cells also provide signals that help regulate B cells and stimulate them to produce antibodies. Specific antibodies mediate the clearance and elimination of soluble toxins and extracellular pathogens. They interact not only with the toxins or the antigens on microbes but also with the Fc region of specific receptors that are expressed by many types of phagocytes. Phagocytes also express receptors for complement proteins that are deposited on microbial surfaces, particularly in the presence of antibody.

Failures of immunity can be caused by genetic defects or by infections that target important components of the immune system. Misdirected immune responses can damage host tissues, as in autoimmune diseases or allergy, or lead to the failure of transplanted organs. While vaccination is still the greatest tool of immunology to fight diseases, modern approaches have added new tools, such as monoclonal antibodies, that have become progressively more important in the clinic since their initial use in the mid-1980s.

Summary to Chapter 1.

The immune system defends the host against infection. Innate immunity serves as a first line of defense but lacks the ability to recognize certain pathogens and to provide the specific protective immunity that prevents reinfection. Adaptive immunity is based on clonal selection from a repertoire of lymphocytes bearing highly diverse antigen-specific receptors that enable the immune system to recognize any foreign antigen. In the adaptive immune response, antigen-specific lymphocytes proliferate and differentiate into clones of effector lymphocytes that eliminate the pathogen. Figure 1.7 summarizes the phases of the immune response and their approximate timings. Host defense requires different recognition systems and a wide variety of effector mechanisms to seek out and destroy the wide variety of pathogens in their various habitats within the body and at its external and internal surfaces. Not only can the adaptive immune response eliminate a pathogen, but, in the process, it also generates increased numbers of differentiated memory lymphocytes through clonal selection, and this allows a more rapid and effective response upon reinfection. The regulation of immune responses, whether to suppress them when unwanted or to stimulate them in the prevention of infectious disease, is the major medical goal of research in immunology.

General references.

Historical background

Burnet, F.M.: *The Clonal Selection Theory of Acquired Immunity.* London: Cambridge University Press, 1959.

Gowans, J.L.: **The lymphocyte—a disgraceful gap in medical knowledge.** *Immunol. Today* 1996, 17:288–291.

Landsteiner, K.: *The Specificity of Serological Reactions*, 3rd ed. Boston: Harvard University Press, 1964.

Metchnikoff, É.: *Immunity in the Infectious Diseases*, 1st ed. New York: Macmillan Press, 1905.

Silverstein, A.M.: *History of Immunology*, 1st ed. London: Academic Press, 1989.

Biological background

Alberts, B., Heald, R., Johnson, A., Morgan, D., Raff, M., Roberts, K., and Walter, P.: *Molecular Biology of the Cell*, 7th ed. New York: W.W. Norton, 2022.

Berg, J.M., Tymoczko, J.L., Gatto, G.J., Jr., and Stryer, L.: *Biochemistry*, 9th ed. New York: W.H. Freeman, 2019.

Geha, R.S., and Notarangelo, L.D.: *Case Studies in Immunology: A Clinical Companion*, 7th ed. New York: W.W. Norton, 2016.

Harper, D.R.: *Viruses: Biology, Applications, Control*. New York: Garland Science, 2012.

Kaufmann, S.E., Sher, A., and Ahmed, R. (eds): *Immunology of Infectious Diseases*. Washington, DC: ASM Press, 2001.

Lodish, H., Berk, A., Kaiser, C.A., Krieger, M., Bretscher, A., Ploegh, H., Martin, K.C., Yaffe, M., and Amon, A.: *Molecular Cell Biology*, 8th ed. New York: W.H. Freeman, 2021.

Lydyard, P., Cole, M., Holton, J., Irving, W., Porakishvili, N., Venkatesan, P., and Ward, K.: *Case Studies in Infectious Disease*. New York: Garland Science, 2009.

Nash, A., Dalziel, R., and Fitzgerald, J.: *Mims' Pathogenesis of Infectious Disease*, 6th ed. London: Academic Press, 2015.

Ryan, K.J. (ed): *Sherris Medical Microbiology*, 7th ed. New York: McGraw-Hill Education, 2018.

Advanced textbooks in immunology, compendia, etc.

Lachmann, P.J., Peters, D.K., Rosen, F.S., and Walport, M.J. (eds): *Clinical Aspects of Immunology*, 5th ed. Oxford: Blackwell Scientific, 1993.

Mak, T.W., and Saunders, M.E.: *The Immune Response: Basic and Clinical Principles*. Burlington, MA: Elsevier/Academic Press, 2006.

Mak, T.W., and Simard, J.J.L.: *Handbook of Immune Response Genes*. New York: Plenum Press, 1998.

Paul, W.E. (ed): *Fundamental Immunology*, 7th ed. New York: Lippincott Williams & Wilkins, 2012.

Roitt, I.M., and Delves, P.J. (eds): *Encyclopedia of Immunology*, 2nd ed. (4 vols). London and San Diego: Academic Press, 1998.

Innate Immunity: The First Lines of Defense

2

As stated in Chapter 1, most microbial invaders can be detected and destroyed within minutes or hours by the body's defense mechanisms of **innate immunity**, which do not rely on expansion of antigen-specific lymphocytes. The innate immune system uses a limited number of secreted proteins and cell-associated receptors to detect infection and to distinguish between pathogens and host tissues. These are called innate receptors because they are inborn; they are encoded by genes directly inherited from an individual's parents and do not need to be generated by the gene rearrangements used to assemble antigen receptors of lymphocytes described in Section 1-11. The importance of innate immunity is illustrated by several immunodeficiencies that result when it is impaired, increasing susceptibility to infection even in the presence of an intact adaptive immune system, as we will discuss in Chapter 13.

As we saw in Fig. 1.5, an infection starts when a pathogen breaches one of the host's anatomic barriers. Some innate immune mechanisms start acting immediately (**Fig. 2.1**). These immediate defenses include several classes of preformed soluble molecules that are present in extracellular fluid, blood, and epithelial secretions and which can either kill the pathogen or weaken its effect. **Antimicrobial enzymes** such as lysozyme begin to digest bacterial cell walls; **antimicrobial peptides** such as the defensins lyse bacterial cell membranes directly; and a system of plasma proteins known as the **complement system** targets pathogens both for lysis and for phagocytosis by cells of the innate immune system, such as macrophages. If these fail, innate immune cells become activated by pattern-recognition receptors (PRRs) that detect molecules called pathogen-associated molecular patterns (PAMPs) that are typical of microbes (see Section 1-5). The activated innate cells can engage various effector mechanisms to eliminate the infection. By themselves, neither the soluble nor the cellular components of innate immunity generate long-term protective immunological memory. If an infectious organism breaches these first two lines of defense, mechanisms will be engaged to induce an adaptive immune response—the third phase of the response to a pathogen. This leads to the expansion of antigen-specific lymphocytes that target the pathogen specifically and to the formation of memory cells that provide long-lasting specific immunity.

This chapter considers the first phase of the innate immune response. We first describe the anatomic barriers that protect the host against infection and examine the immediate innate defenses provided by various secreted soluble

IN THIS CHAPTER

Anatomic barriers and initial chemical defenses.

The complement system and innate immunity.

Fig. 2.1 The response to an initial infection occurs in three phases. These are the innate phase, the induced innate response, and the adaptive immune response. The first two phases rely on the recognition of pathogens by germline-encoded receptors of the innate immune system, whereas adaptive immunity uses variable antigen-specific receptors that are produced as a result of gene segment rearrangements. Adaptive immunity occurs late, because the rare B cells and T cells specific for the invading pathogen must first undergo clonal expansion before they differentiate into effector cells that migrate to the site of infection and clear the infection. The effector mechanisms that remove the infectious agent are similar or identical in each phase.

proteins. The anatomic barriers are fixed defenses against infection and consist of the epithelia that line the internal and external surfaces of the body, along with the phagocytes residing beneath all epithelial surfaces. These phagocytes act directly by engulfing and digesting invading microorganisms. Epithelia are also protected by many kinds of chemical defenses, including antimicrobial enzymes and peptides. Next we describe the complement system, which directly kills some microorganisms and interacts with others to promote their removal by phagocytic cells. The complement system together with other soluble circulating defensive proteins is sometimes referred to as **humoral** innate immunity, from the old word 'humor' for body fluids. If these early defenses fail, the phagocytes at the site of infection help recruit new cells and circulating effector molecules, a process called inflammation, which we will discuss in Chapter 3.

Anatomic barriers and initial chemical defenses.

Microorganisms that cause disease in humans and animals enter the body at different sites and produce disease symptoms by a variety of mechanisms. Microorganisms that cause disease and produce damage, or pathology, to tissues are referred to as **pathogenic microorganisms**, or simply **pathogens**. As innate immunity eliminates most microorganisms that may occasionally cross an anatomic barrier, pathogens are microorganisms that have evolved ways of overcoming the body's innate defenses more effectively than have other microorganisms. Once infection is established, both innate and adaptive immune responses are typically required to eliminate pathogens from the body. Even in these cases, the innate immune system performs a valuable function by reducing pathogen numbers during the time needed for the adaptive immune system to gear up for action. In the first part of this chapter, we briefly describe the different types of pathogens and their invasive strategies and then examine the immediate innate defenses that, in most cases, prevent microorganisms from establishing an infection.

2-1 Infectious diseases are caused by diverse living agents that replicate in their hosts.

The agents that cause disease fall into five groups: viruses, bacteria, fungi, protozoa, and helminths (worms). Protozoa and worms are usually grouped together as parasites and are the subject of the discipline of parasitology, whereas viruses, bacteria, and fungi are the subject of microbiology. **Figure 2.2** lists some examples of the different classes of microorganisms and parasites, and the diseases they cause. The characteristic features of each pathogen are its mode of transmission, its mechanism of replication, its mechanism of **pathogenesis**—the means by which it causes disease—and the response it elicits from the host. The distinct pathogen habitats and life cycles mean that a range of different innate and adaptive immune mechanisms have to be deployed for pathogen destruction.

Infectious agents can grow in all body compartments, as shown schematically in **Fig. 2.3**. We saw in Chapter 1 that two major compartments can be defined: extracellular and intracellular. Both innate and adaptive immune responses have different ways of dealing with pathogens found in these two compartments. Many bacterial pathogens live and replicate in extracellular spaces, either within tissues or on the surface of the epithelia that line body cavities. Extracellular bacteria are usually susceptible to killing by phagocytes, an important arm of the innate immune system, but some pathogens, such as *Staphylococcus* and *Streptococcus* species, achieve a very basic form of

Routes of infection for pathogens				
Route of entry	Mode of transmission	Pathogen	Disease	Type of pathogen
Mucosal surfaces				
Mouth and respiratory tract	Inhalation or ingestion of infective material (e.g., saliva droplets)	Measles virus	Measles	Paramyxovirus
		Influenza virus	Influenza	Orthomyxovirus
		Varicella-zoster	Chickenpox	Herpesvirus
		Epstein–Barr virus	Mononucleosis	Herpesvirus
		Streptococcus pyogenes	Tonsilitis	Gram-positive bacterium
		Haemophilus influenzae	Pneumonia, meningitis	Gram-negative bacterium
		Neisseria meningitidis	Meningococcal meningitis	Gram-negative bacterium
	Spores	*Bacillus anthracis*	Inhalation anthrax	Gram-positive bacterium
Gastrointestinal tract	Contaminated water or food	Rotavirus	Diarrhea	Rotavirus
		Hepatitis A	Jaundice	Picornavirus
		Salmonella enterica ssp. *enteritidis*, *Salmonella enterica* ssp. *typhimurium*	Food poisoning	Gram-negative bacterium
		Vibrio cholerae	Cholera	Gram-negative bacterium
		Salmonella enterica ssp. *typhi*	Typhoid fever	Gram-negative bacterium
		Trichuris trichiura	Trichuriasis	Helminth
Reproductive tract and other routes	Sexual transmission/ infected blood	Hepatitis B virus	Hepatitis B	Hepadnavirus
		Human immunodeficiency virus (HIV)	Acquired immune deficiency syndrome (AIDS)	Retrovirus
	Sexual transmission	*Neisseria gonorrhoeae*	Gonorrhea	Gram-negative bacterium
		Treponema pallidum	Syphilis	Bacterium (spirochete)
Opportunistic infections	Resident microbiota	*Candida albicans*	Candidiasis, thrush	Fungus
	Resident lung microbiota	*Pneumocystis jirovecii*	Pneumonia	Fungus
External epithelia				
External surface	Physical contact	*Trichophyton*	Athlete's foot	Fungus
Wounds and abrasions	Minor skin abrasions	*Bacillus anthracis*	Cutaneous anthrax	Gram-positive bacterium
	Puncture wounds	*Clostridium tetani*	Tetanus	Gram-positive bacterium
	Handling infected animals	*Francisella tularensis*	Tularemia	Gram-negative bacterium
Insect bites	Mosquito bites (*Aedes aegypti*)	Flavivirus	Yellow fever	Virus
	Deer tick bites	*Borrelia burgdorferi*	Lyme disease	Bacterium (spirochete)
	Mosquito bites (*Anopheles*)	*Plasmodium* spp.	Malaria	Protozoan

Fig. 2.2 A variety of microorganisms can cause disease. Pathogenic organisms are of five main types: viruses, bacteria, fungi, protozoa, and helminths (worms). Some well-known pathogens are listed.

Fig. 2.3 Pathogens can be found in various compartments of the body, where they must be combated by different host-defense mechanisms. Virtually all pathogens have an extracellular phase in which they are vulnerable to the circulating molecules and cells of innate immunity and to the antibodies of the adaptive immune response. All these clear the microorganism mainly by promoting its uptake and destruction by the phagocytes of the immune system. Intracellular phases of pathogens such as viruses are not accessible to these mechanisms; instead, the infected cell is attacked by the NK cells of innate immunity or by the cytotoxic T cells of adaptive immunity. Activation of macrophages as a result of NK-cell or T-cell activity can induce the macrophage to kill pathogens that are living inside macrophage vesicles.

	Extracellular		Intracellular	
	Interstitial spaces, blood, lymph	**Epithelial surfaces**	**Cytoplasmic**	**Vesicular**
Site of infection				
Organisms	Viruses Bacteria Protozoa Fungi Worms	*Neisseria gonorrhoeae* *Streptococcus pneumoniae* *Vibrio cholerae* *Helicobacter pylori* *Candida albicans* Worms	Viruses *Chlamydia* spp. *Rickettsia* spp. Protozoa	*Mycobacterium* spp. *Yersinia pestis* *Legionella pneumophila* *Cryptococcus neoformans* *Leishmania* spp.
Protective immunity	Complement Phagocytosis Antibodies	Antimicrobial peptides Antibodies, especially IgA	NK cells Cytotoxic T cells	T cell–dependent and NK cell–dependent macrophage activation

immune evasion by having a protective polysaccharide capsule that resists engulfment. This can be overcome to some extent by the help of another component of innate immunity (complement), which deposits specific molecules on the surface of the bacteria (opsonization), rendering them more susceptible to phagocytosis. In the adaptive immune response, bacteria are rendered more susceptible to phagocytosis by a combination of antibodies and complement.

Infectious diseases differ in their symptoms and outcome depending on where the causal pathogen replicates within the body—the intracellular or the extracellular compartment—and what damage it does to the tissues (**Fig. 2.4**). Pathogens that live intracellularly frequently cause disease by damaging or killing the cells they infect. Obligate intracellular pathogens, such as viruses, must invade host cells to replicate. Facultative intracellular pathogens, such as mycobacteria, can replicate either intracellularly or outside the cell. Two strategies of innate immunity defend against intracellular pathogens. One strategy aims to destroy pathogens before they infect cells and includes soluble defenses such as antimicrobial peptides, as well as phagocytic cells that can engulf and destroy pathogens before they become intracellular. Alternatively, the innate immune system can recognize and kill cells infected by some pathogens. This is the role of the natural killer cells (NK cells), which act to limit certain viral infections before cytotoxic T cells of the adaptive immune system become functional. Intracellular pathogens can be subdivided further into those that replicate freely in the cell, such as viruses and certain bacteria (for example, *Chlamydia*, *Rickettsia*, and *Listeria*), and those that replicate inside intracellular vesicles, such as mycobacteria. Pathogens that live inside macrophage vesicles may become more susceptible to being killed after activation of the macrophage as a result of NK-cell or T-cell actions (see Fig. 2.3).

Many of the most dangerous extracellular bacterial pathogens cause disease by releasing protein toxins; these secreted toxins are called **exotoxins** (see Fig. 2.4). The innate immune system has little defense against such toxins, and highly specific antibodies produced by the adaptive immune system are required to neutralize their action (see Fig. 1.28). The damage caused by a particular infectious agent also depends on where it grows; *Streptococcus*

	Direct mechanisms of tissue damage by pathogens			Indirect mechanisms of tissue damage by pathogens		
	Exotoxin production	Endotoxin	Direct cytopathic effect	Immune complexes	Anti-host antibody	Cell-mediated immunity
Pathogenic mechanism						
Infectious agent	*Streptococcus pyogenes* *Staphylococcus aureus* *Corynebacterium diphtheriae* *Clostridium tetani* *Vibrio cholerae*	*Escherichia coli* *Haemophilus influenzae* *Salmonella enterica* ssp. *typhi* *Shigella* *Pseudomonas aeruginosa* *Yersinia pestis*	Variola Varicella-zoster Hepatitis B virus Polio virus Measles virus Influenza virus Herpes simplex virus Human herpes virus 8 (HHV8)	Hepatitis B virus *Plasmodium* *Streptococcus pyogenes* *Treponema pallidum* Most acute infections	*Streptococcus pyogenes* *Mycoplasma pneumoniae*	Lymphocytic choriomeningitis virus Herpes simplex virus *Mycobacterium tuberculosis* *Mycobacterium leprae* *Borrelia burgdorferi* *Schistosoma mansoni*
Disease	Tonsilitis, scarlet fever Boils, toxic shock syndrome, food poisoning Diphtheria Tetanus Cholera	Gram-negative sepsis Meningitis, pneumonia Typhoid fever Bacillary dysentery Wound infection Plague	Smallpox Chickenpox, shingles Hepatitis Poliomyelitis Measles, subacute sclerosing panencephalitis Influenza Cold sores Kaposi's sarcoma	Kidney disease Vascular deposits Glomerulonephritis Kidney damage in secondary syphilis Transient renal deposits	Rheumatic fever Hemolytic anemia	Aseptic meningitis Herpes stromal keratitis Tuberculosis Tuberculoid leprosy Lyme arthritis Schistosomiasis

Fig. 2.4 Pathogens can damage tissues in a variety of different ways. The mechanisms of damage, representative infectious agents, and the common names of the diseases associated with each are shown. Exotoxins are released by microorganisms and act at the surface of host cells, for example, by binding to receptors. Endotoxins, which are intrinsic components of microbial structure, trigger phagocytes to release cytokines that produce local or systemic symptoms. Many pathogens are cytopathic, directly damaging the cells they infect. Finally, an adaptive immune response to the pathogen can generate antigen:antibody complexes that activate neutrophils and macrophages, antibodies that can cross-react with host tissues, or T cells that kill infected cells. All of these have some potential to damage the host's tissues. In addition, neutrophils, the most abundant cells early in infection, release many proteins and small-molecule inflammatory mediators that both control infection and cause tissue damage.

pneumoniae in the lung causes pneumonia, for example, whereas in the blood it causes a potentially fatal systemic illness, pneumococcal sepsis. In contrast, nonsecreted constituents of bacterial structure that trigger phagocytes to release cytokines with local and systemic effects are called **endotoxins**. An endotoxin of major medical importance is the **lipopolysaccharide (LPS)** of the outer cell membrane of **Gram-negative bacteria**, such as *Salmonella*. Many of the clinical symptoms of infection by such bacteria—including fever, pain, rash, hemorrhage, septic shock—are due largely to LPS.

Most pathogenic microorganisms can overcome innate immune responses and continue to grow, making us ill. An adaptive immune response is required to eliminate them and to prevent subsequent reinfections. Certain pathogens are never entirely eliminated by the immune system and persist in the body for years. But most pathogens are not universally lethal. Those that have lived for thousands of years in the human population are highly evolved to exploit their human hosts; they cannot alter their pathogenicity without upsetting the compromise they have achieved with the human immune system. Rapidly killing every host it infects is no better for the long-term survival of a pathogen than being wiped out by the immune response before the microbe has had time to infect someone else. In short, we have adapted to live with many microbes, and they with us. Nevertheless, highly pathogenic strains of avian influenza, the episode in 2002–2003 of SARS (severe acute respiratory syndrome), a severe pneumonia in humans that is caused by the coronavirus SARS-CoV from bats, and the SARS-CoV-2 pandemic of 2020 all remind us that new and deadly infections can transfer from animal reservoirs to humans. Even though infection with SARS-CoV-2 has a case fatality rate substantially lower than that seen in SARS, the 2020 pandemic has had an enormous negative impact on the global economy. Such transmission appears responsible for the Ebola virus epidemic in West Africa in 2014–2015. These are known as **zoonotic** infections—and we must be on the alert at all times for the emergence of new pathogens and new threats to health. The human immunodeficiency virus that causes AIDS (discussed in Chapter 13) serves as a warning that we remain constantly vulnerable.

Acquired Immune Deficiency Syndrome (AIDS)

2-2 Epithelial surfaces of the body provide the first barrier against infection.

Our body surfaces are composed of epithelia with diverse functions. They can provide a protective physical barrier between the internal milieu and the external world that contains pathogens. Epithelia compose the skin and the linings of the body's tubular structures—the respiratory, urogenital, and gastrointestinal tracts. Epithelia in these locations are specialized for their particular functions and possess unique innate defense strategies against the microbes they typically encounter (**Fig. 2.5** and **Fig. 2.6**). The necessity to carry out various functions in these locations, such as absorption of nutrients or oxygen for example, means that these epithelia are not perfect barriers to infection.

Epithelia can be a layer of single cells or multiple layers of cells with varying geometry. Epithelial cells are held together by tight junctions, which effectively form a seal against the external environment. The body's internal epithelia are known as **mucosal epithelia** because they secrete a viscous fluid called **mucus**, which contains many glycoproteins called **mucins**. Mucus has a number of protective functions. The mucus layer establishes a viscous physical barrier that impedes microbial access to various epithelial surfaces. In the respiratory tract, microorganisms can be expelled in the outward flow of

Fig. 2.5 Many barriers prevent pathogens from crossing epithelia and colonizing tissues. Surface epithelia provide mechanical, chemical, and microbiological barriers to infection. The epithelium of the skin is stratified, having multiple layers. Epithelia in the various locations in the intestine have a single cell layer. The epithelia of the upper airway have a single cell layer, but the cell nuclei are staggered in a way that suggests multiple layers.

		Skin	Gut	Lungs	Eyes/nose/oral cavity
		Stratified epithelium	Single cell layer of columnar epithelium	Upper airway: pseudostratified columnar epithelium Lower airway: single cell layer of columnar epithelium	Pseudostratified columnar epithelium
Mechanical		Epithelial cells joined by tight junctions			
		Longitudinal flow of air or fluid	Longitudinal flow of air or fluid	Movement of mucus by cilia	Tears Nasal cilia
Chemical		Fatty acids	Low pH	Pulmonary surfactant	Enzymes in tears and saliva (lysozyme)
			Enzymes (pepsin)		
		β-defensins Lamellar bodies Cathelicidin	α-defensins (cryptdins) RegIII (lecticidins) Cathelicidin	α-defensins Cathelicidin	Histatins β-defensins
Microbiological		Normal microbiota			

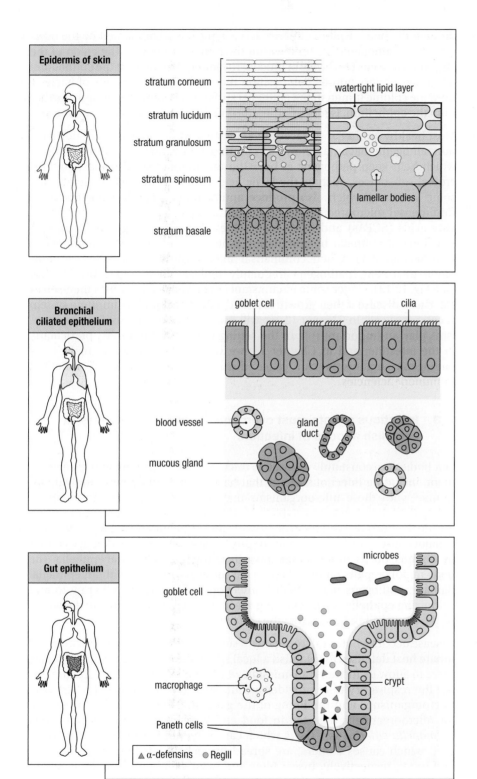

Epidermis of skin

stratum corneum

stratum lucidum

stratum granulosum

stratum spinosum

stratum basale

watertight lipid layer

lamellar bodies

Bronchial ciliated epithelium

goblet cell

cilia

blood vessel

gland duct

mucous gland

Gut epithelium

microbes

goblet cell

macrophage

crypt

Paneth cells

△ α-defensins   ● RegIII

Fig. 2.6 Epithelia form specialized physical and chemical barriers that provide innate defenses in different locations. Top panel: The epidermis has multiple layers of keratinocytes in different stages of differentiation arising from the basal layer of stem cells. Differentiated keratinocytes in the stratum spinosum produce β-defensins and cathelicidins, which are incorporated into secretory organelles called lamellar bodies (yellow) and secreted into the intercellular space to form a waterproof lipid layer (the stratum corneum) containing antimicrobial activity. Center panel: In the lung, the airways are lined with ciliated epithelium. Beating of the cilia moves a continuous stream of mucus (green) secreted by goblet cells outward, trapping and ejecting potential pathogens. Type II pneumocytes in the lung alveoli (not shown) also produce and secrete antimicrobial defensins. Bottom panel: In the intestine, epithelial cells and Paneth cells—specialized cells deep in the epithelial crypts—produce several kinds of antimicrobial proteins: α-defensins (cryptdins) and the antimicrobial RegIII proteins.

mucus driven by the beating of cilia on the mucosal epithelium (**Fig. 2.7**). The importance of mucus flow in clearing infection is illustrated by people with the inherited disease **cystic fibrosis**, in which the mucus becomes abnormally thick and dehydrated because of defects in a gene, *CFTR*, encoding a chloride channel in the epithelium. Such individuals frequently develop lung infections caused by bacteria that colonize the epithelial surface but do not cross it (see Fig. 2.7). Mucus also plays an important role in the gut. Peristalsis is an important mechanism for keeping both food and infectious agents moving

Ciliated respiratory epithelium is covered by a layer of mucus

Mucus

Cilia

Epithelium

Lung of a person with cystic fibrosis

Fig. 2.7 Ciliated respiratory epithelium propels the overlying mucus layer for clearance of environmental microbes. Top panel: The ciliated respiratory epithelium in the airways of the lung is covered by a layer of mucus. The cilia propel the mucus outward and help prevent colonization of the airways by bacteria. Bottom panel: Section of a lung from an individual with cystic fibrosis. The dehydrated mucus layer impairs the ability of cilia to propel it, leading to frequent bacterial colonization and resulting inflammation of the airway.

through the body. Failure of peristalsis is typically accompanied by the overgrowth of pathogenic bacteria within the lumen of the gut. The colon of the large intestine has two layers of mucus. The inner layer, nearest the epithelium, has a denser, less porous composition that excludes the passage of bacteria from the colonic lumen to the epithelial surface. An outer mucus layer, farther from the epithelium, is more porous, forming the habitat for colonic bacteria.

Most healthy epithelial surfaces are associated with populations of normally nonpathogenic bacteria, known as **commensal bacteria** or the **microbiota**, which help keep pathogens at bay. The microbiota can also make antimicrobial substances, such as the lactic acid produced by vaginal lactobacilli, some strains of which also produce antimicrobial peptides (bacteriocins). Commensal microorganisms in the outer mucus layer generate short-chain fatty acids (SCFAs) and other metabolites that can strengthen the barrier functions of epithelia by stimulating production of antimicrobial peptides (see Section 2-4). When commensal microorganisms are killed by antibiotic treatment, pathogens frequently replace them and cause disease (see Fig. 12.13). Under some circumstances commensal microbes themselves can cause disease if their growth is not kept in check or if the immune system is compromised. In Chapter 12, we will discuss how commensal microorganisms play an important role in the setting of normal immunity, particularly in the intestine; and in Chapter 15, we will see how these normally nonpathogenic organisms can cause disease in the context of inherited immunodeficiencies.

2-3 Infectious agents must overcome innate host defenses to establish a focus of infection.

Our bodies are constantly exposed to microorganisms present in our environment, including infectious agents that have been shed by other individuals. Contact with these microorganisms may occur through external or internal epithelial surfaces. To establish an infection, a microorganism must first invade the body by binding to or crossing an epithelium (**Fig. 2.8**). Infection is a major cause of mortality and morbidity in cases of epithelial damage caused by wounds, burns, or loss of the integrity of the body's internal epithelia. The body rapidly repairs damaged epithelial surfaces, but even without epithelial damage, pathogens may establish infection by specifically adhering to and colonizing epithelial surfaces, using the attachment to avoid being dislodged by the flow of air or fluid across the surface.

Disease occurs when a microorganism succeeds in evading or overwhelming innate host defenses to establish a local site of infection, and then replicates there to allow its further transmission within our bodies. The epithelium lining the respiratory tract provides a route of entry into tissues for airborne microorganisms, and the lining of the gastrointestinal tract does the same for microorganisms ingested in food and water. The intestinal pathogens *Salmonella enterica* ssp. *typhi*, which causes typhoid fever, and *Vibrio cholerae*, which causes cholera, are spread through fecally contaminated food and water, respectively. Insect bites and wounds allow microorganisms to penetrate the skin, and direct contact between individuals offers opportunities for infection through the skin, the gut, and the reproductive tract (see Fig. 2.2).

In spite of this exposure, infectious disease is fortunately quite infrequent. Most of the microorganisms that succeed in crossing an epithelial surface are efficiently removed by innate immune mechanisms that function in the underlying tissues, preventing infection from becoming established. It is difficult to know how many infections are repelled in this way, because they cause no symptoms and pass undetected.

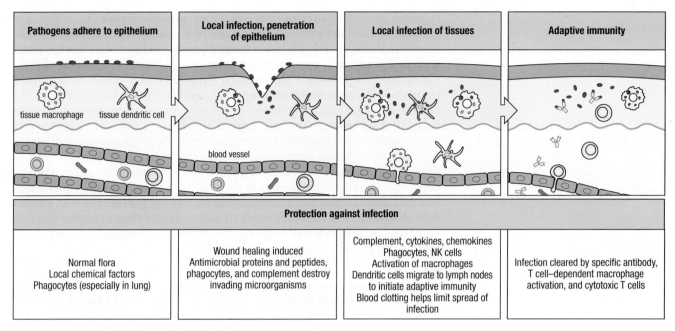

Pathogens adhere to epithelium	Local infection, penetration of epithelium	Local infection of tissues	Adaptive immunity

Protection against infection

| Normal flora
Local chemical factors
Phagocytes (especially in lung) | Wound healing induced
Antimicrobial proteins and peptides, phagocytes, and complement destroy invading microorganisms | Complement, cytokines, chemokines
Phagocytes, NK cells
Activation of macrophages
Dendritic cells migrate to lymph nodes to initiate adaptive immunity
Blood clotting helps limit spread of infection | Infection cleared by specific antibody, T cell–dependent macrophage activation, and cytotoxic T cells |

Fig. 2.8 An infection and the response to it can be divided into a series of stages. These are illustrated here for an infectious microorganism entering through a wound in the skin. The infectious agent must first adhere to the epithelial cells and then cross the epithelium. A local immune response may prevent the infection from becoming established. If not, it helps to contain the infection and also delivers the infectious agent, carried in lymph and inside dendritic cells, to local lymph nodes. This initiates the adaptive immune response and eventual clearance of the infection.

In general, pathogenic microorganisms are distinguished from the mass of microorganisms in the environment by having special adaptations that evade the immune system. In some cases, such as the fungal disease athlete's foot, the initial infection remains local and does not cause significant pathology. In other cases, such as tetanus, the bacterium (*Clostridium tetani* in this case) secretes a powerful neurotoxin, and the infection causes serious illness as it spreads through the lymphatics or the bloodstream, invades and destroys tissues, and disrupts the body's workings.

The spread of a pathogen is often initially countered by an **inflammatory response** that recruits more effector cells and molecules of the innate immune system out of the blood and into the tissues, while inducing clotting in small blood vessels further downstream so that the microbe cannot spread through the circulation (see Fig. 2.8). The cellular responses of innate immunity act over several days. During this time, the adaptive immune response may also begin if antigens derived from the pathogen are delivered to local lymphoid tissues by dendritic cells (see Section 1-15). While an innate immune response may eliminate some infections, an adaptive immune response can target particular strains and variants of pathogens and protect the host against reinfection by using either effector T cells or antibodies to generate immunological memory.

2-4 Epithelial cells and phagocytes produce several kinds of antimicrobial molecules.

Our surface epithelia are more than mere physical barriers to infection; they also produce a wide variety of chemical substances that are microbicidal or that inhibit microbial growth. For example, the acid pH of the stomach and the digestive enzymes, bile salts, fatty acids, and lysolipids present in the upper gastrointestinal tract create a substantial chemical barrier to infection (see Fig. 2.5). One important group of antimicrobial proteins comprises enzymes that attack chemical features specific to bacterial cell walls. Such antimicrobial enzymes include **lysozyme** and **secretory phospholipase A₂,** which are secreted in tears and saliva and by phagocytes. Lysozyme is a glycosidase that breaks a specific chemical bond in the **peptidoglycan** layer of the bacterial cell wall. Peptidoglycan is composed of a network of polymers that consist of alternating residues of *N*-acetylglucosamine (GlcNAc) and *N*-acetylmuramic acid (MurNAc); the peptidoglycan layer is formed by peptide bridges that cross-link these polysaccharide polymers (**Fig. 2.9**). Lysozyme selectively cleaves the β-(1,4) linkage between the two sugars of the polymer and is more effective in acting against Gram-positive bacteria, in which the peptidoglycan cell wall is exposed, than against Gram-negative bacteria, which have an outer layer of LPS covering the peptidoglycan layer. Lysozyme is also produced by **Paneth cells**, specialized epithelial cells in the base of the crypts in the small intestine that secrete many antimicrobial proteins into the gut (see Fig. 2.6). Paneth cells also produce secretory phospholipase A₂, a highly basic enzyme that can enter the bacterial cell wall to access and hydrolyze phospholipids in the cell membrane, killing the bacteria.

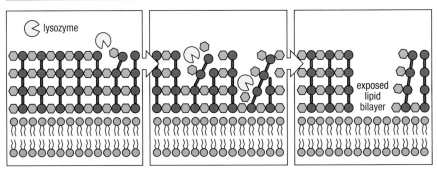

Fig. 2.9 Lysozyme digests the cell walls of Gram-positive and Gram-negative bacteria. Upper panels: The peptidoglycan layer of bacterial cell walls is a dense, three-dimensional network of polymers of alternating residues of β-(1,4)–linked *N*-acetylglucosamine (GlcNAc; large turquoise hexagons) and *N*-acetylmuramic acid (MurNAc; purple circles) that are cross-linked by peptide bridges (red bars). In Gram-positive bacteria (upper left panel), peptidoglycan forms the outer layer in which other molecules are embedded such as teichoic acid and the lipoteichoic acids that link the peptidoglycan layer to the bacterial cell membrane itself. In Gram-negative bacteria (upper right panel), a thin inner wall of peptidoglycan is covered by an outer lipid membrane that contains proteins and lipopolysaccharide (LPS). Lipopolysaccharide is composed of a lipid, lipid A (turquoise circles), to which is attached a polysaccharide core (small turquoise hexagons). Lysozyme (lower panels) cleaves β-(1,4) linkages between GlcNAc and MurNAc, creating a defect in the peptidoglycan layer and exposing the underlying cell membrane to other antimicrobial agents. Lysozyme is more effective against Gram-positive bacteria because of the relatively greater accessibility of the peptidoglycan.

Fig. 2.10 Defensins are amphipathic peptides that disrupt the cell membranes of microbes. The structure of human β₁-defensin is shown in the top panel. It is composed of a short segment of α helix (yellow) resting against three strands of antiparallel β sheet (green), generating an amphipathic peptide with charged and hydrophobic residues residing in separate regions. This general feature is shared by defensins from plants and insects and allows the defensins to interact with the charged surface of the cell membrane and become inserted in the lipid bilayer (center panel). Although the details are still unclear, a transition in the arrangement of the defensins in the membrane leads to the formation of pores and a loss of membrane integrity (bottom panel).

Human β₁-defensin

Electrostatic attraction and the transmembrane electric field bring the defensin into the lipid bilayer

defensin

electric field

Defensin peptides form a pore

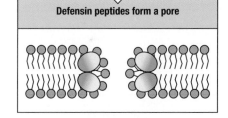

A second group of antimicrobial agents secreted by epithelial cells and phagocytes is the antimicrobial peptides. These represent one of the most ancient forms of defense against infection. These peptides can be produced by phagocytic immune cells, such as neutrophils, where they may be retained within phagocytic granules. They are also produced by epithelial cells, such as in the lung, where they can be secreted onto mucosal surfaces. Three important classes of antimicrobial peptides in mammals are **defensins**, **cathelicidins**, and **histatins**.

Defensins are an ancient, evolutionarily conserved class of antimicrobial peptides made by many eukaryotic organisms, including mammals, insects, and plants (**Fig. 2.10**). They are short cationic peptides of around 30–40 amino acids that usually have three disulfide bonds stabilizing a common **amphipathic** structure—a positively charged region separated from a hydrophobic region. Defensins act within minutes to disrupt the cell membranes of bacteria and fungi, as well as the membrane envelopes of some viruses. The mechanism is thought to involve insertion of the hydrophobic region into the membrane bilayer and the formation of a pore that makes the membrane leaky (see Fig. 2.10). Most multicellular organisms make many different defensins—the plant *Arabidopsis thaliana* produces 13 and the fruit fly *Drosophila melanogaster* at least 15. Human Paneth cells make as many as 21 different defensins, many of which are encoded by a cluster of genes on chromosome 8.

Three subfamilies of defensins—α-, β-, and θ-defensins—are distinguished on the basis of amino acid sequence. Each family has members with distinct activities, some being active against Gram-positive bacteria and some against Gram-negative bacteria, while others are specific for fungal pathogens. All the antimicrobial peptides, including the defensins, are generated by proteolytic processing from inactive **propeptides** (**Fig. 2.11**). In humans, developing neutrophils produce **α-defensins** through the processing of an initial propeptide of about 90 amino acids by cellular proteases to remove an anionic propiece, generating a mature cationic defensin that is stored in so-called **primary granules**. The primary granules of neutrophils are specialized membrane-enclosed vesicles, rather similar to lysosomes, that contain a number of other antimicrobial agents as well as defensins. We will explain in Chapter 3 how these primary granules are induced to fuse with phagocytic vesicles (phagosomes) after the cell has engulfed a pathogen, helping to kill the microbe. The Paneth cells of the gut constitutively produce α-defensins, called **cryptdins**, which are processed by proteases such as the metalloprotease matrilysin in mice or trypsin in humans, before being secreted into the gut lumen. The **β-defensins** lack the long propiece of α-defensins and are generally produced specifically in response to the presence of microbial products. β-Defensins (and some α-defensins) are made by epithelia outside the gut, primarily in the respiratory and urogenital tracts, skin, and tongue. β-Defensins made by keratinocytes in the epidermis and by type II pneumocytes in the lungs are packaged into **lamellar bodies** (see Fig. 2.6), lipid-rich secretory organelles that release their contents into the extracellular space to form a watertight lipid sheet in the epidermis and the pulmonary surfactant layer in the lung. The θ-defensins arose in the primates, but the single human θ-defensin gene has been inactivated by a mutation.

The antimicrobial peptides belonging to the cathelicidin family lack the disulfide bonds that stabilize the defensins. Humans and mice have one

Defensins, cathelicidins, and histatins are activated by proteolysis to release an amphipathic antimicrobial peptide

α-Defensins

cut

Pro-region → AMPH

β-Defensins

cut

→ AMPH

Cathelicidins

cut

Cathelin → AMPH

RegIII 'lecticidins'

cut

→ CTLD/CRD

Fig. 2.11 Defensins, cathelicidins, and RegIII proteins are activated by proteolysis. When α- and β-defensins are first synthesized, they contain a signal peptide (not shown); a pro-region (blue), which is shorter in the β-defensins; and an amphipathic domain (AMPH; green–yellow); the pro-region represses the membrane-inserting properties of the amphipathic domain. After defensins are released from the cell or into phagosomes, they undergo cleavage by proteases, which releases the amphipathic domain in active form. Newly synthesized cathelicidins contain a signal peptide (not shown), a cathelin domain, a short pro-region, and an amphipathic domain; they, too, are activated by proteolytic cleavage. RegIII proteins contain a C-type lectin domain (CTLD), also known as a carbohydrate-recognition domain (CRD). After release of the signal peptide, further proteolytic cleavage of a RegIII protein also regulates its antimicrobial activity.

cathelicidin gene, but some other mammals, including cattle and sheep, have several. Cathelicidins are made constitutively by neutrophils and macrophages, and in response to infection by keratinocytes in the skin and epithelial cells in the lungs and intestine. They are made as inactive propeptides composed of two linked domains and are processed before secretion (see Fig. 2.11). In neutrophils, the inactive cathelicidin propeptides are stored in another type of specialized cytoplasmic granules called **secondary granules**. Cathelicidin is activated by proteolytic cleavage only when primary and secondary granules are induced to fuse with phagosomes, where it is cleaved by **neutrophil elastase** that has been stored in primary granules. Cleavage separates the two domains, and the cleavage products either remain in the phagosome or are released from the neutrophil by exocytosis. The carboxyl-terminal peptide is a cationic amphipathic peptide that disrupts membranes and is toxic to a wide range of microorganisms. The amino-terminal peptide is similar in structure to a protein called **cathelin**, an inhibitor of cathepsin L (a lysosomal enzyme involved in antigen processing and protein degradation), but its role in immune defense is unclear. In keratinocytes, cathelicidins, like β-defensins, are stored and processed in the lamellar bodies.

A class of antimicrobial peptides called histatins are constitutively produced in the oral cavity by the parotid, sublingual, and submandibular glands. These short, histidine-rich, cationic peptides are active against pathogenic fungi such as *Cryptococcus neoformans* and *Candida albicans*. More recently, histatins were found to promote the rapid wound healing that is typical in the oral cavity, but the mechanism of this effect is unclear.

Another type of bactericidal proteins made by epithelia is carbohydrate-binding proteins, or **lectins**. Most **C-type lectins** require calcium for the binding activity of their carbohydrate-recognition domain (CRD), which provides a variable interface for binding carbohydrate structures. C-type lectins of the RegIII family include several bactericidal proteins expressed by intestinal epithelium in humans and mice. However, carbohydrate recognition by RegIII proteins is not calcium dependent, but instead is inhibited by calcium. In mice, **RegIIIγ** is produced by Paneth cells and secreted into the gut, where it binds to peptidoglycans in bacterial cell walls and exerts direct bactericidal activity. Like other bactericidal peptides, RegIIIγ is produced in inactive form but is cleaved by the protease trypsin, which removes a short amino-terminal fragment to activate the bactericidal potential of RegIIIγ within the intestinal lumen (see Fig. 2.11). Human RegIIIα (also called **HIP/PAP** for hepatocarcinoma intestine pancreas/pancreatitis–associated protein) kills bacteria directly by forming a hexameric pore in the bacterial membrane (**Fig. 2.12**). RegIII family

Fig. 2.12 Pore formation by human RegIIIα. Panel a: A model of the RegIIIα pore was generated by docking the human pro-RegIIIα structure (PDB ID: 1UV0), shown as individual purple and turquoise ribbon diagrams, into the cryo-electron microscopic map of the RegIIIα filament. LPS blocks the pore-forming activity of RegIIIα, explaining its selective bactericidal activity against Gram-positive but not Gram-negative bacteria. Panel b: Electron microscopic images of RegIIIα pores assembled in the presence of lipid bilayers.

proteins preferentially kill Gram-positive bacteria, in which the peptidoglycan is exposed on the outer surface (see Fig. 2.9). In fact, the LPS of Gram-negative bacteria inhibits the pore-forming ability of RegIIIα, further enforcing the selectivity of RegIII proteins for Gram-positive bacteria.

Finally, we briefly mention the peptides S100A8 and S100A9, which heterodimerize to form **calprotectin**, which we will discuss in Section 11-11 in the context of production by T cells. Calprotectin acts to sequester magnesium and iron required by microorganisms and exerts an antimicrobial effect at sites of its production. This activity requires binding of calcium to one of calprotectin's two metal-binding sites, which allows its second site to bind other metal ions. Calprotectin is produced in high amounts by neutrophils, and by T cells, but it is also made by intestinal epithelia, and so is part of the innate barrier defense system.

Summary.

The mammalian immune response to invading organisms proceeds in three phases, beginning with immediate innate defenses, then the induced innate defenses, and finally adaptive immunity. The first phase of host defense consists of those mechanisms that are present and ready to resist an invader at any time. Epithelial surfaces provide a physical barrier against pathogen entry, but they also have other, more specialized strategies. Mucosal surfaces have a protective barrier of mucus. Through particular cell-surface interactions, highly differentiated epithelia protect against both microbial colonization and invasion. Defense mechanisms of epithelia include the prevention of pathogen adherence, secretion of antimicrobial enzymes and bactericidal peptides, and the flow caused by the actions of cilia. Antimicrobial peptides and the bactericidal lectins of the RegIII family are made as inactive proproteins that require a proteolytic step to complete their activation, whereupon they become capable of killing microbes by forming pores in the microbial cell membranes. The actions of antimicrobial enzymes and peptides described in this part of the chapter often involve binding to unique glycan/carbohydrate structures on the microbe. Thus, these soluble molecular defenses are both pattern-recognition receptors and effector molecules at the same time, representing the simplest form of innate immunity.

The complement system and innate immunity.

When a pathogen breaches the host's epithelial barriers and initial antimicrobial defenses, it next encounters a major component of innate immunity known as the complement system, or **complement**. Complement is a collection of soluble proteins present in blood and other body fluids. It was discovered in the 1890s by Jules Bordet as a heat-labile substance in normal plasma whose activity could 'complement' the bactericidal activity of immune sera. Part of the process is **opsonization**, which refers to coating a pathogen with antibodies and/or complement proteins so that it can be more readily taken up and destroyed by phagocytic cells. Although complement was first discovered as an effector arm of the antibody response, we now understand that it originally evolved as part of the innate immune system and that it still provides protection early in infection, in the absence of antibodies, through more ancient pathways of complement activation.

The complement system is composed of more than 30 different plasma proteins, which are produced mainly by the liver. In the absence of infection, these proteins circulate in an inactive form. In the presence of pathogens or of antibody bound to pathogens, the complement system becomes 'activated.'

Fig. 2.13 The complement system proceeds in distinct phases in the elimination of microbes. Proteins that can distinguish self from microbial surfaces (yellow) activate a proteolytic amplification cascade that ends in the formation of the critical enzymatic activity (green) of C3 convertase, a family of proteases. This activity is the gateway to the three effector arms of complement, which produce inflammation (purple), enhance phagocytosis of the microbe (blue), and lyse microbial membranes (pink). We will use this color scheme in the figures throughout this chapter to illustrate which activity each complement protein serves.

Particular **complement proteins** interact with each other to form several different pathways of complement activation, all of which have the final outcome of killing the pathogen, either directly or by facilitating its phagocytosis, and inducing inflammatory responses that help to fight infection. There are three pathways of **complement activation**. As the antibody-triggered pathway of complement activation was discovered first, this became known as the classical pathway of complement activation. The next to be discovered, the so-called alternative pathway, can be activated by the presence of the pathogen alone; and the most recently discovered is the lectin pathway, which is activated by lectin-type proteins that recognize and bind to carbohydrates on pathogen surfaces.

We learned in Section 2-4 that proteolysis can be used as a means of activating antimicrobial proteins. In the complement system, activation by proteolysis is inherent, with many of the complement proteins being proteases that successively cleave and activate one another. The proteases of the complement system are synthesized as inactive pro-enzymes, or **zymogens**, which become enzymatically active only after proteolytic cleavage, usually by another complement protein. The complement pathways are triggered by proteins that act as pattern-recognition receptors to detect the presence of pathogens. This detection activates an initial zymogen, triggering a cascade of proteolysis in which complement zymogens are activated sequentially, each becoming an active protease that cleaves and activates many molecules of the next zymogen in the pathway, amplifying the signal as the cascade proceeds. This results in activation of three distinct effector pathways—**inflammation**, **phagocytosis**, and **membrane attack**—that help eliminate the pathogen. In this way, the detection of even a small number of pathogens produces a rapid response that is greatly amplified at each step. This overall scheme for complement is shown in **Fig. 2.13**.

Nomenclature for complement proteins can seem confusing, so we will start by explaining their names. The first proteins discovered belong to the classical pathway, and they are designated by the letter C followed by a number. The native complement proteins—such as the inactive zymogens—have a simple number designation; for example, C1 and C2. Unfortunately, they were named in the order of their discovery rather than the sequence of reactions. The reaction sequence in the classical pathway, for example, is C1, C4, C2, C3, C5, C6, C7, C8, and C9 (note that not all of these are proteases). Products of cleavage reactions are designated by adding a lowercase letter as a suffix. For example, cleavage of C3 produces a small protein fragment called C3a and the remaining larger fragment, C3b. By convention, the larger fragment for other factors is designated by the suffix b. There is an exception to this convention. For **C2**, the larger fragment was originally named **C2a** in the literature by its discoverers. Although there have been discussions regarding changes to this nomenclature, there has not been uniform agreement and so we will preserve the original usage of C2a as the large active fragment of C2. Another exception is the naming of C1q, C1r, and C1s: these are not cleavage products of C1 but are distinct proteins that together compose C1. The proteins of the alternative pathway were discovered later and are designated by different capital letters; for example, factor B and factor D. The factor B cleavage products are also designated by the addition of lowercase a and b; thus, the large fragment of B is called Bb and the small fragment is called Ba. Activated complement components were often designated in the past by a horizontal line, for example, C$\overline{2a}$, but we will not use this convention. All the components of the complement system are listed in **Fig. 2.14**.

Besides acting in innate immunity, complement also influences adaptive immunity. Opsonization of pathogens by complement facilitates their uptake by phagocytic antigen-presenting cells that express complement receptors;

this enhances the presentation of pathogen antigens to T cells, which we discuss in more detail in Chapter 6. B cells express receptors for complement proteins that enhance their responses to complement-coated antigens, as we describe later in Chapter 10. In addition, several of the complement fragments can act to influence cytokine production by antigen-presenting cells, thereby influencing the direction and extent of the subsequent adaptive immune response, as we describe in Chapter 11.

2-5 The complement system recognizes features of microbial surfaces and marks them for destruction by coating them with C3b.

Figure 2.15 gives a highly simplified preview of the initiation mechanisms and outcomes of complement activation. The three pathways of complement activation are initiated in different ways. The **lectin pathway** is initiated by soluble carbohydrate-binding proteins—mannose-binding lectin (MBL) and ficolins—that bind to particular carbohydrate structures on microbial surfaces. Specific proteases, called MBL-associated serine proteases (MASPs), that associate with these recognition proteins trigger the cleavage of complement proteins and activation of the pathway. The **classical pathway** is initiated when complement component 1 (C1), which comprises a recognition protein (C1q) associated with proteases (C1r and C1s), either recognizes a microbial surface directly or binds to antibodies already bound to a pathogen. Finally, the **alternative pathway** can be initiated by spontaneous hydrolysis and activation of complement component 3 (C3), which can then bind directly to microbial surfaces.

These three pathways converge at the central and most important step in complement activation. When any of the pathways interacts with a pathogen surface, the enzymatic activity of a **C3 convertase** is generated. There are various types of C3 convertase, depending on the complement pathway activated, but each is a multi-subunit protein with protease activity that cleaves C3. The C3 convertase is bound covalently to the pathogen surface, where it cleaves C3 to generate large amounts of **C3b**, the main effector molecule of the complement system, and **C3a**, a small peptide that binds to specific receptors and helps induce inflammation. Cleavage of C3 is the critical step in complement activation and leads directly or indirectly to all the effector activities of the complement system (see Fig. 2.15). C3b binds covalently to the microbial surface and acts as an opsonin, enabling phagocytes that carry receptors for complement to take up and destroy the C3b-coated microbe. Later in the chapter, we will describe the different complement receptors that bind C3b and are involved in this function of complement and explain how C3b is degraded by a serum protease into inactive smaller fragments called **C3f** and **C3dg** and C3d. C3b can also bind to the C3 convertases produced by the classical and lectin pathways and form another multi-subunit enzyme, the **C5 convertase**, which cleaves C5, liberating the highly inflammatory peptide **C5a** and generating **C5b**. C5b initiates the 'late' events of complement activation, also called the terminal pathway, in which additional complement proteins interact with C5b to form a **membrane-attack complex (MAC)** on the pathogen surface, creating a pore in the cell membrane that leads to cell lysis (see Fig. 2.15, bottom right).

The key feature of C3b is its ability to form a covalent bond with microbial surfaces, which allows the innate recognition of microbes to be translated into effector responses. Covalent bond formation is due to a highly reactive thioester bond that is hidden inside the folded C3 protein and cannot react until C3 is cleaved. When C3 convertase cleaves C3 and releases the C3a fragment, large conformational changes occur in C3b that allow the thioester bond to react with a hydroxyl or amino group on the nearby microbial surface

Functional protein classes in the complement system	
Binding to antigen:antibody complexes and pathogen surfaces	C1q
Binding to carbohydrate structures such as mannose or GlcNAc on microbial surfaces	MBL Ficolins Properdin (P)
Activating enzymes*	C1r C1s C2a Bb Factor D MASP-1 MASP-2 MASP-3
Surface-binding proteins and opsonins	C4b C3b
Peptide mediators of inflammation	C5a C3a C4a
Membrane-attack proteins	C5b C6 C7 C8 C9
Complement receptors	CR1 CR2 CR3 CR4 CRIg
Complement-regulatory proteins	C1INH C4BP CR1/CD35 MCP/CD46 DAF/CD55 Factor H Factor I Properdin (P) CD59

Fig. 2.14 Functional protein classes in the complement system. *In this book, C2a is used to denote the larger, active fragment of C2.

ANIMATION 2.1

Fig. 2.15 Complement is a system of soluble pattern-recognition receptors and effector molecules that detect and destroy microorganisms. The pathogen-recognition mechanisms of the three complement-activation pathways are shown in the top row, along with the complement components used in the proteolytic cascades leading to formation of a C3 convertase. This enzyme activity cleaves complement component 3 (C3) into a small soluble protein, C3a, and a larger component, C3b, which becomes covalently bound to the pathogen surface (middle row). The components are listed by biochemical function in Fig. 2.14 and are described in detail in later figures. The lectin pathway of complement activation (top left) is triggered by the binding of mannose-binding lectin (MBL) or ficolins to carbohydrate residues in microbial cell walls and capsules. The classical pathway (top center) is triggered by binding of C1 either to the pathogen surface or to antibody bound to the pathogen. In the alternative pathway

(top right), soluble C3 undergoes spontaneous hydrolysis in the fluid phase, generating C3(H_2O), which, in concert with factors B, D, and properdin, propagates the cascade. All pathways thus converge on the formation of C3b bound to a pathogen and lead to all of the effector activities of complement, which are shown in the bottom row. C3b bound to a pathogen acts as an opsonin, enabling phagocytes that express receptors for C3b to ingest the complement-coated microbe more easily (bottom center). C3b can also bind to C3 convertases to produce another enzyme, a C5 convertase (detail not shown here), which cleaves C5 to C5a and C5b. C5b triggers the late events of the complement pathway in which the terminal components of complement—C6 to C9—assemble into a membrane-attack complex (MAC) that can damage the membrane of certain pathogens (bottom right). C3a and C5a act as chemoattractants that recruit immune-system cells to the site of infection and cause inflammation (bottom left).

Fig. 2.16 C3 convertase activates C3 for covalent bonding to microbial surfaces by cleaving it into C3a and C3b and exposing a highly reactive thioester bond in C3b. Top panel: C3 in blood plasma consists of an α chain and a β chain (formed by proteolytic processing from the native C3 polypeptide) held together by a disulfide bond. The thioester-containing domain (TED) of the α chain contains a potentially highly reactive thioester bond (red spot). Bottom left panels: Cleavage by C3 convertase (the lectin and classical pathway convertase C4b2a is shown here) and release of C3a from the amino terminus of the α chain causes a conformational change in C3b that exposes the thioester bond. This can now react with hydroxyl or amino groups on molecules on microbial surfaces, covalently bonding C3b to the surface. Bottom right panels: Schematic view of the thioester reaction. If a bond is not made with a microbial surface, the thioester is rapidly hydrolyzed (that is, cleaved by water), rendering C3b inactive.

(**Fig. 2.16**). If no bond is made, the thioester is rapidly hydrolyzed, inactivating C3b, which is one way that alternative pathway activity is confined to a target area in healthy individuals. As we will see below, some of the individual components of C3 and C5 convertases differ between the various complement pathways; the components that are different are listed in **Fig. 2.17**.

Pathways leading to such potent inflammatory and destructive effects—and which have a series of built-in amplification steps—are potentially dangerous and must be tightly regulated. One important safeguard is that the key activated complement components are rapidly inactivated unless they bind to the pathogen surface on which their activation was initiated. There are also several points in the pathway at which regulatory proteins act to prevent the activation of complement on the surfaces of healthy host cells, thereby protecting them from accidental damage, as we shall see later in the chapter. Complement can, however, be activated by dying cells, such as those at sites of ischemic injury, and by cells undergoing apoptosis, or programmed cell death. In these cases, the complement coating helps phagocytes dispose of the dead and dying cells neatly, thus limiting the risk of cell contents being released and triggering an autoimmune response (discussed in Chapter 15).

Having introduced some of the main complement components, we are ready for a more detailed account of the three pathways. To help indicate the types of functions carried out by each of the complement components in the tables throughout the rest of the chapter, we will use the color code introduced in Fig. 2.13 and Fig. 2.14: yellow for recognition and activation, green for amplification, purple for inflammation, blue for phagocytosis, and pink for membrane attack.

C3 convertase	
Lectin pathway	C4b2a
Classical pathway	C4b2a
Alternative pathway	C3bBb
Fluid phase	C3(H$_2$O)Bb

C5 convertase	
Lectin pathway	C4b2a3b
Classical pathway	C4b2a3b
Alternative pathway	C3b$_2$Bb

Fig. 2.17 C3 and C5 convertases of the complement pathways. Note the C5 convertase of the alternative pathway consists of two C3b subunits and one Bb subunit.

2-6   The lectin pathway uses soluble receptors that recognize microbial surfaces to activate the complement cascade.

Microorganisms typically bear on their surface repeating patterns of molecular structures, known generally as pathogen-associated molecular patterns (PAMPs). The cell walls of Gram-positive and Gram-negative bacteria, for example, are composed of a matrix of proteins, carbohydrates, and lipids in a repetitive array (see Fig. 2.9). The lipoteichoic acids of Gram-positive bacterial cell walls and the lipopolysaccharide of the outer membrane of Gram-negative bacteria are not present on animal cells and are important in the recognition of bacteria by the innate immune system. Similarly, the glycans of yeast surface proteins commonly terminate in mannose residues rather than the sialic acid residues (N-acetylneuraminic acid) that terminate the glycans of vertebrate cells (**Fig. 2.18**). The lectin pathway uses these features of microbial surfaces to detect and respond to pathogens.

The lectin pathway can be triggered by any of four different pattern-recognition receptors that circulate in blood and extracellular fluids and recognize carbohydrates on microbial surfaces. The first such receptor to be discovered was **mannose-binding lectin (MBL)**, which is shown in **Fig. 2.19**, and which is synthesized in the liver. MBL is an oligomeric protein built up from a monomer that contains an amino-terminal collagen-like domain and a carboxyl-terminal C-type lectin domain (see Section 2-4). Proteins of this type are called **collectins**. MBL monomers assemble into trimers through the formation of a triple helix by their collagen-like domains. Trimers then assemble into oligomers by disulfide bonding between the cysteine-rich collagen domains. The MBL present in the blood is composed of two to six trimers, with the major forms of human MBL being trimers and tetramers. A single carbohydrate-recognition domain of MBL has a low affinity for mannose, fucose, and N-acetylglucosamine (GlcNAc) residues, which are common on microbial glycans, but does not bind sialic acid residues, which terminate vertebrate glycans. Thus, multimeric MBL has high total binding strength, or **avidity**, for repetitive carbohydrate structures on a wide variety of microbial surfaces, including Gram-positive and Gram-negative bacteria, mycobacteria, yeasts, and some viruses and parasites, while not interacting with host cells. MBL is present at low concentrations in the plasma of most individuals, but in the presence of infection, its production is increased during the **acute-phase**

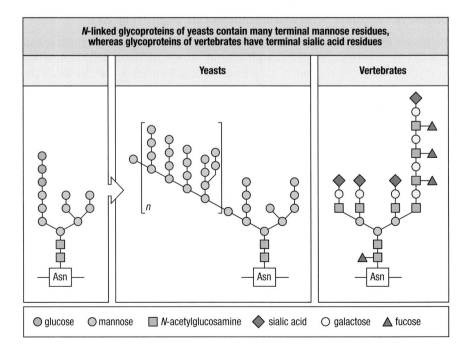

Fig. 2.18 The carbohydrate side chains on yeast and vertebrate glycoproteins are terminated with different patterns of sugars. N-linked glycosylation in fungi and animals is initiated by the addition of the same precursor oligosaccharide, Glc_3-Man_9-$GlcNAc_2$ (left panel), to an asparagine residue. In many yeasts this is processed to high-mannose glycans (middle panel). In contrast, in vertebrates, the initial glycan is trimmed and processed, and the N-linked glycoproteins have terminal sialic acid residues (right panel).

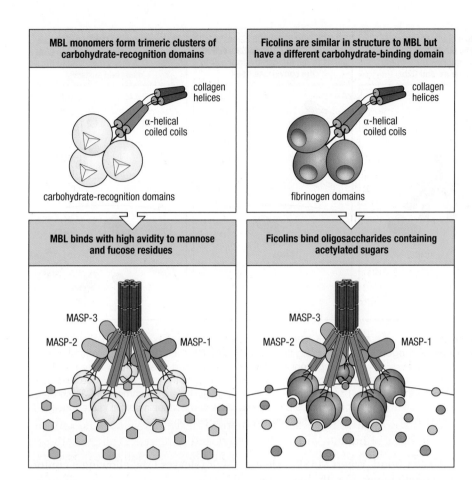

MBL monomers form trimeric clusters of carbohydrate-recognition domains

collagen helices

α-helical coiled coils

carbohydrate-recognition domains

MBL binds with high avidity to mannose and fucose residues

MASP-3

MASP-2   MASP-1

Ficolins are similar in structure to MBL but have a different carbohydrate-binding domain

collagen helices

α-helical coiled coils

fibrinogen domains

Ficolins bind oligosaccharides containing acetylated sugars

MASP-3

MASP-2   MASP-1

Fig. 2.19 Mannose-binding lectin and ficolins form complexes with serine proteases and recognize particular carbohydrates on microbial surfaces. Mannose-binding lectin (MBL; left panels) is an oligomeric protein in which two to six clusters of carbohydrate-binding heads arise from a central stalk that is formed from the collagen-like tails of the MBL monomers. An MBL monomer is composed of a collagen region (red), an α-helical neck region (blue), and a carbohydrate-recognition domain (yellow). Three MBL monomers associate to form a trimer (top left panel), and between two and six trimers assemble to form a mature MBL molecule (bottom left panel). MBL binds to bacterial surfaces that display a particular spatial arrangement of mannose or fucose residues. An MBL molecule associates with the serine proteases MASP-1, MASP-2, and MASP-3, and with the nonenzymatic proteins MAp19 and MAp44 (not shown), and can activate C4 and C2 after binding to carbohydrate molecules present on microbial surfaces. The ficolins (right panels) resemble MBL in their overall structure and activation mechanism. The carbohydrate-binding domain of ficolins is a fibrinogen-like domain, rather than the lectin domain present in MBL.

response. This is part of the induced phase of the innate immune response and is discussed in Chapter 3.

The other pathogen-recognition molecules used by the lectin pathway are known as **ficolins**. Although related in overall shape and function to MBL, they have a fibrinogen-like domain, rather than a lectin domain, attached to the collagen-like stalk (see Fig. 2.19). The fibrinogen-like domain gives ficolins a general specificity for oligosaccharides containing acetylated sugars, but it does not bind mannose-containing carbohydrates. Humans have three ficolins: ficolin-1 (M-ficolin), ficolin-2 (L-ficolin), and ficolin-3 (H-ficolin). Each binds to a spectrum of bacteria. Ficolins are secreted into the blood and tissues by various cells, including cells of the liver and lung, and by neutrophils.

MBL in plasma can bind to five proteins: three **MBL-associated serine proteases**, **MASP-1, MASP-2,** and **MASP-3**, and two nonenzymatic proteins, **MAp19** and **MAp44**. These five proteins are encoded by alternative splice variants of two genes: *MASP1*, which encodes MASP-1, MASP-3, and MAp44, and *MASP2,* which encodes MASP-2 and MAp19. MASP-1 and MASP-3 use different serine protease domains and have different substrate specificity. When MBL bound to MASP-1 and MASP-2 interacts with a pathogen surface, a conformational change occurs in MASP-1 that enables it to cleave and activate a MASP-2 molecule in the same MBL complex. Activated MASP-2 can then cleave complement components 4 and 2 (C4 and C2) to initiate the lectin and classical complement pathways (**Fig. 2.20**). When MBL bound to MASP-3 and MAp44 binds a pathogen surface, MASP-3 cleaves a pro-form of factor D, producing active factor D, which is a key event in the initiation of the alternative complement pathway. Like MBL, ficolins form oligomers that make a complex with MASP-1 and MASP-2, which similarly activate complement upon recognition of a microbial surface by the ficolin. **C4**, like C3, contains a buried

| Activated MASP-2 associated with MBL or ficolin cleaves C4 to C4a and C4b, which binds to the microbial surface | C4b then binds C2, which is cleaved by MASP-2 to C2a, with which it forms the C4b2a complex, and C2b | C4b2a is an active C3 convertase cleaving C3 to C3a and C3b, which binds to the microbial surface or to the convertase itself | One molecule of C4b2a can cleave up to 1000 molecules of C3 to C3b. Many C3b molecules bind to the microbial surface |

Fig. 2.20 The actions of the C3 convertase result in the binding of large numbers of C3b molecules to the pathogen surface. Binding of mannose-binding lectin or ficolins to their carbohydrate ligands on microbial surfaces induces MASP-1 to cleave and activate the serine protease MASP-2. MASP-2 then cleaves C4, exposing the thioester bond in C4b that allows it to react covalently with the pathogen surface. C4b then binds C2, making C2 susceptible to cleavage by MASP-2 and thus generating the C3 convertase C4b2a. C2a is the active protease component of the C3 convertase and cleaves many molecules of C3 to produce C3b, which binds to the pathogen surface, and C3a, an inflammatory mediator. The covalent attachment of C3b and C4b to the pathogen surface is important in confining subsequent complement activity to pathogen surfaces.

thioester bond. When MASP-2 cleaves C4, it releases C4a, allowing a conformational change in C4b that exposes the reactive thioester as described for C3b (see Fig. 2.16). C4b bonds covalently via this thioester to the microbial surface nearby, where it then binds one molecule of C2 (see Fig. 2.20). C2 is cleaved by MASP-2, producing C2a, an active serine protease that remains bound to C4b to form **C4b2a**, which is the C3 convertase of the lectin and classical pathways. (Remember, we use the original convention by which C2a is the active large C2 fragment.) C4b2a now cleaves many molecules of C3 into C3a and C3b. The C3b fragments bond covalently to the nearby pathogen surface, and the released C3a initiates a local inflammatory response. The complement-activation pathway initiated by ficolins proceeds like the MBL lectin pathway (see Fig. 2.20).

Individuals deficient in MBL or MASP-2 experience substantially more respiratory infections by common extracellular bacteria during early childhood, indicating the importance of the lectin pathway for host defense. This susceptibility illustrates the particular importance of innate defense mechanisms in early childhood, when adaptive immune responses are not yet fully developed but the maternal antibodies transferred across the placenta and present in the mother's milk are gone. Other members of the collectin family are the **surfactant proteins A and D (SP-A and SP-D)**, which are present in the fluid that bathes the epithelial surfaces of the lung. There they coat the surfaces of pathogens, making them more susceptible to phagocytosis by macrophages that have left the subepithelial tissues to enter the alveoli. Because SP-A and SP-D do not associate with MASPs, they do not activate complement.

We have used MBL here as our prototype activator of the lectin pathway, but the ficolins are more abundant than MBL in plasma and so may actually be more important. Ficolin-2 recognizes acetylated sugars, such as GlcNAc and *N*-acetylgalactosamine (GalNAc), and particularly recognizes lipoteichoic acid, a component of the cell walls of Gram-positive bacteria that contains

GalNAc. It can also activate complement after binding to a variety of capsulated bacteria. Ficolin-1 also recognizes acetylated sugar residues; ficolin-3 shows a more restricted binding specificity, for D-fucose and D-galactose, and has been linked to activity against the Gram-positive bacterium *Aerococcus viridans*, a cause of bacterial endocarditis.

2-7 The classical pathway is initiated by activation of the C1 complex and is homologous to the lectin pathway.

In its overall scheme, the classical pathway is similar to the lectin pathway, except that it uses a pathogen sensor known as the **C1 complex,** or **C1.** Because C1 interacts directly with some pathogens but can also interact with antibodies, C1 allows the classical pathway to function both in innate immunity, which we describe now, and in adaptive immunity, which we examine in more detail in Chapter 10.

Like the MBL:MASP complex, the C1 complex is composed of a large subunit (**C1q**), which acts as the pathogen sensor, and two serine proteases (**C1r** and **C1s**), which are initially in their inactive form (**Fig. 2.21**). C1q is a hexamer of trimers, composed of monomers that contain an amino-terminal globular domain and a carboxyl-terminal collagen-like domain. The trimers assemble through interactions of the collagen-like domains, bringing the globular domains together to form a globular head. Six of these trimers assemble to form a complete C1q molecule, which has six globular heads held together by their collagen-like tails. C1r and C1s are closely related to MASP-2 and somewhat more distantly related to MASP-1 and MASP-3; all five enzymes are likely to have evolved from the duplication of a gene for a common precursor. C1r and C1s interact noncovalently and form tetramers that fold into the arms of C1q, with at least part of the C1r:C1s complex being external to C1q, as illustrated in Fig. 2.21.

The recognition function of C1 resides in the six globular heads of C1q. When two or more of these heads interact with a ligand, this causes a conformational change in the C1r:C1s complex, which leads to the activation of an autocatalytic enzymatic activity in C1r; the active form of C1r then cleaves its associated C1s to generate an active serine protease. The activated C1s acts on the next two components of the classical pathway, C4 and C2. C1s cleaves C4 to produce C4b, which binds covalently to the pathogen surface as described earlier for the lectin pathway (see Fig. 2.20). C4b then also binds one molecule of C2, which is cleaved by C1s to produce the serine protease C2a. This produces the active C3 convertase C4b2a, which is the C3 convertase of both the lectin and the classical pathways. However, because it was first discovered as part of the classical pathway, C4b2a is often known as the **classical C3 convertase** (see Fig. 2.17). The proteins involved in the classical pathway, along with their active forms, are listed in **Fig. 2.22**.

C1q can attach itself to the surface of pathogens in several different ways. One is by binding directly to surface components on some bacteria, including certain proteins of bacterial cell walls and polyanionic structures, such as the lipoteichoic acid on Gram-positive bacteria. A second is through binding to C-reactive protein, an acute-phase protein in human plasma that binds to phosphocholine residues in bacterial surface molecules such as pneumococcal C polysaccharide—hence the name C-reactive protein. We discuss the acute-phase proteins in detail in Chapter 3. However, a main function of C1q in an immune response is to bind to the constant, or Fc, regions of antibodies (see Section 1-9) that have bound pathogens via their antigen-binding sites. C1q thus links the effector functions of complement to recognition provided by adaptive immunity. This might seem to limit the usefulness of C1q in fighting the first stages of an infection, before the adaptive immune response has

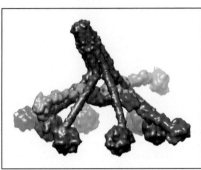

Fig. 2.21 The first protein in the classical pathway of complement activation is C1, which is a complex of C1q, C1r, and C1s. Upper panel: C1q is composed of six identical subunits with globular heads (yellow) and long collagen-like tails (red); it has been described as looking like "a bunch of tulips." The tails combine to bind to two molecules each of C1r and C1s, forming the C1 complex $C1q:C1r_2:C1s_2$. The heads can bind to the constant regions of immunoglobulin molecules or directly to the pathogen surface, causing a conformational change in C1r, which then cleaves and activates the C1s zymogen (proenzyme). The C1 complex is similar in overall structure to the MBL:MASP complex, and it has an identical function, cleaving C4 and C2 to form the C3 convertase C4b2a (see Fig. 2.20). Lower panel: Structure of the C1 complex solved by cryo-electron microscopy (cryo-EM): C1q (red), C1r (green), C1s (blue). Modified from Sharp, T.H., et al.: *Proc. Natl. Acad. Sci. USA* 2019, 116:11900–11905.

Fig. 2.22 The proteins of the classical pathway of complement activation.

Proteins of the classical pathway of complement activation		
Native component	**Active form**	**Function of the active form**
C1 (C1q: C1r$_2$:C1s$_2$)	C1q	Binds directly to pathogen surfaces or indirectly to antibody bound to pathogens, thus allowing autoactivation of C1r
	C1r	Cleaves C1s to active protease
	C1s	Cleaves C4 and C2
C4	C4b	Covalently binds to pathogen and opsonizes it. Binds C2 for cleavage by C1s
	C4a	Peptide mediator of inflammation (weak activity)
C2	C2a	Active enzyme of classical pathway C3/C5 convertase: cleaves C3 and C5
	C2b	Inactive small fragment
C3	C3b	Binds to pathogen surface and acts as opsonin. Initiates amplification via the alternative pathway. Binds C5 for cleavage by C2a
	C3a	Peptide mediator of inflammation (intermediate activity)

generated pathogen-specific antibodies. However, some antibodies, called **natural antibodies**, are produced by the immune system in the apparent absence of infection. These antibodies have a low affinity for many microbial pathogens and are highly cross-reactive, recognizing common membrane constituents such as phosphocholine and even recognizing some antigens of the body's own cells (that is, self antigens). Natural antibodies may be produced in response to commensal microbiota or to self antigens, but do not seem to be the consequence of an adaptive immune response to infection by pathogens. Most natural antibody is of the isotype, or class, known as IgM (see Chapter 5) and represents a considerable amount of the total IgM circulating in humans. IgM is the class of antibody most efficient at binding C1q, making natural antibodies an effective means of activating complement on microbial surfaces immediately after infection and leading to the clearance of bacteria such as *Streptococcus pneumoniae* (the pneumococcus) before they become dangerous.

2-8 Complement activation is largely confined to the surface on which it is initiated.

We have seen that both the lectin and the classical pathways of complement activation are initiated by proteins that bind to pathogen surfaces. During the triggered enzyme cascade that follows, it is important that activating events are confined to this same site, so that C3 activation also occurs on the surface of the pathogen and not in the plasma or on host-cell surfaces. This is achieved principally by the covalent binding of C4b to the pathogen surface. In innate immunity, C4 cleavage is catalyzed by a ficolin or MBL complex that is bound to the pathogen surface, and so the C4b cleavage product can bind adjacent proteins or carbohydrates on the pathogen surface. If C4b does not rapidly form this bond, the thioester bond is cleaved by reaction with water, and C4b is irreversibly inactivated. This helps to prevent C4b from diffusing from its site of activation on the microbial surface and becoming attached to healthy host cells.

C2 becomes susceptible to cleavage by C1s only when it is bound by C4b, and the active C2a serine protease is thereby also confined to the pathogen surface, where it remains associated with C4b, forming the C3 convertase C4b2a. Cleavage of C3 to C3a and C3b is thus also confined to the surface of the pathogen. Like C4b, C3b is inactivated by hydrolysis unless its exposed thioester rapidly makes a covalent bond (see Fig. 2.16), and it therefore opsonizes only the surface on which complement activation has taken place. Opsonization by C3b is more effective when antibodies are also bound to the pathogen surface, as phagocytes have receptors for both complement and Fc receptors that bind the Fc region of antibody (see Sections 1-20 and 10-20). Because the reactive forms of C3b and C4b are able to form a covalent bond with any adjacent protein or carbohydrate, when complement is activated by bound antibody a proportion of the reactive C3b or C4b will become linked to the antibody molecules themselves. Antibody that is chemically cross-linked to complement is likely the most efficient trigger for phagocytosis.

2-9   The alternative pathway is an amplification loop for C3b formation that is accelerated by properdin in the presence of pathogens.

Although probably the most ancient of the complement pathways, the alternative pathway is so named because it was discovered as a second, or 'alternative,' pathway for complement activation after the classical pathway had been defined. Its key feature is its ability to be spontaneously activated. It has a unique C3 convertase, the **alternative pathway C3 convertase**, which differs from the C4b2a convertase of the lectin or classical pathways (see Fig. 2.17). The alternative pathway C3 convertase is composed of C3b itself bound to Bb, which is a cleavage fragment of the plasma protein **factor B**. This C3 convertase, designated **C3bBb**, has a special place in complement activation because, by producing C3b, it can generate more of itself. This means that once some C3b has been formed, by whichever pathway, the alternative pathway can act as an amplification loop to increase C3b production rapidly.

The alternative pathway can be activated in two different ways. The first is by the action of the lectin or classical pathway. C3b generated by either of these pathways and covalently linked to a microbial surface can bind factor B (**Fig. 2.23**). This alters the conformation of factor B, enabling a plasma protease

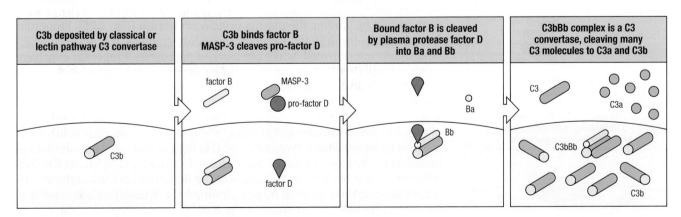

Fig. 2.23 The alternative pathway of complement activation can amplify the classical or the lectin pathway by forming an alternative C3 convertase and depositing more C3b molecules on the pathogen. C3b deposited by the classical or lectin pathway can bind factor B, making it susceptible to cleavage by factor D. MASP-3 cleaves pro-factor D (red circle) to form the active form of factor D (red fan). Cleavage of factor B produces the C3bBb complex, which is the C3 convertase of the alternative pathway of complement activation. This action of this C3 convertase, like that of C4b2a, results in the deposition of many molecules of C3b on the pathogen surface.

Fig. 2.24 The alternative pathway can be activated by spontaneous activation of C3. Complement component C3 hydrolyzes spontaneously in plasma to give $C3(H_2O)$, which binds factor B and enables the bound factor B to be cleaved by factor D (first panel). The resulting 'soluble C3 convertase' cleaves C3 to give C3a and C3b, which can attach to host cells or pathogen surfaces (second panel). Covalently bound to the cell surface, C3b binds factor B; in turn, factor B is rapidly cleaved by factor D to Bb, which remains bound to C3b to form a C3 convertase (C3bBb), and Ba, which is released (third panel). This convertase functions in the alternative pathway as the C3 convertase C4b2a does in the lectin and classical pathways (see Fig. 2.17).

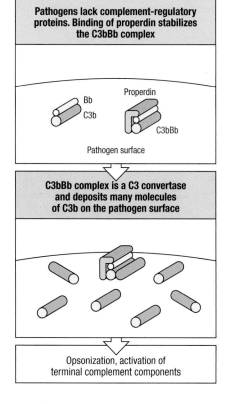

Pathogens lack complement-regulatory proteins. Binding of properdin stabilizes the C3bBb complex

C3bBb complex is a C3 convertase and deposits many molecules of C3b on the pathogen surface

Opsonization, activation of terminal complement components

called **factor D** to cleave it into Ba and Bb. Bb remains stably associated with C3b, forming the C3bBb C3 convertase. The second way of activating the alternative pathway involves the spontaneous hydrolysis (known as '**tickover**') of the thioester bond in C3 to form $C3(H_2O)$, as shown in **Fig. 2.24**. C3 is abundant in plasma, and tickover causes a steady, low-level production of $C3(H_2O)$. This $C3(H_2O)$ can bind factor B, which is then cleaved by factor D, producing a short-lived **fluid-phase C3 convertase, $C3(H_2O)Bb$**. Although formed in only small amounts by C3 tickover, fluid-phase $C3(H_2O)Bb$ can cleave many molecules of C3 to C3a and C3b. Much of this C3b is inactivated by hydrolysis, but some attaches covalently via its thioester bond to the surfaces of any microbes present. C3b formed in this way is no different from C3b produced by the lectin or classical pathways and binds factor B, leading to the formation of C3 convertase and a stepping up of C3b production (see Fig. 2.23).

On their own, the alternative pathway C3 convertases C3bBb and $C3(H_2O)Bb$ are very short-lived (~90 seconds). They are stabilized, however, by around 5- to 10-fold by binding the plasma protein **properdin** (**Fig. 2.25**). Properdin is made by neutrophils and stored in secondary granules. It is released when neutrophils are activated by the presence of pathogens. Properdin may have some properties of a pattern-recognition receptor, as it can bind to some microbial surfaces. Properdin-deficient individuals are particularly susceptible to infections with *Neisseria meningitidis*, the main agent of bacterial meningitis. Properdin's ability to bind to bacterial surfaces may direct the activity of the alternative complement pathway to these pathogens, thus aiding their removal by phagocytosis. Properdin can also bind to mammalian cells that are undergoing apoptosis or have been damaged or modified by ischemia, viral infection, or antibody binding, leading to the deposition of C3b on these cells and facilitating their removal by phagocytosis. The distinctive components of the alternative pathway are listed in **Fig. 2.26**.

Fig. 2.25 Properdin stabilizes the alternative pathway C3 convertase on pathogen surfaces. Bacterial surfaces do not express complement-regulatory proteins and favor the binding of properdin, which stabilizes the C3bBb convertase. This convertase activity is the equivalent of C4b2a of the lectin and classical pathways. C3bBb then cleaves many more molecules of C3, coating the pathogen surface with bound C3b.

Proteins of the alternative pathway of complement activation		
Native component	**Active fragments**	**Function**
C3	C3b	Binds to pathogen surface; binds B for cleavage by D; C3bBb is a C3 convertase and C3b$_2$Bb is a C5 convertase
Factor B (B)	Ba	Small fragment of B, unknown function
	Bb	Bb is the active enzyme of the C3 convertase C3bBb and the C5 convertase C3b$_2$Bb
Factor D (D)	D	Plasma serine protease, cleaves B when it is bound to C3b to Ba and Bb
Properdin (P)	P	Plasma protein that binds to bacterial surfaces and stabilizes the C3bBb convertase

Fig. 2.26 The proteins of the alternative pathway of complement activation.

2-10 Membrane and plasma proteins that regulate the formation and stability of C3 convertases determine the extent of complement activation.

Several mechanisms ensure that complement activation will proceed only on the surface of a pathogen or on damaged host cells, and not on normal host cells and tissues. After initial complement activation by any pathway, the extent of amplification via the alternative pathway is critically dependent on the stability of the C3 convertase C3bBb. This stability is controlled by both positive and negative regulatory proteins. We have already described how properdin acts as a positive regulatory protein on foreign surfaces, such as those of bacteria or damaged host cells, by stabilizing C3bBb.

Several negative regulatory proteins, present in plasma and in host-cell membranes, protect healthy host cells from the injurious effects of inappropriate complement activation on their surfaces. These **complement-regulatory proteins** interact with C3b and either prevent the convertase from forming or promote its rapid dissociation (**Fig. 2.27**). For example, a membrane-attached protein known as **decay-accelerating factor (DAF** or **CD55)** competes with factor B for binding to C3b on the cell surface and can displace Bb from a convertase that has already formed. Convertase formation can also be prevented by cleaving C3b to an inactive derivative, **iC3b**. This is achieved by a plasma protease, **factor I**, in conjunction with C3b-binding proteins that act as cofactors, such as **membrane cofactor of proteolysis (MCP** or **CD46)**, another host-cell membrane protein (see Fig. 2.27). Cell-surface complement receptor type 1 (**CR1**, also known as **CD35**) behaves similarly to DAF and MCP in that it inhibits C3 convertase formation and promotes the catabolism of C3b to inactive products, respectively, but it has a more limited tissue distribution. **Factor H** is another complement-regulatory protein in plasma that binds C3b, and like CR1, it is able to compete with factor B to displace Bb from the convertase; in addition, it acts as a cofactor for factor I. Factor H binds preferentially to C3b bound to vertebrate cells because it has an affinity for the sialic acid residues present on their cell surfaces (see Fig. 2.18). Thus, the amplification loop of the alternative pathway is allowed to proceed on the surface of a pathogen or on damaged host cells, but not on normal host cells or on tissues that express these negative regulatory proteins.

The C3 convertase of the classical and lectin pathways (C4b2a) is molecularly distinct from that of the alternative pathway (C3bBb). However, understanding of the complement system is simplified somewhat by recognition of the close evolutionary relationships between the different complement proteins (**Fig. 2.28**). Thus the complement zymogens factor B and C2 are closely related proteins encoded by homologous genes located in tandem within the major

Fig. 2.27 Complement activation spares host cells, which are protected by complement-regulatory proteins. If C3bBb forms on the surface of host cells, it is rapidly inactivated by complement-regulatory proteins expressed by the host cell: complement receptor 1 (CR1), decay-accelerating factor (DAF), and membrane cofactor of proteolysis (MCP). Host-cell surfaces also favor the binding of factor H from plasma. CR1, DAF, and factor H displace Bb from C3b, and CR1, MCP, and factor H catalyze the cleavage of bound C3b by the plasma protease factor I to produce inactive C3b (known as iC3b).

Fig. 2.28 There is a close evolutionary relationship among the factors of the alternative, lectin, and classical pathways of complement activation. Most of the factors are either identical or the homologous products of genes that have duplicated and then diverged in sequence. The proteins C4 and C3 are homologous and contain the unstable thioester bond by which their large fragments, C4b and C3b, bind covalently to membranes. The genes encoding proteins C2 and factor B are adjacent in the MHC region of the genome and arose by gene duplication. The regulatory proteins factor H, CR1, and C4BP share a repeat sequence common to many complement-regulatory proteins. The greatest divergence between the pathways is in their initiation: in the classical pathway the C1 complex binds either to certain pathogens or to bound antibody, and in the latter circumstance it serves to convert antibody binding into enzyme activity on a specific surface; in the lectin pathway, mannose-binding lectin (MBL) associates with a serine protease, activating MBL-associated serine protease (MASP), to serve the same function as C1r:C1s; in the alternative pathway this enzyme activity is provided by factor D.

Step in pathway	Protein serving function in pathway			Relationship
	Alternative	**Lectin**	**Classical**	
Initiating serine protease	D	MASP	C1s	Homologous (C1s and MASP)
Covalent binding to cell surface	C3b	C4b		Homologous
C3/C5 convertase	Bb	C2a		Homologous
Control of activation	CR1 H	CR1 C4BP		Identical Homologous
Opsonization	C3b			Identical
Initiation of effector pathway	C5b			Identical
Local inflammation	C5a, C3a			Identical
Stabilization	P	None		Unique

histocompatibility complex (MHC) on human chromosome 6. Furthermore, their respective binding partners, C3 and C4, both contain thioester bonds that provide the means of covalently attaching the C3 convertases to a pathogen surface.

Only one component of the alternative pathway seems entirely unrelated to its functional equivalents in the classical and lectin pathways: the initiating serine protease, factor D. Factor D can also be singled out as the only activating protease of the complement system to circulate as an active enzyme rather than a zymogen. This is both necessary for the initiation of the alternative pathway (through the cleavage of factor B bound to spontaneously activated C3) and safe for the host, because factor D has no other substrate than factor B bound to C3b. This means factor D finds its substrate only at pathogen surfaces and at a very low level in plasma, where the alternative pathway of complement activation can be allowed to proceed.

2-11 Complement developed early in the evolution of multicellular organisms.

The complement system was originally known only from vertebrates, but homologs of C3 and factor B and a prototypical 'alternative pathway' have been discovered in nonchordate invertebrates. This is not altogether surprising as C3, which is cleaved and activated by serine proteases, is evolutionarily related to the serine protease inhibitor α_2-macroglobulin, whose first appearance likely was in an ancestor to all modern vertebrates. The amplification loop of the alternative pathway also has an ancestral origin, as it is present in echinoderms (which include sea urchins and sea stars) and is based on a C3 convertase formed by the echinoderm homologs of C3 and factor B. These factors are expressed by phagocytic cells called **amoeboid coelomocytes** present in the coelomic fluid. Expression of C3 by these cells increases when bacteria are present. This simple system seems to function to opsonize bacterial cells and other foreign particles and facilitate their uptake by coelomocytes. C3 homologs in invertebrates are clearly related to each other. They all contain the distinctive thioester linkage and form a family of proteins, the **thioester-containing proteins**, or **TEPs**. In the mosquito *Anopheles*, the production of protein TEP1 is induced in response to infection, and the protein may directly bind to bacterial surfaces to mediate phagocytosis of Gram-negative bacteria. Some form of C3 activity may even predate the evolution of the Bilateria—animals with bilateral symmetry, flatworms being the most primitive modern representatives—because genomic evidence of C3, factor B, and some later-acting complement components has been found in the Anthozoa (corals and sea anemones).

After its initial appearance, the complement system seems to have evolved by the acquisition of new activation pathways that allow specific targeting of microbial surfaces. The first to evolve was likely the ficolin pathway, which is present both in vertebrates and in some closely related invertebrates, such as the urochordates. Evolutionarily, the ficolins may predate the collectins, which are also first seen in the urochordates. Homologs of MBL and of the classical pathway complement component 1q (C1q), both collectins, have been identified in the genome of the ascidian urochordate *Ciona* (sea squirt). Two invertebrate homologs of mammalian MASPs also have been identified in *Ciona*, and it seems likely that they may be able to cleave and activate C3. Thus, the minimal complement system of the echinoderms appears to have been expanded in the urochordates by the recruitment of a specific activation system that may target C3 deposition onto microbial surfaces. This also suggests that when adaptive immunity evolved, much later, the ancestral antibody molecule used an already diversified C1q-like collectin member to activate the complement pathway, and that the complement activation system evolved further by use of this collectin and its associated MASPs to become the initiating components of the classical complement pathway; namely, C1q, C1r, and C1s.

2-12 Surface-bound C3 convertase deposits large numbers of C3b fragments on pathogen surfaces and generates C5 convertase activity.

We now return to the present-day complement system. The formation of C3 convertases is the point at which the three pathways of complement activation converge. The convertase of the lectin and classical pathways, C4b2a, and the convertase of the alternative pathway, C3bBb, initiate the same subsequent events—they cleave C3 to C3b and C3a. C3b binds covalently through its thioester bond to adjacent molecules on the pathogen surface; otherwise it is inactivated by hydrolysis. C3 is the most abundant complement protein in plasma, occurring at a concentration of 1.2 mg/ml, and up to 1000 molecules of C3b can bind in the vicinity of a single active C3 convertase (see Fig. 2.23). Thus the main effect of complement activation is to deposit large quantities of C3b on the surface of the infecting pathogen, where the C3b forms a covalently bonded coat that can signal the ultimate destruction of the pathogen by phagocytes.

The next step in the complement cascade is the generation of the C5 convertases. C5 is a member of the same family of proteins as C3, C4, α_2-macroglobulin, and the thioester-containing proteins of invertebrates. C5 does not form an active thioester bond during its synthesis, but, like C3 and C4, it is cleaved by a specific protease into C5a and C5b fragments, each of which exerts specific downstream actions that are important in propagating the complement cascade. In the classical and the lectin pathways, a C5 convertase is formed by the binding of C3b to C4b2a to yield **C4b2a3b**. The C5 convertase of the alternative pathway is formed by the binding of C3b to the C3bBb convertase to form **C3b$_2$Bb**. A C5 is captured by these C5 convertase complexes through binding to an acceptor site on C3b and is thus rendered susceptible to cleavage by the serine protease activity of C2a or Bb. This reaction, which generates C5b and C5a, is much more limited than cleavage of C3, because C5 can be cleaved only when it binds to C3b that is in turn bound to C4b2a or C3bBb to form the active C5 convertase complex. Thus, complement activated by all three pathways leads to the binding of large numbers of C3b molecules on the surface of the pathogen, the generation of a more limited number of C5b molecules, and the release of C3a and a smaller amount of C5a (**Fig. 2.29**).

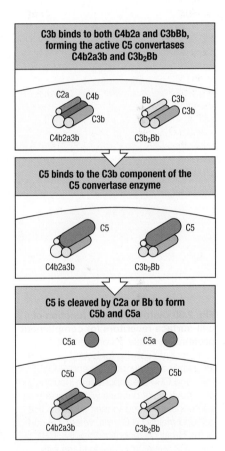

Fig. 2.29 Complement component 5 (C5) is cleaved when captured by a C3b molecule that is part of a C5 convertase complex. As shown in the top panel, C5 convertases are formed when C3b binds either the classical or lectin pathway C3 convertase C4b2a to form C4b2a3b or the alternative pathway C3 convertase C3bBb to form C3b$_2$Bb. C5 binds to C3b in these complexes (center panel). The bottom panel shows that C5 is cleaved by the active enzyme C2a or Bb to form C5b and the inflammatory mediator C5a. Unlike C3b and C4b, C5b is not covalently bound to the cell surface. The production of C5b initiates the assembly of the terminal complement components.

2-13 Ingestion of complement-tagged pathogens by phagocytes is mediated by receptors for the bound complement proteins.

The most important action of complement is to facilitate the uptake and destruction of pathogens by phagocytic cells. This occurs by the specific recognition of bound complement components by **complement receptors (CRs)** on phagocytes. These complement receptors bind pathogens opsonized with complement components: opsonization of pathogens is a major function of C3b and its proteolytic derivatives. C4b also acts as an opsonin but has a relatively minor role, largely because so much more C3b than C4b is generated.

The known receptors for bound complement components and for C5a and C3a are listed, with their functions and distributions, in **Fig. 2.30**. The C3b receptor CR1, described in Section 2-10, is a negative regulator of complement activation (see Fig. 2.27). CR1 is expressed on many types of immune cells, including macrophages and neutrophils. Binding of C3b to CR1 cannot by itself stimulate phagocytosis, but it can lead to phagocytosis in the presence of other immune mediators that activate macrophages. For example, the small complement fragment C5a can activate macrophages to ingest bacteria that are bound to their CR1 receptors (**Fig. 2.31**). C5a accomplishes this by binding to another receptor expressed by macrophages, the **C5a receptor 1** (C5aR1, CD88), which has seven membrane-spanning domains. Receptors of this type transduce their signals via intracellular guanine nucleotide–binding proteins

Fig. 2.30 Distribution and function of cell-surface receptors for complement proteins. A variety of complement receptors are specific for bound C3b and its cleavage products (iC3b and C3dg). CR1 and CR3 are important in inducing the phagocytosis of bacteria with complement components bound to their surface. CR2 is found mainly on B cells, where it is part of the B-cell co-receptor complex. CR1 and CR2 share structural features with the complement-regulatory proteins that bind C3b and C4b. CR3 and CR4 are integrins composed of integrin β2 (also known as CD18, and sometimes gp95) paired with either integrin αM (CD11b) or integrin αX (CD11c), respectively (see eAppendix II, found in the ebook and on the Digital Landing Page for this book); CR3, also called Mac-1, is also important for leukocyte adhesion and migration, as we shall see in Chapter 3, whereas CR4 is only known to function in phagocytosis. The receptors for C5a and C3a are seven-span G protein–coupled receptors. FDCs (follicular dendritic cells) are not involved in innate immunity and are discussed in later chapters.

Receptor	Specificity	Functions	Cell types
CR1 (CD35)	C3b, C4b	Promotes C3b and C4b decay Stimulates phagocytosis (requires C5a) Erythrocyte transport of immune complexes	Erythrocytes, macrophages, monocytes, neutrophils, B cells, FDCs
CR2 (CD21)	C3d, iC3b, C3dg	Enhances B-cell response to antigens bearing C3d, iC3b, or C3dg, part of B-cell co-receptor Epstein–Barr virus receptor	B cells, FDCs
CR3 (Mac-1) (CD11b: CD18)	iC3b	Stimulates phagocytosis	Macrophages, monocytes, polymorphonuclear leukocytes, FDCs
CR4 (gp150, 95) (CD11c: CD18)	iC3b	Stimulates phagocytosis	Macrophages, monocytes, polymorphonuclear leukocytes, dendritic cells
CRIg	C3b, iC3b	Phagocytosis of circulating pathogens	Tissue-resident macrophages Hepatic sinusoid macrophages
C5aR1 (CD88)	C5a	Binding of C5a, activates G protein	Neutrophils, macrophages, endothelial cells, mast cells
C5aR2 (C5L2, GPR77)	C5a	Decoy receptor, regulates C5a receptor	Neutrophils, macrophages
C3a receptor	C3a	Binding of C3a, activates G protein	Macrophages, endothelial cells, mast cells
PAR1 PAR4	C4a	Increases vascular permeability Coagulation	Epithelium, platelets

Fig. 2.31 The anaphylatoxin C5a can enhance the phagocytosis of microorganisms opsonized in an innate immune response. Activation of complement leads to the deposition of C3b on the surface of microorganisms (left panel). C3b can be bound by complement receptor 1 (CR1) on the surface of phagocytes, but this on its own is insufficient to induce phagocytosis (center panel). Phagocytes also express receptors for the anaphylatoxin C5a, and binding of C5a will activate the cell to phagocytose microorganisms bound through CR1 (right panel).

called G proteins and are known generally as **G protein–coupled receptors (GPCRs)**; they are discussed in Section 3-2. **C5a receptor 2** (C5L2, GPR77) is expressed by neutrophils and macrophages, but its function is not firmly established. It is a nonsignaling receptor that may act as a decoy receptor for C5a and regulate activity of the C5a receptor. Proteins associated with the extracellular matrix, such as fibronectin, can also contribute to phagocyte activation; these are encountered when phagocytes are recruited to connective tissue and activated there.

Four other complement receptors—**CR2** (also known as **CD21**), **CR3 (CD11b:CD18)**, **CR4 (CD11c:CD18)**, and **CRIg** (complement receptor of the immunoglobulin superfamily)—bind to forms of C3b that have been cleaved by factor I but that remain attached to the pathogen surface. Like several other key components of complement, C3b is subject to regulatory mechanisms that cleave it into derivatives, such as iC3b, that cannot form an active convertase. C3b bound to the microbial surface can be cleaved by factor I and MCP to remove the small fragment C3f, leaving the inactive iC3b form bound to the surface (**Fig. 2.32**). iC3b is recognized by several complement receptors—CR2, CR3, CR4, and CRIg. Unlike the binding of C3b to CR1, the binding of iC3b to the receptor CR3 is sufficient on its own to stimulate phagocytosis. Factor I and CR1 cleave iC3b to release C3c, leaving C3dg bound to the pathogen. C3dg is recognized only by CR2. CR2 is found on B cells as part of a co-receptor complex that can augment the signal received through the antigen-specific immunoglobulin receptor. Thus, a B cell whose antigen receptor is specific for an antigen of a pathogen will receive a strong signal on binding this antigen if it or the pathogen is also coated with C3dg. The activation of complement can therefore contribute to producing a strong antibody response.

The importance of opsonization by C3b and its inactive fragments in destroying extracellular pathogens can be seen in the effects of various complement deficiencies. For example, individuals deficient in C3 or in molecules that

Fig. 2.32 The cleavage products of C3b are recognized by different complement receptors. After C3b is deposited on the surface of pathogens, it can undergo several conformational changes that alter its interaction with complement receptors. Factor I and MCP can cleave the C3f fragment from C3b, producing iC3b, which is a ligand for the complement receptors CR3, CR4, CRIg, and weakly for CR2, but not CR1. Factor I and CR1 cleave iC3b to release C3c, leaving C3dg bound. C3dg is then recognized by CR2.

catalyze C3b deposition show an increased susceptibility to infection by a wide range of extracellular bacteria, including *Streptococcus pneumoniae.* We describe the effects of various defects in complement and the diseases they cause in Chapter 13.

2-14 The small fragments of some complement proteins initiate a local inflammatory response.

The small complement fragments C3a and C5a act on specific receptors on endothelial cells and mast cells (see Fig. 2.30) to produce local inflammatory responses. Like C5a, C3a also signals through a GPCR family member. When produced in large amounts or injected systemically, C3a and C5a induce a generalized circulatory collapse, producing a shocklike syndrome similar to that seen in a systemic allergic reaction involving antibodies of the IgE class, discussed in Chapter 14. Such a reaction is termed **anaphylactic shock**, and these small fragments of complement are therefore often referred to as **anaphylatoxins**. C5a has the highest specific biological activity, but both C3a and C5a induce the contraction of smooth muscle, increase vascular permeability, and act on the endothelial cells lining blood vessels to induce the synthesis of adhesion molecules. In addition, C3a and C5a can activate the mast cells that populate submucosal tissues to release inflammatory molecules such as histamine and the cytokine tumor necrosis factor-α (TNF-α), which cause similar effects. C4a is also generated during C4 cleavage and is inactive at C3a and C5a receptors. Instead, C4a acts at two other GPCRs, protease-activated receptor 1 (PAR1) and protease-activated receptor 4 (PAR4), which are expressed on endothelial cells and platelets and are also activated by thrombin, a protease activated in the clotting cascade. C4a activates signaling in these cells to increase endothelial-cell permeability and by actions on platelets may link complement activation with the clotting cascade.

The changes induced by C5a, C3a, and C4a combine to recruit antibody, complement, and phagocytic cells to the site of an infection (**Fig. 2.33**). The increased fluid in the tissues hastens the movement of pathogen-bearing antigen-presenting cells to the local lymph nodes, contributing to the prompt initiation of the adaptive immune response. C5a also acts directly on neutrophils and monocytes to increase their adherence to vessel walls, their migration toward sites of antigen deposition, and their ability to ingest particles; it also increases the expression of CR1 and CR3 on the surfaces of these cells. In this way, C5a, and to a lesser extent C3a and C4a, act in concert with other complement components to hasten the destruction of pathogens by phagocytes.

2-15 The terminal complement proteins polymerize to form pores in membranes that can kill certain pathogens.

Deficiency of the
C8 Complement
Component

One of the important effects of complement activation is the assembly of the terminal components of complement (**Fig. 2.34**) to form a membrane-attack complex. The reactions leading to the formation of this complex are shown schematically in **Fig. 2.35**. The end result is a pore in the lipid bilayer membrane that destroys membrane integrity. This is thought to kill the pathogen by destroying the proton gradient across the pathogen's cell membrane.

The first step in the formation of the membrane-attack complex is the cleavage of C5 by a C5 convertase to release C5b (see Fig. 2.29). In the next stages (see Fig. 2.35), C5b initiates the assembly of the terminal complement components and their insertion into the cell membrane. The process begins when one molecule of C5b binds one molecule of **C6**, and the C5b6 complex then binds one molecule of **C7**. This reaction leads to a conformational change that exposes a hydrophobic site on C7, which inserts into the lipid bilayer. Similar

Small complement-cleavage products act on blood vessels to increase vascular permeability and cell-adhesion molecules

C3a   C5a   C4a

Increased permeability allows increased fluid leakage from blood vessels and extravasation of immunoglobulin and complement molecules

IgG

IgM

complement components

Migration of macrophages, neutrophils, and lymphocytes is increased. Microbicidal activity of macrophages and neutrophils is also increased

Fig. 2.33 Local inflammatory responses can be induced by small complement fragments, especially C5a. The small complement fragments are differentially active: C5a is more active than C3a. C5a and C3a cause local inflammatory responses by acting directly on local blood vessels, stimulating an increase in blood flow, increased vascular permeability, and increased binding of phagocytes to endothelial cells. C3a and C5a also activate mast cells (not shown) to release mediators, such as histamine and TNF-α, which contribute to the inflammatory response. C4a binds to receptors expressed on endothelium and platelets that are normally activated by thrombin, PAR1, and PAR4, and so also promotes vascular permeability and local coagulation. In response to all these signals, an increase in vessel diameter and permeability leads to the accumulation of fluid and protein in the surrounding tissue. Fluid accumulation increases lymphatic drainage, bringing pathogens and their antigenic components to nearby lymph nodes. The antibodies, complement, and cells thus recruited participate in pathogen clearance by enhancing phagocytosis. The small complement fragments can also directly increase the activity of the phagocytes.

hydrophobic sites are exposed on the later components **C8** and **C9** when they are bound to the complex, allowing these proteins also to insert into the lipid bilayer. C8 is a complex of two proteins, C8β and C8α-γ. The C8β protein binds to C5b, and this binding of C8β to the membrane-associated C5b67 complex allows the hydrophobic domain of C8α-γ to insert into the lipid bilayer. Finally, C8α-γ induces the polymerization of 10–16 molecules of C9 into a pore-forming structure called the membrane-attack complex. The membrane-attack complex has a hydrophobic external face, allowing it to associate with the lipid bilayer, but a hydrophilic internal channel. The diameter of this channel

The terminal complement components that form the membrane-attack complex		
Native protein	**Active component**	**Function**
C5	C5a	Small peptide mediator of inflammation (high activity)
	C5b	Initiates assembly of the membrane-attack system
C6	C6	Binds C5b; forms acceptor for C7
C7	C7	Binds C5b6; amphiphilic complex inserts into lipid bilayer
C8	C8	Binds C5b67; initiates C9 polymerization
C9	C9$_n$	Polymerizes to C5b678 to form a membrane-spanning channel, lysing the cell

Fig. 2.34 The terminal complement components.

C5b binds C6 and C7	C5b67 complexes bind to membrane via C7	C8 binds to the complex and inserts into the cell membrane	C9 molecules bind to the complex and polymerize	10–16 molecules of C9 bind to form a pore in the membrane

Membrane lesions—end on (rings)	Membrane lesions—side on (tubes)	Schematic representation of the membrane-attack complex pore

Fig. 2.35 Assembly of the membrane-attack complex generates a pore in the lipid bilayer membrane. The sequence of steps and their approximate appearance are shown here in schematic form. C5b triggers the assembly of a complex of one molecule each of C6, C7, and C8, in that order. C7 and C8 undergo conformational changes, exposing hydrophobic domains that insert into the membrane. This complex causes moderate membrane damage in its own right, and also serves to induce the polymerization of C9, again with the exposure of a hydrophobic site. Up to 16 molecules of C9 are then added to the assembly to generate a channel 10 nm in diameter in the membrane. This channel disrupts the bacterial cell membrane, killing the bacterium. The electron micrographs show erythrocyte membranes with membrane-attack complexes in two orientations, end on and side on.

is about 10 nm, allowing the free passage of solutes and water across the lipid bilayer. The pore damage to the lipid bilayer leads to the loss of cellular homeostasis, the disruption of the proton gradient across the membrane, the penetration of enzymes such as lysozyme into the cell, and the eventual destruction of the pathogen.

Although the effect of the membrane-attack complex is very dramatic, particularly in experimental demonstrations in which antibodies against red blood cell membranes are used to trigger the complement cascade, the significance of these components in host defense seems to be quite limited. So far, deficiencies in C5–C9 have been associated with susceptibility only to *Neisseria* species, the bacteria that cause the sexually transmitted disease gonorrhea and a common form of bacterial meningitis. Thus, the opsonizing and inflammatory actions of the earlier components of the complement cascade are clearly more important for host defense against infection. Formation of the membrane-attack complex seems to be important only for the killing of a few pathogens, although, as we will see in Chapter 15, this complex might well have a major role in immunopathology.

2-16 Complement-control proteins regulate all three pathways of complement activation and protect the host from their destructive effects.

Complement activation usually is initiated on a pathogen surface, and the activated complement fragments that are produced usually bind nearby on the pathogen surface or are rapidly inactivated by hydrolysis. Even so, all complement components are activated spontaneously at a low rate in plasma, and these activated complement components will sometimes bind proteins on host cells. Section 2-10 introduced the soluble host proteins factor I and factor H

Regulatory proteins of the classical and alternative pathways			
Soluble factors regulating complement			
Name	**Ligand/ Binding factor**	**Action**	**Pathology if defective**
C1 inhibitor (C1INH)	C1r, C1s (C1); MASP-2 (MBL)	Binds and deactivates C1r, C1s, and MASP-2	Hereditary angiodema
C4-binding protein (C4BP)	C4b	Displaces C2a from C4b cofactor for C4b cleavage by factor I	
CPN1 (Carboxypeptidase N)	C3a, C5a	Inactivates C3a and C5a	Recurrent angioedema
Factor H	C3b	Displaces Bb from C3b, cofactor for C3b cleavage by factor I	Age-related macular degeneration, atypical hemolytic uremic syndrome
Factor I	C3b, C4b	Serine protease, cleaves C3b and C4b	Low C3 levels, atypical hemolytic uremic syndrome
Membrane-bound factors regulating complement			
Name	**Ligand/ Binding factor**	**Action**	**Pathology if defective**
CRIg	C3b, iC3b	Inhibits activation of alternative pathway	Increased susceptibiity to blood-borne infections
Complement receptor 1 (CR1, CD35)	C3b, C4b	Cofactor for factor I; displaces Bb from C3b, and C2a from C4b	
Decay-accelerating factor (DAF, CD55)	C3 convertase	Displaces Bb and C2a from C3b and C4b respectively	Paroxysmal nocturnal hemoglobinuria
Membrane cofactor of proteolysis (MCP, CD46)	C3b, C4b	Cofactor for factor I	Atypical hemolytic uremic syndrome
Protectin (CD59)	C8	Inhibits MAC formation	Paroxysmal nocturnal hemoglobinuria

Fig. 2.36 The soluble and membrane-bound proteins that regulate the activity of complement.

and the membrane-bound proteins MCP and DAF that regulate the alternative pathway of complement activation. In addition, several other soluble and membrane-bound complement-control proteins can regulate the complement cascade at various steps to protect normal host cells while allowing complement activation to proceed on pathogen surfaces (**Fig. 2.36**).

The activation of C1 is controlled by the **C1 inhibitor (C1INH)**, which is a plasma **serine protease inhibitor**, or **serpin**. C1INH binds to the catalytic sites of C1r and C1s and irreversibly inactivates them (**Fig. 2.37**). In this way, C1INH limits cleavage and activation of C4 and C2 by C1. By the same means, C1INH limits the spontaneous activation of C1 in plasma. Its importance can be seen in the C1INH deficiency disease **hereditary angioedema (HAE)**, in which chronic spontaneous complement activation leads to the production of excess cleaved fragments of C4 and C2. The large activated fragments from this cleavage (C2a and C4b), which normally combine to form the C3 convertase, do not damage host cells in such individuals because C4b is rapidly inactivated by hydrolysis in plasma, and the convertase does not form. C1INH also regulates the plasma protease kallikrein, a component of the kinin system (discussed in Section 3-3). Kallikrein is normally activated by tissue damage,

 Hereditary Angioedema

Fig. 2.37 Complement activation is regulated by a series of proteins that serve to protect host cells from accidental damage. These act on different stages of the complement cascade, dissociating complexes or catalyzing the enzymatic degradation of covalently bound complement proteins. Stages in the complement cascade are shown schematically down the left side of the figure, with the regulatory reactions on the right. The alternative pathway C3 convertase is similarly regulated by DAF, CR1, MCP, and factor H.

but in HAE the lack of C1INH leads to increased kallikrein activity and thus to the uncontrolled production of bradykinin. Hereditary angioedema is fully corrected by replacing C1INH. A similar, extremely rare human disease stems from a partial deficiency of **carboxypeptidase N (CPN)**, a metalloproteinase that inactivates the anaphylatoxins C3a and C5a as well as bradykinin and kallikrein. Humans with partial CPN deficiency exhibit recurrent angioedema due to delayed inactivation of serum C3a and bradykinin.

Because the highly reactive thioester bond of activated C3 and C4 cannot distinguish acceptor groups on a host cell from those on the surface of a pathogen, mechanisms have evolved to prevent the small amounts of C3 or C4 molecules deposited on host cells from fully triggering complement activation. We introduced these mechanisms in the context of control of the alternative pathway (see Fig. 2.27), but they are also important regulators of the classical pathway convertase (see Fig. 2.37, second and third rows). Section 2-10 described the proteins that inactivate any C3b or C4b that has bound to host cells. These are the plasma factor I and its cofactors MCP and CR1, which are membrane proteins. Circulating factor I is an active serine protease, but it can cleave C3b and C4b only when they are bound to MCP, factor H, or CR1 (see Fig. 2.27). In these circumstances, factor I cleaves C3b, first into iC3b and then further to C3dg, thus permanently inactivating it. C4b is similarly inactivated by cleavage into C4c and C4d. Microbial cell walls lack MCP and CR1 and thus cannot promote the breakdown of C3b and C4b, which instead act as binding sites for factor B and C2, promoting complement activation. The importance of factor I can be seen in people with genetically determined **factor I deficiency**. Because of uncontrolled complement activation, complement proteins rapidly become depleted, and such people suffer repeated bacterial infections, especially with ubiquitous pyogenic bacteria.

There are also plasma proteins with cofactor activity for factor I, most notably **C4b-binding protein (C4BP)** (see Fig. 2.36). It binds C4b and acts mainly as a regulator of the classical pathway in the fluid phase. Factor H binds C3b in the fluid phase, as well as at cell membranes, and helps to distinguish the C3b that is bound to host cells from that bound to microbial surfaces. The higher affinity of factor H for sialic acid residues on host-membrane glycoproteins allows it to displace factor B in binding to C3b on host cells. Also, C3b at host-cell membranes is bound by cofactor protein MCP. Factor H competes with factor B for binding to C3b bound to host cells, so that the bound C3b is catabolized by factor I into iC3b and C3dg, and complement activation is inhibited. In contrast, microbial membranes do not express MCP and lack the sialic acid modifications that attract factor H, and so factor B is favored for binding C3b on these surfaces. The greater amount of factor B on a microbial surface stimulates formation of more C3bBb, the alternative pathway C3 convertase, and thus amplifies complement activation.

2-17 Genetic and acquired disorders in complement regulation can produce various inflammatory conditions.

The critical balance between the inhibition and the activation of complement on cell surfaces is illustrated in individuals heterozygous for mutations in various complement-regulatory proteins. Several renal diseases are caused by complement dysregulation. A condition known as **atypical hemolytic uremic syndrome (aHUS)** can be caused by relatively rare mutations in factor H, factor I, and MCP. The reduced action of these regulatory factors can increase the alternative pathway activation on the surface of platelets and red blood cells. The damage that this produces can lead to low levels of platelets (thrombocytopenia) and red blood cells (anemia) and can damage the kidneys. aHUS can also be caused by an acquired autoantibody that binds to factor H and reduces its activity, again leading to increased alternative pathway activity. A related condition, called **C3 glomerulopathy**, can be caused by similar mutations in these factors. It is characterized by deposition of C3b in the renal glomerulus but is not associated with thrombocytopenia or anemia. Like aHUS, C3 glomerulopathy is more commonly caused by autoantibodies that inhibit factor H. Such autoantibodies are called **nephritic factors**, as they lead to inflammation in the kidney, and they can be directed at other components of complement. One type of nephritic factor is targeted to C3, and stabilizes the alternative pathway C3 convertase C3bBb, rather than inhibiting a complement regulatory protein.

Another serious health problem related to complement malfunction is a significantly increased risk of **age-related macular degeneration (AMD)**. AMD is the leading cause of blindness in the elderly in developed countries. It has been linked to single-nucleotide polymorphisms in the factor H gene, where tyrosine 402 is changed to histidine (Y402H). This polymorphism in factor H is not the primary cause of AMD, but it influences the response to retinal injury. Cellular debris produced during injury or renewal of photoreceptors, such as oxidized lipids, can activate complement and induce local inflammation. Normal factor H can bind these oxidized lipids and inactivate C3b that would otherwise trigger further complement activation. The Y402H variant of factor H interacts more weakly with oxidized lipids than does normal factor H, and consequently allows a chronic background of complement activation and inflammation to take place, which damages retinal epithelial cells and activates macrophages. Polymorphisms in other complement genes have also been found to be either detrimental or protective for this disease. Thus, even small alterations in the efficiency of either the activation or the regulation of this powerful effector system can contribute to the progression of degenerative or inflammatory disorders.

DAF and MCP also mediate protection against complement through a third mechanism, which augments the dissociation of C4b2a and C3bBb convertases that have already formed. CR1 is among the host-cell membrane molecules that regulate complement through both these mechanisms; that is, by promoting the dissociation of convertase and exhibiting cofactor activity. All the proteins that bind the homologous C4b and C3b molecules contain three or more tandem copies of a structural element called the short consensus repeat (SCR), the complement-control protein (CCP) repeat, or (especially in Japan) the sushi domain.

In addition to the mechanisms for preventing C3 convertase formation and C4 and C3 deposition on cell membranes, there are also inhibitory mechanisms that prevent the inappropriate insertion of the membrane-attack complex (MAC) into membranes. We saw in Section 2-15 that the membrane-attack complex polymerizes onto C5b molecules created by the action of C5 convertase. The membrane-attack complex mainly inserts into cell membranes adjacent to the site of the C5 convertase; that is, close to the site of complement activation on a pathogen. However, some newly formed membrane-attack complexes may diffuse from the site of complement activation and insert into adjacent host-cell membranes. Several plasma proteins, including, notably, **vitronectin** (also known as **S-protein**), bind to the C5b67, C5b678, and C5b6789 complexes and thereby inhibit their random insertion into cell membranes. Host-cell membranes also contain the intrinsic protein **CD59**, or **protectin**, which inhibits the binding of C9 to the C5b678 complex (see Fig. 2.37, bottom row). CD59 and DAF are both linked to the cell surface by a **glycosylphosphatidylinositol (GPI) tail**, like many other peripheral membrane proteins. One of the enzymes involved in the synthesis of GPI tails is encoded by a gene, *PIGA*, on the X chromosome. In people with a somatic mutation in this gene in a clone of hematopoietic cells, both CD59 and DAF fail to function. This causes the disease **paroxysmal nocturnal hemoglobinuria**, which is characterized by episodes of intravascular red blood cell lysis by complement. Red blood cells that lack only CD59 are also susceptible to destruction as a result of spontaneous activation of the complement cascade.

2-18 Pathogens produce several types of proteins that can inhibit complement activation.

Bacterial pathogens have evolved various strategies to avoid activation of complement, and thereby to avoid elimination by this first line of innate defense (**Fig. 2.38**). One strategy that many pathogens employ is to mimic host surfaces by attracting host complement regulators to their own surfaces. A mechanism to achieve this is for the pathogen to express surface proteins that bind to soluble complement-regulatory proteins such as C4BP and factor H; for example, the Gram-negative pathogen *Neisseria meningitidis* produces **factor H binding protein (fHbp)**, which recruits factor H (see Section 2-10), and the outer membrane protein **PorA**, which binds to C4BP. By recruiting factor H and C4BP to the pathogen membrane, the pathogen is able to inactivate C3b that is deposited on its surface and thereby avoid the consequences of complement activation. Complement is important in defense against *Neisseria* species, and several complement deficiencies are associated with increased susceptibility to this pathogen.

Another strategy employed by pathogens is to secrete proteins that directly inhibit components of complement. The Gram-positive pathogen *Staphylococcus aureus* provides several examples of this type of strategy. **Staphylococcal protein A (Spa)** binds to the Fc regions of immunoglobulins and interferes with the recruitment and activation of C1. This binding specificity was used as an early biochemical technique in the purification of antibodies. The staphylococcal protein **staphylokinase (SAK)** acts by cleaving immunoglobulins bound to the pathogen membrane, preventing complement activation and avoiding phagocytosis. The **staphylococcal complement inhibitor (SCIN)** protein binds to the classical C3 convertase, C4b2a, and the alternative pathway C3 convertase, C3bBb, and inhibits their activity. Other stages of complement activation, including formation of the C5 convertase, are targets of inhibition by proteins produced by these and other pathogens.

Pathogen	Evasion molecule	Host target	Mechanism of action
Membrane proteins			
Neisseria meningitidis	Factor H binding protein (fHbp)	Factor H	Inactivates bound C3b
Borrelia burgdorferi	Outer surface protein E (OspE)	Factor H	Inactivates bound C3b
Streptococcus pneumoniae	Pneumococcal surface protein C (PspC)	Factor H	Inactivates bound C3b
Secreted proteins			
Neisseria meningitidis	PorA	C4BP	Inactivates bound C3b
Staphylococcus aureus	Clumping factor A (ClfA)	Factor I	Inactivates bound C3b
Staphylococcus aureus	Staphylococcal protein A (Spa)	Immunoglobulin	Binds to Fc regions and interferes with C1 activation
Staphylococcus aureus	Staphylokinase (SAK)	Immunoglobulin	Cleaves immunoglobulins
Staphylococcus aureus	Complement inhibitor (SCIN, CINB, SCINC)	C3 convertase (C4b2a, C3bBb)	Inhibition of convertase activity

Fig. 2.38 Complement evasion proteins produced by various pathogens.

We will return to this topic of complement regulation in Chapter 13 when we discuss how the immune system sometimes fails or is evaded by pathogens.

Summary.

The complement system is one of the major mechanisms by which pathogen recognition is converted into an effective host defense against initial infection. Complement is a system of plasma proteins that can be activated directly by pathogens or indirectly by pathogen-bound antibody, leading to a cascade of reactions that occurs on the surface of pathogens and generates active components with various effector functions. There are three pathways of complement activation: the lectin pathway, triggered by the pattern-recognition receptors MBL and the ficolins; the classical pathway, triggered directly by antibody binding to the pathogen surface; and the alternative pathway, which utilizes spontaneous C3 deposition onto microbial surfaces, is augmented by properdin, and provides an amplification loop for the other two pathways. The early events in all pathways consist of a sequence of cleavage reactions in which the larger cleavage product binds covalently to the pathogen surface and contributes to the activation of the next component. The pathways converge with the formation of a C3 convertase enzyme, which cleaves C3 to produce the active cleavage product C3b. The binding of large numbers of C3b molecules to the pathogen is the central event in complement activation. Bound complement components, especially bound C3b and its inactive fragments, are recognized by specific complement receptors on phagocytic cells, which engulf pathogens opsonized by C3b and its inactive fragments. The small cleavage fragments of C3, C4, and C5 act on specific trimeric G protein–coupled receptors to recruit phagocytes, such as neutrophils, to sites of infection or to alter local vascular permeability and coagulation. Together, these activities promote the uptake and destruction of pathogens by phagocytes. The molecules of C3b that bind the C3 convertase itself initiate the late events of complement, binding C5 to make it susceptible to cleavage by C2a or Bb. The larger C5b fragment triggers the assembly of a membrane-attack complex, which can result in the lysis of certain pathogens. A system of soluble and membrane-bound complement-regulatory proteins acts to limit complement activation on host tissues, in order to prevent tissue damage from the inadvertent binding of activated complement components to host cells or from the spontaneous activation of complement components in plasma. Many pathogens produce a variety of soluble and membrane-associated proteins that can counteract complement activation and contribute to infection of the host by the microbe.

Summary to Chapter 2.

This chapter has described the preexisting, constitutive components of innate immunity. The body's epithelial surfaces are a constant but imperfect barrier to pathogen entry. In addition to their other specialized functions, epithelia have specialized adaptations, such as cilia, various antimicrobial molecules, and mucus that provide the simplest form of innate immunity. The complement system is a more specialized system that combines direct recognition of microbes with a complex effector system. The lectin pathway relies on pattern-recognition receptors that detect microbial membranes, while the alternative pathway relies on spontaneous complement activation that is down-regulated by host molecules expressed on self membranes. The main event in complement activation is accumulation of C3b on microbial membranes, which is recognized by complement receptors on phagocytic cells to promote microbial clearance by cells recruited to sites of infection by C3a and C5a. In addition, C5b initiates the membrane-attack complex that is able to lyse some microbes directly. The complement cascade is under regulation to prevent attack on host tissues, and genetic variation in regulatory pathways can result in autoimmune syndromes and age-related tissue damage.

Discussion Questions

2.1 What activities and structural features of the skin, lungs, and intestine are used to keep microbes from penetrating beyond the epithelial boundary?

2.2 Most antimicrobial peptides do not exert their actions within the host cells that produce them. What structural features of such peptides prevent their activation within neutrophils and Paneth cells?

2.3 The proteins of the complement cascade all circulate freely within the blood plasma. How is it that complement is normally activated only during an infection?

2.4 Recognition of bacteria by mannose-binding lectin and ficolins leads to their destruction by the same mechanisms as those of recognition of bacteria by antibodies. Explain how this is so. What evolutionary adaptation was necessary to allow for this?

2.5 Spontaneous hydrolysis of the thioester bond in C3 occurs continually at a low rate even in the absence of infection. Contrast the reactions that occur as a consequence of this C3 'tickover' in a healthy person with those that occur in a person infected with bacteria.

2.6 What is the central feature of the amplification loop in the alternative pathway? As this pathway is initiated spontaneously, how are host tissues protected from nonspecific damage by this pathway?

2.7 How do acquired antibodies directed against factor H lead to atypical hemolytic uremic syndrome? What are such antibodies called?

2.8 Age-related macular degeneration is associated with inherited variants of factor H. If this disease is not caused by these polymorphisms, how does this variant contribute to this disease?

Section references.

2-1 Infectious diseases are caused by diverse living agents that replicate in their hosts.

Kauffmann, S.H.E., Sher, A., and Ahmed, R.: *Immunology of Infectious Diseases.* Washington, DC: ASM Press, 2002.

Mandell, G.L., Bennett, J.E., and Dolin, R. (eds): *Principles and Practice of Infectious Diseases*, 4th ed. New York: Churchill Livingstone, 1995.

2-2 Epithelial surfaces of the body provide the first barrier against infection.

Birchenough, G.M., Nyström, E.E., Johansson, M.E., and Hansson, G.C.: A sentinel goblet cell guards the colonic crypt by triggering Nlrp6-dependent Muc2 secretion. *Science* 2016, **352**:1535–1542.

Gallo, R.L., and Hooper, L.V.: Epithelial antimicrobial defense of the skin and intestine. *Nat. Rev. Immunol.* 2012, **12**:503–516.

Johansson, M.E., and Hansson, G.C.: Microbiology. Keeping bacteria at a distance. *Science* 2011, **334**:182–183.

Shan, M., Gentile, M., Yeiser, J.R., Walland, A.C., Bornstein, V.U., Chen, K., He, B., Cassis, L., Bigas, A., Cols, M., et al.: Mucus enhances gut homeostasis and oral tolerance by delivering immunoregulatory signals. *Science* 2013, **342**:447–453.

2-3 Infectious agents must overcome innate host defenses to establish a focus of infection.

Gorbach, S.L., Bartlett, J.G., and Blacklow, N.R. (eds): *Infectious Diseases*, 3rd ed. Philadelphia: Lippincott Williams & Wilkins, 2003.

Hornef, M.W., Wick, M.J., Rhen, M., and Normark, S.: Bacterial strategies for overcoming host innate and adaptive immune responses. *Nat. Immunol.* 2002, **3**:1033–1040.

2-4 Epithelial cells and phagocytes produce several kinds of antimicrobial molecules.

Cash, H.L., Whitham, C.V., Behrendt, C.L., and Hooper, L.H.: Symbiotic bacteria direct expression of an intestinal bactericidal lectin. *Science* 2006, **313**: 1126–1130.

De Smet, K., and Contreras, R.: Human antimicrobial peptides: defensins, cathelicidins and histatins. *Biotechnol. Lett.* 2005, **27**:1337–1347.

Ganz, T.: Defensins: antimicrobial peptides of innate immunity. *Nat. Rev. Immunol.* 2003, **3**:710–720.

Mukherjee, S., Zheng, H., Derebe, M.G., Callenberg, K.M., Partch, C.L., Rollins, D., Propheter, D.C., Rizo, J., Grabe, M., Jiang, Q.X., and Hooper, L.V.: Antibacterial membrane attack by a pore-forming intestinal C-type lectin. *Nature* 2014, **505**:103–107.

Zanetti, M.: The role of cathelicidins in the innate host defense of mammals. *Curr. Issues Mol. Biol.* 2005, **7**:179–196.

2-5 The complement system recognizes features of microbial surfaces and marks them for destruction by coating them with C3b.

Borsos, T., Rapp, H.J.: Chromatographic separation of the first component of complement and its assay on a molecular basis. *J. Immunol.* 1963, **91**:851–858.

Gros, P., Milder, F.J., and Janssen, B.J.: Complement driven by conformational changes. *Nat. Rev. Immunol.* 2008, **8**:48–58.

Janssen, B.J., Christodoulidou, A., McCarthy, A., Lambris, J.D., and Gros, P.: Structure of C3b reveals conformational changes that underlie complement activity. *Nature* 2006, **444**:213–216.

Janssen, B.J., Huizinga, E.G., Raaijmakers, H.C., Roos, A., Daha, M.R., Nilsson-Ekdahl, K., Nilsson, B., and Gros, P.: Structures of complement component C3 provide insights into the function and evolution of immunity. *Nature* 2005, **437**:505–511.

2-6 The lectin pathway uses soluble receptors that recognize microbial surfaces to activate the complement cascade.

Bohlson, S.S., Fraser, D.A., and Tenner, A.J.: Complement proteins C1q and MBL are pattern recognition molecules that signal immediate and long-term protective immune functions. *Mol. Immunol.* 2007, **44**:33–43.

Degn, S.E., Jensen, L., Gál, P., Dobó, J., Holmvad, S.H., Jensenius, J.C., and Thiel, S.: Biological variations of MASP-3 and MAp44, two splice products of the MASP1 gene involved in regulation of the complement system. *J. Immunol. Methods* 2010, **361**:37–50.

Fujita, T.: Evolution of the lectin-complement pathway and its role in innate immunity. *Nat. Rev. Immunol.* 2002, **2**:346–353.

Garred, P., Genster, N., Pilely, K., Bayarri-Olmos, R., Rosbjerg, A., Ma, Y.J., and Skjoedt, M.O.: A journey through the lectin pathway of complement-MBL and beyond. *Immunol. Rev.* 2016, **274**:74–97.

Héja, D., Kocsis, A., Dobó, J., Szilágyi, K., Szász, R., Závodszky, P., Pál, G., and Gál, P.: Revised mechanism of complement lectin-pathway activation revealing the role of serine protease MASP-1 as the exclusive activator of MASP-2. *Proc. Natl. Acad. Sci. USA* 2012, **109**:10498–10503.

2-7 The classical pathway is initiated by activation of the C1 complex and is homologous to the lectin pathway.

McGrath, F.D., Brouwer, M.C., Arlaud, G.J., Daha, M.R., Hack, C.E., and Roos, A.: Evidence that complement protein C1q interacts with C-reactive protein through its globular head region. *J. Immunol.* 2006, **176**:2950–2957.

2-8 Complement activation is largely confined to the surface on which it is initiated.

Cicardi, M., Bergamaschini, L., Cugno, M., Beretta, A., Zingale, L.C., Colombo, M., and Agostoni, A.: Pathogenetic and clinical aspects of C1 inhibitor deficiency. *Immunobiology* 1998, **199**:366–376.

2-9 The alternative pathway is an amplification loop for C3b formation that is accelerated by properdin in the presence of pathogens.

Fijen, C.A., van den Bogaard, R., Schipper, M., Mannens, M., Schlesinger, M., Nordin, F.G., Dankert, J., Daha, M.R., Sjoholm, A.G., Truedsson, L., et al.: Properdin deficiency: molecular basis and disease association. *Mol. Immunol.* 1999, **36**:863–867.

Kemper, C., and Hourcade, D.E.: Properdin: new roles in pattern recognition and target clearance. *Mol. Immunol.* 2008, **45**:4048–4056.

Spitzer, D., Mitchell, L.M., Atkinson, J.P., and Hourcade, D.E.: Properdin can initiate complement activation by binding specific target surfaces and providing a platform for de novo convertase assembly. *J. Immunol.* 2007, **179**:2600–2608.

Xu, Y., Narayana, S.V., and Volanakis, J.E.: Structural biology of the alternative pathway convertase. *Immunol. Rev.* 2001, **180**:123–135.

2-10 Membrane and plasma proteins that regulate the formation and stability of C3 convertases determine the extent of complement activation.

Golay, J., Zaffaroni, L., Vaccari, T., Lazzari, M., Borleri, G.M., Bernasconi, S., Tedesco, F., Rambaldi, A., and Introna, M.: Biologic response of B lymphoma cells to anti-CD20 monoclonal antibody rituximab *in vitro*: CD55 and CD59 regulate complement-mediated cell lysis. *Blood* 2000, **95**:3900–3908.

Spiller, O.B., Criado-Garcia, O., Rodriguez De Cordoba, S., and Morgan, B.P.: Cytokine-mediated up-regulation of CD55 and CD59 protects human hepatoma cells from complement attack. *Clin. Exp. Immunol.* 2000, **121**:234–241.

Varsano, S., Frolkis, I., Rashkovsky, L., Ophir, D., and Fishelson, Z.: Protection of human nasal respiratory epithelium from complement-mediated lysis by cell-membrane regulators of complement activation. *Am. J. Respir. Cell Mol. Biol.* 1996, **15**:731–737.

2-11 Complement developed early in the evolution of multicellular organisms.

Fujita, T.: Evolution of the lectin-complement pathway and its role in innate immunity. *Nat. Rev. Immunol.* 2002, **2**:346–353.

Zhang, H., Song, L., Li, C., Zhao, J., Wang, H., Gao, Q., and Xu, W.: Molecular cloning and characterization of a thioester-containing protein from Zhikong scallop *Chlamys farreri*. *Mol. Immunol.* 2007, **44**:3492–3500.

2-12 Surface-bound C3 convertase deposits large numbers of C3b fragments on pathogen surfaces and generates C5 convertase activity.

Rawal, N., and Pangburn, M.K.: Structure/function of C5 convertases of complement. *Int. Immunopharmacol.* 2001, **1**:415–422.

2-13 Ingestion of complement-tagged pathogens by phagocytes is mediated by receptors for the bound complement proteins.

Gasque, P.: Complement: a unique innate immune sensor for danger signals. *Mol. Immunol.* 2004, **41**:1089–1098.

Helmy, K.Y., Katschke, K.J., Jr., Gorgani, N.N., Kljavin, N.M., Elliott, J.M., Diehl, L., Scales, S.J., Ghilardi, N., and van Lookeren Campagne, M.: CRIg: a macrophage complement receptor required for phagocytosis of circulating pathogens. *Cell* 2006, **124**:915–927.

Kovtun, A., Bergdolt, S., Hägele, Y., Matthes, R., Lambris, J.D., Huber-Lang, M., and Ignatius, A.: Complement receptors C5aR1 and C5aR2 act differentially during the early immune response after bone fracture but are similarly involved in bone repair. *Sci. Rep.* 2017, **7**:14061.

Li, X.X., Lee, J.D., Kemper, C., and Woodruff, T.M.: The complement receptor C5aR2: a powerful modulator of innate and adaptive immunity. *J. Immunol.* 2019, **202**:3339–3348.

2-14 The small fragments of some complement proteins initiate a local inflammatory response.

Barnum, S.R.: C4a: an anaphylatoxin in name only. *J. Innate Immun.* 2015, **7**:333–339.

Kohl, J.: Anaphylatoxins and infectious and noninfectious inflammatory diseases. *Mol. Immunol.* 2001, **38**:175–187.

Schraufstatter, I.U., Trieu, K., Sikora, L., Sriramarao, P., and DiScipio, R.: Complement C3a and C5a induce different signal transduction cascades in endothelial cells. *J. Immunol.* 2002, **169**:2102–2110.

Wang, H., Ricklin, D., and Lambris, J.D.: Complement-activation fragment C4a mediates effector functions by binding as untethered agonist to protease-activated receptors 1 and 4. *Proc. Natl. Acad. Sci. USA* 2017, **114**:10948–10953.

2-15 The terminal complement proteins polymerize to form pores in membranes that can kill certain pathogens.

Hadders, M.A., Beringer, D.X., and Gros, P.: Structure of C8α-MACPF reveals mechanism of membrane attack in complement immune defense. *Science* 2007, **317**:1552–1554.

Parker, C.L., and Sodetz, J.M.: Role of the human C8 subunits in complement-mediated bacterial killing: evidence that C8γ is not essential. *Mol. Immunol.* 2002, **39**:453–458.

Scibek, J.J., Plumb, M.E., and Sodetz, J.M.: Binding of human complement C8 to C9: role of the N-terminal modules in the C8α subunit. *Biochemistry* 2002, **41**:14546–14551.

2-16 Complement-control proteins regulate all three pathways of complement activation and protect the host from their destructive effects.

Ambati, J., Atkinson, J.P., and Gelfand, B.D.: Immunology of age-related macular degeneration. *Nat. Rev. Immunol.* 2013, **13**:438–451.

Jiang, H., Wagner, E., Zhang, H., and Frank, M.M.: Complement 1 inhibitor is a regulator of the alternative complement pathway. *J. Exp. Med.* 2001, **194**:1609–1616.

Miwa, T., Zhou, L., Hilliard, B., Molina, H., and Song, W.C.: Crry, but not CD59 and DAF, is indispensable for murine erythrocyte protection in vivo from spontaneous complement attack. *Blood* 2002, **99**:3707–3716.

2-17 Genetic and acquired disorders in complement regulation can produce various inflammatory conditions.

Atkinson, J.P., and Goodship, T.H.: Complement factor H and the hemolytic uremic syndrome. *J. Exp. Med.* 2007, **204**:1245–1248.

Chauvet, S., Roumenina, L.T., Bruneau, S., Marinozzi, M.C., Rybkine, T., Schramm, E.C., Java, A., Atkinson, J.P., Aldigier, J.C., Bridoux, F., et al.: A familial C3GN secondary to defective C3 regulation by complement receptor 1 and complement factor H. *J. Am. Soc. Nephrol.* 2016, **27**:1665–1677.

Spencer, K.L., Hauser, M.A., Olson, L.M., Schmidt, S., Scott, W.K., Gallins, P., Agarwal, A., Postel, E.A., Pericak-Vance, M.A., and Haines, J.L.: Protective effect of complement factor B and complement component 2 variants in age-related macular degeneration. *Hum. Mol. Genet.* 2007, **16**:1986–1992.

Spencer, K.L., Olson, L.M., Anderson, B.M., Schnetz-Boutaud, N., Scott, W.K., Gallins, P., Agarwal, A., Postel, E.A., Pericak-Vance, M.A., and Haines, J.L.: **C3 R102G polymorphism increases risk of age-related macular degeneration.** *Hum. Mol. Genet.* 2008, **17**:1821–1824.

2-18 Pathogens produce several types of proteins that can inhibit complement activation.

Blom, A.M., Rytkonen, A., Vasquez, P., Lindahl, G., Dahlback, B., and Jonsson, A.B.: **A novel interaction between type IV pili of** *Neisseria gonorrhoeae* **and the human complement regulator C4B-binding protein.** *J. Immunol.* 2001, **166**:6764–6770.

Caine, J.A., and Coburn, J.: **Multifunctional and redundant roles of** *Borrelia burgdorferi* **outer surface proteins in tissue adhesion, colonization, and complement evasion.** *Front. Immunol.* 2016, **7**:442.

Serruto, D., Rappuoli, R., Scarselli, M., Gros, P., and van Strijp, J.A.: **Molecular mechanisms of complement evasion: learning from staphylococci and meningococci.** *Nat. Rev. Microbiol.* 2010, **8**:393–399.

Potempa, M., and Potempa, J.: **Protease-dependent mechanisms of complement evasion by bacterial pathogens.** *Biol. Chem.* 2012, **393**:873–888.

Cellular Mechanisms of Innate Immunity

3

In Chapter 2 we introduced the innate defenses—such as epithelial barriers, secreted antimicrobial proteins, and the complement system—that act immediately upon encounter with microbes to protect the body from infection. We also introduced the phagocytic cells that lie beneath the epithelial barriers and stand ready to engulf and digest invading microorganisms that have been flagged for destruction by complement. These phagocytes also initiate the next phase, the induced innate immune response, leading to an inflammatory reaction that recruits new phagocytic cells and circulating effector molecules to the site of infection.

In this chapter we describe how phagocytic cells of the innate immune system detect microbes or the cellular damage they cause, how they destroy these pathogens, and how they orchestrate downstream inflammatory responses through production of cytokines and chemokines (chemoattractant cytokines). We also introduce other cells of the innate immune system—a diverse array of specialized innate lymphoid cells (ILCs) including the natural killer cells (NK cells)—that contribute to innate host defenses against viruses and other intracellular pathogens. Also in this stage of infection, dendritic cells initiate adaptive immune responses.

Pathogen recognition by cells of the innate immune system.

The basis of the adaptive immune system's enormous capacity for antigen recognition has long been appreciated. In contrast, the basis of recognition of microorganisms by innate immune receptors was discovered only in the late 1990s. Overall, the diversity of features recognized by innate immune receptors is quite limited compared with the diversity of features recognized by antigen receptors of the adaptive immune system. Nevertheless, the innate immune system has the capacity to recognize essentially any microorganism because innate immune receptors recognize conserved molecular features shared by related groups of microbes. These features are often referred to as **pathogen-associated molecular patterns (PAMPs)**, and the receptors that recognize them are called **pattern-recognition receptors (PRRs)**.

We will discuss specific examples of PAMPs and PRRs later in this chapter, but before doing so it is useful to establish some key principles that shape our understanding of innate immunity and distinguish it from adaptive immunity. The general characteristics of PRRs are contrasted with those of the antigen-specific receptors of adaptive immunity in **Fig. 3.1**. One key feature of PRRs is that their specificities are genetically encoded and inherited through the germline, in contrast to the random generation of antigen receptors of the adaptive immune system. Therefore, the specificities of PRRs have been shaped through evolution to recognize PAMPs, which are typically molecules that cannot be mutated without a significant fitness cost to the microbe. This selection of receptors that recognize conserved, largely invariant microbial features is how the innate immune system can recognize the broad diversity of potential pathogens with a limited number of receptors. In general, ligands for PRRs do not occur in healthy host cells, which ensures that immune responses

Fig. 3.1 Comparison of the characteristics of recognition molecules of the innate and adaptive immune systems. The innate immune system uses germline-encoded receptors while the adaptive immune system uses antigen receptors of unique specificity assembled from incomplete gene segments during lymphocyte development. Antigen receptors of the adaptive immune system are clonally expressed on individual lymphocytes and their progeny. Typically, receptors of the innate immune system are expressed nonclonally; that is, they are expressed on many, if not all, the cells of a given cell type.

Receptor characteristic	Innate immunity	Adaptive immunity
Specificity inherited in the genome	Yes	No
Triggers immediate response	Yes	No
Recognizes broad classes of pathogens	Yes	No
Encoded in multiple gene segments	No	Yes
Requires gene rearrangement	No	Yes
Clonal expression	No	Yes
Able to discriminate between even closely related molecular structures	Yes	Yes

are only directed against microbes; however, we will cover some interesting exceptions to this rule later in the chapter. Another critical feature of innate immune recognition is that cells express multiple PRRs, which we refer to as nonclonal expression, to distinguish it from the clonal expression of antigen receptors of the adaptive immune system. Nonclonal expression enables a given cell to respond to a range of pathogens so that large numbers of cells can rapidly mobilize when an infection is first detected. For example, macrophages, neutrophils, and dendritic cells express a variety of PRRs and can therefore respond to many distinct pathogens.

In addition to direct PAMP recognition by PRRs, a more recently appreciated concept is that certain innate immune receptors respond to the consequences of infection. Pathogens often disrupt specific cellular functions while establishing infection, and some innate receptors detect these perturbations. The actions of pathogens can also induce the release or production of self-derived host molecules, which in turn activate innate immune receptors. Such molecules have been termed **damage-associated molecular patterns (DAMPs)**. While the cellular perturbations and DAMPs are often the result of infection, they can also be induced in other contexts, such as tissue damage or neoplastic transformation.

Coordination of the innate immune response relies on the information provided by many types of receptors. Innate immune receptors can be classified into four main groups on the basis of their cellular localization and their function: free receptors in the serum, such as ficolins and histatins (discussed in Chapter 2); membrane-bound phagocytic receptors; membrane-bound signaling receptors; and cytoplasmic signaling receptors. Phagocytic receptors primarily signal for phagocytosis of the microbes they recognize. A diverse group of chemotactic receptors helps to guide cells to sites of infection; other receptors, including PRRs and cytokine receptors, help to control the activity of effector molecules at those sites.

In this part of the chapter we first look at the recognition properties of phagocytic receptors and of signaling receptors that activate phagocytic microbial killing mechanisms. Next, we describe the main PRR families that detect infection, including the Toll-like receptors (TLRs), the first of the innate sensor systems to be discovered, and several families of receptors that detect intracellular infections.

3-1 After entering tissues, many microbes are recognized, ingested, and killed by phagocytes.

If a microorganism crosses an epithelial barrier and begins to replicate in the tissues of the host, in most cases it is immediately recognized by resident phagocytic cells. The main classes of phagocytic cells in the innate immune

ANIMATION 3.1

system are macrophages and monocytes, granulocytes, and dendritic cells. **Macrophages** are the major phagocyte population resident in most normal tissues at homeostasis. They can arise either from progenitor cells that enter the tissues during embryonic development, and then self-renew at steady state during life, or from circulating **monocytes**. Studies suggest that the embryonic progenitors arise from either the fetal liver, the yolk sac, or an embryonic region near the dorsal aorta called the **aorta–gonad–mesonephros (AGM)**, although the relative contribution of these origins is still debated. Macrophages are found in especially large numbers in connective tissue: for example, in the submucosal layer of the gastrointestinal tract; in the submucosal layer of the bronchi and in the lung interstitium—the tissue and intercellular spaces around the air sacs (alveoli)—and in the alveoli themselves; along some blood vessels in the liver; and throughout the spleen, where they remove senescent blood cells. Macrophages in different tissues were historically given different names; for example, **microglial cells** in neural tissue and **Kupffer cells** in the liver. The self-renewal of these two types of cells is dependent on a cytokine called interleukin-34 (IL-34) that is produced in these tissues and acts on the same receptor as macrophage-colony stimulating factor (M-CSF).

During infection or inflammation, macrophages can also arise from monocytes that leave from the circulation to enter into tissues. Monocytes in both mouse and human develop in the bone marrow and circulate in the blood as two main populations. In humans, 90% of circulating monocytes are **'classical' monocytes** that express CD14, a co-receptor for a PRR described later, and function during infection by entering tissues and differentiating into activated inflammatory monocytes or macrophages. In mice, this monocyte population expresses high levels of the surface marker Ly6C. A smaller population of **'patrolling' monocytes** roll along the endothelium rather than circulating freely in the blood. In humans, they express CD14 and CD16, a type of Fc receptor (FcγRIII; see Section 10-21), and are thought to survey for injury to the endothelium, but they do not differentiate into tissue macrophages. In mice, they express low levels of Ly6C.

ANIMATION 3.2

The second major class of phagocytes comprises the granulocytes, which include **neutrophils**, **eosinophils**, and **basophils**. Of these, neutrophils have the greatest phagocytic activity and are the cells most immediately involved in innate immunity against infectious agents. Also called polymorphonuclear neutrophilic leukocytes (PMNs, or polys), they are short-lived cells that are abundant in the blood but are not present in healthy tissues. Macrophages and granulocytes have an important role in innate immunity because they can recognize, ingest, and destroy many pathogens without the aid of an adaptive immune response. Phagocytic cells that scavenge incoming pathogens represent an ancient mechanism of innate immunity, as they are found in both invertebrates and vertebrates.

The third class of phagocytes in the immune system is the immature **dendritic cells** that reside in lymphoid organs and in peripheral tissues. There are two main functional types of dendritic cells: **conventional (or classical) dendritic cells (cDCs)** and **plasmacytoid dendritic cells (pDCs)**. Both types of cells arise from progenitors within the bone marrow, and they migrate via the blood to tissues throughout the body and to peripheral lymphoid organs. Dendritic cells ingest and break down microbes, but, unlike macrophages and neutrophils, their primary role in immune defense is not the frontline, large-scale direct killing of microbes. A major role of cDCs is to process ingested microbes in order to generate peptide antigens that can activate T cells and induce an adaptive immune response. They also produce cytokines in response to microbial recognition (via PRRs) that activate other types of cells against infection. cDCs are thus considered to act as a bridge between innate and adaptive immune responses. pDCs can produce large amounts of a class of cytokines known as type I **interferons**, or antiviral interferons, and are considered to be part of innate immunity; they are discussed in detail later in the chapter.

Because most microorganisms enter the body through the mucosa of the gut and respiratory system, the skin, or the urogenital tract, macrophages in the submucosal tissues are the first cells to encounter most pathogens, but they are soon reinforced by the recruitment of large numbers of neutrophils to sites of infection. Macrophages and neutrophils recognize pathogens by means of cell-surface PRRs that bind PAMPs on the surface of pathogens, as discussed at the beginning of this chapter. Although they are both phagocytic, macrophages and neutrophils have distinct properties and functions in innate immunity.

The process of **phagocytosis** is initiated when certain receptors on the surface of the cell—typically a macrophage, neutrophil, or dendritic cell—interact with the microbial surface. The bound pathogen is first surrounded by the phagocyte plasma membrane and then internalized in a large membrane-enclosed endocytic vesicle known as a **phagosome**. The phagosome fuses with one or more lysosomes to generate a **phagolysosome**, in which the lysosomal contents are released. The phagolysosome also becomes acidified, acquires antimicrobial peptides and enzymes, and undergoes enzymatic processes that produce highly reactive **superoxide radicals** and **nitric oxide radicals**, which together kill the microbe (**Fig. 3.2**). Neutrophils are highly specialized for the intracellular killing of microbes and contain different types of cytoplasmic granules—the **primary granules** and **secondary granules** described in Section 2-4. These granules fuse with phagosomes, releasing additional enzymes and antimicrobial peptides that attack the microbe. Another pathway by which extracellular material, including microbial material, can be taken up into the endosomal compartment of cells and degraded is **receptor-mediated endocytosis**, which is not restricted to phagocytes. Dendritic cells and other phagocytes can also take up pathogens by a nonspecific process called **macropinocytosis**, in which large amounts of extracellular fluid and its contents are ingested.

Macrophages and neutrophils constitutively express a number of cell-surface PRRs that stimulate the phagocytosis and intracellular killing of microbes bound to them, although some also signal through other pathways to trigger responses such as cytokine production. This set of phagocytic PRRs includes several members of the C-type lectin–like family (see Fig. 3.2). For example, **Dectin-1** is strongly expressed by macrophages and neutrophils and recognizes β-(1,3)–linked glucans (polymers of glucose), which are common components of fungal cell walls in particular. Dendritic cells also express Dectin-1, as well as several other C-type lectin–like phagocytic receptors. Another C-type lectin, the **mannose receptor** expressed by macrophages and dendritic cells, recognizes various mannosylated ligands, including some present on fungi, bacteria, and viruses; it was once suspected of having an important role in resistance to microbes. However, experiments with mice that lack this

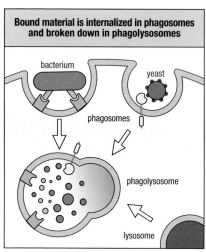

Fig. 3.2 Macrophages express receptors that enable them to take up microbes by phagocytosis. First panel: Macrophages residing in tissues throughout the body are among the first cells to encounter and respond to pathogens. They carry cell-surface receptors that bind to various molecules on microbes, in particular carbohydrates and lipids, and induce phagocytosis of the bound material. Second panel: Dectin-1 is a member of the C-type lectin–like family built around a single C-type lectin–like domain (CTLD). Lectins in general are based on a carbohydrate-recognition domain (CRD). The macrophage mannose receptor contains many CTLDs and has a fibronectin-like domain and a cysteine-rich region at its amino terminus. Class A scavenger receptors, such as MARCO, are built from collagen-like domains and form trimers. The receptor protein CD36 is a class B scavenger receptor that recognizes and internalizes lipids. Various complement receptors bind and internalize complement-coated bacteria. Third panel: In phagocytosis, receptor-bound material is taken into intracellular phagosomes, which fuse with lysosomes to form an acidified phagolysosome in which the ingested material is broken down by lysosomal hydrolases.

receptor do not support this idea. The macrophage mannose receptor is now thought to function mainly as a clearance receptor for host glycoproteins such as β-glucuronidase and lysosomal hydrolases, which have mannose-containing carbohydrate side chains and whose extracellular concentrations are raised during inflammation.

Another set of phagocytic PRRs on macrophages, called **scavenger receptors**, recognize various anionic polymers and acetylated low-density lipoproteins. These receptors are structurally heterogeneous, consisting of at least six different molecular families. Class A scavenger receptors are membrane proteins composed of trimers of collagen domains (see Fig. 3.2). They include **SR-A I**, **SR-A II**, and **MARCO** (<u>ma</u>crophage <u>r</u>eceptor with a <u>co</u>llagenous structure), all of which bind various bacterial cell-wall components and help to internalize bacteria, although the basis of their specificity is poorly understood. Class B scavenger receptors bind high-density lipoproteins, and they internalize lipids. One of these receptors is CD36, which binds many ligands, including long-chain fatty acids.

A third set of receptors of crucial importance in macrophage and neutrophil phagocytosis is the complement receptors and Fc receptors introduced in Chapters 1 and 2. These receptors bind to complement-coated microbes or to antibodies that have bound to the surface of microbes and facilitate the phagocytosis of a wide range of microorganisms.

3-2   G protein–coupled receptors on phagocytes link microbe recognition with increased efficiency of intracellular killing.

Phagocytosis of microbes by macrophages and neutrophils is generally followed by the death of the microbe inside the phagocyte. In addition to the phagocytic receptors described above, macrophages and neutrophils have other receptors that signal to stimulate antimicrobial killing. These receptors belong to the evolutionarily ancient family of **G protein–coupled receptors (GPCRs)**, which are characterized by seven membrane-spanning segments. Members of this family are crucial to immune-system function because they also direct responses to anaphylatoxins such as the complement fragment C5a (see Section 2-14), leukotrienes, and to many chemokines, recruiting phagocytes to sites of infection and promoting inflammation.

The **fMet-Leu-Phe (fMLF) receptor** is a G protein–coupled receptor that senses the presence of bacteria by recognizing a unique feature of bacterial polypeptides. Protein synthesis in bacteria is typically initiated with an *N*-formylmethionine (fMet) residue, an amino acid present in prokaryotes but not in eukaryotes. The fMLF receptor is named after a tripeptide, formylmethionyl-leucyl phenylalanine, for which it has a high affinity, although it also binds other peptide motifs. Bacterial polypeptides binding to this receptor activate intracellular signaling pathways that direct the cell to move toward the most concentrated source of the ligand. Signaling through the fMLF receptor also induces the production of microbicidal **reactive oxygen species (ROS)** in the phagolysosome. The C5a receptor 1 recognizes the small fragment of C5 generated when complement is activated, usually by the presence of microbes (see Section 2-13), and signals by a similar pathway as the fMLF receptor. Thus, stimulation of these receptors both guides monocytes and neutrophils toward a site of infection and leads to increased antimicrobial activity; these cell responses can be activated by directly sensing unique bacterial products or by messengers such as C5a that indicate previous recognition of a microbe.

 ANIMATION 3.3

The G protein–coupled receptors are so named because ligand binding activates a member of a class of intracellular GTP-binding proteins called

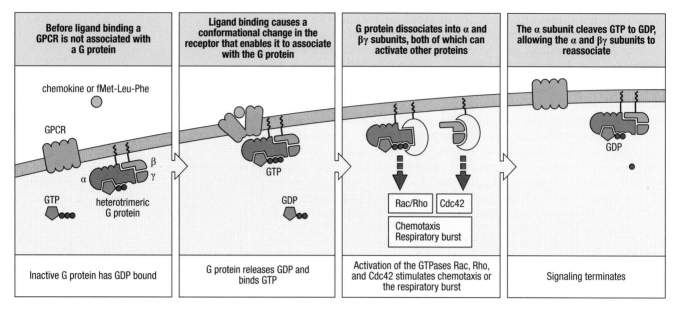

Before ligand binding a GPCR is not associated with a G protein	Ligand binding causes a conformational change in the receptor that enables it to associate with the G protein	G protein dissociates into α and βγ subunits, both of which can activate other proteins	The α subunit cleaves GTP to GDP, allowing the α and βγ subunits to reassociate
Inactive G protein has GDP bound	G protein releases GDP and binds GTP	Activation of the GTPases Rac, Rho, and Cdc42 stimulates chemotaxis or the respiratory burst	Signaling terminates

Fig. 3.3 G protein–coupled receptors signal by coupling with intracellular heterotrimeric G proteins. First panel: G protein–coupled receptors (GPCRs) such as the fMet-Leu-Phe (fMLF) and chemokine receptors signal through GTP-binding proteins known as heterotrimeric G proteins. In the inactive state, the α subunit of the G protein binds GDP and is associated with the β and γ subunits. Second panel: The binding of a ligand to the receptor induces a conformational change that allows the receptor to interact with the G protein, which results in the displacement of GDP and binding of GTP by the α subunit. Third panel: GTP binding triggers the dissociation of the G protein into the α subunit and the βγ subunit, each of which can activate other proteins at the inner face of the cell membrane. In the case of fMLF signaling in macrophages and neutrophils, the α subunit of the activated G protein indirectly activates the GTPases Rac and Rho, whereas the βγ subunit indirectly activates the GTPase Cdc42. The actions of these proteins result in the assembly of NADPH oxidase, resulting in a respiratory burst, a brief spurt in oxygen consumption leading to the production of reactive oxygen species. Chemokine signaling acts by a similar pathway and activates chemotaxis, which is the process whereby a cell migrates toward the source of chemokine. Fourth panel: The activated response ceases when the intrinsic GTPase activity of the α subunit hydrolyzes GTP to GDP, and the α and βγ subunits reassociate. The intrinsic rate of GTP hydrolysis by α subunits is relatively slow, and signaling is regulated by additional GTPase-activating proteins (not shown), which accelerate the rate of GTP hydrolysis.

G proteins, sometimes referred to as **heterotrimeric G proteins** to distinguish them from the family of 'small' GTPases typified by Ras. Heterotrimeric G proteins are composed of three subunits: Gα, Gβ, and Gγ, of which the α subunit is similar to the small GTPases (**Fig. 3.3**). In the resting state, the G protein is inactive, not associated with the receptor, and a molecule of GDP is bound to the α subunit. Ligand binding induces conformational changes in the receptor that allow it to bind the G protein, which results in the displacement of the GDP from the G protein and its replacement with GTP. The active G protein dissociates into two components, the Gα subunit and a complex consisting of a Gβ and a Gγ subunit. Each of these components can interact with other intracellular signaling molecules to transmit and amplify the signal. G proteins can activate a wide variety of downstream enzymatic targets, such as adenylate cyclase, which produces the second messenger cyclic AMP, and phospholipase C, whose activation gives rise to the second messenger inositol 1,4,5-trisphosphate (IP_3) and the release of Ca^{2+} from stores in the endoplasmic reticulum. The subsequent increase in cytosolic Ca^{2+} can induce several signaling pathways, including the activation of protein kinase C (PKC) (see Chapter 7 for a more detailed discussion of these and other signaling pathways).

Signaling by fMLF and C5a receptors influences cell motility, metabolism, gene expression, and cell division through activation of several **Rho family small GTPase proteins**. The α subunit of the activated G protein indirectly activates **Rac** and **Rho**, while the βγ subunit indirectly activates the small GTPase Cdc42 (see Fig. 3.3). Activation of these GTPases is controlled by **guanine nucleotide exchange factors (GEFs)** (see Fig. 7.5), which exchange GTP for GDP bound to the GTPase. The G proteins activated by fMLF activate the GEF protein **PREX1** (phosphatidylinositol 3,4,5-trisphosphate–dependent

Antimicrobial mechanisms of phagocytes		
Class of mechanism	**Macrophage products**	**Neutrophil products**
Acidification	pH ≈ 3.5–4.0, bacteriostatic or bactericidal	
Toxic oxygen–derived products	Superoxide O_2^-, hydrogen peroxide H_2O_2, singlet oxygen $^1O_2^{\bullet}$, hydroxyl radical $^{\bullet}OH$, hypochlorite OCl^-	
Toxic nitrogen oxides	Nitric oxide NO	
Antimicrobial peptides	Cathelicidin, macrophage elastase–derived peptide	α-Defensins (HNP1–4), β-defensin HBD4, cathelicidin, azurocidin, bacterial permeability inducing protein (BPI), lactoferricin
Enzymes	Lysozyme: digests cell walls of some Gram-positive bacteria Acid hydrolases (e.g., elastase and other proteases): break down ingested microbes	
Competitors		Lactoferrin (sequesters Fe^{2+}), vitamin B_{12}–binding protein

Fig. 3.4 Bactericidal agents produced or released by phagocytes after uptake of microorganisms. Most of the agents listed are directly toxic to microbes and can act directly in the phagolysosome. They can also be secreted into the extracellular environment, and many of these substances are toxic to host cells. Other phagocyte products sequester essential nutrients in the extracellular environment, rendering them inaccessible to microbes and hindering microbial growth. Besides being directly bacteriostatic or bactericidal, acidification of lysosomes also activates the many acid hydrolases that degrade the contents of the vacuole.

Rac exchanger 1 protein), which can directly activate Rac. Other GEFs, including members of the Vav family that are controlled by other types of receptors (see Section 7-19), can also activate Rac activity, and their activity synergizes with the actions of fMLF and C5a.

The activation of Rac and Rho helps to increase the microbicidal capacity of macrophages and neutrophils that have ingested pathogens. Upon phagocytosing microbes, macrophages and neutrophils produce a variety of toxic products that help to kill the engulfed microorganism (**Fig. 3.4**). The most important of these are the antimicrobial peptides described in Section 2-4, reactive nitrogen species such as nitric oxide (NO), and ROS such as the superoxide anion (O_2^-) and hydrogen peroxide (H_2O_2). Nitric oxide is produced by a high-output form of nitric oxide synthase, inducible NOS2 (iNOS2), whose expression is induced by a variety of stimuli, including fMLF.

Activation of phagocytic receptors, including the fMLF and C5a receptors, can promote ROS generation by inducing assembly of a multicomponent, membrane-associated **NADPH oxidase**, also called **phagocyte oxidase**. In unstimulated phagocytes, this enzyme is inactive because it is not fully assembled. One set of subunits, the cytochrome b_{558} complex (composed of p22 and gp91), is localized in the plasma membranes of resting macrophages and neutrophils, and it appears in lysosomes after the maturation of phagolysosomes. The other components, p40, p47, and p67, are in the cytosol. Activation of phagocytes induces the cytosolic subunits to join with the membrane-associated cytochrome b_{558} to form a complete, functional NADPH oxidase in the phagolysosome membrane (**Fig. 3.5**). Activation of Rac promotes the movement of the cytosolic components to the membrane to assemble the active NADPH oxidase. Phosphorylation of certain residues of the NADPH oxidase complex also plays a critical role in activation and is mediated by PKC activation downstream of GPCRs. PKC activation can also occur downstream of phagocytic receptors, such as Dectin-1 and Fc receptors, which contain **immunoreceptor tyrosine-based activation motifs (ITAMs)** in their cytosolic tails. The signaling mediated by ITAMs is discussed in greater detail later in this chapter (Section 3-26) as well as in later chapters.

The NADPH oxidase reaction results in a transient increase in oxygen consumption by the cell, which is known as the **respiratory burst**. It generates superoxide anion within the lumen of the phagolysosome, and this is converted

Fig. 3.5 The microbicidal respiratory burst in phagocytes is initiated by activation-induced assembly of the phagocyte NADPH oxidase. First panel: Neutrophils are highly specialized for the uptake and killing of pathogens and contain several different kinds of cytoplasmic granules, such as the primary and secondary granules shown in the first panel. These granules contain antimicrobial peptides and enzymes. Second panel: In resting neutrophils, the cytochrome b_{558} subunits (gp91 and p22) of NADPH oxidase are localized in the plasma membrane; the other oxidase components (p40, p47, and p67) are located in the cytosol. Signaling by phagocytic receptors and by fMLF or C5a receptors synergizes to activate Rac and induce the assembly of the complete, active NADPH oxidase in the membrane of the phagolysosome, which has formed by the fusion of the phagosome with lysosomes and primary and secondary granules. Third panel: Active NADPH oxidase transfers electrons from NADPH to molecular oxygen, forming the superoxide ion O_2^- (blue) and other free oxygen radicals in the lumen of the phagolysosome. Potassium and hydrogen ions are then drawn into the phagolysosome to neutralize the charged superoxide ion, increasing acidification of the vesicle. Acidification dissociates granule enzymes such as cathepsin G and elastase (yellow) from their proteoglycan matrix, leading to their cleavage and activation by lysosomal proteases. O_2^- is converted by superoxide dismutase (SOD) to hydrogen peroxide (H_2O_2), which can kill microorganisms and can be converted by myeloperoxidase, a heme-containing enzyme, to microbicidal hypochlorite (OCl^-) and by chemical reaction with ferrous (Fe^{2+}) ions to the hydroxyl radical ($^{\bullet}OH$).

by the enzyme **superoxide dismutase (SOD)** into H_2O_2. Further chemical and enzymatic reactions produce a range of toxic ROS from H_2O_2, including the hydroxyl radical ($^{\bullet}OH$), hypochlorite (OCl^-), and hypobromite (OBr^-). In this way, the direct recognition of bacterially derived polypeptides or previous pathogen recognition by the complement system activates a potent killing mechanism within macrophages and neutrophils that have ingested microbes via their phagocytic receptors. However, phagocyte activation can also cause extensive tissue damage because hydrolytic enzymes, membrane-disrupting peptides, and reactive oxygen species can be released into the extracellular environment and are toxic to host cells.

Neutrophils use the respiratory burst described above in their role as an early responder to infection. Neutrophils are not tissue-resident cells, and they need to be recruited to a site of infection from the bloodstream. Their main function is to ingest and kill microorganisms, but they also produce cytokines and lipid mediators that promote and orchestrate the inflammatory response. Although neutrophils are eventually present in much larger numbers than macrophages in some types of acute infection, they are short-lived, dying soon after they have accomplished a round of phagocytosis and used up their primary and secondary granules. Dead and dying neutrophils are a major component of the **pus** that forms in abscesses and in wounds infected by certain extracellular capsulated bacteria such as streptococci and staphylococci, which are thus known as **pus-forming, or pyogenic, bacteria**. Macrophages, in contrast, are long-lived cells and continue to generate new lysosomes.

Individuals with a disease called **chronic granulomatous disease (CGD)** have a genetic deficiency of NADPH oxidase, which means their phagocytes do not produce the toxic oxygen derivatives characteristic of the respiratory burst and so are less able to kill ingested microorganisms and clear an infection. The most common form of CGD is an X-linked heritable disease that arises from inactivating mutations in the gene encoding the gp91 subunit of cytochrome b_{558}. People with this defect are unusually susceptible to bacterial and fungal infections, especially in infancy, though they remain susceptible for life. One autosomal recessive form of NADPH oxidase deficiency, p47phox deficiency, has very low but detectable activity and causes a milder form of CGD.

 Chronic Granulomatous Disease

In addition to killing microbes engulfed by phagocytosis, neutrophils use another rather novel mechanism of destruction that is directed at extracellular pathogens. During infection, some activated neutrophils undergo a unique form of cell death in which the nuclear chromatin, rather than being degraded as occurs during apoptosis, is released into the extracellular space and forms a fibril matrix known as **neutrophil extracellular traps, or NETs (Fig. 3.6)**. It has been proposed that NETs act to capture microorganisms, which may then be more efficiently phagocytosed by other neutrophils or macrophages, but the importance of this mechanism during infection remains rather unclear.

 ANIMATION 3.4

Macrophages can phagocytose pathogens and produce the respiratory burst immediately upon encountering an infecting microorganism, and this can be sufficient to prevent an infection from becoming established. In the 19th century, the immunologist Élie Metchnikoff believed that the innate response of macrophages encompassed all host defenses; indeed, invertebrates such as the sea star that he was studying rely entirely on innate immunity to overcome infection. Although this is not the case in humans and other vertebrates, the innate response of macrophages still provides an important front line of defense that must be overcome if a microorganism is to establish an infection that can be passed on to a new host.

Pathogens have, however, developed a variety of strategies to avoid immediate destruction by macrophages and neutrophils. Many extracellular pathogenic bacteria coat themselves with a thick polysaccharide capsule that is not recognized by any phagocytic receptor. In such cases, however, the complement system can recognize microbial surfaces and coat them with C3b, thereby flagging them for phagocytosis via complement receptors, as described in Chapter 2. Other pathogens, for example, mycobacteria, have evolved ways to grow inside macrophage phagosomes by inhibiting their acidification and fusion with lysosomes. Without such strategies, a microorganism must enter the body in sufficient numbers to overwhelm the immediate innate host defenses and to establish a focus of infection.

3-3 Microbial recognition and tissue damage initiate an inflammatory response.

An important effect of the interaction between microbes and tissue macrophages is the activation of macrophages and other immune cells to release small proteins called **cytokines** and **chemokines**, and other chemical mediators, such as lipid mediators. Collectively, these signals induce a state of

Fig. 3.6 Neutrophil extracellular traps (NETs) can trap bacteria and fungi. This scanning electron micrograph of activated human neutrophils infected with a virulent strain of *Shigella flexneri* (pink rods) shows the stimulated neutrophils forming NETs (blue, indicated by arrows). Bacteria trapped within NETs are visible (lower arrow).

| Cytokines and lipid mediators produced by macrophages cause dilation of local small blood vessels | Leukocytes move to periphery of blood vessel as a result of increased expression of adhesion molecules by endothelium | Leukocytes extravasate at site of infection | Blood clotting occurs in the microvessels |

Fig. 3.7 Infection stimulates macrophages to release cytokines and chemokines that initiate an inflammatory response. Cytokines and lipid mediators produced by tissue macrophages at the site of infection cause the dilation of local small blood vessels and changes in the endothelial cells of their walls. These changes lead to the movement of leukocytes, such as neutrophils and monocytes, out of the blood vessel (extravasation) and into the infected tissue; this movement is guided by chemokines produced by the activated macrophages. The blood vessels also become more permeable, allowing plasma proteins and fluid to leak into the tissues. Together, these changes cause the characteristic inflammatory signs of heat, pain, redness, and swelling at the site of infection.

inflammation in the tissue, attract monocytes and neutrophils to the infection, and allow plasma proteins to enter the tissue from the blood. An inflammatory response is usually initiated within minutes to hours of infection or wounding. Macrophages are stimulated to secrete **pro-inflammatory** cytokines, such as TNF-α, and chemokines by interactions between microbes or microbial products and specific receptors expressed by macrophages. We will examine how the cytokines interact with pathogens later in the chapter, but first we describe some general aspects of inflammation and how it contributes to host defense.

Inflammation has three essential roles in combating infection. The first is to deliver additional effector molecules and cells from the blood into sites of infection, and so increase the destruction of invading microorganisms. The second is to induce local blood clotting, which provides a physical barrier to the spread of the infection in the bloodstream. The third is to promote the repair of injured tissue, which occurs during the resolution phase, after the infection has been cleared.

Inflammatory responses are characterized by heat, pain, redness, and swelling at the site of an infection, reflecting four types of change in the local blood vessels, as shown in **Fig. 3.7**. The first is an increase in vascular diameter, leading to increased local blood flow—hence the heat and redness—and a reduction in the velocity of blood flow, especially along the inner walls of small blood vessels. The second change is the activation of endothelial cells lining the blood vessel to express **cell-adhesion molecules** that promote the binding of circulating leukocytes. The combination of slowed blood flow and adhesion molecules allows leukocytes to attach to the endothelium and migrate into the tissues, a process known as **extravasation**. All these changes are initiated by the pro-inflammatory cytokines and chemokines produced by activated macrophages and other cells in the tissue.

Once inflammation has begun, the first white blood cells attracted to the site are neutrophils. These are followed by monocytes (**Fig. 3.8**), which upon activation are called **inflammatory monocytes**. Monocytes can produce various pro-inflammatory cytokines but are distinguishable from macrophages by their lack of expression of the adhesion G protein–coupled receptor E1, commonly called F4/80. Monocytes are also able to give rise to dendritic cells in the tissues, depending on signals that they receive from their environment. In the later stages of inflammation, other leukocytes such as eosinophils and lymphocytes also enter the infected site.

The third major change in local blood vessels is an increase in vascular permeability. Thus, instead of being tightly joined together, the endothelial cells lining the blood vessel walls become separated, leading to an exit of fluid and proteins from the blood and their local accumulation in the tissue. This accounts for the swelling, or **edema**, and pain—as well as the accumulation

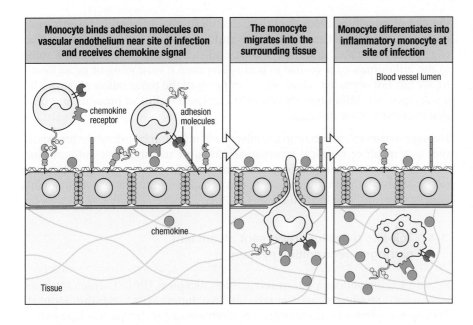

| Monocyte binds adhesion molecules on vascular endothelium near site of infection and receives chemokine signal | The monocyte migrates into the surrounding tissue | Monocyte differentiates into inflammatory monocyte at site of infection |

chemokine receptor

adhesion molecules

Blood vessel lumen

chemokine

Tissue

Fig. 3.8 Monocytes circulating in the blood migrate into infected and inflamed tissues. Adhesion molecules on the endothelial cells of the blood vessel wall capture the monocyte and cause it to adhere to the vascular endothelium. Chemokines bound to the vascular endothelium then signal the monocyte to migrate across the endothelium into the underlying tissue. The monocyte, now differentiating into an inflammatory monocyte, continues to migrate, under the influence of chemokines released during inflammatory responses, toward the site of infection. Monocytes leaving the blood are also able to differentiate into dendritic cells (not shown), depending on the signals that they receive from their environment.

in tissues of plasma proteins such as complement and mannose-binding lectin (MBL) that aid in host defense. The changes that occur in endothelium as a result of inflammation are known generally as **endothelial activation**. The fourth change, clotting in microvessels in the site of infection, prevents the spread of the pathogen via the blood.

These changes are induced by a variety of inflammatory mediators released as a consequence of the recognition of pathogens by macrophages, and later by neutrophils and other white blood cells. Macrophages and neutrophils secrete lipid mediators of inflammation—**prostaglandins**, **leukotrienes**, and **platelet-activating factor (PAF)**—which are rapidly produced by enzymatic pathways that degrade membrane phospholipids. Their actions are followed by those of the chemokines and cytokines that are synthesized and secreted by macrophages and inflammatory monocytes in response to pathogens. The cytokine **tumor necrosis factor-α (TNF-α, also known simply as TNF)**, for example, is a potent activator of endothelial cells. We describe TNF-α and related cytokines in more detail in Section 3-15.

Besides stimulating the respiratory burst in phagocytes and acting as a chemoattractant for neutrophils and monocytes, C5a also promotes inflammation by increasing vascular permeability and inducing the expression of certain adhesion molecules on endothelium. C5a also activates local **mast cells** (see Section 1-4), which are stimulated to release their granules containing the small inflammatory molecule histamine as well as TNF-α and cathelicidins.

If wounding has occurred, the injury to blood vessels immediately triggers two protective enzyme cascades. One is the **kinin system** of plasma proteases that is triggered by tissue damage to generate several polypeptides that regulate blood pressure, coagulation, and pain. Although we will not fully describe its components here, one inflammatory mediator produced is the vasoactive peptide **bradykinin**, which increases vascular permeability to promote the influx of plasma proteins to the site of tissue injury. It also causes pain. Although unpleasant to the victim, pain draws attention to the problem and leads to immobilization of the affected part of the body, which helps to limit the spread of the infection.

The **coagulation system** is another protease cascade that is triggered in the blood after damage to blood vessels, although its full description is also outside our present scope. Its activation leads to the formation of a fibrin clot, whose normal role is to prevent blood loss. With regard to innate immunity, however,

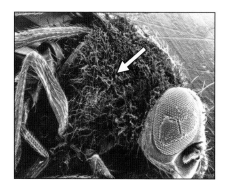

Fig. 3.9 Toll is required for antifungal responses in Drosophila *melanogaster*. Flies that are deficient in the Toll receptor are dramatically more susceptible than wild-type flies to fungal infection. This is illustrated here by the uncontrolled hyphal growth (arrow) of the normally weak pathogen *Aspergillus fumigatus* in a Toll-deficient fly.

ANIMATION 3.5

the clot physically encases the infectious microorganisms and prevents their entry into the bloodstream. The kinin and the coagulation cascades are also triggered by activated endothelial cells, and so they can have important roles in the inflammatory response to pathogens even if wounding or gross tissue injury has not occurred. Thus, within minutes of the penetration of tissues by a pathogen, the inflammatory response causes an influx of proteins and cells that may control the infection.

Damage to tissues can occur in the absence of infection by microbes; for example, as a result of physical trauma, ischemia, or metabolic or autoimmune disorders. In such **sterile injury**, many of the changes associated with infection, such as neutrophil recruitment, can occur, in addition to activation of the kinin system and clot formation.

3-4 Toll-like receptors represent an ancient pathogen-recognition system.

Section 1-5 introduced pattern-recognition receptors (PRRs), which function as sensors for pathogen-associated molecular patterns (PAMPs). The existence of these receptors was predicted by Charles Janeway, Jr., before mechanisms of innate recognition of PAMPs were known, to explain how complex mixtures of microbial molecules, called adjuvants, were able to stimulate adaptive immune responses to purified antigens. The first example of such a receptor was the **Toll** protein, discovered in the fruit fly *Drosophila melanogaster*. Although Toll was identified earlier as a gene controlling the dorso-ventral patterning during development of *Drosophila*, in 1996 Jules Hoffmann discovered that Toll signaling induces the expression of several host-defense mechanisms. The importance of this mechanism was illustrated by the decreased production of antimicrobial peptides and the enhanced susceptibility to infection of adult flies with mutations in the Toll pathway (**Fig 3.9**). For this work, Hoffmann was awarded part of the 2011 Nobel Prize in Physiology or Medicine.

In 1997, Janeway and Ruslan Medzhitov discovered a human homolog of Toll, subsequently termed **Toll-like receptor (TLR)**, and showed that signaling by this receptor activates innate and adaptive immune responses. Subsequently, numerous TLRs associated with resistance to infection by pathogens have been found in humans and other animals. In plants, proteins with domains resembling the ligand-binding regions of TLR proteins are involved in the production of antimicrobial peptides, indicating the ancient association of these domains with host defense.

3-5 Mammalian Toll-like receptors are activated by many different pathogen-associated molecular patterns.

There are 10 expressed TLR genes in humans and 12 in mice. Each TLR recognizes one or more distinct molecular 'patterns' present on microbes, which are referred to as pathogen-associated molecular patterns (PAMPs), as discussed at the beginning of this chapter. These molecules are general components of both pathogenic and nonpathogenic microorganisms and are sometimes called microbial-associated molecular patterns, or MAMPs, to reflect this fact. Collectively, the mammalian TLRs recognize molecules from bacteria, fungi, viruses, and protozoa. The mammalian TLRs and their known microbial ligands are listed in **Fig. 3.10**. Note that in almost all cases the ligands represent highly conserved features that are characteristic of these microbial groups. For example, **lipoteichoic acids** of Gram-positive bacterial cell walls and **lipopolysaccharide (LPS)** of the outer membrane of Gram-negative bacteria (see Fig. 2.9) are recognized by TLRs. In general, these microbial molecules are not found in vertebrate cells, which prevents inappropriate immune recognition of host cells. The major exceptions to this

Innate immune recognition by mammalian Toll-like receptors	
Toll-like receptor	**Ligand**
TLR-1:TLR-2 heterodimer	Lipomannans (mycobacteria) Diacyl and triacyl lipopeptides (bacteria)
TLR-2:TLR-6 heterodimer	Lipoteichoic acids (Gram-positive bacteria) Cell-wall β-glucans (fungi)
TLR-3	Double-stranded RNA (viruses), poly I:C
TLR-4	LPS (Gram-negative bacteria)
TLR-5	Flagellin (bacteria)
TLR-7	Single-stranded RNA (viruses)
TLR-8	Single-stranded RNA (viruses)
TLR-9	DNA with unmethylated CpG (bacteria and DNA viruses)
TLR-10 (human only)	Unknown
TLR-11 (mouse only)	Profilin and profilin-like proteins (*Toxoplasma gondii*, uropathogenic bacteria)
TLR-12 (mouse only)	Profilin (*Toxoplasma gondii*)
TLR-13 (mouse only)	Single-stranded RNA (bacterial ribosomal RNA)

Fig. 3.10 Innate immune recognition by Toll-like receptors. Each of the human or mouse TLRs recognizes one or more microbial molecular patterns, generally by direct interaction with molecules on the pathogen surface. Some Toll-like receptor proteins form heterodimers (for example, TLR-1:TLR-2 and TLR-2:TLR-6). LPS, lipopolysaccharide.

rule, however, are the DNA and RNA ligands for certain TLRs. As discussed later in this section, additional mechanisms are used to distinguish between microbial and host DNA and RNA.

TLRs are sensors for microbes present in extracellular spaces. Some mammalian TLRs are cell-surface receptors, but others are located intracellularly in the membranes of endosomes, where they detect pathogens or their components that have been taken into cells by phagocytosis, receptor-mediated endocytosis, or macropinocytosis (**Fig. 3.11**). TLRs localized to the plasma membrane

Fig. 3.11 The cellular locations of the mammalian Toll-like receptors. TLRs are transmembrane proteins where the extracellular region of the monomer contains 18–25 copies of the leucine-rich repeat (LRR), but these diagrams depict only 9 LRRs in each monomer for simplicity. Some TLRs are located on the cell surface of dendritic cells, macrophages, and other cells, where they are able to detect extracellular pathogen molecules. TLRs are thought to act as dimers. Only those that form heterodimers are shown in dimeric form here; the rest act as homodimers but are shown as monomers for simplicity. TLRs located intracellularly, in the membranes of endosomes, can recognize microbial components, such as DNA or RNA, that are accessible only after the microbe has been broken down. The ectodomains of TLR-3, TLR-7, TLR-8, and TLR-9 undergo proteolytic cleavage once they reach the endosome. This cleavage is required for their function and is thought to prevent responses to self nucleic acids in the extracellular space (see text for further discussion). TLR-11, TLR-12, and TLR-13 (also localized to endosomes) are not shown.

can also be incorporated into phagosomes, which further enables detection of phagocytosed microbes. TLRs are transmembrane proteins in which the extracellular region of the monomer is composed of 18–25 copies of a **leucine-rich repeat (LRR)**. Each LRR of a TLR protein is composed of approximately 20–25 amino acids, and multiple LRRs create a horseshoe-shaped protein scaffold that is adaptable for ligand binding and recognition on both the outer (convex) and inner (concave) surfaces. Signaling by mammalian TLRs is activated when binding of a ligand induces formation of a dimer or induces conformational changes in a preformed TLR dimer. All mammalian TLR proteins have in their cytoplasmic tails a **TIR (for Toll–IL-1 receptor) domain**, which is also found in the cytoplasmic tail of the receptor for the cytokines interleukin-1α (**IL-1α**) and interleukin-1β (**IL-1β**). The TLR TIR domains mediate interaction with other TIR domain–containing signaling molecules, discussed in greater detail in Section 3-7. For years after the discovery of the mammalian TLRs it was not known whether they made direct contact with microbial products or whether they sensed the presence of microbes by some indirect means. *Drosophila* Toll, for example, does not recognize pathogen products directly, but instead is activated when it binds a cleaved version of a self protein, Spätzle. *Drosophila* has other direct pathogen-recognition molecules, and these trigger the proteolytic cascade that ends in the cleavage of Spätzle. In this sense, Toll is not a classical pattern-recognition receptor. However, X-ray crystal structures of several mammalian dimeric TLRs bound to their ligands show that mammalian TLRs make direct contact with microbial ligands.

TLRs are expressed on many cell types, including macrophages, dendritic cells, B cells, stromal cells, and certain epithelial cells, enabling the initiation of antimicrobial responses in many tissues. Mammalian **TLR-1**, **TLR-2**, and **TLR-6** are cell-surface receptors that are activated by various ligands, including lipoteichoic acid from Gram-positive bacteria and **diacyl** and **triacyl lipoproteins** present in both Gram-positive and Gram-negative bacteria. Ligand binding induces the formation of heterodimers of TLR-2 and TLR-1 or of TLR-2 and TLR-6. The X-ray crystal structure of a synthetic triacyl lipopeptide ligand bound to TLR-1 and TLR-2 shows exactly how ligand binding induces dimerization (**Fig. 3.12**). Two of the three lipid chains bind to the convex surface of TLR-2, while the third binds to the convex surface of TLR-1. Dimerization brings the cytoplasmic TIR domains of the TLR chains into close proximity with each other to initiate signaling. Similar interactions are presumed to occur with the diacyl lipopeptide ligands that induce the dimerization of TLR-2 and TLR-6.

TLR-5 is expressed on the cell surface of certain macrophages and dendritic cells and also in intestinal epithelial cells; it recognizes flagellin, a protein subunit of bacterial flagella. TLR-5 recognizes a highly conserved site on flagellin

Fig. 3.12 Direct recognition of pathogen-associated molecular patterns by TLR-1 and TLR-2 induces dimerization of the TLRs and signaling. TLR-1 and TLR-2 are located on cell surfaces (left panel), where they can directly recognize bacterial triacyl lipoproteins (middle panel). The convex surfaces of their extracellular domains have binding sites for the lipid side chains of triacyl lipopeptides. In the crystal structure (right panel), the ligand is a synthetic lipid that can activate TLR-1:TLR-2 dimers; it has three fatty-acid chains bound to a polypeptide backbone. Two fatty-acid chains bind to a pocket on the convex surface of the TLR-2 ectodomain, and the third chain associates with a hydrophobic channel in the convex binding surface of TLR-1, inducing dimerization of the two TLR subunits and bringing their cytoplasmic Toll–IL-1 receptor (TIR) domains together to initiate signaling.

that is buried and inaccessible in the assembled flagellar filament. This means the receptor is activated only by monomeric flagellin, which can be shed during flagellar assembly or when flagella are degraded.

Mice, but not humans, express **TLR-11** and **TLR-12**. TLR-11–deficient mice develop urinary infections caused by uropathogenic strains of *Escherichia coli*, although the bacterial ligand for TLR-11 has not yet been identified. TLR-11 and TLR-12 also both recognize protozoan parasites such as *Toxoplasma gondii* and *Plasmodium falciparum*. They bind to motifs that are present in the protozoan actin-binding protein **profilin** but absent in mammalian profilins. TLR-11 and TLR-12 are both required in macrophages and conventional dendritic cells for activation by *T. gondii* profilin, but TLR-12 plays a more dominant role. Mice lacking TLR-11 develop more severe tissue injury than normal mice on infection with *Toxoplasma*, whereas mice lacking TLR-12 die rapidly after infection.

Five of the mammalian TLRs (TLR3, TLR7, TLR8, TLR9, and TLR13) recognize nucleic acids. These receptors are all localized to endosomes. The endosome lumen is acidic and contains many proteases, which degrade internalized microbes and release their nucleic acids for recognition by TLRs. All microbes possess some form of nucleic acid and so can be recognized by one or more of the nucleic acid–sensing TLRs; however, analysis of mice and humans with defects in one or more of these TLRs indicates that these receptors are most important for detection of viruses. In general, viruses lack other conserved features that could serve as PAMPs.

TLR-7 and **TLR-8** share very similar amino acid sequences, and both receptors are activated by degradation products of **single-stranded RNA (ssRNA)**. Many viruses (for example, orthomyxoviruses such as influenza; flaviviruses such as West Nile virus; and coronaviruses such as SARS-CoV-2) utilize ssRNA genomes, and TLR-7 and TLR-8 bind to small RNA fragments released when viruses are degraded in endosomes. Recent X-ray crystal structures of TLR-7 and TLR-8 have revealed two pairs of binding sites for distinct RNA fragments: guanosine and a short RNA fragment bind TLR-7, while uridine and a short RNA fragment bind TLR-8. Whether differences in the RNA sequences that activate TLR-7 and TLR-8 have consequences for antiviral immunity remains unclear. In mice, TLR-7 plays a dominant role over TLR-8 for detection of ssRNA viruses. For example, mice lacking TLR-7 have impaired immune responses to influenza. A viral detection function for TLR-8 in mice has not been established as clearly. The difference between mice and humans may be based, at least in part, on which cell types express the receptors in each species. In mice, TLR-7 is expressed broadly in many innate immune cell types, but in humans TLR-7 expression is limited to plasmacytoid dendritic cells and B cells, while TLR-8 is expressed more broadly. **TLR-13** also binds RNA but has specificity for certain bacterial ribosomal RNA sequences instead of viral RNA. TLR-13 is present in mice but not humans.

TLR-9 recognizes single-stranded DNA sequences that contain **unmethylated CpG dinucleotides**. In mammals, CpG dinucleotides in genomic DNA are often methylated on the cytosine by DNA methyltransferases. In the genomes of bacteria and many viruses, CpG dinucleotides remain unmethylated, so these sequences serve as ligands for TLR-9. The requirement for unmethylated CpG sequences is thought to limit the potential for recognition of self DNA by TLR-9. The structure of the TLR-9 dimer bound to DNA reveals a ligand-binding modality similar to what was previously described for TLR-7 and TLR-8: two pairs of binding sites within the dimer bind distinct DNA sequences. While the DNA genomes of viruses and bacteria are typically double-stranded, TLR-9 recognizes single-stranded DNA, so the DNA strands of pathogen genomes must be melted apart within endosomes prior to TLR-9 binding.

TLR-3 is expressed by macrophages, conventional dendritic cells, and intestinal epithelial cells; it recognizes **double-stranded RNA (dsRNA)**. Some viruses have genomes composed of dsRNA, but dsRNA is also generated when ssRNA viruses replicate or express genes. dsRNA can be recognized by TLR-3 after direct endocytosis of viruses with double-stranded RNA genomes, such as rotavirus, or by the phagocytosis of dying cells in which viruses are replicating. Crystallographic analysis shows that TLR-3 binds directly to dsRNA. TLR-3 has two contact sites for dsRNA: one on the amino terminus and a second near the membrane-proximal carboxyl terminus. Mutations in the ectodomain of human TLR-3, which produce a dominantly acting loss-of-function mutant receptor, have been associated with encephalitis that is caused by a failure to control the herpes simplex virus. This increased susceptibility is somewhat surprising because herpes simplex virus is a DNA virus; the most likely explanation for sensing by TLR-3 is generation of dsRNA after transcription of overlapping viral genes encoded on opposing strands of DNA.

To reach endosomes, TLR-3, TLR-7, TLR-8, TLR-9, TLR-11, TLR-12, and TLR-13 must interact with a specific protein, **UNC93B1**. UNC93B1, which is composed of 12 transmembrane domains, binds TLRs in the endoplasmic reticulum and shuttles them to endosomes. Mice lacking this protein have defects in signaling by these endosomal TLRs because the receptors cannot exit the endoplasmic reticulum. Rare human mutations in UNC93B1 have been identified as causing susceptibility to herpes simplex encephalitis, similarly to TLR-3 deficiency, but they do not impair immunity to many other viral pathogens, presumably because of the existence of other viral sensors, which are discussed later in this chapter.

Recurrent Herpes Simplex Encephalitis

Sensing of nucleic acids enables broad recognition of diverse pathogens, but, in abnormal settings, TLRs may be activated by self-derived nucleic acids, leading to autoimmunity. In healthy cells, RNA and DNA are normally confined to the nucleus and cytoplasm and are not present in endosomes; however, nucleic acids can be released into the extracellular space during tissue damage or inflammation (for example, NETs). The localization of nucleic acid–sensing TLRs to endosomes reduces the likelihood that these receptors encounter such extracellular RNA and DNA. RNases and DNases in the extracellular space degrade RNA and DNA before they are taken up by endocytosis and delivered to TLRs. Another mechanism that limits TLR activation to endosomes is that the ectodomains of each of the nucleic acid–sensing TLRs must undergo proteolytic cleavage before the receptors can be activated; this cleavage occurs when TLRs arrive in endosomes, which prevents receptors from responding to ligands in other subcellular compartments, such as the cell surface (see Fig. 3.11). The two halves of the cleaved TLR remain associated and both contribute to ligand binding. Without this proteolytic event, the receptor cannot undergo the necessary conformational change required to initiate signaling.

In mouse models of systemic lupus erythematosus (SLE), an autoimmune disease associated with responses to self nucleic acids, TLR-7 and TLR-9 both contribute to disease. Several studies have identified polymorphisms in the human TLR-7 gene that are associated with increased risk of SLE, suggesting a potential role in this disease.

3-6 TLR-4 recognizes bacterial lipopolysaccharide in association with the host accessory proteins MD-2 and CD14.

Not all mammalian TLRs bind their ligands so directly. **TLR-4** is expressed by several types of immune-system cells, including dendritic cells and macrophages, and is important in sensing and responding to numerous bacterial infections. TLR-4 recognizes the LPS of Gram-negative bacteria by a mechanism that is partly direct and partly indirect. LPS varies in composition among different bacteria but essentially consists of a polysaccharide core attached to an amphipathic lipid, lipid A, with a variable number of fatty-acid chains per

| LPS has multiple fatty-acyl chains linked to a glycan head. Five acyl chains can bind to a pocket within MD-2, but one acyl chain is free | The free acyl chain of an LPS molecule then binds to the outer convex surface of another TLR-4 molecule, inducing a dimer |

Fig. 3.13 TLR-4 recognizes LPS in association with the accessory protein MD-2. A side view of the symmetrical complex of TLR-4, MD-2, and LPS. TLR-4 polypeptide backbones are shown in green and purple. The MD-2 protein is shown in light blue. Five of the LPS acyl chains (shown in red) are inserted into a hydrophobic pocket within MD-2. The remainder of the LPS glycan (orange in the crystal structure) and one lipid chain make contact with the convex surface of a second TLR-4 monomer. The crystal structure shows the entire extracellular region of TLR-4, composed of the LRR region (shown in green and purple), but lacks the intracellular signaling domains.

molecule. To recognize LPS, the ectodomain of TLR-4 uses an accessory protein, **MD-2**. MD-2 initially binds to TLR-4 within the cell and is necessary both for the correct trafficking of TLR-4 to the cell surface and for the recognition of LPS. MD-2 associates with the central section of the curved ectodomain of TLR-4, binding off to one side as shown in **Fig. 3.13**. When the TLR-4:MD-2 complex encounters LPS, five lipid chains of LPS bind to a deep hydrophobic pocket of MD-2, but not directly to TLR-4, while a sixth lipid chain remains exposed on the surface of MD-2. This last lipid chain and parts of the LPS polysaccharide backbone can then bind to the convex side of a second TLR-4 ectodomain, inducing TLR-4 dimerization, which activates intracellular signaling pathways.

TLR-4 activation by LPS involves two other accessory proteins besides MD-2. While LPS is normally an integral component of the outer membrane of Gram-negative bacteria, during infections it can become detached from the membrane and be picked up by the host **LPS-binding protein** present in the blood and in extracellular fluid in tissues. LPS is transferred from LPS-binding protein to a second protein, CD14, which is present on the surface of macrophages, neutrophils, and dendritic cells. On its own, CD14 can act as a phagocytic receptor, but on macrophages and dendritic cells it also acts as an accessory protein for TLR-4.

The systemic injection of LPS causes a collapse of the circulatory and respiratory systems, a condition known as **shock**. These dramatic effects of LPS are seen in humans as **septic shock**, which results from an uncontrolled systemic bacterial infection, or **sepsis**. In this case, LPS induces an overwhelming secretion of cytokines, including IL-1β and TNF-α, causing systemic vascular permeability, an undesirable effect of its normal role in containing local infections. Mutant mice lacking TLR-4 function are resistant to LPS-induced septic shock but are highly sensitive to LPS-bearing pathogens such as *Salmonella enterica* ssp. *typhimurium*. In fact, TLR-4 (the first human homolog of Toll discovered by Medzhitov and Janeway, as discussed earlier) was identified as a receptor for LPS by positional cloning of its gene from the LPS-resistant C3H/HeJ mouse strain, which harbors a naturally occurring mutation in the cytoplasmic tail of TLR-4 that interferes with the receptor's ability to signal. For this discovery, the 2011 Nobel Prize in Physiology or Medicine was partly awarded to Bruce Beutler.

3-7   TLRs activate NFκB, AP-1, and IRF transcription factors to induce the expression of inflammatory cytokines and type I interferons.

Signaling by mammalian TLRs in various cell types induces a diverse range of intracellular responses that together result in the production of inflammatory cytokines, chemotactic factors, antimicrobial peptides, and the antiviral cytokines interferon-α (**IFN-α**) and interferon-β (**IFN-β**), the **type I interferons**. TLR signaling achieves this by activating several signaling pathways that each activate different transcription factors. As mentioned earlier, ligand-induced dimerization of two TLR ectodomains brings the cytoplasmic TIR domains together, allowing them to interact with the TIR domains of cytoplasmic adaptor molecules that initiate intracellular signaling. There are five such adaptors used by mammalian TLRs: **MyD88**, **TRIF**, **MAL** (also known as TIRAP), **TRAM**, and **BCAP**. It is significant that the TIR domains of the different TLRs interact with different combinations of these adaptors because the choice of adaptor influences which of several downstream signals will be activated by the TLR. Recruitment of MyD88 and/or TRIF controls most of the signaling downstream of TLR activation, while MAL and TRAM facilitate the recruitment of MyD88 and TRIF, respectively, but do not directly participate in signal transduction. Most TLRs interact with MyD88 and not TRIF. TLR-3 interacts only with TRIF, and TLR-4 interacts with both MyD88 and TRIF. BCAP links TLR activation to distinct signaling pathways, but the details of this signaling are less clear because BCAP was only recently discovered as a TLR adaptor.

Signaling by most TLRs activates the transcription factor **NFκB** (**Fig. 3.14**). Mammalian TLRs also activate several members of the **interferon regulatory factor (IRF)** transcription factor family through a second pathway, and they activate members of the **activator protein 1 (AP-1)** family, such as c-Jun, through yet another signaling pathway involving **mitogen-activated protein kinases (MAPKs)**. NFκB and AP-1 act primarily to induce the expression of pro-inflammatory cytokines and chemotactic factors. The IRF factors IRF3

Fig. 3.14 TLR signaling can activate the transcription factor NFκB, which induces the expression of pro-inflammatory cytokines. First panel: TLRs signal via their cytoplasmic TIR domains, which are brought into proximity to each other by ligand-induced dimerization of their ectodomains. Some TLRs use the adaptor protein MyD88, and others use the MyD88/MAL pair to initiate signaling. The MyD88 death domain recruits the serine/threonine kinases IRAK1 and IRAK4, in association with the ubiquitin E3 ligase TRAF6. IRAK undergoes autoactivation and phosphorylates TRAF6, activating its E3 ligase activity. Second panel: TRAF6 cooperates with an E2 ligase (UBC13) and a cofactor (Uve1A) to generate polyubiquitin scaffolds (yellow triangles) by attachment of ubiquitin through its lysine 63 (K63) residue. This scaffold recruits a complex of proteins composed of the kinase TAK1 (transforming growth factor-β–activated kinase 1) and two

adaptor proteins, TAB1 (TAK1-binding protein 1) and TAB2. TAB1 and TAB2 bind to polyubiquitin, bringing TAK1 into proximity with IRAK to become phosphorylated (red dot). Third panel: Activated TAK1 activates IKK, the IκB kinase complex. First, the IKKγ subunit (NEMO) binds to the polyubiquitin scaffold and brings the IKK complex into proximity to TAK1. TAK1 then phosphorylates and activates IKKβ. IKKβ then phosphorylates IκB, the cytoplasmic inhibitor of NFκB. Fourth panel: Phosphorylated IκB is targeted by a process of ubiquitination (not shown) that leads to its degradation. This releases NFκB, which is composed of two subunits, p50 and p65, into the nucleus, driving the transcription of many genes including those encoding inflammatory cytokines. TAK1 also stimulates activation of the mitogen-activated protein kinases (MAPKs) JNK and p38, which phosphorylate and activate AP-1 transcription factors (not shown).

and IRF7 are particularly important for inducing antiviral type I interferons, whereas a related factor, IRF5, is involved in the production of pro-inflammatory cytokines. Here we will describe how TLR signaling induces the transcription of various cytokine genes; later in the chapter, we will explain how those cytokines exert their various actions.

We consider first the signaling pathway triggered by TLRs that use MyD88. Two protein domains of MyD88 are responsible for its function as an adaptor. MyD88 has a TIR domain at its carboxyl terminus that associates with the TIR domains in the TLR cytoplasmic tails. At its amino terminus, MyD88 has a **death domain**, so named because it was first identified in signaling proteins involved in apoptosis, a type of programmed cell death. The MyD88 death domain associates with a similar death domain present in other intracellular signaling proteins. Both MyD88 domains are required for signaling, and rare mutations in either domain are associated with immunodeficiency characterized by recurrent bacterial infections in humans. The MyD88 death domain recruits and activates two serine/threonine protein kinases—**IRAK4** (IL-1 receptor–associated kinase 4) and **IRAK1**—via their death domains. This IRAK complex performs two functions: it recruits enzymes that produce a **signaling scaffold**, and it uses this scaffold to recruit other molecules that are then phosphorylated by the IRAKs.

Interleukin-1 Receptor–
Associated Kinase 4
Deficiency

To form a signaling scaffold, the IRAK complex recruits the enzyme **TRAF6 (tumor necrosis factor receptor–associated factor 6)**, which is an E3 **ubiquitin ligase** that acts in cooperation with **UBC13**, an E2 ubiquitin ligase, and its cofactor **Uve1A** (together called **TRIKA1**) (see Fig. 3.14). The combined activity of TRAF6 and UBC13 is to ligate (unite with a chemical bond) one ubiquitin molecule to another protein, which can be another ubiquitin molecule, and thereby generate protein polymers. The polyubiquitin involved in signaling contains linkages between the lysine 63 residue on one ubiquitin and the carboxyl terminus of the next, forming **K63 linkages**. This polyubiquitin polymer can be initiated on other proteins, including TRAF6 itself, or produced as free linear ubiquitin polymers, and can be extended to produce **polyubiquitin chains** that act as a platform—or scaffold—to which other signaling molecules bind. Next, the scaffold recruits a signaling complex consisting of the polyubiquitin-binding adaptor proteins **TAB1**, **TAB2**, and the serine/threonine kinase **TAK1** (see Fig. 3.14). By being brought onto the scaffold, TAK1 is phosphorylated by the IRAK complex, and activated TAK1 propagates signaling by activating certain MAPKs, such as c-Jun terminal kinase (JNK) and MAPK14 (p38 MAPK). These then activate AP-1 family transcription factors that transcribe cytokine genes.

TAK1 also phosphorylates and activates the **IκB kinase (IKK)** complex, which is composed of three proteins: IKKα, IKKβ, and IKKγ (the latter also known as **NEMO**, for NFκB essential modifier). IKKγ functions by binding to polyubiquitin chains, which brings the IKK complex into proximity with TAK1. TAK1 phosphorylates and activates IKKβ. IKKβ then phosphorylates **IκB** (inhibitor of κB), which is a distinct molecule whose name should not be confused with IKKβ. IκB is a cytoplasmic protein that constitutively binds to the transcription factor NFκB, which is a family of transcription factors. One version of NFκB is composed of the subunits **p50** and **p65**, but other heterodimers and homodimers also exist. The binding of IκB traps the NFκB proteins in the cytoplasm. Phosphorylation by IKK induces the degradation of IκB, and this releases NFκB into the nucleus, where it can drive transcription of genes for pro-inflammatory cytokines such as TNF-α, IL-1β, and **IL-6**. The actions of these cytokines in the innate immune response are described in the second half of this chapter. The outcome of TLR activation can also vary depending on the cell type in which it occurs.

The ability of TLRs to activate NFκB is crucial to their role of alerting the immune system to the presence of bacterial pathogens. Rare instances of inactivating mutations in IRAK4 in humans cause an immunodeficiency, **IRAK4 deficiency**, which, like MyD88 deficiency, is characterized by recurrent

Fig. 3.15 Expression of antiviral interferons in response to viral nucleic acids can be stimulated by two different pathways from different TLRs. Left panel: TLR-3, expressed by dendritic cells and macrophages, senses double-stranded viral RNA (dsRNA). TLR-3 signaling uses the adaptor protein TRIF, which recruits the E3 ligase TRAF3 to generate K63-linked polyubiquitin chains. This scaffold recruits NEMO and TANK (TRAF family member–associated NFκB activator), which associate with the serine/threonine kinases IKKε (IκB kinase ε) and TBK1 (TANK-binding kinase 1). TBK1 phosphorylates (red dot) the transcription factor IRF3, and IRF3 then enters the nucleus and induces expression of type I interferon genes. Right panel: TLR-7, expressed by plasmacytoid dendritic cells, detects single-stranded RNA (ssRNA) and signals through MyD88. Here, IRAK1 directly recruits and phosphorylates IRF7, which is also highly expressed in plasmacytoid dendritic cells. IRF7 then enters the nucleus to induce expression of type I interferons.

bacterial infections. Mutations in human IKKγ(NEMO) produce a syndrome known as **X-linked hypohidrotic ectodermal dysplasia and immunodeficiency** or **NEMO deficiency**, which is characterized by both immunodeficiency and developmental defects.

TLR signaling also activates several members of the IRF family. IRF proteins reside in the cytoplasm and are inactive until they become phosphorylated on serine and threonine residues in their carboxyl termini. They then move to the nucleus as active transcription factors. Of the nine IRF family members, IRF3 and IRF7 are particularly important for TLR signaling and expression of antiviral type I interferons. For TLR-3, the cytoplasmic TIR domain interacts with the adaptor protein TRIF. TRIF interacts with the E3 ubiquitin ligase **TRAF3**, which, like TRAF6, generates a polyubiquitin scaffold. In TLR-3 signaling, this scaffold recruits a multiprotein complex containing the kinases **IKKε** and **TBK1**, which phosphorylate IRF3 (**Fig. 3.15**). TLR-4 also triggers this pathway by binding TRIF, but the IRF3 response induced by TLR-4 is relatively weak compared with that induced by TLR-3, and its functional role *in vivo* remains elusive. In contrast to TLR-3, the TLRs TLR-7, TLR-8, and TLR-9 use MyD88-dependent signaling to activate IRFs and induce expression of type I interferons. This signaling pathway is particularly relevant in plasmacytoid dendritic cells and represents a good example of how the outcome of TLR signaling can vary depending on the cell type in which it occurs. Upon TLR-7 and TLR-9 signaling in plasmacytoid dendritic cells, the MyD88 TIR domain recruits the IRAK1:IRAK4 complex as described earlier. However, the IRAK complex carries out a distinct function beyond recruiting TRAFs that generate a signaling scaffold. In these cells, IRAK1 can also physically associate with IRF7, which is highly expressed by plasmacytoid dendritic cells. This allows IRF7 to become phosphorylated by IRAK1, leading to induction of type I interferons (see Fig. 3.15). Not all IRF factors regulate type I interferon genes; IRF5, for example, plays a role in the induction of pro-inflammatory cytokines.

The collective ability of TLRs to activate both IRFs and NFκB means that they can stimulate either antiviral or antibacterial responses as needed. TLRs are expressed by different types of cells involved in innate immunity and by some stromal and epithelial cells, and the responses generated will differ in some respects depending on what type of cell is being activated.

3-8   The RIG-I–like receptors detect cytoplasmic viral RNAs and activate MAVS to induce type I interferon production and pro–inflammatory cytokines.

The TLRs, being expressed on the cell's plasma membrane or endocytic vesicles, are primarily sensors of extracellular microbial products. Since the discovery of the mammalian TLRs, additional families of innate sensors have been identified that detect microbial products in the cytosol (**Fig. 3.16**). Certain TLR family members detect extracellular viral RNAs and DNAs that enter the cell from the endocytic pathway. By contrast, viral RNAs produced within a cell are sensed by a separate family of proteins called the **RIG-I–like receptors (RLRs)**. These proteins serve as viral sensors by binding to viral dsRNAs using an RNA helicase–like domain. The first of these sensors to be discovered was **RIG-I (retinoic acid–inducible gene I)**. RIG-I is widely expressed across tissues and cell types. Mice deficient in RIG-I are highly susceptible to infection by several kinds of single-stranded RNA viruses, including paramyxoviruses, rhabdoviruses, orthomyxoviruses, and flaviviruses, but not picornaviruses.

The RLR proteins also contain two amino-terminal **caspase recruitment domains (CARDs)**. CARD was initially recognized in a family of proteases called **caspases** (for cysteine–aspartic acid proteases), which are important in many intracellular pathways, including those leading to cell death by apoptosis. CARD is structurally related to the death domain in MyD88 and can dimerize with CARDs on other proteins to activate signaling to produce type I interferons when viral RNAs are bound (**Fig. 3.17**).

RIG-I discriminates between host and viral RNA by sensing differences at the 5′ end of RNA transcripts. Eukaryotic RNA is transcribed in the nucleus and contains a 5′-triphosphate group on its initial nucleotide that undergoes subsequent enzymatic modification called **capping** by the addition of a 7-methylguanosine to the 5′-triphosphate. Most RNA viruses do not replicate in the nucleus, where capping normally occurs, so their RNA genomes do not undergo this modification. Biochemical and structural studies have determined that RIG-I senses dsRNAs with the unmodified 5′-triphosphate. Many viruses produce dsRNAs with 5′-triphosphate that are detected by RIG-I, either during viral replication or due to hairpins that form when base pairing occurs within the viral RNA. In contrast, the picornaviruses, which include poliovirus and hepatitis A, replicate by a mechanism that involves the covalent attachment of a viral protein to the 5′ end of the viral RNA, so that the 5′-triphosphate is masked, which explains why RIG-I is not involved in sensing them.

MDA-5 (melanoma differentiation–associated 5) is similar in structure to RIG-I, but it senses longer dsRNAs and does not require the 5′-triphosphate for recognition. In contrast to RIG-I–deficient mice, mice deficient in MDA-5 are susceptible to picornaviruses, indicating that these two sensors of viral RNAs have crucial but distinct roles in host defense. The RLR family member **LGP2** (encoded by *DHX58*) contains a helicase domain but lacks CARDs. LGP2 appears to cooperate with RIG-I and MDA-5 in the recognition of viral RNA, as mice lacking LGP2 have impaired antiviral responses normally mediated by RIG-I or MDA-5. This cooperative viral recognition by LGP2 appears to depend on its helicase domain, because in mice, mutations that disrupt the helicase ATPase activity result in impaired IFN-β production in response to various RNA viruses.

Sensing of viral RNAs by RIG-I and MDA-5 activates signaling that leads to type I interferon production appropriate for defense against viral infection (see Fig. 3.17). Upon binding dsRNA, both RIG-I and MDA-5 assemble into filaments along the dsRNA, which promotes the aggregation of CARDs from multiple RIG-I or MDA-5 molecules. For RIG-I, aggregation of the CARDs is facilitated by recruitment of E3 ligases **Riplet** (encoded by *RNF153*) and **TRIM25**, which generate K63-linked polyubiquitin scaffolds (see Section 3-7) that stabilize interactions between the CARDs. The initiation of MDA-5 signaling does not require Riplet or TRIM25, most likely because MDA-5 more readily assembles into filaments along dsRNA, which enables aggregation of the CARDs. The aggregated CARDs interact with a downstream adaptor protein called **MAVS (mitochondrial antiviral signaling protein)**. MAVS is attached to the outer mitochondrial membrane and contains its own CARD that mediates interaction with RIG-I and MDA-5 assembled on dsRNAs. Activated MAVS also forms polymers. In this state, MAVS propagates signals by recruiting various TRAF family E3 ubiquitin ligases, including TRAF2, TRAF3, TRAF5, and TRAF6. The relative importance of each E3 ligase may differ between cell types, but their

Ligand	Recognition strategies
RIG-I	Triphosphate dsRNA
MDA-5	dsRNA
cGAS	DNA
NOD1	γ-Glutamyl diaminopimelic acid (iE-DAP)
NOD2	Muramyl dipeptide (MDP)
NLRP1	Pathogen protease activity
NLRP3	Reduced intracellular potassium, ROS, disruption of lysosomes
NAIP1 with NLRC4 (mouse)	Needle subunit of bacterial T3SS
NAIP2 with NLRC4 (mouse)	Rod subunit of bacterial T3SS
NAIP5 with NLRC4 (mouse)	Flagellin
NAIP with NLRC4 (human)	Flagellin
Pyrin	Inactivation of Rho GTPases
AIM2	DNA

Fig. 3.16 Ligands and recognition strategies for cytosolic innate immune receptors. Some cytosolic innate immune receptors detect pathogens directly, while others are activated by the activities of pathogens. This figure lists the major receptors for which the ligands or mechanisms of activation are known. ROS, reactive oxygen species; T3SS, type 3 secretion system.

Fig. 3.17 RIG-I and other RLRs are cytoplasmic sensors of viral RNA. First panel: Before detecting viral RNA, RIG-I is cytoplasmic and in an inactive, autoinhibited conformation. The adaptor protein MAVS is attached to the mitochondrial outer membrane. Second panel: Detection of uncapped 5′-triphosphate dsRNA by RIG-I leads to assembly of RIG-I proteins along the dsRNA, enabling aggregation of the CARDs and interaction with the amino-terminal CARD of MAVS. This interaction involves the generation of K63-linked polyubiquitin from the E3 ligases Riplet and TRIM25 (the latter not shown). Third panel: The aggregation induces a proline rich region of MAVS to interact with TRAFs (see text) and leads to the generation of additional K63-linked polyubiquitin scaffold. As in TLR signaling, this scaffold recruits TBK1 and IKK complexes (see Figs. 3.14 and 3.15) to activate IRF3 and NFκB, producing type I interferons and pro-inflammatory cytokines, respectively. CTD, C-terminal domain.

further production of K63-linked polyubiquitin leads to activation of TBK1 and IRF3 and production of type I interferons, as described for TLR-3 signaling (see Fig. 3.15), and also to activation of NFκB.

The recognition of specific features of dsRNA (5′-triphosphate for RIG-I and longer dsRNAs for MDA-5) reduces the chance that cellular RNAs will trigger activation of RLRs. However, humans have been identified with mutations in RIG-I and MDA-5 that result in inappropriate activation of the receptors, which manifests as severe diseases such as SLE, Aicardi–Goutières syndrome, and Singleton–Merten syndrome. How these mutations facilitate RIG-I or MDA-5 activation is an area of active investigation, but in some cases they appear to enable the inappropriate activation of the receptors by endogenous RNAs.

3-9 Cytosolic DNA activates the cGAS–STING pathway to induce production of type I interferons.

Innate sensors that recognize cytosolic RNA use specific modifications, such as the 5′ cap, to discriminate between host and viral origin. Host DNA is generally restricted to the nucleus, but viral, microbial, or protozoan DNA may become located in the cytosol during various stages of infection. The fact that introduction of DNA into the cytosol induces the production of type I interferons was known for a number of years before the sensor or signaling proteins that mediate the response were identified. It is now known that the main sensor of cytosolic DNA is an enzyme called **cGAS, for cyclic GAMP synthase**. cGAS binds directly to cytosolic DNA, which stimulates its enzymatic activity to produce a second messenger molecule called **cyclic guanosine monophosphate–adenosine monophosphate (cyclic GMP–AMP), or cGAMP**. cGAMP binds to and activates **STING (stimulator of interferon genes)**, which is a protein encoded by *TMEM173* and localized within the endoplasmic reticulum membrane by an amino-terminal tetraspan transmembrane domain (**Fig. 3.18**). STING exists as an inactive homodimer until

Double-stranded DNA from viruses activates cGAS to produce cGAMP from ATP and GTP

cGAMP or other bacterial-derived cyclic dinucleotides bind to the STING dimer present on the ER membrane and activate its signaling

STING activates the kinase TBK1 to phosphorylate IRF3, which enters the nucleus and induces expression of type I interferon genes

Fig. 3.18 cGAS is a cytosolic sensor of DNA that signals through STING to activate type I interferon production. First panel: cGAS resides in the cytoplasm and serves as a sensor of double-stranded DNA (dsDNA) from viruses. When cGAS binds dsDNA, its enzymatic activity is stimulated, leading to production of cyclic GMP–AMP (cGAMP). Bacteria that infect cells produce second messengers such as cyclic dinucleotides, including cyclic diguanylate monophosphate (c-di-GMP) and cyclic diadenylate monophosphate (c-di-AMP). Second panel: cGAMP and other bacterial dinucleotides can bind and activate the STING dimer present on the endoplasmic reticulum (ER) membrane. Third panel: In this state, STING activates TBK1. Active TBK1 activates IRF3, as described in Fig. 3.15.

cGAMP binding, which induces a conformation change, recruitment of TBK1, activation of IRF3, and production of type I interferons, similarly to signaling by TLR-3 and RLRs (see Figs. 3.15 and 3.17).

cGAMP is a member of a larger family of **cyclic dinucleotides (CDNs)** produced by diverse organisms. In fact, the importance of CDNs was first appreciated in bacteria, where CDNs such as cyclic diguanylate monophosphate (c-di-GMP) and cyclic diadenylate monophosphate (c-di-AMP) are synthesized by bacterial enzymes and function as signaling molecules. Before the discovery of mammalian cGAS and cGAMP, these bacterial CDNs were shown to bind and activate STING directly, suggesting that STING may itself serve as a direct sensor of intracellular bacterial infection.

cGAS and STING are expressed in most immune-cell types and many nonimmune cells, and there is good evidence that detection of DNA by the cGAS–STING pathway is important for the immune response to infection, especially viral infection. Mice harboring inactivated cGAS or STING genes show increased susceptibility to a number of DNA viruses. The cGAS–STING pathway can also be activated during infections with certain intracellular bacterial pathogens, either by bacterial DNA released during infection or by bacterial CDNs that bind STING directly, as discussed above. However, the relevance of cGAS–STING signaling for the host response to bacterial infections remains rather unclear, as the type I interferon response induced by cGAS–STING signaling is predominantly antiviral. In some contexts, the production of type I interferons can impair the response to bacteria, so it is possible that activation of cGAS–STING by some pathogens represents a pathogen-evolved mechanism of immune evasion. It is also possible that STING activation can induce other host-defense mechanisms besides production of type I interferons, such as autophagy, which may help to degrade intracellular bacteria.

As with many of the nucleic acid–sensing PRRs discussed earlier, inappropriate activation of the cGAS–STING pathway can lead to inflammatory diseases. An enzyme called **Trex1** limits activation of cGAS by degrading DNA present in the cytosol. Mice and humans with defective Trex1 develop autoimmune diseases similar to those described earlier for humans with gain-of-function mutations in MDA-5 and RIG-I (see Section 3-8). DNA accumulates in the cytosol of Trex1-deficient cells, where it activates cGAS. Accordingly, loss of cGAS reverses disease symptoms seen in Trex1-mutant mice. The origin of the cytosolic DNA in Trex1-mutant cells is an area of active investigation, but one source appears to be endogenous retroelements, mobile genetic elements present within mammalian genomes. Other individuals have been identified with mutations in STING that result in constitutive signaling, leading to an autoimmune disorder called STING-associated vasculopathy with onset in infancy (SAVI).

3-10 NLRs comprise a large family of intracellular sensors with diverse functions.

One large group of cytosolic innate sensors is collectively called **NOD-like receptors (NLRs)**, and their family members contain a **nucleotide-binding and oligomerization domain (NOD)** and leucine-rich repeats (LRRs) in their structure. Each NLR possesses additional domains that result in diverse functions and, in some instances, enable detection of infection. Some NLRs activate NFκB to initiate the same inflammatory responses as the TLRs, while other NLRs trigger a very different response that leads to cell death and the release of different pro-inflammatory cytokines. We will discuss this second type of response in the next section. Not all NLRs are involved in pathogen detection. For example, NLRC5 and CIITA regulate the transcription of MHC class I and class II genes, respectively.

NOD1 and NOD2 are NLRs that recognize fragments of bacterial cell-wall peptidoglycans, although it is not known whether this occurs through direct binding or via accessory proteins. **NOD1** senses **γ-glutamyl diaminopimelic acid (iE-DAP)**, a breakdown product of peptidoglycans of Gram-negative bacteria such as *Salmonella* and some Gram-positive bacteria such as *Listeria*, whereas **NOD2** recognizes **muramyl dipeptide (MDP)**, which is present in the peptidoglycans of most bacteria. NOD ligands may enter the cytoplasm as a result of intracellular infection, but they may also be transported from materials captured by endocytosis, as mice lacking certain oligopeptide transporters have reduced responses to NOD ligands.

Both NOD1 and NOD2 contain CARDs. When NOD1 or NOD2 is activated, it recruits the CARD-containing serine/threonine kinase **RIP2** (also known as RICK and RIPK2) (**Fig. 3.19**). RIP2 associates with the E3 ligases cIAP1, cIAP2, and XIAP, whose activity generates a polyubiquitin scaffold similar to the scaffold already discussed in the context of TLR signaling. This scaffold recruits TAK1 and IKK and results in activation of NFκB as shown in Fig. 3.14. NFκB then induces the expression of genes for inflammatory cytokines and for enzymes involved in the production of **nitric oxide (NO)**, which is toxic to bacteria and intracellular parasites. In keeping with their role as sensors of bacterial components, NOD proteins are expressed in cells that are routinely exposed to bacteria. These include epithelial cells forming the barrier that bacteria must cross to establish an infection in the body and the macrophages and dendritic cells that ingest bacteria that have succeeded in entering the body. Macrophages and dendritic cells express TLRs as well as NOD1 and NOD2 and are activated by both pathways.

NOD2 seems to have a more specialized role, being strongly expressed in the Paneth cells of the gut, where it regulates the expression of potent antimicrobial peptides such as the α- and β-defensins (see Chapter 2). Loss-of-function mutations in NOD2 in humans are associated with the inflammatory bowel condition known as **Crohn's disease** (discussed in Chapter 15). Lack of NOD2 function is thought to diminish the production of defensins and other antimicrobial peptides, thereby weakening the natural barrier function of the intestinal epithelium and leading to the inflammation characteristic of this disease. Gain-of-function mutations in human NOD2 are associated with the inflammatory disorders **early-onset sarcoidosis** and **Blau syndrome**, which are characterized by spontaneous inflammation in tissues such as the liver or in the joints, eyes, and skin. Activating mutations in the NOD domain seem to promote the signaling cascade in the absence of ligand, leading to an inappropriate inflammatory response in the absence of pathogens.

Crohn's Disease

Hereditary Periodic Fever Syndromes

ANIMATION 3.6

Fig. 3.19 Intracellular NOD proteins sense the presence of bacteria by recognizing bacterial peptidoglycans and activate NFκB to induce the expression of pro-inflammatory genes. First panel: NOD proteins reside in an inactive state in the cytoplasm, where they serve as sensors for various bacterial components. Second panel: Degradation of bacterial cell-wall peptidoglycans produces muramyl dipeptide, which activates NOD2. NOD1 is activated by γ-glutamyl diaminopimelic acid (iE-DAP), a breakdown product of Gram-negative bacterial cell walls. Whether these ligands are recognized directly by NOD1 and NOD2 remains unclear. Activation of NOD1 and NOD2 induces aggregation, allowing CARD-dependent recruitment of the serine/threonine kinase RIP2, which associates with E3 ligases, including XIAP (X-linked inhibitor of apoptosis protein), cIAP1 (cellular inhibitor of apoptosis 1), and cIAP2. This recruited E3 ligase activity produces a polyubiquitin scaffold, as in TLR signaling, and the association of TAK1 and the IKK complex with this scaffold leads to the activation of NFκB, as shown in Fig. 3.14. In this pathway, RIP2 acts as a scaffold to recruit XIAP, and RIP2 kinase activity is not required for signaling.

3-11 Certain NLR proteins react to infection or cellular damage by forming an inflammasome that induces cell death and secretion of inflammatory cytokines.

Some NLR proteins respond to infection or, in some cases, cellular damage in the absence of infection by inducing the formation of a multiprotein complex known as an **inflammasome**. Inflammasomes serve as platforms for the activation of inflammatory caspases such as **caspase 1**, a protease that when activated induces the proteolytic cleavage and release of pro-inflammatory cytokines IL-1β and IL-18. Cleavage of these cytokines converts them into their active forms. Activated caspase 1 also cleaves **gasdermin D**, a cytosolic protein that, once cleaved, inserts into the plasma membrane and assembles into a pore (**Fig. 3.20**). This pore is required for exit of active IL-1β and IL-18 from the cell, as these cytokines lack signal peptides and are otherwise confined to the cytosol. The gasdermin D pore also induces a lytic form of cell death called **pyroptosis** ('fiery death'). While the induction of host-cell death in response to infection may seem counterproductive at first glance, pyroptosis exposes intracellular pathogens that otherwise hide within host cells (for example, macrophages). These pathogens are now visible and thus susceptible to killing by neutrophils and activated macrophages recruited by the inflammatory cytokines produced by inflammasome activation.

Certain NLR proteins function as PRRs by inducing inflammasome assembly after directly binding to molecules produced by pathogens. For example, **NAIPs** (**N**LR family, **a**poptosis **i**nhibitory **p**roteins) assemble into inflammasomes

A priming step (TLR stimulation induces expression of the pro-forms of IL-1β and IL-18)	NLRs respond to PAMPs or pathogen activities and oligomerize into an inflammasome	The assembled inflammasome recruits and activates caspase 1, which in turn cleaves pro-IL-1β, pro-IL-18 and gasdermin D	Formation of a gasdermin D pore allows release of IL-1β and IL-18 and induces pyroptotic cell death

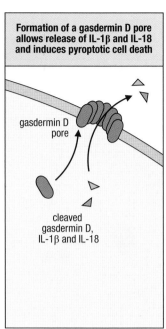

Fig. 3.20 Inflammasomes activate inflammatory caspases, leading to secretion of pro-inflammatory cytokines and pyroptosis. The general steps of inflammasome activation and the downstream events after activation are shown for a 'generic' NLR protein. First panel: The NLR is in an inactive conformation in unstimulated cells. Second and third panels: Some NLRs detect pathogens directly while others respond to pathogen activities. NLR activation leads to a conformation change that enables oligomerization of the NLR and recruitment of the inflammatory protease caspase 1. In unstimulated cells caspase 1 is inactive, but binding to the assembled inflammasome activates its protease activity. Active caspase 1 cleaves pro-IL-1β, pro-IL-18, and gasdermin D, converting these proteins into their active forms. Fourth panel: Cleaved gasdermin D proteins form a pore in the plasma membrane, which allows release of IL-1β and IL-18. The loss of membrane integrity also induces lysis of cells. This form of cell death is called pyroptosis. Most cells require a separate priming step to induce expression of IL-1β or IL-18 (and in some cases inflammasome components themselves). This priming step, which can be achieved through TLR activation, may help prevent accidental inflammasome activation.

Fig. 3.21 NAIP5 and NLRC4 form an inflammasome upon flagellin recognition. A model of the structure of the NAIP5–NLRC4 inflammasome bound to flagellin. Note that NAIP5 (shown in yellow) directly contacts the D0 domain of flagellin (shown in red). This interaction induces a conformation change in NAIP5 that promotes interaction with multiple NLRC4 proteins (shown in blue) and assembly into an inflammasome. The CARDs of NLRC4 (not shown) form an inner ring and are responsible for the recruitment and activation of caspase 1.

with **NLRC4** after recognizing certain bacterial proteins that access the host cytosol. Mice encode a small family of NAIP proteins, each of which recognizes a distinct ligand. For example, **NAIP5** recognizes bacterial flagellin, whereas NAIP1 and **NAIP2** recognize distinct protein subunits of the **type III secretion system (T3SS)**, a needle-like macromolecular machine that bacterial pathogens use to inject proteins into host cells. Humans encode a single NAIP protein that has a broad specificity for flagellin and T3SS proteins. NAIP5 recognizes the highly conserved D0 domain of flagellin, which is distinct from the region of flagellin recognized by TLR-5. As a cell-surface receptor, TLR-5 can detect flagellin from potentially any extracellular flagellated bacterium, including harmless commensal species, whereas cytosolic NAIP5 will respond only to bacteria that have the capacity to invade or access the cytosol—typically only pathogenic species.

Structural analyses of the NAIP5–NLRC4 inflammasome bound to flagellin have confirmed that NAIP5 binds flagellin directly. This binding induces a conformational change in NAIP5, promoting interaction with NLRC4 and formation of an inflammasome (**Fig. 3.21**). NLRC4 contains an N-terminal CARD that, upon inflammasome assembly, interacts with the CARD present in caspase 1 to mediate its dimerization and activation. Active caspase 1 then cleaves multiple substrates, including the pro-forms of IL-1β, IL-18, and gasdermin D, as discussed earlier.

The importance of NAIP–NLRC4 inflammasomes for the host response to infection has been established by studies of cells or mice with disrupted NAIP or NLRC4 genes. Mice lacking NLRC4 are more susceptible to infection by numerous intracellular bacterial pathogens, including *Salmonella enterica* ssp. *typhimurium* and *Legionella pneumophila*. NAIP and NLRC4 genes are highly expressed in intestinal epithelial cells. In these cells, inflammasome activation leads to pyroptotic cell death, which is accompanied by expulsion of the infected cell back into the intestinal lumen, which limits the ability of bacteria to establish infection.

While the NAIPs represent classic PRRs, other NLRs do not recognize pathogens directly but rather assemble inflammasomes in response to the consequences of infection, such as pathogen-induced disruptions of cellular structures. The most studied member of this subgroup of NLRs is **NLRP3** (also known as NALP3 or cryopyrin). In contrast to NLRC4, NLRP3 has a **pyrin** domain at its N terminus, hence its **NLRP** designation (NLRs with CARDs are designated NLR**C**). Pyrin domains are structurally related to CARDs and interact with other pyrin domains. Several seemingly unrelated triggers can induce NLRP3 activation: reduced intracellular potassium, the generation of reactive oxygen species (ROS), or the disruption of lysosomes (for example, via phagocytosis of crystalline material). It remains unclear how such diverse stimuli are sensed by this NLR, but each represents a potential consequence of infection. The loss of intracellular potassium through efflux can occur during infection with, for example, intracellular bacteria such as *Staphylococcus aureus* that produce pore-forming toxins. Also, the death of nearby cells during infection can release ATP into the extracellular space; this ATP can activate the **purinergic receptor P2X7**, which itself is a potassium channel, and allow K^+ ion efflux. As discussed earlier in this chapter, ROS are produced by phagocytes upon infection. Finally, a number of pathogens are known to disrupt or permeabilize the phagosomal membrane as a mechanism of escape or to manipulate the host cell.

While it is still not understood how NLRP3 senses such diverse changes to cellular homeostasis, structural and biochemical approaches have delineated the steps of NLRP3 inflammasome assembly. As mentioned earlier, NLRP3 lacks a CARD, so it cannot recruit caspase 1 directly. Instead, upon activation, NLRP3 oligomerizes, and this aggregation induces the pyrin domains of NLRP3 to interact with pyrin domains of another protein named **ASC** (also called PYCARD). ASC is an adaptor protein composed of an amino-terminal pyrin domain and a carboxyl-terminal CARD. Recruitment of ASC creates a platform for caspase 1 recruitment and activation, via CARD–CARD interactions, as described earlier for the NAIP–NLRC4 inflammasomes. Once caspase 1 is activated, the downstream events are similar for all inflammasomes.

NLRP1 is another NLR that assembles into an inflammasome in response to the activity of pathogens. Specifically, NLRP1 is partially degraded by several different bacterial enzymes; however, instead of inactivating NLRP1, this partial degradation releases a fragment of NLRP1 containing a CARD that assembles into an inflammasome that recruits and activates caspase 1. The best-understood example of this mechanism comes from studies of the **lethal factor protease**, a toxin secreted by the anthrax bacterium, *Bacillus anthracis*. Lethal factor enters into cells and promotes infection by cleaving MAP kinase kinases, which disrupts signaling and the ensuing immune response. However, lethal factor also cleaves NLRP1, leading to its partial degradation and inflammasome formation. Because responses downstream of caspase 1 are effective in preventing anthrax, it appears unlikely that *B. anthracis* evolved to activate NLRP1. Instead, NLRP1 appears to serve as a 'decoy' substrate for pathogen proteases and assembles into an inflammasome when such protease activity is detected.

Inflammasome activation can also be initiated by proteins other than NLRs. As discussed earlier for NLRs, some of these proteins detect pathogen-derived ligands while others sense the consequences of infection. As an example of the former, **AIM2 (absent in melanoma 2)**, a member of the **PYHIN** family of proteins, is activated by direct binding to cytosolic DNA. PYHIN proteins contain an N-terminal pyrin domain but lack the LRR domains present in the NLR family. In place of LRR domains, PYHIN proteins have an HIN (hematopoietic expression, interferon-inducible nature, and nuclear localization) domain. The HIN domain of AIM2 recognizes the DNA genomes of pathogens and triggers caspase 1 activation through pyrin domain interactions with ASC. The protein **Pyrin** (not to be confused with the pyrin domain that is present in multiple proteins and was described earlier) is another inflammasome sensor protein with an N-terminal pyrin domain but no LRRs. Pyrin senses the inactivation of Rho GTPases, enzymes that regulate the cytoskeleton and cell motility (see Section 3-2). Kinases activated by RhoA phosphorylate specific residues in the Pyrin protein, and this phosphorylation keeps Pyrin in an inactive conformation. Certain pathogens, such as *Clostridium difficile*, produce toxins that inactivate RhoA, which correspondingly reduces phosphorylation of Pyrin and enables its activation. Activated Pyrin recruits ASC, leading to caspase 1 activation in a manner analogous to the other inflammasomes discussed above.

Many cell types, including most macrophages, must undergo a priming step before inflammasome activation can lead to release of inflammatory cytokines. This priming step induces the transcription and translation of the mRNAs that encode the pro-forms of IL-1β, IL-18, and other cytokines (see Fig. 3.20). In some cases, inflammasome components themselves (for example, NLRP3) are induced upon priming. TLR signaling can satisfy this priming step, which may help ensure that inflammasome activation proceeds primarily during infections. Priming is not always necessary, however, as some cells in tissues (for example, the intestine) express pro-IL-1 β and pro-IL-18 constitutively.

Caspase 11 (in mice) and **caspase 4** and **caspase 5** (in humans) are pro-inflammatory caspases that also function as cytosolic sensors of LPS. Once activated, these caspases are able to cleave and activate gasdermin D directly, leading to pyroptosis, but they do not appear to directly cleave the pro-forms of IL-1β and IL-18. However, once pyroptosis is initiated, K^+ efflux occurs via gasdermin D pores, resulting in NLRP3 activation, caspase 1 activation, and IL-1β and IL-18 processing and release. This response to LPS has been referred to as a 'noncanonical' inflammasome pathway. The ability of LPS to induce toxic shock in mice is due primarily to activation of caspase 11. TLR-4 is still involved, however, because caspase 11 requires TLR-4 signaling to be transcriptionally induced.

Inappropriate inflammasome activation has been associated with various diseases. **Gout** has been known for many years to cause inflammation in the cartilaginous tissues by the deposition of monosodium urate crystals, but how urate crystals caused inflammation was a mystery. Although the precise mechanism is still unclear, urate crystals are known to activate the NLRP3 inflammasome, which induces the inflammatory cytokines associated with the symptoms of gout. Mutations in NLRs can activate inflammasomes inappropriately, and they are the cause of some inherited **autoinflammatory diseases**, in which inflammation occurs in the absence of infection. Mutations in NLRP3 in humans are associated with hereditary periodic fever syndromes, such as **familial cold autoinflammatory syndrome** and **Muckle–Wells syndrome** (discussed in more detail in Chapter 13). Individuals with activating NLRC4 mutations have also been identified. Macrophages from individuals with these conditions show spontaneous production of inflammatory cytokines such as IL-1β and IL-18. We will discuss how pathogens can interfere with formation of the inflammasome in Chapter 13.

Hereditary Periodic
Fant Syndromes

3-12 Activation of innate sensors in macrophages and dendritic cells triggers changes in gene expression that have far–reaching effects on the immune response.

Besides activating effector functions and cytokine production, another outcome of the activation of innate sensing pathways is the induction of **co-stimulatory molecules** on tissue dendritic cells and macrophages (see

Fig. 3.22 Bacterial LPS induces changes in dendritic cells, stimulating them to migrate and to initiate adaptive immunity by activating T cells. Top panel: Immature dendritic cells in the skin are highly phagocytic and macropinocytic but lack the ability to activate T lymphocytes. Dendritic cells residing in the skin ingest microbes and their products and degrade them. During a bacterial infection, the dendritic cells are activated by various innate sensors, and the activation induces two types of changes. Second panel: The dendritic cells migrate out of the tissues into the lymphatic system and begin to mature. They lose the ability to ingest antigen but gain the ability to stimulate T cells. Third panel: In the regional lymph nodes, they become mature dendritic cells. They change the character of their cell-surface molecules, increasing the number of MHC molecules on their surface and the expression of the co-stimulatory molecules CD80 and CD86.

Section 1-15). We will describe these in more detail later in the book but mention them now because they provide an important link between innate and adaptive immune responses. Two important co-stimulatory molecules are the cell-surface proteins CD80 and CD86, which are induced on macrophages and tissue dendritic cells by innate sensors such as TLRs in response to pathogen recognition (**Fig. 3.22**). CD80 and CD86 are recognized by specific **co-stimulatory receptors** expressed by cells of the adaptive immune response, particularly CD4 T cells, and their activation is an important step in activating adaptive immune responses.

Substances such as LPS that induce co-stimulatory activity have been used for years in mixtures that are co-injected with protein antigens to enhance their immunogenicity. These substances are known as **adjuvants** (see Appendix I, Section A-1), and it was found empirically that the best adjuvants contain microbial components that induce macrophages and tissue dendritic cells to express co-stimulatory molecules and cytokines. We now know that the effect of these microbial components is due to activation of PRRs. As we shall see in Chapters 9 and 11, the cytokines produced in response to infections influence the functional character of the adaptive immune response that develops. In this way, the ability of the innate immune system to discriminate among different types of pathogens is used by the organism to ensure an appropriate module of the adaptive immune response is induced.

3-13 Toll signaling in *Drosophila* is downstream of a distinct set of pathogen-recognition molecules.

Before leaving innate sensing, we shall look briefly at how Toll, TLRs, and NODs are used in invertebrate innate immunity. Although Toll is central to defense against both bacterial and fungal pathogens in *Drosophila*, Toll itself is not a pattern-recognition receptor but is downstream of other proteins that detect pathogens (**Fig. 3.23**). In *Drosophila*, there are 13 genes encoding **peptidoglycan-recognition proteins (PGRPs)** that bind the peptidoglycan components of bacterial cell walls. Another family, the **Gram-negative binding proteins (GNBPs)**, recognizes LPS and β-(1,3)–linked glucans. GNBPs recognize Gram-negative bacteria and fungi rather than Gram-positive bacteria. The family members GNBP1 and PGRP-SA cooperate in the recognition of peptidoglycan from Gram-positive bacteria. They interact with a serine protease called **Grass**, which initiates a proteolytic cascade that terminates in the cleavage of the protein Spätzle. One of the cleaved fragments forms a homodimer that binds to Toll and induces its dimerization, which in turn stimulates the antimicrobial response. A fungus-specific recognition protein, GNBP3, also activates the proteolytic cascade, causing cleavage of Spätzle and activation of Toll.

In *Drosophila*, fat-body cells and hemocytes are phagocytic cells that act as part of the fly's immune system. When the Spätzle dimer binds to Toll, hemocytes synthesize and secrete antimicrobial peptides. The Toll signaling pathway in *Drosophila* activates a transcription factor called DIF, which is related to mammalian NFκB. DIF enters the nucleus and induces the transcription of genes for antimicrobial peptides such as drosomycin. Another

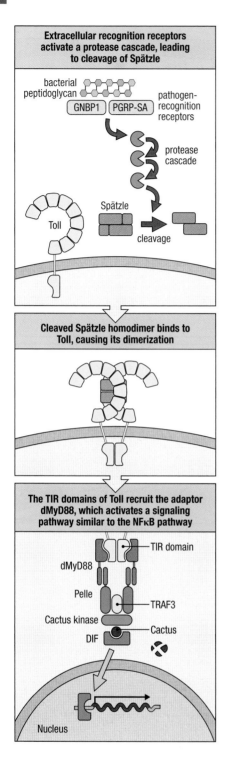

Extracellular recognition receptors activate a protease cascade, leading to cleavage of Spätzle

bacterial peptidoglycan

GNBP1 PGRP-SA

pathogen-recognition receptors

protease cascade

Spätzle

Toll

cleavage

Cleaved Spätzle homodimer binds to Toll, causing its dimerization

The TIR domains of Toll recruit the adaptor dMyD88, which activates a signaling pathway similar to the NFκB pathway

dMyD88

Pelle

Cactus kinase

DIF

TIR domain

TRAF3

Cactus

Nucleus

Fig. 3.23 *Drosophila* Toll is activated as a result of a proteolytic cascade initiated by pathogen recognition. The peptidoglycan-recognition protein PGRP-SA and the Gram-negative binding protein GNBP1 cooperate in the recognition of bacterial pathogens and activate the first protease in a protease cascade that leads to cleavage of the *Drosophila* protein Spätzle (first panel). Cleavage alters the conformation of Spätzle, enabling it to bind Toll and induce Toll dimerization (second panel). Toll's cytoplasmic TIR domains recruit the adaptor protein dMyD88 (third panel), which initiates a signaling pathway very similar to that leading to the release of NFκB from its cytoplasmic inhibitor in mammals. The *Drosophila* version of NFκB is the transcription factor DIF, which enters the nucleus and activates the transcription of genes encoding antimicrobial peptides. Fungal recognition also leads to cleavage of Spätzle and the production of antimicrobial peptides by this pathway.

Drosophila factor in the NFκB family, **Relish**, induces the production of antimicrobial peptides in response to the **Imd (immunodeficiency) signaling pathway**, which is triggered in *Drosophila* by particular PGRPs that recognize Gram-negative bacteria. Relish induces expression of the antimicrobial peptides diptericin, attacin, and cecropin, which are distinct from the peptides induced by Toll signaling. Thus, the Toll and Imd pathways activate effector mechanisms to eliminate infection by different kinds of pathogens. Four mammalian PGRP homologs have been identified but act differently than in *Drosophila*. One, PGLYRP-2, is secreted and functions as an amidase to hydrolyze bacterial peptidoglycans. The others are present in neutrophil granules and exert a bacteriostatic action through interactions with bacterial cell-wall peptidoglycan.

3-14 TLR and NOD genes have undergone extensive diversification in both invertebrates and some primitive chordates.

There are only about a dozen mammalian TLR genes, but some organisms have diversified their repertoire of innate recognition receptors, especially those containing LRR domains, to a much greater degree. The sea urchin *Strongylocentrotus purpuratus* has an unprecedented 222 different TLR genes, more than 200 NOD-like receptor genes, and more than 200 scavenger receptor genes in its genome. The sea urchin also has an increased number of proteins that are likely to be involved in signaling from these receptors, there being, for example, four genes that are similar to the single mammalian MyD88 gene. However, there is no apparent increase in the number of downstream targets, such as the family of NFκB transcription factors, suggesting that the ultimate outcome of TLR signaling in the sea urchin may be very similar to that in other organisms.

Sea urchin TLR genes fall into two broad categories. One is a small set of 11 divergent genes. The other is a large family of 211 genes, which show a high degree of sequence variation within particular LRR regions; this, together with the large number of pseudogenes in this family, indicates rapid evolutionary turnover, suggesting rapidly changing receptor specificities, in contrast with the few stable mammalian TLRs. Although the pathogen specificity of sea urchin TLRs is unknown, the hypervariability in the LRR domains could be used to generate a highly diversified pathogen-recognition system based on Toll-like receptors. A similar expansion of innate receptors has occurred in some chordates, the phylum to which vertebrates belong. Amphioxus (the lancelet) is a nonvertebrate chordate lacking an adaptive immune system. The amphioxus genome contains 71 TLRs, more than 100 NOD-like receptors, and more than 200 scavenger receptors. As we will see in Chapter 5, a primitive vertebrate lineage—the jawless fishes, which lack immunoglobulin-based and T cell–based adaptive immunity—uses somatic gene rearrangement of LRR-containing proteins to provide a version of adaptive immunity (see Section 5-18).

Summary.

Innate immune cells express several receptor systems that recognize microbes and induce rapid defenses as well as delayed cellular responses. Several scavenger and lectin-like receptors on neutrophils, macrophages, and dendritic cells help rapidly eliminate microbes through phagocytosis. G protein–coupled receptors for C5a (which can be produced by activation of the complement system's innate pathogen-recognition ability) and for the bacterial peptide fMLF synergize with phagocytic receptors in activating the NADPH oxidase in phagosomes to generate antimicrobial reactive oxygen intermediates. Toll-like receptors (TLRs) on the cell surface and in the membranes of endosomes detect microbes outside the cell and activate several host-defense signaling pathways. The NFκB and IRF pathways downstream of these receptors induce pro-inflammatory cytokines, including TNF-α, IL-1β, and IL-6, and antiviral cytokines including type I interferons. Other receptor families detect microbial infection in the cytosol. RIG-I and MDA-5 detect viral infection by sensing the presence of viral RNAs and activate the MAVS pathway, while cGAS senses cytosolic DNA and activates the STING pathway; both of these pathways induce type I interferons. NLR proteins detect pathogen products within the cytosol or sense changes to the cell due to pathogen infection. Some NLRs activate NFκB and induce the production of pro-inflammatory cytokines, while others form inflammasomes, leading to secretion of pro-inflammatory cytokines and pyroptotic cell death. The signaling pathways activated by all of these primary sensors of pathogens induce a variety of genes, including those for cytokines, chemokines, and co-stimulatory molecules that have essential roles in immediate defense and in directing the course of the adaptive immune response later in infection.

Consequences of innate immune activation.

We will now examine the responses of innate immunity induced as an immediate consequence of pathogen recognition by the sensors described in the first half of this chapter. We will focus on the major phagocytes—neutrophils, macrophages, and dendritic cells—and the cytokines they produce that induce and maintain inflammation. First, we will introduce the families of cytokines and chemokines that coordinate many cellular responses, such as the recruitment of neutrophils and other immune cells to sites of infection. We will discuss the various adhesion molecules that are induced on immune cells circulating in the blood and on endothelial cells of blood vessels to coordinate movement of cells out of the blood and into infected tissues. We will consider in some detail how macrophage-derived chemokines and cytokines promote the continued destruction of infecting microbes. This is achieved both by stimulating the production and recruitment of fresh phagocytes and by inducing another phase of the innate immune response—the acute-phase response—in which the liver produces proteins that act as opsonizing molecules, helping to augment the actions of complement. We will also look at the mechanism of action of antiviral interferons, the type I interferons, and finally examine the growing class of innate lymphoid cells, or ILCs, which include the NK cells that contribute to innate immune defense against viruses, other intracellular pathogens, and even cancerous cells. ILCs exert a diverse array of effector functions that contribute to a rapid innate immune response to infection. They respond to early cytokine signals provided by innate sensor cells and amplify the response by producing various types of effector cytokines. Some time after induction of the innate response, an adaptive response will ensue that uses many of the same effector mechanisms used by the innate immune system but targets them with much greater precision. The effector mechanisms described here therefore serve as a primer for the focus on adaptive immunity in the later parts of this book.

3-15 Cytokines and their receptors fall into distinct families of structurally related proteins.

Cytokines are small proteins (about 25 kDa) that are released by various cells in the body, usually in response to an activating stimulus, and that induce responses through binding to specific receptors. Cytokines can act in an **autocrine** manner, affecting the behavior of the cell that releases the cytokine, or in a **paracrine** manner, affecting adjacent cells. Some cytokines are even stable enough to act in an **endocrine** manner, affecting distant cells, although this depends on their ability to enter the circulation and on their half-life in the blood. In an attempt to develop a standardized nomenclature for molecules secreted by, and acting on, leukocytes, many cytokines are called by the name **interleukin (IL)** followed by a number (for example, IL-1 or IL-2). However, not all cytokines are included in this system; thus, students of immunology are still faced with a somewhat confusing and difficult task. The cytokines are listed alphabetically, together with their receptors, in eAppendix III.

Cytokines can be grouped by structure into families—the IL-1 family, the hematopoietin superfamily, the interferons (described in Section 3-7), the TNF family, and chemokines—and their receptors can likewise be grouped (**Fig. 3.24**). The **IL-1 family** contains 11 members, notably IL-1α, IL-1β, IL-18, and IL-33. Most members of this family are produced as inactive proproteins that are cleaved (removing an amino-terminal peptide) to produce the mature cytokine. The exception to this rule is IL-1α, for which both the proprotein and its cleaved forms are biologically active. As discussed earlier (see Section 3-11), mature IL-1β and IL-18 are produced by macrophages through the action of caspase 1 in response to TLR signaling and inflammasome activation. The IL-1 family receptors have TIR domains in their cytoplasmic tails and signal by the NFκB pathway described earlier for TLRs. The IL-1 receptor functions in concert with a second transmembrane protein, the IL-1 receptor accessory protein (IL1RAP), which is required for IL-1 signal transduction.

The **hematopoietin superfamily** of cytokines is quite large and includes non-immune-system growth and differentiation factors, such as erythropoietin (which stimulates red blood cell development), as well as interleukins with roles in innate immunity and adaptive immunity. IL-6 is a member of this superfamily, as is the cytokine GM-CSF, which stimulates the production of new monocytes and granulocytes in the bone marrow. Many of the soluble cytokines made by activated T cells are members of the hematopoietin superfamily. The receptors for the hematopoietin cytokines are tyrosine kinase–associated receptors that form dimers when their cytokine ligand binds. Dimerization initiates intracellular signaling from the tyrosine kinases associated with the cytoplasmic domains of the receptor. Some types of cytokine receptors are composed of two identical subunits, but others have two different subunits. An important feature of cytokine signaling is the large variety of different receptor subunit combinations that occur.

These cytokines and their receptors can also be further divided into subfamilies characterized by functional similarities and genetic linkage. For instance, IL-3, IL-4, IL-5, IL-13, and GM-CSF are related structurally, their genes are closely linked in the genome, and they are often produced together by the same kinds of cells. In addition, they bind to closely related receptors, which belong to the family of **class I cytokine receptors**. The IL-3, IL-5, and GM-CSF receptors form a subgroup that shares a **common β chain (β_c)**. Another subgroup of class I cytokine receptors is defined by a **common γ chain (γ_c)** of the IL-2 receptor. This chain is shared by receptors for the cytokines IL-2, IL-4, IL-7, IL-9, IL-15, and IL-21 and is encoded by a gene located on the X chromosome. Mutations

Homodimeric receptors		Receptors for erythropoietin and growth hormone
Heterodimeric receptors with a common chain	β_c	Receptors for IL-3, IL-5, GM-CSF share a common chain, CD131 or β_c (common β chain)
	γ_c	Receptors for IL-2, IL-4, IL-7, IL-9, IL-15, and IL-21 share a common chain, CD132 or γ_c (common γ chain). IL-2 receptor also has a third chain, a high-affinity subunit IL-2Rα (CD25)
Heterodimeric receptors (no common chain)		IL-1 family receptors
		Receptors for IL-13, IFN-α, IFN-β, IFN-γ, IL-10
TNF receptor family		Tumor necrosis factor (TNF) receptors I and II, CD40, Fas (Apo1, CD95), CD30, CD27, nerve growth factor receptor
Chemokine receptor family		CCR1–10, CXCR1–5, XCR1, CX3CR1

Fig. 3.24 Cytokine receptors belong to families of receptor proteins, each with a distinctive structure. Many cytokines signal through receptors of the hematopoietin receptor superfamily, named after its first member, the erythropoietin receptor. The hematopoietin receptor superfamily includes homodimeric and heterodimeric receptors, which are subdivided into families on the basis of protein sequence and structure. Examples of these are given in the first three rows. Heterodimeric class I cytokine receptors have an α chain that often defines the ligand specificity of the receptor; they may share with other receptors a common β or γ chain that confers the intracellular signaling function. Heterodimeric class II cytokine receptors have no common chain and include receptors for interferons or interferon-like cytokines. Many cytokine receptors signal through the JAK–STAT pathway. The IL-1 family receptors have extracellular immunoglobulin domains and signal as dimers through TIR domains in their cytoplasmic tails and through MyD88. Other families of cytokine receptors are the tumor necrosis factor receptor (TNFR) family and the chemokine receptor family, the latter belonging to the very large family of G protein–coupled receptors. The ligands of the TNFR family act as trimers and may be associated with the cell membrane rather than being secreted.

that inactivate γ_c cause an **X-linked severe combined immune deficiency (X-linked SCID)** because of inactivation of the signaling pathways for several cytokines—IL-7, IL-15, and IL-2—that are required for normal lymphocyte development (see Section 13-2). More distantly related, the receptor for IFN-γ is a member of a small family of heterodimeric cytokine receptors with some similarities to the hematopoietin receptor superfamily. These so-called **class II cytokine receptors** (also known as interferon receptors) include the receptors for IFN-α and IFN-β and the IL-10 receptor. The hematopoietin and interferon receptors all signal through the JAK–STAT pathway described in the next section and activate different combinations of STATs with different effects.

The **TNF family**, of which TNF-α is the prototype, contains more than 17 cytokines with important functions in adaptive immunity and innate immunity. Unlike most of the other immunologically important cytokines, many members of the TNF family are transmembrane proteins, a characteristic that gives them distinct properties and limits their range of action. Some, however, can be released from the membrane in some circumstances. They are usually found as homotrimers of a membrane-bound subunit, although

X-linked Severe Combined Immune Deficiency

some heterotrimers consisting of different subunits also occur. TNF-α (sometimes called simply TNF) is initially expressed as a trimeric membrane-bound cytokine but can be released from the membrane. The effects of TNF-α are mediated by either of two **TNF receptors**. TNF receptor I (TNFR-I) is expressed on a wide range of cells, including endothelial cells and macrophages, whereas TNFR-II is expressed largely by lymphocytes. The receptors for cytokines of the TNF family are structurally unrelated to the receptors described above and also have to cluster to become activated. Because TNF family cytokines are produced as trimers, the binding of these cytokines induces the clustering of three identical receptor subunits. The signaling pathway activated by these receptors is described in Chapter 7, where we see that signaling uses members of the TRAF family to activate the so-called non-canonical NFκB pathway.

Members of the chemokine receptor family are listed in eAppendix IV, along with the chemokines they recognize. These receptors have a seven-transmembrane structure and signal by interacting with G proteins as described in Section 3-2.

3-16 Cytokine receptors of the hematopoietin superfamily are associated with the JAK family of tyrosine kinases, which activate STAT transcription factors.

The signaling chains of the hematopoietin superfamily of cytokine receptors are noncovalently associated with protein tyrosine kinases of the **Janus kinase (JAK) family**—so called because they have two tandem kinase-like domains and thus resemble the two-headed mythical Roman god Janus. There are four members of the JAK family: Jak1, Jak2, Jak3, and Tyk2. Because mice deficient for individual JAK family members show different phenotypes, each kinase must have a distinct function. For example, Jak3 is used by γ_c for signaling by several of the cytokines described above. Mutations that inactivate Jak3 cause a form of **SCID** that is not X-linked.

ANIMATION 3.7

The dimerization or clustering of receptor signaling chains brings the JAKs into close proximity, causing phosphorylation of each JAK on a tyrosine residue that stimulates its kinase activity. The activated JAKs then phosphorylate their associated receptors on specific tyrosine residues. This phosphotyrosine, and the specific amino acid sequence surrounding it, creates a binding site that is recognized by **SH2 domains** found in other proteins, in particular members of a family of transcription factors known as **signal transducers and activators of transcription (STATs)** (**Fig. 3.25**).

There are seven STATs (1–4, 5a, 5b, and 6), which reside in the cytoplasm in an inactive form until activated by cytokine receptors. Before activation, most STATs form homodimers, due to a specific homotypic interaction between domains present at the amino termini of the individual STAT monomers. The receptor specificity of each STAT is determined by the recognition of the distinctive phosphotyrosine sequence on each activated receptor by the different SH2 domains within the various STAT proteins. Recruitment of a STAT to the activated receptor brings the STAT close to an activated JAK, which can then phosphorylate the conserved tyrosine residue in the carboxyl terminus of each of the STATs. This leads to a rearrangement of the STAT dimer, in which the phosphotyrosine of each STAT monomer binds to the SH2 domain of the other STAT monomer, forming a configuration that can bind DNA with high affinity. Activated STATs predominantly form homodimers, with a cytokine typically activating one type of STAT. For example, IFN-γ activates STAT1 and generates STAT1 homodimers, whereas IL-4 activates STAT6, generating STAT6 homodimers. Other cytokine receptors can activate several STATs, and some STAT heterodimers can be formed, such as STAT1–STAT2 heterodimers formed downstream of the receptor for

| Cytokine receptors consist of at least two chains, the cytoplasmic domains of which bind Janus kinases (JAKs) | Cytokine binding dimerizes the receptor, bringing together the cytoplasmic JAKs, which activate each other and phosphorylate the receptor | Transcription factors (STATs) bind to the phosphorylated receptors, and are in turn phosphorylated by the activated JAKs | Phosphorylated STATs form dimers that translocate into the nucleus to initiate gene transcription |

Fig. 3.25 Many cytokine receptors signal using a rapid pathway called the JAK–STAT pathway. First panel: Many cytokines act via receptors that are associated with cytoplasmic Janus kinases (JAKs). The receptor consists of at least two chains, each associated with a specific JAK. Second panel: Binding of ligand brings the two chains together, allowing the JAKs to phosphorylate and activate each other, and then to phosphorylate (red dots) specific tyrosines in the receptor tails. Each member of the STAT (signal transducer and activator of transcription) family of proteins has an N-terminal domain that homodimerizes STAT monomers in the cytosol before activation and an SH2 domain that binds to a tyrosine-phosphorylated cytokine receptor tail. Third panel: Upon binding, the STAT homodimers are phosphorylated on a conserved tyrosine residue in their carboxyl terminus by JAKs. Fourth panel: After phosphorylation, the STAT dimer reconfigures into a dimer that is stabilized by the SH2 domain of one monomer binding to a phosphotyrosine residue on the other monomer. They then translocate to the nucleus, where they bind to and activate the transcription of a variety of genes important for adaptive immunity.

IFN-α and IFN-β. The phosphorylated STAT dimer enters the nucleus, where it acts as a transcription factor to initiate the expression of selected genes that can regulate growth, differentiation, and/or survival of particular subsets of lymphocytes.

Because signaling by these receptors depends on tyrosine phosphorylation, dephosphorylation of the receptor complex by **tyrosine phosphatases** is one way that cells can terminate signaling. A variety of tyrosine phosphatases have been implicated in the dephosphorylation of cytokine receptors, JAKs, and STATs. These include the nonreceptor tyrosine phosphatases SHP-1 and SHP-2 (encoded by *PTPN6* and *PTPN11*) and the transmembrane receptor tyrosine phosphatase **CD45**, which is expressed as multiple isoforms on many hematopoietic cells. Cytokine signaling can also be terminated by negative feedback involving specific inhibitors that are induced by cytokine activation. The **suppressor of cytokine signaling (SOCS)** proteins are a class of inhibitors that terminate the signaling of many cytokine and hormone receptors. SOCS proteins contain an SH2 domain that can recruit them to the phosphorylated JAK protein or receptor, and they can inhibit JAK activity directly, or compete for the receptor, and direct the ubiquitination and subsequent degradation of JAKs and STATs. SOCS proteins are induced by STAT activation and thus inhibit receptor signaling after the cytokine has had its effect. Their importance can be seen in SOCS1-deficient mice, which develop a multiorgan inflammatory infiltrate caused by increased signaling from interferon receptors, γ_c-containing receptors, and TLRs. Another class of inhibitory proteins, the **protein inhibitors of activated STAT (PIAS)**, regulate the response to cytokines, as well as other biological pathways, by promoting the degradation of pathway components.

3-17 Chemokines released by macrophages and dendritic cells recruit effector cells to sites of infection.

All the cytokines produced by macrophages in innate immune responses have important local and systemic effects that contribute to both innate and adaptive immunity, and these are summarized in **Fig. 3.26**. The recognition of different classes of pathogens by phagocytes and dendritic cells may involve signaling through different receptors, such as the various TLRs, and can result in some variation in the cytokines expressed by stimulated macrophages and dendritic cells. This is one way in which appropriate immune responses can be selectively activated, as the released cytokines orchestrate the next phase of host defense. In response to activation by PRRs, macrophages and dendritic cells secrete a diverse group of cytokines that includes IL-1β, IL-6, IL-12, TNF-α, and the chemokine CXCL8 (formerly known as IL-8).

Among the cytokines released by tissues in the earliest phases of infection are members of a family of chemoattractant cytokines known as chemokines. These small proteins induce directed **chemotaxis** in nearby responsive cells, resulting in the movement of the cells toward the source of the chemokine. Because chemokines were first detected in functional assays, they were initially given a variety of names, which are listed along with their standardized nomenclature in eAppendix IV. All the chemokines are related in amino acid sequence, and their receptors are G protein–coupled receptors (see Section 3-2). The signaling pathway stimulated by chemokines causes changes in cell adhesiveness and changes in the cell's cytoskeleton that lead to directed migration. Chemokines can be produced and released by many different types of cells, not only those of the immune system. In the immune system they function mainly as chemoattractants for leukocytes, recruiting monocytes, neutrophils, and other effector cells of innate immunity from the blood into sites of

ANIMATION 3.8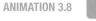

Fig. 3.26 Important cytokines and chemokines secreted by dendritic cells and macrophages in response to bacterial products include IL-1β, IL-6, CXCL8, IL-12, and TNF-α. TNF-α is an inducer of a local inflammatory response that helps to contain infections. It also has systemic effects, many of which are harmful (discussed in Section 3-20). The chemokine CXCL8 is also involved in the local inflammatory response, helping to attract neutrophils to the site of infection. IL-1β, IL-6, and TNF-α have a crucial role in inducing the acute-phase response in the liver and inducing fever, which favors effective host defense in various ways. IL-12 activates natural killer (NK) cells and favors the differentiation of CD4 T cells into the T_H1 subset in adaptive immunity.

infection. They also guide lymphocytes in adaptive immunity, as we will learn in Chapters 9–11. Some chemokines also function in lymphocyte development and migration and in angiogenesis (the growth of new blood vessels). There are more than 50 known chemokines, and this striking multiplicity may reflect their importance in delivering cells to their correct locations, which seems to be their main function in the case of lymphocytes. Some of the chemokines that are produced by or that affect human innate immune cells are listed in **Fig. 3.27**, along with their properties.

Chemokines fall mainly into two related but distinct groups. **CC chemokines** have two adjacent cysteine residues near the amino terminus, whereas in **CXC chemokines** the corresponding two cysteine residues are separated by a single amino acid. The CC chemokines promote the migration of monocytes, lymphocytes, and other cell types. One example relevant to innate immunity is CCL2, which attracts monocytes through the receptor CCR2B, inducing their migration from the bloodstream to become tissue macrophages. In contrast, neutrophil migration is promoted by CXC chemokines. CXCL8, acting through CXCR2, mobilizes neutrophils from bone marrow and induces them to leave the blood and migrate into the surrounding tissues. CCL2 and CXCL8 therefore have similar but complementary functions in the innate immune response, attracting monocytes and neutrophils, respectively.

The role of chemokines in cell recruitment is twofold. First, they act on the leukocyte as it rolls along endothelial cells at sites of inflammation, converting this rolling into stable binding by triggering a change of conformation in the adhesion molecules known as leukocyte integrins. These conformational changes enable integrins to bind strongly to their ligands on the endothelial

Fig. 3.27 Properties of selected human chemokines. Chemokines fall mainly into two related but distinct groups: the CC chemokines, which have two adjacent cysteine residues near the amino terminus; and the CXC chemokines, in which the equivalent cysteine residues are separated by a single amino acid. In humans, the genes for CC chemokines are mostly clustered in one region of chromosome 4. Genes for CXC chemokines are found mainly in a cluster on chromosome 17. The two groups of chemokines act on different sets of receptors, all of which are G protein–coupled receptors. CC chemokines bind to receptors designated CCR1–10. CXC chemokines bind to receptors designated CXCR1–7. Different receptors are expressed on different cell types, and so a particular chemokine can be used to attract a particular cell type. In general, CXC chemokines with a Glu-Leu-Arg tripeptide motif immediately before the first cysteine promote the migration of neutrophils. CXCL8 is an example of this type. Most of the other CXC chemokines, including those that interact with receptors CXCR3, 4, and 5, lack this motif. Fractalkine is unusual in several respects: it has three amino acid residues between the two cysteines, and it exists in two forms, one that is tethered to the membrane of the endothelial and epithelial cells that express it, where it serves as an adhesion protein, and a soluble form that is released from the cell surface and acts as a chemoattractant for a wide range of cell types. A more comprehensive list of chemokines and their receptors is given in eAppendix IV.

Class	Chemokine	Produced by	Receptors	Cells attracted	Major effects
CXC	CXCL8 (IL-8)	Monocytes Macrophages Fibroblasts Epithelial cells Endothelial cells	CXCR1 CXCR2	Neutrophils Naive T cells	Mobilizes, activates, and degranulates neutrophils Angiogenesis
CXC	CXCL7 (PBP, β-TG, NAP-2)	Platelets	CXCR2	Neutrophils	Activates neutrophils Clot resorption Angiogenesis
CXC	CXCL1 (GROα) CXCL2 (GROβ) CXCL3 (GROγ)	Monocytes Fibroblasts Endothelium	CXCR2	Neutrophils Naive T cells Fibroblasts	Activates neutrophils Fibroplasia Angiogenesis
CC	CCL3 (MIP-1α)	Monocytes T cells Mast cells Fibroblasts	CCR1, 3, 5	Monocytes NK and T cells Basophils Dendritic cells	Competes with HIV-1 Antiviral defense Promotes T_H1 immunity
CC	CCL4 (MIP-1β)	Monocytes Macrophages Neutrophils Endothelium	CCR1, 3, 5	Monocytes NK and T cells Dendritic cells	Competes with HIV-1
CC	CCL2 (MCP-1)	Monocytes Macrophages Fibroblasts Keratinocytes	CCR2B	Monocytes NK and T cells Basophils Dendritic cells	Activates macrophages Basophil histamine release Promotes T_H2 immunity
CC	CCL5 (RANTES)	T cells Endothelium Platelets	CCR1, 3, 5	Monocytes NK and T cells Basophils Eosinophils Dendritic cells	Degranulates basophils Activates T cells Chronic inflammation
CXXXC (CX₃C)	CX3CL1 (Fractalkine)	Monocytes Endothelium Microglial cells	CX₃CR1	Monocytes T cells	Leukocyte–endothelial adhesion Brain inflammation

ANIMATION 3.9

cells, which allows the leukocyte to cross the blood vessel walls by squeezing between the endothelial cells. Second, the chemokine directs the migration of the leukocyte along a gradient of chemokine molecules bound to the extracellular matrix and the surfaces of endothelial cells. This gradient increases in concentration toward the site of infection.

Chemokines are produced by a wide variety of cell types in response to bacterial products, viruses, and agents that cause physical damage, such as silica, alum, or the urate crystals that occur in gout. Complement fragments, such as C3a and C5a, and fMLF bacterial peptides also act as chemoattractants for neutrophils. Thus, infection or physical damage to tissues induces the production of chemokine gradients that can direct phagocytes to the sites where they are needed. Neutrophils arrive rapidly in large numbers at a site of infection. The recruitment of monocytes occurs simultaneously, but they accumulate more slowly at the site of infection, perhaps because they are less abundant in the circulation. The complement fragment C5a and the chemokines CXCL8 and CCL2 activate their respective target cells, so that not only are neutrophils and monocytes brought to potential sites of infection, but also, in the process, they are armed to deal with the pathogens they encounter there. In particular, the signaling induced by C5a or CXCL8 in neutrophils serves to augment the respiratory burst that generates oxygen radicals and nitric oxide and to induce the neutrophils to release their stored antimicrobial granule contents (see Section 3-2).

Chemokines do not act alone in cell recruitment. They require the action of vasoactive mediators that bring leukocytes close to the blood vessel wall (see Section 3-3) and cytokines such as TNF-α to induce the necessary adhesion molecules on endothelial cells. We will return to the chemokines in later chapters, where they are discussed in the context of the adaptive immune response. Now, however, we turn to the molecules that enable leukocytes to adhere to the endothelium, and we shall then describe step by step the extravasation process by which monocytes and neutrophils enter infected sites.

3-18 Cell-adhesion molecules control interactions between leukocytes and endothelial cells during an inflammatory response.

The recruitment of activated phagocytes to sites of infection is one of the most important functions of innate immunity. Recruitment occurs as part of the inflammatory response and is mediated by cell-adhesion molecules that are induced on the surface of the endothelial cells of local blood vessels. Here we consider those functions that participate in the recruitment of inflammatory cells in the hours to days after the establishment of an infection.

ANIMATION 3.10

As with the complement components, a significant barrier to understanding the functions of cell-adhesion molecules is their nomenclature. Most adhesion molecules, especially those on leukocytes, which are relatively easy to analyze functionally, were originally named after the effects of specific monoclonal antibodies directed against them. Their names therefore bear no relation to their structural class. For instance, the **leukocyte functional antigens** LFA-1, LFA-2, and LFA-3 are actually members of two different protein families. In **Fig. 3.28**, the adhesion molecules relevant to innate immunity are grouped according to their molecular structure, which is shown in schematic form alongside their different names, sites of expression, and ligands. Three structural families of adhesion molecules are important for leukocyte recruitment. The **selectins** are membrane glycoproteins with a distal lectin-like domain that binds specific carbohydrate groups. Members of this family are induced on activated endothelium and initiate endothelium–leukocyte interactions by binding to fucosylated oligosaccharide ligands on passing leukocytes (see Fig. 3.28).

	Name	Tissue distribution	Ligand
Selectins Bind carbohydrates. Initiate leukocyte–endothelial interaction	P-selectin	P-selectin (PADGEM, CD62P)	Activated endothelium and platelets	PSGL-1, sialyl-Lewis^X
		E-selectin (ELAM-1, CD62E)	Activated endothelium	Sialyl-Lewis^X
Integrins Bind to cell-adhesion molecules and extracellular matrix. Strong adhesion	LFA-1	$\alpha_L\beta_2$ (LFA-1, CD11a:CD18)	Monocytes, T cells, macrophages, neutrophils, dendritic cells, NK cells	ICAM-1, ICAM-2
		$\alpha_M\beta_2$ (CR3, Mac-1, CD11b:CD18)	Neutrophils, monocytes, macrophages, NK cells	ICAM-1, iC3b, fibrinogen
		$\alpha_X\beta_2$ (CR4, p150.95, CD11c:CD18)	Dendritic cells, macrophages, neutrophils, NK cells	iC3b
		$\alpha_5\beta_1$ (VLA-5, CD49d:CD29)	Monocytes, macrophages	Fibronectin
Immunoglobulin superfamily Various roles in cell adhesion. Ligand for integrins	ICAM-1	ICAM-1 (CD54)	Activated endothelium, activated leukocytes	LFA-1, Mac-1
		ICAM-2 (CD102)	Resting endothelium, dendritic cells	LFA-1
		VCAM-1 (CD106)	Activated endothelium	VLA-4
		PECAM (CD31)	Activated leukocytes, endothelial cell–cell junctions	CD31

Fig. 3.28 Adhesion molecules involved in leukocyte interactions. Three structural families of adhesion molecules have a role in leukocyte migration, homing, and cell–cell interactions: the selectins, the integrins, and proteins of the immunoglobulin superfamily. The figure shows schematic representations of an example from each family, a list of other family members that participate in leukocyte interactions, their cellular distribution, and their ligand in adhesive interactions. The family members shown here are limited to those that participate in inflammation and other innate immune mechanisms. The same molecules and others participate in adaptive immunity and will be considered in Chapters 9 and 11. The nomenclature of the different molecules in these families is confusing because it often reflects the way in which the molecules were first identified rather than their related structural characteristics. Alternative names for each of the adhesion molecules are given in parentheses. Sulfated sialyl-Lewis^X, which is recognized by P-selectin and E-selectin, is an oligosaccharide present on the cell-surface glycoproteins of circulating leukocytes.

The next step in leukocyte recruitment depends on tighter adhesion, which is due to the binding of **intercellular adhesion molecules (ICAMs)** on the endothelium to heterodimeric proteins of the **integrin** family on leukocytes. ICAMs are single-pass membrane proteins that belong to the large superfamily of **immunoglobulin-like proteins**, which contain protein domains similar to those of immunoglobulins. The extracellular regions of ICAMs are composed of several immunoglobulin-like domains. An integrin molecule is composed of two transmembrane protein chains, α and β, of which there are numerous different types. Subsets of integrins have a common β chain partnered with different α chains. The leukocyte integrins important for extravasation are **LFA-1** ($\alpha_L\beta_2$, also known as **CD11a:CD18**) and **CR3** ($\alpha_M\beta_2$, complement receptor 3, also known as **CD11b:CD18** or Mac-1). We described CR3 in Section 2-13 as a receptor for iC3b, but it also binds other ligands. Both LFA-1 and CR3 bind to ICAM-1 (**Fig. 3.29**). Even in the absence of infection, circulating monocytes are continually leaving the blood and entering certain tissues, such as the intestine, where they become resident macrophages. LFA-1 also binds to ICAM-2. To navigate out of the blood vessel, monocytes may adhere to ICAM-2, which is expressed at low levels by unactivated endothelium. CR3 also binds to fibrinogen and factor X, both substrates of the coagulation cascade.

Strong adhesion between leukocytes and endothelial cells is promoted by the induction of ICAM-1 on inflamed endothelium together with a conformational change in LFA-1 and CR3 that occurs on the leukocyte. Integrins can switch between an 'active' state, in which they bind strongly to their ligands, and an 'inactive' state, in which binding is easily broken. This enables cells to make and break integrin-mediated adhesions in response to signals received by the cell either through the integrin itself or through other receptors. In the

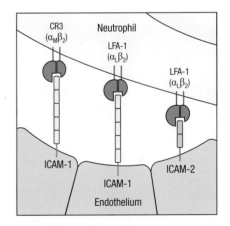

Fig. 3.29 Phagocyte adhesion to vascular endothelium is mediated by integrins. When vascular endothelium is activated by inflammatory mediators it expresses two adhesion molecules, namely ICAM-1 and ICAM-2. These are ligands for integrins expressed by phagocytes—ICAM-1 for $\alpha_M\beta_2$ (also called CR3, Mac-1, or CD11b:CD18), and ICAM-1 and ICAM-2 for $\alpha_L\beta_2$ (also called LFA-1 or CD11a:CD18).

activated state, an integrin molecule is linked via the intracellular protein **talin** to the actin cytoskeleton. In the case of migrating leukocytes, chemokines binding to their receptors on the leukocyte generate intracellular signals that cause talin to bind to the cytoplasmic tails of the β chains of LFA-1 and CR3, forcing the integrin extracellular regions to assume an active binding conformation. The importance of leukocyte integrin function in inflammatory-cell recruitment is illustrated by **leukocyte adhesion deficiencies (LADs)**, which can be caused by defects in the integrins themselves or in the proteins required for modulating adhesion. People with these diseases suffer from recurrent bacterial infections and impaired healing of wounds.

Endothelial activation is driven by macrophage-produced cytokines, particularly TNF-α, which induce the rapid externalization of granules called **Weibel–Palade bodies** in the endothelial cells. These granules contain preformed **P-selectin**, which appears on the surfaces of local endothelial cells just minutes after macrophages have responded to the presence of microbes by producing TNF-α. Shortly after P-selectin gets to the cell surface, mRNA encoding **E-selectin** is synthesized, and within 2 hours the endothelial cells are expressing mainly E-selectin. Both P-selectin and E-selectin interact with **sulfated sialyl-Lewis^X**, a sulfated form of a carbohydrate structure that is also an important blood group antigen. Sulfated sialyl-Lewis^X is present on the surface of neutrophils, and its interactions with P-selectin and E-selectin are important for neutrophil rolling on the endothelium. Mutations in enzymes involved in its synthesis, such as fucosyltransferase, cause defective sialyl-Lewis^X expression that results in an immunodeficiency, **leukocyte adhesion deficiency type 2**.

Integrins are also convenient cell-surface markers for distinguishing different cell types. Dendritic cells, macrophages, and monocytes express different integrin α chains and thus display distinct β2 integrins on their surface. The predominant leukocyte integrin on conventional dendritic cells is $\alpha_X\beta_2$, also known as **CD11c:CD18** or complement receptor 4 (**CR4**) (see Fig. 3.28). This integrin is a receptor for the complement C3 cleavage product iC3b, fibrinogen, and ICAM-1. In contrast to conventional dendritic cells, most monocytes and macrophages express low levels of CD11c and predominantly express the integrin $\alpha_M\beta_2$ (CD11b:CD18; CR3). However, patterns of integrin expression can vary, with some tissue macrophages, such as those in the lung, expressing high levels of CD11c:CD18. In the mouse, the two major branches of conventional dendritic cells can be distinguished by expression of CD11b:CD18: one branch characterized by high expression of CD11b:CD18, and a second branch that lacks CD11b:CD18. Plasmacytoid dendritic cells (pDCs) express lower levels of CD11c but can be distinguished from conventional dendritic cells using other markers; human pDCs express the C-type lectin **BDCA-2 (blood dendritic cell antigen 2)**, and mouse pDCs express **BST2 (bone marrow stromal antigen 2)**, neither of which is expressed by conventional dendritic cells.

3-19 Neutrophils make up the first wave of cells that cross the blood vessel wall to enter an inflamed tissue.

The migration of leukocytes out of blood vessels, the process known as extravasation, occurs in response to signals generated at sites of infection. Under normal conditions, leukocytes travel in the center of small blood vessels, where blood flow is fastest. Within sites of inflammation, the vessels are dilated and the consequent slower blood flow allows leukocytes to interact in large numbers with the vascular endothelium. During an inflammatory response, the induction of adhesion molecules on the endothelial cells of blood vessels within the infected tissue, as well as changes in the adhesion molecules expressed on leukocytes, recruits large numbers of circulating leukocytes to the site of infection. We will describe this process with regard to monocytes and neutrophils (**Fig. 3.30**).

Selectin-mediated adhesion to leukocyte sialyl-Lewisˣ is weak and allows leukocytes to roll along the vascular endothelial surface

blood flow ➤

s-Leˣ

E-selectin

vascular endothelial cell

basement membrane

| Rolling adhesion | Tight binding | Diapedesis | Migration |

CXCL8R (IL-8 receptor)

s-Leˣ

E-selectin

LFA-1 ($\alpha_L\beta_2$)

ICAM-1

CD31

chemokine CXCL8 (IL-8)

Fig. 3.30 Neutrophils leave the blood and migrate to sites of infection in a multistep process involving adhesive interactions that are regulated by macrophage-derived cytokines and chemokines. Top panel: The first step involves the reversible binding of a neutrophil to vascular endothelium through interactions between selectins induced on the endothelium and their carbohydrate ligands on the neutrophil, shown here for E-selectin and its ligand, the sialyl-Lewisˣ moiety (s-Leˣ). This interaction cannot anchor the cells against the shearing force of the flow of blood, and thus they roll along the endothelium, continually making and breaking contact. Bottom panel: The binding does, however, eventually trigger stronger interactions, which result only when binding of a chemokine such as CXCL8 to its specific receptor on the neutrophil triggers the activation of the integrins LFA-1 and CR3 (Mac-1; not shown). Inflammatory cytokines such as TNF-α are also necessary to induce the expression of adhesion molecules such as ICAM-1 and ICAM-2, the ligands for these integrins, on the vascular endothelium. Tight binding between ICAM-1 and the integrins arrests the rolling and allows the neutrophil to squeeze between the endothelial cells forming the wall of the blood vessel (that is, to extravasate). The leukocyte integrins LFA-1 and CR3 are required for extravasation and for migration toward chemoattractants. Adhesion between molecules of CD31, expressed on both the neutrophil and the junction of the endothelial cells, is also thought to contribute to extravasation. The neutrophil also needs to traverse the basement membrane; it penetrates this with the aid of a matrix metalloproteinase enzyme, MMP-9, that it expresses at the cell surface. Finally, the neutrophil migrates along a concentration gradient of chemokines (shown here as CXCL8) secreted by cells at the site of infection.

 ANIMATION 3.12

Extravasation proceeds in four stages. In the first, induction of selectins enables leukocyte rolling along the endothelium. P-selectin appears on endothelial cell surfaces within a few minutes of exposure to leukotriene B4, C5a, or histamine, which is released from mast cells in response to C5a. P-selectin can also be induced by TNF-α or LPS, and both of these induce synthesis of E-selectin, which appears on the endothelial cell surface a few hours later. When the sulfated sialyl-Lewisˣ on monocytes and neutrophils contacts these exposed P- and E-selectins, these cells adhere reversibly to the vessel wall and begin to 'roll' along endothelium (see Fig. 3.30, top panel), permitting stronger interactions of the next step in leukocyte migration. Neutrophils are particularly efficient at rolling along endothelium, even under flow rates that prevent rolling by other cells. Such **shear-resistant rolling** by neutrophils uses long extensions of plasma membrane, termed **slings**, that bind the endothelium and wrap around the cell as it rolls, serving to tether the cell firmly to the endothelium and to promote rapid entry to sites of infection.

The second step depends on interactions between the leukocyte integrins LFA-1 and CR3 and adhesion molecules such as ICAM-1 (which can be induced on endothelial cells by TNF-α) or ICAM-2 on endothelium (see Fig. 3.30, bottom panel). LFA-1 and CR3 normally bind their ligands only weakly, but CXCL8 (or other chemokines), bound to proteoglycans on the surface of endothelial cells, binds to specific chemokine receptors on the leukocyte and signals the cell to trigger a conformational change in LFA-1 and CR3 on

ANIMATION 3.13

the rolling leukocyte; this greatly increases the adhesive properties of the leukocyte, as discussed in Section 3-18. The cell then attaches firmly to the endothelium, and its rolling is arrested.

In the third step the leukocyte extravasates, or crosses the endothelial wall. This step also involves LFA-1 and CR3, as well as a further adhesive interaction involving an immunoglobulin-related molecule called **PECAM**, or **CD31**, which is expressed both on the leukocyte and at the intercellular junctions of endothelial cells. These interactions enable cells to squeeze between the endothelial cells. It then penetrates the basement membrane with the aid of enzymes that break down the extracellular matrix proteins of the basement membrane. The movement through the basement membrane is known as **diapedesis**, and it enables cells to enter the subendothelial tissues.

The fourth and final step in extravasation is the migration of leukocytes through the tissues under the influence of chemokines. Chemokines such as CXCL8 and CCL2 (see Section 3-17) are produced at the site of infection and bind to proteoglycans in the extracellular matrix and on endothelial cell surfaces. In this way, a matrix-associated concentration gradient of chemokines is formed on a solid surface along which the leukocyte can migrate to the focus of infection (see Fig. 3.30). CXCL8 is released by the macrophages that first encounter pathogens; it recruits neutrophils, which enter the infected tissue in large numbers in the early part of the induced response. Their influx usually peaks within the first 6 hours of an inflammatory response. Monocytes are recruited through the action of CCL2 and accumulate more slowly than neutrophils. Once in the inflamed tissue, neutrophils are able to eliminate many pathogens by phagocytosis. In an innate immune response, neutrophils use their complement receptors and the direct pattern-recognition receptors discussed earlier in this chapter (see Section 3-1) to recognize and phagocytose pathogens or pathogen components directly or after opsonization with complement (see Section 2-13). In addition, as we will see in Chapter 10, neutrophils act as phagocytic effectors in humoral adaptive immunity, taking up antibody-coated microbes by means of specific receptors.

The importance of neutrophils in immune defense is dramatically illustrated by diseases or medical treatments that severely reduce neutrophil numbers. Individuals suffering this affliction are said to have **neutropenia**, and they are highly susceptible to deadly infection with a wide range of pathogens and commensal organisms. Restoring neutrophil levels in such individuals by transfusion of neutrophil-rich blood fractions or by stimulating their production with specific growth factors largely corrects this susceptibility.

3-20 TNF-α is an important cytokine that triggers local containment of infection but induces shock when released systemically.

TNF-α acting on endothelial cells stimulates the expression of adhesion molecules and aids the extravasation of cells such as monocytes and neutrophils. Another important action of TNF-α is to stimulate endothelial cells to express proteins that trigger blood clotting in the local small vessels, occluding them and cutting off blood flow. This can be important in preventing the pathogen from entering the bloodstream and spreading through the blood to organs all over the body. The importance of TNF-α in the containment of local infection is illustrated by experiments in which rabbits were infected locally with a bacterium. Normally, the infection would be contained at the site of the inoculation; if, however, an injection of anti-TNF-α antibody was also given to block the action of TNF-α, the infection spread via the blood to other organs. In parallel, the fluid that has leaked into the tissue in the early phases of an infection carries the pathogen, usually enclosed in dendritic cells, via the lymph to the regional lymph nodes, where an adaptive immune response can be initiated.

Once an infection has spread to the bloodstream, however, the same mechanisms by which TNF-α so effectively contains local infection instead become catastrophic (**Fig. 3.31**). Although produced as a membrane-associated cytokine, TNF-α can be cleaved by a protease, **TACE (TNF-α–converting enzyme**, which is encoded by the ADAM17 gene), and released from the membrane as a soluble cytokine. The presence of infection in the bloodstream, or sepsis, is accompanied by a massive release of soluble TNF-α from macrophages in the liver, spleen, and other sites throughout the body. The systemic release of TNF-α into the bloodstream causes vasodilation, which leads to a loss of blood pressure and increased vascular permeability; this in turn

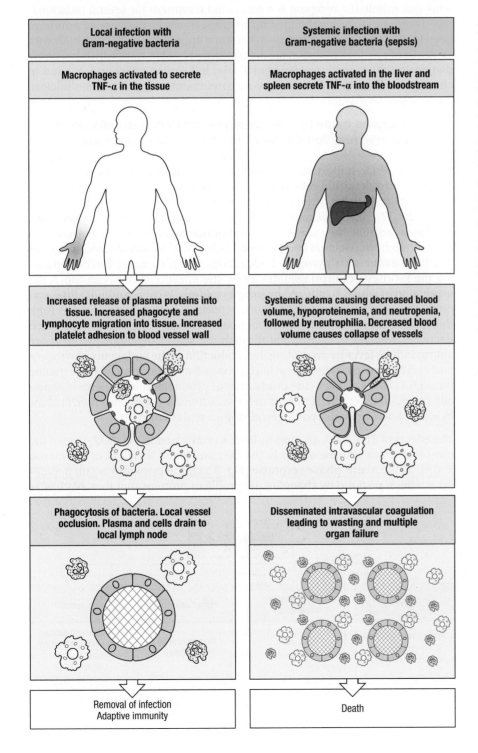

Fig. 3.31 The release of TNF-α by macrophages induces local protective effects, but TNF-α can be damaging when released systemically. The panels on the left show the causes and consequences of local release of TNF-α, and the panels on the right show the causes and consequences of systemic release. In both cases, TNF-α acts on blood vessels, especially venules, to increase blood flow and vascular permeability to fluid, proteins, and cells, and to increase endothelial adhesiveness for leukocytes and platelets (center row). Local release thus allows an influx of fluid, cells, and proteins into the infected tissue, where they participate in host defense. Later, blood clots form in the small vessels (bottom left panel), preventing spread of infection via the blood, and the accumulated fluid and cells drain to regional lymph nodes, where an adaptive immune response is initiated. When there is a systemic infection, or sepsis, with bacteria that elicit TNF-α production, TNF-α is released into the blood by macrophages in the liver and spleen and acts in a similar way on all small blood vessels in the body (bottom right panel). The result is shock, disseminated intravascular coagulation with depletion of clotting factors, and consequent bleeding, multiple organ failure, and frequently death.

leads to a loss of plasma volume and eventually to shock, known in this case as septic shock because the underlying cause is a bacterial infection. The TNF-α released in septic shock also triggers blood clotting in small vessels throughout the body—known as **disseminated intravascular coagulation (DIC)**—which leads to the massive consumption of clotting proteins, so that the individual's blood cannot clot appropriately. Disseminated intravascular coagulation frequently leads to the failure of vital organs such as the kidneys, liver, heart, and lungs, which are quickly compromised by the failure of normal blood perfusion; consequently, septic shock has a very high mortality rate.

Blockade of TNF-α activity, either with specific antibodies or with soluble proteins that mimic the receptor, is a successful treatment for several inflammatory disorders, including rheumatoid arthritis. However, these treatments have been found to reactivate tuberculosis in some apparently well individuals with evidence of previous infection (as demonstrated by skin test), which is a direct demonstration of the importance of TNF-α in keeping infection local and in check. The efficacy of TNF-α blockade as a treatment for sepsis remains unclear.

3-21 Cytokines made by macrophages and dendritic cells induce a systemic reaction known as the acute-phase response.

As well as their important local effects, the cytokines produced by macrophages and dendritic cells have long-range effects that contribute to host defense. One of these is the elevation of body temperature, which is caused mainly by TNF-α, IL-1β, and IL-6. These cytokines are termed **endogenous pyrogens** because they cause fever and derive from an endogenous source rather than from bacterial components such as LPS, which also induces fever and is an **exogenous pyrogen**. Endogenous pyrogens cause fever by inducing the synthesis of prostaglandin E2 by the enzyme cyclooxygenase-2, the expression of which is induced by these cytokines. Prostaglandin E2 then acts on the hypothalamus, resulting in an increase in both heat production from the catabolism of brown fat and heat retention from vasoconstriction, which decreases the loss of excess heat through the skin. Exogenous pyrogens are able to induce fever by promoting the production of the endogenous pyrogens and also by directly inducing cyclooxygenase-2 as a consequence of signaling through TLR-4, leading to the production of prostaglandin E2. Fever is generally considered beneficial to host defense, although the precise mechanisms by which fever facilitates pathogen clearance remain unclear.

The effects of TNF-α, IL-1β, and IL-6 are summarized in **Fig. 3.32**. One of the most important of these occurs in the liver and is the initiation of a response known as the **acute-phase response** (**Fig. 3.33**). The cytokines act on hepatocytes, which respond by changing the profile of proteins that they synthesize

Fig. 3.32 The cytokines TNF-α, IL 1β, and IL-6 have a wide spectrum of biological activities that help to coordinate the body's responses to infection. TNF-α, IL-1β, and IL-6 activate hepatocytes to synthesize acute-phase proteins and activate bone marrow endothelium to release neutrophils. The acute-phase proteins act as opsonins, whereas the disposal of opsonized pathogens is augmented by the enhanced recruitment of neutrophils from the bone marrow. TNF-α, IL-1β, and IL-6 are also endogenous pyrogens, raising body temperature, which is believed to help in eliminating infections. A major effect of these cytokines is to induce synthesis of prostaglandin E2, which acts on the hypothalamus, altering the body's temperature regulation, and on muscle and fat cells, altering energy mobilization to increase the body temperature. At higher temperatures, bacterial and viral replication is less efficient, whereas the adaptive immune response operates more efficiently.

Fig. 3.33 The acute-phase response produces molecules that bind pathogens but not host cells. Acute-phase proteins are produced by liver cells in response to cytokines released by macrophages in the presence of bacteria (top panel). They include serum amyloid protein (SAP) (in mice but not humans), C-reactive protein (CRP), fibrinogen, and mannose-binding lectin (MBL). CRP binds phosphocholine on certain bacterial and fungal surfaces but does not recognize it in the form in which it is found in host-cell membranes (middle panel). SAP and CRP are homologous in structure; both are pentraxins, forming five-membered discs, as shown for SAP (lower panel). SAP both acts as an opsonin in its own right and activates the classical complement pathway by binding C1q to augment opsonization. MBL is a member of the collectin family, which also includes the pulmonary surfactant proteins SP-A and SP-D. Like CRP, MBL can act as an opsonin in its own right, as can SP-A and SP-D.

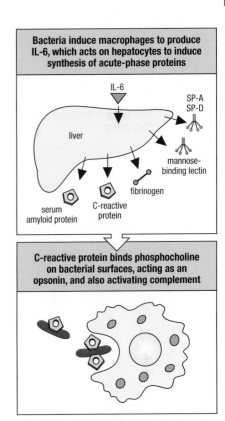

Bacteria induce macrophages to produce IL-6, which acts on hepatocytes to induce synthesis of acute-phase proteins

C-reactive protein binds phosphocholine on bacterial surfaces, acting as an opsonin, and also activating complement

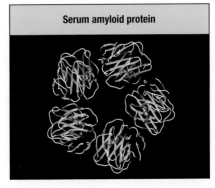

Serum amyloid protein

and secrete into the blood. In the acute-phase response, blood levels of some proteins go down, whereas levels of others increase markedly. The proteins induced by TNF-α, IL-1β, and IL-6 are called the **acute-phase proteins**. Several of these are of particular interest because they mimic the action of antibodies, but unlike antibodies they have broad specificity for pathogen-associated molecular patterns and depend only on the presence of cytokines for their production.

One acute-phase protein, the **C-reactive protein**, is a member of the **pentraxin** protein family, so called because the proteins are formed from five identical subunits. C-reactive protein is yet another example of a multipronged pathogen-recognition molecule, and it binds to the phosphocholine portion of certain bacterial and fungal cell-wall lipopolysaccharides. Phosphocholine is also found in mammalian cell-membrane phospholipids, but it cannot be bound by C-reactive protein. When C-reactive protein binds to a bacterium, it not only is able to opsonize the bacterium but can also activate the complement cascade by binding to C1q, the first component of the classical pathway of complement activation (see Section 2-7). The interaction with C1q involves the collagen-like parts of C1q rather than the globular heads that make contact with pathogen surfaces, but the same cascade of reactions is initiated.

Mannose-binding lectin (MBL) is another acute-phase protein; it serves as an innate recognition molecule that can activate the lectin pathway of complement (see Section 2-6). MBL is present at low levels in the blood of healthy individuals, but it is produced in increased amounts during the acute-phase response. By recognizing mannose residues on microbial surfaces, MBL can act as an opsonin that is recognized by monocytes, which do not express the macrophage mannose receptor. Two other proteins with opsonizing properties that are also produced in increased amounts during an acute-phase response are the **surfactant proteins A and D (SP-A and SP-D)**. These are produced by the liver and a variety of epithelia. They are, for example, found along with macrophages in the alveolar fluid of the lung, where they are secreted by pneumocytes, and are important in promoting the phagocytosis of opportunistic respiratory pathogens such as *Pneumocystis jirovecii* (formerly known as *P. carinii*), one of the main causes of pneumonia in individuals with AIDS.

Thus, within a day or two, the acute-phase response provides the host with several proteins with the functional properties of antibodies but able to bind a broad range of pathogens. However, unlike antibodies, which we describe in Chapters 4 and 10, acute-phase proteins have no structural diversity and are made in response to any stimulus that triggers the release of TNF-α, IL-1β, and IL-6. Therefore, unlike antibodies, their synthesis is not specifically induced and targeted.

A final, distant effect of the cytokines produced by macrophages is to induce **leukocytosis**, an increase in the numbers of circulating neutrophils. The neutrophils come from two sources: the bone marrow, from which mature leukocytes are released in increased numbers; and sites in blood vessels, where they are attached loosely to endothelial cells. Thus, the effects of these cytokines contribute to the control of infection while the adaptive immune response is being developed.

3-22 Interferons induced by viral infection make several contributions to host defense.

Viral infection induces the production of interferons, originally named because of their ability to interfere with viral replication in previously uninfected tissue culture cells. Interferons have a similar role *in vivo*, blocking the spread of viruses to uninfected cells. There are numerous genes encoding antiviral, or type I, interferons. Best understood are the IFN-α family of 12 closely related human genes and IFN-β, the product of a single gene; less well studied are IFN-κ, IFN-ε, and IFN-ω. **IFN-γ** is the sole **type II interferon**.

Type III interferons are a newly classified IFN family composed of the products of three **IFN-λ** genes, also known as IL-28A, IL-28B, and IL-29, which bind a heterodimeric **IFN-λ receptor** composed of a unique IL-28Rα subunit and the β subunit of the IL-10 receptor. While receptors for type I interferons and IFN-γ are widespread in their tissue distribution, type III receptors are more restricted. For example, they are not expressed by fibroblasts but are expressed on epithelial cells.

Type I interferons are inducible and are synthesized by many cell types after infection by diverse viruses. Almost all types of cells can produce IFN-α and IFN-β in response to activation of several innate sensors. For example, type I interferons are induced by RLRs and cGAS–STING signaling (see Sections 3-8 and 3-9). However, some immune cells seem to be specialized for this task. In Section 3-1 we introduced the plasmacytoid dendritic cell (pDC). Also called **interferon-producing cells (IPCs)** or **natural interferon-producing cells**, human plasmacytoid dendritic cells were initially recognized as rare peripheral blood cells that accumulate in peripheral lymphoid tissues during a viral infection and make abundant type I interferons (IFN-α and IFN-β)—up to 1000 times more than that made by other cell types. This abundant production of type I interferons may result from the efficient coupling of viral recognition by TLRs to the pathways of interferon production (see Section 3-7). Plasmacytoid dendritic cells express a subset of TLRs that includes TLR-7 and TLR-9, which are endosomal sensors of viral RNA and DNA (see Fig. 3.11). The requirement for TLR-9 in sensing infections caused by DNA viruses has been demonstrated, for example, by the inability of TLR-9–deficient plasmacytoid dendritic cells to generate type I interferons in response to herpes simplex virus.

Interferons help defend against viral infection in several ways (**Fig. 3.34**). IFN-β induces an antiviral state in cells, which includes making cells more likely to produce IFN-α in response to PRR triggering, thus amplifying the interferon response. IFN-α and IFN-β bind to a common cell-surface receptor, known as the **interferon-α receptor (IFNAR)**, which uses the JAK and STAT pathways described in Section 3-16. IFNAR uses the kinases Tyk2 and Jak1 to activate the factors **STAT1 and STAT2**, which can interact with **IRF9** and form a complex called **ISGF3**, which binds to the promoters of many **interferon-stimulated genes (ISGs)**. The induction of ISGs induces a state of resistance

Interferon-γ Receptor Deficiency

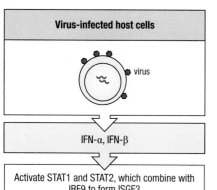

Virus-infected host cells
virus
↓
IFN-α, IFN-β
↓
Activate STAT1 and STAT2, which combine with IRF9 to form ISGF3
Induce resistance to viral replication in all cells by inducing Mx proteins, 2′,5′-linked adenosine oligomers, and the kinase PKR
Enhance sensing of viral infection by increasing expression of PRRs and signaling components
Induce expression of IFIT proteins, which suppress the translation of viral RNA
Increase MHC class I expression and antigen presentation in all cells
Activate dendritic cells and macrophages
Activate NK cells to kill virus-infected cells
Induce chemokines to recruit lymphocytes

Fig. 3.34 Interferons are antiviral proteins produced by cells in response to viral infection. The interferons IFN-α and IFN-β promote antiviral immunity through multiple mechanisms. They induce resistance to viral replication in uninfected cells by activating genes that cause the destruction of mRNA and inhibit the translation of viral proteins and some host proteins. The products of these genes include the Mx proteins, oligoadenylate synthetase, PKR, and IFIT proteins. Interferons can also induce MHC class I expression in most cell types in the body, thus enhancing their resistance to NK cells; they may also induce increased synthesis of MHC class I molecules in cells that are newly infected by virus, thus making them more susceptible to being killed by CD8 cytotoxic T cells (see Chapter 9). In addition, interferons activate NK cells, which then selectively kill virus-infected cells.

to viral replication in all cells. Many of the genes involved in nucleic-acid sensing and signaling are ISGs, including the genes for RIG-I, MDA-5, IRF7, and STING, such that cells exposed to interferons have a heightened ability to recognize viral nucleic acids.

ISGs exert antiviral activities through a variety of mechanisms. One ISG encodes the enzyme **oligoadenylate synthetase**, which polymerizes ATP into 2′,5′-linked oligomers (whereas nucleotides in nucleic acids are normally linked 3′,5′). These 2′,5′-linked oligomers serve as second messengers and activate an endoribonuclease that then degrades viral RNA (note the parallels to cGAMP activation of STING, described in Section 3-9). Another ISG-encoded protein induced by IFN-α and IFN-β is a dsRNA-dependent protein kinase called **PKR**. This serine/threonine kinase phosphorylates the α subunit of eukaryotic initiation factor 2 (eIF2), thus suppressing protein translation and contributing to the inhibition of viral replication. **Mx (myxoma resistant) proteins** are also ISG-encoded proteins induced by type I interferons. Humans and wild mice have two highly similar proteins, Mx1 and Mx2, which are GTPases belonging to the dynamin protein family, but how they interfere with viral replication is not understood.

The **IFIT (IFN-induced protein with tetratricoid repeats)** family of ISG-encoded proteins contains four human and three mouse proteins that function in restraining the translation of viral RNA into proteins. **IFIT1 and IFIT2** can both suppress the translation of normal capped mRNAs by binding to subunits of the **eukaryotic initiation factor 3 (eIF3)** complex, which prevents eIF3 from interacting with eIF2 to form the 43S pre-initiation complex (**Fig. 3.35**). This action may be responsible in part for the reduction in cellular

Fig. 3.35 IFIT proteins act as antiviral effector molecules by inhibiting steps in the translation of RNA. Top left panel: Formation of a 43S pre-initiation complex is an early step in the translation of RNA into protein by the 80S ribosome that involves a charged methionine tRNA, the 40S ribosome subunit, and eukaryotic initiation factors (eIFs) eIF4, eIF2, and eIF3. Middle panel: eIFs and a charged methionine tRNA assemble into a 43S pre-initiation complex. Right panel: The pre-initiation complex mRNA recognizes the 5′ cap structure and joins with the 60S ribosomal subunit, releasing eIF2, eIF3, and eIF4 and forming a functional 80S ribosome. Lower panel: eIF3 has 13 subunits, a–m. IFIT proteins can inhibit several steps in protein translation. Mouse IFIT1 and IFIT2 interact with eIF3C, and human IFIT1 and IFIT2 interact with eIF3E, preventing formation of the 43S pre-initiation complex. IFITs can also interfere with other steps in translation and can bind and sequester uncapped viral mRNAs to prevent their translation (not shown). Expression of IFIT proteins is induced in viral infection by signaling downstream of type I interferons.

proliferation induced by type I interferons. Mice lacking IFIT1 or IFIT2 show increased susceptibility to infection by certain viruses, such as vesicular stomatitis virus.

Another function of IFIT1 is to suppress translation of viral RNA that lacks a normal host modification of the 5′ cap. Recall that the normal mammalian 5′ cap is initiated by linking a 7-methylguanosine nucleotide to the first ribose sugar of the mRNA by a 5′,5′-linked triphosphate bridge to produce a structure called cap-0. This structure is further modified by cytoplasmic methylation of the 2′ hydroxyl groups on the first and second ribose sugars of the RNA. Methylation of the first ribose sugar produces a structure called cap-1; methylation of the second generates cap-2. IFIT1 has a high affinity for cap-0 but much lower affinity for cap-1 and cap-2. Some viruses, such as Sindbis virus (family Togaviridae), lack 2′-O-methylation and therefore are restricted by this action of IFIT1. Many viruses, such as West Nile virus and SARS coronavirus, have acquired a **2′-O-methyltransferase (MTase)** that produces cap-1 or cap-2 on their viral transcripts. These viruses can thus evade restriction by IFIT1.

Members of the **interferon-induced transmembrane protein (IFITM)** family are expressed at a basal level on many types of tissues but are strongly induced by type I interferons. There are four functional IFITM genes in humans and in mice, and these encode proteins that have two transmembrane domains and are localized to various vesicular compartments of the cell. IFITM proteins act to inhibit, or restrict, viruses at early steps of infection. Although the molecular details are unclear, **IFITM1** appears to interfere with the fusion of viral membranes with the membrane of the lysosome, which is required for introducing some viral genomes into the cytoplasm. Viruses that must undergo this fusion event in lysosomes, such as the Ebola virus, are restricted by IFITM1. Similarly, **IFITM3** interferes with membrane fusion in late endosomes, and so restricts the influenza A virus, which undergoes fusion there. The importance of this mechanism is demonstrated by the increased viral load and higher mortality in mice lacking IFITM3 that are infected with the influenza A virus.

Interferons also stimulate production of the chemokines CXCL9, CXCL10, and CXCL11, which recruit lymphocytes to sites of infection. They also increase the expression of MHC class I molecules on all types of cells, which facilitates recognition of virally infected cells by cytotoxic T lymphocytes via the display of viral peptides complexed to MHC class I molecules on the infected cell surface (see Fig. 1.30). Through these effects, interferons indirectly help promote the killing of virus-infected cells by CD8 cytotoxic T cells. Another way in which interferons act is to activate populations of innate immune cells, such as NK cells, that can kill virus-infected cells, as described below.

3-23 Several types of innate lymphoid cells provide protection in early infection.

A defining feature of adaptive immunity is the clonal expression of antigen receptors, produced by somatic gene rearrangements, that provide the extraordinarily diverse specificities of T and B lymphocytes (see Section 1-11). However, for several decades, immunologists have recognized cells with lymphoid characteristics that lack specific antigen receptors. **Natural killer (NK) cells** have been known the longest, but in the past several years other distinct groups of such cells have been identified. Collectively, these are now called **innate lymphoid cells (ILCs)** and include NK cells (**Fig. 3.36**). ILCs develop in the bone marrow from the same **common lymphoid progenitor (CLP)** that gives rise to B and T cells. Expression of the transcription factor Id2 (inhibitor of DNA binding 2) in the CLP represses B- and T-cell fates and is required for the development of all ILCs. ILCs are identified by the absence of T- and B-cell antigen receptor and co-receptor complexes, but they express receptors for common γ-chain cytokines. They migrate from the bone marrow and take up

The major categories of innate lymphoid cells (ILCs) and their properties			
Innate lymphoid subgroup	**Inducing cytokines**	**Effector molecules produced**	**Function**
NK cells	IL-12, IL-18, type I IFN	IFN-γ, perforin, granzyme	Immunity against viruses, intracellular pathogens
ILC1	IL-12, IL-18	IFN-γ	Defense against viruses, intracellular pathogens
ILC2	IL-25, IL-33, TSLP	IL-5, IL-13, amphiregulin, IL-4	Expulsion of extracellular parasites, tissue repair
ILC3 (LTi cells)	IL-1β, IL-23	IL-17, IL-22	Immunity to extracellular bacteria

Fig. 3.36 The major categories of innate lymphoid cells (ILCs) and their properties.

residence in lymphoid tissues and peripheral organs, notably the dermis, liver, small intestine, adipose tissue, and lung.

ILCs function in innate immunity as effector cells that amplify the signals delivered by innate recognition. They are stimulated by cytokines produced by other innate cells, such as macrophages or dendritic cells, or by nonimmune cells, such as epithelial cells, that have been activated by innate sensors of microbial infection or cellular damage. Three major subgroups of ILCs are defined, largely on the basis of the types of cytokines that each produces. **Group 1 ILCs (ILC1s)** generate IFN-γ in response to activation by certain cytokines, in particular IL-12 and IL-18, made by dendritic cells and macrophages, and they function in protection against infection by viruses or intracellular pathogens. NK cells are now considered to be a type of ILC. ILC1s and NK cells are closely related but have distinct functional properties and differ in the cytokines and transcription factors required for their development. For example, both NK and ILC1 cells require the transcription factors Id2 and **Nfil3** for their development, but ILC1s also require the transcription factor PLZF whereas NK cells do not. NK cells require the cytokine IL-15, while liver ILC1 cells require the cytokine IL-7 and the transcription factor **Tbet**. Functionally, NK cells are more similar to CD8 T cells, while ILC1s resemble more closely the T$_H$1 subset of CD4 T cells (see Section 3-24). NK cells can be found within tissues, but they also circulate through the blood, while ILC1 cells appear to be largely noncirculating tissue-resident cells. In the mouse, conventional NK cells express the integrin α2 (CD49b), while ILC1 cells, for example in the liver, lack CD49b but express the surface protein CD49a.

Group 2 ILCs (ILC2s) produce the cytokines IL-4, IL-5, and IL-13 in response to various cytokines, particularly **thymic stromal lymphopoietin (TSLP)**, IL-25, and IL-33. ILC2 cytokines function in promoting mucosal and barrier immunity and aid in protection against parasites. ILC2s also produce amphiregulin, an EGF family member that induces epithelial cell proliferation and differentiation, which facilitates repair of damaged tissues.

Group 3 ILCs (ILC3s) respond to the cytokines IL-1β and IL-23 and produce several cytokines, including IL-17 and IL-22, which increase defenses against extracellular bacteria and fungi. IL-17 functions by stimulating the production of chemokines that recruit neutrophils, while IL-22 acts directly on epithelial cells to stimulate the production of antimicrobial peptides such as RegIIIγ (see Section 2-4).

The classification of ILC subtypes and the analysis of their development and function is still an active area, and studies to define the relative importance of these cells in immune responses are ongoing. The ILC subgroups identified so far appear to be highly parallel in structure to the subsets of effector CD8 and CD4 T cells that were defined over the past three decades. The transcription factors that control the development of different ILC subsets seem, for now at least, to be the same as those that control the corresponding T-cell subsets.

Because of these similarities, we will postpone a detailed description of ILC development until Chapter 9, where we will cover this topic along with the development of T-cell subsets.

3-24 NK cells are activated by type I interferon and macrophage-derived cytokines.

NK cells are larger than naive T and B cells, have distinctive cytoplasmic granules containing cytotoxic proteins, and were functionally identified by their ability to kill certain tumor cell lines *in vitro* without the need for prior immunization. NK cells kill cells by releasing their cytotoxic granules, which are similar to those of cytotoxic T cells and have the same effects (discussed in Chapter 9). In brief, the contents of cytotoxic granules, which contain granzymes and the pore-forming protein perforin, are released onto the surface of the target cell and penetrate the cell membrane and induce programmed cell death. However, unlike T cells, killing by NK cells is triggered by germline-encoded receptors that recognize molecules on the surface of infected or malignantly transformed cells. A second pathway used by NK cells to kill target cells involves the TNF family member known as **TRAIL (tumor necrosis factor–related apoptosis-inducing ligand)**. NK cells express TRAIL on their cell surface. TRAIL interacts with two TNFR superfamily 'death' receptors, **DR4 and DR5** (encoded by *TNFSF10A* and *TNFSF10B*), that are expressed by many types of cells. When NK cells recognize a target cell, TRAIL stimulates DR4 and DR5 to activate the pro-enzyme **caspase 8**, which leads to apoptosis. In contrast to pyroptosis, induced by caspase 1 after inflammasome activation (see Section 3-11), apoptosis is not associated with production of inflammatory cytokines. We will discuss more details of the mechanisms of caspase-induced apoptosis when we discuss killing by cytotoxic T cells in Chapter 9. Finally, NK cells express Fc receptors (see Section 1-20); binding of antibodies to these receptors activates NK cells to release their cytotoxic granules, a process known as **antibody-dependent cell-mediated cytotoxicity, or ADCC**, to which we will return in Chapter 10.

The ability of NK cells to kill target cells can be enhanced by interferons or certain cytokines. NK cells that can kill sensitive targets can be isolated from uninfected individuals, but this activity is increased 20- to 100-fold when NK cells are exposed to IFN-α and IFN-β or to IL-12, a cytokine produced by dendritic cells and macrophages during infection by many types of pathogens. Activated NK cells serve to contain virus infections while the adaptive immune response is generating antigen-specific cytotoxic T cells and neutralizing antibodies that can clear the infection (**Fig. 3.37**). A clue to the physiological function of NK cells in humans comes from rare individuals deficient in these cells, who are frequently susceptible to herpesvirus infection. For example, a selective NK-cell deficiency results from mutations in the human MCM4 (minichromosome maintenance-deficient 4) protein, which is associated with predisposition to viral infections. Similarly, depletion of NK cells in mice, either by antibody or genetically, results in susceptibility to a number of viruses, including herpesviruses.

IL-12, produced by activated macrophages and dendritic cells, acts in synergy with the cytokine IL-18 to stimulate NK cells to secrete large amounts of IFN-γ. This IFN-γ is crucial in controlling certain infections because it precedes the production of IFN-γ by activated CD8 cytotoxic T cells. IFN-γ, whose receptor activates only the STAT1 transcription factor, is quite distinct functionally from the antiviral type I interferons IFN-α and IFN-β and is not directly induced by viral infection. The production of IFN-γ by NK cells early in an immune response can directly activate macrophages to enhance their capacity to kill pathogens, augmenting innate immunity. IFN-γ also influences adaptive immunity through actions on dendritic cells and by regulating the

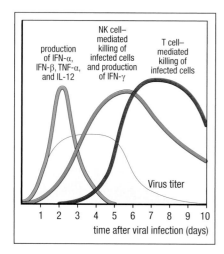

Fig. 3.37 Natural killer cells (NK cells) are an early component of the host response to virus infection. Experiments in mice have shown that IFN-α, IFN-β, and the cytokines TNF-α and IL-12 are produced first after viral infection, and are followed by a wave of NK cells, which together control virus replication via IFN-α secretion and cytotoxicity but do not eliminate the virus. Virus elimination is accomplished when virus-specific CD8 T cells and neutralizing antibodies are produced. Without NK cells, the levels of some viruses are much higher in the early days of the infection, and the infection can be lethal unless treated vigorously with antiviral compounds.

differentiation of CD4 T cells into the pro-inflammatory T$_H$1 subset, which produces IFN-γ. Accordingly, mice deficient for the gene encoding IFN-γ are highly susceptible to viruses and intracellular bacterial pathogens. NK cells also produce TNF-α, **granulocyte–macrophage colony-stimulating factor (GM-CSF)**, and the chemokines CCL3 (MIP-1α), CCL4, and CCL5 (RANTES), which act to recruit and activate macrophages.

3-25 NK cells express activating and inhibitory receptors to distinguish between healthy and infected cells.

For NK cells to defend against viruses or other pathogens, they must be able to distinguish infected cells from uninfected healthy cells. To do this, NK cells use a mechanism distinct from the mechanism of pathogen recognition used by T or B cells. An individual NK cell expresses various combinations of germline-encoded **activating receptors** and **inhibitory receptors**. While the exact details are not clear in every case, it is thought that the overall balance of signaling by these receptors determines whether an NK cell engages and kills a target cell. The receptors on an NK cell are tuned to detect changes in expression of various surface proteins on a target cell, referred to as '**dysregulated self**'. The activating receptors generally recognize cell-surface proteins that are induced on target cells by infection or stress, such as malignant transformation. These induced proteins are referred to as '**stress-induced self**'. A number of cellular perturbations, including DNA damage, signals related to proliferation, and heat shock–related stress, can lead to induction of ligands for activating receptors. Signaling by innate sensors (for example, TLRs) is also capable of inducing such ligands. When activating receptors on NK cells detect stress-induced self ligands, signaling is initiated in the NK cell that results in release of cytokines, such as IFN-γ, and killing of the stimulating cell through the release of cytotoxic granules. However, engagement of activating receptors is not always sufficient to induce NK-cell activation; negative signals imposed by inhibitory receptors must either be lost or overcome, as discussed below.

Inhibitory receptors on NK cells recognize surface molecules that are constitutively expressed at high levels by most healthy cells. As such, NK cells that encounter healthy cells receive signals that inhibit the signals downstream of activating receptors and prevent their activation. However, infection, cellular stress, or transformation can lead to down-regulation of the ligands for inhibitory receptors. The loss of these molecules is referred to as '**missing self**'. Inhibitory receptors can recognize other molecules, but those recognizing **MHC class I molecules** have been best characterized. MHC molecules are glycoproteins expressed on nearly all cells of the body. We will discuss the role of MHC proteins in antigen presentation to T cells in Chapter 6, but for now we need only to introduce the two main classes of MHC molecules. MHC class I molecules are expressed on most of the cells of the body (except, notably, red blood cells), whereas the expression of **MHC class II molecules** is far more restricted, largely to immune cells.

Inhibitory receptors that recognize MHC class I molecules function to prevent NK cells from killing normal host cells. The greater the number of MHC class I molecules on a cell surface, the better protected that cell is against attack by NK cells. Interferons induce expression of MHC class I molecules and protect uninfected host cells from being killed by NK cells, while also activating NK cells to kill virus-infected cells. Viruses and some other intracellular pathogens can cause down-regulation of MHC class I molecules as a strategy to prevent the display of antigens as peptides to T cells, also discussed in Chapter 13. MHC class I molecules are often similarly down-regulated in cancerous cells. Importantly, NK cells are able to sense this reduction in expression of MHC class I molecules through reduced signaling from their inhibitory receptors. Reduction in MHC class I expression is an example of 'missing self' and

Fig. 3.38 Killing by NK cells depends on the balance between activating and inhibitory signals. NK cells have several different activating receptors that signal the NK to kill the bound cell. However, NK cells are prevented from a wholesale attack by another set of inhibitory receptors that recognize MHC class I molecules (which are present on almost all cell types) and that inhibit signaling by the activating receptors. Up-regulation of ligands for activating receptors can overrule this inhibition. Alternatively, activation can occur when inhibitory signals are lost, such as when viruses inhibit MHC class I expression or alter its conformation so as to avoid recognition by CD8 T cells. NK cells may also kill target cells through their expression of the TNF family member TRAIL, which binds to TNFR members DR4 and DR5 expressed by some types of cells. DR4 and DR5 signal through FADD, an adaptor that activates pro-caspase 8, leading to induction of apoptosis of the target cell.

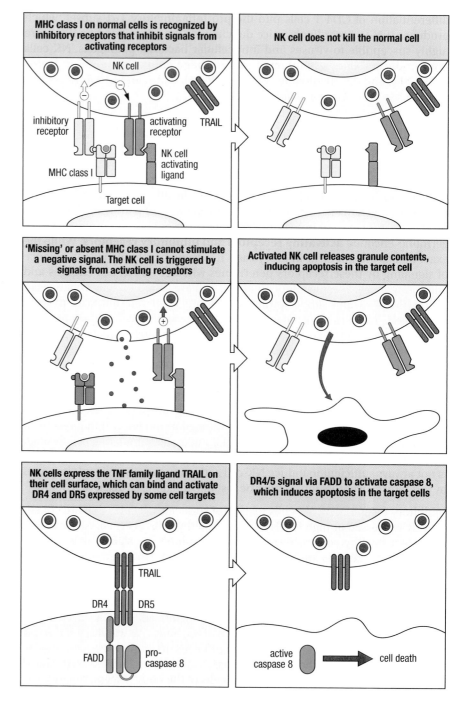

increases the chance that an NK cell will kill the target cell. It is thought that the balance of signals from 'stress-induced self' and 'missing self' determines whether an individual NK cell will be triggered to kill a particular target cell (**Fig. 3.38**). Thus, receptors expressed on NK cells integrate the signals from two types of surface receptors, which together control an NK cell's cytotoxic activity and cytokine production.

3-26 NK-cell receptors belong to several structural families.

The receptors that regulate the activity of NK cells fall into several large families that contain a number of other cell-surface receptors in addition to NK receptors (**Fig. 3.39**). Members of the family of **killer cell immunoglobulin-like**

Fig. 3.39 **The genes that encode NK receptors fall into two large families.** The first, the leukocyte receptor complex (LRC), comprises a large cluster of genes encoding a family of proteins composed of immunoglobulin-like domains. These include the killer cell immunoglobulin-like receptors (KIRs) expressed by NK cells, the ILT (immunoglobulin-like transcript) class, and the leukocyte-associated immunoglobulin-like receptor (LAIR) gene families. The sialic acid–binding Ig-like lectins (SIGLECs) and members of the CD66 family are located nearby. In humans, this complex is located on chromosome 19. The second gene cluster is called the NK receptor complex (NKC) and encodes killer cell lectin-like receptors (KLRs), a receptor family that includes the NKG2 proteins and CD94, with which some NKG2 molecules pair to form a functional receptor. This complex is located on human chromosome 12. The corresponding locus in mice is located on chromosome 6 and also contains the expanded family of Ly49 genes. Some NK receptor genes are found outside these major gene clusters.

receptors (KIRs) have differing numbers of immunoglobulin domains. Some, such as KIR-2D, have two immunoglobulin domains, whereas others, such as KIR-3D, have three. The KIR genes form part of a larger cluster of immunoglobulin-like receptor genes known as the **leukocyte receptor complex (LRC)**. Another family, the **killer cell lectin-like receptors (KLRs)** are C-type lectin–like proteins whose genes reside in a gene cluster called the **NK receptor complex (NKC)**. Mice lack KIR genes and instead predominantly express **Ly49 receptors**, encoded in the NKC on mouse chromosome 6, to control their NK-cell activity. These receptors can be activating or inhibitory and are highly polymorphic between different strains of mice. By contrast, humans lack functional Ly49 genes and rely on KIRs encoded in the LRC to control their NK-cell activity. An important feature of the NK-cell population is that any given NK cell expresses only a subset of the receptors in its potential repertoire, and so not all NK cells in an individual are identical.

Activating and inhibitory receptors are present within the same structural family. Whether a KIR or Ly49 protein is activating or inhibitory depends on the presence or absence of particular signaling motifs in its cytoplasmic domain. Inhibitory KIRs and Ly49s have long cytoplasmic tails that contain an **immunoreceptor tyrosine-based inhibition motif (ITIM)**. The consensus amino acid sequence for the ITIM is V/I/LxYxxL/V, where 'x' stands for any amino acid. For example, the cytoplasmic tails of the inhibitory receptors KIR-2DL and KIR-3DL each contain two ITIMs (**Fig. 3.40**). When ligands associate with an inhibitory KIR, the tyrosine in its ITIM becomes phosphorylated by the action of **Src family protein tyrosine kinases**. When phosphorylated, the ITIM can then bind the intracellular protein tyrosine phosphatases **SHP-1** (Src homology region 2–containing protein tyrosine phosphatase-1) and **SHP-2**, which become localized near the cell membrane. These phosphatases inhibit

Fig. 3.40 **The structural families of NK receptors encode both activating and inhibitory receptors.** The families of killer cell immunoglobulin-like receptors (KIRs) and killer cell lectin-like receptors (KLRs and Ly49 receptors) have members that send activating signals to the NK cell (upper panel) and others that send inhibitory signals to the NK cell (lower panel). KIR family members are designated according to the number of immunoglobulin-like domains they possess and by the length of their cytoplasmic tails. Activating KIRs have short cytoplasmic tails and bear the designation 'S.' These associate with the signaling protein DAP12 via a charged amino acid residue in the transmembrane region. The cytoplasmic tails of DAP12 contain amino acid motifs called ITAMs, which are involved in signaling. NKG2 receptors belong to the KLR family, and, whether activating or inhibitory, form heterodimers with another C-type lectin–like family member, CD94. The inhibitory KIRs have longer cytoplasmic tails and are designated 'L.' Inhibitory KIR and Ly49 family members do not associate constitutively with adaptor proteins but contain a signaling motif called an ITIM, which, when phosphorylated, is recognized by inhibitory phosphatases.

signaling induced by other receptors (for example, the NK activating receptors) by removing phosphates from tyrosine residues on other intracellular signaling molecules.

Activating KIRs have short cytoplasmic tails and are designated, for example, as KIR-2DS and KIR-3DS (see Fig. 3.40). In mice, activating Ly49 proteins similarly have a short cytoplasmic tail that contains no signaling domain. Instead, these activating KIRs and Ly49 receptors have a charged residue in their transmembrane regions that associates with an accessory signaling protein called **DAP12**. DAP12 is a transmembrane protein that contains an immunoreceptor tyrosine-based activation motif (ITAM) with consensus sequence $Yxx[L/I]$ $x_{6-9}Yxx[L/I])$ in its cytoplasmic tail and forms a disulfide-linked homodimer in the membrane. When a ligand binds to an activating KIR or Ly49 receptor, the tyrosine residues in the ITAM of DAP12 become phosphorylated, turning on intracellular signaling pathways that activate the NK cell and lead to release of the cytotoxic granules. The phosphorylated ITAMs bind and activate intracellular tyrosine kinases such as Syk or ZAP-70, leading to further signaling events similar to those described for T cells in Chapter 7.

The KLR family also has both activating and inhibitory members. In mice, inhibitory Ly49 receptors have an ITIM in their cytoplasmic tail that recruits SHP-1. The latter's importance is shown by the failure of Ly49 to inhibit NK activation upon binding to MHC class I in mice carrying the **motheaten** mutation, which inactivates SHP-1 protein. In humans and mice, NK cells express a heterodimer of two different C-type lectin–like receptors, **CD94** and **NKG2**. This heterodimer interacts with nonpolymorphic MHC class I–like molecules, including HLA-E in humans and Qa1 in mice. HLA-E and Qa1 are unusual in that instead of binding peptides derived from pathogens, they bind fragments of the **signal peptide** derived from other MHC class I molecules during processing in the endoplasmic reticulum. This enables CD94:NKG2 to detect the presence of several different MHC class I variants, whose expression may be targeted by viruses, and kill cells in which overall MHC molecule expression is diminished. In humans there are four closely related NKG2 family proteins, NKG2A, C, E, and F (encoded by *KLRC1–4*), and a more distantly related protein, NKG2D (encoded by *KLRK1*). Of these, for example, NKG2A contains an ITIM and is inhibitory, whereas NKG2C has a charged transmembrane residue, associates with DAP12, and is activating (see Fig. 3.40). NKG2D is also activating but quite distinct from the other NKG2 receptors, and we will discuss it separately in the next section.

The overall response of NK cells to differences in MHC expression is further complicated by the extensive polymorphism of KIR genes, with different numbers of activating and inhibitory KIR genes being found in different people. The responsiveness of NK cells is thought to be tuned by their ability to recognize inhibitory ligands during their development. This process, referred to as licensing or education, is likely to underlie the effect of NK cells as a barrier to transplantation, because the NK cells educated in the environment of the recipient may fail to recognize the same inhibitory ligands on donor cells. A similar phenomenon may occur during pregnancy, because of differences between fetal and maternal MHC molecules (see Section 15-26). The advantage of such extensive KIR polymorphism is not yet clear, and some genetic epidemiologic studies even suggest an association between certain alleles of KIR genes and earlier onset (although not absolute frequency) of rheumatoid arthritis. The KIR gene cluster is not present in mice, but some species, including some primates, contain genes of both the KIR and KLR families. This might suggest that both gene clusters are relatively ancient and that for some reason, one or the other gene cluster was lost by mice and humans.

Signaling by the inhibitory NK receptors suppresses the killing activity and cytokine production of NK cells. This means NK cells will not kill healthy, genetically identical cells with normal expression of MHC class I molecules, such as the other cells of the body. Virus-infected cells, however, can become susceptible to being killed by NK cells by a variety of mechanisms. First, some viruses inhibit all protein synthesis in their host cells, so that synthesis of MHC class I proteins would be blocked in infected cells, even while their production in uninfected cells is being stimulated by the actions of type I interferons. The reduced level of MHC class I expression in infected cells would make them correspondingly less able to inhibit NK cells through their MHC-specific receptors, and they would become more susceptible to being killed. Second, many viruses can selectively prevent the export of MHC class I molecules to the cell surface or induce their degradation once there. This might allow the infected cell to evade recognition by cytotoxic T cells but would make it susceptible to being killed by NK cells. Virally infected cells can still be killed by NK cells even if the cells do not down-regulate MHC, provided that ligands for activating receptors are induced. However, some viruses target ligands for the activating receptors on NK cells, thwarting NK-cell recognition and killing of virus-infected cells.

3-27 NK cells express activating receptors that recognize ligands induced on infected cells or tumor cells.

In addition to the KIRs and KLRs, which have a role in sensing the level of MHC class I proteins present on other cells, NK cells also express receptors that more directly sense the presence of infection or other perturbations in a cell. Activating receptors for the recognition of infected cells, tumor cells, and cells injured by physical or chemical damage include the **natural cytotoxicity receptors (NCRs)** NKp30, NKp44, and NKp46, which are immunoglobulin-like receptors, and the C-type lectin–like family members **Ly49H** and **NKG2D** (**Fig. 3.41**). Among NCRs, only NKp46 is conserved in humans and in mice, and it is the most selective marker of NK cells across mammalian species. The ligands recognized by the NCRs are still being defined, but some evidence suggests that they recognize viral proteins. Ly49H is an activating receptor that recognizes the viral protein m157, an MHC class I–like structure encoded by the murine cytomegalovirus. The ligand for NKp30 is a protein named B7-H6, a member of the B7 family of co-stimulatory proteins, further described in Chapters 7 and 9.

NKG2D has a specialized role in activating NK cells. NKG2A, NKG2C, NKG2E, and NKG2F form heterodimers with CD94 and bind the MHC class I molecule HLA-E. In contrast, two NKG2D molecules form a homodimer that binds to several MHC class I–like molecules that are induced by various types of cellular stress. These include the MIC molecules **MIC-A and MIC-B** and the **RAET1** family of proteins, which are similar to the α_1 and α_2 domains of MHC class I molecules (**Fig. 3.42**). The RAET1 family has 10 members, three of which were initially characterized as ligands for the **cytomegalovirus UL16 protein** and are also called **UL16-binding proteins, or ULBPs**. Mice do not have equivalents of the MIC molecules; however, the ligands for mouse NKG2D have a very similar structure to that of the RAET1 proteins and are probably orthologs of them. In fact, these ligands were first identified in mice as the **RAE1 (retinoic acid early inducible 1) protein family** and also include related proteins H60 and MULT1 (see Fig. 6.26). We will return to these MHC-like molecules when we discuss the structure of the MHC molecule in Chapter 6.

The ligands for NKG2D are expressed in response to cellular or metabolic stress, and so are up-regulated on cells infected with intracellular bacteria and most viruses, as well as on incipient tumor cells that have become malignantly transformed. Thus, recognition by NKG2D acts as a generalized alarm signal to the immune system. In addition to expression by a subset of NK cells, NKG2D is expressed by various T cells, including all CD8 T cells and some $\gamma\delta$ T cells and invariant NKT cells (described in Chapter 8). In these

Fig. 3.41 Activating receptors of NK cells include the natural cytotoxicity receptors and NKG2D. The natural cytotoxicity receptors are immunoglobulin-like proteins. NKp30 and NKp44, for example, have an extracellular domain that resembles a single variable domain of an immunoglobulin molecule. NKp30 and NKp46 activate the NK cell through their association with homodimers of the CD3ζ chain or the Fc receptor γ chain (not shown). These signaling proteins also associate with other types of receptors that are described in Chapter 7. NKp44 activates the NK cell through its association with homodimers of DAP12. NKp46 resembles the KIR-2D molecules in having two domains that resemble the constant domains of an immunoglobulin molecule. NKG2D is a member of the C-type lectin–like family and forms a homodimer that associates with DAP10. In mice, an alternatively spliced form of NKG2D also associates with DAP12 (not shown).

The ligands for NKG2D are the MHC-like molecules MIC-A and MIC-B and the RAET1 family members, whose expression is induced by cellular stress

MIC-A or MIC-B

RAET1 family (includes MULT1, ULBPs)

Fig. 3.42 The ligands for the activating NK receptor NKG2D are proteins that are expressed in conditions of cellular stress. Ligands for NKG2D are induced on epithelial and other cells by stress, such as DNA damage, cellular transformation, or infection. The MIC proteins MIC-A and MIC-B are MHC-like molecules. RAET1 family members, including the subset designated as UL16-binding proteins (ULBPs), also resemble a portion of an MHC class I molecule—the α_1 and α_2 domains—and most (but not all) are attached to the cell via a glycosylphosphatidylinositol linkage. Unlike MHC class I molecules, the NKG2D ligands do not bind processed peptides.

cells, recognition of NKG2D ligands provides a potent co-stimulatory signal that enhances their effector functions.

NKG2D differs from other activating receptors on NK cells in the signaling pathway it engages within the cell. The other activating receptors are associated intracellularly with signaling proteins such as the CD3ζ chain, the Fc receptor γ chain, and DAP12, which all contain ITAMs. In contrast, NKG2D binds a different adaptor protein, **DAP10**, which does not contain an ITAM sequence and instead activates the intracellular lipid kinase **phosphatidylinositol 3-kinase (PI 3-kinase)**, initiating a different series of intracellular signaling events in the NK cell (see Section 7-4). Generally, PI 3-kinase is considered to enhance the survival of cells in which it is activated, thereby augmenting the cell's overall effector activity. In NK cells, activation of PI 3-kinase is directly linked to the induction of cytotoxic activity. In mice, the workings of NKG2D are more complicated, because mouse NKG2D is produced in two alternatively spliced forms, one of which binds DAP12 and DAP10, whereas the other binds only DAP10. Mouse NKG2D can thus activate both signaling pathways, whereas human NKG2D seems to signal only through DAP10 to activate the PI 3-kinase pathway. Finally, NK cells express several receptors from the **SLAM (signaling lymphocyte activation molecule)** family, including **2B4**, which recognizes the cell-surface molecule **CD48** expressed by many cells including NK cells. Interactions between 2B4 and CD48 on nearby NK cells can release signals that promote survival and proliferation through **SAP (SLAM-associated protein)** and the Src kinase Fyn.

Summary.

Triggering of innate sensors on various cells—neutrophils, macrophages, and dendritic cells in particular—not only activates these cells' individual effector functions but also stimulates the release of pro-inflammatory chemokines and cytokines that act together to recruit more phagocytic cells to the site of infection. Especially prominent is the early recruitment of neutrophils and monocytes. Furthermore, cytokines released by tissue phagocytic cells can induce more systemic effects, including fever and the production of acute-phase response proteins, such as mannose-binding lectin, C-reactive protein, fibrinogen, and pulmonary surfactant proteins, which add to a general state of augmented innate immunity. These cytokines also mobilize antigen-presenting cells that induce the adaptive immune response. The innate immune system has at its service several recently recognized subtypes of innate lymphoid cells to join the ranks of the long-recognized NK cells. ILCs exhibit specialized effector activity in response to different signals and act to amplify the strength of the innate response. The production of interferons in response to viral infections serves to inhibit viral replication and to activate NK cells. These in turn can distinguish healthy cells from those that are infected by virus or that are transformed or stressed in some way on the basis of expression of MHC class I molecules and MHC-related molecules that are ligands for some NK receptors. As we will see later in the book, cytokines, chemokines, phagocytic cells, and NK cells are all effector mechanisms that are also employed in the adaptive immune response, which uses variable receptors to target specific pathogen antigens.

Summary to Chapter 3.

Innate immunity uses a variety of effector mechanisms to detect infection and eliminate pathogens or to hold them in check until an adaptive immune response develops. These effector mechanisms are all regulated by germline-encoded receptors on many types of cells that can detect molecules of microbial origin or that sense pathogen-induced changes to host cells. The induced responses of the innate immune system are based on several distinct components. After the initial barriers—the body's epithelia and the soluble antimicrobial molecules described in Chapter 2—have been breached, the most important innate defenses rely on tissue macrophages and other tissue-resident sensor cells, such as dendritic cells and ILCs. Macrophages provide a double service: they mediate rapid cellular defense at the borders of infection through phagocytosis and antimicrobial actions, and they also use their various innate sensors to activate the process of inflammation, which involves recruiting additional cells to sites of infection. Innate sensors activate signaling pathways that lead to the production of pro-inflammatory and antiviral cytokines, which in turn stimulate innate effector responses while also helping to initiate an adaptive immune response. The uncovering of the pathogen-sensing mechanisms described in this chapter is still extremely active. It is providing new insights into human autoinflammatory conditions such as lupus, Crohn's disease, and gout. Indeed, the induction of powerful effector mechanisms by innate immune recognition based on germline-encoded receptors clearly has some dangers. It is a double-edged sword, as is illustrated by the effects of the cytokine TNF-α—beneficial when released locally, but disastrous when produced systemically. This illustrates the evolutionary knife edge along which all innate mechanisms of host defense travel. The innate immune system can be viewed as a defense system that mainly frustrates the establishment of a focus of infection; however, even when it proves limited in fulfilling this function, it has already set in motion the initiation of the adaptive immune response, which forms an essential part of human defenses against infection.

Discussion Questions

3.1 The innate immune system uses multiple strategies to identify pathogens.

    a. Give examples of each strategy.

    b. What are the advantages or disadvantages of these different strategies?

3.2 What is the significance of nonclonal expression of pattern-recognition receptors?

3.3 There are a number of cases in which multiple innate immune receptors recognize the same ligand. List some examples. Why might multiple receptors evolve to recognize the same ligand?

3.4 Signaling cascades involving multiple adaptors and numerous intermediate steps seem unnecessarily complex. Why might they have evolved in this way?

3.5 Many signaling cascades used in innate immunity involve the interactions of proteins via specific protein domains. Name the kinds of interaction domains used in TLR signaling. How are the domains of the intermediates used to propagate signals? Also answer this question for RLR and NLR proteins.

3.6 Describe the ways in which interferons interfere with viral replication. Why doesn't the host produce interferons all the time, as a way of preventing viral infection?

3.7 How is it that NK cells can recognize both infected cells and cancerous cells?

3.8 Throughout the chapter we discuss how inappropriate activation of the innate immune system can lead to disease. Select two examples and describe how the inappropriate activation occurs.

Section references.

3-1   After entering tissues, many microbes are recognized, ingested, and killed by phagocytes.

Aderem, A., and Underhill, D.M.: **Mechanisms of phagocytosis in macrophages.** *Annu. Rev. Immunol.* 1999, **17**:593–623.

Auffray, C., Fogg, D., Garfa, M., Elain, G., Join-Lambert, O., Kayal, S., Sarnacki, S., Cumano, A., Lauvau, G., and Geissmann, F.: **Monitoring of blood vessels and tissues by a population of monocytes with patrolling behavior.** *Science* 2007, **317**:666–670.

Cervantes-Barragan, L., Lewis, K.L., Firner, S., Thiel, V., Hugues, S., Reith, W., Ludewig, B., and Reizis, B.: **Plasmacytoid dendritic cells control T-cell response to chronic viral infection.** *Proc. Natl. Acad. Sci. USA* 2012, **109**:3012–3017.

Goodridge, H.S., Wolf, A.J., and Underhill, D.M.: **Beta-glucan recognition by the innate immune system.** *Immunol. Rev.* 2009, **230**:38–50.

Greaves, D.R., and Gordon, S.: **The macrophage scavenger receptor at 30 years of age: current knowledge and future challenges.** *J. Lipid Res.* 2009, **50**:S282–S286.

Greter, M., Lelios, I., Pelczar, P., Hoeffel, G., Price, J., Leboeuf, M., Kündig, T.M., Frei, K., Ginhoux, F., Merad, M., and Becher, B.: **Stroma-derived interleukin-34 controls the development and maintenance of Langerhans cells and the maintenance of microglia.** *Immunity* 2012, **37**:1050–1060.

Harrison, R.E., and Grinstein, S.: **Phagocytosis and the microtubule cytoskeleton.** *Biochem. Cell Biol.* 2002, **80**:509–515.

Lawson, C.D., Donald, S., Anderson, K.E., Patton, D.T., and Welch, H.C.: **P-Rex1 and Vav1 cooperate in the regulation of formyl-methionyl-leucyl-phenylalanine-dependent neutrophil responses.** *J. Immunol.* 2011, **186**:1467–1476.

Lee, S.J., Evers, S., Roeder, D., Parlow, A.F., Risteli, J., Risteli, L., Lee, Y.C., Feizi, T., Langen, H., and Nussenzweig, M.C.: **Mannose receptor-mediated regulation of serum glycoprotein homeostasis.** *Science* 2002, **295**:1898–1901.

Linehan, S.A., Martinez-Pomares, L., and Gordon, S.: **Macrophage lectins in host defence.** *Microbes Infect.* 2000, **2**:279–288.

McGreal, E.P., Miller, J.L., and Gordon, S.: **Ligand recognition by antigen-presenting cell C-type lectin receptors.** *Curr. Opin. Immunol.* 2005, **17**:18–24.

Peiser, L., De Winther, M.P., Makepeace, K., Hollinshead, M., Coull, P., Plested, J., Kodama, T., Moxon, E.R., and Gordon, S.: **The class A macrophage scavenger receptor is a major pattern recognition receptor for *Neisseria meningitidis* which is independent of lipopolysaccharide and not required for secretory responses.** *Infect. Immun.* 2002, **70**:5346–5354.

Podrez, E.A., Poliakov, E., Shen, Z., Zhang, R., Deng, Y., Sun, M., Finton, P.J., Shan, L., Gugiu, B., Fox, P.L., *et al.*: **Identification of a novel family of oxidized phospholipids that serve as ligands for the macrophage scavenger receptor CD36.** *J. Biol. Chem.* 2002, **277**:38503–38516.

3-2   G protein–coupled receptors on phagocytes link microbe recognition with increased efficiency of intracellular killing.

Bogdan, C., Rollinghoff, M., and Diefenbach, A.: **Reactive oxygen and reactive nitrogen intermediates in innate and specific immunity.** *Curr. Opin. Immunol.* 2000, **12**:64–76.

Brinkmann, V., and Zychlinsky, A.: **Beneficial suicide: why neutrophils die to make NETs.** *Nat. Rev. Microbiol.* 2007, **5**:577–582.

Dahlgren, C., and Karlsson, A.: **Respiratory burst in human neutrophils.** *J. Immunol. Methods* 1999, **232**:3–14.

Gerber, B.O., Meng, E.C., Dotsch, V., Baranski, T.J., and Bourne, H.R.: **An activation switch in the ligand binding pocket of the C5a receptor.** *J. Biol. Chem.* 2001, **276**:3394–3400.

Reeves, E.P., Lu, H., Jacobs, H.L., Messina, C.G., Bolsover, S., Gabella, G., Potma, E.O., Warley, A., Roes, J., and Segal, A.W.: **Killing activity of neutrophils is mediated through activation of proteases by K+ flux.** *Nature* 2002, **416**:291–297.

Ward, P.A.: **The dark side of C5a in sepsis.** *Nat. Rev. Immunol.* 2004, **4**:133–142.

3-3   Microbial recognition and tissue damage initiate an inflammatory response.

Chertov, O., Yang, D., Howard, O.M., and Oppenheim, J.J.: **Leukocyte granule proteins mobilize innate host defenses and adaptive immune responses.** *Immunol. Rev.* 2000, **177**:68–78.

Kohl, J.: **Anaphylatoxins and infectious and noninfectious inflammatory diseases.** *Mol. Immunol.* 2001, **38**:175–187.

Mekori, Y.A., and Metcalfe, D.D.: **Mast cells in innate immunity.** *Immunol. Rev.* 2000, **173**:131–140.

Svanborg, C., Godaly, G., and Hedlund, M.: **Cytokine responses during mucosal infections: role in disease pathogenesis and host defence.** *Curr. Opin. Microbiol.* 1999, **2**:99–105.

Van der Poll, T.: **Coagulation and inflammation.** *J. Endotoxin Res.* 2001, **7**:301–304.

3-4   Toll-like receptors represent an ancient pathogen-recognition system.

Lemaitre, B., Nicolas, E., Michaut, L., Reichhart, J.M., and Hoffmann, J.A.: **The dorsoventral regulatory gene cassette spätzle/Toll/cactus controls the potent antifungal response in *Drosophila* adults.** *Cell* 1996, **86**:973–983.

Lemaitre, B., Reichhart, J.M., and Hoffmann, J.A.: **Drosophila host defense: differential induction of antimicrobial peptide genes after infection by various classes of microorganisms.** *Proc. Natl. Acad. Sci. USA* 1997, **94**:14614–14619.

Medzhitov, R., Preston-Hurlburt, P., and Janeway, C.A., Jr.: **A human homologue of the *Drosophila* Toll protein signals activation of adaptive immunity.** *Nature* 1997, **388**:394–397.

3-5   Mammalian Toll-like receptors are activated by many different pathogen-associated molecular patterns.

Alexopoulou, L., Holt, A.C., Medzhitov, R., and Flavell, R.A.: **Recognition of double-stranded RNA and activation of NF-kappaB by Toll-like receptor 3.** *Nature* 2001, **413**:732–738.

Brightbill, H.D., Libraty, D.H., Krutzik, S.R., Yang, R.B., Belisle, J.T., Bleharski, J.R., Maitland, M., Norgard, M.V., Plevy, S.E., Smale, S.T., *et al.*: **Host defense mechanisms triggered by microbial lipoproteins through Toll-like receptors.** *Science* 1999, **285**:732–736.

Diebold, S.S., Kaisho, T., Hemmi, H., Akira, S., and Reis e Sousa, C.: **Innate antiviral responses by means of TLR7-mediated recognition of single-stranded RNA.** *Science* 2004, **303**:1529–1531.

Ewald, S.E., Lee, B.L., Lau, L., Wickliffe, K.E., Shi, G.P., Chapman, H.A., and Barton, G.M.: **The ectodomain of Toll-like receptor 9 is cleaved to generate a functional receptor.** *Nature* 2011, **456**:658–662.

Hayashi, F., Smith, K.D., Ozinsky, A., Hawn, T.R., Yi, E.C., Goodlett, D.R., Eng, J.K., Akira, S., Underhill, D.M., and Aderem, A.: **The innate immune response to bacterial flagellin is mediated by Toll-like receptor 5.** *Nature* 2001, **410**:1099–1103.

Heil, F., Hemmi, H., Hochrein, H., Ampenberger, F., Kirschning, C., Akira, S., Lipford, G., Wagner, H., and Bauer, S.: **Species-specific recognition of single-stranded RNA via Toll-like receptor 7 and 8.** *Science* 2004, **303**:1526–1529.

Hemmi, H., Takeuchi, O., Kawai, T., Kaisho, T., Sato, S., Sanjo, H., Matsumoto, M., Hoshino, K., Wagner, H., Takeda, K., and Akira, S.: **A Toll-like receptor recognizes DNA.** *Nature* 2000, **408**:740–745.

Jin, M.S., Kim, S.E., Heo, J.Y., Lee, M.E., Kim, H.M., Paik, S.G., Lee, H., and Lee, J.O.: **Crystal structure of the TLR1-TLR2 heterodimer induced by binding of a tri-acylated lipopeptide.** *Cell* 2007, **130**:1071–1082.

Kim, Y.M., Brinkman, M.M., Paquet, M.E., and Ploegh, H.L.: **UNC93B1 delivers nucleotide-sensing toll-like receptors to endolysosomes.** *Nature* 2008, **452**:234–238.

Liu, L., Botos, I., Wang, Y., Leonard, J.N., Shiloach, J., Segal, D.M., and Davies, D.R.: **Structural basis of Toll-like receptor 3 signaling with double-stranded RNA.** *Science* 2008, **320**:379–381.

Lund, J.M., Alexopoulou, L., Sato, A., Karow, M., Adams, N.C., Gale, N.W., Iwasaki, A., and Flavell, R.A.: **Recognition of single-stranded RNA viruses by Toll-like receptor 7.** *Proc. Natl. Acad. Sci. USA* 2004, **101**:5598–5603.

Lund, J., Sato, A., Akira, S., Medzhitov, R., and Iwasaki, A.: Toll-like receptor 9-mediated recognition of herpes simplex virus-2 by plasmacytoid dendritic cells. *J. Exp. Med.* 2003, **198**:513–520.

Takeuchi, O., Hoshino, K., Kawai, T., Sanjo, H., Takada, H., Ogawa, T., Takeda, K., and Akira, S.: Differential roles of TLR2 and TLR4 in recognition of gram-negative and gram-positive bacterial cell wall components. *Immunity* 1999, **11**:443-451.

Tanji, H., Ohto, U., Shibata, T., Miyake, K., and Shimizu, T.: Structural reorganization of the Toll-like receptor 8 dimer induced by agonistic ligands. *Science* 2013, **339**:1426–1429.

Yarovinsky, F., Zhang, D., Andersen, J.F., Bannenberg, G.L., Serhan, C.N., Hayden, M.S., Hieny, S., Sutterwala, F.S., Flavell, R.A., Ghosh, S., *et al.*: TLR11 activation of dendritic cells by a protozoan profilin-like protein. *Science* 2005, **308**:1626–1629.

3-6 TLR-4 recognizes bacterial lipopolysaccharide in association with the host accessory proteins MD-2 and CD14.

Beutler, B., and Rietschel, E.T.: Innate immune sensing and its roots: the story of endotoxin. *Nat. Rev. Immunol.* 2003, **3**:169–176.

Kim, H.M., Park, B.S., Kim, J.I., Kim, S.E., Lee, J., Oh, S.C., Enkhbayar, P., Matsushima, N., Lee, H., Yoo, O.J., *et al.*: Crystal structure of the TLR4–MD-2 complex with bound endotoxin antagonist Eritoran. *Cell* 2007, **130**:906–917.

Park, B.S., Song, D.H., Kim, H.M., Choi, B.S., Lee, H., and Lee, J.O.: The structural basis of lipopolysaccharide recognition by the TLR4–MD-2 complex. *Nature* 2009, **458**:1191–1195.

Poltorak, A., He, X., Smirnova, I., Liu, M.Y., Huffel, C.V., Du, X., Birdwell, D., Alejos, E., Silva, M., Galanos, C., *et al.*: Defective LPS signalling in C3H/HeJ and C57BL/10ScCr mice: mutations in Tlr4 gene. *Science* 1998, **282**:2085–2088.

3-7 TLRs activate NFκB, AP-1, and IRF transcription factors to induce the expression of inflammatory cytokines and type I interferons.

Fitzgerald, K.A., McWhirter, S.M., Faia, K.L., Rowe, D.C., Latz, E., Golenbock, D.T., Coyle, A.J., Liao, S.M., and Maniatis, T.: IKKε and TBK1 are essential components of the IRF3 signaling pathway. *Nat. Immunol.* 2003, **4**:491–496.

Häcker, H., Redecke, V., Blagoev, B., Kratchmarova, I., Hsu, L.C., Wang, G.G., Kamps, M.P., Raz, E., Wagner, H., Häcker, G., *et al.*: Specificity in Toll-like receptor signaling through distinct effector functions of TRAF3 and TRAF6. *Nature* 2006, **439**:204–207.

Hiscott, J., Nguyen, T.L., Arguello, M., Nakhaei, P., and Paz, S.: Manipulation of the nuclear factor-κB pathway and the innate immune response by viruses. *Oncogene* 2006, **25**:6844–6867.

Honda, K., and Taniguchi, T.: IRFs: master regulators of signalling by Toll-like receptors and cytosolic pattern-recognition receptors. *Nat. Rev. Immunol.* 2006, **6**:644–658.

Kawai, T., and Akira, S.: The role of pattern-recognition receptors in innate immunity: update on Toll-like receptors. *Nat Immunol.* 2010, **11**:373–384.

Kawai, T., Sato, S., Ishii, K.J., Coban, C., Hemmi, H., Yamamoto, M., Terai, K., Matsuda, M., Inoue, J., Uematsu, S., *et al.*: Interferon-alpha induction through Toll-like receptors involves a direct interaction of IRF7 with MyD88 and TRAF6. *Nat. Immunol.* 2004, **5**:1061–1068.

Puel, A., Yang, K., Ku, C.L., von Bernuth, H., Bustamante, J., Santos, O.F., Lawrence, T., Chang, H.H., Al-Mousa, H., Picard, C., *et al.*: Heritable defects of the human TLR signalling pathways. *J. Endotoxin Res.* 2005, **11**:220–224.

Von Bernuth, H., Picard, C., Jin, Z., Pankla, R., Xiao, H., Ku, C.L., Chrabieh, M., Mustapha, I.B., Ghandil, P., Camcioglu, Y., *et al.*: Pyogenic bacterial infections in humans with MyD88 deficiency. *Science* 2008, **321**:691–696.

3-8 The RIG-I–like receptors detect cytoplasmic viral RNAs and activate MAVS to induce type I interferon production and pro-inflammatory cytokines.

Hornung, V., Ellegast, J., Kim, S., Brzózka, K., Jung, A., Kato, H., Poeck, H., Akira, S., Conzelmann, K.K., Schlee, M., *et al.*: 5′-Triphosphate RNA is the ligand for RIG-I. *Science* 2006, **314**:994–997.

Kato, H., Takeuchi, O., Sato, S., Yoneyama, M., Yamamoto, M., Matsui, K., Uematsu, S., Jung, A., Kawai, T., Ishii, K.J., *et al.*: Differential roles of MDA5 and RIG-I helicases in the recognition of RNA viruses. *Nature* 2006, **441**: 101–105.

Pichlmair, A., Schulz, O., Tan, C.P., Näslund, T.I., Liljeström, P., Weber, F., and Reis e Sousa, C.: RIG-I-mediated antiviral responses to single-stranded RNA bearing 5′-phosphates. *Science* 2006, **314**:935–936.

3-9 Cytosolic DNA activates the cGAS–STING pathway to induce production of type I interferons.

Cai, X., Chiu, Y.H., and Chen, Z.J.: The cGAS-cGAMP-STING pathway of cytosolic DNA sensing and signaling. *Mol. Cell* 2014, **54**:289–296.

Ishikawa, H., and Barber, G.N.: STING is an endoplasmic reticulum adaptor that facilitates innate immune signalling. *Nature* 2008, **455**:674–678.

Li, X.D., Wu, J., Gao, D., Wang, H., Sun, L., and Chen, Z.J.: Pivotal roles of cGAS-cGAMP signaling in antiviral defense and immune adjuvant effects. *Science* 2013, **341**:1390–1394.

Liu, S., Cai, X., Wu, J., Cong, Q., Chen, X., Li, T., Du, F., Ren, J., Wu, Y.T., Grishin, N.V., and Chen, Z.J.: Phosphorylation of innate immune adaptor proteins MAVS, STING, and TRIF induces IRF3 activation. *Science* 2015, **347**:aaa2630.

Liu, Y., Jesus, A.A., Marrero, B., Yang, D., Ramsey, S.E., Sanchez, G.A.M., Tenbrock, K., Wittkowski, H., Jones, O.Y., Kuehn, H.S., *et al.*: Activated STING in a vascular and pulmonary syndrome. *N. Engl. J. Med.* 2014, **371**:507–518.

Stetson, D.B., Ko, J.S., Heidmann, T., and Medzhitov, R.: Trex1 prevents cell-intrinsic initiation of autoimmunity. *Cell* 2008, **134**:587–598.

Sun, L., Wu, J., Du, F., Chen, X., and Chen, Z.J.: Cyclic GMP-AMP synthase is a cytosolic DNA sensor that activates the type I interferon pathway. *Science* 2013, **339**:786–791.

Wu, J., Sun, L., Chen, X., Du, F., Shi, H., Chen, C., and Chen, Z.J.: Cyclic GMP-AMP is an endogenous second messenger in innate immune signalling by cytosolic DNA. *Science* 2015, **339**:826–830.

3-10 NLRs comprise a large family of intracellular sensors with diverse functions.

Caruso, R., Warner, N., Inohara, N. and Nunez, G.: NOD1 and NOD2: signalling, host defense, and inflammatory disease. *Immunity* 2014, **41**:898–908.

Chen, G., Shaw, M.H., Kim, Y.-G., and Nunez, G.: NOD-like receptors: role in innate immunity and inflammatory disease. *Annu. Rev. Pathol.* 2009, **4**:365–398.

Ting, J.P., Duncan, J.A., and Lei, Y.: How the noninflammasome NLRs function in the innate immune system. *Science* 2010, **327**:286–290.

3-11 Certain NLR proteins react to infection or cellular damage by forming an inflammasome that induces cell death and secretion of inflammatory cytokines.

He, W.T., Wan, H., Hu, L., Chen, P., Wang, X., Huang, Z., Yang, Z.H., Zhong, C.Q., and Han, J.: Gasdermin D is an executor of pyroptosis and required for interleukin-1β secretion. *Cell Res.* 2015, **25**:1285–1298.

Hornung, V., Ablasser, A., Charrel-Dennis, M., Bauernfeind, F., Horvath, G., Caffrey, D.R., Latz, E., and Fitzgerald, K.A.: AIM2 recognizes cytosolic dsDNA and forms a caspase-1-activating inflammasome with ASC. *Nature* 2009, **458**:514–518.

Kayagaki, N., Stowe, I.B., Lee, B.L., O'Rourke, K., Anderson, K., Warming, S., Cuellar, T., Haley, B., Roose-Girma, M., Phung, Q.T., *et al.*: Caspase-11 cleaves gasdermin D for non-canonical inflammasome signalling. *Nature* 2015, **526**:666–671.

Kofoed, E.M., and Vance, R.E.: Innate immune recognition of bacterial ligands by NAIPs determines inflammasome specificity. *Nature* 2011, **477**: 592–595.

Martinon, F., Pétrilli, V., Mayor, A., Tardivel, A., and Tschopp, J.: Gout-associated uric acid crystals activate the NALP3 inflammasome. *Nature* 2006, **440**: 237–241.

Muñoz-Planillo, R., Kuffa, P., Martínez-Colón, G., Smith, B.L., Rajendiran, T.M., and Núñez, G.: K⁺ efflux is the common trigger of NLRP3 inflammasome activation by bacterial toxins and particulate matter. *Immunity* 2013, 38: 1142–1153.

Shi, J., Zhao, Y., Wang, Y., Gao, W., Ding, J., Li, P., Hu, L., and Shao, F.: Inflammatory caspases are innate immune receptors for intracellular LPS. *Nature* 2014, **514**:187–192.

Shi, J., Zhao, Y., Wang, K., Shi, X., Wang, Y., Huang, H., Zhuang, Y., Cai, T., Wang, F., and Shao, F.: Cleavage of GSDMD by inflammatory caspases determines pyroptotic cell death. *Nature* 2015, 526:660–665.

Tenthorey, J.L., Haloupek, N., Lopez-Blanco, J.R., Grob, P., Adamson, E., Hartenian, E., Lind, N.A., Bourgeois, N.M., Chacon, P., Nogales, E., and Vance, R.E.: The structural basis of flagellin detection by NAIP5: a strategy to limit pathogen immune evasion. *Science* 2017, 358:888–893.

3-12 Activation of innate sensors in macrophages and dendritic cells triggers changes in gene expression that have far-reaching effects on the immune response.

Schnare, M., Barton, G.M., Holt, A.C., Takeda, K., Akira, S., and Medzhitov, R.: Toll-like receptors control activation of adaptive immune responses. *Nat. Immunol.* 2001, 2:947–950.

3-13 Toll signaling in *Drosophila* is downstream of a distinct set of pathogen-recognition molecules.

Ferrandon, D., Imler, J.L., Hetru, C., and Hoffmann, J.A.: The *Drosophila* systemic immune response: sensing and signalling during bacterial and fungal infections. *Nat. Rev. Immunol.* 2007, 7:862–874.

Gottar, M., Gobert, V., Matskevich, A.A., Reichhart, J.M., Wang, C., Butt, T.M., Belvin, M., Hoffmann, J.A., and Ferrandon, D.: Dual detection of fungal infections in *Drosophila* via recognition of glucans and sensing of virulence factors. *Cell* 2006, 127:1425–1437.

Pili-Floury, S., Leulier, F., Takahashi, K., Saigo, K., Samain, E., Ueda, R., and Lemaitre, B.: *In vivo* RNA interference analysis reveals an unexpected role for GNBP1 in the defense against Gram-positive bacterial infection in *Drosophila* adults. *J. Biol. Chem.* 2004, 279:12848–12853.

Royet, J., and Dziarski, R.: Peptidoglycan recognition proteins: pleiotropic sensors and effectors of antimicrobial defences. *Nat. Rev. Microbiol.* 2007, 5:264–277.

3-14 TLR and NOD genes have undergone extensive diversification in both invertebrates and some primitive chordates.

Rast, J.P., Smith, L.C., Loza-Coll, M., Hibino, T., and Litman, G.W.: Genomic insights into the immune system of the sea urchin. *Science* 2006, **314**: 952–956.

Samanta, M.P., Tongprasit, W., Istrail, S., Cameron, R.A., Tu, Q., Davidson, E.H., and Stolc, V.: The transcriptome of the sea urchin embryo. *Science* 2006, 314:960–962.

3-15 Cytokines and their receptors fall into distinct families of structurally related proteins.

Boulay, J.L., O'Shea, J.J., and Paul, W.E.: Molecular phylogeny within type I cytokines and their cognate receptors. *Immunity* 2003, 19:159–163.

Collette, Y., Gilles, A., Pontarotti, P., and Olive, D.: A co-evolution perspective of the TNFSF and TNFRSF families in the immune system. *Trends Immunol.* 2003, 24:387–394.

Ihle, J.N.: Cytokine receptor signalling. *Nature* 1995, 377:591–594.

Proudfoot, A.E.: Chemokine receptors: multifaceted therapeutic targets. *Nat. Rev. Immunol.* 2002, 2:106–115.

Taniguchi, T., and Takaoka, A.: The interferon-α/β system in antiviral responses: a multimodal machinery of gene regulation by the IRF family of transcription factors. *Curr. Opin. Immunol.* 2002, **14**:111–116.

3-16 Cytokine receptors of the hematopoietin superfamily are associated with the JAK family of tyrosine kinases, which activate STAT transcription factors.

Fu, X.Y.: A transcription factor with SH2 and SH3 domains is directly activated by an interferon α-induced cytoplasmic protein tyrosine kinase(s). *Cell* 1992, 70:323–335.

Krebs, D.L., and Hilton, D.J.: SOCS proteins: negative regulators of cytokine signaling. *Stem Cells* 2001, 19:378–387.

Leonard, W.J., and O'Shea, J.J.: Jaks and STATs: biological implications. *Annu. Rev. Immunol.* 1998, 16:293–322.

Levy, D.E., and Darnell, J.E., Jr.: Stats: transcriptional control and biological impact. *Nat. Rev. Mol. Cell Biol.* 2002, 3:651–662.

Ota, N., Brett, T.J., Murphy, T.L., Fremont, D.H., and Murphy, K.M.: N-domain-dependent nonphosphorylated STAT4 dimers required for cytokine-driven activation. *Nat. Immunol.* 2004, 5:208–215.

Pesu, M., Candotti, F., Husa, M., Hofmann, S.R., Notarangelo, L.D., and O'Shea, J.J.: Jak3, severe combined immunodeficiency, and a new class of immunosuppressive drugs. *Immunol. Rev.* 2005, 203:127–142.

Rytinki, M.M., Kaikkonen, S., Pehkonen, P., Jääskeläinen, T., and Palvimo, J.J.: PIAS proteins: pleiotropic interactors associated with SUMO. *Cell. Mol. Life Sci.* 2009, 66:3029–3041.

Schindler, C., Shuai, K., Prezioso, V.R., and Darnell, J.E., Jr.: Interferon-dependent tyrosine phosphorylation of a latent cytoplasmic transcription factor. *Science* 1992, 257:809–813.

Shuai, K., and Liu, B.: Regulation of JAK-STAT signalling in the immune system. *Nat. Rev. Immunol.* 2003, 3:900–911.

Yasukawa, H., Sasaki, A., and Yoshimura, A.: Negative regulation of cytokine signaling pathways. *Annu. Rev. Immunol.* 2000, 18:143–164.

3-17 Chemokines released by macrophages and dendritic cells recruit effector cells to sites of infection.

Larsson, B.M., Larsson, K., Malmberg, P., and Palmberg, L.: Gram-positive bacteria induce IL-6 and IL-8 production in human alveolar macrophages and epithelial cells. *Inflammation* 1999, 23:217–230.

Luster, A.D.: The role of chemokines in linking innate and adaptive immunity. *Curr. Opin. Immunol.* 2002, 14:129–135.

Matsukawa, A., Hogaboam, C.M., Lukacs, N.W., and Kunkel, S.L.: Chemokines and innate immunity. *Rev. Immunogenet.* 2000, 2:339–358.

Scapini, P., Lapinet-Vera, J.A., Gasperini, S., Calzetti, F., Bazzoni, F., and Cassatella, M.A.: The neutrophil as a cellular source of chemokines. *Immunol. Rev.* 2000, 177:195–203.

Shortman, K., and Liu, Y.J.: Mouse and human dendritic cell subtypes. *Nat. Rev. Immunol.* 2002, 2:151–161.

Svanborg, C., Godaly, G., and Hedlund, M.: Cytokine responses during mucosal infections: role in disease pathogenesis and host defence. *Curr. Opin. Microbiol.* 1999, 2:99–105.

Yoshie, O.: Role of chemokines in trafficking of lymphocytes and dendritic cells. *Int. J. Hematol.* 2000, **72**:399–407.

3-18 Cell-adhesion molecules control interactions between leukocytes and endothelial cells during an inflammatory response.

Alon, R., and Feigelson, S.: From rolling to arrest on blood vessels: leukocyte tap dancing on endothelial integrin ligands and chemokines at sub-second contacts. *Semin. Immunol.* 2002, 14:93–104.

Bunting, M., Harris, E.S., McIntyre, T.M., Prescott, S.M., and Zimmerman, G.A.: Leukocyte adhesion deficiency syndromes: adhesion and tethering defects involving β2 integrins and selectin ligands. *Curr. Opin. Hematol.* 2002, 9:30–35.

D'Ambrosio, D., Albanesi, C., Lang, R., Girolomoni, G., Sinigaglia, F., and Laudanna, C.: Quantitative differences in chemokine receptor engagement generate diversity in integrin-dependent lymphocyte adhesion. *J. Immunol.* 2002, **169**:2303–2312.

Johnston, B., and Butcher, E.C.: Chemokines in rapid leukocyte adhesion triggering and migration. *Semin. Immunol.* 2002, **14**:83–92.

Ley, K.: Integration of inflammatory signals by rolling neutrophils. *Immunol. Rev.* 2002, **186**:8–18.

Vestweber, D.: Lymphocyte trafficking through blood and lymphatic vessels: more than just selectins, chemokines and integrins. *Eur. J. Immunol.* 2003, **33**:1361–1364.

3-19 Neutrophils make up the first wave of cells that cross the blood vessel wall to enter an inflamed tissue.

Bochenska-Marciniak, M., Kupczyk, M., Gorski, P., and Kuna, P.: The effect of recombinant interleukin-8 on eosinophils' and neutrophils' migration *in vivo* and *in vitro*. *Allergy* 2003, **58**:795–801.

Godaly, G., Bergsten, G., Hang, L., Fischer, H., Frendeus, B., Lundstedt, A.C., Samuelsson, M., Samuelsson, P., and Svanborg, C.: Neutrophil recruitment, chemokine receptors, and resistance to mucosal infection. *J. Leukoc. Biol.* 2001, **69**:899–906.

Gompertz, S., and Stockley, R.A.: Inflammation—role of the neutrophil and the eosinophil. *Semin. Respir. Infect.* 2000, **15**:14–23.

Lee, S.C., Brummet, M.E., Shahabuddin, S., Woodworth, T.G., Georas, S.N., Leiferman, K.M., Gilman, S.C., Stellato, C., Gladue, R.P., Schleimer, R.P., *et al.*: Cutaneous injection of human subjects with macrophage inflammatory protein-1α induces significant recruitment of neutrophils and monocytes. *J. Immunol.* 2000, **164**:3392–3401.

Sundd, P., Gutierrez, E., Koltsova, E.K., Kuwano, Y., Fukuda, S., Pospieszalska, M.K., Groisman, A., and Ley, K.: 'Slings' enable neutrophil rolling at high shear. *Nature* 2012, **488**:399–403.

Worthylake, R.A., and Burridge, K.: Leukocyte transendothelial migration: orchestrating the underlying molecular machinery. *Curr. Opin. Cell Biol.* 2001, **13**:569–577.

3-20 TNF-α is an important cytokine that triggers local containment of infection but induces shock when released systemically.

Croft, M.: The role of TNF superfamily members in T-cell function and diseases. *Nat. Rev. Immunol.* 2009, **9**:271–285.

Dellinger, R.P.: Inflammation and coagulation: implications for the septic patient. *Clin. Infect. Dis.* 2003, **36**:1259–1265.

Georgel, P., Naitza, S., Kappler, C., Ferrandon, D., Zachary, D., Swimmer, C., Kopczynski, C., Duyk, G., Reichhart, J.M., and Hoffmann, J.A.: *Drosophila* immune deficiency (IMD) is a death domain protein that activates antibacterial defense and can promote apoptosis. *Dev. Cell* 2001, **1**:503–514.

Pfeffer, K.: Biological functions of tumor necrosis factor cytokines and their receptors. *Cytokine Growth Factor Rev.* 2003, **14**:185–191.

Rutschmann, S., Jung, A.C., Zhou, R., Silverman, N., Hoffmann, J.A., and Ferrandon, D.: Role of *Drosophila* IKKγ in a *toll*-independent antibacterial immune response. *Nat. Immunol.* 2000, **1**:342–347.

3-21 Cytokines made by macrophages and dendritic cells induce a systemic reaction known as the acute-phase response.

Bopst, M., Haas, C., Car, B., and Eugster, H.P.: The combined inactivation of tumor necrosis factor and interleukin-6 prevents induction of the major acute phase proteins by endotoxin. *Eur. J. Immunol.* 1998, **28**:4130–4137.

Ceciliani, F., Giordano, A., and Spagnolo, V.: The systemic reaction during inflammation: the acute-phase proteins. *Protein Pept. Lett.* 2002, **9**:211–223.

He, R., Sang, H., and Ye, R.D.: Serum amyloid A induces IL-8 secretion through a G protein-coupled receptor, FPRL1/LXA4R. *Blood* 2003, **101**:1572–1581.

Horn, F., Henze, C., and Heidrich, K.: Interleukin-6 signal transduction and lymphocyte function. *Immunobiology* 2000, **202**:151–167.

Manfredi, A.A., Rovere-Querini, P., Bottazzi, B., Garlanda, C., and Mantovani, A.: Pentraxins, humoral innate immunity and tissue injury. *Curr. Opin. Immunol.* 2008, **20**:538–544.

Mold, C., Rodriguez, W., Rodic-Polic, B., and Du Clos, T.W.: C-reactive protein mediates protection from lipopolysaccharide through interactions with FcγR. *J. Immunol.* 2002, **169**:7019–7025.

3-22 Interferons induced by viral infection make several contributions to host defense.

Baldridge, M.T., Nice, T.J., McCune, B.T., Yokoyama, C.C., Kambal, A., Wheadon, M., Diamond, M.S., Ivanova, Y., Artyomov, M., and Virgin, H.W.: Commensal microbes and interferon-λ determine persistence of enteric murine norovirus infection. *Science* 2015, **347**:266–269.

Honda, K., Takaoka, A., and Taniguchi, T.: Type I interferon gene induction by the interferon regulatory factor family of transcription factors. *Immunity* 2006, **25**:349–360.

Kawai, T., and Akira, S.: Innate immune recognition of viral infection. *Nat. Immunol.* 2006, **7**:131–137.

Liu, Y.J.: IPC: professional type 1 interferon-producing cells and plasmacytoid dendritic cell precursors. *Annu. Rev. Immunol.* 2005, **23**:275–306.

Meylan, E., and Tschopp, J.: Toll-like receptors and RNA helicases: two parallel ways to trigger antiviral responses. *Mol. Cell* 2006, **22**:561–569.

Pietras, E.M., Saha, S.K., and Cheng, G.: The interferon response to bacterial and viral infections. *J. Endotoxin Res.* 2006, **12**:246–250.

Pott, J., Mahlakõiv, T., Mordstein, M., Duerr, C.U., Michiels, T., Stockinger, S., Staeheli, P., and Hornef, M.W.: IFN-lambda determines the intestinal epithelial antiviral host defense. *Proc. Natl. Acad. Sci. USA* 2011, **108**:7944–7949.

3-23 Several types of innate lymphoid cells provide protection in early infection.

Artis, D., and Spits, H.: The biology of innate lymphoid cells. *Nature* 2015, **517**:293–301.

Cortez, V.S., Robinette, M.L., and Colonna, M.: Innate lymphoid cells: new insights into function and development. *Curr. Opin. Immunol.* 2015, **32**:71–77.

Spits, H., Artis, D., Colonna, M., Diefenbach, A., Di Santo, J.P., Eberl, G., Koyasu, S., Locksley, R.M., McKenzie, A.N., Mebius, R.E., *et al.*: Innate lymphoid cells—a proposal for uniform nomenclature. *Nat. Rev. Immunol.* 2013, **13**:145–149.

3-24 NK cells are activated by type I interferon and macrophage-derived cytokines.

Gineau, L., Cognet, C., Kara, N., Lach, F.P., Dunne, J., Veturi, U., Picard, C., Trouillet, C., Eidenschenk, C., Aoufouchi S., *et al.*: Partial MCM4 deficiency in patients with growth retardation, adrenal insufficiency, and natural killer cell deficiency. *J. Clin. Invest.* 2012, **122**:821–832.

Godshall, C.J., Scott, M.J., Burch, P.T., Peyton, J.C., and Cheadle, W.G.: Natural killer cells participate in bacterial clearance during septic peritonitis through interactions with macrophages. *Shock* 2003, **19**:144–149.

Lanier, L.L.: Evolutionary struggles between NK cells and viruses. *Nat. Rev. Immunol.* 2008, **8**:259–268.

Salazar-Mather, T.P., Hamilton, T.A., and Biron, C.A.: A chemokine-to-cytokine-to-chemokine cascade critical in antiviral defense. *J. Clin. Invest.* 2000, **105**:985–993.

Seki, S., Habu, Y., Kawamura, T., Takeda, K., Dobashi, H., Ohkawa, T., and Hiraide, H.: The liver as a crucial organ in the first line of host defense: the roles of Kupffer cells, natural killer (NK) cells and NK1.1 Ag+ T cells in T helper 1 immune responses. *Immunol. Rev.* 2000, **174**:35–46.

Yokoyama, W.M., and Plougastel, B.F.: Immune functions encoded by the natural killer gene complex. *Nat. Rev. Immunol.* 2003, **3**:304–316.

3-25 NK cells express activating and inhibitory receptors to distinguish between healthy and infected cells.

&

3-26 NK-cell receptors belong to several structural families.

Borrego, F., Kabat, J., Kim, D.K., Lieto, L., Maasho, K., Pena, J., Solana, R., and Coligan, J.E.: Structure and function of major histocompatibility complex (MHC) class I specific receptors expressed on human natural killer (NK) cells. *Mol. Immunol.* 2002, **38**:637–660.

Boyington, J.C., and Sun, P.D.: **A structural perspective on MHC class I recognition by killer cell immunoglobulin-like receptors.** *Mol. Immunol.* 2002, **38**:1007–1021.

Brown, M.G., Dokun, A.O., Heusel, J.W., Smith, H.R., Beckman, D.L., Blattenberger, E.A., Dubbelde, C.E., Stone, L.R., Scalzo, A.A., and Yokoyama, W.M.: **Vital involvement of a natural killer cell activation receptor in resistance to viral infection.** *Science* 2001, **292**:934–937.

Long, E.O.: **Negative signalling by inhibitory receptors: the NK cell paradigm.** *Immunol. Rev.* 2008, **224**:70–84.

Robbins, S.H., and Brossay, L.: **NK cell receptors: emerging roles in host defense against infectious agents.** *Microbes Infect.* 2002, **4**:1523–1530.

Trowsdale, J.: **Genetic and functional relationships between MHC and NK receptor genes.** *Immunity* 2001, **15**:363–374.

Vilches, C., and Parham, P.: **KIR: diverse, rapidly evolving receptors of innate and adaptive immunity.** *Annu. Rev. Immunol.* 2002, **20**:217–251.

Vivier, E., Raulet, D.H., Moretta, A., Caligiuri, M.A., Zitvogel, L., Lanier, L.L., Yokoyama, W.M., and Ugolini, S.: **Innate or adaptive immunity? The example of natural killer cells.** *Science* 2011, **331**:44–49.

Vivier, E., Tomasello, E., Baratin, M., Walzer, T., and Ugolini, S.: **Functions of natural killer cells.** *Nat. Immunol.* 2008, **9**:503–510.

3-27 NK cells express activating receptors that recognize ligands induced on infected cells or tumor cells.

Brandt, C.S., Baratin, M., Yi, E.C., Kennedy, J., Gao, Z., Fox, B., Haldeman, B., Ostrander, C.D., Kaifu, T., Chabannon, C., *et al.*: **The B7 family member B7-H6 is a tumor cell ligand for the activating natural killer cell receptor NKp30 in humans.** *J. Exp. Med.* 2009, **206**:1495–1503.

Diefenbach, A., Tomasello, E., Lucas, M., Jamieson, A.M., Hsia, J.K., Vivier, E., and Raulet, D.H.: **Selective associations with signaling proteins determine stimulatory versus costimulatory activity of NKG2D.** *Nat Immunol.* 2002, **3**:1142–1149.

Gasser, S., Orsulic, S., Brown, E.J., and Raulet, D.H.: **The DNA damage pathway regulates innate immune system ligands of the NKG2D receptor.** *Nature* 2005, **436**:1186–1190.

Gonzalez, S., Groh, V., and Spies, T.: **Immunobiology of human NKG2D and its ligands.** *Curr. Top. Microbiol. Immunol.* 2006, **298**:121–138.

Moretta, L., Bottino, C., Pende, D., Castriconi, R., Mingari, M.C., and Moretta, A.: **Surface NK receptors and their ligands on tumor cells.** *Semin. Immunol.* 2006, **18**:151–158.

Parham, P.: **MHC class I molecules and KIRs in human history, health and survival.** *Nat. Rev. Immunol.* 2005, **5**:201–214.

Raulet, D.H., Gasser, S., Gowen, B.G., Deng, W., and Jung, H.: **Regulation of ligands for the NKG2D activating receptor.** *Annu. Rev. Immunol.* 2013, **31**:413–441.

Upshaw, J.L., and Leibson, P.J.: **NKG2D-mediated activation of cytotoxic lymphocytes: unique signaling pathways and distinct functional outcomes.** *Semin. Immunol.* 2006, **18**:167–175.

Vivier, E., Nunes, J.A., and Vely, F.: **Natural killer cell signaling pathways.** *Science* 2004, **306**:1517–1519.

Antigen Recognition by B-cell and T-cell Receptors

4

Innate immune responses are the body's initial defense against infection, but these work only to control pathogens that have certain molecular patterns or that induce interferons and other nonspecific defenses. To effectively fight the wide range of pathogens an individual will encounter, the lymphocytes of the adaptive immune system have evolved to recognize a great variety of different **antigens** from bacteria, viruses, and other disease-causing organisms. An antigen is any molecule or part of a molecule that is specifically recognized by the highly specialized recognition proteins of lymphocytes. On B cells these proteins are the **immunoglobulins (Igs)**, which these cells produce in a vast range of antigen specificities, each B cell producing immunoglobulins of a single specificity (see Section 1-12). A membrane-bound form of immunoglobulin on the B-cell surface serves as the cell's receptor for antigen and is known as the **B-cell receptor (BCR)**. A secreted form of immunoglobulin of the same antigen specificity is the **antibody** produced by terminally differentiated B cells—plasmablasts and plasma cells. The secretion of antibodies, which bind pathogens or their toxic products in the extracellular spaces of the body (see Fig. 1.28), is the main effector function of B cells in adaptive immunity.

Antibodies were the first proteins involved in specific immune recognition to be characterized and are understood in great detail. The antibody molecule has two separate functions: one is to bind specifically to the pathogen or its products that have elicited the immune response; the other is to recruit other cells and molecules to destroy the pathogen once antibody has bound. For example, binding by antibodies can neutralize viruses and mark pathogens for destruction by phagocytes and complement, as described in Chapters 2 and 3. Recognition and effector functions are structurally separated in the antibody molecule, one part of which specifically binds to the antigen whereas the other engages the elimination mechanisms. The antigen-binding region varies extensively among antibody molecules and is known as the **variable region**, or **V region**. The variability of antibody molecules allows each antibody to bind a different specific antigen, and the total repertoire of antibodies made by a single individual is large enough to ensure that virtually any structure can be recognized. The region of the antibody molecule that engages the

IN THIS CHAPTER

The structure of a typical antibody molecule.

Structural variation in immunoglobulin constant regions.

The interaction of the antibody molecule with specific antigen.

Antigen recognition by T cells.

effector functions of the immune system does not vary in the same way and is known as the **constant region**, or **C region**. It comes in five main forms, called **isotypes**, each of which is specialized for activating different effector mechanisms. The membrane-bound B-cell receptor does not have these effector functions, because the C region remains inserted in the membrane of the B cell. The function of the B-cell receptor is to recognize and bind antigen via the V regions exposed on the surface of the cell, thus transmitting a signal that activates the B cell, leading to clonal expansion and antibody production. To this end, the B-cell receptor is associated with a set of intracellular signaling proteins, which will be described in Chapter 7. Antibodies have become an important class of drug due to their highly specific activities, and we return to discuss their therapeutic uses in Chapter 16.

The antigen-recognition molecules of T cells are made solely as membrane-bound proteins, which are associated with an intracellular signaling complex and function only to signal T cells for activation. These **T-cell receptors (TCRs)** are related to immunoglobulins both in their protein structure—having both V and C regions—and in the genetic mechanism that produces their great variability, which is discussed in Chapter 5. The T-cell receptor differs from the B-cell receptor in an important way, however: it does not recognize and bind antigen by itself but instead recognizes short peptide fragments of protein antigens that are presented to it by proteins known as **MHC molecules** on the surface of host cells.

The MHC molecules are transmembrane glycoproteins encoded in the large cluster of genes known as the **major histocompatibility complex (MHC)**. The most striking structural feature of MHC molecules is a cleft in the extracellular face of the molecule in which peptides can be bound. MHC molecules are highly **polymorphic**—each type of MHC molecule occurs in many different versions—within the population. These are encoded by slightly different versions of individual genes called **alleles**. Most people are therefore heterozygous for the MHC molecules; that is, they express two different alleles for each type of MHC molecule, thus increasing the range of pathogen-derived peptides and self peptides that can be bound. T-cell receptors recognize features of both the peptide antigen and the MHC molecule to which it is bound. This introduces an extra dimension to antigen recognition by T cells, known as **MHC restriction** because any given T-cell receptor is specific for a particular peptide bound to a particular MHC molecule.

In this chapter, we focus on the structure and antigen-binding properties of immunoglobulins and T-cell receptors. Although B cells and T cells recognize foreign molecules in separate distinct fashions, the receptor molecules they use for this task are very similar in structure. We will see how this basic structure can accommodate great variability in antigen specificity, and how it enables immunoglobulins and T-cell receptors to perform their functions as the antigen-recognition molecules of the adaptive immune response. With this foundation, we will return to discuss the impact of MHC polymorphism on T-cell antigen recognition and T-cell development in Chapters 6 and 8, respectively.

The structure of a typical antibody molecule.

Antibodies are the secreted form of the B-cell receptor. Because they are soluble and secreted into the blood in large quantities, antibodies are easily obtained and easily studied. For this reason, most of what we know about the B-cell receptor comes from the study of antibodies.

Fig. 4.1 Structure of an antibody molecule. In panel a, the X-ray crystallographic structure of an IgG antibody is illustrated as a ribbon diagram of the backbones of the polypeptide chains. The two heavy chains are shown in yellow and purple. The two light chains are both shown in red. Three globular regions form an approximate Y shape. The two antigen-binding sites are at the tips of the arms, which are tethered at their other end to the trunk of the Y by a flexible hinge region. The light-chain variable (V_L) and constant (C_L) regions are indicated. The heavy-chain variable region (V_H) and V_L together form the antigen-binding site of the antibody. In panel b, a schematic representation of the same structure denotes each immunoglobulin domain as a separate rectangle. The hinge that tethers each heavy chain's first constant domain (C_H1) to its second (C_H2) is illustrated by a thin purple or yellow line, respectively. The antigen-binding sites are indicated by concave regions in V_L and V_H. Positions of carbohydrate modifications and disulfide linkages are indicated. In panel c, a more simplified schematic is shown that will be used throughout this book with the variable region in red and the constant region in blue. C terminus, carboxyl terminus; N terminus, amino terminus.

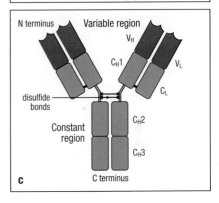

Antibody molecules are roughly Y-shaped, as represented in **Fig. 4.1** using three different schematic styles. This part of the chapter will explain how this structure is formed and allows the antibody molecule to perform its dual tasks of binding to a wide variety of antigens while also binding to effector molecules and to cells that destroy the antigen. Each of these tasks is performed by different parts of the molecule. The ends of the two arms of the Y—the V regions—are involved in antigen binding, and they vary in their detailed structure between different antibody molecules. The stem of the Y—the C region—is far less variable and is the part that interacts with effector molecules and cells. There are five different **classes** of immunoglobulins, distinguished in their being constructed from C regions that have different structures and properties. These are known as **immunoglobulin M (IgM)**, **immunoglobulin D (IgD)**, **immunoglobulin G (IgG)**, **immunoglobulin A (IgA)**, and **immunoglobulin E (IgE)**.

All antibodies are constructed in the same way from paired heavy and light polypeptide chains, and the generic term immunoglobulin is used for all such proteins. More subtle differences confined to the V region account for the specificity of antigen binding. We will use the IgG antibody molecule as an example to describe the general structural features of immunoglobulins.

4-1 IgG antibodies consist of four polypeptide chains.

IgG antibodies are large molecules with a molecular mass of approximately 150 kDa and are composed of two different kinds of polypeptide chains. One, of approximately 50 kDa, is called the **heavy** or **H chain**, and the other, of 25 kDa, is the **light** or **L chain** (**Fig. 4.2**). Each IgG molecule consists of two heavy chains and two light chains. The two heavy chains are linked to each other by disulfide bonds, and each heavy chain is linked to a light chain by a disulfide bond. In any given immunoglobulin molecule, the two heavy chains and the two light chains are identical, giving an antibody molecule two identical antigen-binding sites. This gives the antibody the ability to bind simultaneously to two identical antigens on a surface, thereby increasing the total strength of the interaction, which is called its **avidity**. The strength of the interaction between a single antigen-binding site and its antigen is called its **affinity**.

Two types of light chains, **lambda (λ)** and **kappa (κ)**, are found in antibodies. A given immunoglobulin has either κ chains or λ chains, never one of each. No

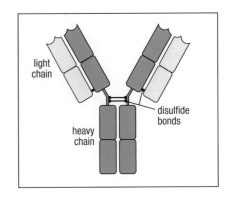

Fig. 4.2 Immunoglobulin molecules are composed of two types of protein chains: heavy chains and light chains. Each immunoglobulin molecule is made up of two hinged heavy chains (green) and two light chains (yellow) joined by disulfide bonds so that each heavy chain is linked to a light chain and the two heavy chains are linked together.

functional difference has been found between antibodies having λ or κ light chains, and either type of light chain can be found in antibodies of any of the five major classes. The ratio of the two types of light chains varies from species to species. In mice, the average κ to λ ratio is 20:1, whereas in humans it is 2:1 and in cattle it is 1:20. The reason for this variation is unknown. Distortions of this ratio can sometimes be used to detect the abnormal proliferation of a B-cell clone, because all progeny of a particular B cell will express an identical light chain. For example, an abnormally high level of λ light chains in a person might indicate the presence of a B-cell tumor that is producing λ chains.

Figure 4.2 depicts a typical IgG molecule; however, not all antibodies in the body are IgG. In addition to IgG, there are four other classes of antibodies that differ in the structures of their heavy chains. These different classes of antibodies are known as isotypes, and they include IgM, IgD, IgG, IgA, and IgE. We will first consider IgG as a typical antibody molecule and then return to discuss the structural and functional properties of the different heavy-chain isotypes in Section 4-6.

The structure of a B-cell antigen receptor on the surface of a B cell is identical to that of its corresponding antibody except for a small portion of the carboxyl terminus of the heavy-chain C region. In the B-cell receptor, the carboxyl terminus is a hydrophobic amino acid sequence that anchors the molecule in the membrane, whereas in the antibody it is a hydrophilic sequence that allows secretion.

4-2 Immunoglobulin heavy and light chains are composed of constant and variable regions.

The amino acid sequences of many immunoglobulin heavy and light chains have been determined and reveal two important features of antibody molecules. First, each chain consists of a series of similar, although not identical, sequences, each about 110 amino acids long. Each of these repeats corresponds to a discrete, compactly folded region of protein known as an **immunoglobulin domain**, or **Ig domain**. The light chain consists of two Ig domains, whereas the heavy chain of the IgG antibody contains four Ig domains (see Fig. 4.2). This suggests that the immunoglobulin chains have evolved by repeated duplication of ancestral gene segments corresponding to a single Ig domain.

The second important feature is that the amino-terminal amino acid sequences of the heavy and light chains vary greatly between different antibodies. The variability is limited to approximately the first 110 amino acids, corresponding to the first Ig domain, whereas the remaining domains are constant between immunoglobulin chains of the same isotype. The amino-terminal **variable Ig domains (V domains)** of the heavy and light chains (V_H and V_L, respectively) together make up the V region of the antibody and determine its antigen-binding specificity, whereas the **constant Ig domains (C domains)** of the heavy and light chains (C_H and C_L, respectively) make up the C region (see Fig. 4.1). The multiple heavy-chain C domains are numbered from the amino-terminal end to the carboxyl terminus; for example, C_H1, C_H2, and so on.

4-3 The domains of an immunoglobulin molecule have similar structures.

Immunoglobulin heavy and light chains are composed of a series of Ig domains that have a similar overall structure. Within this basic structure, there are distinct differences between V and C domains that are illustrated for the light chain in **Fig. 4.3**. Each V or C domain is constructed from two **β sheets**. A β sheet is built from several **β strands**, which are regions of protein where several consecutive polypeptides have their peptide backbone bonds arranged

Light-chain C domain

carboxyl terminus

β strands

disulfide bond

Light-chain V domain

amino terminus

β strands

Arrangement of β strands

disulfide bond

D E B A   G F C

disulfide bond

D E B A   G F C C′ C″

Fig. 4.3 The structure of immunoglobulin constant and variable domains. The upper panels show schematically the folding pattern of the constant (C) and variable (V) domains of an immunoglobulin light chain. Each domain is a barrel-shaped structure in which strands of polypeptide chain (β strands) running in opposite directions (antiparallel) pack together to form two β sheets (shown in yellow and green for the C domain and red and blue for the V domain), which are held together by a disulfide bond. The way in which the polypeptide chain folds to give the final structure can be seen more clearly when the sheets are opened out, as shown in the lower panels. The β strands are lettered sequentially with respect to the order of their occurrence in the amino acid sequence of the domains; the order in each β sheet is characteristic of immunoglobulin domains. The β strands C′ and C″ that are found in the V domains but not in the C domains are indicated by a blue-shaded background. The characteristic four-strand plus three-strand (C-region type domain) or four-strand plus five-strand (V-region type domain) arrangements are typical immunoglobulin superfamily domain building blocks, found in a whole range of other proteins as well as antibodies and T-cell receptors.

in an extended, or flat, conformation. β strands in proteins are sometimes shown as 'ribbons with an arrow' to indicate the direction of the polypeptide backbone (see Fig. 4.3). β strands can pack together in a side-by-side manner, being stabilized laterally by two or three backbone hydrogen bonds between adjacent strands. This arrangement is called a β sheet. The Ig domain has two β sheets that are folded onto each other, like two pieces of bread, into a structure called a β **sandwich**, and are covalently linked by a disulfide bond between cysteine residues from each β sheet. This distinctive structure is known as the **immunoglobulin fold**.

The similarities and differences between V and C domains can be seen in the bottom panels of Fig. 4.3. Here, the Ig domains have been opened out to show how their respective polypeptide chains fold to create each of the β sheets and how each polypeptide chain forms flexible loops between adjacent β strands as it turns to change direction. The main difference between the V and C domains is that the V domain is larger and contains extra β strands, called C′ and C″. In the V domain, the flexible loops formed between some of the β strands contribute to the antigen-binding site of the immunoglobulin molecule.

Many of the amino acids that are common to the C and V domains are present in the core of the immunoglobulin fold and are essential for its stability. Other proteins with sequences similar to those of immunoglobulins have been found to have domains with a similar structure, called **immunoglobulin-like**

domains (Ig-like domains). These domains are present in many proteins of the immune system, such as the KIRs expressed by NK cells described in Chapter 3. They are also frequently involved in cell–cell recognition and adhesion, and together with the immunoglobulins and the T-cell receptors, these proteins make up the extensive **immunoglobulin superfamily**.

4-4 The antibody molecule can readily be cleaved into functionally distinct fragments.

When fully assembled, an antibody molecule comprises three equal-sized globular portions, with its two arms joined to its trunk by a flexible stretch of polypeptide chain known as the **hinge region** (see Fig. 4.1b). Each arm of this Y-shaped structure is formed by the association of a light chain with the amino-terminal half of a heavy chain; the V_H domain is paired with the V_L domain, and the C_H1 domain is paired with the C_L domain. The two antigen-binding sites are formed by the paired V_H and V_L domains at the ends of the two arms of the Y (see Fig. 4.1b). The trunk of the Y is formed by the pairing of the carboxyl-terminal halves of the two heavy chains. The C_H3 domains pair with each other but the C_H2 domains do not interact. Carbohydrate side chains attached to the C_H2 domains lie between the two heavy chains.

Proteolytic enzymes (proteases) were an important tool in early studies of antibody structure, and it is valuable to review the terminology they generated. Limited digestion with the protease papain cleaves antibody molecules into three fragments (**Fig. 4.4**). **Papain** cuts the antibody molecule on the amino-terminal side of the disulfide bonds that link the two heavy chains, releasing the two arms of the antibody molecule as two identical fragments that contain the antigen-binding activity. These are called the **Fab fragments**, for fragment antigen binding. The other fragment contains no antigen-binding activity, but because it crystallized readily, it was named the **Fc fragment** (fragment crystallizable). It corresponds to the paired C_H2 and C_H3 domains. The Fc fragment is the part of the antibody molecule that does not interact with antigen, but rather interacts with effector molecules and cells, and it differs between heavy-chain isotypes. Another protease, **pepsin**, cuts on the carboxyl-terminal side of the disulfide bonds (see Fig. 4.4). This produces a fragment, the **F(ab′)₂ fragment**, in which the two antigen-binding arms of the antibody molecule remain linked. Pepsin cuts the remaining part of the heavy chain into several small fragments. The F(ab′)₂ fragment has exactly the same antigen-binding characteristics as the original antibody but is unable to interact with any effector molecule, such as C1q or Fc receptors, and can be used experimentally to separate the antigen-binding functions from the antibody's other effector functions.

Many antibody-related molecules can be constructed using genetic engineering techniques, and many antibodies and antibody-related molecules are being used therapeutically to treat a variety of diseases. We will return to this topic in Chapter 16, where we discuss the various therapeutic uses of antibodies that have been developed over the past two decades.

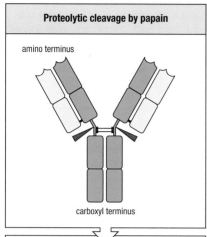

Proteolytic cleavage by papain

amino terminus

carboxyl terminus

Fab   Fab

Fc

Proteolytic cleavage by pepsin

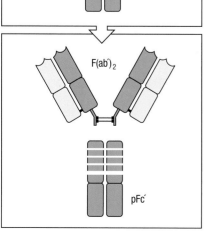

F(ab′)₂

pFc′

Fig. 4.4 The Y-shaped immunoglobulin molecule can be dissected by partial digestion with proteases. Upper panels: Papain cleaves the immunoglobulin molecule into three pieces, two Fab fragments and one Fc fragment. The Fab fragment contains the V regions and binds antigen. The Fc fragment is crystallizable and contains C regions. Lower panels: Pepsin cleaves immunoglobulin to yield one F(ab′)₂ fragment and many small pieces of the Fc fragment, the largest of which is called the pFc′ fragment. F(ab′)₂ is written with a prime because it contains a few more amino acids than Fab, including the cysteines that form the disulfide bonds.

4-5 The hinge region of the immunoglobulin molecule allows flexibility in binding to multiple antigens.

The hinge region between the Fc and Fab portions of the IgG molecule allows for some degree of independent movement of the two Fab arms. For example, in the antibody molecule shown in Fig. 4.1a, not only are the two hinge regions clearly bent differently, but the angle between the V and C domains in each of the two Fab arms is also different. This range of motion has led to the junction between the V and C domains being referred to as a 'molecular ball-and-socket joint.' This flexibility can be revealed by studies of antibodies bound to small antigens known as **haptens**. These are molecules of various types that are typically about the size of a tyrosine side chain. Although haptens are specifically recognized by antibody, they can stimulate the production of anti-hapten antibodies only when linked to a protein (see Appendix I, Section A-1). Two identical hapten molecules joined by a short flexible region can link two or more anti-hapten antibodies, forming dimers, trimers, tetramers, and so on, which can be seen by electron microscopy (**Fig. 4.5**). The shapes formed by these complexes show that antibody molecules are flexible at the hinge region. Some flexibility is also found at the junction between the V and C domains, allowing bending and rotation of the V domain relative to the C domain. Flexibility at both the hinge and the V–C junction enables the two arms of an antibody molecule to bind to sites some distance apart, such as the repeating sites on bacterial cell-wall polysaccharides. Flexibility at the hinge also enables antibodies to interact with the antibody-binding proteins that mediate immune effector mechanisms.

Summary.

The IgG antibody molecule is made up of four polypeptide chains, comprising two identical light chains and two identical heavy chains, and can be thought of as forming a flexible Y-shaped structure. Each of the four chains has a variable (V) region at its amino terminus, which contributes to the antigen-binding site, and a constant (C) region. The light chains are bound to the heavy chains by many noncovalent interactions and by disulfide bonds, and the V regions of the heavy and light chains pair in each arm of the Y to generate two identical

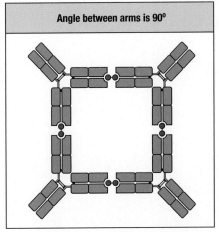

Fig. 4.5 Antibody arms are joined by a flexible hinge. An antigen consisting of two hapten molecules (red balls in diagrams) that can cross-link two antigen-binding sites is used to create antigen:antibody complexes, which can be seen in the electron micrograph. Linear, triangular, and square forms are seen, with short projections or spikes. Limited pepsin digestion removes these spikes (not shown in the figure), which therefore correspond to the Fc portion of the antibody; the F(ab')₂ pieces remain cross-linked by antigen. The interpretation of some of the complexes is shown in the diagrams. The angle between the arms of the antibody molecules varies. In the triangular forms, this angle is 60°, whereas it is 90° in the square forms, showing that the connections between the arms are flexible.

antigen-binding sites, which lie at the tips of the arms of the Y. The possession of two antigen-binding sites allows antibody molecules to cross-link antigens and to bind them much more stably and with higher avidity. The trunk of the Y, also called the Fc fragment, is composed of the carboxyl-terminal domains of the heavy chains, and it is these domains that determine the antibody's isotype. Joining the arms of the Y to the trunk are the flexible hinge regions. The Fc fragment and hinge regions differ in antibodies of different isotypes. Different isotypes have different properties and therefore differ in their interactions with effector molecules and cell types. However, the overall organization of the domains is similar in all isotypes.

Structural variation in immunoglobulin constant regions.

The class or isotype of an antibody is defined by the structure of its heavy-chain constant region. The differences between the antibody isotypes determine the effector functions of the antibody once it has bound antigen. There are five main heavy-chain isotypes, IgM, IgD, IgG, IgA, and IgE, some of which have several subtypes. These heavy-chain proteins are denoted by the lowercase Greek letters μ, δ, γ, α, and ϵ, respectively. For example, the constant region of IgM is denoted by C_μ. IgG is by far the most abundant immunoglobulin in serum. The distinctive functional properties of the different classes of antibodies are conferred by the carboxyl-terminal part of the heavy chain, where this chain is not associated with the light chain. In spite of these differences, the general structural features of all the isotypes are similar, particularly with respect to antigen binding. In this part of the chapter, we will consider the structural differences of the antibody isotypes and the specialized properties of each isotype. For IgM and IgA, individual antibodies form multimers that are secreted from cells. IgM forms pentamers, and IgA forms dimers. This feature aids in binding to repetitive structures, such as those on the surfaces of bacteria or viruses.

4-6 Different classes of immunoglobulins are distinguished by the structure of their heavy-chain constant regions.

The five main classes of immunoglobulins (IgM, IgD, IgG, IgE, and IgA) can occur as transmembrane antigen receptors or secreted antibodies (**Fig. 4.6**). In humans, IgG is found as four subclasses (IgG1, IgG2, IgG3, and IgG4), named by decreasing order of their abundance in serum, and IgA antibodies are found as two subclasses (IgA1 and IgA2). The heavy chains are encoded by different immunoglobulin C_H genes located in a gene cluster that is 3' of the J_H segments as illustrated in Fig. 4.6. The major physical and functional properties of the different classes of human antibody are listed in **Fig. 4.7**.

The functions of the immunoglobulin classes are discussed in detail in Chapter 10, in the context of the humoral immune response; here, we just touch on them briefly. IgM is the first class of immunoglobulin produced after activation of a B cell, and the IgM antibody is secreted as a pentamer (see Section 4-8 and **Fig. 4.8**). This accounts for the high molecular mass of IgM and the fact that it is normally present in the bloodstream but not in tissues. Being a pentamer also increases the avidity of IgM for antigens before its affinity is increased through the process of affinity maturation.

IgG isotypes produced during an immune response are found in the bloodstream and in the extracellular spaces in tissues. IgM and most IgG isotypes can interact with the complement component C1 to activate the classical complement pathway (described in Section 2-7). IgA and IgE do not activate

Fig. 4.6 The immunoglobulin isotypes are encoded by a cluster of immunoglobulin heavy-chain C-region genes. The general structure of the main immunoglobulin isotypes (upper panel) is indicated, with each rectangle denoting an immunoglobulin domain. These isotypes are encoded by separate heavy-chain C-region genes arranged in a cluster in both mouse and human (lower panel). The constant region of the heavy chain for each isotype is indicated by the same color as the C-region gene segment that encodes it. IgM and IgE lack a hinge region, but each contains an extra heavy-chain domain. Note the differences in the number and location of the disulfide bonds (heavy black lines) linking the chains. The isotypes also differ in the distribution of N-linked carbohydrate groups, shown as hexagons. In humans, the gene cluster shows evidence of evolutionary duplication of a unit consisting of two γ genes, an ε gene, and an α gene. One of the ε genes is a nonfunctional gene, called a pseudogene (ψC_ϵ); hence only one subtype of IgE is expressed. For simplicity, other pseudogenes are not illustrated, and the exon details within each C gene are not shown. The classes of immunoglobulins found in mice are called IgM, IgD, IgG1, IgG2a, IgG2b, IgG3, IgA, and IgE.

	Immunoglobulin								
	IgG1	IgG2	IgG3	IgG4	IgM	IgA1	IgA2	IgD	IgE
Heavy chain	γ_1	γ_2	γ_3	γ_4	μ	α_1	α_2	δ	ϵ
Molecular mass (kDa)	146	146	165	146	970	160	160	184	188
Serum level (mean adult mg/ml)	9	3	1	0.5	1.5	3.0	0.5	0.03	5×10^{-5}
Half-life in serum (days)	21	20	7	21	10	6	6	3	2
Classical pathway of complement activation	++	+	+++	–	++++	–	–	–	–
Alternative pathway of complement activation	–	–	–	–	–	+	–	–	–
Placental transfer	+++	+	++	–/+	–	–	–	–	–
Binding to macrophage and phagocyte Fc receptors	+	–	+	–/+	–	+	+	–	+
High-affinity binding to mast cells and basophils	–	–	–	–	–	–	–	–	+++
Reactivity with staphylococcal Protein A	+	+	–/+	+	–	–	–	–	–

Fig. 4.7 The physical and functional properties of the human immunoglobulin isotypes. IgM is so called because of its size: although monomeric IgM is only 190 kDa, it normally forms pentamers, known as macroglobulin (hence the M), of very large molecular mass (see Fig. 4.8). IgA dimerizes to give an approximate molecular mass of around 390 kDa in secretions. IgE antibody is associated with immediate-type hypersensitivity. When fixed to tissue mast cells, IgE has a much longer half-life than its half-life in serum shown here. The relative activities of the various isotypes are compared for several functions, ranging from inactive (–) to most active (++++).

Fig. 4.8 The IgM and IgA molecules can form multimers. IgM and IgA are usually synthesized as multimers in association with an additional polypeptide chain, the J chain. In dimeric IgA (left panel), the monomers have disulfide bonds to the J chain as well as to each other. In pentameric IgM (right panel), the monomers are cross-linked by disulfide bonds to each other and to the J chain. IgM can also form hexamers that lack a J chain (not shown). IgM and IgA in secretions also contain a 'secretory piece,' a part of the receptor that transports the Igs through the cell via transcytosis.

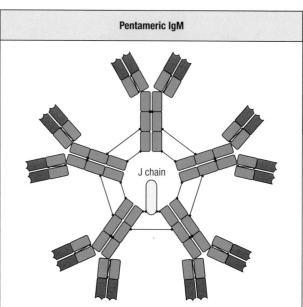

the complement. IgA can be found in the bloodstream, but it also acts in the defense of mucosal surfaces; it is secreted into the gut and respiratory tract and also into mother's milk. IgE is particularly involved in defense against multicellular parasites (for example, schistosomes), but it is also the antibody involved in common allergic diseases such as allergic asthma. IgG and IgE are always monomers, but IgA can be secreted as either a monomer or a dimer (see Fig. 4.8).

Sequence differences in the constant regions of the immunoglobulin heavy chains produce the distinct characteristics of each antibody isotype. These characteristics include the number and location of interchain disulfide bonds, the number of attached carbohydrate groups, the number of C domains, and the length of the hinge region (see Fig. 4.6). IgM and IgE heavy chains contain an extra C domain that replaces the hinge region found in γ, δ, and α chains. The absence of the hinge region does not mean that IgM and IgE molecules lack flexibility; electron micrographs of IgM molecules binding to ligands show that the Fab arms can bend relative to the Fc portion. However, such a difference in structure may have functional consequences that are not yet characterized. Different isotypes and subtypes also differ in their ability to engage various effector functions, as described next.

4-7 The constant region confers functional specialization on the antibody.

Antibodies can protect the body in a variety of ways. In some cases it is enough for the antibody simply to bind antigen. For instance, by binding tightly to a toxin or virus, an antibody can prevent it from recognizing its receptor on a host cell (see Fig. 1.28). The antibody V regions are sufficient for this activity. The C region is essential, however, for recruiting the help of other cells and molecules to destroy and dispose of pathogens to which the antibody has bound.

The Fc region contains C-region domains of the heavy chain and has three main effector functions: Fc-receptor binding, complement activation, and regulation of secretion. First, the Fc region of certain isotypes binds to specialized Fc receptors expressed by immune effector cells. Fcγ receptors expressed on the surface of macrophages and neutrophils bind the Fc portions of IgG1 and IgG3 antibodies, facilitating the phagocytosis of pathogens coated with these antibodies. The Fc region of IgE binds to a high-affinity Fcε receptor on mast cells, basophils, and activated eosinophils, triggering the release of inflammatory mediators in response to antigens. We will return to this topic in Chapter 10.

Second, the Fc regions in antigen:antibody complexes can bind to the C1q complement protein (see Section 2-7) and initiate the classical complement cascade, which recruits and activates phagocytes to engulf and destroy pathogens. Third, the Fc portion can deliver antibodies to places they would not reach without active transport. These include transport of IgA into mucous secretions, tears, and breast milk, and the transfer of IgG from the pregnant mother into the fetal blood circulation. In both cases, the Fc portion of IgA or IgG engages a specific receptor, the poly-Ig receptor (pIgR) or the neonatal Fc receptor (FcRn), respectively, which actively transports the immunoglobulin through cells to reach different body compartments. Podocytes, a specialized cell type in the kidney glomerulus, express FcRn to help remove IgG that has been filtered from the blood and accumulated at the glomerular basement membrane.

The role of the Fc portion in these effector functions has been demonstrated by studying immunoglobulins that have had one or more Fc domains cleaved off enzymatically or modified genetically. Many microorganisms have responded to the destructive potential of the Fc portion by evolving proteins that either bind it or cleave it, and so prevent the Fc region from working; examples are Protein A and Protein G of *Staphylococcus* and Protein D of *Haemophilus*. Researchers have exploited these proteins to help map the Fc region and also as immunological reagents. Not all immunoglobulin classes have the same capacity to engage each of the effector functions (see Fig. 4.7). For example, IgG1 and IgG3 have a higher affinity than IgG2 for the most common type of Fc receptor.

4-8   IgM and IgA can form polymers by interacting with the J chain.

Although all immunoglobulin molecules are constructed from a basic unit of two heavy and two light chains, both IgM and IgA can form multimers of these basic units (see Fig. 4.8). C regions of IgM and IgA can include a 'tailpiece' of 18 amino acids that contains a cysteine residue essential for polymerization. A separate 15-kDa polypeptide chain called the **J chain** promotes polymerization by linking to the cysteine of this tailpiece, which is found only in the secreted forms of the μ and α chains. (This J chain should not be confused with the immunoglobulin J region encoded by a J gene segment; see Section 5-1.) In the case of IgA, dimerization is required for transport through epithelia, as we will discuss in Chapter 10. IgM molecules are found as pentamers, and occasionally hexamers (without J chain), in plasma, whereas IgA is found mainly as a dimer in mucous secretions but as a monomer in plasma.

Immunoglobulin polymerization is also thought to be important in the binding of antibody to repetitive structures. An antibody molecule has at least two identical antigen-binding sites, each of which has a given affinity, or binding strength, for antigen. If the antibody attaches to multiple identical structures on a target antigen, it will dissociate only when all binding sites dissociate. The dissociation rate of the whole antibody will therefore be much slower than the dissociation rate for a single binding site; multiple binding sites thus give the antibody a greater total binding strength, or avidity. This consideration is particularly relevant for pentameric IgM, which has 10 antigen-binding sites.

IgM antibodies frequently recognize repetitive structures such as those on bacterial cell-wall polysaccharides, but individual binding sites are often of low affinity because IgM is made early in immune responses, before somatic hypermutation and affinity maturation. Multisite binding makes up for this, markedly improving the overall functional binding strength. This implies that binding of a single IgM pentamer to a target could be sufficient to mediate biological effector activity, whereas in the case of IgGs, two independent target molecules may need to be located in close proximity.

Summary.

The classes of immunoglobulins are defined by their heavy-chain C regions, with the different heavy-chain isotypes being encoded by different C-region genes. The heavy-chain C-region genes are present in a cluster 3′ to the V, D, and J gene segments. The constant region isotype of an antibody determines its effector functions, including binding to Fc receptors on effector cells such as phagocytes and mast cells, binding to the complement protein C1q, and binding to Fc receptors that mediate transport of antibodies between tissue compartments. Whereas all antibodies have two identical binding sites for antigen, some antibodies form multimeric complexes, thereby increasing their avidity for pathogen binding. Secreted IgM forms pentamers that include a small polypeptide called the J chain, creating a large antibody molecule with 10 antigen-binding sites. IgA that is transported into bodily secretions is a dimer of two IgA monomers plus the J chain. Differences in Fc-receptor binding, complement C1q binding, tissue localization, and antibody avidity are responsible for the specialized effector functions of each antibody isotype.

The interaction of the antibody molecule with specific antigen.

In this part of the chapter we look at the antigen-binding site of an immunoglobulin molecule in more detail. We discuss the different ways in which antigens can bind to antibody and address the question of how variation in the sequences of the antibody V domains determines the specificity for antigen.

4-9   Localized regions of hypervariable sequence form the antigen-binding site.

The V regions of any given antibody molecule differ from those of every other. Sequence variability is not, however, distributed evenly throughout the V region but is concentrated in certain segments, as is clearly seen in a **variability plot** (**Fig. 4.9**), in which the amino acid sequences of many different antibody V regions are compared. Three particularly variable segments can be

Fig. 4.9 There are discrete regions of hypervariability in V domains. The hypervariability regions of both the heavy chain and the light chain contribute to antigen binding of an antibody molecule. A variability plot derived from comparison of the amino acid sequences of several dozen heavy-chain and light-chain V domains is shown. At each amino acid position, the degree of variability is the ratio of the number of different amino acids seen in all of the sequences together to the frequency of the most common amino acid. Three hypervariable regions (HV1, HV2, and HV3) are indicated in red. They are flanked by less variable framework regions (FR1, FR2, FR3, and FR4, shown in blue or yellow).

Fig. 4.10 The hypervariable regions lie in discrete loops of the folded structure.
First panel: The hypervariable regions (red) are positioned on the structure of a map of the coding region of the V domain. Second panel: When shown as a flattened ribbon diagram, hypervariable regions are seen to occur in loops (red) that join particular β strands. Third panel: In the folded structure of the V domain, these loops (red) are brought together to form antigen-binding regions. Fourth panel: In a complete antibody molecule, the pairing of a heavy chain and a light chain brings together the hypervariable loops from each chain to create a single hypervariable surface, which forms the antigen-binding site at the tip of each arm. Because they are complementary to the antigen surface, the hypervariable regions are also commonly known as the complementarity-determining regions (CDRs). C, carboxyl terminus; N, amino terminus.

identified in both the V_H and V_L domains. They are designated **hypervariable regions** and are denoted HV1, HV2, and HV3. In the heavy chains they are located at residues 30 to 36, 49 to 65, and 95 to 103, respectively, while in the light chains they are located at residues 28 to 35, 50 to 56, and 91 to 98, respectively. The most variable part of the domain is in the HV3 region. The regions between the hypervariable regions comprise the rest of the V domain; they show less variability and are termed the **framework regions**. There are four such regions in each V domain, designated FR1, FR2, FR3, and FR4.

The framework regions form the β sheets that provide the structural framework of the immunoglobulin domain. The hypervariable sequences correspond to three loops and are positioned near one another in the folded domain at the outer edge of the β sandwich (**Fig. 4.10**). Thus, not only is diversity concentrated in particular parts of the V domain sequence, but it is also localized to a particular region on the surface of the molecule. When the V_H and V_L immunoglobulin domains are paired in the antibody molecule, the three hypervariable loops from each domain are brought together, creating a single hypervariable site at the tip of each arm of the molecule. This is the **antigen-binding site**, or **antibody-combining site**, which determines the antigen specificity of the antibody. These six hypervariable loops are more commonly termed the **complementarity-determining regions**, or **CDRs**, because the surface they form is complementary to that of the antigen they bind. There are three CDRs from each of the heavy and light chains, namely, CDR1, CDR2, and CDR3. In most cases, CDRs from both V_H and V_L domains contribute to the antigen-binding site; thus it is the combination of the heavy chain and the light chain that usually determines the final antigen specificity (see Fig. 4.9). However, there are some Fab crystal structures that show antigen interaction with just the heavy chain; for example, in one influenza Fab, antigen interaction involves binding mostly to the V_H CDR3 and only minor contacts with other CDRs. Thus, one way in which the immune system is able to generate antibodies of different specificities is by generating different combinations of heavy-chain and light-chain V regions. This is known as combinatorial diversity; we will encounter a second form of **combinatorial diversity** in Chapter 5 when we consider how the genes encoding the heavy-chain and light-chain V regions are created from smaller segments of DNA during the development of B cells in the bone marrow.

4-10 Antibodies bind antigens via contacts in CDRs that are complementary to the size and shape of the antigen.

In early investigations of antigen binding to antibodies, the only available sources of large quantities of a single type of antibody molecule were tumors of antibody-secreting cells. The antigen specificities of these antibodies were unknown, and therefore many compounds had to be screened to identify ligands that could be used to study antigen binding. In general, the substances found to bind to these antibodies were haptens (see Section 4-5) such as phosphocholine or vitamin K_1. Structural analysis of complexes of antibodies with their hapten ligands provided the first direct evidence that the hypervariable regions form the antigen-binding site and demonstrated the structural basis of specificity for the hapten. Subsequently, with the discovery of methods of generating **monoclonal antibodies** (see Appendix I, Section A-8), it became possible to make large amounts of pure antibody specific for a given antigen. This has provided a more general picture of how antibodies interact with their antigens, confirming and extending the view of antibody–antigen interactions derived from the study of haptens.

The surface of the antibody molecule formed by the juxtaposition of the CDRs of the heavy and light chains is the site to which an antigen binds. The amino acid sequences of the CDRs are different in different antibodies, and so too are the shapes and properties of the surfaces created by these CDRs. As a general principle, antibodies bind ligands whose surfaces are complementary to that of the antigen-binding site. A small antigen, such as a hapten or a short peptide, generally binds in a pocket or groove lying between the heavy-chain and light-chain V domains (**Fig. 4.11a and b**). Some antigens, such as proteins, can be the same size as or larger than the antibody itself. In these cases, the interface between antigen and antibody is often an extended surface that involves all the CDRs and, in some cases, part of the framework region as well (**Fig. 4.11c**). This surface need not be concave but can be flat, undulating, or

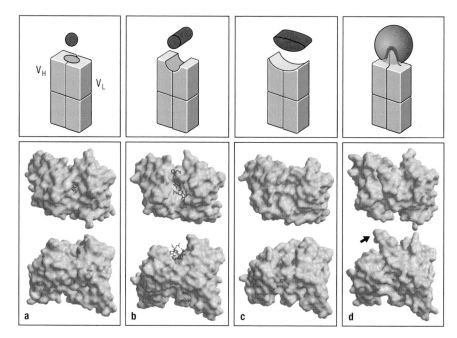

Fig. 4.11 Antigens can bind in pockets, or grooves, or on extended surfaces in the binding sites of antibodies. The panels in the top row show schematic representations of the different types of binding sites in a Fab fragment of an antibody: first panel, pocket; second panel, groove; third panel, extended surface; and fourth panel, protruding surface. Below are examples of each type. Panel a: The top image shows the molecular surface of the interaction of a small hapten with the complementarity-determining regions (CDRs) of a Fab fragment as viewed looking into the antigen-binding site. The ferrocene hapten, shown in red, is bound into the antigen-binding pocket (yellow). In the bottom image (and in those of panels b, c, and d), the molecule has been rotated by about 90° to give a side-on view of the binding site. Panel b: In a complex of an antibody with a peptide from the human immunodeficiency virus (HIV), the peptide (red) binds along a groove (yellow) formed between the heavy-chain and light-chain V domains. Panel c: Shown is a Fab fragment of an antibody specific for hen egg-white lysozyme (HyHel5). The surface on the antibody that comes into contact with the lysozyme is colored yellow. All six CDRs of the antigen-binding site are involved in the binding. Panel d: An antibody molecule against the HIV gp120 antigen has an elongated CDR3 loop (arrow) that protrudes into a recess on the side of the antigen. The structure of the complex between this antibody and gp120 has been solved, and in this case, only the heavy chain interacts with gp120.

even convex. In some cases, antibody molecules with elongated CDR3 loops can protrude a 'finger' into recesses in the surface of the antigen, as shown in **Fig. 4.11d**, where an antibody binding to the HIV gp120 antigen projects a long loop into its target.

4-11 Antibodies bind to conformational shapes on the surfaces of antigens using a variety of noncovalent forces.

The biological function of antibodies is to bind to pathogens and their products and to facilitate their removal from the body. An antibody generally recognizes only a small region on the surface of a large molecule such as a polysaccharide or protein. The structure recognized by an antibody is called an **antigenic determinant**, or **epitope**. Some of the most important pathogens have polysaccharide coats, and antibodies that recognize epitopes formed by the sugar subunits of these molecules are essential in providing immune protection against such pathogens. In many cases, however, the antigens that provoke an immune response are proteins. For example, many protective antibodies against viruses recognize viral coat proteins. In all such cases, the structures recognized by the antibody are located on the surface of the protein. Such sites are likely to be composed of amino acids from different parts of the polypeptide chain that have been brought together by protein folding. Antigenic determinants of this kind are known as **conformational** or **discontinuous epitopes** because the structure recognized is composed of segments of the protein that are discontinuous in the amino acid sequence of the antigen but are brought together in the three-dimensional structure (**Fig. 4.12**). In contrast, an epitope composed of a single segment of polypeptide chain is termed a **continuous** or **linear epitope**. Although most antibodies raised against intact, fully folded proteins recognize discontinuous epitopes, some will bind to peptide fragments of the protein. Conversely, antibodies raised against peptides of a protein or against synthetic peptides corresponding to part of its sequence are occasionally found to bind to the natural folded protein. This makes it possible, in some cases, to use synthetic peptides in vaccines that aim to raise antibodies against a pathogen's protein.

The interaction between an antibody and its antigen can be disrupted by high salt concentrations, by extremes of pH, by detergents, and sometimes by competition with high concentrations of the pure epitope itself. The binding is therefore a reversible noncovalent interaction. The forces, or bonds, involved in these noncovalent interactions are outlined in **Fig. 4.13**. **Electrostatic interactions** occur between charged amino acid side chains, as in salt bridges. Most antibody–antigen interactions involve at least one electrostatic interaction. Interactions also occur between electric dipoles, as in hydrogen bonds, or can involve short-range van der Waals forces. High salt concentrations and extremes of pH disrupt antigen–antibody binding by weakening electrostatic interactions and/or hydrogen bonds. This principle is employed in the purification of antigens by using affinity columns of immobilized antibodies (or in the purification of antibody by using antigens in a like manner) (see Appendix I, Section A-3). **Hydrophobic interactions** occur when two hydrophobic surfaces come together to exclude water. The strength of a hydrophobic interaction is proportional to the surface area that is hidden from water, and for some antigens, hydrophobic interactions probably account for most of the binding energy. In some cases, water molecules are trapped in pockets in the interface between antigen and antibody. These trapped water molecules, especially those between polar amino acid residues, may also contribute to binding and hence to the specificity of the antibody.

The contribution of each of these forces to the overall interaction depends on the particular antibody and antigen involved. A striking difference between antibody interactions with protein antigens and most other natural protein–protein interactions is that antibodies often have many aromatic amino acids

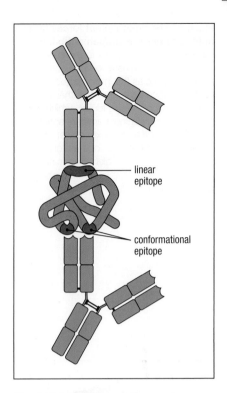

linear epitope

conformational epitope

Fig. 4.12 Antibodies can recognize linear or conformational determinants in folded proteins. In a folded protein, antibodies can recognize amino acid sequences that are discontinuous in the linear amino acid sequence of the protein, but are brought into proximity in the three-dimensional structure. These are known as conformational or discontinuous epitopes. Antibodies can also bind to peptides that are continuous in the linear amino acid sequence of the protein and these are known as linear or continuous epitopes.

Fig. 4.13 The noncovalent forces that hold together the antigen:antibody complex. Partial charges found in electric dipoles are shown as δ+ or δ−. Electrostatic forces diminish as the inverse square of the distance separating the charges, whereas van der Waals forces, which are more numerous in most antigen–antibody contacts, fall off as the sixth power of the separation and therefore operate only over very short ranges. Covalent bonds never occur between antigens and naturally produced antibodies.

Noncovalent forces	Origin	
Electrostatic forces	Attraction between opposite charges	$-\overset{\oplus}{NH_3}$ $\overset{\ominus}{OOC}-$
Hydrogen bonds	Hydrogen shared between electronegative atoms (N, O)	$>\underset{\delta^-}{N}\,-\,\underset{\delta^+}{H}\,--\,\underset{\delta^-}{O}=C<$
Van der Waals forces	Fluctuations in electron clouds around molecules polarize neighboring atoms oppositely	$\delta^+ \rightleftharpoons \delta^-$ $\delta^- \rightleftharpoons \delta^+$
Hydrophobic forces	Hydrophobic groups interact unfavorably with water and tend to pack together to exclude water molecules. The attraction also involves van der Waals forces	
Cation-pi interaction	Noncovalent interaction between a cation and an electron cloud of a nearby aromatic group	Na^+

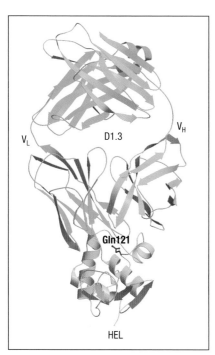

V_L   D1.3   V_H

Gln121

HEL

V_L Phe91

V_L Tyr32   V_H Tyr101

V_L Trp92

V_L Ser93   HEL Asp119

HEL Arg125

in their antigen-binding sites. These amino acids participate mainly in van der Waals and hydrophobic interactions, and sometimes in hydrogen bonds and **cation-pi interactions**. Tyrosine, for example, can take part in both hydrogen bonding and hydrophobic interactions; it is therefore particularly suitable for providing diversity in antigen recognition and is overrepresented in antigen-binding sites. In general, the hydrophobic and van der Waals forces operate over very short ranges and serve to pull together two surfaces that are complementary in shape: hills on one surface must fit into valleys on the other for good binding to occur. In contrast, electrostatic interactions between charged side chains as well as hydrogen bonds bridging oxygen and/or nitrogen atoms accommodate more specific chemical interactions while strengthening the interaction overall. The side chains of aromatic amino acids such as tyrosine can interact noncovalently through their pi-electron system with nearby cations, including nitrogen-containing side chains that may be in a protonated cationic state.

4-12 Antibody interaction with intact antigens is influenced by steric constraints.

An example of an antibody–antigen interaction involving a specific amino acid in the antigen can be seen in the complex of hen egg-white lysozyme with the antibody D1.3 (**Fig. 4.14**). In this structure, strong hydrogen bonds are formed

Fig. 4.14 The complex of lysozyme with the antibody D1.3. Top panel: The interaction of the Fab fragment of D1.3 with hen egg-white lysozyme (HEL) is shown. HEL is depicted in yellow, the heavy chain (V_H) in turquoise, and the light chain (V_L) in green. Bottom panel: A glutamine residue (Gln121) that protrudes from HEL (yellow) extends its side chain (shown in red) between the V_L (green) and V_H (turquoise) domains of the antigen-binding site and makes hydrogen bonds with the hydroxyl group (purple dots) of the indicated amino acids of both domains. These hydrogen bonds are important to the antigen–antibody binding.

Fig. 4.15 Steric hindrance occludes the binding of antibody to native antigen in the intact West Nile viral particle. Top panel: The monoclonal antibody E16 recognizes DIII, one of the three structural domains in the West Nile virus (WNV) glycoprotein E. Shown is a crystal structure of the E16 Fab bound to the DIII epitope. Bottom left panel: Cryo-electron microscopy (cryo-EM) reconstruction of saturating E16 Fab bound to West Nile virion confirmed the predicted steric hindrance. The vertices of the triangle shown in the figure indicate the icosahedral symmetry axes. Bottom right panel: A computer model was used to dock E16 Fab to the mature West Nile virion. E16 Fabs were able to bind 120 of the 180 DIII epitopes. Sixty of the fivefold clustered DIII epitopes are sterically hindered by the binding of Fab to four nearby DIII epitopes within that cluster. An example of an occluded epitope is the blue area indicated by the arrow.

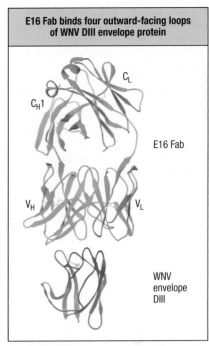

E16 Fab binds four outward-facing loops of WNV DIII envelope protein

C_L

C_H1

E16 Fab

V_H V_L

WNV envelope DIII

between the antibody and a particular glutamine in the lysozyme molecule that protrudes between the V_H and V_L domains. Lysozymes from partridge and turkey have another amino acid in place of the glutamine and do not bind to this antibody. Overall surface complementarity must have an important role in antigen–antibody interactions, but in most antibodies that have been studied at this level of detail, only a few residues make a major contribution to the binding energy and hence to the final specificity of the antibody. Although many antibodies naturally bind their ligands with high affinity (in the nanomolar range), genetic engineering by site-directed mutagenesis can tailor an antibody to bind even more strongly to its epitope.

Even when antibodies have high affinity for antigens on a larger structure, such as an intact viral particle, antibody binding may be prevented by their particular arrangement. For example, the intact West Nile virion is built from an icosahedral scaffold that has 90 homodimers of a membrane-anchored envelope glycoprotein, E, which has three domains, DI, DII, and DIII. The DIII domain has four polypeptide loops that protrude outward from the viral particle. A neutralizing antibody against West Nile virus, E16, recognizes these loops of DIII, as shown in **Fig. 4.15**. In theory, there should be 180 possible antigen-binding sites for the E16 antibody on the West Nile viral particle. However, a combination of crystallographic and electron micrographic studies show that even with an excess of the E16 Fab fragment, only about 120 of the total 180 DIII domains of E are able to bind the E16 Fab fragment (see Fig. 4.14). This appears to result from steric hindrance, with the presence of one Fab blocking the ability of another Fab to bind to some nearby E protein sites. Presumably, such steric hindrance would become more severe with intact antibody than is evident with the smaller Fab fragment. This study also showed that the Fab binds to the DIII region with only one of its antigen-binding arms, indicating that antibodies may not always bind to antigens with both antigen-binding sites. Therefore, the orientation of the antigens being recognized on the pathogen places constraints that impact the ability of antibodies to neutralize their targets.

Cryo-EM reconstruction of E16 Fab bound to mature WNV particle

Molecular model of E16 Fab bound to mature WNV particle

4-13 Some species generate antibodies with alternative structures.

Our focus in this chapter has been on the structure of antibodies produced by humans, which is generally similar in most mammalian species, including mice, an important model system for immunology research. However, some mammals have the ability to produce an alternative form of antibody that is based on the ability of a single V_H domain to interact with antigen in the absence of a V_L domain (**Fig. 4.16**). It has been known for some time that the serum of camels contains abundant immunoglobulin-like material composed of heavy-chain dimers that lack associated light chains but retain the capacity to bind antigens. These antibodies are called **heavy-chain-only IgGs (hcIgGs)**. This property is shared by other camelids, including llamas and alpacas. These species have retained the genes for the immunoglobulin light chains, and some IgG-like material in their sera remains associated with light

Fig. 4.16 Camelid and shark antibody can consist of heavy chain only. In the camelid heavy-chain-only antibody, a splicing event of the mature heavy chain can delete the exon encoding the C_H1 region and thereby create an in_frame hinge region linking the V_H to the C_H2 region. In the shark, the heavy-chain-only Ig molecule retains the C_H1 region, suggesting that this form of antibody may predate the evolution of light chains. For both, the repertoire of antigen-binding sites involves extensive variations in long CDR3 regions of the V_H domain relative to other types of antibody.

Human IgG

Camelid IgG

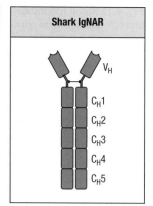

Shark IgNAR

chains, and so it is unclear what led to this particular adaptation during their evolution. In camelids, the ability to produce hcIgGs arises from mutations that allow the alternative splicing of the heavy-chain mRNA, with loss of the C_H1 exon and thus the joining of the V_H directly to the C_H2 domain in the protein. Other mutations stabilize this structure in the absence of V_L domains.

Cartilaginous fish, in particular the shark, also have an antibody molecule that differs substantially from human or murine antibodies (see Fig. 4.16). Like camelids, the shark also has genes encoding both immunoglobulin heavy and light chains and does produce immunoglobulins containing both heavy and light chains. But sharks also produce an **immunoglobulin new antigen receptor (IgNAR)**, a heavy-chain-only antibody in which the V_H is spliced to the C_H1 exon, rather than the C_H1 exon being spliced out as in camelids. These differences suggest that hcIgG production by camelids and sharks represents an event of convergent evolution. The ability of camelid V_H domains to interact efficiently with antigens is the basis for producing so-called **single-chain antibody**. The simplification of using only a single domain for antigen recognition has prompted recent interest in single-chain monoclonal antibodies as an alternative to standard monoclonal antibodies, which we will discuss more in Chapter 16.

Summary.

X-ray crystallographic analyses of antigen:antibody complexes have shown that the hypervariable loops (complementarity-determining regions; CDRs) of immunoglobulin V regions determine the binding specificity of an antibody. Contact between an antibody molecule and a protein antigen usually occurs over a broad area of the antibody surface that is complementary to the surface recognized on the antigen. Electrostatic interactions, hydrogen bonds, van der Waals forces, and hydrophobic and cation-pi interactions can all contribute to binding. Depending on the size of the antigen, amino acid side chains in most or all of the CDRs make contact with antigen and determine both the specificity and the affinity of the interaction. Other parts of the V region normally play little part in the direct contact with the antigen, but they provide a stable structural framework for the CDRs and help to determine their position and conformation. Antibodies raised against intact proteins usually bind to the surface of the protein and make contact with residues that are discontinuous in the primary structure of the molecule; they may, however, occasionally bind peptide fragments of the protein, and antibodies raised against peptides derived from a protein can sometimes be used to detect the native protein molecule. Peptides binding to antibodies usually bind in a cleft or pocket between the V regions of the heavy and light chains, where they make specific contact with some, but not necessarily all, of the CDRs. This is also the usual mode of binding for carbohydrate antigens and small molecules such as haptens.

Antigen recognition by T cells.

In contrast to the immunoglobulins, which interact with pathogens and their toxic products in the extracellular spaces of the body, T cells recognize foreign antigens only when they are displayed on the surface of the body's own cells. These antigens can derive from pathogens such as viruses or intracellular bacteria, which replicate within cells, or from pathogens or their products that have been internalized by endocytosis from the extracellular fluid.

T cells detect the presence of an intracellular pathogen because the infected cells display peptide fragments of the pathogen's proteins on their surface. These foreign peptides are delivered to the cell surface by specialized host-cell glycoproteins—the MHC molecules. These are encoded in a large cluster of genes that were first identified by their powerful effects on the immune response to transplanted tissues. For that reason, the gene complex was called the major histocompatibility complex (MHC), and the peptide-binding glycoproteins are known as MHC molecules. The recognition of antigen as a small peptide fragment bound to an MHC molecule and displayed at the cell surface is one of the most distinctive features of T cells and will be the focus of this part of the chapter. How the peptide fragments of antigen are generated and become associated with MHC molecules will be described in Chapter 6.

We describe here the structure and properties of the T-cell receptor (TCR). As might be expected from the function of T-cell receptors as highly variable antigen-recognition structures, the genes for TCRs are closely related to those for immunoglobulins. There are, however, important differences between T-cell receptors and immunoglobulins, and these differences reflect the special features of antigen recognition by T cells.

4-14 The TCRαβ heterodimer is very similar to a Fab fragment of immunoglobulin.

T-cell receptors were first identified by using monoclonal antibodies that bound to a single cloned T-cell line: such antibodies either specifically inhibit antigen recognition by the clone or specifically activate it by mimicking the antigen (see Appendix I, Section A-21). These **clonotypic** antibodies were then used to show that each T cell bears about 30,000 identical antigen receptors on its surface, each receptor consisting of two different polypeptide chains, termed the **T-cell receptor α (TCRα)** and **β (TCRβ)** chains. Each chain of the **αβ heterodimer** is composed of two Ig domains, and the two chains are linked by a disulfide bond, similar to the structure of the Fab fragment of an immunoglobulin molecule (**Fig. 4.17**). Also similar to the antibody Fab fragment, the T-cell receptor αβ heterodimer is the antigen-binding portion of the T-cell receptor. On the surface of T cells, the αβ heterodimer is always found in a large multiprotein complex that contains six additional subunits: CD3γ, CD3δ, two copies of CD3ε, and two copies of the T-cell receptor ζ chain (Fig 4.17). These additional subunits function in signal transduction, rather than in antigen recognition, and unlike the αβ heterodimer, they do not vary between T cells. The functions of these receptor signaling subunits will be discussed in Chapter 7.

The TCRα and TCRβ chains of the αβ heterodimer account for antigen recognition by most T cells. A minority of T cells bear an alternative, but structurally similar, receptor made up of a different pair of polypeptide chains designated γ and δ. The **γδ T-cell receptors** have different antigen-recognition properties from the **αβ T-cell receptors**, and the functions of γδ T cells in immune responses are still being clarified as the various ligands they recognize are identified (see Section 6-20). In the rest of this chapter and elsewhere in the book, we use the term T-cell receptor to mean the αβ receptor, except

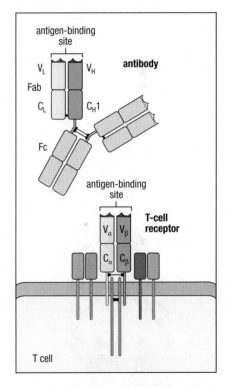

Fig. 4.17 The T-cell receptor resembles a membrane-bound Fab fragment. The Fab fragment of an antibody molecule is a disulfide-linked heterodimer, each chain of which contains one immunoglobulin C domain and one V domain; the juxtaposition of the V domains forms the antigen-binding site (see Section 4-6). The antigen-binding subunits of the T-cell receptor also form a disulfide-linked heterodimer, with each chain containing an immunoglobulin C-like domain and an immunoglobulin V-like domain. This heterodimer is always associated with six additional polypeptides (shown in gray) that form the complete membrane-bound T-cell receptor. As in the Fab fragment, the juxtaposition of the T-cell receptor V_α and V_β domains forms the site for antigen recognition.

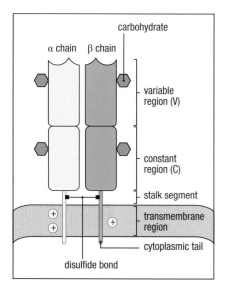

Fig. 4.18 Structure of the T-cell receptor. The T-cell receptor heterodimer is composed of two transmembrane glycoprotein chains, α and β. The extracellular portion of each chain consists of two domains, resembling immunoglobulin V and C domains, respectively. Both chains have carbohydrate side chains attached to each domain. A short stalk segment, analogous to an immunoglobulin hinge region, connects the Ig-like domains to the membrane and contains the cysteine residue that forms the interchain disulfide bond. The transmembrane helices of both chains are unusual in containing positively charged (basic) residues within the hydrophobic transmembrane segment. The α chain carries two such residues; the β chain has one. These basic residues are required for assembly of the T-cell receptor αβ heterodimer with the additional polypeptides that form the complete membrane-bound T-cell receptor complex.

where specified otherwise. Both types of T-cell receptors differ from the membrane-bound immunoglobulin that serves as the B-cell receptor in two main ways. A T-cell receptor has only one antigen-binding site, whereas a B-cell receptor has two, and T-cell receptors are never secreted, whereas immunoglobulins can be secreted as antibodies.

Further insights into the structure and function of the αβ T-cell receptor came from studies of cloned cDNA encoding the receptor chains. The amino acid sequences predicted from the cDNA showed that both chains of the T-cell receptor have an amino-terminal variable (V) region with sequence homology to an immunoglobulin V domain, a constant (C) region with homology to an immunoglobulin C domain, and a short stalk segment containing a cysteine residue that forms the interchain disulfide bond (**Fig. 4.18**). Each chain spans the lipid bilayer by a hydrophobic transmembrane domain and ends in a short cytoplasmic tail. These close similarities of T-cell receptor chains to the heavy and light immunoglobulin chains first enabled prediction of the structural resemblance of the T-cell receptor heterodimer to a Fab fragment of immunoglobulin.

The three-dimensional structure of the T-cell receptor αβ heterodimer determined by X-ray crystallography, illustrated in **Fig. 4.19a**, shows that T-cell

Fig. 4.19 The crystal structure of an αβ T-cell receptor resolved at 0.25 nm. In panels a and b, the α chain is shown in pink and the β chain in blue. Disulfide bonds are shown in green. In panel a, the T-cell receptor is viewed from the side as it would sit on a cell surface, with the CDR loops that form the antigen-binding site (labeled 1, 2, and 3) arrayed across its relatively flat top. In panel b, the Cα and Cβ domains are shown. The Cα domain does not fold into a typical Ig-like domain; the face of the domain away from the Cβ domain is mainly composed of irregular strands of polypeptide rather than β sheet. The intramolecular disulfide bond (far left) joins a β strand to this segment of α helix. The interaction between the Cα and Cβ domains is assisted by carbohydrate (colored gray and labeled), with a sugar group from the Cα domain making hydrogen bonds to the Cβ domain. In panel c, the T-cell receptor is shown

aligned with the antigen-binding sites from three different antibodies. This view is looking down into the binding site. The Vα domain of the T-cell receptor is aligned with the VL domains of the antigen-binding sites of the antibodies, and the Vβ domain is aligned with the VH domains. The CDRs of the T-cell receptor and immunoglobulin molecules are colored, with CDRs 1, 2, and 3 of the TCR shown in red and the HV4 loop in orange. For the immunoglobulin V domains, the CDR1 loops of the heavy chain (H1) and light chain (L1) are shown in light and dark blue, respectively, and the CDR2 loops (H2, L2) in light and dark purple, respectively. The heavy-chain CDR3 loops (H3) are in yellow; the light-chain CDR3 loops (L3) are in bright green. The HV4 loops of the TCR (orange) have no hypervariable counterparts in immunoglobulins.

receptor chains fold in much the same way as the regions comprising the Fab fragment shown in Fig. 4.1a. There are, however, some distinct structural differences between T-cell receptors and Fab fragments. The most striking is in the C_α domain, where the fold is unlike that of any other Ig-like domain. The half of the C_α domain that is juxtaposed with the C_β domain forms a β sheet similar to that found in other Ig-like domains, but the other half of the domain is formed of loosely packed strands and a short segment of α helix (**Fig. 4.19b**). In a C_α domain the intramolecular disulfide bond, which in Ig-like domains normally joins two β strands, joins a β strand to this segment of α helix.

There are also differences in the way in which the domains interact. The interface between the V and C domains of both T-cell receptor chains is more extensive than in most antibodies. The interaction between the C_α and C_β domains is distinctive, as it might be assisted by carbohydrates, with a sugar group from the C_α domain making a number of hydrogen bonds to the C_β domain (see Fig. 4.19b). Finally, a comparison of the variable binding sites shows that although the CDR loops align fairly closely with those of antibody molecules, there is some relative displacement (**Fig. 4.19c**). This is particularly marked in the V_α CDR2 loop, which is oriented at roughly right angles to the equivalent loop in antibody V domains, as a result of a shift in the β strand that anchors one end of the loop from one face of the domain to the other. A strand displacement also causes a change in the orientation of the V_β CDR2 loop in some V_β domains. These differences with antibodies influence the ability of the T-cell receptor to recognize their specific ligands, as we will discuss in the next section. In addition to the three hypervariable regions shared with immunoglobulins, the T-cell receptor has a fourth hypervariability region, HV4, in both of its chains (see Fig. 4.19c). These regions occur away from the antigen-binding face of the receptor and have been implicated in other functions of the TCR, such as superantigen binding, which we will describe in Section 6-14.

4-15 A T-cell receptor recognizes antigen in the form of a complex of a foreign peptide bound to an MHC molecule.

Antigen recognition by T-cell receptors clearly differs from recognition by B-cell receptors and antibodies. The immunoglobulin on B cells binds directly to the intact antigen, and, as discussed in Section 4-11, antibodies typically bind to the surface of protein antigens, contacting amino acids that are discontinuous in the primary structure but are brought together in the folded protein. In contrast, αβ T cells respond to short, continuous amino acid sequences. As we described in Section 1-10, these peptide sequences are often buried within the native structure of the protein. Thus, antigens cannot be recognized directly by T-cell receptors unless the protein is unfolded and processed into peptide fragments (**Fig. 4.20**) and then presented by an MHC molecule (see Fig. 1.15). We will discuss this process in Chapter 6.

The nature of the antigen recognized by T cells became clear with the realization that the peptides that stimulate T cells are recognized only when bound

Fig. 4.20 Differences in the recognition of hen egg-white lysozyme by immunoglobulins and T-cell receptors. Antibodies can be shown by X-ray crystallography to bind epitopes on the surface of proteins, as shown in panel a, where the epitopes for three antibodies are shown in different colors (red, yellow, purple) on the surface of hen egg-white lysozyme (see also Fig. 4.11). In contrast, the epitopes recognized by T-cell receptors need not lie on the surface of the molecule, because the T-cell receptor recognizes not the antigenic protein itself but a peptide fragment of the protein. The peptides corresponding to two T-cell epitopes of lysozyme are shown in panel b. One epitope, shown in blue, lies on the surface of the protein, but a second, shown in red, lies mostly within the core and is inaccessible in the folded protein. This indicates that T-cell receptors do not recognize their epitopes in the native protein.

Fig. 4.21 The structure of an MHC class I molecule determined by X-ray crystallography. Panel a shows a computer-generated representation of a human MHC class I molecule, HLA-A2, which has been cleaved from the cell surface by the enzyme papain. The surface of the molecule is shown, colored according to the domains shown in panels b–d and described below. Panels b and c each show a ribbon diagram of the structure. Shown schematically in panel d, the MHC class I molecule is a heterodimer of a membrane-spanning α chain (molecular mass 43 kDa) bound noncovalently to β$_2$-microglobulin (12 kDa), which does not span the membrane. The α chain folds into three domains: α$_1$, α$_2$, and α$_3$. The α$_3$ domain and β$_2$-microglobulin show similarities in amino acid sequence to immunoglobulin C domains and have similar folded structures, whereas the α$_1$ and α$_2$ domains are part of the same polypeptide and fold together into a single structure consisting of two separated α helices lying on a sheet of eight antiparallel β strands. The folding of the α$_1$ and α$_2$ domains creates a long cleft or groove, which is the site at which peptide antigens bind to the MHC molecules. For class I molecules, this groove is open at only one end. The transmembrane region and the short stretch of peptide that connects the external domains to the cell surface are not seen in panels a and b because they have been removed by the digestion with papain. As can be seen in panel c, looking down on the molecule from above, the sides of the cleft are formed from the inner faces of the two α helices; the β pleated sheet formed by the pairing of the α$_1$ and α$_2$ domains creates the floor of the cleft.

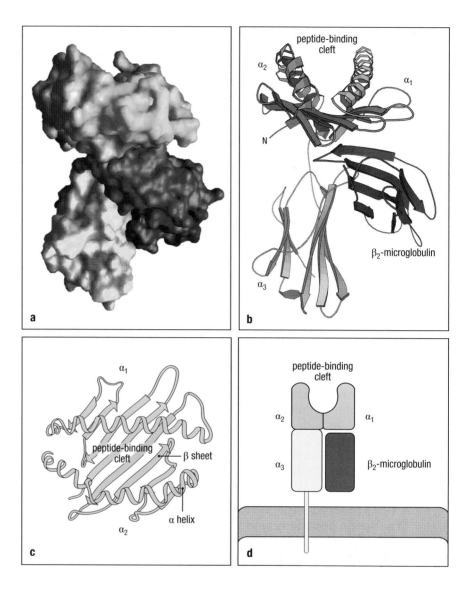

to an MHC molecule. The ligand recognized by the T cell is thus a complex of peptide and MHC molecule. The evidence for involvement of the MHC in T-cell recognition of antigen was indirect at first, but it has been proven conclusively by stimulating T cells with purified peptide:MHC complexes. The T-cell receptor interacts with this ligand by making contacts with both the MHC molecule and the antigen peptide.

4-16 There are two classes of MHC molecules with distinct subunit compositions but similar three-dimensional structures.

There are two classes of MHC molecules—**MHC class I** and **MHC class II**—and they differ in both their structure and their expression pattern in the tissues of the body. As shown in **Figs. 4.21** and **4.22**, MHC class I and MHC class II molecules are closely related in overall structure but differ in their subunit composition. In both classes, the two paired protein domains nearest to the membrane resemble immunoglobulin domains, whereas the two domains furthest away from the membrane fold together to create a long cleft, or groove, which is the site at which a peptide binds. Purified peptide:MHC class I and peptide:MHC class II complexes have been characterized structurally, allowing us to describe in detail both the MHC molecules themselves and the way in which they bind peptides.

Fig. 4.22 MHC class II molecules resemble MHC class I molecules in overall structure. The MHC class II molecule is composed of two transmembrane glycoprotein chains, α (34 kDa) and β (29 kDa), as shown schematically in panel d. Each chain has two domains, and the two chains together form a compact four-domain structure similar to that of the MHC class I molecule (compare with panel d of Fig. 4.21). Panel a shows a computer-generated representation of the surface of the MHC class II molecule, in this case the human protein HLA-DR1, and panel b shows the equivalent ribbon diagram. N, amino terminus; C, carboxyl terminus. The α_2 and β_2 domains, like the α_3 and β_2-microglobulin domains of the MHC class I molecule, have amino acid sequence and structural similarities to immunoglobulin C domains; in the MHC class II molecule the two domains forming the peptide-binding cleft are contributed by different chains and are therefore not joined by a covalent bond (see panels c and d). Another important difference, not apparent in this diagram, is that the peptide-binding groove of the MHC class II molecule is open at both ends.

MHC class I molecules (see Fig. 4.21) consist of two polypeptide chains. One chain, the α chain, is encoded in the MHC (on chromosome 6 in humans) and is noncovalently associated with a smaller chain, **β_2-microglobulin**, which is encoded on a different chromosome—chromosome 15 in humans. Only the class I α chain spans the membrane. The complete MHC class I molecule has four domains, three formed from the MHC-encoded α chain, and one contributed by β_2-microglobulin. The α_3 domain and β_2-microglobulin closely resemble Ig-like domains in their folded structure. The folded α_1 and α_2 domains form the walls of a cleft on the surface of the molecule; because this is where the peptide binds, this part of the MHC molecule is known as the **peptide-binding cleft** or **peptide-binding groove**. The MHC molecules are highly polymorphic, and the major differences between the different allelic forms are located in the peptide-binding cleft, influencing which peptides will bind and thus the specificity of the peptide:MHC antigen presented to T cells. By contrast, β_2-microglobulin, which does not contribute directly to peptide binding, is not polymorphic.

An MHC class II molecule consists of a noncovalent complex of two chains, α and β, both of which span the membrane (see Fig. 4.22). The MHC class II α chain is a different protein from the class I α chain. The MHC class II α and β chains are both encoded within the MHC. The crystallographic structure of the MHC class II molecule shows that it is folded very much like the MHC class

Fig. 4.23 MHC molecules bind peptides tightly within the cleft. When MHC molecules are crystallized with a single synthetic peptide antigen, the details of peptide binding are revealed. In MHC class I molecules (panels a and c), the peptide is bound in an elongated conformation with both ends tightly bound at either end of the cleft. In MHC class II molecules (panels b and d), the peptide is also bound in an elongated conformation, but the ends of the peptide are not tightly bound and the peptide extends beyond the cleft. The upper surface of the peptide:MHC complex is recognized by T cells and is composed of residues of the MHC molecule and the peptide. The amino acid side chains of the peptide insert into pockets in the peptide-binding groove of the MHC molecule; these pockets are lined with residues that are polymorphic within the MHC. In representations c and d, the surfaces of the different pockets for the different amino acids are depicted as areas of different colors.

I molecule, but the peptide-binding cleft is formed by two domains from different chains, the α_1 and β_1 domains. The major differences lie at the ends of the peptide-binding cleft, which are more open in MHC class II than in MHC class I molecules. Consequently, the ends of a peptide bound to an MHC class I molecule are substantially buried within the molecule, whereas the ends of peptides bound to MHC class II molecules are not. In both MHC class I and class II molecules, bound peptides are sandwiched between the two α-helical segments of the MHC molecule (**Fig. 4.23**). The T-cell receptor interacts with this compound ligand, making contacts with both the MHC molecule and the peptide antigen. As in the case of MHC class I molecules, the sites of major polymorphism in MHC class II molecules are located in the peptide-binding cleft.

4-17 Peptides are stably bound to MHC molecules and also serve to stabilize the MHC molecule on the cell surface.

An individual can be infected by a wide variety of pathogens, whose proteins will not generally have peptide sequences in common. For T cells to be able to detect the widest possible array of infections, the MHC molecules (both class I and class II) of an individual should be able to bind stably to many different peptides. This behavior is quite distinct from that of other peptide-binding receptors, such as those for peptide hormones, which usually bind only a single type of peptide. The crystal structures of peptide:MHC complexes have helped to show how a single binding site can bind a peptide with high affinity while retaining the ability to bind a wide variety of different peptides.

An important feature of the binding of peptides to MHC molecules is that the peptide is bound as an integral part of the MHC molecule's structure, and MHC molecules are unstable when peptides are not bound. This dependence on bound peptide applies to both MHC class I and MHC class II molecules. Stable peptide binding is important, because otherwise peptide exchanges occurring at the cell surface would prevent peptide:MHC complexes from being reliable indicators of infection or of uptake of a specific antigen. When MHC molecules are purified from cells, their stably bound peptides co-purify with them, and this fact has allowed the peptides bound by particular MHC molecules to be analyzed. Peptides are released from the MHC molecules by denaturing the complex in acid, and they are then purified and sequenced. Pure synthetic peptides can also be incorporated into empty MHC molecules and the structure of the complex determined, revealing details of the contacts between the MHC molecule and the peptide. From such studies a detailed picture of the binding interactions has been built up. We discuss the peptide-binding properties of MHC class I molecules first.

4-18 MHC class I molecules bind short peptides of 8–10 amino acids by both ends.

Binding of a peptide to an MHC class I molecule is stabilized at both ends of the peptide-binding cleft by contacts between atoms in the free amino and carboxyl termini of the peptide and invariant sites that are found at each end of the cleft in all MHC class I molecules (**Fig. 4.24**). These are thought to be the main stabilizing contacts for peptide:MHC class I complexes, because synthetic peptide analogs lacking terminal amino and carboxyl groups fail to bind stably to MHC class I molecules. Other residues in the peptide serve as additional anchors. Peptides that bind to MHC class I molecules are usually 8–10 amino acids long. However, longer peptides are thought to bind, particularly if they can bind at their carboxyl terminus, but they are subsequently shortened to 8–10 amino acids through cleavage by exopeptidases present in the endoplasmic reticulum, which is where MHC class I molecules bind peptides. The peptide lies in an elongated conformation along the cleft; variations in peptide length seem to be accommodated, in most cases, by the peptide bulging out of the binding groove. However, in some cases, length variation can also be accommodated in MHC class I molecules by allowing the peptide to extend out of the cleft at the carboxyl terminus.

These interactions give MHC class I molecules a broad peptide-binding specificity. In addition, MHC molecules are highly polymorphic. As mentioned earlier, MHC genes are highly polymorphic, and there are hundreds of different

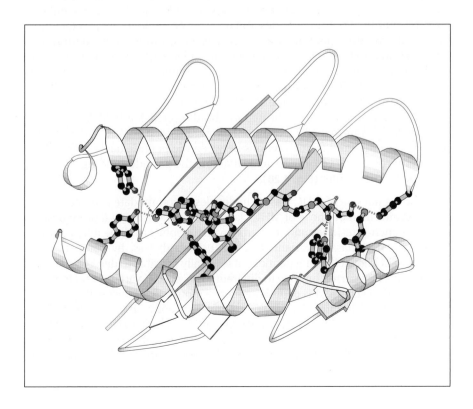

Fig. 4.24 Peptides are bound to MHC class I molecules by their ends. MHC class I molecules interact with the backbone of a bound peptide (shown in yellow) through a series of hydrogen bonds and ionic interactions (shown as dotted blue lines) at each end of the peptide. The amino terminus of the peptide is to the left, the carboxyl terminus to the right. Black circles are carbon atoms; red are oxygen; blue are nitrogen. The amino acid residues in the MHC molecule that form these bonds are common to all MHC class I molecules, and their side chains are shown in full (in gray) on a ribbon diagram of the MHC class I groove. A cluster of tyrosine residues common to all MHC class I molecules forms hydrogen bonds to the amino terminus of the bound peptide, while a second cluster of residues forms hydrogen bonds and ionic interactions with the peptide backbone at the carboxyl terminus and with the carboxyl terminus itself.

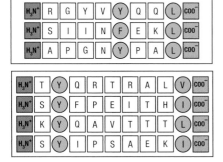

Fig. 4.25 Peptides bind to MHC molecules through structurally related anchor residues. The sequences of two sets of peptides eluted from two different MHC class I molecules are shown in the upper and lower panels. The anchor residues (green) differ for peptides that bind different allelic variants of MHC class I molecules but are similar for all peptides that bind to the same MHC molecule. The anchor residues that bind a particular MHC molecule need not be identical but are always related; for example, phenylalanine (F) and tyrosine (Y) are both aromatic amino acids, whereas valine (V), leucine (L), and isoleucine (I) are all large hydrophobic amino acids. Peptides also bind to MHC class I molecules through their amino (blue) and carboxyl (red) termini.

allelic variations of the MHC class I genes in the human population. Each individual carries only a small selection of these variants. The main differences between allelic MHC variants are found at certain sites in the peptide-binding cleft, resulting in different amino acids in key peptide-interaction sites. For this reason, different MHC variants preferentially bind different peptides. The peptides that can bind to a given MHC variant have the same or very similar amino acid residues at two or three particular positions along the peptide sequence. The amino acid side chains at these positions insert into pockets in the MHC molecule that are lined by the polymorphic amino acids. Because this binding anchors the peptide to the MHC molecule, the peptide residues involved are called the **anchor residues**, as illustrated in **Fig. 4.25**. Both the position and identity of these anchor residues can vary, depending on the particular MHC class I variant that is binding the peptide. However, most peptides that bind to MHC class I molecules have a hydrophobic (or sometimes basic) residue at the carboxyl terminus that also serves to anchor the peptide in the groove. Whereas changing an anchor residue will in most cases prevent the peptide from binding, not every synthetic peptide of suitable length that contains these anchor residues will bind the appropriate MHC class I molecule, and so the overall binding must also depend on the nature of the amino acids at other positions in the peptide. In some cases, particular amino acids are preferred in certain positions, whereas in others the presence of particular amino acids prevents binding. These additional amino acid positions are called 'secondary anchors.' These features of peptide binding enable an individual MHC class I molecule to bind a wide variety of different peptides, yet allow different MHC class I allelic variants to bind different sets of peptides. As we will see in Chapter 15, MHC polymorphisms also impact the binding of peptides derived from self proteins and can influence the susceptibility of an individual to various autoimmune diseases.

4-19 The length of the peptides bound by MHC class II molecules is not constrained.

Like MHC class I molecules, MHC class II molecules that lack bound peptide are unstable. Peptide binding to MHC class II molecules has also been analyzed by elution of bound peptides and by X-ray crystallography, and it differs in several ways from peptide binding to MHC class I molecules. Natural peptides that bind to MHC class II molecules are at least 13 amino acids long and can be much longer. The clusters of conserved residues that bind the two ends of a peptide in MHC class I molecules are not found in MHC class II molecules, and the ends of the peptide are not bound. Instead, the peptide lies in an extended conformation along the peptide-binding cleft. It is held there both by peptide side chains that protrude into shallow and deep pockets lined by polymorphic residues and by interactions between the peptide backbone and the side chains of conserved amino acids that line the peptide-binding cleft in all MHC class II molecules (**Fig. 4.26**).

The binding pockets of MHC class II molecules accommodate a greater variety of side chains than do those of MHC class I molecules, making it more difficult to define anchor residues and to predict which peptides will be able to bind a particular MHC class II variant (**Fig. 4.27**). Nevertheless, by comparing the sequences of known binding peptides, it is usually possible to detect patterns of amino acids that permit binding to different MHC class II variants and to model how the amino acids of this peptide sequence motif will interact with the amino acids of the peptide-binding cleft. For example, structural data show that amino acid side chains at residues 1, 4, 6, and 9 of peptides bound to HLA-DR3 are held in pockets lining the binding site (see Fig. 4.27). Because the peptide is bound by its backbone and allowed to emerge from both ends of the binding groove, there is, in principle, no upper limit to the length of peptides that could bind to MHC class II molecules. An example is the protein known as **invariant chain**, part of

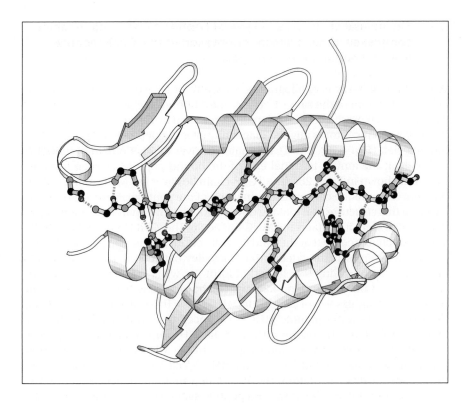

Fig. 4.26 Peptides bind to MHC class II molecules by interactions along the length of the binding groove. A peptide (yellow; shown as the peptide backbone only, with the amino terminus to the left and the carboxyl terminus to the right) is bound by an MHC class II molecule through a series of hydrogen bonds (dotted blue lines) that are distributed along the length of the peptide. The hydrogen bonds toward the amino terminus of the peptide are made with the backbone of the MHC class II polypeptide chain, whereas throughout the peptide's length, bonds are made with residues that are highly conserved in MHC class II molecules. The side chains of these residues are shown in gray on the ribbon diagram of the MHC class II groove.

which lies entirely across the peptide-binding groove of nascent MHC class II molecules during their synthesis in the endoplasmic reticulum. We will return in Chapter 6 to the role of the invariant chain in the loading of peptides onto MHC class II molecules. In most cases, long peptides bound to MHC class II molecules are trimmed by peptidases to a length of around 13–17 amino acids.

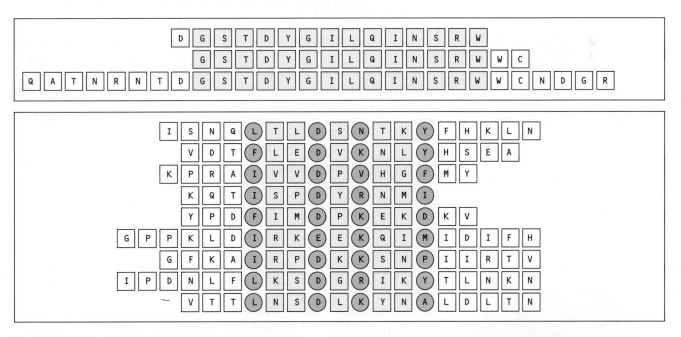

							D	G	S	T	D	Y	G	I	L	Q	I	N	S	R	W				
								G	S	T	D	Y	G	I	L	Q	I	N	S	R	W	W	C		
Q	A	T	N	R	N	T	D	G	S	T	D	Y	G	I	L	Q	I	N	S	R	W	W	C	N	D	G	R

		I	S	N	Q	(L)	T	L	(D)	S	(N)	T	K	(Y)	F	H	K	L	N
		V	D	T	(F)	L	E	(D)	V	(K)	N	L	(Y)	H	S	E	A	
		K	P	R	A	(I)	V	V	(D)	P	(V)	H	G	(F)	M	Y		
		K	Q	T	(I)	S	P	(D)	Y	(R)	N	M	(I)					
		Y	P	D	(F)	I	M	(D)	P	K	E	K	(D)	K	V			
G	P	P	K	L	D	(I)	R	K	(E)	E	(K)	Q	I	(M)	I	D	I	F	H
	G	F	K	A	(I)	R	P	(D)	K	(K)	S	N	(P)	I	I	R	T	V
I	P	D	N	L	F	(L)	K	S	(D)	G	(R)	I	K	(Y)	T	L	N	K	N
	—	V	T	T	(L)	N	S	(D)	L	(K)	Y	N	(A)	L	D	L	T	N

Fig. 4.27 Peptides that bind MHC class II molecules are variable in length, and their anchor residues lie at various distances from the ends of the peptide. The sequences of a set of peptides that bind to the mouse MHC class II A^k protein are shown in the upper panel. All contain the same core sequence (shaded) but differ in length. In the lower panel, different peptides binding to the human MHC class II protein HLA-DR3 are shown. Anchor residues are shown as green circles. The lengths of these peptides can vary, and so by convention the first anchor residue is denoted as residue 1. Note that all of the peptides share a hydrophobic residue in position 1, a negatively charged residue [aspartic acid (D) or glutamic acid (E)] in position 4, and a tendency to have a basic or polar residue [lysine (K), arginine (R), histidine (H), glutamine (Q), or asparagine (N)] in position 6 and a hydrophobic residue [for example, tyrosine (Y), leucine (L), or phenylalanine (F)] in position 9.

a

b

4-20 The crystal structures of several peptide:MHC:T-cell receptor complexes show a similar orientation of the T-cell receptor over the peptide:MHC complex.

When the first X-ray crystallographic structure of a T-cell receptor was published, a structure of the same T-cell receptor bound to a peptide:MHC class I ligand was also produced. The orientation revealed by these structures showed that the T-cell receptor is aligned diagonally over the peptide and the peptide-binding cleft (**Fig. 4.28**). The TCRα chain lies over the α_2 domain of the MHC molecule at the amino-terminal end of the bound peptide, as seen from the side view shown in Fig. 4.28a. The TCRβ chain lies over the MHC molecule's α_1 domain, closer to the carboxyl-terminal end of the peptide. Figure 4.27b shows a view of this structure as if looking down through a transparent T-cell receptor to indicate where it contacts the MHC molecule. The CDR3 loops of both TCRα and TCRβ chains come together and lie over central amino acids of the peptide. The T-cell receptor is threaded through a valley between the two high points on the two surrounding α helices that form the walls of the peptide-binding cleft. This can be seen in **Fig. 4.29**, which shows a view from the end of the peptide-binding groove of a peptide:MHC class II:T-cell receptor complex. Comparison of various peptide:MHC:T-cell receptor complexes shows that the axis of the TCR as it binds the surface of the MHC molecule is rotated somewhat relative to the peptide-binding groove of the MHC molecule, with some variation between individual peptide:MHC:T-cell receptor complexes (see Fig. 4.28b). In this orientation, the V_α domain makes contact primarily with the amino-terminal half of the bound peptide, whereas the V_β domain contacts primarily the carboxyl-terminal half. Both chains also interact with the α helices of the MHC class I molecule (see Fig. 4.28). The T-cell receptor contacts are not symmetrically distributed over the MHC molecule: whereas the V_α CDR1 and CDR2 loops are in close contact with the helices of the peptide:MHC complex around the amino terminus of the bound peptide, the β-chain CDR1 and CDR2 loops, which interact with the complex at the carboxyl terminus of the bound peptide, have variable contributions to the binding.

Comparison of the three-dimensional structure of an unliganded T-cell receptor and the same T-cell receptor complexed to its peptide:MHC ligand shows that the binding results in some degree of conformational change, or 'induced fit,' particularly within the V_α CDR3 loop. Subtle variations at amino acids that contact the T-cell receptor can have strikingly different effects on the recognition of an otherwise identical peptide:MHC ligand by the same T cell. The flexibility in the CDR3 loop demonstrated by these two structures helps to explain how the T-cell receptor can adopt conformations that recognize related, but different, peptide ligands.

The specificity of T-cell recognition involves both the peptide and its presenting MHC molecule. Simply changing a leucine to isoleucine in the peptide,

Fig. 4.28 The T-cell receptor binds to the peptide:MHC complex. Panel a: The T-cell receptor binds to the top of a peptide:MHC class I molecule, touching both the α_1 and α_2 domain helices. The CDRs of the T-cell receptor are shown in color: the CDR1 and CDR2 loops of the β chain are light and dark blue, respectively, and the CDR1 and CDR2 loops of the α chain are light and dark purple, respectively. The α-chain CDR3 loop is yellow, and the β-chain CDR3 loop is green. The β-chain HV4 loop is in red. The thick yellow line P1–P8 is the bound peptide. Panel b: The outline of the T-cell receptor's antigen-binding site (thick black line) is superimposed over the top surface of the peptide:MHC complex (the peptide is shaded dull yellow). The T-cell receptor lies at a somewhat diagonal angle across the peptide:MHC complex, with the α and β CDR3 loops of the T-cell receptor (3α, 3β, yellow and green, respectively) contacting the center of the peptide. The α-chain CDR1 and CDR2 loops (1α, 2α, light and dark purple, respectively) contact the MHC helices at the amino terminus of the bound peptide, whereas the β-chain CDR1 and CDR2 loops (1β, 2β, light and dark blue, respectively) make contact with the helices at the carboxyl terminus of the bound peptide.

Fig. 4.29 The T-cell receptor interacts with MHC class I and MHC class II molecules in a similar fashion. Shown is the structure of a T-cell receptor, specific for a peptide derived from chicken cytochrome *c*, bound to an MHC class II molecule. This T-cell receptor's binding is at a site and orientation similar to that of the T-cell receptor bound to the MHC class I molecule shown in Fig. 4.28. The α and β chains of the T-cell receptor are colored in light and dark blue, respectively. The cytochrome *c* peptide is light orange. The T-cell receptor sits in a shallow saddle formed between the α-helical regions of the MHC class II α (brown) and β (yellow) chains at roughly 90° to the long axis of the MHC class II molecule and the bound peptide. Structure derived from PDB 3QIB.

for example, is sufficient to alter a T-cell response from strong killing to no response at all. Mutations of single residues in the presenting MHC molecules can have the same effect. This dual specificity for T-cell recognition of antigen underlies the MHC restriction of T-cell responses, a phenomenon that was observed long before the peptide-binding properties of MHC molecules were known. Another consequence of this dual specificity is a need for T-cell receptors to exhibit some inherent specificity for MHC molecules in order to be able to interact appropriately with the antigen-presenting surface of MHC molecules. We will return to these issues in Chapter 6, where we recount the discovery of MHC restriction in the context of T-cell recognition and MHC polymorphisms, and in Chapter 8, where we discuss the impact of these phenomena on T-cell development in the thymus.

4-21 The CD4 and CD8 cell-surface proteins of T cells directly contact MHC molecules and are required to make an effective response to antigen.

As we introduced in Section 1-21, T cells fall into two major classes distinguished by the expression of the cell-surface proteins **CD4** and **CD8**. CD8 is expressed by cytotoxic T cells, while CD4 is expressed by T cells whose function is to activate other cells. CD4 and CD8 were known as markers for these functional sets for some time before it became clear that the distinction was based on the ability of T cells to recognize different classes of MHC molecules. We now know that CD8 recognizes MHC class I molecules and CD4 recognizes MHC class II. During antigen recognition, CD4 or CD8 (depending on the type of T cell) associates with the T-cell receptor on the T-cell surface and binds to invariant sites on the MHC portion of the composite peptide:MHC ligand, away from the peptide-binding site. This binding contributes to the overall effectiveness of the T-cell response, and so CD4 and CD8 are called **co-receptors**.

CD4 is a single-chain protein composed of four Ig-like domains (**Fig. 4.30**). The first two domains (D1 and D2) are packed tightly together to form a rigid rod about 6 nm long, which is joined by a flexible hinge to a similar rod formed by the third and fourth domains (D3 and D4). The MHC-binding region on CD4 is located mainly on a lateral face of the D1 domain, and CD4 binds to a hydrophobic crevice formed at the junction of the α_2 and β_2 domains of the MHC class II molecule (**Fig. 4.31a**). This site is well away from the site where the T-cell receptor binds, as shown by the complete crystal structure of a T-cell receptor bound to peptide:MHC class II with bound CD4 (**Fig. 4.32**). This structure demonstrates that the CD4 molecule and the T-cell receptor can bind simultaneously to the same peptide:MHC class II complex. CD4 enhances sensitivity to antigen, as the T cell is about 100-fold more sensitive to the antigen when CD4 is present. The enhancement process results from the ability of the intracellular portion of CD4 to bind to a cytoplasmic tyrosine kinase called **Lck**. As we will discuss in detail Chapter 7, bringing Lck into proximity with the T-cell receptor complex helps activate the signaling cascade induced by antigen recognition.

Fig. 4.30 The structures of the CD4 and CD8 co-receptor molecules. The CD4 molecule contains four Ig-like domains, shown in schematic form in panel a and as a ribbon diagram from the crystal structure in panel b. The amino-terminal domain, D1, is similar in structure to an immunoglobulin V domain. The second domain, D2, although related to an immunoglobulin domain, is different from both V and C domains and has been termed a C2 domain. The first two domains of CD4 form a rigid rodlike structure that is linked to the two carboxyl-terminal domains by a flexible link. The binding site for MHC class II molecules involves mainly the D1 domain. The CD8 molecule is a heterodimer of an α and a β chain covalently linked by a disulfide bond. An alternative form of CD8 exists as a homodimer of α chains. The heterodimer is depicted in panel a, whereas the ribbon diagram in panel b is of the homodimer. CD8α and CD8β chains have very similar structures, each having a single domain resembling an immunoglobulin V domain and a stretch of polypeptide chain, believed to be in a relatively extended conformation, that anchors the V-like domain to the cell membrane.

The structure of CD8 is quite different. It is a disulfide-linked dimer of two different chains, called α and β, each containing a single Ig-like domain linked to the membrane by a segment of extended polypeptide (see Fig. 4.30). This segment is extensively glycosylated, which is thought to maintain it in an extended conformation and protect it from cleavage by proteases. CD8α chains can form homodimers, although these are usually not found when CD8β is expressed. Naive T cells express CD8αβ, but the CD8αα homodimer can be expressed by highly activated effector and memory T cells. CD8αα is also expressed by a population of intraepithelial lymphocytes known as **mucosal associated invariant T cells (MAIT cells)**; these cells recognize metabolites of folic acid that are produced by bacteria in association with the nonclassical MHC class I molecule **MR1**, which we will describe in Chapter 6.

CD8αβ binds weakly to an invariant loop site in the α_3 domain of an MHC class I molecule (**Fig. 4.31b**). The CD8β chain interacts with residues in the base of the α_2 domain of the MHC class I molecule, while the α chain is in a lower position interacting with the α_3 domain of the MHC class I molecule. The strength of binding of CD8 to the MHC class I molecule is influenced by the glycosylation state of the CD8 molecule; increasing the number of sialic acid residues on CD8 carbohydrate structures decreases the strength of the interaction. The pattern of sialylation of CD8 changes during the maturation of T cells in the thymus and also on activation, and this likely has a role in modulating antigen recognition.

Fig. 4.31 The binding sites for CD4 and CD8 on MHC class II and class I molecules lie in the Ig-like domains. The binding sites for CD4 and CD8 on the MHC class II and class I molecules, respectively, lie in the Ig-like domains nearest to the membrane and distant from the peptide-binding cleft. The binding of CD4 to an MHC class II molecule is shown as a ribbon structure in panel a and schematically in panel c. The α chain of the MHC class II molecule is shown in pink, and the β chain in white, while CD4 is in gold. Only the D1 and D2 domains of the CD4 molecule are shown in panel a. The binding site for CD4 lies at the base of the β_2 domain of an MHC class II molecule, in the hydrophobic crevice between the β_2 and α_2 domains. The binding of CD8$\alpha\beta$ to an MHC class I molecule is shown in panel b and schematically in panel d. The class I heavy chain and β_2-microglobulin are shown in white and pink, respectively, and the two chains of the CD8 dimer are shown in light (CD8β) and dark (CD8α) purple. The binding site for CD8 on the MHC class I molecule lies in a similar position to that of CD4 in the MHC class II molecule, but CD8 binding also involves the base of the α_1 and α_2 domains, and thus the binding of CD8 to MHC class I is not completely equivalent to the binding of CD4 to MHC class II. The cylindrical shapes in panels a and b represent the α helices lining the peptide-binding sites of MHC class II and MHC class I, respectively. Structures derived from PDB 3S4S (CD4/MHC class II) and PDB 3DMM (CD8$\alpha\beta$/MHC class I).

Fig. 4.32 CD4 and the T-cell receptor bind to distinct regions of the MHC class II molecule. A ribbon diagram is shown from a crystal structure of a complete αβ TCR:peptide-MHC:CD4 ternary complex. The α and β chains of the T-cell receptor (TCR) are blue and red, respectively. The peptide-MHC class II complex is green. CD4 is shown in orange. Structure derived from PDB 3T0E.

Fig. 4.33 CD8 binds to a site on MHC class I molecules that is distant from where the T-cell receptor binds. The relative binding positions of both the T-cell receptor and CD8 molecules can be seen in this hypothetical reconstruction of their interaction with MHC class I (α chain in dark green and β2-microglobulin in light green). The α and β chains of the T-cell receptor are shown in brown and purple, respectively. The CD8αβ heterodimer is shown bound to the MHC class I α3 domain. The CD8 α chain is in blue, and the CD8β chain is in red.

Like the interactions with MHC class II molecules, the T-cell receptor and CD8 can interact simultaneously with one MHC class I molecule (**Fig. 4.33**). Like CD4, CD8 binds Lck through the cytoplasmic tail of the α chain, and CD8αβ increases the sensitivity of T cells to antigen presented by MHC class I molecules about 100-fold. Although the molecular details are unclear, the CD8αα homodimer appears to function less efficiently than CD8αβ as a co-receptor and may negatively regulate activation. In contrast to CD8, CD4 is not thought to dimerize.

4-22 The two classes of MHC molecules are expressed differentially on cells.

MHC class I and MHC class II molecules have distinct distributions among cells, and these reflect the different effector functions of the T cells that recognize them (**Fig. 4.34**). MHC class I molecules present peptides from pathogens, commonly viruses, to CD8 cytotoxic T cells, which are specialized to kill any cell that they specifically recognize. Because viruses can infect any nucleated cell, almost all such cells express MHC class I molecules, although the level of constitutive expression varies from one cell type to the next. For example, cells of the immune system express abundant MHC class I on their surface, whereas liver cells (hepatocytes) express relatively low levels (see Fig. 4.34). Nonnucleated cells, such as mammalian red blood cells, express little or no MHC class I, and thus the interior of red blood cells is a site in which an infection can go undetected by cytotoxic T cells. Because red blood cells cannot support viral replication, this is of no great consequence for viral infection, but it might be the absence of MHC class I that allows the *Plasmodium* parasites that cause malaria to live in this privileged site.

In contrast, a major function of the CD4 T cells that recognize MHC class II molecules is to activate other effector cells of the immune system. Thus, MHC class II molecules are normally found on dendritic cells, B lymphocytes, and macrophages—antigen-presenting cells that participate in immune responses—but not on other tissue cells (see Fig. 4.34). The peptides presented by MHC class II molecules expressed by dendritic cells can function to activate naive CD4 T cells. When previously activated CD4 T cells recognize peptides bound to MHC class II molecules on B cells, the T cells secrete cytokines that can influence the isotype of antibody that those B cells will choose to produce. Upon recognizing peptides bound to MHC class II molecules on macrophages, CD4 T cells activate these cells, again in part through cytokines, to destroy the pathogens in their intracellular vesicles.

The expression of both MHC class I and MHC class II molecules is regulated by cytokines, in particular, interferons, released in the course of an immune response. Interferon-α (IFN-α) and IFN-β increase the expression of MHC class I molecules on all types of cells, whereas IFN-γ increases the expression of both MHC class I and MHC class II molecules and can induce the expression of MHC class II molecules on certain cell types that do not normally express them. Interferons also enhance the antigen-presenting function of MHC class I molecules by inducing the expression of key components of the intracellular machinery that enables peptides to be loaded onto the MHC molecules.

4-23 A distinct subset of T cells bears an alternative receptor made up of γ and δ chains.

During the search for the gene for the TCRα chain, another T-cell receptor–like gene was unexpectedly discovered. This gene was named TCRγ, and its discovery led to a search for further T-cell receptor genes. Another receptor chain was identified by using antibody against the predicted sequence of the γ chain and was called the δ chain. It was soon discovered that a minority population of T cells in lymphoid organs bore a distinct type of T-cell receptor made up of $\gamma\delta$ heterodimers rather than $\alpha\beta$ heterodimers. The development of these cells is described in Sections 8-17 and 8-18.

Like $\alpha\beta$ T cells, $\gamma\delta$ T cells can be found in the lymphoid tissues of all vertebrates, but they are more prominent as populations of intraepithelial lymphocytes, particularly in the skin and female reproductive tracts, where their receptors display very limited diversity. Unlike $\alpha\beta$ T cells, $\gamma\delta$ T cells do not generally recognize antigen as peptides presented by MHC molecules, and $\gamma\delta$ T-cell receptors are not restricted by the 'classical' MHC class I and class II molecules that function in binding and presenting peptides to T cells. Instead, $\gamma\delta$ T-cell receptors seem to recognize their target antigens directly and thus probably are able to recognize and respond rapidly to molecules expressed by many different cell types. Their ligands have been difficult to identify, but several have now been described and seem to indicate that $\gamma\delta$ T cells play an intermediate, or transitional, role between wholly innate and fully adaptive immune responses.

Like NK-cell receptor ligands, such as the proteins MIC and RAET1 (see Section 3-27), many of the ligands seen by $\gamma\delta$ T cells are induced by cellular stress or damage that is a consequence of infection or malignancy, rather than being pathogen- or tumor-specific antigens themselves. Some $\gamma\delta$ T cells also bind antigens presented by 'nonclassical' **MHC class Ib molecules**, which we will discuss in Chapter 6. These proteins are related structurally to the MHC proteins we have already discussed, but have functions besides binding peptides for presentation to T cells. Additional ligands may include heat-shock proteins and nonpeptide ligands such as phosphorylated ligands or mycobacterial lipid antigens. One well-studied subset of human $\gamma\delta$ T cells recognizes a class of pyrophosphate metabolites, called phosphoantigens, that are

Tissue	MHC class I	MHC class II
Lymphoid tissues		
T cells	+++	+*
B cells	+++	+++
Macrophages	+++	++
Dendritic cells	+++	+++
Epithelial cells of thymus	+	+++
Other nucleated cells		
Neutrophils	+++	–
Hepatocytes	+	–
Kidney	+	–
Brain	+	–†
Nonnucleated cells		
Red blood cells	–	–

Fig. 4.34 The expression of MHC molecules varies among tissues. MHC class I molecules are expressed on all nucleated cells, although they are most highly expressed in hematopoietic cells. MHC class II molecules are normally expressed only by a subset of hematopoietic cells and by thymic stromal cells, although they may be expressed by other cell types on exposure to the inflammatory cytokine IFN-γ. *In humans, activated T cells express MHC class II molecules, whereas in mice all T cells are MHC class II–negative. †In the brain, most cell types are MHC class II–negative, but microglia, which are related to macrophages, are MHC class II–positive.

produced by microbial pathogens or malignant cells. In this case, recognition of the phosphoantigen is not direct, but requires an interaction between the phosphoantigen and a protein of the butyrophilin family expressed on human cells. Currently the precise details of butyrophilin-mediated phosphoantigen recognition by these γδ T cells remains unclear.

The crystallographic structure of a γδ T-cell receptor reveals that, as expected, it is similar in shape to αβ T-cell receptors. **Figure 4.35** shows a crystal structure of a γδ T-cell receptor complex bound to one of the nonclassical MHC class I molecules, called **T22**. This structure shows that the overall orientation of the γδ T-cell receptor with the MHC molecule is strikingly different from that of an αβ T-cell receptor, in that it interacts primarily with one end of the T22 molecule. However, the CDR3 regions of the γδ T-cell receptor still play a critical role in recognition, similar to that of antibodies and of αβ T-cell receptors. Further, the CDR3 of the γδ T-cell receptor is longer than either of these other two antigen receptors, and this could have implications for the type of ligand that the γδ T-cell receptor recognizes, as there is enormous combinatorial diversity from the CDR3 within the γδ T-cell receptor repertoire. We will return to discuss further the ligands and the development of γδ T cells in Chapters 6 and 8.

Summary.

The receptor for antigen on most T cells, the αβ T-cell receptor, is composed of two protein chains, TCRα and TCRβ, and resembles in many respects a single Fab fragment of immunoglobulin. αβ T-cell receptors are always membrane-bound and recognize a composite ligand of a peptide antigen bound to an MHC molecule. Each MHC molecule binds a wide variety of different peptides, but the different variants of MHC each preferentially recognize sets of peptides with particular sequences and physical features. The peptide antigen is generated intracellularly and is bound stably in a peptide-binding cleft on the surface of the MHC molecule. There are two classes of MHC molecules, and these are bound in their nonpolymorphic domains by CD8 and CD4 molecules that distinguish two different functional classes of αβ T cells. CD8 binds MHC class I molecules and can bind simultaneously to the same peptide:MHC class I complex being recognized by a T-cell receptor, thus acting as a co-receptor and enhancing the T-cell response; CD4 binds MHC class II molecules and acts as a co-receptor for T-cell receptors that recognize peptide:MHC class II ligands. A T-cell receptor interacts directly both with the antigenic peptide and with polymorphic features of the MHC molecule that displays it, and this dual specificity underlies the MHC restriction of T-cell responses. A second type of T-cell receptor, composed of a γ and a δ chain, is structurally similar to the αβ T-cell receptor, but it binds to different ligands, including nonpeptide ligands, nonpolymorphic nonclassical MHC molecules, and certain lipids. The receptor is thought not to be MHC-restricted and is found on a minority population of lymphoid and intraepithelial T cells, the γδ T cells.

Summary to Chapter 4.

B cells and T cells use different but structurally similar molecules to recognize antigen. The antigen-recognition molecules of B cells are immunoglobulins and are made both as a membrane-bound receptor for antigen, the B-cell receptor, and as secreted antibodies that bind antigens and elicit humoral effector functions. The antigen-recognition molecules of T cells, in contrast, are made only as cell-surface receptors and so elicit only cellular effector functions. Immunoglobulins and T-cell receptors are highly variable molecules, with the variability concentrated in that part of the molecule—the variable (V) region—that binds to antigen. Immunoglobulins bind a wide variety of chemically different antigens, whereas the major type of T-cell receptor, the αβ T-cell receptor, predominantly recognizes peptide fragments of foreign proteins bound to MHC molecules, which are ubiquitous on cell surfaces.

Fig. 4.35 Structures of γδ T-cell receptor bound to the nonclassical MHC class I molecule T22. The γδ T-cell receptor has a similar overall structure to the αβ T-cell receptor and the Fab fragment of an immunoglobulin. The C_δ domain is more like an immunoglobulin domain than is the corresponding C_α domain of the αβ T-cell receptor. In this structure, the overall orientation of the γδ T-cell receptor with respect to the nonclassical MHC molecule T22 is very different from the orientation of an αβ T-cell receptor with either MHC class I or class II molecules. Rather than lying directly over the peptide-binding groove, the γδ T-cell receptor is engaged with one end much more than the other; this is consistent with a lack of peptide contact and absence of MHC-restricted recognition.

Binding of antigen by immunoglobulins has chiefly been studied with antibodies. The binding of antibody to its antigen is highly specific and is determined by the shape and physicochemical properties of the antigen-binding site. Located at the other end of the antibody from the antigen-binding site is the constant, or Fc, region, which influences the types of effector function the antibody can elicit. There are five main functional classes of antibodies, each encoded by a different type of constant region. As we will see in Chapter 10, these interact with different components of the immune system to incite an inflammatory response and eliminate the antigen.

T-cell receptors differ in several respects from the B-cell immunoglobulins. One is the absence of a secreted form of T-cell receptor, reflecting the functional differences between T cells and B cells. B cells deal with pathogens and their protein products circulating within the body; secretion of a soluble antigen-recognition molecule enables the B cell to act in the clearance of antigen effectively throughout the extracellular spaces of the body. T cells, in contrast, are specialized for active surveillance of pathogens, and T-cell recognition does not involve a soluble, secreted receptor. Some T cells, such as CD8 T cells, are able to detect intracellular infections and are able to kill infected cells that bear foreign antigenic peptides on their surface. Others, such as CD4 T cells, interact with cells of the immune system that have taken up foreign antigen and are displaying it on the cell surface.

T-cell receptors also recognize a composite ligand made up of the foreign peptide bound to a self MHC molecule and do not recognize intact antigen. This means T cells can interact only with a body cell displaying the antigen, not with the intact pathogen or protein. Each T-cell receptor is specific for a particular combination of peptide and a self MHC molecule. MHC molecules are encoded by a family of highly polymorphic genes. Expression of multiple variant MHC molecules, each with a different peptide-binding repertoire, helps to ensure that T cells from an individual will be able to recognize at least some peptides generated from nearly every pathogen.

Discussion Questions

4.1 When a mixture of IgG antibodies is treated with the proteolytic enzyme papain, each antibody is cleaved into three pieces. One of these pieces, the Fc fragment, was found to crystallize readily, indicating that the sequence of this fragment did not vary between individual antibody molecules, as did the Fab portion. Why is it important that the variability in amino acid sequence between different antibody molecules is restricted to the Fab portion of each antibody?

4.2 The initial antibody produced by an activated B cell is IgM. As an immune response progresses, B cells specific for the antigen can produce other antibody isotypes. What important functions are provided by antibodies of the IgG, IgA, or IgE class compared to IgM?

4.3 What advantage is conferred by antibodies that form multimers compared to those that are monomers?

4.4 Amino acid sequence variability (that is, the differences in sequence between many different antibodies) in antibody V_H and V_L domains is predominantly found in three short regions of sequence, known as CDR1, CDR2, and CDR3. Why is it important that the V_H and V_L domain sequences outside of these CDRs remain constant in all antibodies?

4.5 Unlike antibodies, T-cell antigen receptors only recognize foreign antigens that are displayed on the surface of the body's own cells. How does this mode of T-cell antigen recognition fit with the known functions of T lymphocytes? Why are T-cell receptor αβ heterodimers never secreted by T cells?

4.6 MHC molecules are among the most polymorphic genes in the human population. For some human MHC genes, there are hundreds of different alleles. Where in the protein structure are most of the differences in amino acid sequence between the allelic forms? What are the consequences of these amino acid differences?

4.7 Many protein–protein interactions, such as an antibody binding to a protein antigen, are highly specific. Often, a single amino acid change in one of the proteins will abolish the binding to the second protein. In contrast, peptide binding to MHC proteins is much more promiscuous. Why is this lack of specificity an important aspect of peptide:MHC binding?

4.8 How do the CD4 and CD8 co-receptors contribute to peptide:MHC binding by T cells?

4.9 Why do MHC class I and MHC class II molecules have very different expression patterns among cells in the body? Which type of MHC molecule is more widely expressed and why?

General references.

Garcia, K.C., Degano, M., Speir, J.A., and Wilson, I.A.: Emerging principles for T cell receptor recognition of antigen in cellular immunity. *Rev. Immunogenet.* 1999, **1**:75–90.

Garcia, K.C., Teyton, L., and Wilson, I.A.: Structural basis of T cell recognition. *Annu. Rev. Immunol.* 1999, **17**:369–397.

Moller, G. (ed): Origin of major histocompatibility complex diversity. *Immunol. Rev.* 1995, **143**:5–292.

Poljak, R.J.: Structure of antibodies and their complexes with antigens. *Mol. Immunol.* 1991, **28**:1341–1345.

Rudolph, M.G., Stanfield, R.L., and Wilson, I.A: How TCRs bind MHCs, peptides, and coreceptors. *Annu. Rev. Immunol.* 2006, **24**:419–466.

Sundberg, E.J., and Mariuzza, R.A.: Luxury accommodations: the expanding role of structural plasticity in protein-protein interactions. *Structure* 2000, **8**:R137–R142.

Section references.

4-1   IgG antibodies consist of four polypeptide chains.

Edelman, G.M.: Antibody structure and molecular immunology. *Scand. J. Immunol.* 1991, **34**:4–22.

Faber, C., Shan, L., Fan, Z., Guddat, L.W., Furebring, C., Ohlin, M., Borrebaeck, C.A.K., and Edmundson, A.B.: Three-dimensional structure of a human Fab with high affinity for tetanus toxoid. *Immunotechnology* 1998, **3**:253–270.

Harris, L.J., Larson, S.B., Hasel, K.W., Day, J., Greenwood, A., and McPherson, A.: The three-dimensional structure of an intact monoclonal antibody for canine lymphoma. *Nature* 1992, **360**:369–372.

4-2   Immunoglobulin heavy and light chains are composed of constant and variable regions.

&

4-3   The domains of an immunoglobulin molecule have similar structures.

Barclay, A.N., Brown, M.H., Law, S.K., McKnight, A.J., Tomlinson, M.G., and van der Merwe, P.A. (eds): *The Leukocyte Antigen Factsbook*, 2nd ed. London: Academic Press, 1997.

Brummendorf, T., and Lemmon, V.: Immunoglobulin superfamily receptors: *cis*-interactions, intracellular adapters and alternative splicing regulate adhesion. *Curr. Opin. Cell Biol.* 2001, **13**:611–618.

Marchalonis, J.J., Jensen, I., and Schluter, S.F.: Structural, antigenic and evolutionary analyses of immunoglobulins and T cell receptors. *J. Mol. Recognit.* 2002, **15**:260–271.

Ramsland, P.A., and Farrugia, W.: Crystal structures of human antibodies: a detailed and unfinished tapestry of immunoglobulin gene products. *J. Mol. Recognit.* 2002, **15**:248–259.

4-4   The antibody molecule can readily be cleaved into functionally distinct fragments.

Porter, R.R.: Structural studies of immunoglobulins. *Scand. J. Immunol.* 1991, **34**:382–389.

Yamaguchi, Y., Kim, H., Kato, K., Masuda, K., Shimada, I., and Arata, Y.: Proteolytic fragmentation with high specificity of mouse IgG—mapping of proteolytic cleavage sites in the hinge region. *J. Immunol. Methods.* 1995, **181**:259–267.

4-5   The hinge region of the immunoglobulin molecule allows flexibility in binding to multiple antigens.

Gerstein, M., Lesk, A.M., and Chothia, C.: Structural mechanisms for domain movements in proteins. *Biochemistry* 1994, **33**:6739–6749.

Jimenez, R., Salazar, G., Baldridge, K.K., and Romesberg, F.E.: Flexibility and molecular recognition in the immune system. *Proc. Natl. Acad. Sci. USA* 2003, **100**:92–97.

Saphire, E.O., Stanfield, R.L., Crispin, M.D., Parren, P.W., Rudd, P.M., Dwek, R.A., Burton, D.R., and Wilson, I.A.: Contrasting IgG structures reveal extreme asymmetry and flexibility. *J. Mol. Biol.* 2002, **319**:9–18.

4-6   Different classes of immunoglobulins are distinguished by the structure of their heavy-chain constant regions.

Davies, D.R., and Metzger, H.: Structural basis of antibody function. *Annu. Rev. Immunol.* 1983, **1**:87–117.

4-7   The constant region confers functional specialization on the antibody.

Helm, B.A., Sayers, I., Higginbottom, A., Machado, D.C., Ling, Y., Ahmad, K., Padlan, E.A., and Wilson, A.P.M.: Identification of the high affinity receptor binding region in human IgE. *J. Biol. Chem.* 1996, **271**:7494–7500.

Nimmerjahn, F., and Ravetch, J.V.: Fc-receptors as regulators of immunity. *Adv. Immunol.* 2007, **96**:179–204.

Sensel, M.G., Kane, L.M., and Morrison, S.L.: Amino acid differences in the N-terminus of C_H2 influence the relative abilities of IgG2 and IgG3 to activate complement. *Mol. Immunol.* **34**:1019–1029.

4-8   IgM and IgA can form polymers by interacting with the J chain.

Hendrickson, B.A., Conner, D.A., Ladd, D.J., Kendall, D., Casanova, J.E., Corthesy, B., Max, E.E., Neutra, M.R., Seidman, C.E., and Seidman, J.G.: Altered hepatic transport of IgA in mice lacking the J chain. *J. Exp. Med.* 1995, **182**:1905–1911.

Niles, M.J., Matsuuchi, L., and Koshland, M.E.: Polymer IgM assembly and secretion in lymphoid and nonlymphoid cell-lines—evidence that J chain is required for pentamer IgM synthesis. *Proc. Natl. Acad. Sci. USA* 1995, **92**:2884–2888.

4-9   Localized regions of hypervariable sequence form the antigen-binding site.

Chitarra, V., Alzari, P.M., Bentley, G.A., Bhat, T.N., Eiselé, J.-L., Houdusse, A., Lescar, J., Souchon, H., and Poljak, R.J.: Three-dimensional structure of a heteroclitic antigen-antibody cross-reaction complex. *Proc. Natl. Acad. Sci. USA* 1993, **90**:7711–7715.

Decanniere, K., Muyldermans, S., and Wyns, L.: Canonical antigen-binding loop structures in immunoglobulins: more structures, more canonical classes? *J. Mol. Biol.* 2000, **300**:83–91.

Gilliland, L.K., Norris, N.A., Marquardt, H., Tsu, T.T., Hayden, M.S., Neubauer, M.G., Yelton, D.E., Mittler, R.S., and Ledbetter, J.A.: Rapid and reliable cloning of antibody variable regions and generation of recombinant single-chain antibody fragments. *Tissue Antigens* 1996, **47**:1–20.

Johnson, G., and Wu, T.T.: Kabat Database and its applications: 30 years after the first variability plot. *Nucleic Acids Res.* 2000, **28**:214–218.

Wu, T.T., and Kabat, E.A.: An analysis of the sequences of the variable regions of Bence Jones proteins and myeloma light chains and their implications for antibody complementarity. *J. Exp. Med.* 1970, **132**:211–250.

Xu, J., Deng, Q., Chen, J., Houk, K.N., Bartek, J., Hilvert, D., and Wilson, I.A.: Evolution of shape complementarity and catalytic efficiency from a primordial antibody template. *Science* 1999, **286**:2345–2348.

4-10   Antibodies bind antigens via contacts in CDRs that are complementary to the size and shape of the antigen.

&

4-11   Antibodies bind to conformational shapes on the surfaces of antigens using a variety of noncovalent forces.

Ban, N., Day, J., Wang, X., Ferrone, S., and McPherson, A.: Crystal structure of an anti-anti-idiotype shows it to be self-complementary. *J. Mol. Biol.* 1996, **255**:617–627.

Davies, D.R., and Cohen, G.H.: Interactions of protein antigens with antibodies. *Proc. Natl. Acad. Sci. USA* 1996, **93**:7–12.

Decanniere, K., Desmyter, A., Lauwereys, M., Ghahroudi, M.A., Muyldermans, S., and Wyns, L.: A single-domain antibody fragment in complex with RNase A: non-canonical loop structures and nanomolar affinity using two CDR loops. *Structure Fold. Des.* 1999, **7**:361–370.

Padlan, E.A.: Anatomy of the antibody molecule. *Mol. Immunol.* 1994, **31**:169–217.

Saphire, E.O., Parren, P.W., Pantophlet, R., Zwick, M.B., Morris, G.M., Rudd, P.M., Dwek, R.A., Stanfield, R.L., Burton, D.R., and Wilson, I.A.: Crystal structure of a neutralizing human IgG against HIV-1: a template for vaccine design. *Science* 2001, **293**:1155–1159.

Stanfield, R.L., and Wilson, I.A.: Protein–peptide interactions. *Curr. Opin. Struct. Biol.* 1995, **5**:103–113.

Tanner, J.J., Komissarov, A.A., and Deutscher, S.L.: Crystal structure of an antigen-binding fragment bound to single-stranded DNA. *J. Mol. Biol.* 2001, **314**:807–822.

Wilson, I.A., and Stanfield, R.L.: Antibody–antigen interactions: new structures and new conformational changes. *Curr. Opin. Struct. Biol.* 1994, **4**:857–867.

4-12 Antibody interaction with intact antigens is influenced by steric constraints.

Braden, B.C., Goldman, E.R., Mariuzza, R.A., and Poljak, R.J.: Anatomy of an antibody molecule: structure, kinetics, thermodynamics and mutational studies of the antilysozyme antibody D1.3. *Immunol. Rev.* 1998, **163**:45–57.

Braden, B.C., and Poljak, R.J.: Structural features of the reactions between antibodies and protein antigens. *FASEB J.* 1995, **9**:9–16.

Diamond, M.S., Pierson, T.C., and Fremont, D.H.: The structural immunology of antibody protection against West Nile virus. *Immunol Rev.* 2008, **225**:212–225.

Lok, S.M., Kostyuchenko, V., Nybakken, G.E., Holdaway, H.A., Battisti, A.J., Sukupolvi-Petty, S., Sedlak, D., Fremont, D.H., Chipman, P.R., Roehrig, J.T., *et al.*: Binding of a neutralizing antibody to dengue virus alters the arrangement of surface glycoproteins. *Nat. Struct. Mol. Biol.* 2008, **15**:312–317.

Ros, R., Schwesinger, F., Anselmetti, D., Kubon, M., Schäfer, R., Plückthun, A., and Tiefenauer, L.: Antigen binding forces of individually addressed single-chain Fv antibody molecules. *Proc. Natl. Acad. Sci. USA* 1998, **95**:7402–7405.

4-13 Some species generate antibodies with alternative structures.

Hamers-Casterman, C., Atarhouch, T., Muyldermans, S., Robinson, G., Hamers, C., Songa, E.B., Bendahman, N., and Hamers, R.: Naturally occurring antibodies devoid of light chains. *Nature* 1993, **363**:446–448.

Muyldermans, S.: Nanobodies: natural single-domain antibodies. *Annu. Rev. Biochem.* 2013, **82**:775–797.

Nguyen, V.K., Desmyter, A., and Muyldermans, S.: Functional heavy-chain antibodies in Camelidae. *Adv. Immunol.* 2001, **79**:261–296.

4-14 The TCRαβ heterodimer is very similar to a Fab fragment of immunoglobulin.

Al-Lazikani, B., Lesk, A.M., and Chothia, C.: Canonical structures for the hypervariable regions of T cell αβ receptors. *J. Mol. Biol.* 2000, **295**:979–995.

Kjer-Nielsen, L., Clements, C.S., Brooks, A.G., Purcell, A.W., McCluskey, J., and Rossjohn, J.: The 1.5 Å crystal structure of a highly selected antiviral T cell receptor provides evidence for a structural basis of immunodominance. *Structure* 2002, **10**:1521–1532.

Machius, M., Cianga, P., Deisenhofer, J., and Ward, E.S.: Crystal structure of a T cell receptor Vα11 (AV11S5) domain: new canonical forms for the first and second complementarity determining regions. *J. Mol. Biol.* 2001, **310**:689–698.

4-15 A T-cell receptor recognizes antigen in the form of a complex of a foreign peptide bound to an MHC molecule.

Garcia, K.C., and Adams, E.J.: How the T cell receptor sees antigen—a structural view. *Cell* 2005, **122**:333–336.

Hennecke, J., and Wiley, D.C.: Structure of a complex of the human αβ T cell receptor (TCR) HA1.7, influenza hemagglutinin peptide, and major histocompatibility complex class II molecule, HLA-DR4 (DRA*0101 and DRB1*0401): insight into TCR cross-restriction and alloreactivity. *J. Exp. Med.* 2002, **195**:571–581.

Luz, J.G., Huang, M., Garcia, K.C., Rudolph, M.G., Apostolopoulos, V., Teyton, L., and Wilson, I.A.: Structural comparison of allogeneic and syngeneic T cell receptor–peptide–major histocompatibility complex complexes: a buried alloreactive mutation subtly alters peptide presentation substantially increasing V_β interactions. *J. Exp. Med.* 2002, **195**:1175–1186.

Reinherz, E.L., Tan, K., Tang, L., Kern, P., Liu, J., Xiong, Y., Hussey, R.E., Smolyar, A., Hare, B., Zhang, R., *et al.*: The crystal structure of a T cell receptor in complex with peptide and MHC class II. *Science* 1999, **286**:1913–1921.

Rudolph, M.G., Stanfield, R.L., and Wilson, I.A.: How TCRs bind MHCs, peptides, and coreceptors. *Annu. Rev. Immunol.* 2006, **24**:419–466.

4-16 There are two classes of MHC molecules with distinct subunit compositions but similar three-dimensional structures.

&

4-17 Peptides are stably bound to MHC molecules and also serve to stabilize the MHC molecule on the cell surface.

Bouvier, M.: Accessory proteins and the assembly of human class I MHC molecules: a molecular and structural perspective. *Mol. Immunol.* 2003, **39**:697–706.

Dessen, A., Lawrence, C.M., Cupo, S., Zaller, D.M., and Wiley, D.C.: X-ray crystal structure of HLA-DR4 (DRA*0101, DRB1*0401) complexed with a peptide from human collagen II. *Immunity* 1997, **7**:473–481.

Fremont, D.H., Hendrickson, W.A., Marrack, P., and Kappler, J.: Structures of an MHC class II molecule with covalently bound single peptides. *Science* 1996, **272**:1001–1004.

Fremont, D.H., Matsumura, M., Stura, E.A., Peterson, P.A., and Wilson, I.A.: Crystal structures of two viral peptides in complex with murine MHC class 1 H-2K^b. *Science* 1992, **257**:919–927.

Fremont, D.H., Monnaie, D., Nelson, C.A., Hendrickson, W.A., and Unanue, E.R.: Crystal structure of I-Ak in complex with a dominant epitope of lysozyme. *Immunity* 1998, **8**:305–317.

Macdonald, W.A., Purcell, A.W., Mifsud, N.A., Ely, L.K., Williams, D.S., Chang, L., Gorman, J.J., Clements, C.S., Kjer-Nielsen, L., Koelle, D.M., *et al.*: A naturally selected dimorphism within the HLA-B44 supertype alters class I structure, peptide repertoire, and T cell recognition. *J. Exp. Med.* 2003, **198**:679–691.

Zhu, Y., Rudensky, A.Y., Corper, A.L., Teyton, L., and Wilson, I.A.: Crystal structure of MHC class II I-Ab in complex with a human CLIP peptide: prediction of an I-Ab peptide-binding motif. *J. Mol. Biol.* 2003, **326**:1157–1174.

4-18 MHC class I molecules bind short peptides of 8–10 amino acids by both ends.

Bouvier, M., and Wiley, D.C.: Importance of peptide amino and carboxyl termini to the stability of MHC class I molecules. *Science* 1994, **265**:398–402.

Govindarajan, K.R., Kangueane, P., Tan, T.W., and Ranganathan, S.: MPID: MHC-Peptide Interaction Database for sequence–structure–function information on peptides binding to MHC molecules. *Bioinformatics* 2003, **19**:309–310.

Saveanu, L., Fruci, D., and van Endert, P.: Beyond the proteasome: trimming, degradation and generation of MHC class I ligands by auxiliary proteases. *Mol. Immunol.* 2002, **39**:203–215.

Weiss, G.A., Collins, E.J., Garboczi, D.N., Wiley, D.C., and Schreiber, S.L.: A tricyclic ring system replaces the variable regions of peptides presented by three alleles of human MHC class I molecules. *Chem. Biol.* 1995, **2**:401–407.

4-19 The length of the peptides bound by MHC class II molecules is not constrained.

Conant, S.B., and Swanborg, R.H.: MHC class II peptide flanking residues of exogenous antigens influence recognition by autoreactive T cells. *Autoimmun. Rev.* 2003, **2**:8–12.

Guan, P., Doytchinova, I.A., Zygouri, C., and Flower, D.R.: **MHCPred: a server for quantitative prediction of peptide–MHC binding.** *Nucleic Acids Res.* 2003, **31**:3621–3624.

Lippolis, J.D., White, F.M., Marto, J.A., Luckey, C.J., Bullock, T.N., Shabanowitz, J., Hunt, D.F., and Engelhard, V.H.: **Analysis of MHC class II antigen processing by quantitation of peptides that constitute nested sets.** *J. Immunol.* 2002, **169**:5089–5097.

Park, J.H., Lee, Y.J., Kim, K.L., and Cho, E.W.: **Selective isolation and identification of HLA-DR-associated naturally processed and presented epitope peptides.** *Immunol. Invest.* 2003, **32**:155–169.

Rammensee, H.G.: **Chemistry of peptides associated with MHC class I and class II molecules.** *Curr. Opin. Immunol.* 1995, **7**:85–96.

Rudensky, A.Y., Preston-Hurlburt, P., Hong, S.C., Barlow, A., and Janeway, C.A., Jr.: **Sequence analysis of peptides bound to MHC class II molecules.** *Nature* 1991, **353**:622–627.

Sercarz, E.E., and Maverakis, E.: **MHC-guided processing: binding of large antigen fragments.** *Nat. Rev. Immunol.* 2003, **3**:621–629.

Sinnathamby, G., and Eisenlohr, L.C.: **Presentation by recycling MHC class II molecules of an influenza hemagglutinin-derived epitope that is revealed in the early endosome by acidification.** *J. Immunol.* 2003, **170**:3504–3513.

4-20 The crystal structures of several peptide:MHC:T-cell receptor complexes show a similar orientation of the T-cell receptor over the peptide:MHC complex.

Buslepp, J., Wang, H., Biddison, W.E., Appella, E., and Collins, E.J.: **A correlation between TCR Vα docking on MHC and CD8 dependence: implications for T cell selection.** *Immunity* 2003, **19**:595–606.

Ding, Y.H., Smith, K.J., Garboczi, D.N., Utz, U., Biddison, W.E., and Wiley, D.C.: **Two human T cell receptors bind in a similar diagonal mode to the HLA-A2/Tax peptide complex using different TCR amino acids.** *Immunity* 1998, **8**:403–411.

Garcia, K.C., Degano, M., Pease, L.R., Huang, M., Peterson, P.A., Leyton, L., and Wilson, I.A.: **Structural basis of plasticity in T cell receptor recognition of a self peptide-MHC antigen.** *Science* 1998, **279**:1166–1172.

Kjer-Nielsen, L., Clements, C.S., Purcell, A.W., Brooks, A.G., Whisstock, J.C., Burrows, S.R., McCluskey, J., and Rossjohn, J.: **A structural basis for the selection of dominant αβ T cell receptors in antiviral immunity.** *Immunity* 2003, **18**:53–64.

Newell, E.W., Ely, L.K., Kruse, A.C., Reay, P.A., Rodriguez, S.N., Lin, A.E., Kuhns, M.S., Garcia, K.C., and Davis, M.M.: **Structural basis of specificity and cross-reactivity in T cell receptors specific for cytochrome c-I-E(k).** *J. Immunol.* 2011, **186**:5823–5832.

Reiser, J.B., Darnault, C., Gregoire, C., Mosser, T., Mazza, G., Kearney, A., van der Merwe, P.A., Fontecilla-Camps, J.C., Housset, D., and Malissen, B.: **CDR3 loop flexibility contributes to the degeneracy of TCR recognition.** *Nat. Immunol.* 2003, **4**:241–247.

Sant'Angelo, D.B., Waterbury, G., Preston-Hurlburt, P., Yoon, S.T., Medzhitov, R., Hong, S.C., and Janeway, C.A., Jr.: **The specificity and orientation of a TCR to its peptide-MHC class II ligands.** *Immunity* 1996, **4**:367–376.

Teng, M.K., Smolyar, A., Tse, A.G.D., Liu, J.H., Liu, J., Hussey, R.E., Nathenson, S.G., Chang, H.C., Reinherz, E.L., and Wang, J.H.: **Identification of a common docking topology with substantial variation among different TCR–MHC–peptide complexes.** *Curr. Biol.* 1998, **8**:409–412.

4-21 The CD4 and CD8 cell-surface proteins of T cells directly contact MHC molecules and are required to make an effective response to antigen.

Chang, H.C., Tan, K., Ouyang, J., Parisini, E., Liu, J.H., Le, Y., Wang, X., Reinherz, E.L., and Wang, J.H.: **Structural and mutational analyses of CD8αβ heterodimer and comparison with the CD8αα homodimer.** *Immunity* 2005, **6**:661–671.

Cheroutre, H., and Lambolez, F.: **Doubting the TCR coreceptor function of CD8αα.** *Immunity* 2008, **28**:149–159.

Gao, G.F., Tormo, J., Gerth, U.C., Wyer, J.R., McMichael, A.J., Stuart, D.I., Bell, J.I., Jones, E.Y., and Jakobsen, B.Y.: **Crystal structure of the complex between human CD8αα and HLA-A2.** *Nature* 1997, **387**:630–634.

Gaspar, R., Jr., Bagossi, P., Bene, L., Matko, J., Szollosi, J., Tozser, J., Fesus, L., Waldmann, T.A., and Damjanovich, S.: **Clustering of class I HLA oligomers with CD8 and TCR: three-dimensional models based on fluorescence resonance energy transfer and crystallographic data.** *J. Immunol.* 2001, **166**:5078–5086.

Kim, P.W., Sun, Z.Y., Blacklow, S.C., Wagner, G., and Eck, M.J.: **A zinc clasp structure tethers Lck to T cell coreceptors CD4 and CD8.** *Science* 2003, **301**:1725–1728.

Moody, A.M., North, S.J., Reinhold, B., Van Dyken, S.J., Rogers, M.E., Panico, M., Dell, A., Morris, H.R., Marth, J.D., and Reinherz, E.L.: **Sialic acid capping of CD8β core 1-O-glycans controls thymocyte-major histocompatibility complex class I interaction.** *J. Biol. Chem.* 2003, **278**:7240–7260.

Walker, L.J., Marrinan, E., Muenchhoff, M., Ferguson, J., Kloverpris, H., Cheroutre, H., Barnes, E., Goulder, P., and Klenerman, P.: **CD8αα expression marks terminally differentiated human CD8+ T cells expanded in chronic viral infection.** *Front. Immunol.* 2013, **4**:223.

Wang, J.H., and Reinherz, E.L.: **Structural basis of T cell recognition of peptides bound to MHC molecules.** *Mol. Immunol.* 2002, **38**:1039–1049.

Wang, R., Natarajan, K., and Margulies, D.H.: **Structural basis of the CD8αβ/MHC class I interaction: focused recognition orients CD8β to a T cell proximal position.** *J. Immunol.* 2009, **183**:2554–2564.

Wang, X.X., Li, Y., Yin, Y., Mo, M., Wang, Q., Gao, W., Wang, L., and Mariuzza, R.A.: **Affinity maturation of human CD4 by yeast surface display and crystal structure of a CD4-HLA-DR1 complex.** *Proc. Natl. Acad. Sci. USA* 2011, **108**:15960–15965.

Wu, H., Kwong, P.D., and Hendrickson, W.A.: **Dimeric association and segmental variability in the structure of human CD4.** *Nature* 1997, **387**:527–530.

Yin, Y., Wang, X.X., and Mariuzza, R.A.: **Crystal structure of a complete ternary complex of T-cell receptor, peptide-MHC, and CD4.** *Proc. Natl. Acad. Sci. USA* 2012, **109**:5405–5410.

Zamoyska, R.: **CD4 and CD8: modulators of T cell receptor recognition of antigen and of immune responses?** *Curr. Opin. Immunol.* 1998, **10**:82–86.

4-22 The two classes of MHC molecules are expressed differentially on cells.

Steimle, V., Siegrist, C.A., Mottet, A., Lisowska-Grospierre, B., and Mach, B.: **Regulation of MHC class II expression by interferon-γ mediated by the transactivator gene CIITA.** *Science* 1994, **265**:106–109.

4-23 A distinct subset of T cells bears an alternative receptor made up of γ and δ chains.

Adams, E.J., Chien, Y.H., and Garcia, K.C.: **Structure of a γδ T cell receptor in complex with the nonclassical MHC T22.** *Science* 2005, **308**:227–231.

Allison, T.J., and Garboczi, D.N.: **Structure of γδ T cell receptors and their recognition of non-peptide antigens.** *Mol. Immunol.* 2002, **38**:1051–1061.

Allison, T.J., Winter, C.C., Fournie, J.J., Bonneville, M., and Garboczi, D.N.: **Structure of a human γδ T-cell antigen receptor.** *Nature* 2001, **411**:820–824.

Das, H., Wang, L., Kamath, A., and Bukowski, J.F.: **Vγ2Vδ2 T-cell receptor-mediated recognition of aminobisphosphonates.** *Blood* 2001, **98**:1616–1618.

Gu, S., Borowska, M.T., Boughter, C.T., and Adams, E.J.: **Butyrophilin3A proteins and Vγ9Vδ2 T cell activation.** *Semin. Cell. Dev. Biol.* 2018, **84**:65–74.

Luoma, A.M., Castro, C.D., Mayassi, T., Bembinster, L.A., Bai, L., Picard, D., Anderson, B., Scharf, L., Kung, J.E., Sibener, L.V., *et al.*: **Crystal structure of Vδ1 T cell receptor in complex with CD1d-sulfatide shows MHC-like recognition of a self-lipid by human γδ T cells.** *Immunity* 2013, **39**:1032–1042.

Vantourout, P., and Hayday, A.: **Six-of-the-best: unique contributions of γδ T cells to immunology.** *Nat. Rev. Immunol.* 2013, **13**:88–100.

Wilson, I.A., and Stanfield, R.L.: **Unraveling the mysteries of γδ T cell recognition.** *Nat. Immunol.* 2001, **2**:579–581.

Wingren, C., Crowley, M.P., Degano, M., Chien, Y., and Wilson, I.A.: **Crystal structure of a γδ T cell receptor ligand T22: a truncated MHC-like fold.** *Science* 2000, **287**:310–314.

Wu, J., Groh, V., and Spies, T.: **T cell antigen receptor engagement and specificity in the recognition of stress-inducible MHC class I-related chains by human epithelial γδ T cells.** *J. Immunol.* 2002, **169**:1236–1240.

The Generation of Lymphocyte Antigen Receptors

5

A lymphocyte expresses many exact copies of a single antigen receptor that has a unique antigen-binding site (see Section 1-12). The clonal expression of antigen receptors means that each lymphocyte is unique among the billions of lymphocytes that each person possesses. Chapter 4 described the structural features of immunoglobulins and T-cell receptors, the antigen receptors on B cells and T cells, respectively. We saw that the vast repertoire of antigen receptors results from variations in the amino acid sequence at the antigen-binding site, which is composed of the two **variable regions** from the two chains of the receptor. In immunoglobulins these are the **heavy-chain variable region (V_H)** and the **light-chain variable region (V_L)**, and in T-cell receptors they are the **V_α** and **V_β** regions. The immunoglobulin domains of these regions contain three loops that comprise three **hypervariable regions**, or **complementarity-determining regions (CDRs)** (see Section 4-9), that determine the receptor's antigen binding site and allow for seemingly limitless diversity in specificity.

In the 1960s and 1970s, immunologists recognized that the limited size of the genome (at roughly 3 billion nucleotides) meant that the genome could not directly encode a sufficient number of genes to account for the observed diversity of antigen receptors. For example, encoding each distinct antibody by its own gene could easily fill the genome with nothing but antibody genes. As we will see, variable regions of the receptor chains are not directly encoded as a complete immunoglobulin domain by a single DNA segment. Instead, the variable regions are encoded by **gene segments** that each encode only a part of the immunoglobulin domain. During the development of each lymphocyte, these gene segments are rearranged by a process of **somatic DNA recombination** to form a complete and unique variable-region coding sequence. This process is known generally as **gene rearrangement**. A fully assembled variable region sequence is produced by combining two or three types of gene segments, each of which is present in multiple copies in the germline genome. The final diversity of the receptor repertoire is the result of assembling complete antigen receptors from the many different gene segments of each type during the development of each individual lymphocyte. This process gives each new lymphocyte only one of many possible combinations of antigen receptors, providing the repertoire of diverse antigen specificities of naive B cells and T cells.

The first part of this chapter describes the gene rearrangements that generate the primary repertoire of immunoglobulins. This part includes a brief explanation of the molecular mechanism that allows activated B cells to transition from production of transmembrane immunoglobulins to become plasma cells, which secrete their immunoglobulin proteins; the secreted form of an immunoglobulin is called an antibody. The second part of this chapter describes the gene rearrangements that generate the repertoire of T-cell receptors. Unlike immunoglobulins, T-cell receptors exist only as transmembrane receptors and are never secreted. The last part of this chapter briefly examines alternative evolutionary forms of gene rearrangements that give rise to different forms of adaptive immunity in other species.

IN THIS CHAPTER

Primary immunoglobulin gene rearrangements and expression.

T-cell receptor gene rearrangement.

Evolution of the adaptive immune response.

Primary immunoglobulin gene rearrangements and expression.

Virtually any substance can be the target of an antibody response, and the response to even a single epitope comprises many different antibody molecules, each with a subtly different specificity for the epitope and a unique **affinity**, or binding strength. The total number of antibody specificities available to an individual is known as the **antibody repertoire** or **immunoglobulin repertoire**, and in humans the repertoire is at least 10^{11} and probably several orders of magnitude greater. However, the number of antibody specificities present at any one time is limited by the total number of B cells in an individual, as well as by each individual's previous encounters with antigens.

Before it was possible to examine the immunoglobulin genes directly, there were two main hypotheses for the origin of this diversity. The **germline theory** held that there is a separate gene for each different immunoglobulin chain and that the antibody repertoire is largely inherited. In contrast, **somatic diversification theories** proposed that the observed repertoire is generated from a limited number of inherited V-region sequences that undergo alteration within B cells during the individual's lifetime. Cloning of the immunoglobulin genes revealed that elements of both theories were correct and that the DNA sequence encoding each variable region is generated by rearrangements of a relatively small group of inherited gene segments. Diversity is further enhanced by the process of **somatic hypermutation** in mature activated B cells. Thus, somatic diversification theory was essentially correct, although the germline theory concept of the existence of multiple germline genes also proved true.

5-1 Complete immunoglobulin genes are generated by the somatic recombination of separate gene segments.

Figure 5.1 shows the relationships between a light-chain variable region's antigen-binding site, its domain structure, and the gene that encodes it. The variable regions of immunoglobulin heavy and light chains are based on the **immunoglobulin fold**, which is composed of nine β strands, forming two β sheets held together by a disulfide bond. The antibody-binding site is formed by three loops of amino acids known as hypervariable regions HV1, HV2, and HV3, or CDR1, CDR2, and CDR3 (see Fig. 5.1a). These loops are located between the pairs of β strands B and C, C′ and C″, and F and G (see Fig. 5.1b). In a mature B cell, the variable region for either a heavy or a light chain is encoded by a single exon; within a given heavy- or light-chain variable-region exon, the sequences encoding each of the three CDRs are not contiguous sequences, but are separated from one another within the exon (see Fig. 5.1c). This exon is the gene's second exon (exon 2). The first exon of the variable regions encodes the antibody's leader sequence, which directs the antibody into the endoplasmic reticulum for surface expression or secretion.

Immunoglobulin variable region

a

b

D E B A | G F C C′ C″

Variable exon region

HV1 HV2 HV3
A B C C′ C″ D E F G
FR1 FR2 FR3 FR4

c

Fig. 5.1 Three hypervariable regions are encoded within a single V-region exon.
Panel a: The variable region is based on the immunoglobulin (Ig) fold that is supported by framework regions (yellow) composed of nine β strands and contains three hypervariable (HV) regions (red) that determine its antigen specificity. Panel b: The three HV regions exist as loops of amino acids on the same face between the β strands of B and C, between C′ and C″, and between F and G. The dotted line separates the β strands forming each of the two β sheets composing the Ig fold. The black bar indicates the disulfide bond holding the two β sheets together. Panel c: A complete variable region in a lymphocyte is encoded within a single exon of the full antigen-receptor gene. The three HV regions are interspersed between four framework regions (FRs) made up of the β strands of the Ig domain and the loops on the face opposite of the CDRs.

Fig. 5.2 The CDR3 region originates from two or more individual gene segments that are joined during lymphocyte development. Panel a: A complete light-chain variable region encoding the CDR1, CDR2, and CDR3 loops resides in a single exon. Panel b: The complete variable region is derived from distinct germline DNA sequences. A V gene segment encodes the CDR1 and CDR2 loops, and the CDR3 loop is formed by sequences from the end of the V gene segment and the beginning of the J gene segment, and by nucleotides added or lost when these gene segments are joined during lymphocyte development. The coding region of the CDR3 loop of the heavy chain is formed by the joining of sequences from V, D, and J gene segments and additional nucleotides added at random (not shown).

Unlike most genes, the complete DNA sequence of the variable-region exon is not present in the germline of the individual, but is originally encoded by separate DNA segments, as illustrated in **Fig. 5.2**. The rearrangements that produce the complete immunoglobulin light-chain and heavy-chain genes are shown in **Fig. 5.3**. For the light chain, the joining of a **variable or V gene**

Fig. 5.3 V regions are constructed from gene segments.
Light-chain V regions are constructed from two segments (center panel). A variable (V) and a joining (J) gene segment in the genomic DNA are joined to form a complete light-chain V-region exon. Immunoglobulin chains are extracellular proteins, and the V gene segment is preceded by an exon encoding a leader peptide (L), which directs the protein into the cell's secretory pathways and is then cleaved. The light-chain C region is encoded in a separate exon and is joined to the V-region exon by splicing of the light-chain RNA to remove the L-to-V and the J-to-C introns. Heavy-chain V regions are constructed from three gene segments (right panel). First, the diversity (D) and J gene segments join, and then the V gene segment joins to the combined DJ sequence, forming a complete V_H exon. A heavy-chain C region is encoded by several exons. The C-region exons, together with the leader sequence, are spliced to the V-domain sequence during processing of the heavy-chain RNA transcript. The leader sequence is removed after translation, and the disulfide bonds that link the polypeptide chains are formed. The hinge region is shown in purple. Only one V, one D, and one J segment is shown for each locus for simplicity; there are actually multiple gene segments of each type in the genome.

segment (denoted V_L for light-chain variable gene segment) and a **joining or J gene segment** (J_L in the case of the light chain) creates an exon that encodes the whole light-chain V_L region. In the unrearranged DNA, the V_L gene segments are located relatively far away from the exons encoding the constant region of the light chain (C_L region). The J_L gene segments are located close to the C_L region, however, and the joining of a V_L gene segment to a J_L gene segment also brings the V_L gene segment close to a C_L-region sequence. The J_L gene segment of the rearranged V_L region is separated from a C_L-region sequence only by a short intron. To make a complete immunoglobulin light-chain messenger RNA, the V-region exon is joined to the C-region sequence by RNA splicing after transcription.

For the heavy chain, there is one additional complication. The heavy-chain V region (V_H) is encoded in three gene segments, rather than two. In addition to the V and J gene segments (denoted V_H and J_H to distinguish them from the light-chain V_L and J_L), the heavy chain uses a third gene segment called the **diversity or D_H gene segment**, which lies between the V_H and J_H gene segments. The recombination process that generates a complete heavy-chain V region is shown in Fig. 5.3 (right panel) and occurs in two separate stages. First, a D_H gene segment is joined to a J_H gene segment; then a V_H gene segment rearranges and joins to DJ_H to make a complete V_H-region exon. As with the light-chain genes, RNA splicing joins the assembled V-region sequence to the neighboring C-region gene.

When this process is complete, the rearranged heavy- and light-chain loci each contain an exon (exon 2) that encodes the entire variable region. The first 95–101 amino acids of the variable region, encoding β strands A–F and the first two complete hypervariable regions, originate from the V_H or V_L gene segment (see Fig. 5.2). This segment also contributes part of the third hypervariable region. Other parts of the third hypervariable region, and the remainder of the variable region including β strand G (up to 13 amino acids), originate from D and J, or from J, gene segments in the heavy- or light-chain locus, respectively. By convention, we will refer to the exon encoding the complete variable region formed by the rearrangement of these gene segments as the **V-region gene**.

5-2 Multiple contiguous V gene segments are present at each immunoglobulin locus.

For simplicity we have discussed the formation of a complete V region as though there were only a single copy of each gene segment. In fact, there are multiple copies of the V, D, and J gene segments in germline DNA. It is the random selection of just one gene segment of each type that produces the great diversity of V regions among immunoglobulins. The number of functional gene segments of each type in the human genome, as determined by gene cloning and sequencing, are shown in **Fig. 5.4**. Not all the gene segments discovered are functional, as some have accumulated mutations that prevent them from encoding a functional protein. Such genes are termed **pseudogenes**. Because there are many V, D, and J gene segments in germline DNA, no single gene segment is essential, resulting in a relatively large number of pseudogenes. Because some of these can undergo rearrangement just like a functional gene segment, a significant proportion of rearrangements incorporate a pseudogene and thus will be nonfunctional.

We saw in Section 4-1 that there are three sets of immunoglobulin chains—the heavy chain and two equivalent types of light chains, the κ **and** λ **chains**. The immunoglobulin gene segments that encode these chains are organized into three clusters or **genetic loci**—the κ, λ, and heavy-chain loci—each of which can assemble a complete V-region sequence. Each locus is on a different chromosome and is organized differently, as shown for the human loci in **Fig. 5.5**. At the λ light-chain locus, located on human chromosome 22, a cluster of Vλ

Number of functional gene segments in human immunoglobulin loci		
Segment	**Light chains**	**Heavy chain**
	κ	λ	H
Variable (V)	31–35	29–32	38–46
Diversity (D)	0	0	23
Joining (J)	5	4–5	6
Constant (C)	1	4–5	9

Fig. 5.4 The number of functional gene segments for the human heavy- and light-chain genes. The numbers shown are derived from exhaustive cloning and sequencing of DNA from one individual and exclude all pseudogenes (mutated and nonfunctional versions of a gene sequence). As a result of genetic polymorphism, the numbers vary for different people.

λ light-chain locus

κ light-chain locus

Heavy-chain locus

Fig. 5.5 The germline organization of the human immunoglobulin heavy- and light-chain loci. Depending on the individual, the genetic locus for the λ light chain (chromosome 22) has between 29 and 33 functional V_λ gene segments and four or five pairs of functional J_λ gene segments and C_λ genes. The κ locus (chromosome 2) is organized in a similar way, with about 49 functional Vκ gene segments accompanied by a cluster of 5 Jκ gene segments but with a single Cκ gene. In approximately 50% of individuals, the entire cluster of Vκ gene segments has undergone an increase by duplication (not shown, for simplicity). The heavy-chain locus (chromosome 14) has about 40 functional V_H gene segments and a cluster of around 23 D_H segments lying between these V_H gene segments and 6 J_H gene segments. The heavy-chain locus also contains a large cluster of C_H genes (see Fig. 4.6). For simplicity, all V gene segments have been shown in the same chromosomal orientation; only the first C_H gene (for C_μ) is shown, without illustrating its separate exons; and all pseudogenes have been omitted. This diagram is not to scale: the total length of the heavy-chain locus is more than 2 megabases (2 million bases), whereas some of the D gene segments are only 6 bases long.

gene segments is followed by four (or in some individuals five) sets of Jλ gene segments each linked to a single Cλ gene. In the κ light-chain locus, on chromosome 2, the cluster of Vκ gene segments is followed by a cluster of Jκ gene segments, and then by a single Cκ gene.

The organization of the heavy-chain locus, on chromosome 14, contains separate clusters of V_H, D_H, and J_H gene segments and of C_H genes. The heavy-chain locus differs in one important way: instead of a single C region, it contains a series of C regions arrayed one after the other, each of which corresponds to a different immunoglobulin isotype (see Fig. 4.6). While the Cλ locus contains several distinct C regions, these encode similar proteins, which function similarly, whereas the different heavy-chain isotypes are structurally quite distinct and have different functions, as outlined in Section 4-7.

B cells initially express the heavy-chain isotypes μ and δ, which is accomplished by alternative mRNA splicing and which leads to the expression of immunoglobulins IgM and IgD, as we shall see in Section 5-8. The expression of other isotypes, such as γ (giving IgG), occurs through DNA rearrangements referred to as **class switching** and takes place at a later stage, after a B cell has been activated by antigen in an immune response. We describe class switching in Chapter 10.

The human V gene segments can be grouped into families in which each member shares at least 80% DNA sequence identity with all others in the family. Both the heavy-chain and the κ-chain V gene segments can be subdivided into seven families, and there are eight families of V_λ gene segments. The families can be grouped into clans, made up of families that are more similar to each other than to families in other clans. Human V_H gene segments fall into three clans. All the V_H gene segments identified from amphibians, reptiles, and mammals also fall into the same three clans, suggesting that these clans existed in a common ancestor of these modern animal groups. Thus, the

V gene segments that we see today have arisen by a series of gene duplications and diversification through evolutionary time.

5-3 Rearrangement of V, D, and J gene segments is guided by flanking DNA sequences.

For a complete immunoglobulin or T-cell receptor chain to be expressed, DNA rearrangements must take place at the correct locations relative to the V, D, or J gene segment coding regions. In addition, these DNA rearrangements must be regulated such that a V gene segment is joined to a D or a J and not joined to another V gene segment. DNA rearrangements are guided by conserved noncoding DNA sequences, called **recombination signal sequences (RSSs)**, that are found adjacent to the points at which recombination takes place. The structure and arrangements of the RSSs are shown in **Fig. 5.6** for the λ and κ light-chain loci and the heavy-chain locus. An RSS consists of a conserved block of seven nucleotides—the **heptamer** 5′CACAGTG3′, which is always contiguous with the coding sequence; followed by a nonconserved region known as the **spacer**, which is either 12 or 23 base pairs (bp) long; followed by a second conserved block of nine nucleotides, the **nonamer** 5′ACAAAAACC3′.

The sequences given here are the consensus sequences, but they can vary substantially from one gene segment to another, even in the same individual, as there is some flexibility in the recognition of these sequences by the enzymes that carry out the recombination. The heptamer–spacer–nonamer sequence motif—the RSS—is always found directly adjacent to the coding sequence of

Fig. 5.6 Recombination signal sequences (RSSs) are conserved heptamer and nonamer sequences that flank the gene segments encoding the V, D, and J gene segments of immunoglobulins. Recombination signal sequences (RSSs) are composed of heptamer (CACAGTG) and nonamer (ACAAAAACC) sequences that are separated by either 12 bp or approximately 23 bp of nucleotides. The heptamer–12-bp spacer–nonamer motif is depicted here as an orange arrowhead; the motif that includes the 23-bp spacer is depicted as a purple arrowhead. Heptamers are found directly adjacent to the 3′ end of V segments, the 5′ end of J segments, and on both sides of D segments. Joining of gene segments almost always involves a 12-bp RSS and a 23-bp RSS—the 12/23 rule. The arrangement of RSSs in the V (red), D (green), and J (yellow) gene segments of heavy (H) and light (λ and κ) chains of immunoglobulin is shown here. The RAG-1 recombinase (see Section 5-4) cuts the DNA precisely between the last nucleotide of the V gene segment and the first C of the heptamer or between the last G of the heptamer and the first nucleotide of the D or J gene segment. Note that according to the 12/23 rule, the arrangement of RSSs in the immunoglobulin heavy-chain gene segments precludes direct V-to-J joining.

V, D, or J gene segments. Recombination normally occurs between gene segments located on the same chromosome. A gene segment flanked by an RSS with a 12-bp spacer typically can be joined only to one flanked by a 23-bp spacer RSS. This principle is known as the **12/23 rule**.

It is important to recognize that the pattern of 12- and 23-bp spacers used by the various gene segments is different between the λ, κ, and heavy-chain loci (see Fig. 5.6). Thus, for the heavy chain, a D_H gene segment can be joined to a J_H gene segment and a V_H gene segment to a D_H gene segment, but V_H gene segments cannot be joined to J_H gene segments directly, as both V_H and J_H gene segments are flanked by 23-bp spacers. However, they can be joined with a D_H gene segment between them, as D_H segments have 12-bp spacers on both sides (see Fig. 5.6).

In the antigen-binding region of an immunoglobulin, CDR1 and CDR2 are encoded directly in the V gene segment (see Fig. 5.2). For the light chain, CDR3 is encoded by the additional DNA sequence that is created by the joining of the V and J gene segments; for the heavy chain, CDR3 is encoded by the V, D, and J gene segments. Further diversity in the antibody repertoire can be supplied by CDR3 regions that result from the joining of one D gene segment to another D gene segment, before being joined by a J gene segment. Such D–D joining is infrequent and seems to violate the 12/23 rule, suggesting that such violations of the 12/23 rule can occur at low frequency. In humans, D–D joining is found in approximately 5% of antibodies and is the major mechanism accounting for the unusually long CDR3 loops found in some heavy chains.

The mechanism of DNA rearrangement is similar for the heavy- and light-chain loci, although only one joining event is needed to generate a light-chain gene but two are required for a heavy-chain gene. When two gene segments are in the same transcriptional orientation in the germline DNA, their rearrangement involves the looping out and deletion of the DNA between them. This looped out DNA is a circular piece of **extrachromosomal DNA** (**Fig. 5.7**, left panels), which is lost from the genome when the cell divides. The V and J gene segments, which remain on the chromosome, join to form what is called the **coding joint**.

By contrast, when the gene segments have opposite transcriptional orientations, the rearrangement retains the intervening DNA in the chromosome but with an inverted orientation (Fig. 5.7, right panels). This mode of recombination is less common, but it accounts for about half of all Vκ to Jκ joins in humans because the orientation of half of the Vκ gene segments is opposite to that of the Jκ gene segments. After recombination of gene segments in this orientation, the RSSs are retained within the chromosome, and the region of DNA between the V gene segment and the RSS of the J gene segment is inverted to form the coding joint. This situation leads to **rearrangement by inversion**. As we shall see later, the coding joint junction in all cases is imprecise, meaning that nucleotides can be added or lost between joined segments during the rearrangement process. This imprecise nature of coding joint formation adds to the variability in the V-region sequence, called **junctional diversity**.

 ANIMATION 5.1

The overall enzymatic mechanisms involved in V-region rearrangement, or **V(D)J recombination**, are illustrated in **Fig. 5.8**. Two RSSs are brought together by interactions between proteins that specifically recognize the length of the spacers and thus enforce the 12/23 rule for recombination. The DNA molecule is then precisely cleaved by endonuclease activity at two locations and is then rejoined in a different configuration. The ends of the heptamer sequences are joined in a head-to-head fashion to form a **signal joint**. In the majority of cases, no nucleotides are lost or added between the two heptamer sequences, creating a double-heptamer sequence 5′CACAGTGCACAGTG3′ within the DNA molecule.

Fig. 5.7 V gene segments are joined by recombination. Top panel: In every V-region recombination event, the recombination signal sequences (RSSs) flanking the gene segments are brought together to allow recombination to take place. The 12-bp-spaced RSSs are shown in orange, the 23-bp-spaced RSSs in purple. For simplicity, the recombination of a light-chain gene is illustrated; for a heavy-chain gene, two separate recombination events are required to generate a functional V region. Left panels: In most cases, the two segments undergoing rearrangement (the V and J gene segments in this example) are arranged in the same transcriptional orientation in the chromosome, and juxtaposition of the RSSs results in the looping out of the intervening DNA. Recombination occurs at the ends of the heptamer sequences in the RSSs, creating the so-called signal joint and releasing the intervening DNA in the form of a closed circle. Subsequently, the joining of the V and J gene segments creates the coding joint in the chromosomal DNA. Right panels: In other cases, the V and J gene segments are initially oriented in opposite transcriptional directions. In this case, alignment of the RSSs requires the coiled configuration shown, rather than a simple loop, so that joining the ends of the two heptamer sequences now results in the inversion and integration of the intervening DNA into a new position on the chromosome. Again, the joining of the V and J segments creates a functional V-region exon.

5-4 The reaction that recombines V, D, and J gene segments involves both lymphocyte-specific and ubiquitous DNA-modifying enzymes.

The complex of enzymes that act in concert to carry out somatic V(D)J recombination is termed the **V(D)J recombinase**. The lymphoid-specific components of the recombinase are called **RAG-1** and **RAG-2**, and they are encoded by two recombination-activating genes, *RAG1* and *RAG2*. This pair of genes is essential for V(D)J recombination, and they are expressed in developing lymphocytes only while the lymphocytes are engaged in assembling their antigen receptors, as described in more detail in Chapter 8. Indeed, the RAG genes

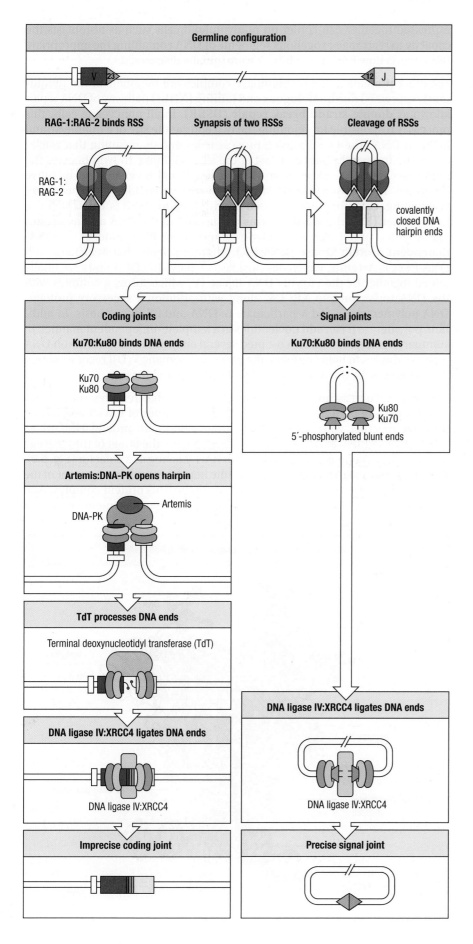

Germline configuration

RAG-1:RAG-2 binds RSS

RAG-1:
RAG-2

Synapsis of two RSSs

Cleavage of RSSs

covalently closed DNA hairpin ends

Coding joints

Ku70:Ku80 binds DNA ends

Ku70
Ku80

Artemis:DNA-PK opens hairpin

Artemis

DNA-PK

TdT processes DNA ends

Terminal deoxynucleotidyl transferase (TdT)

DNA ligase IV:XRCC4 ligates DNA ends

DNA ligase IV:XRCC4

Imprecise coding joint

Signal joints

Ku70:Ku80 binds DNA ends

Ku80
Ku70

5′-phosphorylated blunt ends

DNA ligase IV:XRCC4 ligates DNA ends

DNA ligase IV:XRCC4

Precise signal joint

Fig. 5.8 Enzymatic steps in RAG-dependent V(D)J rearrangement.
Recombination of gene segments containing recombination signal sequences (RSSs; triangles) begins with the binding of a complex of RAG-1 (purple), RAG-2 (blue), and high-mobility group (HMG) proteins (not shown) to one of the RSSs flanking the coding sequences to be joined (second row). The RAG complex then recruits the other RSS. In the cleavage step, the endonuclease activity of RAG makes single-strand cuts in the DNA backbone precisely between each coding segment and its RSS. At each cutting point this creates a 3′-OH group, which then reacts with a phosphodiester bond on the opposite DNA strand to generate a hairpin (see Fig. 5.11 for details), leaving a blunt double-strand break at the end of the RSS. These two types of DNA ends (hairpin and blunt) are resolved in different ways. At the coding ends (left panels), essential repair proteins such as Ku70:Ku80 (green) bind to the hairpin. Ku70:Ku80 forms a ring structure encircling the DNA. The Artemis:DNA-PK complex (purple) then joins the complex, and its endonuclease activity opens the DNA hairpin. The cut end is then modified by terminal deoxynucleotidyl transferase (TdT; pink) and the nuclease action of the Artemis:DNA-PK complex, which randomly add and remove nucleotides, respectively (this step is shown in more detail in Fig. 5.11). The two coding ends are finally ligated by DNA ligase IV in association with XRCC4 (turquoise). At the signal ends (right panels), Ku70:Ku80 binds to the RSS but the ends are not further modified. Instead, a complex of DNA ligase IV:XRCC4 joins the two ends to form the signal joint.

expressed together can confer on nonlymphoid cells such as fibroblasts the capacity to rearrange exogenous segments of DNA containing the appropriate RSSs; this is how RAG-1 and RAG-2 were initially discovered.

The other proteins in the recombinase complex are members of the ubiquitously expressed **nonhomologous end joining (NHEJ)** pathway of DNA repair known as **double-strand break repair (DSBR)**. In all noncycling cells, this process is responsible for rejoining the two ends at the site of a double-strand break in DNA. The DSBR joining process is imprecise, meaning that nucleotides are frequently gained or lost at the site of joining. In lymphocytes the imprecise nature of DSBR is critical for junctional diversity and adaptive immunity. Thus, this may be the driving pressure for NHEJ to mediate imprecise joining. One ubiquitous protein contributing to DSBR is **Ku**, which is a heterodimer (Ku70:Ku80); this forms a ring around the DNA and associates tightly with a protein kinase catalytic subunit, DNA-PKcs, to form the **DNA-dependent protein kinase (DNA-PK)**. Another protein that associates with DNA-PKcs is **Artemis**, which has nuclease activity. The DNA ends are finally joined together by the enzyme **DNA ligase IV**, which forms a complex with the DNA repair protein **XRCC4**, along with additional accessory proteins. DNA polymerases μ and λ participate in DNA-end fill-in synthesis. In addition, polymerase μ can add nucleotides in a template-independent manner. In summary, lymphocytes have co-opted several enzymes used in common DNA repair pathways to help complete the process of somatic V(D)J recombination that is initiated by the RAG-1 and RAG-2 V(D)J recombinases.

The first reaction is an endonucleolytic cleavage that requires the coordinated activity of both RAG proteins. Initially, a complex of RAG-1 and RAG-2 proteins, together with high-mobility group chromatin protein HMGB1 or HMGB2, recognizes and aligns the two RSSs that are the target of the cleavage reaction. RAG-1 operates as a dimer, with RAG-2 acting as a cofactor (**Fig. 5.9**). RAG-1 specifically recognizes and binds the heptamer and the nonamer of the RSS and contains the endonuclease activity of the RAG protein complex. As a dimer, RAG-1 aligns the two RSSs that will undergo rearrangement. Structural

Fig. 5.9 RAG-1 and RAG-2 form a heterotetramer capable of binding to two RSSs. Shown as ribbon diagrams, the RAG-1:RAG-2 complex contains two RAG-1 (light green) and two RAG-2 (purple) proteins. The heterotetramer of RAG-1 and RAG-2 is synapsed with a pair of RSS elements. The heptamers of each RSS are shown in red, and the nonamers are in blue. The 12-bp spacer of one RSS (orange) is in front, and the 23-bp spacer of the second RSS (gray) is in back. This asymmetry in the spacer lengths creates a bend in the orientation of the nonamer-binding domains (NBDs) of each RAG-1 monomer relative to the rest of the structure.

Structure of RAG-1:RAG-2 complex binding RSS DNA

Cryo-EM map of RAG-1:RAG-2 complex	Conformational change when RSSs bind RAG complex

Fig. 5.10 The 12/23 base pair rule may result from asymmetric binding of RSSs to the RAG-1:RAG-2 dimer. Left panel: A space-filling model of the RAG-1:RAG-2 heterotetramer synapsed with a pair of 12-RSS and 23-RSS sequences that is based on the cryo-electron microscopy (cryo-EM) structure. One RAG-1 is shown in green, the second in blue. Both molecules of RAG-2 are in purple. The 12-RSS and 23-RSS are shown as red and orange, respectively. Middle panel: prior to RSS binding, the RAG-1:RAG-2 heterotetramer has a symmetrical structure. Right panel: Upon RSS engagement, the nonamer-binding domain (NBD) dimer tilts toward the 12-RSS and away from the 23-RSS because of induced asymmetry. In this image, the heptamers of each RSS are shown in red, and the nonamers in dark blue.

data show that the 12/23 rule is established because an essential asymmetric orientation of the RAG-1:RAG-2 complex induces a preference for binding to RSS elements of different types (**Fig. 5.10**). The bound RAG complex makes a single-strand DNA break at the nucleotide just 5′ of the heptamer of the RSS, thus creating a free 3′-OH group at the end of the coding segment. This nucleophilic 3′-OH group then attacks the phosphodiester bond on the opposite DNA strand, making a double-strand break and creating a DNA 'hairpin' at the coding region and a flush double-strand break at the end of the heptamer sequence. This cutting process occurs twice, once for each gene segment being joined, producing four ends: two hairpin ends at the coding regions and two flush ends at both heptamer sequences (see Fig. 5.8). These DNA ends do not float apart, however, but are held tightly in the complex until the joining step has been completed. The blunt ends of the heptamer sequence are precisely joined to form the signal joint.

Formation of the coding joint is more complex. The two coding hairpin ends are each bound by Ku, which recruits the DNA-PKcs subunit. Artemis is recruited into this complex and is phosphorylated by DNA-PK. Artemis then opens the DNA hairpins by making a single-strand nick in the DNA. This nicking can happen at various points along the hairpin, which leads to sequence variability in the final joint. The DNA repair enzymes in the complex modify the opened hairpins by removing nucleotides, while at the same time the lymphoid-specific enzyme **terminal deoxynucleotidyl transferase (TdT)**, which is also part of the recombinase complex, adds nucleotides randomly to the single-strand ends. Addition and deletion of nucleotides can occur in any order, and one does not necessarily precede the other. Finally, DNA ligase IV joins the processed ends together, thus reconstituting a chromosome that includes the rearranged gene. This repair process creates diversity in the joint between gene segments while ensuring that the RSS ends are ligated without modification and that unintended genetic damage such as a chromosome break is avoided. Despite the use of some ubiquitous mechanisms of DNA repair, adaptive immunity based on the RAG-mediated generation of antigen receptors by somatic recombination seems to be unique to the jawed vertebrates, and its evolution is discussed in the last part of this chapter.

The *in vivo* roles of the enzymes involved in V(D)J recombination have been established through both natural and artificially induced mutations. Mice lacking TdT have about 10% of the normal level of non-templated nucleotides added to the joints between gene segments. This small remainder may result from the template-independent activity of DNA polymerase μ.

Mice in which one of the RAG genes has been inactivated or which lack DNA-PKcs, Ku, or Artemis suffer a complete block in lymphocyte development at the gene-rearrangement stage or make only trivial numbers of B and T cells. They are said to suffer from **severe combined immune deficiency (SCID)**.

 Omenn Syndrome

The original *scid* mutation was discovered some time before the components of the recombination pathway were identified and was subsequently identified as a mutation in DNA-PKcs. In humans, mutations in *RAG1* or *RAG2* that result in partial V(D)J recombinase activity are responsible for an inherited disorder called **Omenn syndrome**, which is characterized by an absence of circulating B cells and an infiltration of skin by activated oligoclonal T lymphocytes. Mice deficient in components of ubiquitous DNA repair pathways, such as DNA-PKcs, Ku, or Artemis, are defective in double-strand break repair in general and are therefore also hypersensitive to ionizing radiation (which produces double-strand breaks). Defects in Artemis in humans produce a combined immunodeficiency of B and T cells that is associated with increased radiosensitivity. SCID caused by mutations in DNA repair pathways is called **radiation-sensitive SCID (RS-SCID)** to distinguish it from SCID due to lymphocyte-specific defects.

Another genetic condition in which radiosensitivity is associated with some degree of immunodeficiency is **ataxia telangiectasia**, which is due to mutations in the protein kinase **ATM** (ataxia telangiectasia mutated). Ataxia telangiectasia is associated with cerebellar degeneration, increased radiation sensitivity, and cancer risk. ATM is a serine/threonine kinase, like DNA-PKcs, and functions during V(D)J recombination to promote stabilization of the cleaved DNA ends in the RAG complex. This function of ATM greatly reduces the probability that the free DNA ends are prematurely released from the complex and available to participate in chromosomal translocations. Consequently, individuals with ATM deficiencies have a strong predisposition to develop B-cell and T-cell malignancies characterized by chromosomal translocations involving the antigen-receptor gene loci. However, ATM is not absolutely required for V(D)J recombination, as individuals with ataxia telangiectasia show substantial variability in the severity of their immune deficiencies, with some individuals having low numbers of B and T cells and/or a deficiency in antibody class switching that is less severe than that seen in patients with SCID. Evidence that ATM and DNA-PKcs are partially redundant in their functions comes from the observation that B cells lacking both kinases show much more severely abnormal signal joining sequences compared with B cells lacking either enzyme alone.

Ataxia Telangiectasia

5-5 The diversity of the immunoglobulin repertoire is generated by four main processes.

The gene rearrangements that combine gene segments to form a complete V-region exon generate diversity in two ways. First, there are multiple different copies of each type of gene segment, and different combinations of gene segments can be used in different rearrangement events. This **combinatorial diversity** is responsible for a substantial part of the diversity of V regions. Second, junctional diversity is introduced at the joints between the different gene segments as a result of the addition and subtraction of nucleotides by the recombination process. A third source of diversity is also combinatorial, arising from the many possible different combinations of heavy- and light-chain V regions that pair to form the antigen-binding site in the immunoglobulin molecule. The two means of generating combinatorial diversity alone could give rise, in theory, to approximately 3×10^6 different antibody molecules, as we will see below. Coupled with junctional diversity, it is estimated that at least 10^{11} different receptors could make up the repertoire of receptors expressed by naive B cells, and diversity could even be several orders of magnitude greater, depending on how one calculates junctional diversity. Finally, somatic hypermutation, which we describe in Chapter 10, occurs only in B cells after the initiation of an immune response and introduces point mutations into the rearranged V-region genes. This process generates further diversity in the antibody repertoire that can be selected for enhanced binding to antigen.

5-6   The multiple inherited gene segments are used in different combinations.

There are multiple copies of the V, D, and J gene segments, each of which can contribute to an immunoglobulin V region. Many different V regions can therefore be made by selecting different combinations of these segments. For human κ light chains, there are approximately 30 functional Vκ gene segments and 5 Jκ gene segments, and thus potentially 150 different combinations of complete Vκ regions. For λ light chains, there are approximately 30 functional V_λ gene segments and 4–5 J_λ gene segments, yielding at least 120 possible V_λ regions (see Fig. 5.4). So, in all, 270 different light chains can be made as a result of combining different light-chain gene segments. For the heavy chains of humans, there are approximately 40 functional V_H gene segments, 23 D_H gene segments, and 6 J_H gene segments, and thus around 5500 different possible V_H regions ($40 \times 23 \times 6 = 5520$). During B-cell development, rearrangement at the heavy-chain gene locus to produce a heavy chain is followed by several rounds of cell division before light-chain gene rearrangement takes place, resulting in the same heavy chain being paired with different light chains in different cells. Because both the heavy- and the light-chain V regions contribute to antibody specificity, each of the 270 different light chains could be combined with each of the approximately 5500 heavy chains to give around 1.5×10^6 different antibody specificities.

This theoretical estimate of combinatorial diversity is based on the number of germline V gene segments contributing to functional antibodies (see Fig. 5.4); the total number of V gene segments is larger, but the additional gene segments are pseudogenes and do not appear in expressed immunoglobulin molecules. In practice, combinatorial diversity is likely to be less than one might expect from the calculations above. One reason is that not all V gene segments are used at the same frequency; some are common in antibodies, while others are found only rarely. Factors such as chromosomal architecture, DNA accessibility, and differences in RSS sequences contribute to biases in V gene segment usage. Also, not every heavy chain can pair with every light chain: certain combinations of V_H and V_L regions will not form a stable molecule. Cells in which heavy and light chains fail to pair may undergo further light-chain gene rearrangement until a suitable chain is produced or they will be eliminated. Nevertheless, it is thought that most heavy and light chains can pair with each other, and that this type of combinatorial diversity has a major role in forming an immunoglobulin repertoire with a wide range of specificities.

5-7   Variable addition and subtraction of nucleotides at the junctions between gene segments contributes to the diversity of the third hypervariable region.

As noted earlier, of the three hypervariable loops in an immunoglobulin chain, CDR1 and CDR2 are encoded within the V gene segment. CDR3, however, falls at the joint between the V gene segment and the J gene segment, and in the heavy chain it is partly encoded by the D gene segment. In both heavy and light chains, the diversity of CDR3 is significantly increased by the addition and deletion of nucleotides at two steps in the formation of the junctions between gene segments. The added nucleotides are known as P-nucleotides and N-nucleotides, and their addition is illustrated in **Fig. 5.11**.

P-nucleotides are so called because they make up palindromic sequences added to the ends of the gene segments. As described in Section 5-4, the RAG proteins generate DNA hairpins at the coding ends of the V, D, or J segments, after which Artemis catalyzes a single-strand cleavage at an asymmetric site in the hairpin bubble. This generates a single-strand tail including a few nucleotides of the coding sequence plus the complementary nucleotides

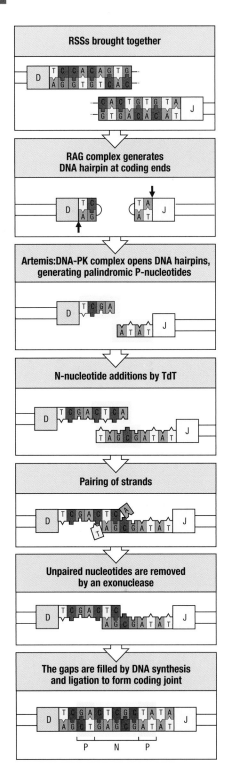

Fig. 5.11 The introduction of P- and N-nucleotides diversifies the joints between gene segments during immunoglobulin gene rearrangement. The process is illustrated for a D_H to J_H rearrangement (first panel); however, the same steps occur in V_H to D_H and in V_L to J_L rearrangements. After formation of the DNA hairpins (second panel), the two heptamer sequences are ligated to form the signal joint (not shown here), while the Artemis:DNA-PK complex cleaves the DNA hairpin at a random site (indicated by the arrows) to yield a single-strand DNA end (third panel). Depending on the site of cleavage, this single-stranded DNA may contain nucleotides that were originally complementary in the double-stranded DNA and which therefore form short DNA palindromes, such as TCGA and ATAT, as indicated by the light blue–shaded box. For example, the sequence GA at the end of the D segment shown is complementary to the preceding sequence TC. Such stretches of nucleotides that originate from the complementary strand are known as P-nucleotides. Where the enzyme terminal deoxynucleotidyl transferase (TdT) is present, nucleotides are added at random to the ends of the single-strand segments (fourth panel); these non-templated, or N, nucleotides are indicated by the shaded box. The two single-strand ends then pair (fifth panel). Exonuclease trimming of unpaired nucleotides (sixth panel) and repair of the coding joint by DNA synthesis and ligation (bottom panel) leaves both P- and N-nucleotides (indicated by light blue shading) in the final coding joint. The randomness of insertion of P- and N-nucleotides makes an individual P–N region virtually unique and a valuable marker for following an individual B-cell clone as it develops, for instance in studies of somatic hypermutation.

from the other DNA strand (see Fig. 5.11). In many light-chain gene rearrangements, DNA repair enzymes then fill in complementary nucleotides on the single-strand tails, which would leave short palindromic sequences (the P-nucleotides) at the joint if the ends were rejoined without any further exonuclease activity.

In heavy-chain gene rearrangements and in a proportion of human light-chain gene rearrangements, **N-nucleotides** are added by a quite different mechanism before the ends are rejoined. N-nucleotides are so called because they are non-template-encoded. They are added by the enzyme TdT to the ends of the coding DNA after hairpin cleavage. After the addition of up to 20 nucleotides, single-strand stretches may have some complementary base pairs. Repair enzymes then trim off nonmatching nucleotides, synthesize complementary DNA to fill in the remaining single-strand gaps, and ligate the new DNA to the palindromic region (see Fig. 5.11). TdT is maximally expressed during the period in B-cell development when the heavy-chain gene is being assembled, and so N-nucleotides are common in heavy-chain V–D and D–J junctions. N-nucleotides are less common in light-chain genes, which undergo rearrangement after heavy-chain genes, when TdT expression has been shut off, as we will explain further in Chapter 8 when discussing the specific developmental stages of B and T cells.

Nucleotides can also be deleted at gene segment junctions. This is accomplished by nucleases, and although these have not yet been identified, Artemis has dual endonuclease and exonuclease activity and so could well be involved in this step. Thus, a heavy-chain CDR3 can be shorter than even the smallest D segment. In some instances it is difficult, if not impossible, to recognize the D segment that contributed to CDR3 formation because of the excision of most of its nucleotides. Deletions may also erase the traces of P-nucleotide palindromes introduced at the time of hairpin opening. For this reason, many completed VDJ joins do not show obvious evidence of P-nucleotides. As the total number of nucleotides added by these processes is random, the added nucleotides often disrupt the reading frame of the coding sequence beyond the joint. Such frameshifts will lead to a nonfunctional protein, and DNA rearrangements leading to such disruptions are known as **nonproductive rearrangements**. As roughly two in every three rearrangements will be nonproductive, many B-cell progenitors never succeed in producing functional immunoglobulin and therefore never become mature B cells. Thus, junctional diversity is achieved only at the expense of considerable loss of cells during B-cell development. In Chapter 8, we return to this topic when we discuss the cellular stages of B-cell development and how they relate to the temporal sequence of rearrangement of the V, D, and J gene segments of the antigen-receptor chains.

5-8   IgM and IgD are derived from the same pre-mRNA transcript and are both expressed on the surface of mature B cells.

Once a progenitor B completes its heavy- and light-chain gene rearrangements, it will express the transmembrane form of the immunoglobulin protein. Recall from Chapter 4 (Section 4-6) that the heavy-chain locus encodes different C regions (C_H) that are present as separate genes located downstream of the V-region segments. This C_H gene cluster spans about 200 kb to the 3′ side of the J_H gene segments (see Fig. 4.6). Each C_H gene is split into several exons (not shown in the figure), with each exon corresponding to an individual immunoglobulin domain in the folded C region. Initially, B cells express two of these C_H genes, the C_μ and C_δ genes, each of which is expressed along with the associated assembled V-region sequence on the surface of the same B cell, producing transmembrane IgM and IgD. The gene encoding the C_μ region lies closest to the J_H gene segments, and therefore closest to the assembled V_H-region exon (VDJ exon) after DNA rearrangement. Once rearrangement has been completed, transcription from a promoter just 5′ to the leader sequence exon adjacent to the rearranged VDJ exon produces a complete μ heavy-chain transcript. Any J_H gene segments remaining between the assembled V gene and the C_μ gene are removed during RNA processing to generate the mature mRNA. The μ heavy chains are therefore the first to be expressed, and IgM is the first immunoglobulin to be produced during B-cell development.

Immediately 3′ to the μ gene lies the δ gene, which encodes the C region of the IgD heavy chain (see Fig. 4.6). IgD is coexpressed with IgM on the surface of almost all mature B cells but is secreted in only small amounts by plasma cells. The unique function of IgD is still unclear and a matter of active research. Because IgD has hinge regions that are more flexible than those in IgM, IgD has been suggested to be an auxiliary receptor that may facilitate the binding of antigens by naive B cells. Mice lacking the C_δ exons show normal B-cell development and can generate largely normal antibody responses but show a delay in the process of affinity maturation of antibody for antigens. We return to this topic in Chapter 10, when we discuss somatic hypermutation.

B cells expressing IgM and IgD have not undergone class switching, which requires irreversible changes to the DNA. Instead, these B cells produce a long primary mRNA transcript that is differentially spliced to yield either of two distinct mRNA molecules (**Fig. 5.12**). In one transcript, the VDJ exon is spliced to the C_μ exons and undergoes polyadenylation from a nearby site (pA_2) to encode a complete membrane-bound IgM molecule. The second RNA transcript extends well beyond this site and includes the downstream C_δ exons. In this transcript, the VDJ exon is spliced to these C_δ exons, and polyadenylation occurs at a separate site downstream (pA_4). This transcript encodes a membrane-bound IgD molecule.

It has been known since the 1980s that the processing of the long mRNA transcript is developmentally regulated, with immature B cells making mostly the μ transcript and mature B cells making mostly the δ along with some μ, although there was little to no molecular explanation until recently. A forward genetic screen of *N*-ethyl-*N*-nitrosourea (ENU)-induced mutagenesis in mice identified a gene involved in IgD expression that regulates the alternative splicing process. The gene encodes **ZFP318**, a protein structurally related to the U1 small nuclear ribonucleoprotein of the spliceosome, the RNA:protein complex that is required for mRNA splicing. ZFP318 is not expressed in immature B cells, where the IgD transcript is not produced, but becomes expressed in mature and activated B cells that coexpress IgD with

Fig. 5.12 Coexpression of IgD and IgM is regulated by RNA processing. In mature B cells, transcription initiated at the V_H promoter extends through both C_μ and C_δ exons. This long primary transcript is then processed by cleavage and polyadenylation (AAA) and by splicing. Cleavage and polyadenylation at the μ site (pA$_2$) and splicing between C_μ exons yields an mRNA encoding the μ heavy chain (top panel). Cleavage and polyadenylation at the δ site (pA$_4$) and a different pattern of splicing that joins the V region exon to the C_δ exons and removes the C_μ exons yields mRNA encoding the complete δ heavy chain (bottom panel).

IgM. ZFP318 functions by suppressing transcription termination and polyadenylation at the pA$_2$ site (see Fig.5.12) and by this mechanism promotes transcript elongation and polyadenylation at the pA$_4$ site. The longer pre-mRNA is preferentially spliced to eliminate the C_μ exons and include the C_δ exons instead. As a consequence, cells expressing ZFP318 express high levels of IgD and lower levels of IgM.

5-9   Transmembrane and secreted forms of immunoglobulin are generated from different heavy-chain mRNA transcripts.

Each of the immunoglobulin isotypes can be produced either as a membrane-bound receptor or as secreted antibodies. B cells initially express the transmembrane form of IgM; after stimulation by antigen, some of their progeny differentiate into plasma cells producing IgM antibodies, whereas others undergo class switching to express transmembrane immunoglobulins of a different class, followed by the production of secreted antibody of the new class. The membrane-bound forms of all immunoglobulin classes are monomers comprising two heavy and two light chains. IgM and IgA polymerize only when they have been secreted. The membrane-bound form of the immunoglobulin heavy chain has at the carboxyl terminus a hydrophobic transmembrane domain of about 25 amino acid residues that anchors it to the surface of the B lymphocyte. The secreted form replaces this transmembrane domain with a carboxyl terminus composed of a hydrophilic secretory tail. These two forms of carboxyl termini are encoded by different exons found at the end of each C_H gene as these exons undergo alternative RNA processing.

For example, the IgM heavy-chain gene contains four exons—$C_{\mu 1}$ to $C_{\mu 4}$—that encode its four heavy-chain Ig domains (**Fig. 5.13**). The end of the $C_{\mu 4}$ exon also encodes the carboxyl terminus for the secreted form. Two additional downstream exons, M_1 and M_2, encode the transmembrane region and cytoplasmic tail. If the primary transcript is cleaved at the polyadenylation site (pA_1) located just downstream of the $C_{\mu 4}$ exon but before the last two exons, then only the secreted molecule can be produced. If the polymerase transcribes through this first polyadenylation site, then splicing can occur from a non-consensus splice-donor site within the $C_{\mu 4}$ exon to the M_1 exon. In this case, polyadenylation occurs at a downstream site (pA_2), and the cell-surface form of immunoglobulin can be produced. This alternative splicing is incompletely understood but may involve the regulation of RNA polymerase activity as the polymerase transcribes through the IgM locus. One factor that regulates the polyadenylation of RNA transcripts is a **cleavage stimulation factor** subunit, **CstF-64**, which favors production of the transcript for secreted IgM. The transcription elongation factor **ELL2**, which is induced in plasma cells, also promotes polyadenylation at the pA_1 site and favors the secreted form. CstF-64 and ELL2 co-associate with RNA polymerase within the immunoglobulin locus. This differential RNA

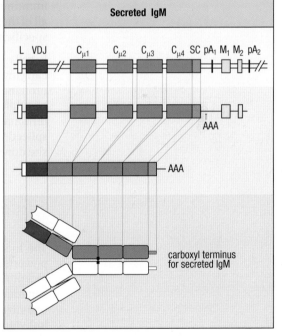

Fig. 5.13 Transmembrane and secreted forms of immunoglobulins are derived from the same heavy-chain sequence by alternative RNA processing. At the end of a heavy-chain C gene, there are two exons (M_1 and M_2; yellow) that together encode the transmembrane region and cytoplasmic tail of the transmembrane form. Within the last C-domain exon, a secretion-coding (SC) sequence (orange) encodes the carboxyl terminus of the secreted form. In the case of IgD, the SC sequence is in a separate exon (not shown), but for all other isotypes, including IgM as shown here, the SC sequence is contiguous with the last C-domain exon. The events that dictate whether a heavy-chain RNA will result in a secreted or a transmembrane immunoglobulin occur during processing of the pre-mRNA transcript. Each heavy-chain C gene has two potential polyadenylation sites (shown as pA_1 and pA_2 for C_μ). Left panel: The transcript is cleaved and polyadenylated (AAA) at the second site (pA_2). Splicing occurs from a site located within the last $C_{\mu 4}$ exon just upstream of the SC sequence (orange) to a second site at the 5′ end of the M_1 exons (yellow). This results in removal of the SC sequence and joining of the $C_{\mu 4}$ exon to the exons M_1 and M_2 and generates the transmembrane form of the heavy chain. Right panel: Polyadenylation occurs at the first poly(A) addition site (pA_1), and transcription terminates before the exons M_1 and M_2, preventing the generation of the transmembrane form of the heavy chain and producing the secreted form.

processing is illustrated for C_μ in Fig. 5.13, but it occurs in the same way for all isotypes. In activated B cells that differentiate to become antibody-secreting plasma cells, most of the transcripts are spliced to yield the secreted rather than the transmembrane form of whichever heavy-chain isotype the B cell is expressing.

Summary.

The extraordinary diversity of the immunoglobulin repertoire is achieved in several ways. Perhaps the most important factor enabling this diversity is that V regions are encoded by separate gene segments (V, D, and J gene segments), which are brought together by a somatic recombination process—V(D)J recombination—to produce a complete V-region exon. Many different gene segments are present in the genome of an individual, thus providing a heritable source of diversity that this combinatorial mechanism can use. Unique lymphocyte-specific recombinases, the RAG proteins, are absolutely required to catalyze this rearrangement, and the evolution of RAG proteins coincided with the appearance of the modern vertebrate adaptive immune system. Another substantial fraction of the functional diversity of immunoglobulins comes from the imprecise nature of the joining process itself. Variability at the coding joints between gene segments is generated by the insertion of random numbers of P- and N-nucleotides and by the variable deletion of nucleotides at the ends of some segments. These are brought about by the opening of the hairpin by Artemis and by the actions of TdT. The association of different light- and heavy-chain V regions to form the antigen-binding site of an immunoglobulin molecule contributes further diversity. The combination of all of these sources of diversity generates a vast primary repertoire of antibody specificities.

B cells initially coexpress IgM and IgD as transmembrane receptors, each carrying the same heavy-chain V-region sequence and the same light-chain protein. The coexpression of these two antibody isotypes is due to the use of two different polyadenylation sites in the heavy-chain pre-mRNA. Transcript termination and polyadenylation at a site downstream of C_μ generates a spliced mRNA encoding IgM, whereas termination and polyadenylation at a site downstream of C_δ generates the mRNA encoding IgD.

T-cell receptor gene rearrangement.

The mechanism by which B-cell antigen receptors are generated is such a powerful means of creating diversity that it is not surprising that the antigen receptors of T cells bear structural resemblances to immunoglobulins and are generated by the same mechanism. In this part of the chapter, we describe the organization of the T-cell receptor loci and the generation of the genes for the individual T-cell receptor chains.

5-10 The T-cell receptor gene segments are arranged in a pattern similar to that of immunoglobulin gene segments and are rearranged by the same enzymes.

Like immunoglobulin light and heavy chains, T-cell receptor (TCR) α and β chains each consist of a variable (V) amino-terminal region and a constant (C) region (see Section 4-14). The organization of the TCRα and TCRβ loci is shown in **Fig. 5.14**. The organization of the gene segments is broadly homologous to that of the immunoglobulin gene segments (see Sections 5-2 and 5-3).

Fig. 5.14 The germline organization of the human T-cell receptor α and β loci.
The arrangement of the gene segments for the T-cell receptor resembles that at the
immunoglobulin loci, with separate variable (V), diversity (D), and joining (J) gene segments
and constant (C) genes. The TCRα locus (chromosome 14) consists of 70–80 V_α gene
segments, each preceded by an exon encoding the leader sequence (L). How many of these
V_α gene segments are functional is not known exactly. A cluster of 61 J_α gene segments
is located a considerable distance from the V_α gene segments. The J_α gene segments
are followed by a single C gene, which contains separate exons for the constant and
hinge domains and a single exon encoding the transmembrane and cytoplasmic regions
(not shown). The TCRβ locus (chromosome 7) has a different organization, with a cluster
of 52 functional V_β gene segments located distant from two separate clusters that each
contain a single D gene segment together with six or seven J gene segments and a single
C gene. Each TCRβ C gene has separate exons encoding the constant domain, the hinge,
the transmembrane region, and the cytoplasmic region (not shown). The TCRα locus is
interrupted between the J and V gene segments by another T-cell receptor locus—the TCRδ
locus (not shown here; see Fig. 5.19).

The TCRα locus, like the loci of the immunoglobulin light chains, contains V
and J gene segments (V_α and J_α). The TCRβ locus, like the locus of the immunoglobulin heavy chain, contains D gene segments in addition to V_β and J_β
gene segments. The T-cell receptor gene segments rearrange during T-cell
development to form complete V-domain exons (**Fig. 5.15**). T-cell receptor
gene rearrangement takes place in the thymus; the order and regulation of
the rearrangements are dealt with in detail in Chapter 8. Essentially, however,
the mechanics of gene rearrangement are similar for B and T cells. The T-cell
receptor gene segments are flanked by 12-bp and 23-bp spacer recombination
signal sequences (RSSs) that are homologous to those flanking immunoglobulin gene segments (**Fig. 5.16**; see Section 5-3) and are recognized by the same
enzymes. The DNA circles resulting from gene rearrangement (see Fig. 5.7) are
known as **T-cell receptor excision circles (TRECs)** and are used as markers
for T cells that have recently emigrated from the thymus. All known defects
in genes that control V(D)J recombination affect T cells and B cells equally,
and animals with these genetic defects lack functional B and T lymphocytes
altogether (see Section 5-4). A further shared feature of immunoglobulin and
T-cell receptor gene rearrangement is the presence of P- and N-nucleotides in
the junctions between the V, D, and J gene segments of the rearranged TCRβ
gene. In T cells, P- and N-nucleotides are also added between the V and J
gene segments of all rearranged TCRα genes, whereas only about half of the

Fig. 5.15 T-cell receptor α- and β-chain gene rearrangement and expression.
The TCRα-chain and TCRβ-chain genes are composed of discrete segments that are joined by somatic recombination during development of the T cell. Functional α- and β-chain genes are generated in the same way that complete immunoglobulin genes are created. For the α chain (upper part of figure), a V_α gene segment rearranges to a J_α gene segment to create a functional V-region exon. Transcription and splicing of the VJ_α exon to C_α generates the mRNA that is translated to yield the T-cell receptor α-chain protein. For the β chain (lower part of figure), like the immunoglobulin heavy chain, the variable domain is encoded in three gene segments, V_β, D_β, and J_β. Rearrangement of these gene segments generates a functional VDJ_β V-region exon that is transcribed and spliced to join to C_β; the resulting mRNA is translated to yield the T-cell receptor β chain. The α and β chains pair soon after their synthesis to yield the αβ T-cell receptor heterodimer. Not all J gene segments are shown, and the leader sequences preceding each V gene segment are omitted for simplicity.

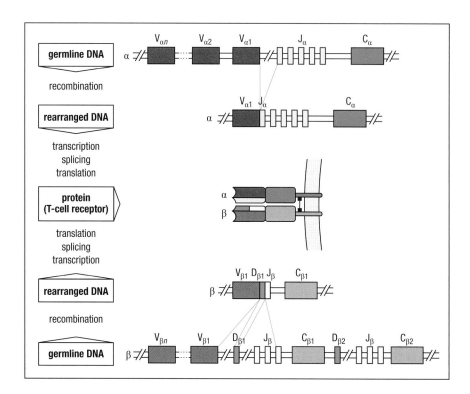

V–J joints in immunoglobulin light-chain genes are modified by N-nucleotide addition, and these are often left without any P-nucleotides as well (**Fig. 5.17**; see Section 5-7).

The main differences between the immunoglobulin genes and those encoding T-cell receptors reflect the differences in how B cells and T cells function. All the effector functions of B cells depend on secreted antibodies whose different heavy-chain C-region isotypes trigger distinct effector mechanisms. The effector functions of T cells, in contrast, depend on cell–cell contact and are not mediated directly by the T-cell receptor, which serves only for antigen recognition. Thus, the C regions of the TCRα and TCRβ loci are much simpler than

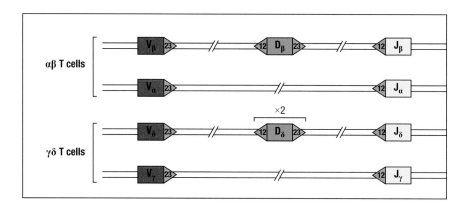

Fig. 5.16 Recombination signal sequences flank T-cell receptor gene segments. As in the immunoglobulin gene loci (see Fig. 5.6), the individual gene segments at the TCRα and TCRβ loci are flanked by heptamer–spacer–nonamer recombination signal sequences (RSSs). RSS motifs containing 12-bp spacers are depicted here as orange arrowheads, and those containing 23-bp spacers are shown in purple. Joining of gene segments almost always follows the 12/23 rule. Because of the disposition of heptamer and nonamer RSSs in the TCRβ and TCRδ loci, direct V_β to J_β joining is in principle allowed by the 12/23 rule (unlike in the immunoglobulin heavy-chain gene), although this occurs very rarely owing to other types of regulation.

Element	Immunoglobulin		αβ T-cell receptors	
	H	κ+λ	β	α
Number of variable segments (V)	~40	~60	~30	~100
Number of diversity segments (D)	23	0	2	0
Number of D segments read in three frames	rarely	–	often	–
Number of joining segments (J)	6	5(κ) 4(λ)	12	~50
Number of joints with N- and P-nucleotides	2 (VD and DJ)	50% of joints	2 (VD and DJ)	1 (VJ)
Number of V gene pairs	1.5×10^6		2.7×10^6	
Total diversity with nucleotide addition and deletion	$\sim 5 \times 10^{13}$		$\sim 10^{18}$	

Fig. 5.17 The number of human T-cell receptor gene segments and the sources of T-cell receptor diversity compared with those of immunoglobulins. Note that only about half of human κ chains contain N-nucleotides. Somatic hypermutation as a source of diversity is not included in this figure because it does not occur in T cells.

those of the immunoglobulin heavy-chain locus. There is only one C_α gene, and although there are two C_β genes, they are very closely homologous and there is no known functional distinction between their products. The T-cell receptor C-region genes encode only transmembrane polypeptides.

Another difference between the rearrangement of immunoglobulin genes and T-cell receptor genes is in the nature of the RSSs surrounding the D gene segments. For the immunoglobulin heavy chain, the D segment is surrounded by two RSSs, both with a 12-bp spacing (see Fig. 5.6), whereas the D segments in the TCRβ and TCRδ loci have a 5′ 12-bp RSS and a 3′ 23-bp RSS (see Fig. 5.16). The arrangement in the immunoglobulin locus naturally enforces the inclusion of D segments in the heavy-chain V region, because direct V to J joining would violate the 12/23 rule. However, in the T-cell receptor loci, direct V to J joining would not violate this rule, because the 23-bp RSS of the V_β or V_δ segment is compatible with the 12-bp RSS of the J gene segment, and yet normally, little direct joining is observed. Instead, regulation of gene rearrangements appears to be controlled by mechanisms beyond the 12/23 rule, and these mechanisms are still being investigated.

5-11 T-cell receptors concentrate diversity in the third hypervariable region.

The three-dimensional structure of the antigen-recognition site of a T-cell receptor looks much like that of the antigen-recognition site of an antibody molecule (see Sections 4-10 and 4-20, respectively). In an antibody, the center of the antigen-binding site is formed by the CDR3 loops of the heavy and light chains. The structurally equivalent third hypervariable loops of the T-cell receptor α and β chains, to which the D and J gene segments contribute, also form the center of the antigen-binding site of a T-cell receptor; the periphery of the site consists of the CDR1 and CDR2 loops, which are encoded within the germline V gene segments for the α and β chains. The extent and pattern of variability in T-cell receptors and immunoglobulins reflect the distinct nature of their ligands. Whereas the antigen-binding sites of immunoglobulins must conform to the surfaces of an almost infinite variety of different antigens, and thus come in a wide variety of shapes and chemical properties, the ligand for the major class of human T-cell receptors (αβ) is always a peptide bound to an MHC molecule. As a group, the antigen-recognition sites of T-cell receptors would therefore be predicted to have a less variable shape, with most of the

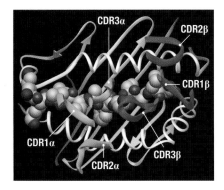

Fig. 5.18 The most variable parts of the T-cell receptor interact with the peptide of a peptide:MHC complex. The CDR loops of a T-cell receptor are shown as colored tubes, which in this figure are superimposed on the peptide:MHC complex (MHC, gray; peptide, yellow-green with O atoms in red and N atoms in blue). The CDR loops of the α chain are in green, while those of the β chain are in purple. The CDR3 loops lie in the center of the interface between the T-cell receptor and the peptide:MHC complex and make direct contact with the antigenic peptide.

variability focused on the bound antigenic peptide occupying the center of the surface in contact with the receptor. Indeed, the less variable CDR1 and CDR2 loops of a T-cell receptor mainly contact the relatively less variable MHC component of the ligand, whereas the highly variable CDR3 regions mainly contact the unique peptide component (**Fig. 5.18**).

5-12 γδ T-cell receptors are also generated by gene rearrangement.

A minority of T cells bear T-cell receptors composed of γ and δ chains (see Section 4-23). The organization of the TCRγ and TCRδ loci (**Fig. 5.19**) resembles that of the TCRα and TCRβ loci, although there are important differences. The cluster of gene segments encoding the δ chain is found entirely within the TCRα locus, between the V_α and the J_α gene segments. V_δ genes are interspersed with the V_α genes but are located primarily in the 3′ region of the locus.

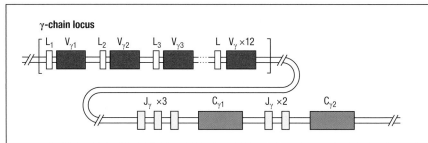

Fig. 5.19 The organization of the T-cell receptor γ- and δ-chain loci in humans. The TCRγ and TCRδ loci, like the TCRα and TCRβ loci, have discrete V, D, and J gene segments as well as C genes. Uniquely, the locus encoding the δ chain is located entirely within the α-chain locus. The three D_δ gene segments, four J_δ gene segments, and the single δ C gene lie between the cluster of V_α gene segments and the cluster of J_α gene segments. There are two V_δ gene segments (not shown) located near the δ C gene, one just upstream of the D regions and one in inverted orientation just downstream of the C gene. In addition, there are six V_δ gene segments interspersed among the V_α gene segments. Five are shared with V_α and can be used by either locus, and one is unique to the δ locus. The human TCRγ locus resembles the TCRβ locus in having two C genes, each with its own set of J gene segments. The mouse γ locus (not shown) has a more complex organization and there are three functional clusters of γ gene segments, each containing V and J gene segments and a C gene. Rearrangement at the γ and δ loci proceeds as for the other T-cell receptor loci, with the exception that during TCRδ rearrangement, two D segments can be used in the same complete V gene. The use of two D segments greatly increases the variability of the δ chain, mainly because N-region nucleotides can be added at the junction between the two D gene segments as well as at the V–D and D–J junctions.

Because all V_α gene segments are oriented such that rearrangement will delete the intervening DNA, any rearrangement at the α locus results in the loss of the δ locus (Fig. 5.20). There are substantially fewer V gene segments at the TCRγ and TCRδ loci than at either the TCRα or TCRβ loci or any of the immunoglobulin loci. Increased junctional variability in the δ chains may compensate for the small number of V gene segments and has the effect of focusing almost all the variability in the $\gamma\delta$ receptor in the junctional region. As we have seen for the $\alpha\beta$ T-cell receptors, the amino acids encoded by the junctional regions lie at the center of the T-cell receptor binding site. T cells bearing $\gamma\delta$ receptors are a distinct lineage of T cells, and as discussed in Chapter 4, some $\gamma\delta$ T cells recognize nonclassical MHC class I molecules and other molecules whose expression may be an indication of cellular damage or infection. As we saw in Section 4-23, the CDR3 of a $\gamma\delta$ T cell is frequently longer than the CDR3 in an $\alpha\beta$ T-cell receptor; this permits the CDR3 of $\gamma\delta$ T cell receptors to interact directly with ligand and also contributes to the great diversity of these receptors.

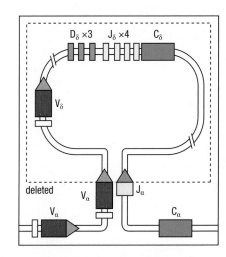

Fig. 5.20 Deletion of the TCRδ locus is induced by rearrangement of a V_α to J_α gene segment. The TCRδ locus is entirely contained within the chromosomal region containing the TCRα locus. When any V region in the V_α/V_δ region rearranges to any one of the J_α segments, the intervening region, and the entire V_δ locus, is deleted. Thus, V_α rearrangement prevents any continued expression of a V_δ gene and precludes lineage development down the γδ pathway.

Summary.

T-cell receptors are structurally similar to immunoglobulins and are encoded by homologous genes. T-cell receptor genes are assembled by somatic recombination from sets of gene segments in the same way that the immunoglobulin genes are. Diversity is distributed differently, however, in immunoglobulins and T-cell receptors: the T-cell receptor loci have roughly the same number of V gene segments as the immunoglobulin loci but more J gene segments, and there is greater diversification of the junctions between gene segments during the process of gene rearrangement. Thus, the greatest diversity of the T-cell receptor is in the central part of the receptor, within the CDR3, which, in the case of $\alpha\beta$ T-cell receptors, contacts the bound peptide fragment of the ligand. Most of the diversity among $\gamma\delta$ T-cell receptors is also within the CDR3, which is frequently longer than the CDR3 of $\alpha\beta$ T-cell receptors and can also directly interact with ligands recognized by the $\gamma\delta$ T cells.

Evolution of the adaptive immune response.

The form of adaptive immunity that we have discussed so far in this book depends on the action of the RAG-1:RAG-2 recombinase to generate an enormously diverse clonally distributed repertoire of immunoglobulins and T-cell receptors. This system is found only in the jawed vertebrates, the **gnathostomes**, which split off from the other vertebrates around 500 million years ago. Adaptive immunity seems to have arisen abruptly in evolution. Even the cartilaginous fishes, the earliest group of jawed fishes to survive to the present day, have organized lymphoid tissue, T-cell receptors, and immunoglobulins, as well as the ability to mount adaptive immune responses. The diversity generated within the vertebrate adaptive immune system was once viewed as unique among animal immune systems. But we now know that organisms as different as insects, echinoderms, and mollusks use a variety of genetic mechanisms to increase their repertoires of pathogen-detecting molecules, although they do not achieve true adaptive immunity. Nearer to home, it has been found that the surviving species of jawless vertebrates, the **agnathans**—the lampreys and hagfish—have a form of adaptive or 'anticipatory' immunity that is based on non-immunoglobulin antibody-like proteins and involves a system of somatic gene rearrangement that is quite distinct from RAG-dependent V(D)J rearrangement. So we should now view our adaptive immune system as only one solution to the problem of generating highly diverse systems for pathogen recognition.

5-13 Some invertebrates generate extensive diversity in a repertoire of immunoglobulin-like genes.

Until recently, it was thought that invertebrate immunity was limited to an innate system that had limited diversity in recognizing pathogens. This idea was based on the knowledge that innate immunity in vertebrates relies on around 10 distinct Toll-like receptors and a similar number of other receptors that also recognize PAMPs, and also on the assumption that the number of receptors in invertebrates was no greater. Recent studies have, however, uncovered at least two invertebrate examples of extensive diversification of an immunoglobulin superfamily member, which could potentially provide an extended range of recognition of pathogens.

In *Drosophila*, fat-body cells and hemocytes act as part of the immune system. Fat-body cells secrete proteins, such as the antimicrobial defensins (see Chapter 2), into the hemolymph. Another protein found in hemolymph is the **Down syndrome cell adhesion molecule (Dscam)**, a member of the immunoglobulin superfamily. Dscam was originally discovered in the fly as a protein involved in specifying neuronal wiring. It is also made in fat-body cells and hemocytes, which can secrete it into the hemolymph, where it is thought to recognize invading bacteria and aid in their engulfment by phagocytes.

The Dscam protein contains multiple, usually 10, immunoglobulin-like domains. However, the gene that encodes Dscam has evolved to contain a large number of alternative exons for several of these domains (**Fig. 5.21**). Exon 4 of the gene encoding the Dscam protein can be any 1 of 12 different exons, each specifying an immunoglobulin domain of differing sequence. Exon cluster 6 has 48 alternative exons, cluster 9 another 33, and cluster 17 a further 2; it is estimated that the Dscam gene could encode around 38,000 protein isoforms. A role for Dscam in immunity was proposed when it was found that *in vitro* phagocytosis of *Escherichia coli* by isolated hemocytes lacking Dscam was less efficient than by normal hemocytes. These observations suggest that at least some of this extensive repertoire of alternative exons may have evolved to diversify insects' ability to recognize pathogens. This role for Dscam has been confirmed in the mosquito *Anopheles gambiae*, in which silencing of the *Dscam* homolog *AgDscam* has been shown to weaken the mosquito's normal

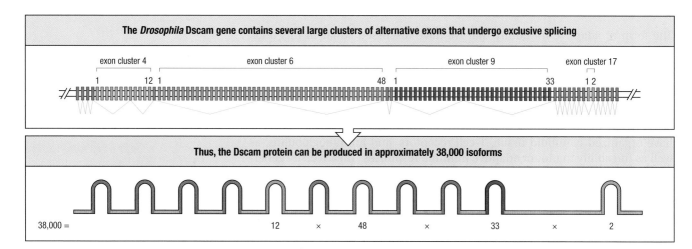

Fig. 5.21 The Dscam protein of *Drosophila* innate immunity contains multiple immunoglobulin domains and is highly diversified through alternative splicing. The gene encoding Dscam in *Drosophila* contains several large clusters of alternative exons. The clusters encoding exon 4 (green), exon 6 (light blue), exon 9 (red), and exon 17 (orange) contain 12, 48, 33, and 2 alternative exons, respectively. For each of these clusters, only one alternative exon is used in the complete *Dscam* mRNA. There is some differential usage of exons in neurons, fat-body cells, and hemocytes. All three cell types use the entire range of alternative exons for exons 4 and 6. For exon 9, there is restricted use of alternative exons in hemocytes and fat-body cells. The combinatorial use of alternative exons in the Dscam gene makes it possible to generate more than 38,000 protein isoforms.

resistance to bacteria and to the malaria parasite *Plasmodium*. There is also evidence from the mosquito that some Dscam exons have specificity for particular pathogens. It is not clear whether Dscam isoforms are expressed in a clonal manner.

Another invertebrate, this time a mollusk, uses a different strategy to diversify an immunoglobulin superfamily protein for use in immunity. The freshwater snail *Biomphalaria glabrata* expresses a small family of **fibrinogen-related proteins (FREPs)** thought to have a role in innate immunity. FREPs have one or two immunoglobulin domains at their amino-terminal end and a fibrinogen domain at their carboxyl terminus. The immunoglobulin domains may interact with pathogens, while the fibrinogen domain may confer on the FREP lectin-like properties that help precipitate the complex. FREPs are produced by hemocytes and secreted into the hemolymph. Their concentration increases when the snail is infected by parasites—it is, for example, the intermediate host for the parasitic schistosomes that cause human schistosomiasis.

The *B. glabrata* genome contains many copies of FREP genes that can be divided into approximately 13 subfamilies. A study of the sequences of expressed FREP3 subfamily members has revealed that the FREPs expressed in an individual organism are extensively diversified compared with the germline genes. There are fewer than five genes in the FREP3 subfamily, but an individual snail was found to generate more than 45 distinct FREP3 proteins, all with slightly different sequences. An analysis of the protein sequences suggested that this diversification was due to the accumulation of point mutations in one of the germline FREP3 genes. Although the precise mechanism of this diversification, and the cell type in which it occurs, are not yet known, it does suggest some similarity to somatic hypermutation that occurs in the immunoglobulins. Both the insect and *Biomphalaria* examples seem to represent a way of diversifying molecules involved in immune defense, but although they resemble in some ways the strategy of an adaptive immune response, there is no evidence of clonal selection—the cornerstone of true adaptive immunity.

5-14 Agnathans possess an adaptive immune system that uses somatic gene rearrangement to diversify receptors built from LRR domains.

Since the early 1960s it has been known that certain jawless fishes, the hagfish and the lamprey, could mount a form of accelerated rejection of transplanted skin grafts and exhibit a kind of immunological delayed-type hypersensitivity. Their serum also seemed to contain an activity that behaved as a specific agglutinin, meaning that after immunization with an antigen, the serum would cause aggregation of the antigen when the two were mixed together *in vitro*, a process known as **agglutination**. Importantly, this agglutination activity increased in titer after secondary immunization, similar to antibody responses in higher vertebrates. Although these phenomena seemed reminiscent of adaptive immunity, there was no evidence of a thymus or of immunoglobulins, but these animals did have cells that could be considered to be genuine lymphocytes on the basis of morphological and molecular analysis. Analysis of the genes expressed by lymphocytes of the sea lamprey *Petromyzon marinus* revealed none related to T-cell receptor or immunoglobulin genes. However, these cells expressed large amounts of mRNAs from genes encoding proteins with multiple leucine-rich repeat (LRR) domains, the same protein domain from which the pathogen-recognizing Toll-like receptors (TLRs) are built (see Section 3-5).

This might simply have meant that these cells are specialized for recognizing and reacting to pathogens, but the LRR proteins expressed had some surprises in store. Instead of being present in a relatively few forms (like the invariant TLRs), they were found to have highly variable amino acid sequences, with a large number of variable LRR units placed between less variable amino-terminal and carboxyl-terminal LRR units. These LRR-containing proteins, called **variable lymphocyte receptors (VLRs)**, have an invariant stalk region connecting them to the plasma membrane by a glycosylphosphatidylinositol linkage, and they can either be tethered to the cell or be secreted into the blood, like antibodies.

Analysis of the expressed lamprey VLR genes indicates that they are assembled by a process of somatic gene rearrangement (**Fig. 5.22**). In the germline configuration, there are three incomplete VLR genes, *VLRA*, *VLRB*, and *VLRC*, each encoding a signal peptide, a partial amino-terminal LRR unit, and a partial carboxyl-terminal LRR unit, but these three blocks of coding sequence are

Fig. 5.22 Somatic recombination of an incomplete germline variable lymphocyte receptor (VLR) gene generates a diverse repertoire of complete VLR genes in the lamprey. Top panel: An incomplete germline copy of a lamprey VLR gene contains a framework (right) for the complete gene: the portion encoding the signal peptide (SP), part of an amino-terminal LRR unit (NT, dark blue), and a carboxyl-terminal LRR unit that is split into two parts (LRR, light red; and CT, red) by intervening noncoding DNA sequences. Nearby flanking regions (left) contain multiple copies of VLR gene 'cassettes' with single or double copies of variable LRR domains (green) and cassettes that encode part of the amino-terminal LRR domains (light blue, yellow). Middle panel: Somatic recombination causes various LRR units to be copied into the original VLR gene. This creates a complete VLR gene that contains the assembled amino-terminal LRR cassette (LRR NT) and first LRR (yellow), followed by several variable LRR units (green) and the completed carboxyl-terminal LRR unit, and ends with the portion that encodes the stalk region of the VLR receptor. The cytidine deaminases PmCDA1 and PmCDA2 from the lamprey *P. marinus* are candidates for enzymes that may initiate this gene rearrangement. Expression of the rearranged gene results in a complete receptor that can be attached to the cell membrane by glycosylphosphatidylinositol (GPI) linkage of its stalk. Bottom panel: An individual lymphocyte undergoes somatic gene rearrangement to produce a unique VLR receptor. These receptors can be tethered to the surface of the lymphocyte via the GPI linkage or can be secreted into the blood as decamers. Unique somatic rearrangement events in each developing lymphocyte generate a repertoire of VLR receptors of differing specificities.

separated by noncoding DNA that contains neither typical signals for RNA splicing nor the RSSs present in immunoglobulin genes (see Section 5-3). Instead, the regions flanking the incomplete VLR genes include a large number of DNA 'cassettes' that contain LRR units—one, two, or three LRR domains at a time. Each mature lamprey lymphocyte expresses a complete and unique VLR gene, either *VLRA, VLRB*, or *VLRC*, which has undergone recombination of these flanking regions with the germline VLR gene.

The creation of a complete VLR gene is currently thought to occur during replication of lamprey lymphocyte DNA by a 'copy-choice' mechanism that is similar, but not identical, to gene conversion (described in Section 5-16). During DNA replication, LRR units flanking the VLR gene are copied into the VLR gene—presumably when a DNA strand being synthesized switches templates and copies sequences from one of these LRR units. Although final proof is still lacking, this template-switching mechanism may be triggered by enzymes of the AID-APOBEC family that are expressed by lamprey lymphocytes, and whose **cytidine deaminase activity (CDA)** could cause the single-strand DNA breaks that can start the copy-choice process. Lampreys possess a family of such enzymes. The first discovered members, CDA1 and CDA2, are expressed in *VLRA/VLRC*-lineage and *VLRB*-lineage lymphocytes, respectively. The final VLR gene contains a complete amino-terminal capping LRR subunit, followed by the addition of up to seven internal LRR domains, each 24 amino acids long, and the removal of the internal noncoding regions to complete the formation of the carboxyl-terminal LRR domain (see Fig. 5.22).

It is estimated that this somatic rearrangement mechanism can generate as much diversity in the VLR proteins as is possible for immunoglobulins. Indeed, the crystal structure of a VLR protein shows that the concave surface formed by the series of LRR repeats interacts with a variable insert in the carboxyl-terminal LRR to form a surface capable of interacting with a great diversity of antigens. Thus, the diversity of the anticipatory repertoire of agnathans may be limited not by the numbers of possible receptors they can generate but by the number of lymphocytes present in any individual, as in the adaptive immune system of their evolutionary cousins, the gnathostomes. As noted above, each lamprey lymphocyte rearranges only one of the three germline VLR genes, expressing a complete VLRA, VLRB, or VLRC protein. Whereas VLRB-expressing cells share characteristics with mammalian B lymphocytes, VLRA- and VLRC-expressing cells resemble αβ T-cell receptor–expressing and γδ T-cell receptor–expressing lymphocytes, respectively. These parallels between lamprey VLR-expressing cell subsets and the subsets of mammalian lymphocytes is reinforced by findings that identify key lineage-associated transcription factors expressed by each cell subset. For example, VLRA-expressing lymphocytes transcribe the lamprey orthologs of TCF1, NOTCH1, and BCL11B; VLRB-expressing lymphocytes, the orthologs of E2A, PAX5, and BLIMP1; whereas VLRC-expressing lymphocytes produce the ortholog of SOX13, a key factor in γδ T-cell lineage determination. In addition, VLR-expressing cell subsets also transcribe genes related to mammalian cytokine and antigen-receptor signaling genes in a pattern that correlates with their mammalian lymphocyte counterparts. Overall, these observations support the conclusion of identical functions in lamprey and our own adaptive immune cells.

5-15 RAG-dependent adaptive immunity based on a diversified repertoire of immunoglobulin-like genes appeared abruptly in the cartilaginous fishes.

Within the vertebrates, we can trace the development of immune functions from the agnathans through the cartilaginous fishes (sharks, skates, and rays) to the bony fishes, then to the amphibians, to reptiles and birds, and finally to mammals. RAG-dependent V(D)J recombination has not been found in agnathans, other chordates, or any invertebrate. The origins of RAG-dependent adaptive immunity are now becoming clearer as the genome sequences of many more animals become available. The first clue was that RAG-dependent recombination shares many features with the transposition mechanism of **DNA transposons**—mobile genetic elements that encode their own **transposase**, an enzymatic activity that allows them to excise from one site in the genome and reinsert themselves elsewhere. The mammalian RAG complex can act as a transposase *in vitro*, and even the structure of the RAG genes, which lie close together in the chromosome and lack the usual introns of mammalian genes, is reminiscent of a transposon. In addition, a transposable element was recently discovered in lancelets, a fish-like vertebrate lineage that diverged from the other two chordate lineages more than half a billion years ago. This transposable element, named ProtoRAG, is flanked by terminal repeat sequences that resemble RSS elements; between these inverted repeats lie *RAG1*- and *RAG2*-like genes, suggesting that ProtoRAG may be an ancestor of the RAG recombination system active in vertebrate immune cells. These findings provoked speculation that the origin of RAG-dependent adaptive immunity was the invasion of a DNA transposon into a gene similar to an immunoglobulin or a T-cell receptor V-region gene, an event that would have occurred in some ancestor of the jawed vertebrates (**Fig. 5.23**). Subsequent duplication, reduplication, and recombination of the immune-receptor gene and its inserted RSSs eventually led to the separation of the RAG genes from the rest of the relic transposon and to the multi-segmented immunoglobulin and T-cell receptor loci of present-day vertebrates.

The earliest origins of the RSSs, the RAG-1 catalytic core, and possibly RAG-2 are now thought to lie in the **Transib** superfamily of DNA transposons, and genome sequencing has led to the discovery of sequences related to *RAG1* in animals as distantly related to vertebrates as the sea anemone *Nematostella*. Additionally, a *RAG1*–*RAG2*-related gene cluster was recently discovered in sea urchins, invertebrate relatives of the chordates. Sea urchins themselves show no evidence of immunoglobulins, T-cell receptors, or adaptive immunity, but the proteins expressed by the sea-urchin RAG genes form a complex with each other and with RAG proteins from the bull shark (*Carcharhinus leucas*), a primitive jawed vertebrate, but not with those from mammals. This suggests that these proteins could indeed be related to the vertebrate RAGs, and that RAG-1 and RAG-2 were already present in a common ancestor of chordates and echinoderms (the group to which sea urchins belong), presumably

Fig. 5.23 Integration of a transposon into a V-type immunoglobulin receptor gene is thought to have given rise to the T-cell receptor and immunoglobulin genes. First panel: A DNA transposon in an ancestor of the deuterostomes (the large group of phyla to which the chordates belong) is thought to have had genes related to *RAG1* and *RAG2*—prototype *RAG1* (purple) and *RAG2* (blue), which acted as its transposase. DNA transposons are bounded by terminal repeat (TR) sequences that are inverted relative to one another as indicated by the directionality of the arrowheads. Second panel: To excise a transposon from DNA, the transposase proteins (purple and blue) bind the TRs, bringing them together, and the transposase enzymatic activity cuts the transposon out of the DNA, leaving a footprint in the host DNA that resembles the TRs. After excision from one site, the transposon reinserts elsewhere in the genome, in this case into a V-type immunoglobulin receptor (green). The enzymatic activity of the transposase enables the transposon to insert into DNA in a reaction that is the reverse of the excision reaction. Third panel: The integration of the *RAG1/2*-like transposon into the middle of the gene for a V-type immunoglobulin receptor splits the V exon into two parts. Fourth and fifth panels: In the evolution of the immunoglobulin and T-cell receptor genes, the initial integration event has been followed by DNA rearrangements that separate the transposase genes (now known as *RAG1* and *RAG2*) from the transposon TRs, which we now term the recombination signal sequences (RSSs). The purple sea urchin (an invertebrate deuterostome) has a *RAG1/2*-like gene cluster (not shown) and expresses proteins similar to RAG-1 and RAG-2 proteins, but does not have immunoglobulins, T-cell receptors, or adaptive immunity. The RAG-like proteins presumably retain some other cellular function (so far unknown) in this animal.

fulfilling some other cellular function. Current models propose that a Transib family transposon was present in this ancestral species and that ProtoRAG, the *RAG1–RAG2*-related genes in sea urchins, and the vertebrate *RAG1–RAG2* all descended from this primitive transposable element.

The evidence indicating the transposon origin of the RAG recombination system raises questions concerning the identities of the genes this transposon inserted into. Proteins containing Ig-like domains are ubiquitous throughout the plant, animal, and bacterial kingdoms, making this one of the most abundant protein superfamilies; in species whose genomes have been fully sequenced, the immunoglobulin superfamily is one of the largest families of protein domains in the genome. The functions of the members of this superfamily are very disparate, and they are a striking example of natural selection taking a useful structure—the basic Ig-domain fold—and adapting it to different purposes. The immunoglobulin superfamily domains can be divided into four families on the basis of differences in the structure and sequence of the immunoglobulin domain. These are V (resembling an immunoglobulin variable domain), C1 and C2 (resembling constant-region domains), and a type of immunoglobulin domain called an I domain (for intermediate). The target of the RSS-containing element is likely to have been a gene encoding a cell-surface receptor containing an Ig-like V domain, most probably a type similar to present-day VJ domains. These domains are found in some invariant receptor proteins and are so called because of the resemblance of one of the strands to a J segment. It is possible to imagine how transposon movement into such a gene could produce separate V and J gene segments (see Fig. 5.23). On the basis of phylogenetic analysis, **agnathan paired receptors resembling Ag receptors,** or **APARs,** which are encoded by a multigene family found in hagfish and lamprey, are currently the best candidates for being relatives of the ancestor of the antigen receptor. Their DNA sequences predict single-pass transmembrane proteins with a single extracellular VJ domain and a cytoplasmic region containing signaling modules. APARs are expressed in leukocytes.

5-16 Different species generate immunoglobulin diversity in different ways.

Most of the vertebrates we are familiar with generate a large part of their antigen-receptor diversity in the same way as mice and humans, by putting together gene segments in different combinations. There are exceptions, however, even within the mammals. Some animals use gene rearrangement to always join together the same V and J gene segment initially, and then diversify this recombined V region. In birds, rabbits, cows, pigs, sheep, and horses, there is little or no germline diversity in the V, D, and J gene segments that are rearranged to form the genes for the initial B-cell receptors, and the rearranged V-region sequences are identical or similar in most immature B cells. These immature B cells migrate to specialized microenvironments—the **bursa of Fabricius** in the gut of chickens, and another intestinal lymphoid organ in rabbits. Here, B cells proliferate rapidly, and their rearranged immunoglobulin genes undergo further diversification.

In birds and rabbits this diversification occurs mainly by gene conversion, a process by which short sequences in the expressed rearranged V-region gene are replaced with sequences from an upstream V gene segment pseudogene. The germline arrangement of the chicken heavy-chain locus is a single set of rearranging V, J, D, and C gene segments and multiple copies of V-segment pseudogenes. Diversity in this system is created by gene conversion in which sequences from the V_H pseudogenes are copied into the single rearranged V_H gene (**Fig. 5.24**). It seems that gene conversion is related to somatic hypermutation in its mechanism, because gene conversion in a chicken B-cell line has been shown to require the enzyme **activation-induced cytidine deaminase (AID)**.

Activation-Induced
Cytidine Deaminase
Deficiency

Fig. 5.24 The diversification of chicken immunoglobulins occurs through gene conversion. In chickens, the immunoglobulin diversity that can be created by V(D)J recombination is extremely limited. Initially, there are only one active V, one J, and 15 D gene segments at the chicken heavy-chain locus and one active V and one J gene segment at the single light-chain locus (top left panel). Primary gene rearrangement can thus produce only a very limited number of receptor specificities (second panels). Immature B cells expressing this receptor migrate to the bursa of Fabricius, where the cross-linking of surface immunoglobulin (sIg) induces cell proliferation (second panels). The chicken genome contains numerous pseudogenes with a pre-rearranged VH–D structure. Gene conversion events introduce sequences from these adjacent V gene segment pseudogenes into the expressed gene, creating diversity in the receptors (third panels). Some of these gene conversions will inactivate the previously expressed gene (not shown). If a B cell can no longer express sIg after such a gene conversion, it is eliminated. Repeated gene conversion events can continue to diversify the repertoire (bottom panels).

In Chapter 10, we will see that this same enzyme is involved in class switching and affinity maturation of the antibody response. For gene conversion, it is thought that single-strand cuts in DNA generated by the endonuclease **apurinic/apyrimidinic endonuclease-1 (APE1)** after the actions of AID are the signal that initiates a homology-directed repair process in which a homologous V pseudogene segment is used as the template for the DNA replication that repairs the V-region gene.

In sheep and cows, immunoglobulin diversification is the result of somatic hypermutation, which occurs in an organ known as the ileal Peyer's patch. Somatic hypermutation, independent of T cells and a particular driving antigen, also contributes to immunoglobulin diversification in birds, sheep, and rabbits.

A more fundamentally different organization of immunoglobulin genes is found in the cartilaginous fishes, the most primitive jawed vertebrates. Sharks have multiple copies of discrete V_L–J_L–C_L and V_H–D_H–J_H–C_H cassettes and activate rearrangement within individual cassettes (**Fig. 5.25**). Although this

Fig. 5.25 The organization of immunoglobulin genes is different in different species, but all can generate a diverse repertoire of receptors. The organization of the immunoglobulin heavy-chain genes in mammals, in which there are separated clusters of repeated V, D, and J gene segments, is not the only solution to the problem of generating a diverse repertoire of receptors. Other vertebrates have found alternative solutions. In 'primitive' groups, such as the sharks, the locus consists of multiple repeats of a basic unit composed of a V gene segment, one or two D gene segments, a J gene segment, and a C gene segment. A more extreme version of this organization is found in the κ-like light-chain locus of some cartilaginous fishes such as the rays and the carcharhine sharks, in which the repeated unit consists of already rearranged VJ–C genes, from which a random choice is made for expression. In chickens, there is a single rearranging set of gene segments at the heavy-chain locus but there are multiple copies of pre-integrated V_H–D segment pseudogenes. Diversity in this system is created by gene conversion, in which sequences from the V_H–D pseudogenes are copied onto the single rearranged V_H gene.

is somewhat different from the kind of combinatorial gene rearrangement of higher vertebrates, in most cases there is still a requirement for a RAG-mediated somatic rearrangement event. As well as rearranging genes, cartilaginous fishes have multiple 'rearranged' V_L regions (and sometimes rearranged V_H regions) in the germline genome (see Fig. 5.25) and apparently generate diversity by activating the transcription of different copies. Even here, some diversity is also contributed by combinatorial means by the subsequent pairing of heavy and light chains.

This 'germline-joined' organization of the light-chain loci is unlikely to represent an intermediate evolutionary stage, because in that case the heavy-chain and light-chain genes would have had to independently acquire the capacity for rearrangement by convergent evolution. It is much more likely that, after the divergence of the cartilaginous fishes, some immunoglobulin loci became rearranged in the germline of various ancestors through activation of the RAG genes in germ cells, with the consequent inheritance of the rearranged loci by the offspring. In these species, the rearranged germline loci might confer some advantages, such as ensuring rapid responses to common pathogens by producing a preformed set of immunoglobulin chains.

The IgM antibody isotype is thought to go back to the origins of adaptive immunity. It is the predominant form of immunoglobulin in cartilaginous fishes and bony fishes. The cartilaginous fishes also have at least two other heavy-chain isotypes not found in more recently evolved species. One, **IgW**, has a constant region composed of six immunoglobulin domains, whereas the second, **IgNAR**, which we described in Section 4-13, seems to be related to IgW but has lost the first constant-region domain and does not pair with light chains. Instead, it forms a homodimer in which each heavy-chain V domain forms a separate antigen-binding site. IgW seems to be related to IgD (which is first found in bony fishes) and, like IgM, seems to go back to the origin of adaptive immunity.

5-17 Both αβ and γδ T-cell receptors are present in cartilaginous fishes.

Neither the T-cell receptors nor the immunoglobulins have been found in any species evolutionarily earlier than the cartilaginous fishes, in which they have essentially the same form that we see in mammals. The identification of TCR β-chain and δ-chain homologs from sharks and of distinct TCR α, β, γ, and δ chains from a skate show that even at the earliest time that these adaptive immune system receptors can be identified, they had already diversified into at least two recognition systems. Moreover, each lineage shows diversity resulting from combinatorial somatic rearrangement. The identification of many ligands recognized by γδ T cells has helped clarify their role in the immune response. Although a complete list is still lacking, the trend appears to be more similar to a kind of innate sensing rather than the fine peptide specificity of the αβ T cells. Ligands of γδ T cells include various lipids that may derive from microbes and nonclassical MHC class Ib molecules whose expression may be an indication of infection or cellular stress (see Section 6-17). Even certain αβ T cells appear to participate in a form of innate recognition, such as the mucosal associated invariant T cells described in Section 4-21. This could indicate that early in the evolution of RAG-dependent adaptive immunity, the receptors generated by excision of the primordial DNA transposon were useful in innate sensing of infections, and this role has persisted in certain minor T-cell populations to this day. In any case, the very early divergence of these two classes of T-cell receptors and their conservation through subsequent evolution suggests an important early separation of functions.

5-18 MHC class I and class II molecules are also first found in the cartilaginous fishes.

One would expect to see the specific ligands of T-cell receptors, the MHC molecules, emerge at around the same time in evolution as the receptors. Indeed, MHC molecules are present in the cartilaginous fishes and in all higher vertebrates, but, like the T-cell receptors, they have not been found in agnathans or invertebrates. Both MHC class I and class II α-chain and β-chain genes are present in sharks, and their products seem to function in an identical way to mammalian MHC molecules. The key residues of the peptide-binding cleft that interact with the ends of the peptide in MHC class I molecules or with the central region of the peptide in MHC class II molecules are conserved in shark MHC molecules.

Moreover, the MHC genes are also polymorphic in sharks, with multiple alleles of class I and class II loci. In some species, more than 20 MHC class I alleles have been identified so far. For the shark MHC class II molecules, both the class II α and the class II β chains are polymorphic. Thus, not only has the function of the MHC molecules in selecting peptides for presentation evolved during the divergence of the agnathans and the cartilaginous fishes, but the continuous selection imposed by pathogens has also resulted in the polymorphism that is a characteristic feature of the MHC.

Section 4-23 introduced the division between **classical MHC class I genes** (sometimes called class Ia) and the **nonclassical MHC class Ib genes**, which will be discussed in Chapter 6. This division is also present in cartilaginous fishes, because the class I genes of sharks include some that resemble mammalian class Ib molecules. However, it is thought that the shark class Ib genes are not the direct ancestors of the mammalian class Ib genes. For the class I genes, it seems that within each of the five major vertebrate lineages studied (cartilaginous fishes, lobe-finned fishes, ray-finned fishes, amphibians, and mammals), these genes have independently separated into classical and nonclassical loci.

Thus, the characteristic features of the MHC molecules are all present when these molecules are first encountered, and there are no intermediate forms to guide our understanding of their evolution. Although we can trace the evolution of the components of the innate immune system, the origin of the adaptive immune system remains largely mysterious. Although we may not have a sure answer to the question of what selective forces led to RAG-dependent elaboration of adaptive immunity, it has never been clearer that, as Charles Darwin remarked about evolution in general, "from so simple a beginning endless forms most beautiful and most wonderful have been, and are being, evolved."

Summary.

Evolution of RAG-dependent adaptive immunity in jawed vertebrates was once considered a wholly unique and inexplicable 'immunological Big Bang.' However, we now understand that adaptive immunity has also evolved independently at least one other time during evolution. Our close vertebrate cousins, the jawless fishes, have evolved an adaptive immune system built on a completely different basis—the diversification of LRR domains rather than immunoglobulin domains—but otherwise seem to have the essential features of clonal expression of receptors produced through a somatic rearrangement and with a form of immunological memory, all features of an adaptive immune system. We now appreciate that evolution of the RAG-dependent adaptive immune system is probably related to the insertion of a transposon into a member of a primordial immunoglobulin superfamily gene, which must have occurred in a germline cell in an ancestor of the vertebrates. By chance, the transposon terminal sequences, the forerunners of the RSSs, were placed in an appropriate location within this primordial antigen-receptor gene to enable intramolecular somatic recombination, thus paving the way for the full-blown somatic gene rearrangement seen in present-day immunoglobulin and T-cell receptor genes. The MHC molecules that are the ligands for T-cell receptors first appear in the cartilaginous fishes, suggesting coevolution with RAG-dependent adaptive immunity. The transposase genes (the RAG genes) could have already been present and active in some other function in the genome of this ancestor. Both *RAG1* and *RAG2* have very ancient origins, as related sequences have been found in a wide variety of animal genomes.

Summary to Chapter 5.

The antigen receptors of lymphocytes are remarkably diverse, and developing B cells and T cells use the same basic mechanism to achieve this diversity. In each cell, functional genes for the immunoglobulin and T-cell receptor chains are assembled by somatic recombination from sets of separate gene segments that together encode the V region. The substrates for the joining process are arrays of V, D, and J gene segments, which are similar in all the antigen-receptor gene loci. The lymphoid-specific proteins RAG-1 and RAG-2 direct the site-specific cleavage of DNA at RSSs flanking the V, D, and J segments to form double-strand breaks that initiate the recombination process in both T and B cells. These proteins function in concert with ubiquitous DNA-modifying enzymes acting in the double-strand break repair pathway, and with at least one other lymphoid-specific enzyme, TdT, to complete the gene rearrangements. As each type of gene segment is present in multiple, slightly different versions, the random selection of one gene segment from each set is a source of substantial potential diversity. During assembly, the imprecise joining mechanisms at the coding junctions create a high degree of diversity concentrated in the CDR3 loops of the receptor, which lie at the center of the antigen-binding sites. The independent association of the two chains of immunoglobulins or T-cell receptors to form a complete antigen receptor multiplies the overall diversity available. An important difference between immunoglobulins and T-cell receptors is that immunoglobulins exist in both membrane-bound forms (B-cell receptors) and secreted forms (antibodies). The ability to express both a secreted and a membrane-bound form of the same molecule is due to alternative splicing of the heavy-chain mRNA to include exons that encode different forms of the carboxyl terminus. Heavy-chain C regions of immunoglobulins contain three or four domains, whereas the T-cell receptor chains have only one. Other species have developed strategies to diversify receptors involved in immunity, and the agnathans use a system of VLRs that undergo somatic rearrangement that has some specific similarities to our own adaptive immune system. Adaptive immunity in jawed vertebrates—gnathostomes—appears to have arisen by the integration of a DNA transposon that encoded prototype RAG1/2 genes into a preexisting V-type immunoglobulin-like gene that subsequently diversified to generate T- and B-cell receptor genes.

Discussion Questions

5.1 Antibody heavy-chain V regions are encoded by a series of gene segments that are separated in the genome. After somatic rearrangement, these gene segments can potentially create about 5000 different antibody V_H sequences. Approximately 300 V_L sequences can be generated by somatic rearrangement of light-chain gene segments. After random pairing of one light chain and one heavy chain, approximately 1 million different antibody specificities can be generated. Yet, estimates indicate that the final repertoire of antibodies that can be created by V(D)J recombination is of the order 10^{13} different sequences. How is all of the 'extra' diversity created during antibody heavy- and light-chain gene segment rearrangement?

5.2 Antibody and T-cell receptor gene segment rearrangement is guided by DNA sequences flanking each gene segment. Early studies identified 'the 12/23 rule' on the basis of observations that gene segments flanked by recombination signal sequences (RSSs) containing a 12-bp spacer were always joined to a gene segment flanked by an RSS containing a 23-bp spacer. How does the three-dimensional structure of the RAG-1:RAG-2 complex bound to DNA explain this rule?

5.3 There are both lymphocyte-specific and ubiquitous (that is, expressed in all cell types) enzymes involved in the process of V(D)J recombination. Name two examples of each category of enzyme and describe their function in V(D)J recombination.

5.4 Some inherited immunodeficiency disorders are caused by mutations in genes important in V(D)J recombination.

Several of these also cause patients to be hypersensitive to ionizing radiation. What is the reason for the sensitivity to radiation in this class of immunodeficiency patients?

5.5 Mature B cells express membrane-bound IgM and IgD molecules that share the same specificity on their cell surface. How does a B cell express both IgM and IgD heavy-chain proteins with the same V_H sequences present in both?

5.6 Deficiencies in RAG-1 or RAG-2 cause a form of SCID in which patients lack both B cells and T cells. Why is this the case?

5.7 Mature T cells never express both $\alpha\beta$ and $\gamma\delta$ T-cell receptor heterodimers on their surface. What aspect of the T-cell antigen-receptor gene loci accounts for this finding?

5.8 Several invertebrate species have been found to express antigen-binding proteins and cellular receptors with a high degree of diversity similar to the antibody and T-cell receptor repertoires in vertebrates. Yet the antigen-binding proteins in invertebrates bear no resemblance to immunoglobulin proteins or immunoglobulin superfamily members. Describe one of these alternative systems of antigen-binding proteins in an invertebrate and how repertoire diversity is generated in this system.

5.9 In some vertebrate species, such as rabbits and birds, antibody diversity is generated by a mechanism distinct from the V(D)J recombination system used in humans and mice. Describe this mechanism of antibody sequence diversification and name the key enzyme and its function that is required for this process.

General references.

Fugmann, S.D., Lee, A.I., Shockett, P.E., Villey, I.J., and Schatz, D.G.: **The RAG proteins and V(D)J recombination: complexes, ends, and transposition.** *Annu. Rev. Immunol.* 2000, 18:495–527.

Jung, D., Giallourakis, C., Mostoslavsky, R., and Alt, F.W.: **Mechanism and control of V(D)J recombination at the immunoglobulin heavy chain locus.** *Annu. Rev. Immunol.* 2006, 24:541–570.

Schatz, D.G.: **V(D)J recombination.** *Immunol. Rev.* 2004, 200:5–11.

Schatz, D.G., and Swanson, P.C.: **V(D)J recombination: mechanisms of initiation.** *Annu. Rev. Genet.* 2011, 45:167–202.

Section references.

5-1   Complete immunoglobulin genes are generated by the somatic recombination of separate gene segments.

Early, P., Huang, H., Davis, M., Calame, K., and Hood, L.: **An immunoglobulin heavy chain variable region gene is generated from three segments of DNA: V_H, D and J_H.** *Cell* 1980, 19:981–992.

Hozumi, N., and Tonegawa, S.: **Evidence for somatic rearrangement of immunoglobulin genes coding for variable and constant regions.** *Proc. Natl. Acad. Sci. USA* 1976, 73:3628–3632.

Seidman, J.G., and Leder, P.: **The arrangement and rearrangement of antibody genes.** *Nature* 1978, 276:790–795.

Tonegawa, S., Brack, C., Hozumi, N., and Pirrotta, V.: **Organization of immunoglobulin genes.** *Cold Spring Harb. Symp. Quant. Biol.* 1978, 42:921–931.

Tonegawa, S., Maxam, A.M., Tizard, R., Bernard, O., and Gilbert, W.: **Sequence of a mouse germ-line gene for a variable region of an immunoglobulin light chain.** *Proc. Natl. Acad. Sci. USA* 1978, 75:1485–1489.

5-2   Multiple contiguous V gene segments are present at each immunoglobulin locus.

Maki, R., Traunecker, A., Sakano, H., Roeder, W., and Tonegawa, S.: **Exon shuffling generates an immunoglobulin heavy chain gene.** *Proc. Natl. Acad. Sci. USA* 1980, 77:2138–2142.

Matsuda, F., and Honjo, T.: **Organization of the human immunoglobulin heavy-chain locus.** *Adv. Immunol.* 1996, 62:1–29.

Thiebe, R., Schable, K.F., Bensch, A., Brensing-Kuppers, J., Heim, V., Kirschbaum, T., Mitlohner, H., Ohnrich, M., Pourrajabi, S., Roschenthaler, F., *et al.*: **The variable genes and gene families of the mouse immunoglobulin kappa locus.** *Eur. J. Immunol.* 1999, 29:2072–2081.

5-3   Rearrangement of V, D, and J gene segments is guided by flanking DNA sequences.

Grawunder, U., West, R.B., and Lieber, M.R.: **Antigen receptor gene rearrangement.** *Curr. Opin. Immunol.* 1998, 10:172–180.

Lieber, M.R.: **The mechanism of human nonhomologous DNA end joining.** *J. Biol. Chem.* 2008, 283:1–5.

Sakano, H., Huppi, K., Heinrich, G., and Tonegawa, S.: **Sequences at the somatic recombination sites of immunoglobulin light-chain genes.** *Nature* 1979, 280:288–294.

5-4   The reaction that recombines V, D, and J gene segments involves both lymphocyte-specific and ubiquitous DNA-modifying enzymes.

Agrawal, A., and Schatz, D.G.: **RAG1 and RAG2 form a stable postcleavage synaptic complex with DNA containing signal ends in V(D)J recombination.** *Cell* 1997, 89:43–53.

Ahnesorg, P., Smith, P., and Jackson, S.P.: **XLF interacts with the XRCC4-DNA ligase IV complex to promote nonhomologous end-joining.** *Cell* 2006, 124:301–313.

Blunt, T., Finnie, N.J., Taccioli, G.E., Smith, G.C.M., Demengeot, J., Gottlieb, T.M., Mizuta, R., Varghese, A.J., Alt, F.W., Jeggo, P.A., and Jackson, S.P.: **Defective DNA-dependent protein kinase activity is linked to V(D)J recombination and DNA repair defects associated with the murine scid mutation.** *Cell* 1995, 80:813–823.

Buck, D., Malivert, L., deChasseval, R., Barraud, A., Fondaneche, M.-C., Xanal, O., Plebani, A., Stephan, J.-L., Hufnagel, M., le Diest, F., *et al.*: **Cernunnos, a novel nonhomologous end-joining factor, is mutated in human immunodeficiency with microcephaly.** *Cell* 2006, 124:287–299.

Jung, D., Giallourakis, C., Mostoslavsky, R., and Alt, F.W.: **Mechanism and control of V(D)J recombination at the immunoglobulin heavy chain locus.** *Annu. Rev. Immunol.* 2006, 24:541–570.

Kim, M.S., Lapkouski, M., Yang, W., and Gellert, M.: **Crystal structure of the V(D)J recombinase RAG1-RAG2.** *Nature* 2015, 518:507–511.

Li, Z.Y., Otevrel, T., Gao, Y.J., Cheng, H.L., Seed, B., Stamato, T.D., Taccioli, G.E., and Alt, F.W.: **The XRCC4 gene encodes a novel protein involved in DNA double-strand break repair and V(D)J recombination.** *Cell* 1995, 83:1079–1089.

Ma, Y., Pannicke, U., Schwarz, K., and Lieber, M.R.: **Hairpin opening and over-hang processing by an Artemis:DNA-PKcs complex in V(D)J recombination and in nonhomologous end joining.** *Cell* 2002, 108:781–794.

Mizuta, R., Varghese, A.J., Alt, F.W., Jeggo, P.A., and Jackson, S.P.: **Defective DNA-dependent protein kinase activity is linked to V(D)J recombination and DNA-repair defects associated with the murine scid mutation.** *Cell* 1995, 80:813–823.

Moshous, D., Callebaut, I., de Chasseval, R., Corneo, B., Cavazzana-Calvo, M., le Deist , F., Tezcan, I., Sanal, O., Bertrand, Y., Philippe, N., *et al.*: **Artemis, a novel DNA double-strand break repair/V(D)J recombination protein, is mutated in human severe combined immune deficiency.** *Cell* 2001, 105:177–186.

Oettinger, M.A., Schatz, D.G., Gorka, C., and Baltimore, D.: **RAG-1 and RAG-2, adjacent genes that synergistically activate V(D)J recombination.** *Science* 1990, 248:1517–1523.

Villa, A., Santagata, S., Bozzi, F., Giliani, S., Frattini, A., Imberti, L., Gatta, L.B., Ochs, H.D., Schwarz, K., Notarangelo, L.D., *et al.*: **Partial V(D)J recombination activity leads to Omenn syndrome.** *Cell* 1998, 93:885–896.

Yin, F.F., Bailey, S., Innis, C.A., Ciubotaru, M., Kamtekar, S., Steitz, T.A., and Schatz, D.G.: **Structure of the RAG1 nonamer binding domain with DNA reveals a dimer that mediates DNA synapsis.** *Nat. Struct. Mol. Biol.* 2009, 16:499–508.

5-5   The diversity of the immunoglobulin repertoire is generated by four main processes.

Weigert, M., Perry, R., Kelley, D., Hunkapiller, T., Schilling, J., and Hood, L.: **The joining of V and J gene segments creates antibody diversity.** *Nature* 1980, 283:497–499.

5-6   The multiple inherited gene segments are used in different combinations.

Lee, A., Desravines, S., and Hsu, E.: **IgH diversity in an individual with only one million B lymphocytes.** *Dev. Immunol.* 1993, 3:211–222.

5-7   Variable addition and subtraction of nucleotides at the junctions between gene segments contributes to the diversity of the third hypervariable region.

Gauss, G.H., and Lieber, M.R.: **Mechanistic constraints on diversity in human V(D)J recombination.** *Mol. Cell. Biol.* 1996, 16:258–269.

Gilfillan, S., Dierich, A., Lemeur, M., Benoist, C., and Mathis, D.: **Mice lacking TdT: mature animals with an immature lymphocyte repertoire.** *Science* 1993, 261:1755–1759.

Komori, T., Okada, A., Stewart, V., and Alt, F.W.: **Lack of N regions in antigen receptor variable region genes of TdT-deficient lymphocytes.** *Science* 1993, 261:1171–1175.

Weigert, M., Gatmaitan, L., Loh, E., Schilling, J., and Hood, L.: **Rearrangement of genetic information may produce immunoglobulin diversity.** *Nature* 1978, 276:785–790.

5-8   IgM and IgD are derived from the same pre-mRNA transcript and are both expressed on the surface of mature B cells.

Abney, E.R., Cooper, M.D., Kearney, J.F., Lawton, A.R., and Parkhouse, R.M.: Sequential expression of immunoglobulin on developing mouse B lymphocytes: a systematic survey that suggests a model for the generation of immunoglobulin isotype diversity. *J. Immunol.* 1978, **120**:2041–2049.

Blattner, F.R., and Tucker, P.W.: The molecular biology of immunoglobulin D. *Nature* 1984, **307**:417–422.

Enders, A., Short, A., Miosge, L.A., Bergmann, H., Sontani, Y., Bertram, E.M., Whittle, B., Balakishnan, B., Yoshida, K., Sjollema, G., *et al.*: Zinc-finger protein ZFP318 is essential for expression of IgD, the alternatively spliced Igh product made by mature B lymphocytes. *Proc. Natl. Acad. Sci. USA* 2014, **111**:4513–4518.

Goding, J.W., Scott, D.W., and Layton, J.E.: Genetics, cellular expression and function of IgD and IgM receptors. *Immunol. Rev.* 1977, **37**:152–186.

5-9   Transmembrane and secreted forms of immunoglobulin are generated from different heavy-chain mRNA transcripts.

Early, P., Rogers, J., Davis, M., Calame, K., Bond, M., Wall, R., and Hood, L.: Two mRNAs can be produced from a single immunoglobulin μ gene by alternative RNA processing pathways. *Cell* 1980, **20**:313–319.

Martincic, K., Alkan, S.A., Cheatle, A., Borghesi, L., and Milcarek, C.: Transcription elongation factor ELL2 directs immunoglobulin secretion in plasma cells by stimulating altered RNA processing. *Nat. Immunol.* 2009, **10**:1102–1109.

Peterson, M.L., Gimmi, E.R., and Perry, R.P.: The developmentally regulated shift from membrane to secreted μ mRNA production is accompanied by an increase in cleavage-polyadenylation efficiency but no measurable change in splicing efficiency. *Mol. Cell. Biol.* 1991, **11**:2324–2327.

Rogers, J., Early, P., Carter, C., Calame, K., Bond, M., Hood, L., and Wall, R.: Two mRNAs with different 3′ ends encode membrane-bound and secreted forms of immunoglobulin μ chain. *Cell* 1980, **20**:303–312.

Takagaki, Y., and Manley, J.L.: Levels of polyadenylation factor CstF-64 control IgM heavy chain mRNA accumulation and other events associated with B cell differentiation. *Mol. Cell.* 1998, **2**:761–771.

Takagaki, Y., Seipelt, R.L., Peterson, M.L., and Manley, J.L.: The polyadenylation factor CstF-64 regulates alternative processing of IgM heavy chain pre-mRNA during B cell differentiation. *Cell* 1996, **87**:941–952.

5-10   The T-cell receptor gene segments are arranged in a pattern similar to that of immunoglobulin gene segments and are rearranged by the same enzymes.

Bassing, C.H., Alt, F.W., Hughes, M.M., D'Auteuil, M., Wehrly, T.D., Woodman, B.B., Gärtner, F., White, J.M., Davidson, L., and Sleckman, B.P.: Recombination signal sequences restrict chromosomal V(D)J recombination beyond the 12/23 rule. *Nature* 2000, **405**:583–586.

Bertocci, B., DeSmet, A., Weill, J.-C., and Reynaud, C.A. Non-overlapping functions of polX family DNA polymerases, pol μ, pol λ, and TdT, during immunoglobulin V(D)J recombination *in vivo*. *Immunity* 2006, **25**:31–41.

Lieber, M.R.: The polymerases for V(D)J recombination. *Immunity* 2006, **25**:7–9.

Rowen, L., Koop, B.F., and Hood, L.: The complete 685-kilobase DNA sequence of the human β T cell receptor locus. *Science* 1996, **272**:1755–1762.

Shinkai, Y., Rathbun, G., Lam, K.P., Oltz, E.M., Stewart, V., Mendelsohn, M., Charron, J., Datta, M., Young, F., Stall, A.M., *et al.*: RAG-2 deficient mice lack mature lymphocytes owing to inability to initiate V(D)J rearrangement. *Cell* 1992, **68**:855–867.

5-11   T-cell receptors concentrate diversity in the third hypervariable region.

Davis, M.M., and Bjorkman, P.J.: T-cell antigen receptor genes and T-cell recognition. *Nature* 1988, **334**:395–402.

Garboczi, D.N., Ghosh, P., Utz, U., Fan, Q.R., Biddison, W.E., and Wiley, D.C.: Structure of the complex between human T-cell receptor, viral peptide and HLA-A2. *Nature* 1996, **384**:134–141.

Hennecke, J., Carfi, A., and Wiley, D.C.: Structure of a covalently stabilized complex of a human αβ T-cell receptor, influenza HA peptide and MHC class II molecule, HLA-DR1. *EMBO J.* 2000, **19**:5611–5624.

Hennecke, J., and Wiley, D.C.: T cell receptor–MHC interactions up close. *Cell* 2001, **104**:1–4.

Jorgensen, J.L., Esser, U., Fazekas de St. Groth, B., Reay, P.A., and Davis, M.M.: Mapping T-cell receptor–peptide contacts by variant peptide immunization of single-chain transgenics. *Nature* 1992, **355**:224–230.

5-12   γδ T-cell receptors are also generated by gene rearrangement.

Chien, Y.H., Iwashima, M., Kaplan, K.B., Elliott, J.F., and Davis, M.M.: A new T-cell receptor gene located within the alpha locus and expressed early in T-cell differentiation. *Nature* 1987, **327**:677–682.

Lafaille, J.J., DeCloux, A., Bonneville, M., Takagaki, Y., and Tonegawa, S.: Junctional sequences of T cell receptor gamma delta genes: implications for gamma delta T cell lineages and for a novel intermediate of V-(D)-J joining. *Cell* 1989, **59**:859–870.

Tonegawa, S., Berns, A., Bonneville, M., Farr, A.G., Ishida, I., Ito, K., Itohara, S., Janeway, C.A., Jr., Kanagawa, O., Kubo, R., *et al.*: Diversity, development, ligands, and probable functions of gamma delta T cells. *Adv. Exp. Med. Biol.* 1991, **292**:53–61.

5-13   Some invertebrates generate extensive diversity in a repertoire of immunoglobulin-like genes.

Dong, Y., Taylor, H.E., and Dimopoulos, G.: AgDscam, a hypervariable immunoglobulin domain-containing receptor of the *Anopheles gambiae* innate immune system. *PLoS Biol.* 2006, **4**:e229.

Loker, E.S., Adema, C.M., Zhang, S.M., and Kepler, T.B.: Invertebrate immune systems—not homogeneous, not simple, not well understood. *Immunol. Rev.* 2004, **198**:10–24.

Watson, F.L., Puttmann-Holgado, R., Thomas, F., Lamar, D.L., Hughes, M., Kondo, M., Rebel, V.I., and Schmucker, D.: Extensive diversity of Ig-superfamily proteins in the immune system of insects. *Science* 2005, **309**:1826–1827.

Zhang, S.M., Adema, C.M., Kepler, T.B., and Loker, E.S.: Diversification of Ig superfamily genes in an invertebrate. *Science* 2004, **305**:251–254.

5-14   Agnathans possess an adaptive immune system that uses somatic gene rearrangement to diversify receptors built from LRR domains.

Boehm, T., McCurley, N., Sutoh, Y., Schorpp, M., Kasahara, M., and Cooper, M.D.: VLR-based adaptive immunity. *Annu. Rev. Immunol.* 2012, **30**:203–220.

Finstad, J., and Good, R.A.: The evolution of the immune response. 3. Immunologic responses in the lamprey. *J. Exp. Med.* 1964, **120**:1151–1168.

Guo, P., Hirano, M., Herrin, B.R., Li, J., Yu, C., Sadlonova, A., and Cooper, M.D.: Dual nature of the adaptive immune system in lampreys. *Nature* 2009, **459**:796–801. [Erratum: *Nature* 2009, **460**:1044.]

Han, B.W., Herrin, B.R., Cooper, M.D., and Wilson, I.A.: Antigen recognition by variable lymphocyte receptors. *Science* 2008, **321**:1834–1837.

Hirano, M., Guo, P., McCurley, N., Schorpp, M., Das, S., Boehm, T., and Cooper, M.D.: Evolutionary implications of a third lymphocyte lineage in lampreys. *Nature* 2013, **501**:435–438.

Litman, G.W., Finstad, F.J., Howell, J., Pollara, B.W., and Good, R.A.: The evolution of the immune response. 3. Structural studies of the lamprey immunoglobulin. *J. Immunol.* 1970, **105**:1278–1285.

5-15   RAG-dependent adaptive immunity based on a diversified repertoire of immunoglobulin-like genes appeared abruptly in the cartilaginous fishes.

Fugmann, S.D., Messier, C., Novack, L.A., Cameron, R.A., and Rast, J.P.: An ancient evolutionary origin of the *Rag1/2* gene locus. *Proc. Natl. Acad. Sci. USA* 2006, **103**:3728–3733.

Kapitonov, V.V., and Jurka, J.: **RAG1 core and V(D)J recombination signal sequences were derived from Transib transposons.** *PLoS Biol.* 2005, **3**:e181.

Litman, G.W., Rast, J.P., and Fugmann, S.D.: **The origins of vertebrate adaptive immunity.** *Nat. Rev. Immunol.* 2010, **10**:543–553.

Suzuki, T., Shin-I, T., Fujiyama, A., Kohara, Y., and Kasahara, M.: **Hagfish leukocytes express a paired receptor family with a variable domain resembling those of antigen receptors.** *J. Immunol.* 2005, **174**:2885–2891.

5-16   Different species generate immunoglobulin diversity in different ways.

Becker, R.S., and Knight, K.L.: **Somatic diversification of immunoglobulin heavy chain VDJ genes: evidence for somatic gene conversion in rabbits.** *Cell* 1990, **63**:987–997.

Knight, K.L., and Crane, M.A.: **Generating the antibody repertoire in rabbit.** *Adv. Immunol.* 1994, **56**:179–218.

Kurosawa, K., and Ohta, K.: **Genetic diversification by somatic gene conversion.** *Genes* (Basel) 2011, **2**:48–58.

Reynaud, C.A., Bertocci, B., Dahan, A., and Weill, J.C.: **Formation of the chicken B-cell repertoire—ontogeny, regulation of Ig gene rearrangement, and diversification by gene conversion.** *Adv. Immunol.* 1994, **57**:353–378.

Reynaud, C.A., Garcia, C., Hein, W.R., and Weill, J.C.: **Hypermutation generating the sheep immunoglobulin repertoire is an antigen independent process.** *Cell* 1995, **80**:115–125.

Vajdy, M., Sethupathi, P., and Knight, K.L.: **Dependence of antibody somatic diversification on gut-associated lymphoid tissue in rabbits.** *J. Immunol.* 1998, **160**:2725–2729.

Winstead, C.R., Zhai, S.K., Sethupathi, P., and Knight, K.L.: **Antigen-induced somatic diversification of rabbit IgH genes: gene conversion and point mutation.** *J. Immunol.* 1999, **162**:6602–6612.

5-17   Both αβ and γδ T-cell receptors are present in cartilaginous fishes.

Rast, J.P., Anderson, M.K., Strong, S.J., Luer, C., Litman, R.T., and Litman, G.W.: **α, β, γ, and δ T-cell antigen receptor genes arose early in vertebrate phylogeny.** *Immunity* 1997, **6**:1–11.

Rast, J.P., and Litman, G.W.: **T-cell receptor gene homologs are present in the most primitive jawed vertebrates.** *Proc. Natl. Acad. Sci. USA* 1994, **91**:9248–9252.

5-18   MHC class I and class II molecules are also first found in the cartilaginous fishes.

Hashimoto, K., Okamura, K., Yamaguchi, H., Ototake, M., Nakanishi, T., and Kurosawa, Y.: **Conservation and diversification of MHC class I and its related molecules in vertebrates.** *Immunol. Rev.* 1999, **167**:81–100.

Kurosawa, Y., and Hashimoto, K.: **How did the primordial T cell receptor and MHC molecules function initially?** *Immunol. Cell Biol.* 1997, **75**:193–196.

Ohta, Y., Okamura, K., McKinney, E.C., Bartl, S., Hashimoto, K., and Flajnik, M.F.: **Primitive synteny of vertebrate major histocompatibility complex class I and class II genes.** *Proc. Natl. Acad. Sci. USA* 2000, **97**:4712–4717.

Okamura, K., Ototake, M., Nakanishi, T., Kurosawa, Y., and Hashimoto, K.: **The most primitive vertebrates with jaws possess highly polymorphic MHC class I genes comparable to those of humans.** *Immunity* 1997, **7**:777–790.

Antigen Presentation to T Lymphocytes

6

Vertebrate adaptive immune cells possess two types of antigen receptors: the immunoglobulins that serve as antigen receptors on B cells, and the T-cell receptors. While immunoglobulins can recognize native antigens, T cells recognize only antigens that are displayed by MHC complexes on cell surfaces. The conventional **αβ T cells** recognize antigens as peptide:MHC complexes (see Section 4-15). The peptides recognized by αβ T cells can be derived from the normal turnover of self proteins, or from proteins derived from intracellular pathogens such as viruses, or from the extracellular fluids. Various tolerance mechanisms normally prevent self peptides from initiating an immune response; when these mechanisms fail, self peptides can become the target of autoimmune responses, as discussed in Chapter 15. Other classes of T cells, such as **NKT cells**, **MAIT cells**, and **γδ T cells** (see Section 4-23), recognize different types of surface molecules whose expression may indicate infection or cellular stress.

The first part of this chapter describes the cellular pathways used by various types of cells to generate peptide:MHC complexes recognized by αβ T cells. This process participates in adaptive immunity in at least two different ways. In somatic cells, peptide:MHC complexes can signal the presence of an intracellular pathogen for elimination by armed effector T cells. In dendritic cells and B lymphocytes, which may not themselves be infected, peptide:MHC complexes serve to activate antigen-specific effector T cells. We will also introduce mechanisms by which certain pathogens defeat adaptive immunity by blocking the production of peptide:MHC complexes.

The second part of this chapter focuses on the MHC class I and class II genes and their tremendous variability. The MHC molecules are encoded within a large cluster of genes that were first identified by their powerful effects on the immune response to transplanted tissues and were therefore called the major histocompatibility complex (MHC). There are several different MHC molecules in each class, and each of their genes is highly polymorphic, with many variants present in the population. MHC polymorphism has a profound effect on antigen recognition by T cells, and the combination of multiple genes and polymorphism greatly extends the range of peptides that can be presented to T cells in each individual and in populations as a whole, thus enabling individuals to respond to the wide range of potential pathogens they will encounter. The MHC also contains genes other than those for the MHC molecules; some of these genes are involved in the processing of antigens to produce peptide:MHC complexes.

The last part of the chapter discusses the ligands for unconventional classes of T cells. We will examine a group of proteins similar to MHC class I molecules that have limited polymorphism and that were called **nonclassical MHC class I proteins** in the past. Some are encoded within the MHC; others are encoded outside the MHC. These MHC class I–like proteins serve various functions, with some acting as ligands for γδ T-cell receptors or as ligands for NKG2D expressed by T cells and NK cells. We also discuss a special subset of αβ T cells called NKT cells, which recognize nonpeptide ligands, including microbial lipid antigens that are presented by several MHC class I–like proteins.

IN THIS CHAPTER

The generation of αβ T-cell receptor ligands.

The major histocompatibility complex and its function.

Recognition of nonpeptide ligands by unconventional T-cell subsets.

The generation of αβ T-cell receptor ligands.

The protective function of T cells depends on their recognition of cells harboring intracellular pathogens or that have internalized their products. As we saw in Chapter 4, the ligand recognized by an αβ T-cell receptor is a peptide bound to an MHC molecule and displayed on a cell surface. The generation of peptides from native proteins is commonly referred to as **antigen processing**, while peptide display at the cell surface by the MHC molecule is referred to as **antigen presentation**. We have already described the structure of MHC molecules and seen how they bind peptide antigens in a cleft, or groove, on their outer surface (see Sections 4-15 to 4-20). We will now look at how peptides are generated from the proteins derived from pathogens and how they are loaded onto MHC class I or MHC class II molecules.

6-1 Antigen presentation functions both in arming effector T cells and in triggering their effector functions to attack pathogen-infected cells.

The processing and presentation of pathogen-derived antigens has two distinct purposes: expanding cohorts of effector T cells, and then activating these effector functions at sites where antigens are encountered. MHC class I molecules bind peptides that are recognized by CD8 T cells, and MHC class II molecules bind peptides that are recognized by CD4 T cells, a pattern of recognition determined by specific binding of the TCR and the CD8 or CD4 co-receptor molecules to the respective MHC molecules (see Section 4-21). The importance of this specificity of recognition lies in the different distributions of MHC class I and class II molecules on cells throughout the body and the cellular locations from which their antigens are derived. MHC class I molecules are expressed by nearly all somatic cells (except red blood cells), and consequently, CD8 T cells are primarily responsible for surveillance and cytolysis of somatic cells. Also called **cytotoxic T cells**, effector CD8 T cells kill the cells on which they recognize antigen and help eliminate cells infected with viruses or bacteria that live only in the cytosol. They can also recognize allogeneic MHC class I expressed on organ transplants and cause their rejection or recognize mutated self proteins on cancer cells and help eliminate them.

In contrast, MHC class II molecules are expressed primarily on cells of the immune system, and particularly by dendritic cells, macrophages, B cells, and thymic cortical epithelial cells; they can also be induced on many cells in response to the cytokine IFN-γ. Activated human T cells also express MHC class II molecules. Thus, during their development, CD4 T cells recognize antigens presented by cells in the thymus, and later, they recognize antigens presented only by certain types of immune cells or somatic cells under specific inflammatory conditions. **Effector CD4 T cells** comprise several subsets with different activities. Importantly, naive CD8 and CD4 T cells can become armed effector cells only after encountering their cognate antigen once it has been processed and presented by activated dendritic cells.

In considering antigen processing, it is important to distinguish between the various cellular compartments from which antigens can be derived (**Fig. 6.1**). These compartments, which are separated by membranes, include the **cytosol** and the various **vesicular compartments** involved in endocytosis and secretion. Peptides derived from the cytosol are transported into the endoplasmic reticulum and either further cut by peptidases or directly loaded onto newly synthesized MHC class I molecules on the same cell for recognition by T cells, as we will discuss later in greater detail. Because viruses and some bacteria replicate in the cytosol or in the contiguous nuclear compartment, peptides

Fig. 6.1 There are two categories of major intracellular compartments, separated by membranes. One compartment is the cytosol, which communicates with the nucleus via pores in the nuclear membrane. The other is the vesicular (also vacuolar) system, which comprises the vesicular compartments: the endoplasmic reticulum, Golgi apparatus, endosomes, lysosomes, and other intracellular vesicles. The vesicular system can be thought of as being continuous with the extracellular fluid. Secretory vesicles bud off from the endoplasmic reticulum and are transported via fusion with Golgi membranes to move vesicular contents out of the cell. Extracellular material is taken up by endocytosis or phagocytosis into endosomes or phagosomes, respectively. The fusion of incoming and outgoing vesicles is important both for pathogen destruction in cells such as neutrophils and for antigen presentation. Autophagosomes surround components in the cytosol and deliver them to lysosomes in a process known as autophagy.

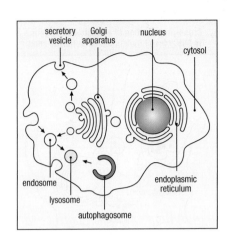

from their components can be loaded onto MHC class I molecules by this process (**Fig. 6.2**, first panel). This pathway of recognition is sometimes referred to as **direct presentation** and can identify both somatic and immune cells that are infected by a pathogen.

Certain pathogenic bacteria and protozoan parasites can survive ingestion by macrophages and are able to replicate inside the intracellular vesicles of the endosomal–lysosomal system (Fig. 6.2, second panel). Antigens derived from such pathogens are processed for presentation by MHC class II molecules. Similarly, pathogenic bacteria that proliferate outside of cells can be taken up, along with their toxic products, by phagocytosis, receptor-mediated endocytosis, or macropinocytosis into endosomes and lysosomes, where they are broken down by digestive enzymes. Receptor-mediated endocytosis by B cells can efficiently internalize extracellular antigens through B-cell receptors, which are then processed and presented by MHC class II molecules (Fig. 6.2, third panel). Virus particles and parasite antigens in extracellular fluids can also be taken up by these routes and degraded, and their peptides presented to T cells.

Some pathogens may infect somatic cells without directly infecting phagocytes, such as dendritic cells. In this case, dendritic cells must acquire antigens from exogenous sources in order to process and present a pathogen's antigens to T cells. For example, for a virus that infects only epithelial cells, the activation of virus-specific CD8 T cells requires that dendritic cells process viral proteins acquired from the virally infected cells and load peptides derived from them onto MHC class I molecules. This exogenous pathway of loading MHC class I molecules is called **cross-presentation** and is carried out very efficiently by

Fig. 6.2 Cells become targets of T-cell recognition by acquiring antigens from either the cytosolic or the vesicular compartments. First panel: Viruses and some bacteria replicate in the cytosolic compartment. Their antigens (shown as red dots) are presented by MHC class I molecules to activate killing by cytotoxic CD8 T cells. Second panel: Other bacteria and some parasites are taken up into endosomes, usually by specialized phagocytic cells such as macrophages. Here they are killed and degraded or in some cases are able to survive and proliferate within the vesicle. Their antigens are presented by MHC class II molecules to activate cytokine production by CD4 T cells. Third panel: Proteins derived from extracellular pathogens may bind to cell-surface receptors and enter the vesicular system by endocytosis, illustrated here for antigens bound by the surface immunoglobulin of B cells. These antigens are presented by MHC class II molecules to CD4 helper T cells, which can then stimulate the B cells to produce antibody.

	Cytosolic pathogens	Intravesicular pathogens	Extracellular pathogens and toxins
	any cell	macrophage	B cell
Degraded in	Cytosol	Endocytic vesicles (low pH)	Endocytic vesicles (low pH)
Peptides bind to	MHC class I	MHC class II	MHC class II
Presented to	Effector CD8 T cells	Effector CD4 T cells	Effector CD4 T cells
Effect on presenting cell	Cell death	Activation of macrophage to kill intravesicular bacteria and parasites	Activation of B cells to secrete Ig to eliminate extracellular bacteria/toxins/viruses

Cross-presentation of exogenous antigens by MHC class I molecules on dendritic cells

Fig. 6.3 Cross-presentation of extracellular antigens on MHC class I molecules by dendritic cells. Certain subsets of dendritic cells, especially cDC1, are efficient in capturing exogenous proteins from necrotic cells and loading peptides (red) derived from them onto MHC class I molecules. Evidence derived largely from studies of cells *in vitro* suggests that several cellular pathways may be involved. One route may involve the translocation of ingested proteins from the phagolysosome into the cytosol for degradation by the proteasome, with the resultant peptides then passing through a TAP transporter (see Section 6-3) and into the endoplasmic reticulum (ER) or phagosome, where they load onto MHC class I molecules in the usual way. Another route may involve direct transport of antigens into a phagolysosome—without passage through the cytosol—where they are processed into peptides and allowed to be bound to either mature MHC class I molecules or peptide-loading complexes that have been delivered there. These are called the cytosolic and vacuolar (or vesicular) pathways, respectively.

some specialized types of dendritic cells (**Fig. 6.3**). The activation of naive T cells by this pathway is called **cross-priming**. Cross-presentation and cross-priming are also important in CD8 T cells' responses to many tumors.

For loading peptides onto MHC class II molecules, dendritic cells, macrophages, and B cells are able to capture exogenous proteins via endocytic vesicles and through specific cell-surface receptors. For B cells, this process of antigen capture can include the B-cell receptor. The peptides that are derived from these proteins are loaded onto MHC class II molecules in specially modified endocytic compartments in these antigen-presenting cells, which we will discuss in more detail later. In dendritic cells, this pathway operates to activate naive CD4 T cells to become effector T cells. Macrophages take up particulate material by phagocytosis and mainly present pathogen-derived peptides on MHC class II molecules. In macrophages, such antigen presentation may also indicate the presence of a pathogen within its own vesicular compartment. Effector CD4 T cells, on recognizing antigen, produce cytokines that can stimulate the macrophage to destroy the pathogen. Some intravesicular pathogens have adapted to resist intracellular killing, and the macrophages in which they live require stimulation by cytokines in order to kill these pathogens. This is one of the roles of the T_H1 subset of CD4 T cells, which we will elaborate in Section 11-6. Other CD4 T-cell subsets have roles in regulating other aspects of the immune response. In B cells, antigen presentation by MHC class II molecules may recruit help from CD4 T cells that recognize peptides derived from the same protein recognized and by the surface immunoglobulin of a B cell. The B cell takes up such proteins by endocytosis, processes and presents peptides derived from them on MHC class II molecules, and thereby can activate CD4 T cells that will serve in turn as helper T cells for the production of antibodies against that antigen.

Beyond the presentation of exogenous proteins, MHC class II molecules can also be loaded with peptides derived from cytosolic proteins by a ubiquitous pathway of **autophagy**, in which cytoplasmic proteins are delivered into the endocytic system for degradation in lysosomes (**Fig. 6.4**). This pathway can serve in the presentation of self-cytosolic proteins for the induction of tolerance to self antigens, and also as a means for presenting antigens from pathogens that have accessed the cell's cytosol, such as herpes simplex virus.

Presentation of cellular antigens by MHC class II molecules

Fig. 6.4 Autophagy pathways can deliver cytosolic antigens for presentation by MHC class II molecules. In the process of autophagy, portions of the cytoplasm are taken into autophagosomes, which are specialized double-membrane vesicles that are fused with endocytic vesicles and eventually with lysosomes, where the contents are catabolized. Some of the resulting peptides of this process can be bound to MHC class II molecules and presented on the cell surface. In dendritic cells and macrophages, this can occur in the absence of activation, so that immature dendritic cells may express self peptides in a tolerogenic context, rather than inducing T-cell responses to self antigens. CLIP, class II–associated invariant chain peptide; MIIC, MHC class II compartment.

6-2 Peptides are generated from ubiquitinated proteins in the cytosol by the proteasome.

Proteins in cells are continually being degraded and replaced with newly synthesized proteins. Much cytosolic protein degradation is carried out by a large, multicatalytic protease complex called the **proteasome** (**Fig. 6.5**). A typical proteasome is composed of one **20S catalytic core** and two **19S regulatory caps**, one at each end; both the core and the caps are multi-subunit complexes of proteins. The 20S core is a large cylindrical complex of some 28 subunits, arranged in four stacked rings of seven subunits each around a hollow core. The two outer rings are each composed of seven distinct α subunits and are noncatalytic. The two inner rings of the 20S proteasome core are each composed of seven distinct β subunits. The constitutively expressed **proteolytic subunits are β1, β2, and β5**, which form a part of the catalytic chamber. The 19S regulator is composed of a base containing nine subunits that binds directly to the α ring of the 20S core particle and a lid that has up to 10 different subunits. The association of the 20S core with a 19S cap requires ATP as well as the ATPase activity of many of the cap's subunits. One of the 19S caps binds and delivers proteins into the proteasome, while the other keeps them from exiting prematurely.

Proteins in the cytosol are tagged for degradation via the **ubiquitin–proteasome system (UPS)**. This begins with the attachment of a chain of several ubiquitin molecules to the target protein, a process called **ubiquitination**. First, a lysine residue on the targeted protein is chemically linked to the glycine at the carboxyl terminus of one ubiquitin molecule. Ubiquitin chains are then formed by linking the lysine at residue 48 (K48) of the first ubiquitin to the carboxyl-terminal glycine of a second ubiquitin, and so on until at least four ubiquitin molecules are bound. This K48-linked type of ubiquitin chain is recognized by the 19S cap of the proteasome, which then unfolds the tagged protein so that it can be introduced into the proteasome's catalytic core. There the protein chain is degraded with a general lack of sequence specificity into short peptides, which are subsequently released into the cytosol. The general degradative functions of the proteasome have been co-opted for antigen presentation, so that MHC molecules have evolved to work with the peptides that the proteasome can produce.

The proteasome is the set of cytosolic proteases responsible for generating the majority of MHC I–presented peptides, but it is possible that some peptides are generated by other proteases. Moreover, not only can the proteasome cleave proteins, but it can also splice some resulting peptides back together by the action of a transpeptidase reaction to generate novel fused sequences. Such spliced sequences can be presented on MHC I molecules and be recognized by CD8 T cells.

The constitutive β1, β2, and β5 subunits of the catalytic chamber of the proteasome are sometimes replaced by three alternative catalytic subunits to form the **immunoproteasome**. These induced subunits are called **β1i (or LMP2), β2i (or MECL-1), and β5i (or LMP7)** and are constitutively expressed in dendritic cells and lymphocytes but induced in other cells by interferons. Both β1i and β5i are encoded by the genes *PSMB9* and *PSMB8*, which are located in the MHC locus, whereas β2i is encoded by *PSMB10* outside the MHC locus. Thus, the proteasome can exist both as a constitutive proteasome present in all cells and as the immunoproteasome present in dendritic cells, lymphocytes, and other cells stimulated with interferons. The two types of proteasome produce some non-overlapping peptides. A particular cell will have the standard proteasome with a number of immunoproteasomes that vary with cell type and interferon exposure. The replacement of the β subunits by their interferon-inducible counterparts alters the enzymatic specificity of the proteasome such that there is increased cleavage of polypeptides after hydrophobic and basic residues and decreased cleavage after acidic residues. This produces peptides with carboxyl-terminal residues that are preferred anchor residues for binding to most MHC class I molecules (see Chapter 4) and are also the preferred substrate for transport into the endoplasmic reticulum by a heterodimeric peptide transporter called TAP (see Section 6-3).

Another substitution for a β subunit in the catalytic chamber has been found to occur in cells in the thymus. Epithelial cells of the thymic cortex (**cTECs**) express a unique β subunit, called **β5t**, which is encoded by *PSMB11*. In cTECs, β5t becomes a component of the proteasome in association with β1i and β2i, and this specialized type of proteasome is called the **thymoproteasome**. Mice lacking expression of β5t have reduced numbers of CD8 T cells, indicating that the peptide:MHC complexes produced by the thymoproteasome are important in CD8 T-cell development in the thymus.

Fig. 6.5 Cytosolic proteins are degraded by the ubiquitin–proteasome system into short peptides. The proteasome is composed of a 20S catalytic core, which consists of four multi-subunit rings (see text), and two 19S regulatory caps, one on either end. Proteins (red) that are targeted become covalently tagged with K48-linked polyubiquitin chains (yellow) through the actions of various E3 ligases (see Section 3-7). The 19S regulatory cap recognizes polyubiquitin and draws the tagged protein inside the catalytic chamber; there, the protein is degraded, giving rise to small peptide fragments that are released back into the cytoplasm.

The boxed figure labels:

One 20S core combines with two 19S regulatory caps to form a proteasome in the cytosol

19S   20S   19S

α β β α

Polyubiquitinated proteins are bound by the 19S cap and degraded within the catalytic core, releasing peptides into the cytosol

protein

ubiquitin

peptide fragments

Fig. 6.6 The PA28 proteasome activator binds to either end of the proteasome. Panel a: In this side-view cross section, the heptamer rings of the PA28 proteasome activator (yellow) interact with the α subunits (pink) at either end of the core proteasome (the β subunits that make up the catalytic cavity of the core are in blue). Within this region is the α-annulus (green), a narrow ringlike opening that is normally blocked by other parts of the α subunits (shown in red). Panel b: A close-up view from the top, looking into the α-annulus without PA28 bound. Panel c: With the same perspective, the binding of PA28 to the proteasome changes the conformation of the α subunits, moving those parts of the molecule that block the α-annulus, and opening the end of the cylinder. For simplicity, PA28 is not shown.

Interferon-γ (IFN-γ) can further influence the production of some antigenic peptides by inducing expression of the **PA28 proteasome-activator complex** that binds to the proteasome. PA28 is a six- or seven-membered ring composed of two proteins, PA28α and PA28β, both of which are induced by IFN-γ. The PA28 ring can bind to either end of the 20S proteasome core in place of the 19S regulatory cap (**Fig. 6.6**). The exact function of the PA28:20S proteasome complex is still unclear, but it may increase the presentation of some peptides. PA28 does not affect rates of protein hydrolysis by the proteasome but may reduce the size of peptides generated.

Translation of self or pathogen-derived mRNAs in the cytoplasm generates not only properly folded proteins but also a significant quantity—possibly up to 30%—of peptides and proteins that are known as **defective ribosomal products (DRiPs)**. These include peptides translated from introns in improperly spliced mRNAs, translations of frameshifts, improperly folded cytoplasmic proteins, and membrane or secreted proteins that fail to enter the endoplasmic reticulum. Such proteins are tagged by ubiquitin for degradation by the proteasome. This seemingly wasteful process might help to generate peptide substrates from self proteins and proteins derived from pathogens for eventual presentation by MHC class I proteins.

6-3   Peptides from the cytosol are transported by TAP into the endoplasmic reticulum and further processed before binding to MHC class I molecules.

The polypeptide chains of proteins destined for the cell surface, such as the two chains of MHC molecules, are translocated during synthesis into the lumen of the endoplasmic reticulum, where two chains fold correctly and assemble with each other. This means the peptide-binding site of the MHC class I molecule is formed in the lumen of the endoplasmic reticulum and is never exposed to the cytosol. However, the antigen fragments that bind to MHC class I molecules are typically derived from proteins made in the cytosol. This raises the question: How are these peptides able to bind to MHC class I molecules and be delivered to the cell surface?

The answer was discovered through studies of mutant cell lines that had a defect in antigen presentation by MHC class I molecules. These cells expressed far fewer MHC class I proteins than normal on their surface despite normal synthesis of these molecules in the cytoplasm. The addition of synthetic peptides to the culture medium restored surface expression of MHC class I proteins, and it was hypothesized that these cells may have a defect in supplying peptides to MHC class I molecules during their assembly. These mutant cells were discovered to have defects in two genes that were members of the **ATP-binding cassette (ABC)** family of proteins that mediate the ATP-dependent transport of ions, sugars, amino acids, and peptides across membranes.

 MHC Class I Deficiency

The defective genes were named **Transporters associated with antigen processing-1 and -2 (*TAP1* and *TAP2*)**, and their protein products are normally associated with the endoplasmic reticulum membrane. Transfection of the mutant cells with correct versions of the defective genes restored the presentation of peptides by MHC class I molecules. The two TAP proteins form a heterodimer in the membrane (**Fig. 6.7**), and mutations in either TAP gene can prevent antigen presentation by MHC class I molecules. The genes *TAP1* and *TAP2* are located in the MHC locus (see Section 6-10), near *PSMB9* and *PSMB8*, and their basal level of expression is further enhanced by interferons produced in response to viral infection, similar to MHC class I and β1i, β2i, and β5i subunits of the proteasome. This induction results in increased delivery of cytosolic peptides into the endoplasmic reticulum. When this delivery of peptides is disrupted, as in *TAP*-mutant cells, newly synthesized MHC class I molecules are retained in a partially folded state in the endoplasmic reticulum. Rare human individuals with immunodeficiency due to defects in *TAP1* and *TAP2* also have few MHC class I molecules on their cell surfaces, a condition known as **MHC class I deficiency**.

Microsomal vesicles from nonmutant cells can mimic the endoplasmic reticulum in assays *in vitro* by internalizing peptides that then bind to MHC class I molecules present in the lumen of the microsome. In contrast, vesicles from TAP-1–deficient or TAP-2–deficient cells do not take up peptides. Peptide transport into normal microsomes requires ATP hydrolysis, confirming that the TAP-1:TAP-2 complex is an ATP-dependent peptide transporter. The TAP complex will transport peptides of between 8 and 16 amino acids in length and prefers to transport peptides that have hydrophobic or basic residues at the carboxyl terminus. Such residues at the carboxyl terminus are precisely the ones preferentially generated by the proteasome and needed for binding to MHC class I molecules (see Section 4-18). In addition to its carboxyl-terminal residue preference, the TAP transporter has a bias against proline in the first three amino acid residues; otherwise, there is no other known peptide-sequence specificity. Cytosolic peptides are short lived, and the vast majority

Fig. 6.7 TAP-1 and TAP-2 form a peptide transporter in the endoplasmic reticulum membrane. Upper panel: TAP-1 and TAP-2 are individual polypeptide chains, each with one hydrophobic and one ATP-binding domain. The two chains assemble into a heterodimer to form a four-domain transporter typical of the ATP-binding cassette (ABC) family. The hydrophobic transmembrane domains have multiple transmembrane regions (not shown here). The ATP-binding domains lie within the cytosol, whereas the hydrophobic domains project through the membrane into the lumen of the endoplasmic reticulum (ER) to form a channel through which peptides can pass. The middle and lower panels show surface representations of the TAP-1:TAP-2 heterodimer as determined by cryo-electron microscopy (cryo-EM), viewed from the side (middle panel) and from the cytoplasm (lower panel), the latter revealing a hollow channel through which peptides can pass.

Schematic diagram of the TAP complex

Lumen of ER

TAP-1   TAP-2

hydrophobic transmembrane domain

ER membrane

ATP-binding cassette (ABC) domain

Cytosol

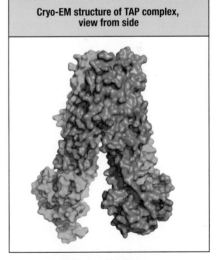

Cryo-EM structure of TAP complex, view from side

Cryo-EM structure of TAP complex, view from cytoplasm

of peptides generated by the proteasome are eventually destroyed. The discovery of TAP explained how viral peptides from proteins synthesized in the cytosol gain access to the lumen of the endoplasmic reticulum and are swiftly presented by MHC class I molecules.

The carboxyl terminus of peptide antigens appears to be produced by cleavage in the proteasome. However, the amino terminus of peptides that are too long to bind MHC class I molecules can be trimmed by an enzyme called the **endoplasmic reticulum aminopeptidase associated with antigen processing (ERAAP)**, also called **ERAP1**, and in humans by a second enzyme, **ERAP2**. Like other components of the antigen-processing pathway, expression of ERAP1 is increased by IFN-γ stimulation. ERAP1 strongly prefers peptides that are 9–16 residues in length, precisely those that are efficiently transported by TAP into the endoplasmic reticulum, but spares peptides of 8–9 amino acids. Mice lacking ERAP1 have an altered repertoire of peptides loaded onto MHC class I molecules. Although the loading of some peptides is not affected by the absence of ERAP1, other peptides fail to load normally, and many unstable and immunogenic peptides not normally present are found bound to MHC molecules on the cell surface, leading to defects in antigen presentation. Polymorphisms in the human ERAP1 gene are significant risk factors in some autoimmune diseases.

6-4 Newly synthesized MHC class I molecules are retained in the endoplasmic reticulum until they bind a peptide.

Binding a peptide is an important step in the assembly of a stable MHC class I molecule. The folding and assembly of a complete MHC class I molecule (see Fig. 4.16) requires that the MHC class I α chain, or heavy chain, associate first with β2-microglobulin and then with peptide. This process involves a number of accessory proteins with chaperone-like functions. Only after binding with peptide is the MHC class I molecule released from the endoplasmic reticulum and transported to the cell surface.

Newly synthesized MHC class I α chains that enter the endoplasmic reticulum membranes bind to **calnexin**, a general-purpose chaperone protein that retains the MHC class I molecule in a partly folded state (**Fig. 6.8**). Calnexin also associates with partly folded T-cell receptors, immunoglobulins, and MHC class II molecules, and so has a central role in the assembly of many immunological as well as non-immunological proteins. When β2-microglobulin binds to the α chain, the partly folded MHC class I α:β2-microglobulin heterodimer dissociates from calnexin and binds to an assembly of proteins called the MHC class I **peptide-loading complex (PLC)** (**Fig. 6.9**). One component of the PLC—**calreticulin**—is similar to calnexin and probably also has a general chaperone function, like calnexin. A second component of the complex is the TAP-associated protein **tapasin**, encoded by a gene within the MHC. Tapasin forms a bridge between MHC class I molecules and TAP, allowing the partly folded α:β2-microglobulin heterodimer to await the transport of a suitable peptide from the cytosol. A third component of this complex is the chaperone **ERp57**, a thiol oxidoreductase that forms a stable disulfide-linked heterodimer with tapasin (Fig. 6.9). While being covalently bound to tapasin, ERp57 plays a structural role in making additional interaction with calreticulin. Tapasin seems to be a component of the PLC that is specific to antigen processing, while calnexin, ERp57, and calreticulin bind various other glycoproteins assembling in the endoplasmic reticulum and seem to be part of the cell's general quality-control machinery. TAP itself is the final component of the PLC, and it delivers peptides to the partially folded MHC class I molecule.

ANIMATION 6.1

The loading of peptides into newly synthesized MHC class I relies on the glycoprotein quality-control machinery of the endoplasmic reticulum. This complex system of enzymes detects and modifies the state of *N*-linked glycans placed

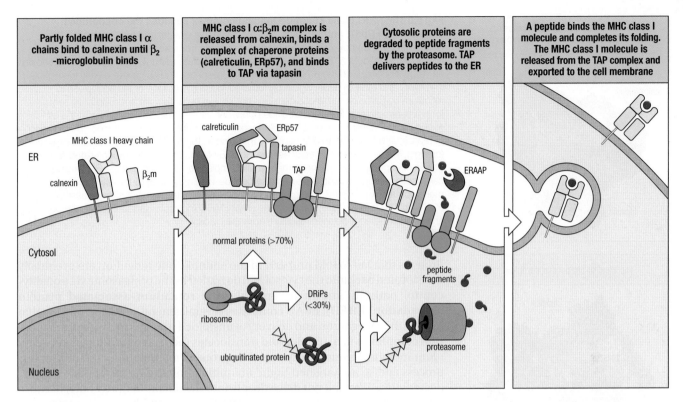

| Partly folded MHC class I α chains bind to calnexin until β₂-microglobulin binds | MHC class I α:β₂m complex is released from calnexin, binds a complex of chaperone proteins (calreticulin, ERp57), and binds to TAP via tapasin | Cytosolic proteins are degraded to peptide fragments by the proteasome. TAP delivers peptides to the ER | A peptide binds the MHC class I molecule and completes its folding. The MHC class I molecule is released from the TAP complex and exported to the cell membrane |

Fig. 6.8 MHC class I molecules do not leave the endoplasmic reticulum unless they bind peptides. Newly synthesized MHC class I α chains assemble in the endoplasmic reticulum (ER) with the membrane-bound protein calnexin. When this complex binds β₂-microglobulin (β₂m), the MHC class I α:β₂m heterodimer dissociates from calnexin, and the partly folded MHC class I molecule then binds to the TAP-associated protein tapasin. Two MHC:tapasin complexes may bind with the TAP dimer at the same time. The chaperone molecules ERp57 (which forms a heterodimer with tapasin) and calreticulin also bind to form the MHC class I peptide-loading complex. The MHC class I molecule is retained within the ER until released by the binding of a peptide, which completes the folding of the MHC molecule. Even in the absence of infection, there is a continual flow of peptides from the cytosol into the ER. Defective ribosomal products (DRiPs) and proteins marked for destruction by K48-linked polyubiquitin (yellow triangles) are degraded in the cytoplasm by the proteasome to generate peptides (red circles and teardrops) that are transported into the lumen of the endoplasmic reticulum by TAP. Some of these peptides will bind to MHC class I molecules. The aminopeptidase ERAAP (ERAP1) trims some peptides at their amino termini, allowing peptides that are too long (red teardrops) to bind to MHC class I molecules and thereby increasing the repertoire of potential peptides for presentation. Once a peptide has bound to the MHC molecule, the peptide:MHC complex leaves the endoplasmic reticulum and is transported through the Golgi apparatus and finally to the cell surface.

on newly synthesized proteins. The initial complex glycans placed on the MHC class I molecule are trimmed by enzymes into a **monoglucosylated glycan** that is the substrate for binding to calreticulin of the PLC. While bound to the PLC, the empty MHC molecule is receptive to binding peptides. Peptides binding with low affinity are continually exchanged for peptides of higher affinity in a process called **peptide editing**. This process continues until a peptide binds that allows for proper folding of the MHC class I molecule when it is released from the PLC. Properly folded peptide:MHC complexes are recognized by the enzyme **glucosidase II (GlsII)**, which then fully deglucosylates the MHC molecule. In this state, the peptide:MHC complex is no longer a substrate for binding to calreticulin, and it leaves the endoplasmic reticulum and is transported to the cell surface.

Recently, a second protein was discovered that functions in quality control of peptide:MHC complexes. This protein, called **TAPBPR** (encoded by the human TAPBPL gene), acts in the Golgi as a secondary sensor for proper protein folding in cooperation with the enzyme **UDP-glucose:glycoprotein glucosyltransferase 1 (UGT1)**. When TAPBPR binds an imperfectly folded peptide:MHC complex, it directs UGT1 to re-glucosylate the MHC, which causes the MHC to be transported back to the endoplasmic reticulum for further peptide editing by the PLC.

Side view of the calreticulin, tapasin, ERp57, and MHC chaperone complex

P domain

ERp57

calreticulin

MHC

tapasin

a

Top view of chaperone complex

tapasin

ERp57

MHC

calreticulin

b

Fig. 6.9 The MHC class I peptide-loading complex includes the chaperones calreticulin, ERp57, and tapasin. This model shows side (a) and top (b) views of the peptide-loading complex (PLC) oriented as it extends from the luminal surface of the endoplasmic reticulum. The newly synthesized MHC class I and β_2-microglobulin are shown as yellow ribbons, with the α helices of the MHC peptide-binding groove clearly identifiable. The MHC and tapasin (blue) would be tethered to the membrane of the endoplasmic reticulum by carboxyl-terminal extensions not shown here. Tapasin and ERp57 (green) form a heterodimer linked by a disulfide bond, and tapasin makes contacts with the MHC molecule that stabilize the empty conformation of the peptide-binding groove. The function of tapasin and ERp57 is to edit peptides that bind to the MHC class I molecule. Calreticulin (orange), like the calnexin it replaces (see Fig. 6.8), binds to the monoglucosylated N-linked glycan at asparagine 86 of the immature MHC molecule. The long, flexible P domain of calreticulin extends around the top of the peptide-binding groove of the MHC molecule to make contact with ERp57. The transmembrane region of tapasin (not shown) associates the PLC with TAP (see Fig. 6.8), bringing the empty MHC molecules into proximity with peptides arriving into the endoplasmic reticulum from the cytosol.

Proteins that fail to fold properly in the endoplasmic reticulum are eventually translocated back into the cytosol and degraded by the proteasome via a quality-control pathway known as **endoplasmic reticulum–associated protein degradation (ERAD)**. ERAD comprises several general cellular pathways that involve the recognition and delivery of misfolded proteins to a **retrotranslocation complex**, which unfolds and translocates them across endoplasmic reticulum membrane into the cytosol. The proteins are ubiquitinated during this process and so are targeted to the ubiquitin–proteasome system for eventual degradation. We shall not delve deeply into the details of ERAD here, because these pathways are not unique to MHC class I assembly or antigen processing. However, we will see in Chapter 13 how many viral pathogens co-opt the ERAD pathways to block assembly of MHC class I molecules as a way to evade recognition by CD8 T cells.

In uninfected cells, peptides derived from self proteins fill the peptide-binding groove of the mature MHC class I molecules and are carried to the cell surface. In normal cells, MHC class I molecules are retained in the endoplasmic reticulum for some time, which suggests that they are present in excess of peptide. This is important for the immunological function of MHC class I molecules, which must be immediately available to transport viral peptides to the cell surface if the cell becomes infected. In order for MHC class I molecules to display peptides derived largely from cytosolic proteins, it is important that peptides not dissociate and allow extracellular peptides to bind in the empty peptide-binding site. Fortunately, loss of peptides from MHC class I molecules causes them to dissociate from β_2-microglobulin and be internalized and degraded. Thus, empty MHC class I molecules are quickly lost from the cell surface, helping ensure that primed T cells target infected cells while sparing surrounding healthy cells.

6-5   Dendritic cells use cross-presentation to present exogenous proteins on MHC class I molecules so as to prime CD8 T cells.

The pathway described above explains how proteins synthesized in the cytosol can generate peptides that become displayed as complexes with MHC class I molecules on the cell surface. This pathway allows for the detection and destruction of pathogen-infected cells by cytotoxic T cells. But these cytotoxic T cells must first be activated and expanded by interacting with dendritic cells that express the same peptide:MHC class I complexes produced on infected cells. However, many pathogens exhibit a restricted **tropism** for different cell types, and not all viruses will infect dendritic cells. To help induce responses against such pathogens, some dendritic cells are able to generate peptide:MHC class I complexes from antigens that are derived from extracellular sources through a process called cross-presentation.

Cross-presentation was first observed in studies of **minor histocompatibility antigens**, which are polymorphic non-MHC molecules that can elicit strong responses between mice of different genetic backgrounds. In other words, polymorphic proteins from one background harbor peptides that are recognized as foreign by T cells in a second background. These studies used two different genetic backgrounds of mice, B10 and BALB, which differed in many such minor histocompatibility antigens. When spleen cells from B10 mice of MHC type H-2^b were injected into BALB mice of MHC type H-2$^{b \times d}$ (which express both b and d MHC types), the BALB mice generated cytotoxic T cells reactive against minor antigens of the B10 background. Some of these cytotoxic T cells recognized minor antigens presented by (or restricted by) the H-2^b B10 cells used for immunization (see Section 4-15). This result is expected if BALB T cells were directly activated by B10 antigen-presenting cells. But other cytotoxic T cells recognized minor B10 antigens presented only by H-2^d MHC cells. This meant that these CD8 T cells had been activated *in vivo* by minor B10 antigens presented by the BALB host's own H-2^d molecules. In other words, minor histocompatibility antigens from the original immunizing B10 cells must have been transferred to the BALB host's dendritic cells and processed for MHC class I presentation. We now know that cross-presentation by MHC class I molecules occurs not only for antigens on tissue or cell grafts, as in the original experiment described above, but also for viral and bacterial antigens, as well as tumor antigens.

The capacity for cross-presentation is not equally distributed across all antigen-presenting cells. The antigen-presenting cells that are responsible for activation and expansion of naive T cells are the conventional dendritic cells (cDCs), which exist in both humans and mice as two major lineages, now called cDC1 and cDC2. These two lineages rely on different factors for their development and express distinct sets of functional surface proteins, discussed in Chapter 9. In human and mouse, the cDC1 lineage is the major cross-presenting dendritic cell and is required for CD8 T-cell responses to many viruses and to tumors. This subset requires the transcription factor **BATF3** for its development, and mice lacking a functional BATF3 gene lack cDC1 and are also unable to generate normal CD8 T-cell responses to many viruses, including herpes simplex virus.

The biochemical pathways for cross-presentation by cDC1 *in vivo* are still unclear, but there is evidence supporting at least two pathways. In the cytosolic pathway, proteins captured by phagocytic receptors and taken into endosomes are transported into the cytosol by unknown mechanisms and degraded by the proteasome into peptides that then pass through TAP into the endoplasmic reticulum. Some evidence supports a **vacuolar pathway**, in which peptides are generated by unknown mechanisms within the endocytic compartment and loaded onto MHC class I molecules in phagosomes. In each case, one important specialization of cDC1 for cross-presentation is the efficient capture of cell-associated antigens by surface receptors. One such receptor is **CLEC9A**, which is selectively expressed by cDC1 and binds to actin filaments exposed on necrotic cells. This pathway may direct the efficient uptake and processing of viral proteins from cells killed during viral infections for cross-presentation to CD8 T cells.

6-6 Peptide:MHC class II complexes are generated in acidified endocytic vesicles from proteins obtained through endocytosis, phagocytosis, and autophagy.

The immunological function of MHC class II molecules is to bind peptides generated in the intracellular vesicles of dendritic cells, macrophages, and B cells, and to present these peptides to CD4 T cells. The purpose of this pathway is different for each cell type. Dendritic cells primarily are concerned with activating and expanding naive CD4 T cells, while macrophages and B cells elicit various forms of helper activities from these activated CD4 T cells. For example, the intracellular vesicles of macrophages are the sites of replication for several types of pathogens, including the protozoan parasite *Leishmania* and the mycobacteria that cause leprosy and tuberculosis. Because these pathogens reside in membrane-enclosed vesicles, the proteins of these pathogens are not usually accessible to proteasomes in the cytosol. Instead, proteins derived from the pathogens are degraded by intravesicular proteases into peptide fragments that can bind to MHC class II molecules that pass through this compartment on their way from the endoplasmic reticulum to the cell surface. In this compartment, peptide:MHC class II complexes are formed and are then delivered to the cell surface, where they can be recognized by CD4 T cells. Section 11-6 describes in great detail how this interaction helps macrophages to contain and eliminate these intracellular pathogens.

Antigen processing for MHC class II molecules begins when extracellular pathogens and proteins are internalized into endocytic vesicles (**Fig. 6.10**). Proteins that bind to surface immunoglobulin on B cells and are internalized by receptor-mediated endocytosis are processed by this pathway. Larger particulate materials, such as fragments of dead cells, are internalized by phagocytosis, particularly by macrophages and dendritic cells. Soluble proteins, such as secreted toxins, are taken up by macropinocytosis. These proteins are delivered to endosomes, which become increasingly acidic as they progress into the interior of the cell, eventually fusing with lysosomes. Acidification of endosomes and lysosomes results from the action of a multimeric protein complex called a **V-type ATPase**. This complex resides on the cytosolic side of endosomes and lysosomes and contains membrane-associated components that allow the energy of ATP hydrolysis to drive protons from the cytosol into the endosome and lysosome, leading to their acidification.

Endosomes and lysosomes contain proteases, known as acid proteases, that are activated at low pH. Drugs such as chloroquine that prevent acidification of endosomes also inhibit the presentation of intravesicular antigens, suggesting that acid proteases are responsible for processing such antigens. These proteases include the cysteine proteases—so called because they use a cysteine in their catalytic site—known as **cathepsins** B, S, and L, of which L is the most active. Cathepsins S and L may be the predominant proteases in the processing of vesicular antigens; mice that lack cathepsin B or cathepsin D process antigens normally, whereas mice with no cathepsin S show some deficiencies, including in the vacuolar pathway of cross-presentation. Asparagine endopeptidase (AEP), a cysteine protease cleaving after asparagines, is important for processing some antigens, such as the tetanus toxin antigen for MHC class II presentation, but is not required in all cases where antigens contain asparagine residues near their relevant epitopes. It is likely that the overall

Fig. 6.10 Peptides that bind to MHC class II molecules are generated in acidified endocytic vesicles. In the case illustrated here, extracellular foreign antigens (red), such as bacteria or bacterial antigens, have been taken up by an antigen-presenting cell such as a macrophage or an immature dendritic cell (first panel). In other cases, the source of the peptide antigen may be bacteria or parasites that have invaded the cell to replicate in endocytic/phagocytic vesicles. In both cases, the antigen-processing pathway is the same. The pH of the early endosome containing the engulfed pathogens is neutral, unlike the acidic pH of the lysosome, which is acidic and contains active protease (second panel). By the action of a V-type ATPase (green), a multimeric assembly of many subunits (not shown), H+ ions are delivered into the early endosome, thereby activating proteases within the vesicle to degrade the engulfed material (third panel). At some point on their pathway to the cell surface, newly synthesized MHC class II molecules pass through such acidified vesicles and bind peptide fragments of the antigen, transporting the peptides to the cell surface (fourth panel).

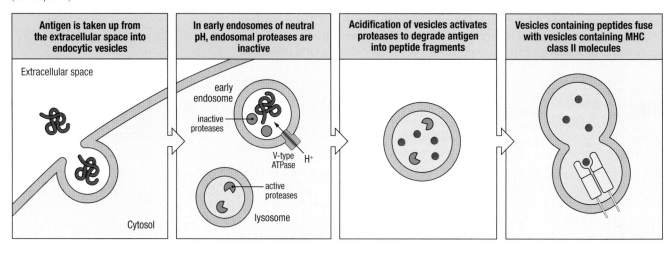

| Antigen is taken up from the extracellular space into endocytic vesicles | In early endosomes of neutral pH, endosomal proteases are inactive | Acidification of vesicles activates proteases to degrade antigen into peptide fragments | Vesicles containing peptides fuse with vesicles containing MHC class II molecules |

repertoire of peptides produced within the vesicular pathway reflects the activities of the many proteases present in endosomes and lysosomes. The breaking of intramolecular disulfide bonds also facilitates the proteolysis of proteins, which is carried out by the enzyme **IFN-γ–induced lysosomal thiol reductase (GILT)** present in endosomes. The various endosomal proteases act in a largely redundant and nonspecific manner to digest regions of the polypeptide that have become accessible to proteolysis by denaturation and previous steps of degradation. The peptides generated vary in sequence and abundance throughout the endocytic pathway, so that MHC class II molecules can bind and present many different peptides from these compartments. Self peptides bound to MHC class II molecules arise from common proteins in the cytosol, including cell membrane proteins. Cytosolic proteins can be processed for MHC class II presentation by the natural process of protein turnover known as autophagy, in which damaged organelles and cytosolic proteins are delivered to lysosomes for degradation. Here their peptides could encounter MHC class II molecules present in the lysosome membranes, and the resulting peptide:MHC class II complex could be transported to the cell surface via endolysosomal tubules (see Fig. 6.4). Autophagy has been shown to be involved in the processing of the Epstein–Barr virus nuclear antigen 1 (EBNA-1) for presentation on MHC class II molecules. Such presentation enables cytotoxic CD4 T cells to recognize and kill B cells infected with Epstein–Barr virus.

6-7 The invariant chain directs newly synthesized MHC class II molecules to acidified intracellular vesicles.

The biosynthetic pathway for MHC class II molecules begins with their translocation into the endoplasmic reticulum. However, the endoplasmic reticulum also contains peptides transported there by TAP as well as unfolded and partly folded polypeptide chains. To prevent premature binding of these peptides to newly synthesized MHC class II molecules, a specific membrane protein known as the MHC class II–associated **invariant chain (Ii, CD74)** is expressed in dendritic cells, macrophages, and B cells. Ii is a type II membrane glycoprotein; its amino terminus resides in the cytosol, and its transmembrane region spans the membrane of the endoplasmic reticulum (**Fig. 6.11**). The remainder of Ii and its carboxyl terminus reside within the endoplasmic reticulum. Ii has a unique cylindrical domain that mediates formation of stable Ii trimers. Near

Fig. 6.11 The invariant chain is cleaved to leave a peptide fragment, CLIP, bound to the MHC class II molecule. A model of the trimeric invariant chain bound to MHC class II αβ heterodimers is shown on the left. The CLIP portion is shown in purple, the rest of the invariant chain is shown in green, and the MHC class II molecules are shown in yellow (model, and leftmost of the three panels). In the endoplasmic reticulum, the invariant chain (Ii) binds to MHC class II molecules with the CLIP section of its polypeptide chain lying along the peptide-binding groove. After transport into an acidified vesicle, Ii is cleaved, initially just at one side of the MHC class II molecule (center panel), first by non-cysteine proteases to give a remaining portion of Ii known as the leupeptin-induced peptide LIP22 (not shown) and then by cysteine protease to give the LIP10 fragment shown. LIP10 retains the transmembrane and cytoplasmic segments that contain the signals that target Ii:MHC class II complexes to the endosomal pathway. Subsequent cleavage (right panel) of LIP10 leaves only a short peptide still bound by the MHC class II molecule; this peptide is the CLIP fragment.

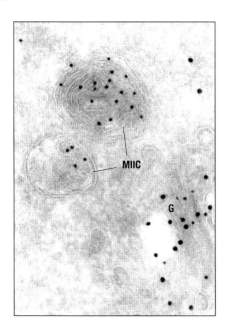

Fig. 6.12 MHC class II molecules are loaded with peptide in a late endosomal compartment. MHC class II molecules are transported from the Golgi apparatus (labeled G in this electron micrograph of an ultrathin section of a B cell) to the cell surface via intracellular vesicles each of which is called an MHC class II compartment (MIIC). These vesicles have a complex morphology, showing internal vesicles and sheets of membrane. This image used antibodies labeled with different-sized gold particles to identify the presence of both MHC class II molecules (visible as small dark spots) and the invariant chain (large dark spots). Large and small spots are seen in the Golgi, indicating both proteins are present there. In contrast, only MHC class II molecules are detectable in the MIIC. This compartment is thought to be a late endosome, an acidified compartment of the endocytic system (pH 4.5–5) in which the invariant chain is cleaved and peptide loading occurs. Magnification ×135,000.

this domain, Ii contains a peptide sequence, the **class II–associated invariant chain peptide (CLIP)**, with which each Ii subunit of the trimer binds noncovalently to an MHC class II αβ heterodimer. Each Ii subunit binds to an MHC class II molecule with CLIP lying within the peptide-binding groove, thus blocking the groove and preventing the binding of either peptides or partly folded proteins. The binding site of an MHC class II molecule is relatively open compared to the binding site of an MHC class I molecule. This allows MHC class II molecules to allow the CLIP region of Ii to pass through their binding sites more easily. While this complex is being assembled in the endoplasmic reticulum, its component parts are associated with calnexin. Only when a nine-chain complex—three Ii chains, three α chains, and three β chains—has been assembled is the complex released from calnexin for transport out of the endoplasmic reticulum. As part of the nine-chain complex, the MHC class II molecules cannot bind peptides or unfolded proteins, so that peptides present in the endoplasmic reticulum are not usually presented by MHC class II molecules. There is evidence that in the absence of Ii, many MHC class II molecules become aggregated and are retained in the endoplasmic reticulum as complexes with misfolded proteins.

Trafficking of membrane proteins is controlled by cytosolic sorting tags. In this regard, Ii has a second function, which is to target delivery of the MHC class II molecules to a low-pH endosomal compartment where peptide loading can occur. The complex of MHC class II αβ heterodimers with Ii trimers is retained for 2–4 hours in this compartment (see Fig. 6.11). During this time, the Ii molecule undergoes an initial cleavage by acid proteases to remove the trimerization domain, generating a truncated 22-kDa fragment of Ii called **LIP22**. LIP22 is further cleaved by cysteine proteases into a 10-kDa fragment called **LIP10**, which is composed of CLIP at one end and a transmembrane region at the other. The CLIP segment binds to the MHC class II molecule while its transmembrane region retains it in the proteolytic compartment. A subsequent cleavage of LIP10 releases CLIP, which remains bound to the MHC class II molecule. This cleavage is carried out by cathepsin S in most MHC class II–positive cells but by cathepsin L in thymic epithelial cells. Because CLIP does not carry the Ii-encoded signals that retain the complex in the endocytic compartment, the MHC:CLIP complex is now free to escape this compartment, but it cannot yet bind other peptides.

Newly synthesized MHC class II molecules are brought toward the cell surface in vesicles, most of which fuse with incoming endosomes at some point. However, some MHC class II:Ii complexes can first be transported to the cell surface and reinternalized into endosomes. In each case, MHC class II:Ii complexes enter the endosomal pathway, where they encounter and bind peptides derived from either internalized pathogen proteins or self proteins. Initially, specialized endosomal compartments were thought to exist for antigen-presenting cells. One was an early endosomal compartment in dendritic cells that was called the **CIIV (MHC class II vesicle)**. Another, a late endosomal compartment containing Ii and MHC class II molecules, was called the **MHC class II compartment, or MIIC (Fig. 6.12)**. The current view is that MHC class II molecules use many common endocytic compartments, including lysosomes, to allow for the exchange of CLIP for other peptides. MHC class II molecules that do not bind peptide after dissociation from CLIP are unstable in the acidic pH after fusion with lysosomes, and they are rapidly degraded.

6-8 The MHC class II–like molecules HLA-DM and HLA-DO regulate exchange of CLIP for other peptides.

To allow other peptides to bind to the MHC class II molecule, CLIP must either dissociate or be displaced. Antigen-presenting cells possess a mechanism that facilitates this process, which was discovered by studies of mutant human

| Invariant chain (Ii) forms a complex with MHC class II molecule, blocking the binding of peptides and misfolded proteins | Ii is cleaved in an acidified endosome, leaving a short peptide fragment, CLIP, still bound to the MHC class II molecule | Endocytosed antigens are degraded to peptides in endosomes, but the CLIP peptide blocks the binding of peptides to MHC class II molecules | HLA-DM binds to the MHC class II molecule, releasing CLIP and allowing other peptides to bind. The MHC class II molecule then travels to the cell surface |

Fig. 6.13 HLA-DM facilitates the loading of antigenic peptides onto MHC class II molecules. First panel: The invariant chain (Ii) binds to newly synthesized MHC class II molecules and blocks peptides from binding class II molecules in the endoplasmic reticulum and during their transport to acidified endosomes. Second panel: In late endosomes, proteases cleave the invariant chain, leaving CLIP bound to the MHC class II molecules. Third panel: Pathogens and their proteins are broken down into peptides within acidified endosomes, but these peptides cannot bind to MHC class II molecules that are occupied by CLIP. Fourth panel: The class II–like molecule HLA-DM binds to MHC class II:CLIP complexes, catalyzing the release of CLIP and the binding of antigenic peptides.

B-cell lines with a defect in antigen presentation. MHC class II molecules in these mutant cells assemble correctly with Ii and seem to follow the normal vesicular route, but fail to bind peptides derived from internalized proteins and often arrive at the cell surface with the CLIP peptide still bound. The defect in these cells lies in an MHC class II–like molecule called **HLA-DM** in humans (**H-2DM** in mice). The HLA-DM genes, *HLA-DMA* and *HLA-DMB*, encode an α chain and a β chain, respectively, which form a heterodimer closely resembling other MHC class II molecules. The HLA-DM molecule is not present at the cell surface, however, but is found predominantly in the endosomal compartment that contains Ii and MHC class II molecules. HLA-DM binds to and stabilizes empty MHC class II molecules and catalyzes the release of CLIP, thus allowing the binding of other peptides to the empty MHC class II molecule (**Fig. 6.13**). The HLA-DM molecule does not contain the open groove found in other MHC class II molecules, so it does not bind peptides. Instead, HLA-DM binds to the α chain of the MHC class II molecule near the region of the floor of the peptide-binding site (**Fig. 6.14**). This binding induces changes in the

Fig. 6.14 HLA-DM and HLA-DO regulate loading of peptides into MHC class II molecules. First panel: The HLA-DM dimer, composed of α (green) and β (turquoise) chains, binds to the HLA-DR MHC class II molecule (side view). HLA-DM contacts the MHC molecule near the peptide-binding groove where the peptide amino terminus would reside. Second panel: HLA-DO binds to HLA-DM in a similar configuration as HLA-DR, thus blocking HLA-DM's peptide-editing activity. Third panel: Top view of HLA-DR with bound peptide in the absence of HLA-DM. Fourth panel: Top view of HLA-DR with HLA-DM bound. The amino-terminal end of the MHC peptide-binding groove is open and devoid of bound peptide, enabling peptide exchange.

| HLA-DM bound to HLA-DR | HLA-DM bound to HLA-DO | HLA-DR binding a peptide | HLA-DM bound to HLA-DR |

ANIMATION 6.2

structure of the MHC class II molecule and holds this part of the peptide-binding groove in a partially 'open' configuration (see Fig. 6.14, right panel). In this way, HLA-DM catalyzes the release of CLIP from MHC class II molecules and the exchange for other peptides contained in the endosomal compartment.

In the presence of a mixture of peptides capable of binding to MHC class II molecules, HLA-DM forms a stable complex that lacks a bound peptide. Peptides rapidly bind to and then release from this complex, but only high-affinity peptides can induce DM dissociation from MHC class II proteins. Antigens presented by MHC class II molecules may have to persist on the surface of antigen-presenting cells for some days before encountering T cells able to recognize them. The ability of HLA-DM to remove unstably bound peptides, sometimes called peptide editing (see Section 6-4), ensures that the peptide:MHC class II complexes displayed on the surface of the antigen-presenting cell can survive long enough to stimulate the appropriate CD4 T cells. During this process, it is likely that some peptides are captured first as longer polypeptides that undergo amino-terminal trimming by exopeptidases, further increasing the number of possible peptides that can be bound.

Binding of longer polypeptides is probably more prominent in early endosomal compartments where antigen degradation is more limited. Allowing the binding of epitopes contained in long polypeptides also helps protects them from degradation.

A second atypical MHC class II molecule, called **HLA-DO** in humans (**H-2O** in mice), is produced in thymic epithelial cells, B cells, and dendritic cells. This molecule is a heterodimer of the HLA-DOα chain and the HLA-DOβ chain. HLA-DO is not present at the cell surface, being found only in intracellular vesicles, and it does not seem to bind peptides. HLA-DO acts as a negative regulator of HLA-DM. HLA-DO binds to HLA-DM in the same manner as MHC class II molecules (see Fig. 6.14), and it must be bound to HLA-DM in order to leave the endoplasmic reticulum. When the DM–DO dimer reaches an acidified endocytic compartment, HLA-DO appears to dissociate slowly from HLA-DM, which is then free to catalyze peptide editing for MHC class II molecules. Moreover, IFN-γ increases the expression of HLA-DM, but not of the HLA-DOβ chain. Thus, during inflammatory responses, IFN-γ produced by T cells and NK cells can increase the expression of HLA-DM, and so overcome the inhibitory effects of HLA-DO. The loss of HLA-DO in mice does not dramatically alter adaptive immunity but does cause a spontaneous production of autoantibodies with age. Proteins captured by the B-cell receptor (BCR) are normally delivered to acidic endosomal compartments where, in the absence of HLA-DO, HLA-DM facilitates the loading of peptides from these proteins onto MHC class II molecules. But loss of HLA-DO may allow loading of peptides derived from proteins not captured by the BCR. Further, because thymic epithelial cells function in the selection of developing CD4 T cells, their expression of HLA-DO may influence the repertoire of self peptides that these T cells encounter at different stages, as discussed further in Chapter 8.

The peptide editing conferred by HLA-DM and the removal of unstable MHC class II molecules provide important safeguards. To reveal the presence of an intracellular pathogen, the peptide:MHC complex must be stable at the cell surface. If peptides were to dissociate too readily, an infected cell could escape detection, and if peptides could too easily be acquired from other cells, then healthy cells might be mistakenly targeted for destruction. Tight binding of peptides to MHC molecules reduces the chance of these unwanted outcomes.

Just as specialized mechanisms for loading peptides onto MHC molecules have evolved, pathogens have evolved strategies to inhibit the loading of peptides onto MHC molecules. We will return to these topics in Chapter 13 when we discuss pathogen immunoevasion mechanisms.

6-9 Cessation of MHC class II antigen processing occurs after dendritic-cell activation through reduced expression of the MARCH-1 E3 ligase.

To enhance the presentation of peptides derived from pathogens, there is a specific mechanism that prolongs the lifetime of peptide:MHC complexes being formed at the same time as innate signals are received indicating possible infection. Dendritic cells that have not yet been activated by infection carry out active surveillance of the antigens in their location; for example, through macropinocytosis of soluble proteins. Peptides derived from such proteins are continually processed and loaded onto MHC class II molecules for expression on the cell surface. These peptide:MHC complexes are continually being endocytosed from the cell surface. They can be recycled to the surface again, but the majority is degraded by ubiquitination and proteasomal degradation. To support ubiquitination, MHC class II molecules contain a conserved lysine residue in the cytoplasmic tails of the β chain; this lysine residue is a target of an **E3 ligase** (see Section 3-7) called **membrane-associated ring finger (C3HC4) 1, or MARCH-1**, expressed in B cells, dendritic cells, and macrophages. MARCH-1 is expressed constitutively in B cells and induced by the cytokine IL-10 in other cells. It resides in the membrane of a recycling endosomal compartment, where it ubiquitinates the cytoplasmic tail of MHC class II molecules, leading to their eventual degradation in lysosomes, thereby regulating their steady-state level of expression (**Fig. 6.15**). MARCH-1–dependent degradation targets even high-affinity peptide:MHC complexes, so that the peptides represented on the cell surface are continually renewed. Thymic epithelial cells (TECs) also express MHC class II molecules but use MARCH-8 to regulate its degradation. In TECs, the membrane protein CD83 binds to MARCH-8 and prevents its degradation of MHC class II. Mice lacking CD83 have reduced expression of MHC class II protein on the surface of TECs, causing reduced positive selection of CD4 T cells (see Section 6-13 and Chapter 8). This effect illustrates why fine-tuning surface expression and half-life of MHC II molecules is important.

Fig. 6.15 Activation of dendritic cells reduces MARCH-1 expression, thus increasing the lifetime of MHC molecules. Before activation by innate recognition of pathogens, dendritic cells express the membrane-associated E3 ligase MARCH-1, which resides in the recycling endosomes compartment. There it attaches K48-linked ubiquitin chains to the β chain of MHC class II molecules. This causes MHC molecules to move out of the recycling endosomes and eventually to be degraded, leading to a reduced overall half-life and level of MHC expression on the cell surface. Signals emanating from innate sensors, such as TLR-4, reduce the level of MARCH-1 mRNA, and with the half-life of MARCH-1 now being short, MHC molecules are free to accumulate on the cell surface. Because innate signaling also triggers acidification of endocytic compartments and activates caspases associated with antigen processing, the MHC molecules that accumulate on the cell surface will bear peptides from the pathogens captured around the time of innate activation of the dendritic cells.

| In immature dendritic cells, MARCH-1 ubiquitinates MHC molecules, targeting them for degradation | Activation stops transcription of the MARCH-1 gene, increasing the lifetime of MHC molecules | MHC molecules accumulate on the cell surface, presenting peptides they acquired at the time of dendritic-cell activation |

When dendritic cells sense the presence of a pathogen in a peripheral tissue, they must first migrate to local lymph nodes in order to activate naive T cells (see Section 9-8); this may take many hours. Because continuous recycling limits the lifetime of peptide:MHC complexes on the cell surface, pathogen-derived peptide:MHC complexes might be lost during this migration, preventing T-cell activation. To prevent this situation, activated dendritic cells undergo a process of maturation in which transcription of the MARCH-1 gene is shut off. Because the MARCH-1 protein half-life is only around 30 minutes, activated dendritic cells soon accumulate peptide:MHC complexes on their cell surface produced at the time of encounter with pathogen. Another gene turned off during dendritic-cell maturation is the transcriptional activator CIITA (see Section 6-10), which is required for expression of MHC class genes. Shutting off CIITA therefore helps prevent the production of new MHC molecules after the dendritic cell leaves the site of infection.

In addition to regulating MHC class II expression in dendritic cells, MARCH-1 similarly regulates expression in dendritic cells of the co-stimulatory molecule (see Section 1-15) **CD86** (or **B7-2**), which like MHC class II molecules is also regulated by ubiquitination. This means by the time dendritic cells arrive at lymph nodes, they express peptides derived from the pathogens that activated them and have higher CD86 levels that provide signals for greater CD4 T-cell activation. However, we will see in Chapter 13 that viral pathogens have taken advantage of this pathway by producing MARCH-1–like proteins, which primarily down-regulate MHC class I molecules in the endoplasmic reticulum as a means of evading adaptive immunity.

Summary.

The ligand recognized by the T-cell receptor is a peptide bound to an MHC molecule. MHC class I and MHC class II molecules acquire peptides at different intracellular sites and activate CD8 and CD4 T cells, respectively. Infected cells presenting peptides derived from virus replication in the cytosol are thus recognized by cytotoxic CD8 T cells, which are specialized to kill any cells displaying foreign antigens. MHC class I molecules are synthesized in the endoplasmic reticulum and typically acquire their peptides at this location. The peptides loaded onto MHC class I molecules are derived from proteins degraded in the cytosol by the proteasome, transported into the endoplasmic reticulum by the heterodimeric ATP-binding protein TAP, and further processed by the aminopeptidase ERAP1 before being loaded onto the MHC molecules. Peptide binding to MHC class I molecules is required for them to be released from chaperones in the endoplasmic reticulum and to travel to the cell surface. A specific type of dendritic cell, the cDC1, is able to load peptides derived from exogenous proteins onto MHC class I molecules in a process known as cross-presentation. This ability ensures that CD8 T cells can be expanded and activated against even those pathogens that may not directly infect dendritic cells.

MHC class II molecules do not acquire their peptide ligands in the endoplasmic reticulum, because the invariant chain (Ii) first inserts CLIP into their peptide-binding groove. Association with Ii targets these MHC molecules to an acidic endosomal compartment where active proteases cleave Ii, and HLA-DM helps to catalyze dissociation of CLIP. The MHC molecules can then associate with peptides derived from proteins that have entered the vesicular compartments of macrophages, dendritic cells, or B cells. The process of autophagy can deliver cytosolic proteins to the vesicular system for presentation by MHC class II molecules. The CD4 T cells that recognize peptide:MHC class II complexes have a variety of specialized effector activities. Subsets of CD4 T cells activate macrophages to kill the intravesicular pathogens they harbor, help B cells to secrete immunoglobulins against foreign molecules, and regulate immune responses. Dendritic cells possess mechanisms that help prolong the lifetime of peptide:MHC complexes produced at the time of infection. MARCH-1 expressed by immature dendritic cells causes the continual turnover of peptide:MHC class II molecules. MARCH-1 expression is shut off when a dendritic cell senses infection, leading to increased lifetime and levels of peptide:MHC class II molecules representative of antigens present when pathogens were initially detected.

The major histocompatibility complex and its function.

The function of MHC molecules is to bind peptide fragments derived from pathogens and display them on the cell surface for recognition by the appropriate T cells. The consequences are almost always deleterious to the pathogen—virus-infected cells are killed, macrophages are activated to kill bacteria living in their intracellular vesicles, and B cells are activated to produce antibodies that eliminate or neutralize extracellular pathogens. Thus, there is strong selective pressure in favor of any pathogen that has mutated in such a way that it escapes presentation by an MHC molecule.

Two separate properties of the MHC make it difficult for pathogens to evade immune responses in this way. First, the MHC is **polygenic**: it contains several different MHC class I and MHC class II genes, so that every individual possesses a set of MHC molecules with different ranges of peptide-binding specificities. Second, the MHC is highly **polymorphic**; that is, there are multiple variants, or alleles, of each gene within the population as a whole. The MHC genes are, in fact, the most polymorphic genes known. In this part of the chapter we describe the organization of the genes in the MHC and discuss how the variation in MHC molecules arises. We also consider how the effect of polygeny and polymorphism on the range of peptides that can be bound contributes to the ability of the immune system to respond to the multitude of different and rapidly evolving pathogens.

6-10 Many proteins involved in antigen processing and presentation are encoded by genes within the MHC.

The MHC is located on chromosome 6 in humans and chromosome 17 in the mouse and extends over at least 4 million base pairs. In humans, it contains more than 200 genes. As work continues to define the genes within and around the MHC, it becomes difficult to establish precise boundaries for this genetic region, which is now thought to span as many as 7 million base pairs. The genes encoding the α chains of MHC class I molecules and the α and β chains of MHC class II molecules are linked within the complex. **Figure 6.16** shows the general organization of the MHC class I and class II genes in human and mouse. In humans, these genes are called **human leukocyte antigen (HLA)** genes, because they were first discovered through antigenic differences between white blood cells from different individuals; in the mouse they are known as the **H-2 genes**. The mouse MHC class II genes were in fact first identified as genes that controlled whether an immune response was made to a given antigen and were originally called **Ir (immune response) genes**. Consequently, the mouse MHC class II A and E genes were referred to as *I-A* and *I-E* in the past. Although this terminology could be confused with MHC class I genes, it is still in use. Several genes encoding proteins primarily dedicated to antigen presentation are located outside the MHC, including genes for β_2-microglobulin, invariant chain, TAPBPR, cathepsin S, and MARCH-1.

Fig. 6.16 The genetic organization of the major histocompatibility complex (MHC) in humans and mice. The organization of the MHC genes is shown. In humans, the cluster is called HLA (short for human leukocyte antigen) and is on chromosome 6, and in mice, it is called H-2 (for histocompatibility) and is on chromosome 17. The organization is similar in both species, with separate clusters of MHC class I genes (red) and MHC class II genes (yellow). In mice, the MHC class I gene *H-2K* has been translocated relative to the human MHC, splitting the class I region in two. Both species have three main class I genes, which are called *HLA-A, HLA-B,* and *HLA-C* in humans, and *H-2K, H-2D,* and *H-2L* in the mouse. These encode the α chain of the respective MHC class I proteins, HLA-A, HLA-B, and so on. The other subunit of an MHC class I molecule, β₂-microglobulin, is encoded by a gene located on a different chromosome—chromosome 15 in humans and chromosome 2 in the mouse. The class II region includes the genes for the α and β chains (designated *A* and *B*) of the MHC class II molecules HLA-DR, -DP, and -DQ (*H-2A* and *H-2E* in the mouse). Also in the MHC class II region are the genes for the TAP-1:TAP-2 peptide transporter, the PSMB (or LMP) genes that encode proteasome subunits, the genes encoding the DMα and DMβ chains (*DMA* and *DMB*), the genes encoding the α and β chains of the DO molecule (*DOA* and *DOB*, respectively), and the gene encoding tapasin (*TAPBP*). The so-called class III genes encode various other proteins with functions in immunity (see Fig. 6.17). Several genes that encode proteins primarily or solely dedicated to antigen presentation but are located outside the MHC include genes for TAPBPR, cathepsin S, and MARCH-1.

There are three class I α-chain genes in humans, called *HLA-A, -B,* and *-C*. There are also three pairs of MHC class II α- and β-chain genes, called *HLA-DR, -DP,* and *-DQ*. In many people, however, the HLA-DR cluster contains an extra β-chain gene whose product can pair with the DRα chain. This means the three sets of genes can give rise to four types of MHC class II molecules. All the MHC class I and class II molecules can present peptides to T cells, but each protein binds a different range of peptides (see Sections 4-18 and 4-19). Thus, the presence of several different genes for each MHC class means that any one individual is equipped to present a much broader range of peptides than if only one MHC molecule of each class were expressed at the cell surface.

Figure 6.17 shows a more detailed map of the human MHC region. Many genes within this locus participate in antigen processing or antigen presentation or have other functions related to the innate or adaptive immune response. The two TAP genes lie in the MHC class II region near the proteasome PSMB8 and PSMB9 genes, whereas the gene encoding tapasin (*TAPBP*) lies at the edge of the MHC nearest the centromere. The genetic linkage of the MHC class I genes, whose products deliver cytosolic peptides to the cell surface, with the TAP, tapasin, and proteasome (*PSMB8, PSMB9, LMP2,* and *LMP5*) genes, whose products deliver cytosolic peptides into the endoplasmic reticulum, suggests that the entire MHC has been selected during evolution for antigen processing and presentation.

When cells are treated with the interferons IFN-α, -β, or -γ, there is a marked increase in the transcription of MHC class I α-chain and β₂-microglobulin genes and of the immunoproteasome, tapasin, and TAP genes. Type I interferons (IFN-α and IFN-β) are produced early in viral infections as part of the innate immune response (see Section 3-7), while IFN-γ is produced during T_H1 responses (see Section 9-14). The increase in MHC expression they produce helps all cells to process viral proteins and present the resulting virus-derived peptides on their surface (except for red blood cells). On dendritic cells, this helps to activate the appropriate T cells and initiate the adaptive immune response to the virus. The coordinated regulation of the genes encoding these components may be facilitated by the linkage of many of them in the MHC.

The HLA-DMA and HLA-DMB genes encoding the subunits of the HLA-DM molecule are clearly related to the MHC class II genes, as are the HLA-DOA and HLA-DOB genes encoding the subunits of HLA-DO. However, unlike

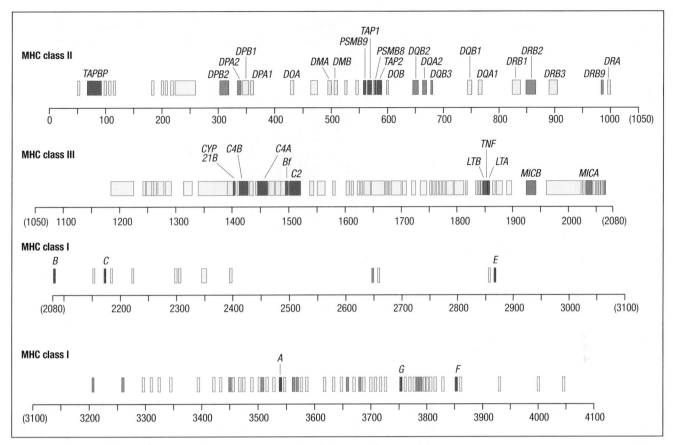

Fig. 6.17 Detailed map of the human MHC. The organization of the class I, class II, and class III regions of the human MHC is shown, with approximate genetic distances given in thousands of base pairs. Most of the genes in the class I and class II regions are mentioned in the text. The additional genes indicated in the class I region (for example, E, F, and G) are class I–like genes encoding class Ib molecules; the additional class II genes are pseudogenes. The genes shown in the class III region encode the complement proteins C4 (two genes, shown as *C4A* and *C4B*), C2, and factor B (shown as *Bf*), as well as the cytokines tumor necrosis factor-α (*TNF*) and lymphotoxin (*LTA*, *LTB*). Closely linked to the C4 genes is the gene encoding 21-hydroxylase (shown as *CYP 21B*), an enzyme involved in steroid biosynthesis. Immunologically important functional protein-coding genes identified in the text are color coded: the MHC class I genes are shown in red, except for the MHC class Ib (MIC) genes, which are shown in blue; these are distinct from the other class I–like genes and are under different transcriptional control. The immunologically important MHC class II genes are shown in yellow. Genes in the MHC region that have immune functions but are not related to the MHC class I and class II genes are shown in purple. Genes in dark gray are pseudogenes related to immune-function genes. Unnamed genes unrelated to immune function are shown in light gray.

conventional MHC genes, the genes encoding HLA-DM and HLA-DO are nonpolymorphic. These genes are found near the TAP and PSMB8/9 genes in the MHC class II region (see Fig. 6.16). Gene expression of the classical MHC class II proteins, along with the invariant chain, HLA-DMA, HLA-DMB, and HLA-DOA, but not HLA-DOB, is coordinately increased by IFN-γ, produced by T_H1 cells, CD8 T cells, and NK cells. This form of regulation allows dendritic cells and macrophages to increase processing of intravesicular antigens when presenting to T cells and NK cells. Expression of all these molecules is induced by IFN-γ (but not by IFN-α or -β) via the production of a protein known as **MHC class II transactivator (CIITA)**, which is a transcriptional co-activator of MHC class II genes. An absence of CIITA causes severe immunodeficiency due to the nonproduction of MHC class II molecules, a condition called **MHC class II deficiency**. Finally, the MHC contains many '**nonclassical' MHC genes**, so called because, while they resemble MHC genes in structure, their products do not function in presenting peptides to conventional αβ T cells. Many of these genes are now referred to as MHC class Ib genes, and their protein products have a variety of different functions, which we will describe later in Section 6-16, after we discuss the conventional MHC genes.

 MHC Class II Deficiency

Fig. 6.18 Human MHC genes are highly polymorphic. With the notable exception of the DRα locus, which is functionally monomorphic, each gene locus has many alleles. The number of functional proteins encoded is less than the total number of alleles. Shown in this figure as the heights of the bars are the number of different HLA proteins assigned by the WHO Nomenclature Committee for Factors of the HLA System as of September 2018.

6-11 The protein products of MHC class I and class II genes are highly polymorphic.

Because of the polygeny of the MHC, every person expresses at least three different MHC class Ia molecules and three (or sometimes four) MHC class II molecules on his or her cells. In fact, the number of different MHC molecules expressed by most people is greater because of the extreme polymorphism of the MHC (**Fig. 6.18**).

The term **polymorphism** comes from the Greek *poly*, meaning many, and *morphe*, meaning shape or structure. As used here, it means within-species variation at a gene, and thus in the gene's protein product; the variant genes that can occupy the locus are termed **alleles**. For several MHC class I and class II genes, there are more than 1000 alleles in the human population, vastly more than for any other gene in the genome. Because there are so many allelic variants present in the human population, there is only a small chance that an individual will have the same allele for a particular MHC gene on both homologous chromosomes; most individuals will be **heterozygous** for the genes encoding MHC class I and class II molecules. The particular combination of MHC alleles found on a single chromosome is known as an **MHC haplotype**. Expression of MHC alleles is **codominant**, meaning that the protein products of both of the alleles at a locus are expressed equally in the cell, and both gene products can present antigens to T cells. The number of known MHC alleles that do not code for a functional protein is remarkably small. The extensive polymorphism at each locus thus has the potential to double the number of different MHC molecules expressed in an individual and thereby increase the diversity already available through polygeny (**Fig. 6.19**). In fully heterozygous individuals, further diversity of MHC class II molecules arises from different allelic forms of the α chain pairing with the various allelic forms of the β chain.

The polymorphic nature of the MHC class II proteins causes their affinity for binding Ii and CLIP to vary among different MHC class II allotypes. Some allotypes do not require cathepsin S and/or HLA-DM to allow peptide binding and can replace LIP10 and CLIP with peptides without the sequence of events described in the several previous sections of this chapter. Thus some MHC class II alleles may be able to bind peptides/polypeptides in compartments where cathepsin S and HLA-DM activity or abundance is low, further increasing the repertoire of antigens available for sampling by MHC molecules.

Polymorphism	Polygeny	Polymorphism and polygeny

Fig. 6.19 Polymorphism and polygeny both contribute to the diversity of MHC molecules expressed by an individual. The high polymorphism of the classical MHC genes ensures diversity in MHC gene expression in the population as a whole. However, no matter how polymorphic a gene is, no individual can express more than two alleles at a single gene locus. Polygeny, the presence of several different related genes with similar functions, ensures that each individual produces a number of different MHC molecules. The combination of polymorphism and polygeny produces the diversity of MHC molecules seen both within an individual and in the population at large. Not shown in this figure are additional variations that result from the pairing of different alleles of α and β chains in the assembly of MHC class II molecules.

Because most individuals are heterozygous, most matings will produce off-spring that receive one of four possible combinations of the parental MHC haplotypes. Thus siblings are also likely to differ in the MHC alleles they express, there being one chance in four that an individual will share both hap-lotypes with a sibling. Sharing of alleles between unrelated individuals is even less frequent. Cells expressing different MHC alleles from a host are highly immunogenic. Therefore, one consequence of this extensive polymorphism is the difficulty of finding suitable donors for tissue transplantation, even among siblings (see Chapter 15).

All MHC class I and II proteins are polymorphic to a greater or lesser extent, with the exception of the DRα chain and its mouse homolog, Eα. These chains do not vary in sequence between different individuals and are said to be **monomorphic**. This might indicate a functional constraint that prevents vari-ation in the DRα and Eα proteins, but no such special function has been found. Many mice, both domestic and wild, have a mutation in the Eα gene that pre-vents synthesis of the Eα protein. They thus lack cell-surface H-2E molecules, so if H-2E does have a special function it is unlikely to be essential.

MHC polymorphisms at individual MHC genes seem to have been strongly selected by evolutionary pressures. Several genetic mechanisms contribute to the generation of new alleles. Some new alleles arise by point mutations and others by gene conversion, a process in which a sequence in one gene is replaced, in part, by sequences from a different gene (**Fig. 6.20.** The effects of selective pressure in favor of polymorphism can be seen clearly in the pattern of point mutations in the MHC genes. Point mutations can be clas-sified as replacement substitutions, which change an amino acid, or silent

Fig. 6.20 Gene conversion can create new alleles by copying sequences from one MHC gene to another. Multiple MHC genes of generally similar structure were derived over evolutionary time by duplication of an unknown ancestral MHC gene (gray) followed by genetic divergence. Further interchange between these genes can occur by a process known as gene conversion, in which sequences can be transferred from part of one gene to a similar gene. For this to happen, the two genes must become apposed during meiosis. This can occur as a consequence of the misalignment of the two paired homologous chromosomes when there are many copies of similar genes arrayed in tandem—somewhat like buttoning in the wrong buttonhole. During the process of crossing-over and DNA recombination, a DNA sequence from one chromosome is sometimes copied to the other, replacing the original sequence. In this way, several nucleotide changes can be inserted all at once into a gene and can cause several simultaneous amino acid changes in the gene product. Because of the similarity of the MHC genes to each other and their close linkage, gene conversion has occurred many times in the evolution of MHC alleles.

substitutions, which simply change the codon but leave the amino acid the same. Replacement substitutions occur within the MHC at a higher frequency relative to silent substitutions than would be expected, providing evidence that polymorphism has been actively selected for in the evolution of the MHC.

6-12 MHC polymorphism affects antigen recognition by T cells by influencing both peptide binding and the contacts between the T-cell receptor and MHC molecule.

The next few sections describe how MHC polymorphisms benefit the immune response and how pathogen-driven selection can account for the large number of MHC alleles. The products of individual MHC alleles, often known as protein **isoforms**, can differ from one another by up to 20 amino acids, making each variant protein quite distinct. Most of the differences are localized to exposed surfaces of the extracellular domain farthest from the membrane, and to the peptide-binding groove in particular (**Fig. 6.21**). We have seen that peptides bind to MHC class I and class II molecules through the interaction of specific anchor residues with peptide-binding pockets in the peptide-binding groove (see Sections 4-18 and 4-19). Non-anchor peptide residues can vary between all 20 amino acids. Many of the polymorphisms in MHC molecules alter the amino acids that line these pockets and thus change the pockets' binding specificities. This in turn changes the anchor residues of peptides that can bind to each MHC isoform. The set of anchor residues that allows binding

Fig. 6.21 Allelic variation in MHC molecules occurs predominantly within the peptide-binding region. Variability plots of the amino acid sequences of MHC molecules show that the variation arising from genetic polymorphism is restricted to the amino-terminal domains (α_1 and α_2 domains of MHC class I molecules and α_1 and β_1 domains of MHC class II molecules). The amino acid sequence is indicated across the bottom of each graph. Regions of high variability are indicated in red. Shown at the top are ribbon diagrams and schemata of the domains that form the peptide-binding groove and the MHC surface that interacts with the T-cell receptor (TCR). Allelic variability is clustered in specific sites within the amino-terminal domains, lying in positions that line the peptide-binding groove, either on the floor of the groove or inward from the walls, and on the helical surface that interacts with the TCR. For the MHC class II molecule, the variability of the HLA-DR alleles is shown. For HLA-DR, and its homologs in other species, the α chain is essentially invariant and only the β chain shows significant polymorphism (see Fig. 6.18). This is the exception; the α chains of HLA-DP and HLA-DQ are highly polymorphic.

to a given isoform of an MHC class I or class II molecule is called a **sequence motif**, and this can be used to predict peptides within a protein that might bind that variant (**Fig. 6.22**). Such predictions may be very important in designing peptide vaccines, as we will see in Chapter 16, where we discuss recent progress in cancer immunotherapy.

In rare cases, the processing of a protein does not generate any peptides with a suitable sequence motif for binding to any of the MHC molecules expressed by an individual. This individual fails to respond to the antigen. Such failures in responsiveness to simple antigens were first reported in inbred animals and were called Ir (immune response) gene defects. These defects were mapped to genes within the MHC long before the structure or

K^b MHC molecule binding ovalbumin peptide

	P1	P2	P3	P4	—	P5	P6	P7	P8
Ovalbumin (257–264)	S	I	I	N		F	E	K	L
HBV surface antigen (208–215)	I	L	S	P		F	L	P	L
Influenza NS2 (114–121)	R	T	F	S		F	Q	L	I
LCMV NP (205–212)	Y	T	V	K		Y	P	N	L
VSV NP (52–59)	R	G	Y	V		Y	Q	G	L
Sendai virus NP (324–332)	F	A	P	G	N	Y	P	A	L

K^d MHC molecule binding influenza virus peptide

	P1	P2	P3	P4	P5	P6	P7	P8	P9
Influenza NP (147–155)	T	Y	Q	R	T	R	A	L	V
ERK4 (136–144)	Q	Y	I	H	S	A	N	V	L
P198 (14–22)	K	Y	Q	A	V	T	T	T	L
P. yoelii CSP (280–288)	S	Y	V	P	S	A	E	Q	I
P. berghei CSP (25)	G	Y	I	P	S	A	E	K	I
JAK1 (367–375)	S	Y	F	P	E	I	T	H	I

Fig. 6.22 Different allelic variants of an MHC class I molecule bind different peptides. Shown are cutaway views of (a) ovalbumin peptide bound to the mouse H-2K^b MHC class I molecule and (b) influenza nucleoprotein (NP) peptide bound to the H-2K^d MHC class I molecule. The solvent-accessible surface of the MHC molecules is shown as a blue dotted surface. Class I MHC molecules typically have six pockets in the peptide-binding groove, which are conventionally called A–F. The bound peptides, shown as space-filling models, fit into the peptide-binding groove, with side chains from the anchor residues extending to fill the pockets. H-2K^b is binding SIINFEKL (single-letter amino acid code), a peptide of eight residues (P1–8) from ovalbumin, and H-2K^d is binding TYQRTRALV, a peptide of nine residues (P1–9) from the influenza nucleoprotein. Anchor residues (shown in yellow) may be primary or secondary in their influence on peptide binding. For H-2K^b, the sequence motif is determined by two primary anchors,

P5 and P8; the C pocket binds the P5 side chain of the peptide [a tyrosine (Y) or a phenylalanine (F)], and the F pocket binds the P8 residue [a nonaromatic hydrophobic side chain from leucine (L), isoleucine (I), methionine (M), or valine (V)]. The B pocket binds P2, a secondary anchor residue in H-2K^b. For H-2K^d, the sequence motif is primarily determined by the two primary anchors, P2 and P9. The B pocket accommodates a tyrosine side chain. The F pocket binds leucine, isoleucine, or valine. Beneath the structures are shown sequence motifs from peptides that are known to bind to the MHC molecule. CSP, circumsporozoite antigen; ERK4, extracellular signal-related kinase 4; HBV, hepatitis B virus; JAK1, Janus kinase 1; LCMV, lymphocytic choriomeningitis virus; NS2, NS2 protein; P198, modified tumor-cell antigen; *P. berghei*, *Plasmodium berghei*; *P. yoelii*, *Plasmodium yoelii*; VSV, vesicular stomatitis virus. An extensive collection of motifs can be found at http://www.syfpeithi.de.

function of MHC molecules was understood, and they were the first clue to the antigen-presenting function of MHC molecules. We now understand that Ir gene defects are common in inbred strains of mice because the mice are **homozygous** at all their MHC gene loci, which limits the range of peptides they can present to T cells. Ordinarily, MHC polymorphism guarantees a sufficient number of different MHC molecules in a single individual to make this type of nonresponsiveness unlikely, even to relatively simple antigens such as small toxins.

Early evidence linking Ir gene defects to the MHC was genetic; the MHC genotype determined whether guinea pigs could produce a T-cell response against a particular polypeptide. Likewise, mice of one MHC genotype could make antibody in response to a particular antigen, whereas mice of a different MHC genotype, but otherwise genetically identical, could not. The MHC genotype was somehow controlling the ability of the immune system to detect or respond to specific antigens. For their discovery of the MHC's relationship to Ir genes, Baruj Benacerraf, with George Davis Snell and Jean Dausset, were awarded the 1980 Nobel Prize.

However, it was not clear at the time how the immune responses were controlled by MHC molecules. Later experiments showed that the antigen specificity of T-cell recognition was controlled by MHC molecules. The immune responses affected by the Ir genes were known to depend on T cells, and this led to a series of experiments in mice to ascertain how MHC polymorphism might control T-cell responses. The earliest of these experiments showed that T cells could be activated only by macrophages or B cells that shared MHC alleles with the mouse in which the T cells originated. This was the first evidence that antigen recognition by T cells depends on the presence of specific MHC molecules in the antigen-presenting cell—the phenomenon we now know as **MHC restriction**.

We first mentioned MHC restriction in Section 4-20 in the context of the crystal structure of the T-cell receptor bound to peptide:MHC complexes. But the phenomenon of MHC restriction was discovered much earlier and is illustrated by the studies of virus-specific cytotoxic T cells carried out by Peter C. Doherty and Rolf M. Zinkernagel, for which they received the Nobel Prize in 1996. When mice are infected with a virus, they generate cytotoxic T cells that kill the virus-infected cells while sparing both uninfected cells and cells infected with unrelated viruses. The cytotoxic T cells are thus virus specific. The additional and striking outcome of these experiments was the demonstration that the ability of cytotoxic T cells to kill virus-infected cells was also affected by the polymorphism of MHC molecules. Cytotoxic T cells induced by viral infection in mice of MHC genotype a (MHC^a) would kill any MHC^a cell infected with that virus. But these same T cells would not kill cells of MHC genotype b, or c, and so on, even if they were infected with the same virus. In other words, cytotoxic T cells kill cells infected by virus only if those cells express the same MHC by which the T cells were primed. Because the MHC genotype 'restricts' the antigen specificity of the T cells, this effect was called MHC restriction. Together with the earlier studies on both B cells and macrophages, this work showed that MHC restriction is a critical feature of antigen recognition by all functional classes of T cells.

We now know that MHC restriction is due to the fact that the binding specificity of an individual T-cell receptor is not for its peptide antigen alone but for the complex of peptide and MHC molecule, as discussed in Section 4-15. MHC restriction is explained in part by the fact that different MHC molecules bind different peptides. In addition, some of the polymorphic amino acids in MHC molecules are located in the α helices that flank the peptide-binding groove but have side chains oriented toward the exposed surface of the peptide:MHC complex that can directly contact the T-cell receptor (see Figs. 6.21 and 4.28). In retrospect, then, it is not surprising

MHC restriction

T cell	T cell	T cell
TCR	TCR	TCR
MHCᵃ — x	MHCᵇ — x	MHCᵃ — y
antigen-presenting cell	antigen-presenting cell	antigen-presenting cell
Recognition	No recognition	No recognition

Fig. 6.23 T-cell recognition of antigens is MHC restricted. The antigen-specific T-cell receptor (TCR) recognizes a complex consisting of an antigenic peptide and a self MHC molecule. One consequence of this is a T cell specific for peptide x and an MHC molecule that is the product of a particular MHC allele, MHCᵃ (left panel), will usually not recognize the complex of peptide x bound to a different MHC allele product, MHCᵇ (center panel), or the complex of a different peptide, peptide y, bound to MHCᵃ (right panel). The co-recognition of a foreign peptide and an MHC molecule is known as MHC restriction because the particular MHC allele product is said to restrict the ability of the T cell to recognize antigen. This restriction is the result of the TCR binding the surface of the MHC and its bound peptides, which are highly variable because of MHC polymorphisms.

that T cells can distinguish between a peptide bound to MHCᵃ and the same peptide bound to MHCᵇ. This restricted recognition may sometimes be caused both by differences in the conformation of the bound peptide imposed by the different MHC molecules and by direct recognition of polymorphic amino acids in the MHC molecule itself. Thus, the specificity of a T-cell receptor is defined both by the peptide it recognizes and by the MHC molecule bound to it (**Fig. 6.23**).

6-13 Alloreactive T cells recognizing nonself MHC molecules are very abundant.

The discovery of MHC restriction also helped to explain the otherwise puzzling phenomenon of recognition of nonself MHC in the rejection of organs and tissues transplanted between members of the same species. Transplanted organs from donors bearing MHC molecules that differ from those of the recipient—even by as little as one amino acid—are rapidly rejected owing to the presence in any individual of large numbers of T cells that react to nonself, or **allogeneic**, MHC molecules. Early studies on T-cell responses to allogeneic MHC molecules used the **mixed lymphocyte reaction**, in which T cells from one individual are mixed with lymphocytes from a second individual. If the T cells of this individual recognize the other individual's MHC molecules as 'foreign,' the T cells will divide and proliferate. The lymphocytes from the second individual are usually prevented from dividing by irradiation or treatment with the cytostatic drug mitomycin C. Such studies have shown that roughly 1–10% of all T cells in an individual will respond to stimulation by cells from another, unrelated, member of the same species. This type of T-cell response is called an **alloreaction or alloreactivity**, because it represents the recognition of allelic polymorphisms in MHC molecules.

Before the role of the MHC molecules in antigen presentation was understood, it was a mystery why so many T cells should recognize nonself MHC molecules, as there is no reason that the immune system should have evolved a defense against tissue transplants. Once it was realized that T-cell receptors have evolved to recognize foreign peptides in combination with polymorphic MHC molecules, alloreactivity became easier to explain. We now know of at least two processes that can contribute to the high frequency of alloreactive T cells. The first is the process of **positive selection**. When developing in the thymus, T cells whose T-cell receptors interact weakly with the self MHC molecules receive survival signals, and so are favored for representation in the peripheral repertoire. It is thought that T-cell receptors that interact with one type of MHC molecule are more likely to cross-react with other (nonself) MHC variants. We discuss positive selection in greater detail in Chapter 8.

But positive selection is not the only basis for alloreactivity. This conclusion was implied by observations that T cells artificially driven to mature in animals lacking MHC class I and class II, in which positive selection in the thymus cannot occur, still display frequent alloreactivity. It appears that T-cell receptor genes encode the inherent ability to recognize MHC molecules. X-ray crystallographic studies of T-cell receptors bound to MHC molecules provide a structural basis for an inherent binding interaction (**Fig. 6.24**). Specific amino acid residues within the germline-encoded region of certain TCRβ genes interact with conserved features of the MHC molecule, implying a type of germline-encoded affinity. Given the large number of variable-region sequences in T-cell receptors, each T-cell receptor may bind MHC molecules in its own idiosyncratic way using both germline-encoded regions and variable regions.

In principle, alloreactivity of T cells against nonself MHC might depend on recognizing either a foreign peptide antigen bound to MHC or just the nonself MHC molecule alone; these options were called 'peptide-dependent' and 'peptide-independent' allorecognition. But as the number of individual alloreactive T-cell clones studied has increased, it seems that most alloreactive T cells actually recognize both; that is, most individual alloreactive T-cell clones respond to a foreign MHC molecule only when a particular peptide is bound to it. In this sense, the structural basis of allorecognition may be quite similar to normal MHC-restricted peptide recognition and dependent on contacts with both peptide and MHC molecule (see Fig. 6.23, left panel), but in this case, the MHC molecule is foreign. In practice, alloreactive responses against a transplanted organ are likely to represent the combined activity of many different alloreactive T cells. While it is not possible to determine what peptides from the donor might be involved in recognition by the alloreactive T cells, these would be an example of the minor histocompatibility antigens described in

Fig. 6.24 Germline-encoded residues in CDR1 and CDR2 of V-region genes confer on T-cell receptors an inherent affinity for MHC molecules. Shown is the structure for several T-cell receptors bound to a class II MHC molecule. Conserved residues (Lys39, Gln57, and Gln61) within the α₁ helix of the MHC (green) make an extended hydrogen-bonded network with germline-encoded and nonpolymorphic residues located in the CDR1 (Asn31) and CDR2 (Glu56, Tyr50) regions of the Vβ 8.2 gene, respectively. The configuration of these contacts is very similar between different structures, implying that the germline sequence of the CDR1 and CDR2 confers an inherent bias for T-cell receptor affinity for MHC.

Section 6-5. We will return to alloreactivity when we discuss organ transplantation in more detail in Chapter 15.

6-14   Many T cells respond to superantigens.

Superantigens are a distinct class of antigens that stimulate a primary T-cell response similar in magnitude to a response to allogeneic MHC molecules. Such responses were first observed in mixed lymphocyte reactions using lymphocytes from strains of mice that were MHC-identical but otherwise genetically distinct. The antigens provoking this reaction were originally designated as **minor lymphocyte stimulating (Mls) antigens**, and it seemed reasonable to suppose that they might be functionally similar to the MHC molecules themselves. We now know that this is not true. The Mls antigens in these mouse strains are encoded by retroviruses, such as the mouse mammary tumor virus, that have become stably integrated at various sites in the mouse chromosomes. Superantigens are produced by many different pathogens, including bacteria, mycoplasmas, and viruses, and the responses they provoke are helpful to the pathogen rather than the host.

Mls proteins act as superantigens because they have a distinctive mode of binding to both MHC and T-cell receptor molecules that enables them to stimulate very large numbers of T cells. Superantigens are unlike other protein antigens in that they are recognized by T cells without being processed into peptides that are captured by MHC molecules. Indeed, fragmentation of a superantigen destroys its biological activity, which depends on binding as an intact protein to the outside surface of an MHC class II molecule that has already bound peptide. In addition to binding MHC class II molecules, superantigens are able to bind the V_β region of many T-cell receptors (**Fig. 6.25**). Bacterial superantigens bind mainly to the V_β CDR2 loop and, to a lesser extent, to the V_β CDR1 loop and an additional loop called the hypervariable 4 (or HV4) loop. The HV4 loop is the predominant binding site for viral superantigens, at least for the Mls antigens encoded by the endogenous mouse mammary tumor viruses. Thus, the α-chain V region and the CDR3 of the β chain of the T-cell receptor have little effect on superantigen recognition, which is determined largely by the germline-encoded V gene segments that encode the expressed V_β chain. Each superantigen is specific for one or a few of the different V_β gene products, of which there are 20–50 in mice and humans; a superantigen can thus stimulate 2–20% of all T cells.

This mode of stimulation does not prime an adaptive immune response specific for the pathogen. Instead, it causes a massive production of cytokines by CD4 T cells, the predominant responding population of T cells. These cytokines have two effects on the host: systemic toxicity and suppression of the adaptive immune response. Both these effects contribute to microbial pathogenicity. Among the bacterial superantigens are the **staphylococcal enterotoxins (SEs)**, which cause food poisoning, and the **toxic shock syndrome toxin-1 (TSST-1)** of *Staphylococcus aureus*, the etiologic principle in **toxic shock syndrome**, which can be caused by a localized infection with toxin-producing strains of the bacterium. The role of viral superantigens in human disease is less clear.

 Toxic Shock Syndrome

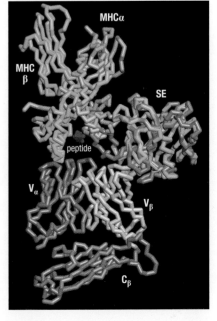

Fig. 6.25 Superantigens bind directly to T-cell receptors and to MHC molecules. Superantigens can bind independently to MHC class II molecules and to T-cell receptors. As shown in the top panels, the superantigens (red bars) can bind to the V_β domain of the T-cell receptor (TCR), away from the complementarity-determining regions, and to the outer faces of the MHC class II molecule, outside the peptide-binding site. In the bottom panel, a reconstruction of the interaction between a T-cell receptor, an MHC class II molecule, and a staphylococcal enterotoxin (SE) superantigen is shown by superimposing separate structures of an enterotoxin:MHC class II complex onto an enterotoxin:T-cell receptor complex. The two enterotoxin molecules (actually SEC3 and SEB) are shown in turquoise and blue, binding to the α chain of the MHC class II molecule (yellow) and to the β chain of the T-cell receptor (colored gray for the V_β domain and pink for the C_β domain).

6-15   MHC polymorphism extends the range of antigens to which the immune system can respond.

Most polymorphic genes encode proteins that vary by only one or a few amino acids, whereas the allelic variants of MHC proteins differ from each other by up to 20 amino acids. The extensive polymorphism of the MHC proteins has almost certainly evolved to outflank the evasive strategies of pathogens. The requirement that pathogen antigens must be presented by an MHC molecule provides two possible ways in which pathogens could evolve to evade detection. One is through mutations that eliminate from the pathogen's proteins all peptides able to bind MHC molecules. The Epstein–Barr virus provides an example. There are small isolated populations in southeast China and Papua New Guinea in which about 60% of the people carry the HLA-A11 allele. Many isolates of the Epstein–Barr virus obtained from these populations have mutations in a dominant peptide epitope normally presented by HLA-A11; the mutant peptides no longer bind to HLA-A11 and cannot be recognized by HLA-A11–restricted T cells. This strategy is clearly much less successful if there are many different MHC molecules, and the polygeny of the MHC may have evolved in response.

In addition, in large outbred populations, polymorphism at each locus can greatly increase the number of different MHC molecules expressed by an individual, as most individuals will be heterozygotes. Polymorphism has the additional advantage that individuals in a population will differ in the combinations of MHC molecules that they express and will therefore present different sets of peptides from each pathogen. This makes it unlikely that all individuals in a population will be equally susceptible to a given pathogen, and its spread will therefore be limited. The fact that exposure to pathogens over an evolutionary timescale can select for particular MHC alleles is indicated by the strong association of the HLA-B53 allele with recovery from a potentially lethal form of malaria. This allele is very common in people from West Africa, where malaria is endemic, and rare elsewhere, where lethal malaria is uncommon.

Similar arguments apply to a second strategy by which pathogens could evade recognition. Pathogens that can block the presentation of their peptides by MHC molecules can avoid the adaptive immune response. Adenoviruses encode a protein that binds to MHC class I molecules in the endoplasmic reticulum and prevents their transport to the cell surface, thus preventing the recognition of viral peptides by cytotoxic CD8 T cells. This viral MHC-binding protein interacts with a polymorphic region of the MHC class I molecule, as some allelic variants are retained in the endoplasmic reticulum by the adenoviral protein, whereas others are not. Increasing the variety of MHC molecules expressed reduces the likelihood that a pathogen will be able to block presentation by all of them and completely evade an immune response.

These arguments raise a question: If having three MHC class I loci is better than having one, why are there not far more? The probable explanation is that each time a distinct MHC molecule is added to the repertoire, all T cells that can respond to self peptides bound to that MHC molecule must be removed to maintain self-tolerance. It seems that the number of MHC genes present in humans and mice is about optimal to balance the advantages of presenting an increased range of foreign peptides with the disadvantages of losing T cells from the repertoire.

Summary.

The major histocompatibility complex (MHC) of genes consists of a linked set of genetic loci encoding many of the proteins involved in antigen presentation to T cells, most notably the MHC class I and class II glycoproteins (the MHC molecules) that present peptides to the T-cell receptor. The outstanding feature of the MHC molecules is their extensive polymorphism. This polymorphism is of critical importance in antigen recognition by T cells. A T cell recognizes antigen as a peptide bound by a particular allelic variant of an MHC molecule and will not recognize the same peptide bound to other MHC molecules. This behavior of T cells is called MHC restriction. Most MHC alleles differ from one another by multiple amino acid substitutions, and these differences are focused on the peptide-binding site and the surface-exposed regions that make direct contact with the T-cell receptor. At least three properties of MHC molecules are affected by MHC polymorphism: the range of peptides bound; the conformation of the bound peptide; and the direct interaction of the MHC molecule with the T-cell receptor. Thus, the highly polymorphic nature of the MHC has functional consequences, and the evolutionary selection for this polymorphism suggests that it is critical to the role of the MHC molecules in the immune response. Powerful genetic mechanisms generate the variation that is seen among MHC alleles, and a compelling argument can be made that selective pressure to maintain a wide variety of MHC molecules in the population comes from infectious agents. As a consequence, the immune system is highly individualized—each individual responds differently to a given antigen.

Recognition of nonpeptide ligands by unconventional T-cell subsets.

So far we have focused on how peptide:MHC complexes—the ligands for αβ T cells—are generated. We now turn to the question of how other types of T cells recognize their ligands and how these ligands are generated. Our current knowledge in this area is still incomplete, and this is perhaps most apparent in the area of γδ T cells, where a growing list of ligands for individual γδ T cells suggests an innate-like pattern of recognition. The recent discovery that mucosal-associated invariant T cells (MAIT cells; see Section 4-21) recognize microbial metabolites when they are presented by a nonpolymorphic MHC class I–like molecule solved a long-standing mystery regarding the specificity of this particular T-cell subset. Another subset, the invariant NKT cells, provides a system for detecting and responding to lipid rather than peptide antigens. These unconventional T cells respond rapidly, without the need for clonal expansion, and therefore operate somewhere between innate and adaptive immunity. In this part of the chapter, we will discuss the ligands they recognize and what is known about how they are generated or expressed.

6-16   A variety of genes with specialized functions in immunity are also encoded in the MHC.

In addition to the highly polymorphic 'classical' MHC class Ia proteins described earlier, there is a group of structurally related MHC class I–like proteins, the so-called 'nonclassical' MHC or MHC class Ib proteins. Some of these are encoded by genes located within the MHC, and others reside outside the MHC. By comparison with MHC class Ia proteins, MHC class Ib genes show little polymorphism. Many of these have yet to be assigned a function, and their exact number varies greatly among species and even among members of the same species. Like MHC class I proteins, many, but not all, associate with β_2-microglobulin when expressed on the cell surface. Their expression on cells is variable, both in the amount present at the cell surface and in tissue distribution. The characteristics of several MHC class Ib gene products are shown in **Fig. 6.26**.

One mouse MHC class Ib molecule, **H2-M3**, can present peptides with *N*-formylated amino termini, which is of interest because all bacteria initiate protein synthesis with *N*-formylmethionine (fMet). Cells infected with cytosolic bacteria can be killed by CD8 T cells that recognize *N*-formylated

	Class Ib molecule					Receptors or interacting proteins			
Human	Mouse	Expression pattern	Associates with β_2m	Poly-morphism	Ligand	T-cell receptor	NK receptor	Other	Biological function
HLA-C (class Ia)		Ubiquitous	Yes	High	Peptide	TCR	KIRs		Activate T cells / Inhibit NK cells
	H2-M3	Limited	Yes	Low	fMet peptide	TCR			Activate CTLs with bacterial peptides
	T22 T10	Splenocytes	Yes	Low	None	γδ TCR			Regulation of activated splenocytes
HLA-E	Qa-1	Ubiquitous	Yes	Low	MHC leader peptides (Qdm)		NKG2A NKG2C		NK-cell inhibition
HLA-F		Widely expressed	Yes	Low	Peptide?		LILRB1 LILRB2		Unknown
HLA-G		Maternal–fetal interface	Yes	Low	Peptide	TCR	LILRB1 LILRB2		Modulate maternal–fetal interaction
MIC-A MIC-B		Widely expressed	No	Moderate	None		NKG2D		Stress-induced activation of NK cells, γδ and CD8 T cells
	TL	Small intestine epithelium	Yes	Low	None	CD8αα			Potential modulation of T-cell activation
	M10	Vomeronasal neurons	Yes	Low	Unknown			Vomeronasal receptor V2R	Pheromone detection
ULBPs	MULT1, H60, Rae1	Limited	No	Low	None		NKG2D		Induced NK-cell–activating ligand
MR1	MR1	Ubiquitous	Yes	None	Riboflavin metabolites (vit B$_2$, vit B$_9$)	αβ TCR			Control of antimicrobial response
CD1a–CD1e	CD1d	Lymphocytes	Yes	None	Lipids glycolipids	αβ TCR			Activate T cells against bacterial lipids
	Mill1 Mill2	Ubiquitous	Yes?	Low	Unknown	Unknown			Unknown
HFE	HFE	Liver and gut	Yes	Low	None			Transferrin receptor	Iron homeostasis
FcRn	FcRn	Maternal–fetal interface	Yes	Low	None			Fc (IgG)	Shuttle maternal IgG to fetus (passive immunity)
ZAG	ZAG	Bodily fluid	No	None	Fatty acid				Lipid homeostasis
EPCR	EPCR	Endothelial cells	No	Low		γδ TCR		Protein C	Blood coagulation

(MHC encoded: rows HLA-C through M10; Non-MHC encoded: rows ULBPs through EPCR)

Fig. 6.26 Mouse and human MHC class Ib proteins and their functions. MHC class Ib proteins are encoded both within the MHC region and on other chromosomes. The functions of some MHC class Ib proteins are unrelated to the adaptive immune response, but many have a role in innate immunity by interacting with receptors on NK cells (see the text and Section 3-25). HLA-C, which is a classical MHC molecule (class Ia), is included here because, in addition to presenting peptides to T-cell receptors, all HLA-C isoforms interact with the KIR class of NK-cell receptors to regulate NK-cell function in the innate immune response. CTLs are cytotoxic T lymphocytes. FcRn, the neonatal Fc receptor, is discussed in Chapters 5 and 10, and TL (thymus leukemia antigen) is discussed in Chapter 12. The role of Mill1 (MHC I–like leukocyte 1) and Mill2 is still under investigation.

bacterial peptides bound to H2-M3. Whether an equivalent MHC class Ib molecule exists in humans is not known.

Two other closely related mouse MHC class Ib genes, *T22* and *T10*, are expressed by activated lymphocytes and are recognized by a subset of $\gamma\delta$ T cells. Although the precise purpose remains unclear, it has been proposed that this interaction allows $\gamma\delta$ T cells to regulate activated lymphocytes expressing T22 and T10 proteins.

The other genes that map within the MHC include some that encode complement components (for example, C2, C4, and factor B) and some that encode cytokines (for example, tumor necrosis factor and lymphotoxin)—all of which have important functions in immunity. These genes lie in the so-called 'MHC class III' region (see Fig. 6.17).

Many studies have established associations between susceptibility to certain diseases and particular alleles of MHC genes (see Chapter 15), and we now have considerable insight into how polymorphism in the classical MHC class I and class II genes can affect disease resistance or susceptibility. Most MHC-influenced traits or diseases are known or suspected to have an immunological cause, but this is not so for all of them: some genes residing within the MHC have no known or suspected immunological function. For example, the class Ib gene *M10* encodes a protein that functions in the vomeronasal organ as a chaperone to escort certain types of pheromone receptors to the cell surface. *M10* could potentially influence mating preference, a trait that has been linked to the MHC region in rodents.

The gene *HFE*, encoding the **hemochromatosis protein**, lies some 4 million base pairs from HLA-A. Its protein product is expressed in cells of the intestinal tract and acts in iron metabolism by regulating the uptake of dietary iron into the body. It seems to interact with the transferrin receptor and decrease the receptor's affinity for iron-loaded transferrin. Individuals defective for this gene have an iron-storage disease, **hereditary hemochromatosis**, in which an abnormally high level of iron is retained in the liver and other organs. Mice lacking β_2-microglobulin have defective expression of all class I molecules and thus also show a similar iron overload. Another MHC gene with a nonimmune function encodes the enzyme **21-hydroxylase**, which, when deficient, causes congenital adrenal hyperplasia and, in severe cases, salt-wasting syndrome. Even where a disease-related gene is clearly homologous to immune-system genes, as is the case with *HFE*, the disease mechanism may not be immune related. Disease associations mapping to the MHC must therefore be interpreted with caution, in the light of a detailed understanding of its genetic structure and the functions of its individual genes. Much remains to be learned about the significance of all the genetic variation localized within the MHC. For instance, the human complement component 4 (C4) comes in two versions, C4A and C4B, not to be confused with the C4 convertase cleavage products C4a and C4b, and different individuals have variable numbers of the gene for each type in their genomes, but the adaptive significance of this genetic variability is not well understood.

6-17   Specialized MHC class I molecules act as ligands for the activation and inhibition of NK cells and unconventional T-cell subsets.

In Sections 3-24 to 3-27, we introduced NK cells and briefly discussed their activation by members of the MIC gene family expressed by humans. These MHC class Ib genes are regulated differently from MHC class Ia genes and are induced in response to cellular stress (such as heat shock). There are seven MIC genes, but only two are expressed and produce protein products, **MIC-A and MIC-B** (see Fig. 6.26). They are expressed in fibroblasts and epithelial cells, particularly in intestinal epithelial cells, and have a role in innate immunity or in the induction of immune responses in circumstances in which interferons are not produced. The MIC-A and MIC-B proteins are recognized by the NKG2D receptor expressed by NK cells. But NKG2D is also expressed by γδ T cells and some CD8 T cells, and it can activate these cells to kill MIC-expressing targets. NKG2D is an 'activating' member of the NKG2 family of NK-cell receptors (see Fig. 3.40); its cytoplasmic domain lacks the inhibitory sequence motif found in other members of this family, which act as inhibitory receptors (see Section 3-26). NKG2D is coupled to the adaptor protein DAP10, which transmits the signal into the interior of the cell by interacting with and activating intracellular phosphatidylinositol 3-kinase.

Even more distantly related to MHC class I genes is a small family of proteins known in humans as the **UL16-binding proteins (ULBPs**; UL16 is a human cytomegalovirus protein) or the **RAET1** proteins (see Fig. 6.26); the homologous proteins in mice are known as Rae1 (retinoic acid early inducible 1) and H60. These proteins also bind NKG2D (see Section 3-27). They seem to be expressed under conditions of cellular stress, such as when cells are infected with pathogens or have undergone transformation to tumor cells. By expressing ULBPs, stressed or infected cells can bind and activate NKG2D molecules expressed on NK cells, γδ T cells, and cytotoxic CD8 αβ T cells, and so be recognized and eliminated.

The human MHC class Ib molecule HLA-E and its mouse counterpart Qa-1 (see Fig. 6.26) have an unusual and somewhat puzzling role in cell recognition by NK cells and CD8 T cells. HLA-E and Qa-1 bind a very restricted subset of nonpolymorphic peptides, called **Qa-1 determinant modifiers (Qdm)**, which are derived from the leader peptides of other HLA class I molecules. These peptide:HLA-E complexes can bind to the inhibitory receptor NKG2A:CD94 expressed on NK cells, and so should inhibit the cytotoxic activity of NK cells. This function might seem redundant, because expression of other MHC class I molecules by cells should prevent NK-cell activation (see Section 3-25). Nonetheless, it has been shown that Qa-1 expression by activated CD4 T cells protects them from lysis by NK cells, and so Qa-1 expression by other host cells may provide them with additional protection from being killed by NK cells. HLA-E and Qa-1 can also bind leader peptides from the heat-shock protein Hsp60, and CD8 T cells that are specific for these complexes have been identified in mice and humans. Some recent evidence suggests that CD8 T cells restricted by HLA-E/Qa-1 may help maintain self-tolerance by killing or suppressing potentially autoreactive T cells.

In Section 3-26, we introduced the **killer cell immunoglobulin-like receptors (KIRs)** expressed by human NK cells. Members of the KIRs recognize the classical class Ia MHC molecules HLA-A, -B, and -C, which present a diverse repertoire of peptides to CD8 T cells. HLA-C is specialized for regulating NK cells in humans, as all HLA-C alleles express proteins that bind KIRs, while only a few HLA-A and HLA-B alleles do so. Although KIRs interact with the same face of the MHC class I molecule as do T-cell receptors, the KIRs bind only at one end, and not over the whole area recognized by the T-cell receptor. KIRs themselves are highly polymorphic, and they have undergone rapid evolution in humans.

Two other MHC class Ib molecules, HLA-F and HLA-G (see Fig. 6.26), can also inhibit cell killing by NK cells. HLA-G is expressed on fetus-derived placental cells that migrate into the uterine wall. These cells express no classical MHC class I molecules and cannot be recognized by CD8 T cells, but, unlike other cells lacking such proteins, they are not killed by NK cells. This seems to be because HLA-G is recognized by two other inhibitory receptors on NK cells, the leukocyte immunoglobulin-like receptor subfamily B member 1 (LILRB1; also called ILT-2 or LIR-1) and by LILRB2.

HLA-G expressed by placental cells prevents their being killed by NK cells. HLA-F is expressed in a variety of tissues, although it is usually not detected at the cell surface, except, for example, on some monocyte cell lines or on virus-transformed lymphoid cells. HLA-F is also thought to interact with LILRB1.

6-18 Members of the CD1 family of MHC class I–like molecules present lipid-based antigens to NKT cells.

Some MHC class I–like genes map outside the MHC region. One small family of such genes is called **CD1** and is expressed on dendritic cells, monocytes, thymocytes, and lymphocytes including T and B cells. Humans have five CD1 genes, CD1a through e, whereas mice and rats have only two highly homologous versions of CD1d, namely CD1d1 and CD1d2. CD1 proteins can present antigens to T cells, but they have two features that distinguish them from classical MHC class I molecules. The first is that CD1, although similar to an MHC class I molecule in its subunit organization and association with β_2-microglobulin, behaves like an MHC class II molecule. It is not retained within the endoplasmic reticulum by association with the TAP complex but is targeted to vesicles, where it binds its ligand. The second unusual feature is that, unlike MHC class I, CD1 molecules have a hydrophobic pocket specialized for binding hydrocarbon alkyl chains. This confers CD1 molecules an ability to bind and present a variety of lipid-based antigens.

CD1 molecules are classified into group 1, comprising CD1a, CD1b, and CD1c, and group 2, containing only CD1d; CD1e is considered intermediate. CD1d expression is constitutive, while expression of all others is inducible during immune responses. Group 1 molecules bind various **microbial glycolipids**, phospholipids, and **lipopeptide antigens**, such as the mycobacterial membrane components mycolic acid, glucose monomycolate, phosphoinositol mannosides, and lipoarabinomannan (**Fig. 6.27**). CD1d molecules can bind self lipid antigens such as **sphingolipids** and **diacylglycerols** but also microbial lipid-based antigens, for example from *Borrelia burgdorferi*, the agent that causes Lyme disease.

Structural studies show that the CD1 molecule has a deep binding groove into which the glycolipid antigens bind (**Fig. 6.28**). Unlike the binding of peptide to MHC, in which the peptide takes on a linear, extended conformation, CD1 molecules bind their antigens by anchoring the alkyl chains in the hydrophobic groove, which orients the variable hydrophilic parts of these molecules, such as a phosphate or carbohydrate group, to protrude from the binding groove, allowing recognition by the T-cell receptors on CD1-restricted T cells. In contrast to other CD1 molecules, CD1e is not bound to the cell membrane and so is not recognized by T cells but may act in the transfer of intracellular lipids.

The T cells that recognize lipids presented by CD1 molecules can vary in their expression of the co-receptors CD4 and CD8; some express CD4, but others are negative for CD4 and CD8 expression. Most of the T cells recognizing lipids presented by group 1 CD1 molecules have a diverse repertoire of $\alpha\beta$ receptors and respond to these lipids presented by CD1a, CD1b, and CD1c. CD1d-restricted T cells are less diverse, with many using the same TCRα chain

MPM from Mtb

MPM bound to CD1c (top view)

α_1

α_2

MPM bound to CD1c (side view)

α_1 α_2

Fig. 6.27 CD1c binds microbial lipids for presentation to iNKT cells. Top panel: The structure of mannosyl-β1-phosphomycoketides (MPMs) from the cell walls of *Mycobacterium tuberculosis* (Mtb) (R = C_7H_{15}) and *M. avium* (R = C_5H_{11}). Middle panel: MPM (stick figure) bound to CD1c (purple) as viewed from the top, facing the surface of the cell bearing CD1c. Bottom panel: Side view of MPM bound to CD1c. The general resemblance with peptide:MHC complexes is apparent. Note: The long acyl chain of MPM extends deep into the binding groove of CD1c, to beneath the α_1 helical domain.

C8PhF bound to CD1d (top view)

C8PhF bound to CD1d (side view)

Fig. 6.28 Structure of CD1 binding to a lipid antigen. Shown are top and side views of the structure of mouse CD1d bound to C8PhF, a synthetic lipid that is an analog of α-GalCer. The helical side chains of CD1d (blue) form a binding pocket that is generally similar in shape to the binding pockets of MHC class I and class II molecules. However, the C8PhF (red) ligand binds to CD1 molecules in a distinctly different conformation from that of peptides. The two long alkyl side chains extend deep inside the binding groove (see side view), where they make contacts with hydrophobic residues. This orientation of the alkyl side chains places the carbohydrate component of α-GalCer to the outer surface of CD1, where it can be recognized by the T-cell receptor. In addition, the CD1 molecule contains an endogenous lipid molecule (yellow) derived from cellular sources and which binds to a distinct region within the groove and prevents a large pocket adjacent to the α-GalCer–binding region from collapsing. The ability to incorporate additional ligands into the binding groove may provide flexibility to CD1d in accommodating a variety of exogenous glycosphingolipids from microorganisms.

(Vα24–Jα18 in humans). Many also express NK-cell receptors, such as NK1.1. In fact, CD1d-restricted T cells were originally called **invariant NKT (iNKT) cells**. However, CD1d-restricted T cells have a diverse TCRβ repertoire, and some are now known to have a more diverse TCRα chain repertoire as well. A new nomenclature uses **type 1 NKT cells** to refer to CD1d-restricted T cells with a restricted TCRα chain and **type 2 NKT cells** to refer to those with a more diverse TCRα repertoire. A recently discovered population of CD1b-restricted human T cells uses a near-invariant TCRα chain (Vα1–2 and Jα9). These cells, which recognize the mycobacterial lipid antigen glucose monomycolate, are called **GEM** (germline-encoded mycolyl lipid-reactive) T cells.

One ligand recognized by CD1d-restricted NKT cells is **α-galactosylceramide (α-GalCer)**, which was isolated from an extract of marine sponge. Related glycosphingolipids are produced by various bacteria, including *Bacteroides fragilis*, which is present in the normal human microbiota. When α-galactosylceramide is bound to CD1d, it forms a structure that is recognized by many NKT cells. Unlike conventional αβ T cells that require several days of activation and expansion in order to acquire effector function, NKT cells can produce cytokines rapidly after they recognize lipid-based antigens presented by CD1d molecules. In this way, they are similar to innate lymphocytes such as NK cells. Their recognition of limited types of antigens is also a characteristic of cells of the innate immune system.

Similar to the theme of loading peptides onto classical MHC proteins from various cellular locations, the various CD1 proteins are transported differently through the endocytic compartments, providing them with access to different lipid antigens. Transport is regulated by an amino acid sequence motif at the terminus of the cytoplasmic domain of the CD1 protein through interaction with the adaptor-protein (AP) complexes AP-2 and AP-3. CD1a lacks this binding motif and moves to the cell surface, where it is transported only through the early endocytic compartment. CD1b, CD1c, and CD1d have motifs that interact with the adaptor AP-2 and are transported through early and late endosomes. CD1b and mouse CD1d bind AP-2 and AP-3 and can be transported through late endosomes, lysosomes, and the MIIC. Thus, CD1 proteins can bind lipids delivered into and processed within the endocytic pathway, such as by the internalization of mycobacteria or the ingestion of mycobacterial glycolipids (such as lipoarabinomannans), mediated by mannose receptors.

CD1a is highly expressed on human **Langerhans cells**, a specialized immune cell that has similarities to macrophages and dendritic cells and which resides in the epidermis. The epidermis is protected in part by the production of sebum, containing various lipids, including wax esters and squalene (see Section 2-2). CD1a-restricted T cells survey human skin for the "headless" lipid-based antigens presented by the CD1a expressed by Langerhans cells, which may indicate a breach of skin tissue. CD1a-restricted T cells also respond to injury caused by bee and wasp venom, presumably in response to ligands generated by the venom's lipid-modifying phospholipases.

MHC class Ib genes evolved before the divergence of cartilaginous fishes from the vertebrate line and are likely to have homologs in all vertebrates. Other MHC class I genes have evolved independently into classical and nonclassical loci within the vertebrate lineages that have been studied (for example, cartilaginous fishes, lobe-finned fishes, ray-finned fishes, amphibians, and mammals). Sequence data have also revealed homologs of the mammalian MHC class I and MHC class II gene families in virtually all jawed vertebrates including sharks, bony fishes, reptiles, and birds. In contrast, CD1 genes may not be as old as other MHC class Ib genes. They have been found only in a subset of these animal groups and appear to be missing in fishes. This pattern of CD1 occurrence in the genomes of living species suggests the emergence of CD1 in an early terrestrial vertebrate.

6-19   The nonclassical MHC class I molecule MR1 presents microbial riboflavin metabolites to MAIT cells.

Another nonclassical MHC class I–like molecule is **MR1 (MHC-related protein 1)**. MR1 is the most highly conserved MHC class I antigen-presenting molecule across many mammalian species and is linked to the CD1 genes on human chromosome 1, suggesting an important function. MR1 associates with β_2-microglobulin and is encoded outside the MHC. The function of MR1 was originally known only in relation to a conserved population of $\alpha\beta$ T cells known as mucosal-associated invariant T cells (MAIT cells), which we introduced in Section 4-21. MAIT cells are uniquely characterized by expression of an invariant α chain of the T-cell receptor, specifically human $V_\alpha 7.2$ and $J_\alpha 33$, and in mouse, $V_\alpha 19$, $J_\alpha 33$, or occasionally $J_\alpha 12$ or $J_\alpha 20$. These α chains pair with a limited number of V_β chains, typically $V_\beta 2$ or $V_\beta 13$. MAIT cells are very abundant in human tissues and can compose up to 10% of lymphocytes in peripheral blood and up to 40% of lymphocytes in liver. They are also present in mesenteric lymph nodes and the mucosa of the intestine, lungs, and all locations where other T cells reside.

When MAIT cells were identified in the 1990s, it was unclear what ligand, if any, they recognized. Studies indicated that development of MAIT cells required MR1 and that they could be activated by a wide spectrum of microbes, including diverse bacteria and yeast. Structural studies of the MR1 protein uncovered an important clue: The MR1 protein produced by cell lines *in vitro* was yellow; chemical analysis revealed that a small molecule, the folate derivative 6-formylpterin (6-FP) was covalently bound to Lys43 of the MR1 protein. Further X-ray crystallographic studies showed that 6-FP bound within the central groove of the MR1 molecule. However, most MAIT cells were not activated by cells expressing the 6-FP:MR1 complex, suggesting that other molecules might be the physiological ligands that activate MAIT cells. Analysis of MR1 proteins that were refolded in the presence of supernatants from cultures of *Salmonella enterica* ssp. *typhimurium* eventually led to the identification of several riboflavin (vitamin B_2) metabolites that are formed by biosynthetic pathways in most bacteria and yeast. One key antigen for MAIT-cell activation is the short-lived metabolite 5-(2-oxopropylideneamino)-6-d-ribitylaminouracil (5-OP-RU) formed by microbial biosynthetic pathways. These metabolites, captured from the extracellular environment or from phagosomes harboring bacteria, find their way to the endoplasmic reticulum, where empty MR1 is being retained. There they bind and stabilize MR1, induce its surface expression, and cause activation of MAIT cells. Thus, the surface expression of MR1 is a sensor of microbial riboflavin metabolism, and MAIT cells are activated in response to infection by organisms that produce it. Like NKT cells, MAIT cells use a TCR assembled by somatic gene rearrangement to recognize a molecular structure that falls within the definition of a PAMP (pathogen-associated molecular pattern; see Section 3-1). Also like NKT cells, MAIT cells produce cytokines rapidly after activation, without the need for priming and expansion by dendritic cells.

6-20 γδ T cells can recognize a variety of diverse ligands.

γδ T cells and αβ T cells have been known to be distinct developmental lineages almost since the T-cell receptor genes were identified. But unlike αβ T cells, the function of γδ T cells has remained somewhat obscure, due primarily to difficulty in identifying the ligands they recognize. Yet the abundance of γδ T cells across vertebrate species, their rapid expansion to form more than 50% of the blood lymphocytes during infections, and their abundant cytokine production all argue for an important role in immunity. They are also the cell type that most favorably correlates with a good prognosis in human tumors. Over time, many different ligands recognized by γδ T-cell clones have been identified (**Fig. 6.29**), and their diversity suggests that, like NKT cells and MAIT cells, they play an intermediate role in the spectrum of innate versus adaptive immunity.

In Section 4-23, we discussed how one γδ T-cell receptor binds to the non-classical MHC class I molecule T22. Instead of binding centrally over the MHC binding groove, similar to an αβ T-cell receptor, the γδ T-cell receptor interacts obliquely from one side of the T22 molecule. However, fewer than 1% of γδ T cells recognize this ligand. Other antigens recognized by murine γδ T cells are the protein **phycoerythrin (PE)** from algae, the inner mitochondrial membrane lipid **cardiolipin**, glycoprotein I (gI) of herpes simplex virus, and a peptide derived from the hormone insulin. Other antigens that can activate human γδ T cells are the nonclassical MHC class I proteins MIC-A and **ULBP4** and the **endothelial protein C receptor (EPCR)**, which is expressed by endothelial cells. Like MIC-A and ULBPs, EPCR appears to be induced by stress, such as infection of cells by cytomegalovirus, suggesting that reactive γδ T cells could serve in an innate capacity similar to that of NK cells activated by stress-induced nonclassical MHC class Ib molecules. Also, some γδ T cells can recognize α-galactosylceramide and the sulfated glycolipid sulfatide (3-*O*-sulfogalactosylceramide) presented by CD1d. A subset of γδ T cells

Ligands that activate γδ T cells		
Ligands	**Species**	**γδ subset**
T22, T10	Mouse	Various
H2-E (MHC class II)	Mouse	Clones
Phycoerythrin (PE)	Mouse	Various
Cardiolipin	Mouse	Various
Keratinocytes	Mouse	DETC $V_\gamma 5V_\delta 1$
HSV-gI	Mouse	Clone
Skint-1	Mouse	$V_\gamma 5V_\delta 1$
MIC-A/MIC-B	Human	Clones
ULBP4	Human	$V_\gamma 9V_\delta 2$
CD1-sulfatide, CD1d-αGalCer	Human	$V_\delta 1$
EPCR (endothelial protein C receptor)	Human	Clones
Phosphoantigens, amino-bisphosphonates, BTN3A1	Human	$V_\gamma 9V_\delta 2$
Alkylamines	Human	$V_\gamma 9V_\delta 2$

Fig. 6.29 **Ligands that activate γδ T cells.**

expressing a Vγ9Vδ2 TCR respond to small phosphate-containing antigens (for example, hydroxymethyl but-2-enyl pyrophosphate) in a manner requiring a cell-surface receptor BTN3A1, a member of the **butyrophilin (BTN)** family. BTNs are type 1 cell-surface transmembrane proteins having two or more extracellular immunoglobulin domains; humans have 11 BTN family members. The mechanism of antigen presentation by BTNs to γδ T cells is still a matter of active research, but some evidence suggests that different BTNs may function in heterodimeric pairs.

Several other antigens can activate human γδ T cells (see Fig. 6.29), although there is still limited structural information about their interaction with the T-cell receptor, and even reservations about whether such an interaction is always the basis for activation. Among these activating antigens is **Skint-1** (selection and upkeep of intraepithelial T cells 1), an immunoglobulin superfamily member related to the butyrophilins that is expressed by thymic epithelial cells and by keratinocytes. Skint-1 seems to be required in mice for the generation of a subset of Vγ5Vδ1 T cells that develop in the thymus and home to the skin to become **dendritic epidermal T cells (DETCs)**. Some evidence suggests a direct interaction between Skint-1 and the γδ T-cell receptor, although structural studies are not yet available. Conceivably, DETCs localize to the skin because their T-cell receptor recognizes Skint-1 expressed by keratinocytes. There DETCs might provide a 'transitional' mode of immune defense, becoming activated through innate receptors that are triggered locally during infections.

Summary.

Antigen presentation to various nonconventional T-cell subsets and γδ T cells generally does not involve the generation of peptide:MHC complexes. Instead, these cells recognize surface proteins, such as ULBPs and RAET1 proteins (which may indicate cellular stress, transformation, or intracellular infection), or nonpeptide antigens; NKT cells recognize various microbial glycolipids presented by CD1 molecules; and MAIT cells recognize microbe-specific riboflavin metabolites presented by MR1. The MHC region contains many genes whose structure is closely related to the MHC class I molecules—the so-called nonclassical, or class Ib, MHC. Some of these genes serve purposes that are unrelated to the immune system, but many are involved in recognition by activating and inhibitory receptors expressed by NK cells, γδ T cells, and αβ T cells. MHC class I–like proteins called CD1 molecules are encoded outside the MHC region. CD1a, CD1c, and CD1d can bind lipids and glycolipid antigens for presentation to NKT cells. The T-cell population called MAIT cells, which are abundant in humans, recognizes vitamin B_2 metabolites presented by the MR1 MHC class I–like molecule, suggesting that the MAIT cells have a 'transitional' role between innate and adaptive immunity. Likewise, many antigens that activate γδ T cells may be indicators of stress or infection, and these cells are able to generate cytokines that amplify immune-defense pathways.

Summary to Chapter 6.

T-cell receptors on conventional αβ T cells recognize peptides bound to MHC molecules. In the absence of infection, MHC molecules are occupied by self peptides, which do not normally provoke a T-cell response because of various tolerance mechanisms. But during infections, pathogen-derived peptides bind to MHC molecules and are displayed on the cell surface, where they can be recognized by T cells that have been previously activated and armed for the specific peptide:MHC complex. Naive T cells become activated when they encounter their specific peptide antigen presented by MHC molecules of activated dendritic cells. MHC class I molecules in most cells bind to peptides derived from proteins that have been synthesized and then degraded in the cytosol of the same cell. Some dendritic cells, the cDC1 subset, can capture exogenous antigens using cell-surface receptors such as CLEC9A and process them for loading onto MHC class I molecules. This process of cross-presentation is important for priming CD8 T cells to many viral infections as well as to antigens expressed by tumors.

Through assembly with the invariant chain (Ii), MHC class II molecules bind peptides derived from proteins degraded in endocytic vesicles, including extracellular proteins that are internalized, or endogenous intracellular proteins that are delivered to endosomes by autophagy or other protein-targeting mechanisms. Stable peptides are bound after a process of peptide editing in the endocytic compartment involving HLA-DM and HLA-DO. CD8 T cells recognize peptide:MHC class I complexes and are activated to kill cells displaying foreign peptides derived from cytosolic pathogens, such as viruses. CD4 T cells recognize peptide:MHC class II complexes expressed by dendritic cells, macrophages, or B cells; naive CD4 T cells become activated when recognizing antigen on dendritic cells, and activated CD4 T cells provide help when recognizing antigen presented to macrophages and B cells.

For each class of MHC molecule, there are several genes arranged in clusters within a larger region known as the major histocompatibility complex (MHC). Within the MHC, the genes encoding MHC molecules are closely linked to genes involved in the degradation of proteins into peptides, the formation of the peptide:MHC complex, and the transport of these complexes to the cell surface. Because the varied genes for the MHC class Ia and class II molecules are highly polymorphic and are expressed in a codominant fashion, each individual expresses a number of different MHC class Ia and class II molecules. Each different MHC molecule can bind stably to a range of different peptides, and thus the MHC repertoire of each individual can recognize and bind many different peptide antigens. Because the T-cell receptor binds a combined peptide:MHC ligand, T cells show MHC-restricted antigen recognition, such that a given T cell is specific for a particular peptide bound to a particular MHC molecule.

Unconventional T-cell subsets include NKT cells, MAIT cells, and γδ T cells, which recognize nonpeptide ligands of various types. CD1 molecules bind self lipids and pathogen-derived lipid-based antigens and present them to NKT cells. MAIT cells recognize microbial-specific riboflavin metabolites presented by MR1. γδ T cells are activated by a diverse array of ligands, including MHC class Ib molecules and EPCR, that are induced by infection or cellular stress. These unconventional T-cell subsets function in the transitional area between innate and adaptive immunity, relying on a repertoire of receptors produced by somatic gene rearrangement but recognizing ligands in a manner somewhat similar to the way PAMPs are recognized by TLRs and other fully innate receptors.

Discussion Questions

6.1 MHC class I and class II molecules are structurally and functionally homologous, yet have dissimilar pathways of assembly and delivery to the cell surface. (a) Describe how these differences in assembly and delivery are related to the different functions of class I and class II molecules. (b) What kinds of cells typically recognize antigens presented by MHC class I molecules? What kinds of cells present antigens to these cells, and what is the purpose in each case? (c) What types of cells present antigens on MHC class II molecules, and for what purpose(s)?

6.2 Different types of antigen-presenting cells carry out cross-presentation and MHC class II processing to varying degrees of efficiency. (a) What would the theoretical consequence be for the loss of cross-presentation by dendritic cells? (b) What would the theoretical consequence be for the loss of MHC class II antigen processing?

6.3 Many of the proteins encoded within the MHC exist in the population in multiple forms, or allelic variants. (a) What genetic events give rise to this variation, and what are the functional consequences? (b) In some cases, particular combinations of alleles of the different MHC genes are found to be present at far higher frequency than chance would predict. What are the possible mechanisms that could explain this finding? (c) MHC proteins are the most polymorphic proteins known. What benefit, if any, does this provide and how?

6.4 Many genes outside the MHC region encode proteins that are structurally and functionally related to class I MHC proteins. (a) Discuss the cell types that recognize various 'nonclassical' MHC proteins and what their functions are. (b) Discuss the kinds of ligands that are presented by various members of these proteins. (c) Compare and contrast the nature of the ligands with the ligand recognized by the TLR proteins, and describe their role in the immune response.

General references.

Godfrey, D.I., Uldrich, A.P., McCluskey, J., Rossjohn, J., and Moody, D.B.: **The burgeoning family of unconventional T cells.** *Nat Immunol.* 2015, **16**:1114–1123.

Moller, G. (ed): **Origin of major histocompatibility complex diversity.** *Immunol. Rev.* 1995, **143**:5–292.

Trombetta, E.S., and Mellman, I.: **Cell biology of antigen processing** *in vitro* and *in vivo. Annu. Rev. Immunol.* 2005, **23**:975–1028.

Unanue, E.R., Turk, V., and Neefjes, J.: **Variations in MHC class II antigen processing and presentation in health and disease.** *Annu. Rev. Immunol.* 2016, **34**:265–297.

Section references.

6-1 Antigen presentation functions both in arming effector T cells and in triggering their effector functions to attack pathogen-infected cells.

Lee, H.K., Mattei, L.M., Steinberg, B.E., Alberts, P., Lee, Y.H., Chervonsky, A., Mizushima, N., Grinstein, S., and Iwasaki, A.: *In vivo* **requirement for Atg5 in antigen presentation by dendritic cells.** *Immunity* 2010, **32**:227–239.

Neefjes, J., Jongsma, M.L.M, Paul, P., and Bakke, O.: **Towards a systems understanding of MHC class I and MHC class II antigen presentation.** *Nat. Rev. Immunol.* 2011, **11**:823–836.

Segura, E., and Amigorena, S.: **Cross-presentation in mouse and human dendritic cells.** *Adv. Immunol.* 2015, **127**:1–31.

Vyas, J.M., Van der Veen, A.G., and Ploegh, H.L.: **The known unknowns of antigen processing and presentation.** *Nat. Rev. Immunol.* 2008, **8**:607–618.

6-2 Peptides are generated from ubiquitinated proteins in the cytosol by the proteasome.

Basler, M., Kirk, C.J., and Groettrup, M.: **The immunoproteasome in antigen processing and other immunological functions.** *Curr. Opin. Immunol.* 2013, **25**:74–80.

Brocke, P., Garbi, N., Momburg, F., and Hammerling, G.J.: **HLA-DM, HLA-DO and tapasin: functional similarities and differences.** *Curr. Opin. Immunol.* 2002, **14**:22–29.

Cascio, P.: **PA28αβ: the enigmatic magic ring of the proteasome?** *Biomolecules* 2014, **4**:566–884.

Chen, X., and Jensen, P.E.: **Biological function of HLA-DO (H2-O).** *Crit. Rev. Immunol.* 2014, **34**:215–225.

de Graaf, N., van Helden, M.J., Textoris-Taube, K., Chiba, T., Topham, D.J., Kloetzel, P.M., Zaiss, D.M., and Sijts, A.J.: **PA28 and the proteasome immunosubunits play a central and independent role in the production of MHC class I-binding peptides in vivo.** *Eur. J. Immunol.* 2011, **41**:926–935.

Goldberg, A.L., Cascio, P., Saric, T., and Rock, K.L.: **The importance of the proteasome and subsequent proteolytic steps in the generation of antigenic peptides.** *Mol. Immunol.* 2002, **39**:147–164.

Hammer, G.E., Gonzalez, F., Champsaur, M., Cado, D., and Shastri, N.: **The aminopeptidase ERAAP shapes the peptide repertoire displayed by major histocompatibility complex class I molecules.** *Nat. Immunol.* 2006, **7**:103–112.

Hammer, G.E., Gonzalez, F., James, E., Nolla, H., and Shastri, N.: **In the absence of aminopeptidase ERAAP, MHC class I molecules present many unstable and highly immunogenic peptides.** *Nat. Immunol.* 2007, **8**:101–108.

Murata, S., Takahama, Y., Kasahara, M., and Tanaka, K.: **The immunoproteasome and thymoproteasome: functions, evolution and human disease.** *Nat. Immunol.* 2018, **19**:923–931.

Raule, M., Cerruti, F., Benaroudj, N., Migotti, R., Kikuchi, J., Bachi, A., Navon, A., Dittmar, G., and Cascio, P.: **PA28αβ reduces size and increases hydrophilicity of 20S immunoproteasome peptide products.** *Chem. Biol.* 2014, **21**:470–480.

Serwold, T., Gonzalez, F., Kim, J., Jacob, R., and Shastri, N.: **ERAAP customizes peptides for MHC class I molecules in the endoplasmic reticulum.** *Nature* 2002, **419**:480–483.

Warren, E.H., Vigneron, N.J., Gavin, M.A., Coulie, P.G., Stroobant, V., Dalet, A., Tykodi, S.S., Xuereb, S.M., Mito, J.K., Riddell, S.R., and Van den Eynde, B.J.: **An antigen produced by splicing of noncontiguous peptides in the reverse order.** *Science* 2006, **313**:1444–1447.

6-3 Peptides from the cytosol are transported by TAP into the endoplasmic reticulum and further processed before binding to MHC class I molecules.

Chang, S.C., Momburg, F., Bhutani, N., and Goldberg, A.L.: **The ER aminopeptidase, ERAP1, trims precursors to lengths of MHC class I peptides by a "molecular ruler" mechanism.** *Proc. Natl. Acad. Sci. USA* 2005, **102**:17107–17112.

Gorbulev, S., Abele, R., and Tampe, R.: **Allosteric crosstalk between peptide-binding, transport, and ATP hydrolysis of the ABC transporter TAP.** *Proc. Natl Acad. Sci. USA* 2001, **98**:3732–3737.

Kelly, A., Powis, S.H., Kerr, L.A., Mockridge, I., Elliott, T., Bastin, J., Uchanska-Ziegler, B., Ziegler, A., Trowsdale, J., and Townsend, A.: **Assembly and function of the two ABC transporter proteins encoded in the human major histocompatibility complex.** *Nature* 1992, **355**:641–644.

Neefjes, J.J., Momburg, F., and Hammerling, G.J.: **Selective and ATP-dependent translocation of peptides by the MHC-encoded transporter.** *Science* 1993, **261**:769–771.

Powis, S.J., Townsend, A.R., Deverson, E.V., Bastin, J., Butcher, G.W., and Howard, J.C.: **Restoration of antigen presentation to the mutant cell line RMA-S by an MHC-linked transporter.** *Nature* 1991, **354**:528–531.

Reits, E., Griekspoor, A., Neijssen, J., Groothuis, T., Jalink, K., van Veelen, P., Janssen, H., Calafat, J., Drijfhout, J.W., and Neefjes, J.: **Peptide diffusion, protection, and degradation in nuclear and cytoplasmic compartments before antigen presentation by MHC class I.** *Immunity* 2003, **18**:97–108.

Roelse, J., Gromme, M., Momburg, F., Hammerling, G., and Neefjes, J.: **Trimming of TAP-translocated peptides in the endoplasmic reticulum and in the cytosol during recycling.** *J. Exp. Med.* 1994, **180**:1591–1597.

Townsend, A., Ohlen, C., Foster, L., Bastin, J., Lunggren, H.G., and Karre, K.: **A mutant cell in which association of class I heavy and light chains is induced by viral peptides.** *Cold Spring Harb. Symp. Quant. Biol.* 1989, **54**:299–308.

6-4 Newly synthesized MHC class I molecules are retained in the endoplasmic reticulum until they bind a peptide.

Blees, A., Januliene, D., Hofmann, T., Koller, N., Schmidt, C., Trowitzsch, S., Moeller, A., and Tampé, R.: **Structure of the human MHC-I peptide-loading complex.** *Nature* 2017, **551**:525–528.

Boyle, L.H., Hermann, C., Boname, J.M., Porter, K.M., Patel, P.A., Burr, M.L., Duncan, L.M., Harbour, M.E., Rhodes, D.A., Skjødt, K., *et al.*: **Tapasin-related protein TAPBPR is an additional component of the MHC class I presentation pathway.** *Proc. Natl. Acad. Sci. USA* 2013, **110**:3465–3470.

de la Salle, H., Hanau, D., Fricker, D., Urlacher, A., Kelly, A., Salamero, J., Powis, S.H., Donato, L., Bausinger, H., Laforet, M., *et al.*: Homozygous human TAP peptide transporter mutation in HLA class I deficiency. *Science* 1994, **265**:237–241.

Peaper, D.R., and Cresswell, P.L.: The redox activity of ERp57 is not essential for its functions in MHC class I peptide loading. *Proc. Natl. Acad. Sci. USA* 2008, **105**:10477–10482.

Thomas, C., and Tampé, R.: Structure of the TAPBPR-MHC I complex defines the mechanism of peptide loading and editing. *Science* 2017, **358**:1060–1064.

Williams, A.P., Peh, C.A., Purcell, A.W., McCluskey, J., and Elliott, T.: Optimization of the MHC class I peptide cargo is dependent on tapasin. *Immunity* 2002, **16**:509–520.

Zhang, W., Wearsch, P.A., Zhu, Y., Leonhardt, R.M., and Cresswell P.: A role for UDP-glucose glycoprotein glucosyltransferase in expression and quality control of MHC class I molecules. *Proc. Natl. Acad. Sci. USA* 2011, **108**:4956–4961.

6-5 Dendritic cells use cross-presentation to present exogenous proteins on MHC class I molecules so as to prime CD8 T cells.

Bevan, M.J.: Minor H antigens introduced on H-2 different stimulating cells cross-react at the cytotoxic T cell level during *in vivo* priming. *J. Immunol.* 1976, **117**:2233–2238.

Hildner, K., Edelson, B.T., Purtha, W.E., Diamond, M., Matsushita, H., Kohyama, M., Calderon, B., Schraml, B.U., Unanue, E.R., Diamond, M.S., *et al.*: Batf3 deficiency reveals a critical role for CD8α+ dendritic cells in cytotoxic T cell immunity. *Science* 2008, **322**:1097–1100.

Joffre, O.P., Segura, E., Savina. A., and Amigorena, S.: Cross-presentation by dendritic cells. *Nat. Rev. Immunol.* 2012, **12**:557–569.

Sancho, D., Joffre, O.P., Keller, A.M., Rogers, N.C., Martínez, D., Hernanz-Falcón, P., Rosewell, I., and Reis e Sousa, C.: Identification of a dendritic cell receptor that couples sensing of necrosis to immunity. *Nature* 2009, **458**:899–903.

Segura, E., and Villadangos, J.A.: A modular and combinatorial view of the antigen cross-presentation pathway in dendritic cells. *Traffic* 2011, **12**:1677–1685.

6-6 Peptide:MHC class II complexes are generated in acidified endocytic vesicles from proteins obtained through endocytosis, phagocytosis, and autophagy.

Beers, C., Burich, A., Kleijmeer, M.J., Griffith, J.M., Wong, P., and Rudensky, A.Y.: Cathepsin S controls MHC class II-mediated antigen presentation by epithelial cells in vivo. *J. Immunol.* 2005, **174**:1205–1212.

Dengjel, J., Schoor, O., Fischer, R., Reich, M., Kraus, M., Müller, M., Kreymborg, K., Altenberend, F., Brandenburg, J., Kalbacher, H., *et al.*: Autophagy promotes MHC class II presentation of peptides from intracellular source proteins. *Proc. Natl. Acad. Sci. USA* 2005, **102**:7922–7927.

Godkin, A.J., Smith, K.J., Willis, A., Tejada-Simon, M.V., Zhang, J., Elliott, T., and Hill, A.V.: Naturally processed HLA class II peptides reveal highly conserved immunogenic flanking region sequence preferences that reflect antigen processing rather than peptide–MHC interactions. *J. Immunol.* 2001, **166**:6720–6727.

Hiltbold, E.M., and Roche, P.A.: Trafficking of MHC class II molecules in the late secretory pathway. *Curr. Opin. Immunol.* 2002, **14**:30–35.

Hsieh, C.S., deRoos, P., Honey, K., Beers, C., and Rudensky, A.Y.: A role for cathepsin L and cathepsin S in peptide generation for MHC class II presentation. *J. Immunol.* 2002, **168**:2618–2625.

Li, P., Gregg, J.L., Wang, N., Zhou, D., O'Donnell, P., Blum, J.S., and Crotzer, V.L.: Compartmentalization of class II antigen presentation: contribution of cytoplasmic and endosomal processing. *Immunol. Rev.* 2005, **207**:206–217.

Maric, M., Arunachalam, B., Phan, U.T., Dong, C., Garrett, W.S., Cannon, K.S., Alfonso, C., Karlsson, L., Flavell, R.A., and Cresswell, P.: Defective antigen processing in GILT-free mice. *Science* 2001, **294**:1361–1365.

Mindell, J.A.: Lysosomal acidification mechanisms. *Annu. Rev. Physiol.* 2012, **74**:69–86.

Pluger, E.B., Boes, M., Alfonso, C., Schroter, C.J., Kalbacher, H., Ploegh, H.L., and Driessen, C.: Specific role for cathepsin S in the generation of antigenic peptides in vivo. *Eur. J. Immunol.* 2002, **32**:467–476.

6-7 The invariant chain directs newly synthesized MHC class II molecules to acidified intracellular vesicles.

Gregers, T.F., Nordeng, T.W., Birkeland, H.C., Sandlie, I., and Bakke, O.: The cytoplasmic tail of invariant chain modulates antigen processing and presentation. *Eur. J. Immunol.* 2003, **33**:277–286.

Kleijmeer, M., Ramm, G., Schuurhuis, D., Griffith, J., Rescigno, M., Ricciardi-Castagnoli, P., Rudensky, A.Y., Ossendorp, F., Melief, C.J., Stoorvogel, W., *et al.*: Reorganization of multivesicular bodies regulates MHC class II antigen presentation by dendritic cells. *J. Cell Biol.* 2001, **155**:53–63.

Neefjes, J.J., Stollorz, V., Peters, P.J., Geuze, H.J., and Ploegh, H.L.: The biosynthetic pathway of MHC class II but not class I molecules intersects the endocytic route. *Cell* 1990, **61**:171–183.

van Lith, M., van Ham, M., Griekspoor, A., Tjin, E., Verwoerd, D., Calafat, J., Janssen, H., Reits, E., Pastoors, L., and Neefjes, J.: Regulation of MHC class II antigen presentation by sorting of recycling HLA-DM/DO and class II within the multivesicular body. *J. Immunol.* 2001, **167**:884–892.

6-8 The MHC class II–like molecules HLA-DM and HLA-DO regulate exchange of CLIP for other peptides.

Alfonso, C., and Karlsson, L.: Nonclassical MHC class II molecules. *Annu. Rev. Immunol.* 2000, **18**:113–142.

Apostolopoulos, V., McKenzie, I.F., and Wilson, I.A.: Getting into the groove: unusual features of peptide binding to MHC class I molecules and implications in vaccine design. *Front. Biosci.* 2001, **6**:D1311–D1320.

Buslepp, J., Zhao, R., Donnini, D., Loftus, D., Saad, M., Appella, E., and Collins, E.J.: T cell activity correlates with oligomeric peptide-major histocompatibility complex binding on T cell surface. *J. Biol. Chem.* 2001, **276**:47320–47328.

Denzin, L.K., Khan, A.A., Virdis, F., Wilks, J., Kane, M., Beilinson, H.A., Dikiy, S., Case, L.K., Roopenian, D., Witkowski, M., *et al.*: Neutralizing antibody responses to viral infections are linked to the non-classical MHC class II gene H2-Ob. *Immunity.* 2017, **47**:310–322.

Gu, Y., Jensen, P.E., and Chen, X.: Immunodeficiency and autoimmunity in H2-O-deficient mice. *J. Immunol.* 2013, **190**:126–137.

Mellins, E.D., and Stern, L.J.: HLA-DM and HLA-DO, key regulators of MHC-II processing and presentation. *Curr. Opin. Immunol.* 2014, **26**:115–122.

Pathak, S.S., Lich, J.D., and Blum, J.S.: Cutting edge: editing of recycling class II:peptide complexes by HLA-DM. *J. Immunol.* 2001, **167**:632–635.

Pos, W., Sethi, D.K., Call, M.J., Schulze, M.S., Anders, A.K., Pyrdol, J., and Wucherpfennig, K.W.: Crystal structure of the HLA-DM-HLA-DR1 complex defines mechanisms for rapid peptide selection. *Cell* 2012, **151**:1557–1568.

Qi, L., and Ostrand-Rosenberg, S.: H2-O inhibits presentation of bacterial superantigens, but not endogenous self antigens. *J. Immunol.* 2001, **167**:1371–1378.

Su, R.C., and Miller, R.G.: Stability of surface H-2Kb, H-2Db, and peptide-receptive H-2Kb on splenocytes. *J. Immunol.* 2001, **167**:4869–4877.

van Ham, M., van Lith, M., Lillemeier, B., Tjin, E., Gruneberg, U., Rahman, D., Pastoors, L., van Meijgaarden, K., Roucard, C., Trowsdale, J., *et al.*: Modulation of the major histocompatibility complex class II-associated peptide repertoire by human histocompatibility leukocyte antigen (HLA)-DO. *J. Exp. Med.* 2000, **191**:1127–1136.

Zarutskie, J.A., Busch, R., Zavala-Ruiz, Z., Rushe, M., Mellins, E.D., and Stern, L.J.: The kinetic basis of peptide exchange catalysis by HLA-DM. *Proc. Natl. Acad. Sci. USA* 2001, **98**:12450–12455.

6-9 Cessation of MHC class II antigen processing occurs after dendritic-cell activation through reduced expression of the MARCH-1 E3 ligase.

Ardouin, L., Luche, H., Chelbi, R., Carpentier, S., Shawket, A., Montanana Sanchis, F., Santa Maria, C., Grenot, P., Alexandre, Y., Grégoire, C., *et al.*: Broad and largely concordant molecular changes characterize tolerogenic and immunogenic dendritic cell maturation in thymus and periphery. *Immunity* 2016, **45**:305–318.

Baravalle, G., Park, H., McSweeney, M., Ohmura-Hoshino, M., Matsuki, Y., Ishido, S., and Shin, J.S.: Ubiquitination of CD86 is a key mechanism in regulating antigen presentation by dendritic cells. *J. Immunol.* 2011, **187**:2966–2973.

De Gassart, A., Camosseto, V., Thibodeau, J., Ceppi, M., Catalan, N., Pierre, P., and Gatti, E.: **MHC class II stabilization at the surface of human dendritic cells is the result of maturation-dependent MARCH I down-regulation.** *Proc. Natl. Acad. Sci. USA* 2008, **105**:3491–3496.

Ma, J.K., Platt, M.Y., Eastham-Anderson, J., Shin, J.S., and Mellman, I.: **MHC class II distribution in dendritic cells and B cells is determined by ubiquitin chain length.** *Proc. Natl. Acad. Sci. USA* 2012, **109**:8820–8827.

Ohmura-Hoshino, M., Matsuki, Y., Mito-Yoshida, M., Goto, E., Aoki-Kawasumi, M., Nakayama, M., Ohara, O., and Ishido, S.: **Cutting edge: requirement of MARCH-I-mediated MHC II ubiquitination for the maintenance of conventional dendritic cells.** *J. Immunol.* 2009, **183**:6893–6897.

Walseng, E., Furuta, K., Bosch, B., Weih, K.A., Matsuki, Y., Bakke, O., Ishido, S., and Roche, P.A.: **Ubiquitination regulates MHC class II-peptide complex retention and degradation in dendritic cells.** *Proc. Natl. Acad. Sci. USA* 2010, **107**:20465–20470.

6-10 Many proteins involved in antigen processing and presentation are encoded by genes within the MHC.

Aguado, B., Bahram, S., Beck, S., Campbell, R.D., Forbes, S.A., Geraghty, D., Guillaudeux, T., Hood, L., Horton, R., Inoko, H., *et al.* (the MHC Sequencing Consortium): **Complete sequence and gene map of a human major histocompatibility complex.** *Nature* 1999, **401**:921–923.

Chang, C.H., Gourley, T.S., and Sisk, T.J.: **Function and regulation of class II transactivator in the immune system.** *Immunol. Res.* 2002, **25**:131–142.

Kumnovics, A., Takada, T., and Lindahl, K.F.: **Genomic organization of the mammalian MHC.** *Annu. Rev. Immunol.* 2003, **21**:629–657.

Lefranc, M.P.: **IMGT, the international ImMunoGeneTics database.** *Nucleic Acids Res.* 2003, **31**:307–310.

6-11 The protein products of MHC class I and class II genes are highly polymorphic.

Gaur, L.K., and Nepom, G.T.: **Ancestral major histocompatibility complex DRB genes beget conserved patterns of localized polymorphisms.** *Proc. Natl .Acad. Sci. USA* 1996, **93**:5380–5383.

Marsh, S.G.: **Nomenclature for factors of the HLA system, update December 2002.** *Eur. J. Immunogenet.* 2003, **30**:167–169.

Robinson, J., and Marsh, S.G.: **HLA informatics. Accessing HLA sequences from sequence databases.** *Methods Mol. Biol.* 2003, **210**:3–21.

6-12 MHC polymorphism affects antigen recognition by T cells by influencing both peptide binding and the contacts between T-cell receptor and MHC molecule.

Falk, K., Rotzschke, O., Stevanovic, S., Jung, G., and Rammensee, H.G.: **Allele-specific motifs revealed by sequencing of self-peptides eluted from MHC molecules.** *Nature* 1991, **351**:290–296.

Garcia, K.C., Degano, M., Speir, J.A., and Wilson, I.A.: **Emerging principles for T cell receptor recognition of antigen in cellular immunity.** *Rev. Immunogenet.* 1999, **1**:75–90.

Katz, D.H., Hamaoka, T., Dorf, M.E., Maurer, P.H., and Benacerraf, B.: **Cell interactions between histoincompatible T and B lymphocytes. IV. Involvement of immune response (Ir) gene control of lymphocyte interaction controlled by the gene.** *J. Exp. Med.* 1973, **138**:734–739.

Kjer-Nielsen, L., Clements, C.S., Brooks, A.G., Purcell, A.W., Fontes, M.R., McCluskey, J., and Rossjohn, J.: **The structure of HLA-B8 complexed to an immunodominant viral determinant: peptide-induced conformational changes and a mode of MHC class I dimerization.** *J. Immunol.* 2002, **169**:5153–5160.

Wang, J.H., and Reinherz, E.L.: **Structural basis of T cell recognition of peptides bound to MHC molecules.** *Mol. Immunol.* 2002, **38**:1039–1049.

Zinkernagel, R.M., and Doherty, P.C.: **Restriction of *in vivo* T-cell mediated cytotoxicity in lymphocytic choriomeningitis within a syngeneic or semiallogeneic system.** *Nature* 1974, **248**:701–702.

6-13 Alloreactive T cells recognizing nonself MHC molecules are very abundant.

Felix, N.J., and Allen, P.M.: **Specificity of T-cell alloreactivity.** *Nat. Rev. Immunol.* 2007, **7**:942–953.

Feng, D., Bond, C.J., Ely, L.K., Maynard, J., and Garcia, K.C.: **Structural evidence for a germline-encoded T cell receptor–major histocompatibility complex interaction 'codon.'** *Nat. Immunol.* 2007, **8**:975–993.

Hennecke, J., and Wiley, D.C.: **Structure of a complex of the human α/β T cell receptor (TCR) HA1.7, influenza hemagglutinin peptide, and major histocompatibility complex class II molecule, HLA-DR4 (DRA*0101 and DRB1*0401): insight into TCR cross-restriction and alloreactivity.** *J. Exp. Med.* 2002, **195**:571–581.

Jankovic, V., Remus, K., Molano, A., and Nikolich-Zugich, J.: **T cell recognition of an engineered MHC class I molecule: implications for peptide-independent alloreactivity.** *J. Immunol.* 2002, **169**:1887–1892.

Nesic, D., Maric, M., Santori, F.R., and Vukmanovic, S.: **Factors influencing the patterns of T lymphocyte allorecognition.** *Transplantation* 2002, **73**:797–803.

Reiser, J.B., Darnault, C., Guimezanes, A., Gregoire, C., Mosser, T., Schmitt-Verhulst, A.M., Fontecilla-Camps, J.C., Malissen, B., Housset, D., and Mazza, G.: **Crystal structure of a T cell receptor bound to an allogeneic MHC molecule.** *Nat. Immunol.* 2000, **1**:291–297.

Rötzschke, O., Falk, K., Faath, S., and Rammensee, H.G.: **On the nature of peptides involved in T cell alloreactivity.** *J. Exp. Med.* 1991, **174**:1059–1071.

Speir, J.A., Garcia, K.C., Brunmark, A., Degano, M., Peterson, P.A., Teyton, L., and Wilson, I.A.: **Structural basis of 2C TCR allorecognition of H-2Ld peptide complexes.** *Immunity* 1998, **8**:553–562.

6-14 Many T cells respond to superantigens.

Kappler, J.W., Staerz, U., White, J., and Marrack, P.: **T cell receptor Vb elements which recognize Mls-modified products of the major histocompatibility complex.** *Nature* 1988, **332**:35–40.

Rammensee, H.G., Kroschewski, R., and Frangoulis, B.: **Clonal anergy induced in mature Vβ6⁺ T lymphocytes on immunizing Mls-1b mice with Mls-1a expressing cells.** *Nature* 1989, **339**:541–544.

Spaulding, A.R., Salgado-Pabón, W., Kohler, P.L., Horswill, A.R., Leung, D.Y., and Schlievert, P.M.: **Staphylococcal and streptococcal superantigen exotoxins.** *Clin. Microbiol. Rev.* 2013, **26**:422–447.

Sundberg, E.J., Li, H., Llera, A.S., McCormick, J.K., Tormo, J., Schlievert, P.M., Karjalainen, K., and Mariuzza, R.A.: **Structures of two streptococcal superantigens bound to TCR β chains reveal diversity in the architecture of T cell signaling complexes.** *Structure* 2002, **10**:687–699.

Torres, B.A., Perrin, G.Q., Mujtaba, M.G., Subramaniam, P.S., Anderson, A.K., and Johnson, H.M.: **Superantigen enhancement of specific immunity: antibody production and signaling pathways.** *J. Immunol.* 2002, **169**:2907–2914.

White, J., Herman, A., Pullen, A.M., Kubo, R., Kappler, J.W., and Marrack, P.: **The Vβ-specific super antigen staphylococcal enterotoxin B: stimulation of mature T cells and clonal deletion in neonatal mice.** *Cell* 1989, **56**:27–35.

6-15 MHC polymorphism extends the range of antigens to which the immune system can respond.

Hill, A.V., Elvin, J., Willis, A.C., Aidoo, M., Allsopp, C.E.M., Gotch, F.M., Gao, X.M., Takiguchi, M., Greenwood, B.M., Townsend, A.R.M., *et al.*: **Molecular analysis of the association of B53 and resistance to severe malaria.** *Nature* 1992, **360**:435–440.

Martin, M.P., and Carrington, M.: **Immunogenetics of viral infections.** *Curr. Opin. Immunol.* 2005, **17**:510–516.

Messaoudi, I., Guevara Patino, J.A., Dyall, R., LeMaoult, J., and Nikolich-Zugich, J.: **Direct link between MHC polymorphism, T cell avidity, and diversity in immune defense.** *Science* 2002, **298**:1797–1800.

Potts, W.K., and Slev, P.R.: **Pathogen-based models favouring MHC genetic diversity.** *Immunol. Rev.* 1995, **143**:181–197.

6-16 A variety of genes with specialized functions in immunity are also encoded in the MHC.

Alfonso, C., and Karlsson, L.: **Nonclassical MHC class II molecules.** *Annu. Rev. Immunol.* 2000, **18**:113–142.

Hofstetter, A.R., Sullivan, L.C., Lukacher, A.E., and Brooks, A.G.: **Diverse roles of non-diverse molecules: MHC class Ib molecules in host defense and control of autoimmunity.** *Curr. Opin. Immunol.* 2011, 23:104–110.

Loconto, J., Papes, F., Chang, E., Stowers, L., Jones, E.P., Takada, T., Kumánovics, A., Fischer Lindahl, K., and Dulac, C.: **Functional expression of murine V2R pheromone receptors involves selective association with the M10 and M1 families of MHC class Ib molecules.** *Cell* 2003, 112:607–118.

Powell, L.W., Subramaniam, V.N., and Yapp, T.R.: **Haemochromatosis in the new millennium.** *J. Hepatol.* 2000, 32:48–62.

6-17 Specialized MHC class I molecules act as ligands for the activation and inhibition of NK cells and unconventional T-cell subsets.

Borrego, F., Kabat, J., Kim, D.K., Lieto, L., Maasho, K., Pena, J., Solana, R., and Coligan, J.E.: **Structure and function of major histocompatibility complex (MHC) class I specific receptors expressed on human natural killer (NK) cells.** *Mol. Immunol.* 2002, 38:637–660.

Boyington, J.C., Riaz, A.N., Patamawenu, A., Coligan, J.E., Brooks, A.G., and Sun, P.D.: **Structure of CD94 reveals a novel C-type lectin fold: implications for the NK cell-associated CD94/NKG2 receptors.** *Immunity* 1999, 10:75–82.

Braud, V.M., Allan, D.S., O'Callaghan, C.A., Söderström, K., D'Andrea, A., Ogg, G.S., Lazetic, S., Young, N.T., Bell, J.I., Phillips, J.H., *et al.*: **HLA-E binds to natural killer cell receptors CD94/NKG2A, B and C.** *Nature* 1998, 391:795–799.

Braud, V.M., and McMichael, A.J.: **Regulation of NK cell functions through interaction of the CD94/NKG2 receptors with the nonclassical class I molecule HLA-E.** *Curr. Top. Microbiol. Immunol.* 1999, 244:85–95.

Jiang, H., Canfield, S.M., Gallagher, M.P., Jiang, H.H., Jiang, Y., Zheng, Z., and Chess, L.: **HLA-E-restricted regulatory CD8(+) T cells are involved in development and control of human autoimmune type 1 diabetes.** *J. Clin. Invest.* 2010, 120:3641–3650.

Lanier, L.L.: **NK cell recognition.** *Annu. Rev. Immunol.* 2005, 23:225–274.

Lopez-Botet, M., Llano, M., Navarro, F., and Bellon, T.: **NK cell recognition of non-classical HLA class I molecules.** *Semin. Immunol.* 2000, 12:109–119.

Lu, L., Ikizawa, K., Hu, D., Werneck, M.B., Wucherpfennig, K.W., and Cantor, H.: **Regulation of activated CD4+ T cells by NK cells via the Qa-1-NKG2A inhibitory pathway.** *Immunity* 2007, 26:593–604.

Pietra, G., Romagnani, C., Moretta, L., and Mingari, M.C.: **HLA-E and HLA-E-bound peptides: recognition by subsets of NK and T cells.** *Curr. Pharm. Des.* 2009, 15:3336–3344.

Rodgers, J.R., and Cook, R.G.: **MHC class Ib molecules bridge innate and acquired immunity.** *Nat. Rev. Immunol.* 2005, 5:459–471.

6-18 Members of the CD1 family of MHC class I–like molecules present lipid-based antigens to NKT cells.

Dasgupta, S., and Kumar, V.: **Type II NKT cells: a distinct CD1d-restricted immune regulatory NKT cell subset.** *Immunogenetics.* 2016, 68:665–676.

de Jong, A., Peña-Cruz, V., Cheng, T.Y., Clark, R.A., Van Rhijn, I., and Moody, D.B.: **CD1a-autoreactive T cells are a normal component of the human αβ T cell repertoire.** *Nat. Immunol.* 2010, 11:1102–1109.

de Lalla, C., Lepore, M., Piccolo, F.M., Rinaldi, A., Scelfo, A., Garavaglia, C., Mori, L., De Libero, G., Dellabona, P., and Casorati, G.: **High-frequency and adaptive-like dynamics of human CD1 self-reactive T cells.** *Eur. J. Immunol.* 2011, 41:602–610.

Godfrey, D.I., Uldrich, A.P., McCluskey, J., Rossjohn, J., and Moody, D.B.: **The burgeoning family of unconventional T cells.** *Nat. Immunol.* 2015, 16:1114–1123.

Hava, D.L., Brigl, M., van den Elzen, P., Zajonc, D.M., Wilson, I.A., and Brenner, M.B.: **CD1 assembly and the formation of CD1-antigen complexes.** *Curr. Opin. Immunol.* 2005, 17:88–94.

Kumar, V., and Delovitch, T.L.: **Different subsets of natural killer T cells may vary in their roles in health and disease.** *Immunology* 2014, 42:321–336.

Kim, J.H., Hu, Y., Yongqing, T., Kim, J., Hughes, V.A., Le Nours, J., Marquez, E.A., Purcell, A.W., Wan, Q., Sugita, M., *et al.*: **CD1a on Langerhans cells controls inflammatory skin disease.** *Nat. Immunol.* 2016, 17:1159–1166.

Moody, D.B., and Besra, G.S.: **Glycolipid targets of CD1-mediated T-cell responses.** *Immunology* 2001, 104:243–251.

Moody, D.B., and Cotton, R.N.: **Four pathways of CD1 antigen presentation to T cells.** *Curr. Opin. Immunol.* 2017, 46:127–133.

Scharf, L., Li, N.S., Hawk, A.J., Garzón, D., Zhang, T., Fox, L.M., Kazen, A.R., Shah, S., Haddadian, E.J., Gumperz, J.E., *et al.*: **The 2.5Å structure of CD1c in complex with a mycobacterial lipid reveals an open groove ideally suited for diverse antigen presentation.** *Immunity* 2010, 33:853–862.

Van Rhijn, I., Kasmar, A., de Jong, A., Gras, S., Bhati, M., Doorenspleet, M.E., de Vries, N., Godfrey, D.I., Altman, J.D., de Jager, W., *et al.*: **A conserved human T cell population targets mycobacterial antigens presented by CD1b.** *Nat. Immunol.* 2013, 14:706–713.

Zajonc, D.M., and Girardi, E.: **Recognition of microbial glycolipids by natural killer T cells.** *Front. Immunol.* 2015, 6:400.

6-19 The nonclassical MHC class I molecule MR1 presents microbial riboflavin metabolites to MAIT cells.

Keller, A.N., Corbett, A.J., Wubben, J.M., McCluskey, J., and Rossjohn, J.: **MAIT cells and MR1-antigen recognition.** *Curr. Opin. Immunol.* 2017, 46:66–74.

Kjer-Nielsen, L., Patel, O., Corbett, A.J., Le Nours, J., Meehan, B., Liu, L., Bhati, M., Chen, Z., Kostenko, L., Reantragoon, R., *et al.*: **MR1 presents microbial vitamin B metabolites to MAIT cells.** *Nature* 2012, 491:717–723.

López-Sagaseta, J., Dulberger, C.L., Crooks, J.E., Parks, C.D., Luoma, A.M., McFedries, A., Van Rhijn, I., Saghatelian, A., and Adams, E.J.: **The molecular basis for mucosal-associated invariant T cell recognition of MR1 proteins.** *Proc. Natl. Acad. Sci. USA* 2013, 110:E1771–1778.

6-20 γδ T cells can recognize a variety of diverse ligands.

Chien, Y.H., Meyer, C., and Bonneville, M.: **γδ T cells: first line of defense and beyond.** *Annu. Rev. Immunol.* 2014, 32:121–155.

Gentles, A.J., Newman, A.M., Liu, C.L., Bratman, S.V., Feng, W., Kim, D., Nair, V.S., Xu, Y., Khuong, A., Hoang, C.D., *et al.*: **The prognostic landscape of genes and infiltrating immune cells across human cancers.** *Nat. Med.* 2015, 21:938–945.

Harly, C., Guillaume, Y., Nedellec, S., Peigné, C.M., Mönkkönen, H., Mönkkönen, J., Li, J., Kuball, J., Adams, E.J., Netzer, S., Déchanet-Merville, J., *et al.*: **Key implication of CD277/butyrophilin-3 (BTN3A) in cellular stress sensing by a major human γδ T-cell subset.** *Blood* 2012, 120:2269–2279.

Nielsen, M.M., Witherden, D.A., and Havran, W.L.: **γδ T cells in homeostasis and host defence of epithelial barrier tissues.** *Nat. Rev. Immunol.* 2017, 17:733–745.

Turchinovich, G., and Hayday, A.C.: **Skint-1 identifies a common molecular mechanism for the development of interferon-γ-secreting versus interleukin-17-secreting γδ T cells.** *Immunity* 2011, 35:59–68.

Uldrich, A.P., Le Nours, J., Pellicci, D.G., Gherardin, N.A., McPherson, K.G., Lim, R.T., Patel, O., Beddoe, T., Gras, S., Rossjohn, J., *et al.*: **CD1d-lipid antigen recognition by the γδ TCR.** *Nat. Immunol.* 2013, 14:1137–1145.

Vantourout, P., Laing, A., Woodward, M.J., Zlatareva, I., Apolonia, L., Jones, A.W., Snijders, A.P., Malim, M.H., and Hayday, A.C.: **Heteromeric interactions regulate butyrophilin (BTN) and BTN-like molecules governing γδ T cell biology.** *Proc. Natl. Acad. Sci. USA* 2018, 115:1039–1044.

Willcox, C.R., Pitard, V., Netzer, S., Couzi, L., Salim, M., Silberzahn, T., Moreau, J.F., Hayday, A.C., Willcox, B.E., and Déchanet-Merville, J.: **Cytomegalovirus and tumor stress surveillance by binding of a human γδ T cell antigen receptor to endothelial protein C receptor.** *Nat. Immunol.* 2012, 13:872–879.

Lymphocyte Receptor Signaling

7

T and B lymphocytes are cells of the adaptive immune system, each of which expresses a unique antigen receptor. After exiting the thymus (T cells) and bone marrow (B cells), these cells circulate through the blood, the lymph, and the secondary lymphoid organs, where they survey antigen-presenting cells for their specific antigen. Once that antigen is encountered, signals from the antigen receptor stimulate several downstream pathways, activating enzymes that promote the conversion of nondividing naive lymphocytes into activated cells that reorganize their actin cytoskeleton, activate transcription factors, and synthesize a wide range of new proteins. As a result of these events, naive T and B cells undergo rapid cell division and differentiate into armed effector cells, thus expanding lymphocyte populations during an immune response and equipping these cells with the machinery to combat infections (**Fig. 7.1**).

We begin by discussing some general principles of intracellular signaling and then outline the pathways activated when a naive lymphocyte encounters its specific antigen. Next, we briefly discuss the co-stimulatory signaling that is necessary to activate naive T cells and, in most cases, naive B cells. In this last part of the chapter we also discuss inhibitory receptors and their roles in down-regulating signaling pathways in T and B cells.

General principles of signal transduction and propagation.

In this part of the chapter we review briefly some general principles of receptor action and signal transduction that are common to many of the pathways discussed here. All cell-surface receptors that have a signaling function either are transmembrane proteins themselves or form parts of protein complexes that link the extracellular environment and the interior of the cell. Different classes of receptors transduce extracellular signals in a variety of ways. A common theme among the receptors covered in this chapter is that ligand binding results in the activation of an intracellular enzymatic activity.

IN THIS CHAPTER

General principles of signal transduction and propagation.

Antigen receptor signaling and lymphocyte activation.

Co-stimulatory and inhibitory receptors modulate antigen receptor signaling in T and B lymphocytes.

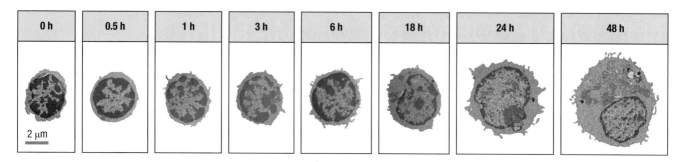

Fig. 7.1 Lymphocyte activation converts small nondividing cells into effector cells. Transmission electron microscopy was used to view resting naive T cells before and after stimulation with anti-CD3 antibodies. Among the changes that can be seen are the increased size of the cell, the expanded volume of the cell cytoplasm, and the decondensation of the chromatin in the cell nucleus.

T-cell receptor strength				
None	**Low**	**Medium low**	**Medium high**	**High**
–	+	++	+++	+++
–	++	+++	+++	+++
–	+	+	++	+++
–	–	–	++	+++
–	–	–	–	++
–	–	–	–	+++

Expression	
Low	High

Fig. 7.2 Antigen receptor signaling can produce varying patterns of gene expression. Receptor-stimulated signaling responses in lymphocytes are complex networks of positive- and negative-feedback pathways that can produce various outcomes. An example illustrated here is a set of genes, each one represented by a row of boxes. Depending on the strength of stimulation through the T-cell receptor, each gene shows a unique pattern of expression.

7-1 Transmembrane receptors convert extracellular signals into intracellular biochemical events.

The enzymes most commonly associated with receptor activation are the **protein kinases**, enzymes that catalyze the covalent attachment of a phosphate group to a protein, a reversible process called **phosphorylation**. In animals, protein kinases phosphorylate proteins on tyrosine, serine, or threonine, and more rarely, on histidine. In the case of the antigen receptors on B lymphocytes and T lymphocytes, the transmembrane receptors themselves have no intrinsic enzymatic activity. Instead these receptors associate with intracellular **protein tyrosine kinases**. Ligand binding to the extracellular domain of such receptors causes tyrosine phosphorylation of intracellular proteins, including the cytoplasmic domains of the receptor subunits.

For many cytokine receptors, ligand binding causes dimerization or clustering of individual receptor molecules, bringing the associated kinases together and enabling them to phosphorylate the cytoplasmic tail of adjacent receptors—thus initiating an intracellular signal. In the case of the lymphocyte antigen receptors, association with cytoplasmic tyrosine kinases occurs after ligand binding but is unlikely to be due to a simple clustering mechanism. Instead, the actions of co-receptors are required: these bring cytoplasmic tyrosine kinases into proximity with the cytoplasmic regions of the antigen receptor, a complex process that we will describe later.

Signaling is usually not a simple 'on or off' switch. Depending on the affinity of the receptor for the ligand, the abundance of the ligand, the concentrations of intracellular signaling components, and a complex network of positive- and negative-feedback pathways, receptor activation and downstream signaling occur when a minimum threshold determined by all of these factors is exceeded. These features are often merged into the simple term 'signal strength.' It is important to keep in mind that variations in signal strength will determine the magnitude of cellular responses—some will be all-or-nothing, whereas others will increase as the strength of signaling increases (**Fig. 7.2**).

The role of protein kinases in cell signaling is not confined to receptor activation, as they act at many different stages in intracellular signaling pathways. Protein kinases figure largely in cell signaling because phosphorylation and **dephosphorylation**—the removal of a phosphate group—are the means of regulating the activity of many enzymes, transcription factors, and other proteins. Equally important to the workings of signaling pathways is the fact that phosphorylation generates sites on proteins to which other signaling proteins can bind.

Phosphate groups are removed from proteins by a large class of enzymes called **protein phosphatases**. Like protein kinases, protein phosphatases can also be soluble cytosolic proteins or transmembrane receptors. Different classes of protein phosphatases remove phosphate groups from phosphotyrosine or from phosphoserine/phosphothreonine, or both (as in dual-specificity phosphatases). Specific dephosphorylation by phosphatases is one important means of regulating signaling pathways by resetting a protein to its original state and thus switching signaling off. Dephosphorylation does not always inhibit a protein's activity. In many instances the removal of a particular phosphate group by a specific phosphatase is needed to activate an enzyme. In other cases, the extent of phosphorylation of an enzyme determines its activity and represents a balance between the activity of kinases and phosphatases.

7-2 Intracellular signal propagation is mediated by large multiprotein signaling complexes.

As we learned in Chapter 3, the binding of a ligand to its receptor can initiate a cascade of biochemical events involving intracellular proteins that sequentially act in a signaling pathway. The unique enzymes and other components assembled into a particular multiprotein receptor complex will determine the specific biochemical and cellular changes that result from each segment of the pathway. These components may be shared by several receptor pathways or they may be exclusive to one receptor pathway, thus allowing distinct signaling pathways to be built up from a relatively limited number of components. The assembly of multi-subunit signaling complexes involves specific interactions of a number of distinct types of **protein-interaction domains**, or **protein-interaction modules**, carried by the signaling proteins. Signaling proteins in general contain at least one such protein-interaction domain, but many contain multiple domains. **Figure 7.3** gives a few examples of such domains.

For the pathways considered in this chapter, an important mechanism underlying the formation of signaling complexes is the phosphorylation of protein tyrosine residues. Phosphotyrosines are binding sites for a number of protein-interaction domains, including the **SH2 (Src homology 2) domain** (see Fig. 7.3). SH2 domains, built from approximately 100 amino acids, are present in many intracellular signaling proteins, where they are frequently linked to enzymatic or other functional domains. SH2 domains recognize the phosphorylated tyrosine (pY) and, typically, the amino acid three positions away (pYXXZ, where X is any amino acid and Z is a specific amino acid); they bind in a sequence-specific fashion, with different SH2 domains preferring different combinations of amino acids. In this way, the unique SH2 domain of a signaling molecule can promote inducible and specific association with a protein that contains the appropriate pY-containing

Protein domain	Found in	Ligand class	Example of ligand
SH2	Lck, ZAP-70, Fyn, Src, Grb2, PLC-γ, STAT, Cbl, Btk, Itk, SHIP, Vav, SAP, PI3K, Syk, Lyn	phosphotyrosine	pYXXZ
SH3	Lck, Fyn, Src, Grb2, Btk, Itk, Tec, Fyb, Nck, Gads	proline	PXXP
PH	Tec, PLC-γ, Akt, Btk, Itk, Sos	phosphoinositides	PIP$_3$
PX	P40^{phox}, P47^{phox}, PLD	phosphoinositides	PI(3)P
PDZ	CARMA1	C termini of proteins	IESDV, VETDV
C1	RasGRP, PKC-θ	membrane lipid	diacylglycerol (DAG) phorbol ester
NZF	TAB2	polyubiquitin (K63-linked)	polyubiquitinated RIP, TRAF6, or NEMO
G domain	Ras, Rho, Cdc42, Rap1	guanine nucleotide	GTP, GDP

Fig. 7.3 Signaling proteins interact with each other and with lipid signaling molecules via modular protein domains. A few of the most common protein domains used by immune-system signaling proteins are listed, together with some proteins that contain them and the general class of ligand bound by the interaction domain. The right-hand column lists specific examples of a protein motif (in single-letter amino acid code) or, for the phosphoinositide-binding domains, the particular phosphoinositide that they bind. All these domains are used in many other nonimmune signaling pathways as well.

Fig. 7.4 Assembly of signaling complexes is mediated by adaptor proteins. Assembly of signaling complexes is an important aspect of signal transduction. This is often achieved through adaptor proteins. In some cases, adaptor proteins have numerous sites of phosphorylation that function to bring many different signaling proteins together. Adaptors may also function to promote membrane localization, to bring enzymes into close proximity with their substrates, and to induce conformational changes in proteins that regulate their functions. Some adaptor proteins function more simply, bringing two different proteins together.

amino acid sequence, an interaction that only occurs after tyrosine phosphorylation of the SH2 domain's binding partner.

Tyrosine kinase–associated receptors can assemble multiprotein signaling complexes by using proteins called **adaptors**. Adaptors lack enzymatic activity, and they function by recruiting other proteins into a signaling complex so that interactions among these proteins can take place (**Fig. 7.4**). The adaptor proteins Grb2 and Gads, for example, each contain an SH2 domain and two copies of another module called the SH3 domain. This arrangement of modules can be used to link tyrosine phosphorylation of a receptor to molecules acting in the next stage of signaling. As we will see later, antigen receptor signaling pathways make extensive use of this mechanism to assemble a variety of distinct multiprotein complexes, each of which functions to activate a different enzyme that contributes to overall lymphocyte responses.

7-3 Small G proteins act as molecular switches in many different signaling pathways.

Another biochemical mechanism important in the signaling pathways leading from many tyrosine kinase–associated receptors is the use of monomeric GTP-binding proteins known as **small G proteins, or small GTPases**. The small GTPases are distinct from the larger heterotrimeric G proteins associated with G protein–coupled receptors such as the chemokine receptors discussed in Chapter 3. The superfamily of small GTPases comprises more than 100 different proteins, and many are important in lymphocyte signaling. One of these, **Ras**, is involved in many pathways leading to cell proliferation. Other small GTPases include Rac, Rho, and Cdc42, which control changes in the actin cytoskeleton caused by signals received through the T-cell receptor or B-cell receptor. We will describe their actions in more detail in Section 7-19.

Small GTPases exist in two states, depending on whether they are bound to GTP or to GDP. The GDP-bound form is inactive but is converted into the active form by exchange of the GDP for GTP. This reaction is mediated by proteins known as **guanine nucleotide exchange factors, or GEFs**, which cause the GTPase to release GDP and to bind the more abundant GTP (**Fig. 7.5**). One

Fig. 7.5 Small G proteins are switched from inactive to active states by guanine nucleotide exchange factors (GEFs) and the binding of GTP. Ras is a small GTP-binding protein with intrinsic GTPase activity. In its resting state, Ras is bound to GDP. Receptor signaling activates GEFs, such as Sos, which can bind to small G proteins such as Ras and increase the rate of exchange of GDP for GTP (center panels). The GTP-bound form of Ras can then bind to a large number of effectors, recruiting them to the membrane. Over time, the intrinsic GTPase activity of Ras will result in the hydrolysis of GTP to GDP. GTPase-activating proteins (GAPs) can accelerate the hydrolysis of GTP to GDP, thus shutting off the signal more rapidly.

of the GEFs for Ras, Sos, is recruited to signaling pathways by the adaptor Grb2. The binding of GTP induces a conformational change in the small GTPase that enables it to bind to and induce effector activity in a variety of target proteins. Thus, GTP binding functions as an on/off switch for small GTPases.

This GTP-bound form does not remain permanently active but is eventually converted into the inactive GDP-bound form by the intrinsic GTPase activity in the G protein, which removes a phosphate group from the bound GTP. Regulatory cofactors known as **GTPase-activating proteins (GAPs)** accelerate the conversion of GTP to GDP, thus rapidly down-regulating the activity of the small GTPase. Because of GAP activity, small GTPases are usually present in the inactive GDP-bound state and are activated only transiently in response to a signal from an activated receptor. *RAS* is frequently mutated in cancer cells, and the mutated Ras protein is thought to be a significant contributor to the cancerous state. The importance of GAPs in signaling regulation is indicated by the fact that some mutations in Ras found in cancer act by preventing GAP from enhancing the intrinsic GTPase activity of Ras, thus prolonging the duration for which Ras exists in the active GTP-bound state.

GEFs are the key to G-protein activation and are recruited to the site of receptor activation at the cell membrane by binding to adaptor proteins or to lipid metabolites produced by receptor activation. Once recruited, they are able to activate Ras or other small G proteins, which are localized to the inner surface of the plasma membrane via fatty acid or polybasic motifs that bind acidic lipids. Thus, G proteins act as molecular switches, becoming switched on when a cell-surface receptor is activated and then being switched off. Each G protein has its own specific GEFs and GAPs, which help to confer specificity on the pathway.

7-4 Signaling proteins are recruited to the membrane by a variety of mechanisms.

We have seen how receptors can recruit intracellular signaling proteins to the plasma membrane through tyrosine phosphorylation of the receptor itself or of an associated adaptor, followed by recruitment of SH2 domain–containing signaling proteins and additional adaptors, such as Grb2 (**Fig. 7.6**). A second mechanism for membrane recruitment of signaling proteins is via binding to small GTPases, such as Ras, after their activation. As described in Section 7-3, small GTPases are constitutively bound to the cytoplasmic surface of the plasma membrane because of their fatty acid modifications. Once activated by exchange of GDP for GTP, the activated GTPases bind to signaling proteins such as Raf, relocalizing the bound proteins to the plasma membrane (see Fig. 7.6).

Another way in which receptors can recruit signaling molecules to the plasma membrane is by the local production of modified membrane lipids. These lipids are produced by phosphorylation of the membrane phospholipid

Fig. 7.6 Signaling proteins can be recruited to the membrane in a variety of ways. Recruitment of signaling proteins to the plasma membrane is important in signal propagation because this is where receptors are usually located. Left panel: Tyrosine phosphorylation of membrane-associated proteins, such as the adaptor LAT, recruits phosphotyrosine-binding proteins. This can also protect the adaptor from dephosphorylation by tyrosine phosphatases, which inhibit signaling. Second panel: Small G proteins such as Ras can associate with the membrane by having lipid modifications (shown in red). When activated, they can bind a variety of signaling proteins. Right two panels: Modifications to the membrane itself that result from receptor activation can recruit signaling proteins. In this example the membrane lipid PIP$_3$ has been produced in the inner leaflet of the plasma membrane by the phosphorylation of PIP$_2$ by PI 3-kinase. PIP$_3$ is recognized by the pleckstrin homology (PH) domains of signaling proteins such as the protein kinases Akt and Itk.

Binding to phosphorylated sites on a membrane-associated protein

Recognition of activated small G proteins

PI 3-kinase phosphorylates PIP$_2$ to generate PIP$_3$

Binding to membrane lipids

phosphatidylinositol by enzymes known as **phosphatidylinositol kinases**, which are activated as a result of receptor signaling. The inositol headgroup of phosphatidylinositol is a carbohydrate ring that can be phosphorylated at one or more positions to generate a wide variety of derivatives. The ones that we will focus on in this chapter are phosphatidylinositol 4,5-bisphosphate (PIP_2) and phosphatidylinositol 3,4,5-trisphosphate (PIP_3), the latter of which is generated from PIP_2 by the enzyme **phosphatidylinositol 3-kinase (PI 3-kinase)** (see Fig. 7.6). PI 3-kinase is often recruited by binding of the SH2 domain of its regulatory subunit to phosphotyrosines in a receptor tail or an adaptor protein, bringing its catalytic subunit into proximity with inositol phospholipid substrates in the membrane. In this way, membrane phosphoinositides such as PIP_3 are rapidly produced after receptor activation. This, combined with their short life span, makes them ideal signaling molecules. PIP_3 is recognized specifically by proteins containing a pleckstrin homology (PH) domain or, less commonly, a PX domain (see Fig. 7.3), and one of its functions is to recruit such proteins to the membrane and in some cases contribute to enzyme activation.

7-5 Post-translational modifications of proteins can both activate and inhibit signaling responses.

Protein phosphorylation is a common mechanism for transducing signals from cellular receptors to downstream pathways. These signals are terminated by the action of protein phosphatases, which dephosphorylate signaling intermediates (**Fig. 7.7**). The importance of protein phosphatases in terminating signaling is underscored by the existence of diseases, such as autoimmunity and cancer, which may result from absent or deficient protein phosphatase activity. However, protein dephosphorylation can also function as a mechanism of activation. Dephosphorylation can regulate protein–protein interactions, protein subcellular localization, or nucleic acid binding, thereby promoting downstream signaling events.

Another general mechanism of protein regulation by post-translational modification is the covalent attachment of one or more molecules of the small protein **ubiquitin**. Ubiquitination is a potent means of signal termination, as it often leads to protein degradation. Ubiquitin is attached by its carboxyl-terminal glycine to lysine residues of target proteins in a multistep process. First, an E1 ubiquitin-activating enzyme promotes attachment of ubiquitin to an E2 ubiquitin-conjugating enzyme. The ubiquitin is then transferred to the protein substrate by an enzyme known as an E3 **ubiquitin ligase**. Ubiquitin ligases can continue to add ubiquitin molecules to form polyubiquitin chains.

Fig. 7.7 Signaling must be turned off as well as turned on. The inability to terminate a signaling pathway can result in serious diseases such as autoimmunity or cancer. Because a significant proportion of signaling events depend on protein phosphorylation, protein phosphatases, such as SHP, have an important part in shutting down signaling pathways (left panel). Another common mechanism for terminating signaling is regulated protein degradation (center and right panels). Phosphorylated proteins recruit ubiquitin ligases, such as Cbl, that add the small protein ubiquitin to proteins, thus targeting them for degradation. Cytoplasmic proteins are targeted for destruction in the proteasome by the addition of polyubiquitin chains, linked through lysine 48 (K48) of ubiquitin (center panel). Membrane receptors that become ubiquitinated by individual ubiquitin molecules or di-ubiquitin are internalized and transported to the lysosome for destruction (right panel).

Dephosphorylation of phosphorylated substrates

SHP

Ubiquitin-mediated degradation by proteasome

Cbl

K48 polyubiquitin

proteasome

Ubiquitin-mediated degradation in the lysosome

Cbl

lysosome

Importantly, different ubiquitin ligases add the carboxyl terminus of one ubiquitin molecule to different lysine residues of the conjugated ubiquitin, typically either lysine 48 (K48) or lysine 63 (K63). These different forms of polyubiquitination produce divergent outcomes for signaling pathways.

When polyubiquitin chains are formed using K48 linkages, the outcome is to target the protein to the proteasome, a large protein complex responsible for degradation of cellular proteins (see Fig. 7.7). An important ubiquitin ligase of this kind in lymphocytes is Cbl, which selects its targets via its SH2 domain. Cbl can thus bind to specific tyrosine-phosphorylated targets, causing them to become ubiquitinated via K48 linkages, resulting in target protein degradation. Membrane proteins such as receptors can be tagged by single ubiquitin molecules or by di-ubiquitin. These are not recognized by the proteasome but instead are recognized by specific ubiquitin-binding proteins that target proteins for degradation in lysosomes or for release from cells in small membrane vesicles known as exosomes (see Fig. 7.7). Thus, ubiquitination of proteins can inhibit signaling. Unlike inhibition by phosphatases, which is reversible, inhibition by ubiquitin-mediated protein degradation is a longer-lasting means of terminating signaling.

Ubiquitination can also activate signaling pathways. We have already discussed this mechanism in Section 3-7 in connection with the NFκB signaling pathway from TLRs. There, the ubiquitin ligase TRAF6 produces K63-linked polyubiquitin chains on TRAF6 and NEMO. In lymphocytes, K63-linked polyubiquitination is a key step in signaling through tumor necrosis factor (TNF) receptor family members, as will be discussed in Section 7-24 (and Fig. 7.33). This form of polyubiquitination is recognized by specific domains in signaling proteins that recruit additional signaling molecules to the pathway (see Fig. 3.14). Thus, like tyrosine phosphorylation, K63-linked ubiquitination functions as a protein–protein interaction motif to promote the formation of multiprotein signaling complexes (see Fig. 7.3).

7-6 The activation of many receptors generates small-molecule second messengers.

In many cases, intracellular signaling involves the activation of enzymes that produce small-molecule biochemical mediators known as **second messengers** (Fig. 7.8). These mediators can diffuse throughout the cell, enabling the signal to activate a variety of target proteins. The enzymatic production of second messengers also serves the dual purpose of achieving concentrations of them sufficient to activate the next stage of the pathway and of amplifying the signaling cascade. The second messengers generated by receptors

Fig. 7.8 Signaling pathways amplify the initial signal. Amplification of the initial signal is an important element of most signal transduction pathways. One means of amplification is a kinase cascade (left panel), in which protein kinases successively phosphorylate and activate each other. In this example, taken from a common kinase cascade (see Fig. 7.20), activation of the kinase Raf results in the phosphorylation and activation of a second kinase, Mek, that phosphorylates yet another kinase, Erk. Because each kinase can phosphorylate many different substrate molecules, the signal is amplified at each step, resulting in a huge amplification of the initial signal. Another method of signal amplification is the generation of second messengers (center and right panels). In this example, signaling results in the release of the second messenger calcium (Ca^{2+}) from intracellular stores into the cytosol or its influx from the extracellular environment. Ca^{2+} release from the endoplasmic reticulum (ER) is shown here. The sharp increase in free Ca^{2+} in the cytoplasm can potentially activate many downstream signaling molecules, such as the calcium-binding protein calmodulin. Calcium binding induces a conformational change in calmodulin, which allows it to bind to and regulate a variety of effector proteins.

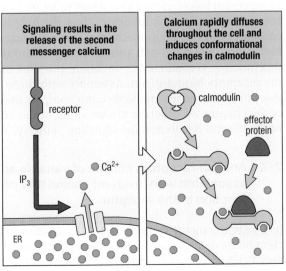

that signal via tyrosine kinases include calcium ions (Ca^{2+}) and a variety of membrane lipids and their soluble derivatives. Although some of these lipid messengers are confined to membranes, they can move within them. A second messenger binding to its target protein typically induces a conformational change that allows the protein to be activated, and can also participate in recruitment of proteins to cellular locations where they function.

Summary.

Cell-surface receptors serve as the front line of a cell's interaction with its environment; they sense extracellular events and convert them into biochemical signals for the cell. Because most receptors sit in the plasma membrane, a critical step in the transduction of extracellular signals to the interior of the cell is recruitment of intracellular proteins to the membrane and changes in the composition of the membrane surrounding the receptor. Many immune receptors operate by activating tyrosine kinases to transmit their signals onward, often using adaptors to form large multiprotein signaling complexes. Both the qualitative and quantitative changes that take place in the composition of these signaling complexes determine the character of the response and biological outcomes. Formation of signaling complexes is mediated by a wide variety of protein-interaction domains, or modules, including the SH2, SH3, and PH domains found in proteins. In many cases, the increase in enzymatically produced small-molecule signaling intermediates called second messengers regulates and amplifies the signaling cascade. Termination of signaling involves protein dephosphorylation as well as ubiquitin-mediated protein degradation.

Antigen receptor signaling and lymphocyte activation.

The ability of T cells and B cells to recognize and respond to their specific antigen is central to adaptive immunity. As described in Chapters 4 and 5, the B-cell antigen receptor (BCR) and the T-cell antigen receptor (TCR) are made up of antigen-binding chains—the heavy and light immunoglobulin chains in the B-cell receptor, and the TCRα and TCRβ chains in the T-cell receptor on conventional T cells. These variable chains have exquisite specificity for antigen, allowing each lymphocyte to detect the presence of one type of pathogen. However, binding of antigen to the antigen receptor is not sufficient for a lymphocyte to respond—the information that antigen receptor engagement has occurred also needs to be transduced into the intracellular compartment of the lymphocyte. Thus, the fully functional antigen receptor complex must include proteins that can transduce a signal across the plasma membrane. For the B-cell antigen receptor and the T-cell antigen receptor, this function is mediated by invariant proteins that initiate signaling when the receptors bind antigen. Assembly with these signaling subunits is also essential for transport of the receptor complex to the cell surface. In this part of the chapter we describe the structure of the antigen receptor complexes on T cells and B cells and the signaling pathways that lead from them.

7-7 Antigen receptors consist of variable antigen-binding chains associated with invariant chains that carry out the signaling function of the receptor.

In T cells, the highly variable TCRαβ heterodimer (see Chapter 5) is not sufficient on its own to make up a complete cell-surface antigen receptor. When non-T cells were transfected with cDNAs encoding the TCRα and TCRβ chains,

Fig. 7.9 The T-cell receptor complex is made up of variable antigen-recognition proteins and invariant signaling proteins. Upper panel: The functional T-cell receptor (TCR) complex is composed of the antigen-binding TCRαβ heterodimer associated with six signaling chains: two ε, one δ, and one γ, collectively called CD3, plus a homodimer of ζ. Cell-surface expression of the antigen-binding chains requires assembly of TCRαβ with the signaling subunits. Each CD3 chain has one immunoreceptor tyrosine-based activation motif (ITAM), shown as a yellow segment, whereas each ζ chain has three. The transmembrane regions of each chain have unusual acidic (–) or basic (+) residues as shown. Lower panel: The transmembrane regions of the various TCR subunits are represented in cross section. It is thought that one of the positive charges, from a lysine (K) of the α chain, interacts with the two negative charges of aspartic acid (D) of the CD3δε dimer (1), while the other positive charge, of arginine (R), interacts with aspartic acids of the ζ homodimer (3). The positive lysine (K) charge of the β chain interacts with the negative charges of aspartic acid and glutamic acid (E) in the CD3γε dimer (2).

the heterodimers formed were degraded and did not appear on the cell surface. This implied that other molecules are required for the T-cell receptor to be expressed on the cell surface. In the T-cell receptor, the other required molecules are the CD3γ, CD3δ, and CD3ε chains, which together form the **CD3 complex**, and the **ζ chain**, which is present as a disulfide-linked homodimer (**Fig. 7.9**). The CD3 proteins have an extracellular immunoglobulin-like domain, whereas the ζ chain contains only a short extracellular domain. Throughout the remainder of the chapter, we will use the term 'T-cell receptor' to refer to the entire T-cell receptor complex, including antigen-binding proteins and the signaling subunits.

The stoichiometry of the complete T-cell receptor is shown in Fig. 7.9. The T-cell receptor consists of one receptor α chain that interacts with one CD3δ:CD3ε dimer and with one ζ dimer, and one receptor β chain that interacts with one CD3γ:CD3ε dimer. These interactions are mediated by reciprocal charge interactions between basic and acidic intramembrane amino acids of the receptor subunits. There are two positive charges in the TCRα transmembrane region and one in the TCRβ transmembrane domain. Negative charges in the CD3 and ζ transmembrane domains interact with the positive charges in α and β. Assembly of CD3 and a ζ dimer with the αβ heterodimer stabilizes the α and β dimer during its production in the endoplasmic reticulum and allows the complex to be transported to the plasma membrane. These associations ensure that all T-cell receptors present on the plasma membrane are properly assembled.

Signaling from the T-cell receptor is initiated by tyrosine phosphorylation within cytoplasmic regions called **immunoreceptor tyrosine-based activation motifs (ITAMs)** in the CD3ε, CD3γ, CD3δ, and ζ chains. CD3γ, CD3δ, and CD3ε each contain one ITAM, and each ζ chain contains three, giving the T-cell receptor a total of 10 ITAMs. This motif is also present in the signaling chains of the B-cell receptor and in the NK-cell receptors described in Chapter 3, as well as in the receptors for the immunoglobulin constant region (Fc receptors) that are present on mast cells, macrophages, monocytes, neutrophils, and NK cells (see Section 7-11).

Each ITAM contains two tyrosine residues that become phosphorylated by specific protein tyrosine kinases when the receptor binds its ligand, providing sites for the recruitment of the SH2 domains of signaling proteins as described earlier in the chapter. Two YXXL/I motifs are separated by about six to nine amino acids within each ITAM, so the canonical ITAM sequence is . . . YXX[L/I]X_{6-9}YXX[L/I]. . ., where Y is tyrosine, L is leucine, I is isoleucine, and X represents any amino acid. The two tyrosines of the ITAM make it particularly efficient in recruiting signaling proteins that contain tandem SH2 domains (**Fig. 7.10**). When both tyrosines of the ITAM are phosphorylated, tandem SH2 domain–containing proteins Syk or ZAP-70 are recruited. This leads to the phosphorylation of Syk or ZAP-70, an essential step in the activation of these kinases, as will be discussed further later (see Section 7-10).

Autoinhibited conformation of ZAP-70	Phosphorylation of the ITAM recruits ZAP-70, which is then activated by phosphorylation

Fig. 7.10 ITAMs recruit signaling proteins that have tandem SH2 domains. The ITAMs of the T-cell receptor (TCR) and B-cell receptor (BCR) contain tyrosine residues within the motif . . . YXX[L/I]X$_{6-9}$YXX[L/I]. . . . The spacing between the tyrosines is important in binding to tandem SH2-containing proteins such as Syk and ZAP-70. Left panel: Prior to TCR or BCR stimulation, these kinases are in an inactive conformation, known as the autoinhibited conformation. The autoinhibited conformation is stabilized by interactions between the tandem SH2 domain–kinase domain linker region and the kinase domain that hold the enzyme in a catalytically inactive state. Right panel: After phosphorylation of both tyrosines within one ITAM (here depicted as two tyrosines separated by 9–12 amino acids), the tandem SH2 domains of Syk or ZAP-70 can dock cooperatively to both phosphotyrosines, as shown here for ZAP-70. By being recruited into the active signaling complex, ZAP-70 can itself be phosphorylated, so that it becomes an active kinase that can then phosphorylate its substrates. This final step of ZAP-70 activation requires phosphorylation on two tyrosines in the ZAP-70 linker region between the tandem SH2 domains and the kinase domain, together with phosphorylation of a tyrosine in the catalytic site of the ZAP-70 kinase domain.

The antigen-binding immunoglobulin on the B-cell surface is also associated with invariant protein chains that mediate signaling. These two polypeptides, called **Igα** and **Igβ**, are required for transport of the receptor to the surface and for B-cell receptor signaling (**Fig. 7.11**). Igα and Igβ are each composed of an extracellular immunoglobulin-like domain connected by a transmembrane domain to a cytoplasmic tail. They form a disulfide-linked heterodimer that becomes associated with immunoglobulin heavy chains and enables their transport to the cell surface. The Igα:Igβ dimer associates with the B-cell receptor through hydrophilic rather than charge interactions between their transmembrane regions. The complete B-cell receptor is thought to be a complex of six chains—two identical light chains, two identical heavy chains, and one associated heterodimer of Igα and Igβ. Like CD3 and the ζ chains of the T-cell receptor, Igα and Igβ have ITAMs, but just one each, and these are essential for the ability of the B-cell receptor to signal.

7-8 Antigen recognition by the T-cell receptor and its co-receptors transduces a signal across the plasma membrane to initiate signaling.

To make an effective immune response, T cells and B cells must be able to respond to their specific antigen even when it is present at extremely low levels. This is especially important for T cells, as an antigen-presenting cell will display on its surface many different peptides from both self and foreign

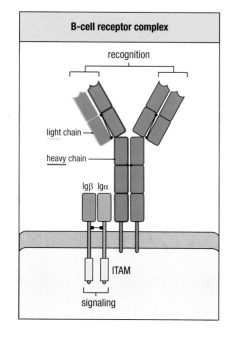

Fig. 7.11 The B-cell receptor complex is made up of cell-surface immunoglobulin with one each of the invariant signaling proteins Igα and Igβ. The immunoglobulin recognizes and binds antigen but cannot itself generate a signal. It is associated with antigen-nonspecific signaling molecules—Igα and Igβ. These each have a single ITAM (yellow segment) in their cytosolic tails that enables them to signal when the B-cell receptor is ligated with antigen. Igα and Igβ form a disulfide-linked heterodimer that is noncovalently associated with the heavy chains.

proteins, and the number of peptide:MHC complexes specific for a particular T-cell receptor is likely to be very low. Some estimates suggest that naive T cells can become activated by one or a few antigenic peptide:MHC complexes displayed by an antigen-presenting cell. B cells become activated when about 20 B-cell receptors are engaged. These estimates are based on *in vitro* studies and may not be precise for cells *in vivo*, but it is clear that the antigen receptors on T cells and B cells confer remarkable sensitivity to antigen.

For a peptide:MHC complex to activate T cells, it must bind directly to the T-cell receptor (**Fig. 7.12**, upper panel, and see Fig. 4.27). Although it remains unclear precisely how this extracellular recognition event is transmitted across the T-cell membrane to initiate signaling, several components of this process have now been established.

Biophysical experiments indicate that mechanical force changes contribute to the initiation of T-cell receptor signaling. When T-cell receptors on the surface of T cells bind to peptide:MHC complexes present on an opposing surface, the application of a force pulling the T cell away from the interaction activates T-cell receptor signaling. This physical force applied to the T-cell receptor is thought to elicit conformational changes in the associated signaling subunits, exposing the ITAM sequences of their cytoplasmic domains to phosphorylation by tyrosine kinases. When T cells encounter peptide:MHC complexes on antigen-presenting cells in a lymph node, the movement of the T cell over the antigen-presenting cell surface as it scans the peptide:MHC complexes on that cell is the most likely source of this mechanical force.

Another component promoting T-cell receptor signal initiation is the formation of higher-order receptor oligomers or clusters on the T cell surface. The contribution of receptor clustering to signaling has long been appreciated, as early studies showed that antibodies that bind to and cross-link T-cell receptors can activate T cells. Because antigenic peptides are vastly outnumbered by other peptides displayed on the surface of the antigen-presenting cell, it is unlikely that physiologic amounts of antigen induce conventional oligomerization as observed with antibodies. However, assemblies of small numbers of T-cell receptors called **microclusters** have been observed in the zone of contact between the T cell and the antigen-presenting cell. These microclusters form rapidly after TCR stimulation and quickly merge with microclusters containing downstream signaling components, such as adaptors. Current evidence indicates that signaling is initiated in these microclusters, which may include T-cell receptor interactions with self-peptide:MHC complexes. Although T-cell receptor binding to self-peptide:MHC is likely to be very low affinity, these interactions may contribute to T-cell receptor clustering and hence to T-cell signaling. This contribution of weak T-cell receptor binding to self-peptide:MHC complexes may explain the ability of T cells to be activated by antigen-presenting cells carrying one or a few antigenic peptide:MHC complexes. Another aspect of the T-cell receptor microclusters that form rapidly after T-cell receptor stimulation is their exclusion of inhibitory signaling proteins. Prior to TCR signaling, activating and inhibitory enzymes are in a balanced equilibrium; the initiation of signaling occurs when this equilibrium is perturbed in favor of the activating modifications.

In addition to studies dissecting the mechanism of T-cell receptor signal transduction across the membrane, substantial effort has been focused on determining the biochemical and biophysical parameters that determine when a T-cell receptor interaction with peptide:MHC will result in T-cell activation. Precise measurements of T-cell receptor:peptide:MHC binding affinities and kinetics and correlation of these measurements with T-cell activation responses have yielded a working model that postulates a parameter known as T-cell receptor dwell time or T-cell receptor occupancy. In this model, the individual binding affinity of the T-cell receptor for peptide:MHC as well as the density or abundance of specific peptide:MHC complexes on the

Fig. 7.12 Engagement of co-receptors with the T-cell receptor enhances phosphorylation of the ITAMs. Upper panel: For simplicity, we show the CD4 co-receptor engaging the same MHC molecule as the T-cell receptor (TCR), although signaling within receptor microclusters may differ from this arrangement. When T-cell receptors and co-receptors are brought together by binding to peptide:MHC complexes on the surface of an antigen-presenting cell, recruitment of the co-receptor–associated kinase Lck leads to phosphorylation of ITAMs in CD3γ, CD3δ, and CD3ε, and in the ζ chains. Lower panel: The tyrosine kinase ZAP-70 binds to phosphorylated ITAMs through its SH2 domains, enabling ZAP-70 to be phosphorylated and activated by Lck. ZAP-70 then phosphorylates other intracellular signaling molecules.

antigen-presenting cell surface both contribute to the average time, usually measured in seconds, that T-cell receptors in a cluster remain engaged with peptide:MHC complexes. When comparisons of many different T-cell receptors are made, the estimated T-cell receptor dwell time provides the best predictor of successful T-cell activation.

The concept of T-cell receptor dwell time as a key determinant of T-cell activation fits well with a popular model called the **kinetic proofreading model**. In this model, T-cell receptor interactions with peptide:MHC that persist for a sufficient time induce T-cell activation, whereas dissociation of T-cell receptor:peptide:MHC interactions before that time elapses produce transient, easily reversible signaling events. Successful T-cell activation depends on the signaling pathway progressing to a step that is no longer reversible. For instance, tyrosine phosphorylation of ITAM motifs or of adaptor proteins may be readily reversed by the action of protein phosphatases as soon as the T-cell receptor dissociates from peptide:MHC. In contrast, the production of second messengers, a later event in T-cell receptor signaling, may represent an irreversible step of the pathway. Once produced, these second messengers will exert their activity regardless of whether the T-cell receptor remains engaged with peptide:MHC. In this way, the T cell can 'measure' the T-cell receptor dwell time and use this measurement to determine whether T-cell activation should proceed or not.

7-9 Antigen recognition by the T-cell receptor and its co-receptors leads to phosphorylation of ITAMs by Src family kinases, generating the first intracellular signal in a signaling cascade.

Early biochemical studies performed in T-cell tumor lines indicated that the first intracellular signal generated after the T cell has detected its specific antigen, or, in some cases, a self-peptide:MHC complex, is the phosphorylation of both tyrosines in the ITAMs of the T-cell receptor. Using these cultured T-cell lines, the basic steps of the T-cell receptor signaling pathway were elucidated, leading to the following general model. In response to T-cell receptor engagement, ITAM phosphorylation is initiated with the help of the CD4 and CD8 co-receptors, which bind to MHC class II molecules and class I molecules, respectively, via their extracellular domains (see Section 4-21), and associate with **nonreceptor kinases** via their intracellular domains. The Src family kinase **Lck** is constitutively associated with the cytoplasmic domains of CD4 and CD8 and is thought to be the kinase primarily responsible for phosphorylation of the ITAMs of the T-cell receptor (see Fig. 7.12).

Evidence suggests that binding of the co-receptor to the peptide:MHC complex that binds the T-cell receptor enhances the recruitment of Lck to the engaged T-cell receptor, leading to more efficient phosphorylation of the T-cell receptor ITAMs. The importance of this event is demonstrated by the loss of T-cell receptor signaling in T-cell tumor lines lacking Lck and by the profound reduction in T-cell development in Lck-deficient mice. This indicates the essential role of Lck in T-cell receptor signaling during the selection of developing T cells in the thymus (discussed in Chapter 8). Lck is important for T-cell receptor signaling in naive T cells and effector T cells but is less important for the activation or maintenance of memory CD8 T cells by their specific antigen. A related tyrosine kinase, **Fyn**, is weakly associated with the ITAMs of the T-cell receptor and may have some role in signaling. Whereas mice lacking Fyn develop normal CD4 and CD8 T cells that respond in essentially normal fashion to antigen, mice lacking both Lck and Fyn show a more complete loss of T-cell development than mice lacking Lck alone. Overall, the activity of a Src family kinase is required, as all T-cell receptor signaling is abolished when T cells are treated with an inhibitor that blocks both Lck and Fyn.

The Lck bound to the cytoplasmic tails of CD4 or CD8 is brought near its substrate ITAMs in the T-cell receptor when the co-receptor binds the

Fig. 7.13 Lck activity is regulated by tyrosine phosphorylation and dephosphorylation. Src kinases such as Lck contain SH3 (blue) and SH2 (orange) domains preceding the kinase domain (green). Lck also contains a unique amino-terminal motif (yellow) with two cysteine residues that bind a Zn ion that is also bound to a similar motif in the cytoplasmic domain of CD4 or CD8. Upper panel: In inactive Lck, the two lobes of the kinase domain are constrained by interactions with both the SH2 and SH3 domains. The SH2 domain interacts with a phosphorylated tyrosine (red) at the carboxyl-terminal end of the kinase domain. The SH3 domain interacts with a proline-rich sequence in the linker between the SH2 domain and the kinase domain. Middle panel: Dephosphorylation of the carboxyl-terminal tyrosine by the phosphatase CD45 (not shown) releases the SH2 domain. Binding of other ligands to the SH3 region can facilitate release of the linker region (not shown). Lower panel: Full activation of Lck catalytic activity requires autophosphorylation on the activation loop in the kinase domain. Active Lck can then phosphorylate ITAMs in the signaling chains of the nearby T-cell receptor. Rephosphorylation of the carboxyl-terminal tyrosine by the C-terminal Src kinase (Csk) or loss of the SH3 ligand returns Lck to the inactive state.

Lck is inactive when its C-terminal tyrosine is phosphorylated and binds the SH2 domain and the linker region binds the SH3 domain

inactive Lck

Lck activation is initiated when its C-terminal tyrosine is dephosphorylated and its SH3 domain releases the linker region

primed Lck

Lck is fully activated when its activation loop tyrosine in the kinase domain is autophosphorylated

active Lck

receptor:peptide:MHC complex (see Fig. 7.12). CD4 or CD8 binding to MHC adds another level of fidelity to the signaling process by ensuring the coincident binding of the T-cell receptor and co-receptor to the same ligand and avoiding T-cell receptor signaling initiation to non-MHC ligands. Lck's kinase activity is also regulated confirmationally by phosphorylation of a tyrosine in its carboxyl terminus by the **C-terminal Src kinase (Csk)**. The resulting phosphotyrosine interacts with Lck's SH2 domain and helps maintain Lck in a closed conformation, resulting in a catalytically inactive state (**Fig. 7.13**). The absence of Csk during T-cell development causes T cells to mature autonomously in the thymus without needing to bind peptide:MHC, presumably as a result of abnormal activation of TCR signaling by hyperactive Lck in Csk-deficient thymocytes. Full activation of catalytic activity also requires Lck autophosphorylation of a tyrosine in its kinase domain. In nonstimulated lymphocytes, phosphorylation of Lck is counteracted by a **tyrosine phosphatase, CD45**, which can dephosphorylate both of the Lck tyrosine phosphorylation sites.

7-10 Phosphorylated ITAMs recruit and activate the tyrosine kinase ZAP-70.

The precise spacing of the two YXXL/I motifs in an ITAM suggests that the ITAM is a binding site for a signaling protein with two SH2 domains. In the case of the T-cell receptor, this protein is the tyrosine kinase ZAP-70 (ζ chain–associated protein), which carries the activation signal onward. ZAP-70 has tandem SH2 domains that can be simultaneously engaged by the two phosphorylated tyrosines in an ITAM (see Fig. 7.10). The affinity of the phosphorylated YXXL sequence for a single SH2 domain is low; furthermore, one of the ZAP-70 SH2 domains is incomplete and requires the second SH2 domain to complete its phosphotyrosine binding pocket. This ensures ZAP-70 specificity for fully phosphorylated ITAM sequences. Unlike the low levels of ITAM phosphorylation in unstimulated tumor T cell lines, T cells isolated directly from mice have substantial levels of constitutive ITAM phosphorylation and have constitutive ZAP-70 binding; however, the ZAP-70 protein bound to the ITAMs in nonstimulated T cells is not enzymatically active.

Once bound, ZAP-70 is activated by phosphorylation by Lck. This phosphorylation occurs at three tyrosine residues, two in the linker region between the tandem SH2 domains and the kinase domain, and a third residue in the catalytic domain. Together these phosphorylations activate ZAP-70 by disrupting the autoinhibited form of inactive ZAP-70, allowing the ZAP-70 kinase domain to adopt the active conformation (**Fig. 7.14**). In addition, the Lck SH2 domain binds to one of phosphorylated tyrosines in the ZAP-70 linker region (pY319), thereby stabilizing active Lck at the T-cell receptor complex.

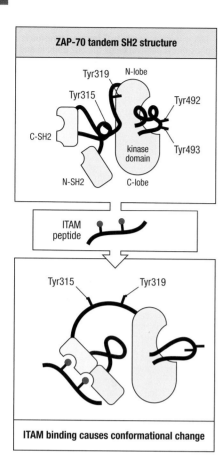

ZAP-70 tandem SH2 structure

Tyr319 N-lobe
Tyr315
Tyr492
C-SH2
kinase domain
Tyr493
N-SH2 C-lobe

ITAM peptide

Tyr315 Tyr319

ITAM binding causes conformational change

ANIMATION 7.1

Fig. 7.14 ITAM binding induces a conformational change in ZAP-70. Prior to binding to a phosphorylated ITAM in the T-cell receptor complex, the ZAP-70 kinase is in the inactive conformation through interactions between the tandem SH2 domain–kinase domain linker region (shown in orange) and the kinase domain. These interactions stabilize ZAP-70 in a catalytically inactive state, referred to as the autoinhibited form of ZAP-70, by locking the kinase domain in an inactive conformation. After ITAM binding, the linker region is released and can be phosphorylated by Lck on two tyrosine residues, Y315 and Y319. Lck also phosphorylates two tyrosine residues in the catalytic (kinase) domain. When Y315 and Y319 and the kinase domain are phosphorylated, ZAP-70 is stabilized in the active conformation.

7-11 ITAMs are also found in other receptors on leukocytes that signal for cell activation.

The signaling subunits of the T-cell receptor and the B-cell receptor each contain ITAMs, which are essential for T-cell receptor and B-cell receptor signaling. Phosphorylation of both tyrosines in the ITAM functions to recruit a tyrosine kinase with tandem SH2 domains—ZAP-70 in the case of T cells, and a closely related kinase, Syk, in B cells. Other immune-system receptors also use ITAM-containing accessory chains to transduce activating signals (**Fig. 7.15**). One example is **FcγRIII** (CD16), a receptor for IgG that triggers antibody-dependent cell-mediated cytotoxicity (ADCC) by NK cells, which we consider in Chapter 11. CD16 is also found on macrophages and neutrophils, where it facilitates the uptake and destruction of antibody-bound pathogens. To signal, FcγRIII must associate either with the ζ chain found also in the T-cell receptor or with another member of the same protein family known as the Fcγ chain. The Fcγ chain is also the signaling component of another Fc receptor—the Fcε receptor I (FcεRI) on mast cells. As we discuss in Chapter 14, this receptor binds IgE antibodies, and on cross-linking by allergens, it triggers the degranulation of mast cells. Last, many activating receptors on NK cells are associated with DAP12, another ITAM-containing protein (see Section 3-26). Each of these additional ITAM-containing signaling chains becomes tyrosine phosphorylated after stimulation of its associated receptor, leading to the recruitment of a tyrosine kinase, either Syk or ZAP-70. With the exception of T cells, Syk is broadly expressed in all leukocyte subsets; in contrast, in healthy individuals, ZAP-70 has been found only in T cells, NK cells, and innate lymphoid cells (ILCs).

Several viral pathogens seem to have acquired ITAM-containing receptors from their hosts. These include the Epstein–Barr virus (EBV), whose LMP2A gene encodes a membrane protein with a cytoplasmic tail containing an ITAM. This enables EBV to trigger B-cell survival by the signaling pathways discussed in Section 7-20, an important step in the development of EBV-induced malignancies. Another virus that expresses an ITAM-containing protein is the Kaposi's sarcoma herpesvirus (KSHV or HHV8), which causes malignant transformation and proliferation of the cells it infects.

NK cells Macrophages Neutrophils	NK cells	Mast cells Basophils
FcγRIII (CD16) FcγRIV	NKG2C, D, E (CD94)	FcεRI
		α β
γ or ζ	DAP12	γ

Receptors other than antigen receptors also associate with ITAM-containing chains that deliver activating signals

Fig. 7.15 Other receptors that pair with ITAM-containing chains can deliver activating signals. Cells other than B and T cells have receptors that pair with accessory chains containing ITAMs, which are phosphorylated when the receptor is cross-linked. These receptors deliver activating signals. The Fcγ receptor III (FcγRIII, or CD16) is found on NK cells, macrophages, and neutrophils. Binding of IgG to this receptor activates the killing function of the NK cell, leading to the process known as antibody-dependent cell-mediated cytotoxicity (ADCC). Activating receptors on NK cells, such as NKG2C, NKG2D, and NKG2E, also associate with ITAM-containing signaling chains. The Fcε receptor (FcεRI) is found on mast cells and basophils. The α subunit binds to IgE antibodies with very high affinity. The β subunit is a four-spanning transmembrane protein. When antigen subsequently binds to the IgE, the mast cell is triggered to release granules containing inflammatory mediators. The γ chain associated with the Fc receptors, and the DAP12 chain that associates with the NK killer-activating receptors, also contain one ITAM per chain and are present as homodimers. Some Fc receptors, such as CD16, can associate with the T-cell receptor ζ homodimer rather than with γ.

7-12 Activated ZAP-70 phosphorylates adaptor proteins and promotes PI 3-kinase activation.

As described in Section 7-10, phosphorylation of the tyrosines in the T-cell receptor ITAMs leads to the recruitment and activation of ZAP-70. This provides ZAP-70 proximity to the cell membrane, where it phosphorylates the adaptor protein **LAT (linker for activation of T cells)**, a transmembrane protein with a large cytoplasmic domain (**Fig. 7.16**). ZAP-70 also phosphorylates another adaptor protein, **SLP-76**. LAT and SLP-76 can be linked by the adaptor protein Gads; this three-protein complex, referred to as the LAT:Gads:SLP-76 complex, plays a central role in T-cell activation. This is illustrated by the profound TCR signaling and T-cell development defects seen in mice lacking any one of these components and in humans lacking ZAP-70. A second essential event that occurs rapidly after ZAP-70 activation is the recruitment and activation of the enzyme PI 3-kinase (see Section 7-4); currently, the detailed mechanism linking PI 3-kinase activation to T-cell receptor stimulation is not understood.

After formation of the LAT:Gads:SLP-76 complex and the activation of PI 3-kinase, the T-cell receptor signaling pathway branches into several downstream modules, each of which induces cellular changes that contribute to optimal T-cell activation (see Fig. 7.16). Together, these signals lead to profound changes in the T cell. A small resting naive T cell that has little cytoplasm expands in size and content and prepares for the rapid rounds of cell division that will begin approximately 30–36 hours after activation. Each

Fig. 7.16 ZAP-70 phosphorylates LAT and SLP-76, initiating four downstream signaling modules. Activated ZAP-70 phosphorylates the adaptor proteins LAT and SLP-76 and recruits them to the activated T-cell receptor (TCR) complex. Another adaptor protein, Gads, holds the tyrosine-phosphorylated LAT and SLP-76 together. The multiple binding sites on these scaffold proteins recruit several additional adaptors and enzymes that initiate four essential downstream signaling modules. One key component required for several of these modules is the activation of PI 3-kinase, which phosphorylates PIP_2 in the plasma membrane to generate PIP_3. These four modules include the activation of the serine/threonine kinase Akt, which promotes enhanced cellular metabolic activity; the activation of PLC-γ, which leads to transcription factor activation; the activation of Vav, which induces actin polymerization and cytoskeletal reorganization; and the recruitment of ADAP, an adaptor protein that promotes enhanced integrin adhesiveness and clustering.

Activated ZAP-70 phosphorylates LAT and SLP-76, initiating four signaling molecules

SLP-76
ZAP-70
LAT

| Akt activation leads to increased cellular metabolic activity | PLC-γ activation leads to transcription factor activation | Vav activation leads to actin polymerization and cytoskeletal reorganization | ADAP recruitment leads to enhanced integrin adhesiveness and clustering |

PIP_3
PH domain
Akt

PLC-γ
Gads

Vav

ADAP

T-Cell Signaling Defects

module is initiated by the recruitment of a key intermediate to the active signaling complexes, either via binding to the LAT:Gads:SLP-76 complex, to the PIP$_3$ generated by PI 3-kinase, or to both. In brief, these modules lead to the activation of phospholipase C-γ (PLC-γ), which affects transcription; the activation of the serine/threonine kinase Akt, which affects metabolism, among other things; the recruitment of the adaptor protein ADAP, which up-regulates cell adhesion; and the activation of the protein Vav, which initiates actin polymerization. Each of these four modules will be described in detail in the sections that follow.

7-13 Activated PLC-γ generates the second messengers diacylglycerol and inositol trisphosphate that lead to transcription factor activation.

One important module of T-cell receptor signaling is the activation of the enzyme **phospholipase C-γ (PLC-γ)**. First, PLC-γ is brought to the inner face of the plasma membrane by the binding of its PH domain to the PIP$_3$ that has been formed by the phosphorylation of PIP$_2$ by PI 3-kinase. It then binds to phosphorylated LAT and SLP-76. The actions of PLC-γ produce two second messengers that activate three distinct terminal branches of the T-cell receptor pathway leading to transcription factor activation.

Because of this crucial role in T-cell activation, PLC-γ activation is controlled at several different levels. Recruitment to the membrane, while necessary, is not sufficient to activate PLC-γ. PLC-γ activation requires phosphorylation by Itk, a member of the Tec family of cytoplasmic tyrosine kinases. Like PLC-γ, Tec kinases contain PH, SH2, and SH3 domains and are recruited to the plasma membrane by interactions via these domains; specifically, the PH domain interacts with PIP$_3$ on the inner face of the membrane (**Fig. 7.17**), and the SH2 and SH3 domains interact with SLP-76. These interactions serve to localize Itk in close proximity to its substrate, PLC-γ, leading to direct binding of Itk to PLC-γ, via one of the PLC-γ SH2 domains, followed by Itk phosphorylation of PLC-γ.

Fig. 7.17 The recruitment of phospholipase C-γ by LAT and SLP-76, and its phosphorylation and activation by the protein kinase Itk, are crucial steps in T-cell activation. ZAP-70 phosphorylates the adaptor proteins LAT and SLP-76, which are brought together to form a complex at the activated T-cell receptor by the adaptor protein Gads. This complex also promotes the activation of PI 3-kinase, leading to the production of PIP$_3$ (formed by the phosphorylation of PIP$_2$ by PI 3-kinase). PLC-γ is recruited to the membrane by its PH domain binding to PIP$_3$ and then binds to phosphorylated sites in LAT and to the proline-rich domain of SLP-76. To be activated, PLC-γ must be phosphorylated by the Tec-family kinase Itk. Itk is recruited to the membrane by interaction of its PH domain with PIP$_3$, and by interactions with phosphorylated SLP-76. Once phosphorylated by Itk, PLC-γ is active.

Fig. 7.18 Phospholipase C-γ cleaves inositol phospholipids to generate two important signaling molecules. Top panel: Phosphatidylinositol 4,5-bisphosphate (PIP$_2$) is a component of the inner leaflet of the plasma membrane. When PLC-γ is activated by phosphorylation, it cleaves PIP$_2$ into two parts: inositol 1,4,5-trisphosphate (IP$_3$), which diffuses away from the membrane into the cytosol, and diacylglycerol (DAG), which stays in the membrane. Both of these molecules are important in signaling. Middle panel: There are two phases of calcium release. IP$_3$ binds to a receptor in the endoplasmic reticulum (ER) membrane, opening calcium channels (yellow) and allowing the early phase of calcium ions (Ca^{2+}) to enter the cytosol from the ER. The depletion of Ca^{2+} stores in the ER causes the aggregation of an ER calcium sensor, STIM1. Bottom panel: Aggregated STIM1 stimulates the second phase of calcium entry by binding to and opening calcium channels called ORAI1 in the plasma membrane. This further increases cytosolic calcium and restores ER Ca^{2+} stores. DAG binds and recruits signaling proteins to the membrane, most important the Ras GEF called RasGRP and a serine/threonine kinase called protein kinase C-θ (PKC-θ). Recruitment of RasGRP to the plasma membrane activates Ras, and PKC-θ activation results in the activation of the transcription factor NFκB.

Once PLC-γ has been recruited to the inner face of the plasma membrane and has been activated, it can catalyze the breakdown of the membrane lipid PIP$_2$ (see Section 7-4 and Fig. 7.6) to generate two products, the membrane lipid **diacylglycerol (DAG)** and the diffusible second messenger **inositol 1,4,5-trisphosphate (IP$_3$)** (not to be confused with the membrane lipid PIP$_3$) (**Fig. 7.18**). DAG is confined to the membrane but diffuses in the plane of the membrane and serves as a molecular target that recruits other signaling molecules to the membrane. IP$_3$ signaling relies on the very low concentrations of calcium ions (Ca^{2+}) normally found in the cytoplasm of resting cells. After release from the membrane lipid, IP$_3$ diffuses into the cytosol and binds to IP$_3$ receptors on the endoplasmic reticulum (ER) membrane. These receptors are Ca^{2+} channels, which open and release calcium stored in the ER into the cytosol. The loss of calcium from the ER then causes a conformational change in the transmembrane protein **STIM1**, promoting its clustering within the ER membrane. The STIM1 oligomers bind to the plasma membrane, where they interact directly with ORAI1, the plasma membrane calcium channel (also known as the **CRAC channel**: calcium release-activated calcium channel). Binding of STIM1 to ORAI1 triggers calcium channel opening, allowing extracellular calcium to flow into the cell to activate further signaling pathways and to replenish ER calcium stores.

The activation of PLC-γ marks an important step in T-cell activation, because after this point the PLC-γ signaling module splits into three distinct branches—the stimulation of Ca^{2+} entry, the activation of Ras, and the activation of **protein kinase C-θ (PKC-θ)**—each of which ends in the activation of a different transcription factor. These signaling pathways are utilized by many cell types, in addition to lymphocytes. Their importance in T-cell activation is shown by the observation that treatment of T cells with phorbol myristate acetate (an analog of DAG) and ionomycin (a pore-forming drug that allows extracellular calcium to flow into the cell) can reconstitute many of the effects of T-cell receptor stimulation. Additionally, deficiencies in several of these signaling components, including Lck, ZAP-70, Itk, CD45, CARMA1, and ORAI1, have been found to be the cause of severe combined immune deficiency (SCID).

7-14   Ca^{2+} entry activates the transcription factor NFAT.

One of the three signaling pathways leading from PLC-γ results in an influx of calcium ions into the cytosol. An important outcome of the increased cytosolic Ca^{2+} resulting from T-cell receptor signaling via PLC-γ is the activation of a family of transcription factors called **NFAT (nuclear factor of activated T cells)**. NFAT is something of a misnomer, because the five members of this family are expressed in many different tissues. In the absence of activating signals, NFAT is kept in the cytosol of resting T cells by phosphorylation on serine/threonine residues. This phosphorylation is mediated by serine/threonine kinases,

Fig. 7.19 The transcription factor NFAT is regulated by calcium signaling. Left panel: NFAT is maintained in the cytoplasm by phosphorylation on serine and threonine residues. Center panel: After antigen receptor stimulation, calcium enters the cytosol, first from the endoplasmic reticulum (not shown; see Fig. 7.18) and later from the extracellular space (shown). After entering the cytosol, calcium binds to calmodulin, and the Ca^{2+}:calmodulin complex binds to the serine/threonine phosphatase calcineurin, activating it to dephosphorylate NFAT. Right panel: Once dephosphorylated, NFAT moves into the nucleus, where it binds to promoter elements and activates the transcription of various genes.

| Phosphorylation on serine and threonine residues keeps NFAT in the cytoplasm of unstimulated cells | Calcium entry activates the serine phosphatase calcineurin, which dephosphorylates NFAT, allowing it to enter the nucleus | Dephosphorylated NFAT enters the nucleus and activates gene transcription |

including glycogen synthase kinase 3 (GSK3) and casein kinase 2 (CK2). When phosphorylated, the nuclear localization sequence of NFAT is not recognized by nuclear transporters, and NFAT is unable to enter into the nucleus (**Fig. 7.19**).

The cytoplasmic Ca^{2+} resulting from T-cell receptor signaling binds to and induces a conformational change in a protein called **calmodulin**, which is then able to bind to and activate a wide range of different target enzymes. In T cells, an important target of calmodulin is **calcineurin**, a protein phosphatase that acts on NFAT. Dephosphorylation of NFAT by calcineurin allows the nuclear localization sequence to be recognized by nuclear transporters, and NFAT enters the nucleus (see Fig. 7.19). There it participates in turning on many of the genes crucial for T-cell activation, such as the gene for the cytokine interleukin-2 (IL-2).

The importance of NFAT in T-cell activation is illustrated by the effects of selective inhibitors of calcineurin called **cyclosporin A (CsA)** and **tacrolimus** (also known as **FK506**). CsA forms a complex with the protein cyclophilin A, and this complex binds to and inhibits calcineurin. Tacrolimus binds a different protein, FK-binding protein (FKBP), making a complex that similarly inhibits calcineurin. By inhibiting calcineurin, these drugs prevent the formation of active NFAT after T-cell receptor stimulation. T cells express low levels of calcineurin, so they are more sensitive to inhibition of this pathway than are many other cell types. NFAT is an important regulator of numerous genes in T cells, including those for cytokines, cytokine receptors, adhesion molecules, and transcription factors. As a consequence of this broad function for NFAT, both cyclosporin A and tacrolimus act as effective immunosuppressants and are widely used to prevent the rejection of organ transplants (see Section 16-2).

7-15   Ras activation stimulates the mitogen-activated protein kinase (MAPK) relay and induces expression of the transcription factor AP-1.

ANIMATION 7.2

A second branch of the PLC-γ signaling module is the activation of the small GTPase Ras. This can occur by various means. The most efficient mechanism for Ras activation in T cells is via the DAG generated by PLC-γ, which diffuses in the plasma membrane and activates a variety of proteins. One of these is the protein RasGRP, which is a guanine nucleotide exchange factor (GEF) that specifically activates Ras. RasGRP contains a protein-interaction module called a C1 domain that binds to DAG. This interaction recruits RasGRP to the membrane near active signaling complexes (**Fig. 7.20**), where it activates Ras by promoting the exchange of GDP for GTP. Ras is also activated in the T-cell

| Ras is initially inactive. TCR signaling produces DAG, which recruits RasGRP to the membrane where it activates Ras | Active Ras binds to Sos, enhancing Sos activity and amplifying Ras activation | Ras activates Raf, which phosphorylates Mek, which phosphorylates Erk | Activated Erk enters the nucleus and activates transcription factors such as Elk-1 |

Fig. 7.20 DAG activates MAPK cascades, leading to transcription factor activation. All MAPK cascades are initiated by the activation of small G proteins, such as Ras in this example. Ras is switched from an inactive state (first panel) to an active state (second panel) by a guanine nucleotide exchange factor (GEF), RasGRP, which is recruited to the membrane by DAG. Active Ras binds to an allosteric pocket in a second Ras GEF called Sos, which is recruited by its PH domain binding PIP$_3$ and its proline-rich region binding to Grb2 on LAT. Once Sos is bound to a molecule of active Ras, Sos activity is enhanced by 75-fold, leading to the production of many molecules of active Ras. Ras activates the first enzyme of the cascade, a protein kinase called Raf, a MAP3K (third panel). Raf phosphorylates Mek, a MAP2K, which in turn phosphorylates and activates Erk, a MAPK. Phosphorylation and activation of Erk releases it from the complex so that it can diffuse within the cell and enter the nucleus (fourth panel). Phosphorylation of transcription factors by Erk results in new gene transcription.

receptor signaling pathway by the GEF Sos, which is recruited by the adaptor protein Grb2 (see Sections 7-2 and 7-3), which has itself been recruited by binding to phosphorylated LAT and SLP-76. An efficient positive feedback loop contributes to robust Ras activation after T-cell receptor signaling. Once a small amount of GTP-bound Ras is generated by RasGRP, this activated Ras binds to a regulatory pocket on a second Ras GEF called Sos. Sos is recruited to the site of T-cell receptor signaling when its PH domain binds to PIP$_3$ and a proline-rich region in Sos binds to the LAT:Grb2 complex (see Fig 7.20). When the Sos protein binds a molecule of active Ras (Ras GTP), this enhances the activity of Sos by 75-fold. This dramatic enhancement of Sos activity after binding Ras GTP generates an all-or-nothing pattern of Ras activation, such that low levels of antigen receptor signaling can induce maximal Ras activation.

Activated Ras triggers a three-kinase relay that ends in the activation of a serine/threonine kinase known as a **mitogen-activated protein kinase** or **MAP kinase (MAPK)** (see Fig. 7.20). In the case of antigen receptor signaling, the first member of the relay is a MAPK kinase kinase (MAP3K) called **Raf**. Raf is a serine/threonine kinase that phosphorylates the next member of the series, a MAPK kinase (MAP2K) called **Mek1**. Mek1 is a dual-specificity protein kinase that phosphorylates a tyrosine and a threonine residue on the last member of the relay, a MAPK which in T cells and B cells is **Erk (extracellular signal-related kinase)**.

As predicted by the positive feedback loop regulating Ras activation, measurements of Erk activation in T cells demonstrate a bimodal (all-or-nothing) pattern of response (**Fig 7.21**).

Fig 7.21. Signaling responses can be graded or all-or-nothing. T cells stimulated by differing intensities of T-cell receptor signaling can produce distinct patterns of responses. These patterns can be visualized by flow cytometry experiments that individually measure the response in each cell and then display a histogram of the entire cell population. For these histograms, the x-axis indicates the magnitude of the response, and the y-axis indicates the number of cells displaying a response of that magnitude. Graded responses act like dials, in which the entire population of cells show a response that is proportional to the T-cell receptor signal intensity. Bimodal responses act like on/off switches, in which the signal intensity determines the relative proportion of cells in the population that respond; for these responses, increasing the signal intensity increases the proportion of responding cells, but the magnitude of the response does not vary. Because of the positive feedback loop for Ras activation in response to T-cell receptor stimulation, activation of the Erk MAPK displays on/off switchlike behavior.

Fig. 7.22 The transcription factor AP-1 is formed as a result of the Ras–MAPK signaling pathway. Left panel: Phosphorylation of the MAPK Erk activated as a result of the Ras–MAPK cascade allows Erk to enter the nucleus, where it phosphorylates the transcription factor Elk-1. Elk-1, along with serum response factor (SRF), binds to the serum response element (SRE) in the promoter of the gene (*FOS*) for the transcription factor c-Fos, stimulating its transcription. Right panel: The protein kinase PKC-θ can induce the phosphorylation of another MAPK called Jun kinase (JNK). This enables JNK to enter the nucleus and phosphorylate the transcription factor c-Jun, which forms a dimer with c-Fos. The phosphorylated c-Jun:Fos dimer is an active AP-1 transcription factor that binds to AP-1 sites and promotes transcription of many target genes.

An important function of MAPKs is to phosphorylate and activate transcription factors that can then induce new gene expression. Erk acts indirectly to generate the transcription factor **AP-1**, which is a heterodimer composed of one monomer each from the Fos and Jun families of transcription factors (**Fig. 7.22**). Active Erk phosphorylates the transcription factor Elk-1, which cooperates with a transcription factor called serum response factor (SRF) to initiate transcription of the *FOS* gene. Fos protein then associates with Jun to form the AP-1 heterodimer, but this remains transcriptionally inactive until another MAPK called **Jun N-terminal kinase (JNK)** phosphorylates Jun. Similar to NFAT, AP-1 participates in turning on transcription of many genes important for T-cell activation, including the genes encoding the cytokine IL-2 and the cell-cycle protein cyclin D1.

7-16 Protein kinase C activates the transcription factors NFκB and AP-1.

The third signaling pathway leading from PLC-γ results in the activation of PKC-θ, an isoform of protein kinase C that is restricted to T cells and muscle. Mice lacking PKC-θ develop T cells in the thymus, but their mature T cells have a defect in the activation of two crucial transcription factors, NFκB and AP-1, in response to signaling by the T-cell receptor and CD28. These transcription factors also participate in turning on genes required for T-cell activation. For example, transcription of the gene for IL-2 requires NFκB in addition to NFAT and AP-1, making PKC-θ activation an important component of T-cell activation.

PKC-θ has a C1 domain and is recruited to the membrane when DAG is generated by activated PLC-γ (see Fig. 7.18). In this location, the kinase activity of PKC-θ initiates a series of steps that results in the activation of NFκB (**Fig. 7.23**). PKC-θ phosphorylates the large membrane-localized adaptor protein CARMA1, causing it to oligomerize and form a multi-subunit complex with other proteins. This complex recruits and activates TRAF6, the same

| DAG recruits PKC-θ to the membrane where it phosphorylates CARMA1 | Phosphorylated CARMA1 creates a scaffold with BCL10 and MALT1 | TRAF-6 is recruited and makes a polyubiquitin scaffold on itself and on NEMO | TAK1, recruited by TAB1/2, phosphorylates IKKβ, which phosphorylates IκB, inducing IκB ubiquitination and degradation | Degradation of IκB releases NFκB, which activates transcription in the nucleus |

protein that we encountered in Chapter 3 in its role in activating NFκB in the TLR signaling pathway (see Fig. 3.14).

NFκB is the general name for a member of a family of homodimeric and heterodimeric transcription factors made up of the Rel family of proteins. The most common NFκB activated in lymphocytes is a heterodimer of p50:p65Rel. The dimer is held in an inactive state in the cytoplasm by binding to an inhibitory protein called inhibitor of κB (IκB). As described for TLR signaling (see Fig. 3.14), TRAF6 stimulates the degradation of IκB by first activating the kinase TAK1, which activates a complex of serine kinases—IκB kinase (IKK). IKK phosphorylates IκB, causing its ubiquitination and subsequent degradation, and the consequent release and entry into the nucleus of active NFκB. Inherited deficiency of the IKKγ subunit (also called **NEMO**) leads to a syndrome known as **X-linked hypohidrotic ectodermal dysplasia and immunodeficiency**, which is characterized by developmental defects in ectodermal structures such as skin and teeth, as well as immunodeficiency.

PKC-θ can also activate JNK and might be able to activate the transcription factor AP-1 by this route. However, T cells lacking PKC-θ have a defect in AP-1 activation in addition to their defect in NFκB activation, but no defect in JNK activation, indicating that our understanding of this pathway is still incomplete.

7-17 PI 3-kinase activation up-regulates cellular metabolic pathways via the serine/threonine kinase Akt.

While the activation of transcription factors is an important outcome of antigen receptor signaling, a productive T-cell response also requires substantial changes in cellular metabolism, which are needed to accommodate the energetic and macromolecular demands of rapidly dividing cells. The PI 3-kinase pathway plays a central role in this response via the recruitment and activation of the second important T-cell receptor signaling module, initiated by the serine/threonine kinase Akt (also known as protein kinase B). Akt, via its PH domain, binds to PIP$_3$ in the membrane, which is generated by PI 3-kinase (**Fig. 7.24**; see also Fig. 7.6). In that location, Akt is phosphorylated by PDK1 and, once activated, phosphorylates a variety of downstream proteins. One of its effects is to promote cell survival by inhibiting cell death via multiple mechanisms. A major mechanism is the phosphorylation of the pro-apoptotic protein Bad. When phosphorylated, Bad can no longer bind to and inhibit the anti-apoptotic (pro-survival) protein Bcl-2 (see Fig. 7.24).

Another effect of activated Akt is to regulate the expression of homing and adhesion receptors that orchestrate the migratory properties of activated T cells. Briefly, activated T cells down-regulate surface receptors that promote

Fig. 7.23 Activation of the transcription factor NFκB by antigen receptors is mediated by protein kinase C. Diacylglycerol (DAG), produced as a result of T-cell receptor signaling activating PLC-γ, recruits a protein kinase C (PKC-θ) to the membrane, where it phosphorylates an adaptor protein called CARMA1. This forms a complex with BCL10 and MALT1 that recruits the E3 ubiquitin ligase TRAF6. As described in Fig. 3.14, the kinase TAK1 is recruited by the polyubiquitin scaffold produced by TRAF6 and phosphorylates the IκB kinase (IKK) complex [IKKα:IKKb:IKKγ (NEMO)]. IKK phosphorylates IκB, stimulating its ubiquitination, which targets IκB for degradation by the proteasome. This releases NFκB to enter the nucleus and stimulate transcription of its target genes. A defect in IKKγ (NEMO) that prevents NFκB activation causes immunodeficiency that results in susceptibility to extracellular bacterial infections, along with a skin disease known as ectodermal dysplasia.

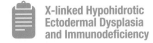

X-linked Hypohidrotic Ectodermal Dysplasia and Immunodeficiency

Fig. 7.24 The serine/threonine kinase Akt is activated by TCR signaling and promotes cell survival and enhanced metabolic activity via mTOR. First panel: T-cell receptor (TCR) signaling activates PI 3-kinase (not shown), generating PIP$_3$ in the plasma membrane; PIP$_3$ recruits and activates the kinase PDK1. Akt, a second serine/threonine kinase, binds to PIP$_3$ via its PH domain and is phosphorylated and activated by PDK1. Second panel: Active Akt phosphorylates the pro-apoptotic protein Bad, which is binding to and inhibiting the anti-apoptotic protein Bcl-2 at the mitochondrial membrane. Third panel: Phosphorylated Bad binds to 14-3-3, releasing Bcl-2 to promote cell survival. Fourth panel: A second function of active Akt is to phosphorylate the TSC1/2 complex, a GAP for the small GTPase Rheb. Fifth panel: When TSC1/2 is phosphorylated, it releases the inactive Rheb protein, leading to Rheb activation. Active Rheb binds to and activates mTOR (mammalian target of rapamycin). Once activated, mTOR acts on multiple pathways that lead to increased lipid production, ribosome biosynthesis, mRNA synthesis, and protein translation.

T-cell entry into lymph nodes and up-regulate chemokine receptors and integrins that direct T-cell migration from the blood into the tissues, particularly at sites of inflammation or infection (discussed in detail in Chapters 9 and 11). In this context, Akt functions to inactivate the transcription factors expressed in naive T cells, factors that maintain expression of receptors required for lymph node homing and T cell recirculation in the blood.

Activated Akt also functions to stimulate the cell's metabolism by increasing the utilization of glucose; this is mediated by increasing the activity of glycolytic enzymes and by inducing the up-regulation of nutrient transporters, such as the glucose transporter Glut 1, on the T-cell membrane. While resting T cells depend primarily on oxidative metabolism to generate energy, activated T cells switch their metabolism to favor aerobic glycolysis, a less efficient pathway for ATP production, but one that provides an abundant source of carbon for the biosynthesis of amino acids and nucleic acids used for protein and DNA/RNA synthesis, respectively. This switch to glycolytic metabolism is essential to support the rapid rate of cell division of activated T cells, which must duplicate their cellular contents once every 4–8 hours.

Yet another important function of activated Akt is to stimulate the **mTOR (mammalian target of rapamycin)** pathway, a key regulator of macromolecular biosynthesis (see Fig. 7.24). In this case, Akt phosphorylates and inactivates the TSC1/2 complex, a GAP for the small GTPase Rheb. As no GEF for Rheb has yet been identified, it is presumed that inactivation of TSC is sufficient for Rheb activation. Rheb activation, in turn, leads to the activation of mTOR. The mTOR pathway has multiple effects on cellular metabolism; these changes include up-regulating the activities and/or expression of molecules that promote protein synthesis, nucleotide synthesis, mitochondrial biogenesis, lipid biosynthesis, and glucose uptake and glycolysis. At the same time, mTOR also represses protein degradation, in part through the inhibition of the ubiquitin–proteasome system. Collectively, these changes are essential to provide the raw materials needed to carry out the increased gene expression, protein production, DNA/RNA synthesis, and lipid synthesis required for the rapid cell divisions that accompany T-cell activation.

7-18   T-cell receptor signaling leads to enhanced integrin-mediated cell adhesion.

The third signaling module induced by T-cell receptor stimulation leads to enhanced integrin adhesion. Together with cytoskeletal changes (discussed in the next section), this process promotes stability of the T cell–antigen-presenting cell (APC) interaction and localizes active signaling complexes into a structure known as the 'immune synapse' described in Section 7-19 (and see Fig. 7.27). The **immune synapse**, the region of the T-cell membrane that is in direct and stable contact with the APC or target cell, is formed within minutes of T-cell receptor recognition of peptide:MHC ligands. One important component of this is increased adhesiveness of the T-cell integrin LFA-1. On nonstimulated T cells, LFA-1 resides in a low-affinity state and is well dispersed on the T-cell membrane, resulting in weak binding to its ligand, ICAM-1. After T-cell receptor stimulation, LFA-1 molecules aggregate at the synapse and also undergo a conformational change that converts each LFA-1 molecule into a high-affinity binding partner for ICAM-1. Together, these changes lead to enhanced adhesion between the T cell and the APC and to stabilization of this cell–cell interaction. These effects on LFA-1 are induced by the recruitment of the adaptor protein ADAP to the LAT:Gads:SLP-76 complex (**Fig. 7.25**). In turn, ADAP recruits two additional proteins, SKAP and RIAM. The ADAP:SKAP:RIAM complex binds to the small GTPase Rap1, and, together with the Rap1 guanine nucleotide exchange factor (GEF) C3G and the adaptor protein CrkL, activates Rap1 at the site of T-cell receptor signaling. An additional Rap1 GEF known as CALDAG-GEF1 may also contribute to Rap1 activation. GTP-bound Rap1 then promotes LFA-1 aggregation and the conformational change that converts LFA-1 into a high-affinity binding partner for ICAM-1. The observation that ADAP-deficient T cells show impaired proliferation and cytokine production after T-cell receptor stimulation demonstrates the importance of this pathway in providing a positive feedback loop to promote T-cell activation.

7-19   T-cell receptor signaling induces cytoskeletal reorganization by activating the small GTPase Cdc42.

The fourth T-cell receptor signaling module, also involved in the formation of a stable immune synapse, leads to reorganization of the actin cytoskeleton. Without this process, integrin aggregation would not occur, interactions between the T cell and the APC would not stabilize, and, in fact, T-cell activation would completely fail. A major component of this T-cell receptor signal is transduced by Vav, a GEF that activates Rho family GTPases, including Cdc42. Like PLC-γ and Itk, Vav is recruited to the site of receptor activation by

Fig. 7.25 Recruitment of ADAP to the LAT:Gads:SLP-76 complex activates integrin adhesion and aggregation. Left panel: Prior to T-cell receptor (TCR) signaling, the integrin LFA-1 is present on the T-cell membrane in a low-affinity conformation that binds weakly to ICAM-1 on antigen-presenting-cells. Middle panel: After TCR signaling, the adaptor protein ADAP is recruited to the LAT:Gads:SLP-76 complex by an interaction between tyrosine-phosphorylated ADAP and the SH2 domain of SLP-76. ADAP then recruits a complex of SKAP and RIAM (Rap1-GTP-interacting adaptor molecule), activating the small GTPase Rap1. Right panel: Active Rap1 induces aggregation of LFA-1 and a conformational change in LFA-1 that leads to high-affinity binding to ICAM-1.

Fig. 7.26 Recruitment of Vav to the LAT:Gads:SLP-76 complex induces activation of Cdc42, leading to actin polymerization. Left panel: Vav, a guanine nucleotide exchange factor (GEF) for the small GTPase Cdc42, is recruited to the activated T-cell receptor (TCR) complex by binding via its PH domain to PIP₃ in the membrane and by binding to phosphorylated SLP-76. The small adaptor protein Nck binds to an adjacent phosphorylated tyrosine on SLP-76 and recruits the inactive form of the protein WASp. Middle panel: Vav activates Cdc42, which binds to and activates WASp. Right panel: Active WASp binds to WIP, recruiting Arp2/3 and inducing actin polymerization. The importance of this pathway is illustrated by the discovery of WASp as the protein encoded by the gene responsible for the human immunodeficiency disease Wiskott–Aldrich syndrome.

Wiskott–Aldrich Syndrome

interactions of the Vav PH domain with PIP₃ and of the Vav SH2 domain with the LAT:Gads:SLP-76 scaffold complex (**Fig. 7.26**). When Cdc42 is activated by Vav, the GTP-bound Cdc42 induces a conformational change in the protein **WASp** (**Wiskott–Aldrich syndrome protein**), which is also recruited to the LAT:Gads:SLP-76 scaffold complex by binding to the small adaptor protein Nck. This active form of WASp binds to WIP, named for its ability to interact with WASp (WASp-interacting protein). Together, WASp and WIP recruit Arp2/3, leading to actin polymerization. The importance of this pathway is underscored by the fact that defects in WASp are the basis for the immunodeficiency disease Wiskott–Aldrich syndrome. Because of expression of WASp in all lineages of hematopoietic cells, individuals suffering from this disease have impairments in multiple immune cell types, all of which depend on WASp-dependent actin polymerization for their functions. One major defect in this disease is a significant reduction in platelet numbers in the blood, called thrombocytopenia, leading to impaired blood clotting at sites of injury. Additionally, individuals with Wiskott–Aldrich syndrome have defects in T cell–dependent antibody responses because of the requirement for actin polymerization to ensure effective interactions between CD4 T cells and B cells. Thus, the failure of WASp-deficient T cells to provide adequate 'help' to B cells most likely results from a defect in the formation of the immune synapse, which is normally required to ensure directed secretion of cytokines from the T cell onto the B-cell membrane (**Fig. 7.27**).

The immune synapse is a structure observed by microscopic imaging of T cells interacting with antigen-presenting cells, such as B cells, or cytotoxic T cells interacting with target cells. It forms 10–15 minutes after cell–cell contact and is characterized by the reorganization of T-cell membrane proteins into discrete topological domains. The T-cell receptor along with signaling molecules such as Lck, ZAP-70, PKC-θ, and LAT coalesce to form a central domain known as the cSMAC, for central **supramolecular activation complex**. The cSMAC is surrounded by a ring of adhesion molecules, such as the integrin LFA-1, that forms the peripheral SMAC, known as the pSMAC (see Fig. 7.27). This organized site of interaction on the T-cell membrane can

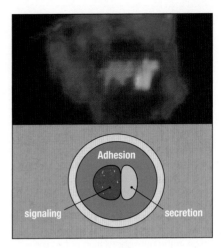

Fig. 7.27 The immune synapse provides a structure for directed secretion of T-cell cytokines. When the T-cell receptors (TCRs) on a T cell recognize peptide:MHC on an antigen-presenting cell, a process of receptor reorganization takes place on the plasma membranes of the two interacting cells. Left panel: When a CD8 T cell recognizes its peptide:MHC ligand on a target cell, the immune synapse functions to direct T cell–secreted cytokines and cytotoxic molecules onto the target-cell surface at the site of closest contact between the plasma membranes of the two cells. The right top panel shows a confocal microscopy image of the TCR signaling complex (Lck, shown in red), granzyme to mark secretory vesicles (shown in green), and actin (shown in blue) to identify the zone of cell adhesion molecules; the right bottom panel provides an illustration of this organizational structure. The central accumulation of the TCR signaling complexes and the secretory vesicles is known as the central supramolecular activation complex (cSMAC), and the ring of adhesion molecules is known as the peripheral supramolecular activation complex (pSMAC).

persist for hours after initial contact and signal initiation and is thought to aid in promoting ongoing T-cell receptor signaling. When the immune synapse is visualized during cytotoxic T cell killing of target cells, the organization of the cSMAC is not symmetric. Instead, the signaling molecules in the cSMAC are segregated to one area of this central domain, while cytotoxic granules are secreted by the cytotoxic T cell from an adjacent area of the cSMAC. This topological organization is thought to allow ongoing T-cell receptor signaling in a cytotoxic T cell that is simultaneously releasing granules to kill a target cell (see Fig 7.27).

7-20 The logic of B-cell receptor signaling is similar to that of T-cell receptor signaling, but some of the signaling components are specific to B cells.

There are many similarities between signaling from T-cell receptors and signaling from B-cell receptors. As with the T-cell receptor, the B-cell receptor is composed of antigen-specific chains associated with ITAM-containing signaling chains, in this case Igα and Igβ (see Fig. 7.11). In B cells, three protein tyrosine kinases of the Src family—Fyn, Blk, and Lyn—are thought to be responsible for phosphorylation of the ITAMs (**Fig. 7.28**). These kinases associate with resting receptors via a low-affinity interaction with unphosphorylated ITAMs in Igα and Igβ. After the receptors have bound antigen, the receptor-associated kinases are activated and phosphorylate the tyrosine residues in the ITAMs. Signal

Fig. 7.28 Src family kinases are associated with B-cell receptors and phosphorylate the tyrosines in ITAMs to create binding sites for Syk and Syk activation via transphosphorylation. The membrane-bound Src family kinases Fyn, Blk, and Lyn associate with the B-cell antigen receptor by binding to ITAMs, either (as shown in the figure) through their amino-terminal domains or by binding a single phosphorylated tyrosine through their SH2 domains. After ligand binding and receptor clustering, the associated kinases phosphorylate tyrosines in the ITAMs on the cytoplasmic tails of Igα and Igβ. Subsequently, Syk binds to the phosphorylated ITAMs of the Igβ chain. Because there are at least two receptor complexes in each cluster, Syk molecules become bound in close proximity and can activate each other by transphosphorylation, thus initiating further signaling.

Fig. 7.29 B-cell antigen receptor plus co-receptor engagement activate downstream signaling modules leading to activation of Akt, PLC-γ, and WASp. B-cell receptor (BCR) signaling is greatly enhanced when the antigen is tagged by complement fragments, engaging the B-cell co-receptor together with the B-cell antigen receptor. Cleavage of the antigen-bound complement component C3 to C3dg (see Fig. 2.30) allows the C3dg tag of the pathogen to bind to the cell-surface protein CD21 (complement receptor 2; CR2), a component of the B-cell co-receptor complex, which also includes CD19 and CD81 (TAPA-1). Cross-linking and clustering of the co-receptor with the antigen receptor result in the phosphorylation of tyrosine residues in the ITAM sequences of the cytoplasmic domains of the BCR signaling subunits, Igα and Igβ. The Src family kinase also phosphorylates tyrosine residues in the cytoplasmic domain of CD19. The phosphorylated ITAMs in Igα and Igβ recruit and activate the tyrosine kinase Syk, which functions similarly to ZAP-70 in T cells. The phosphorylated tail of CD19 recruits PI 3-kinase (PI3K), leading to PIP$_3$ generation in the plasma membrane. Activated Syk phosphorylates the membrane-associated scaffold protein SLP-65, which associates with the plasma membrane by binding Cin85. PIP$_3$ recruits PDK1 and Akt, leading to Akt activation. Phosphorylated SLP-65 and PIP$_3$ recruit the Tec family tyrosine kinase Btk and PLC-γ, leading to Btk phosphorylation and activation of PLC-γ. Phosphorylated SLP-65 and PIP$_3$ also recruit Vav, Nck, and inactive WASp. Vav activates small GTPases that activate WASp, leading to actin polymerization; the activated GTPases also induce integrin aggregation and conversion of LFA-1 to the high-affinity binding state.

initiation at the B-cell receptor is induced by multiple receptors binding to a multivalent antigen, a process that leads to receptor clustering. Alternatively, when the antigen is membrane associated, B-cell receptor signaling can be initiated by monovalent antigen binding (see Fig. 7.28). B cells do not express ZAP-70; instead, a closely related tyrosine kinase, **Syk**, containing tandem SH2 domains organized as in ZAP-70, is recruited to the phosphorylated ITAM. In contrast to ZAP-70, which requires additional phosphorylation for activation, Syk can be activated simply by its binding to the phosphorylated site.

For B cells, accessory receptor functions are combined into one complex of cell-surface proteins—**CD19**, **CD21**, and **CD81**—often referred to as the **B-cell co-receptor** (**Fig. 7.29**). As with T cells, antigen-dependent signaling from the B-cell receptor is enhanced if this complex is simultaneously bound by its ligand and clusters with the antigen receptor. CD21 (also known as complement receptor 2; CR2) is a receptor for the C3dg fragment of complement. The role of the CD81 (TAPA-1) component of the B-cell receptor complex is as yet unknown. The presence of CD21 in this receptor complex means that antigens, such as bacterial pathogens, on which C3dg is bound (see Fig. 7.29) can cross-link the B-cell receptor with the CD21:CD19:CD81 complex. This induces phosphorylation of the cytoplasmic tail of CD19 by B-cell receptor–associated tyrosine kinases, which in turn leads to the binding of additional Src family kinases, the augmentation of signaling through the B-cell receptor itself, and the recruitment of PI 3-kinase (see Section 7-4). Some molecules of CD19 are present on the B-cell membrane as monomers, rather than in a complex with

CD21 and CD81. This allows CD19 to associate with activated B-cell receptors and amplify signaling even in the absence of complement deposition on the antigen. Overall, this receptor activates PI 3-kinase, thereby enhancing the signaling pathways leading from the B-cell receptor (see Fig. 7.29).

Once activated, Syk phosphorylates the adaptor protein **SLP-65** (also known as **BLNK**), In B cells, SLP-65 combines the functions of LAT and SLP-76 in T cells. SLP-65 provides multiple sites for tyrosine phosphorylation and the recruitment of a variety of SH2-containing proteins, including enzymes and additional adaptor proteins. Several distinct multiprotein signaling complexes can form on individual SLP-65 molecules, and these different complexes act in concert to promote signaling. As in T cells, a key signaling protein is the phospholipase PLC-γ, which is activated with the aid of the B cell–specific Tec kinase **Bruton's tyrosine kinase (Btk)** and hydrolyzes PIP_2 to form DAG and IP_3 (see Fig. 7.29). As discussed for the T-cell receptor, signaling by calcium and DAG leads to the activation of downstream transcription factors. A deficiency in Btk (which is encoded by a gene on the X chromosome) prevents the development and functioning of B cells, resulting in the disease **X-linked agammaglobulinemia**, which is characterized by a lack of antibodies. Besides Btk, mutations in other signaling molecules in B cells, including receptor chains and SLP-65, have been linked to B-cell immunodeficiencies (see Chapter 8).

X-linked
Agammaglobulinemia

Several other downstream pathways described for TCR signaling are also shared with BCR signaling and are dependent on the adaptor protein SLP-65. These include the Vav-dependent induction of actin polymerization by Cdc42 and WASp, and the recruitment and activation of small GTPases that promote integrin adhesion (see Fig. 7.27). In the case of B-cell recognition of membrane-bound antigen, B-cell receptor signaling also produces an immune synapse that localizes signaling complexes to the cell–cell interface. One key function of the immune synapse in B cells is to promote antigen uptake by the B cell, a prerequisite to presenting that antigen in the form of peptide:MHC complexes to CD4 T cells.

B-cell receptor signaling also induces metabolic changes in activated B cells. As is the case for T cells, this response is dependent on the action of PI 3-kinase, whose activation leads to formation of the membrane phosphoinositide PIP_3 at the site of the activated B-cell receptor. This response is augmented by combined signaling through the B-cell receptor plus the B-cell co-receptor component CD19. PIP_3 recruits Akt, which is then phosphorylated and activated, leading to downstream activation of mTOR, as well as additional Akt-dependent pathways promoting cell survival and proliferation (see Fig. 7.29).

7-21 Antigen receptor signaling is a dynamic process that evolves over time.

Early biochemical experiments defined the protein–protein interactions and key signaling modules activated by B-cell and T-cell receptor stimulation. These studies provided 'snapshots' of the multiprotein complexes induced by receptor stimulation and identified many of the enzyme–substrate relationships in the pathway, such as the tyrosine phosphorylation of ITAMs by the Src family kinases and the tyrosine phosphorylation of adaptors by the Syk family kinases. However, we now appreciate that these signaling pathways are not static, but involve large-scale changes in protein localization and the assembly and disassembly of protein complexes that vary over time.

High-resolution imaging studies first revealed many of the dynamic movements of membrane proteins after antigen receptor stimulation, as described earlier for the formation of the immune synapse. More recent experiments utilizing affinity purification followed by mass spectrometry have yielded quantitative profiling of signaling complexes from primary lymphocytes at

Fig. 7.30 Summary of antigen receptor signaling pathways. As outlined in this part of the chapter, the signal transduction pathways downstream of the T-cell and B-cell receptors occur in an orchestrated series of stages involving many categories of proteins that produce widespread changes in the cells. The first detectable events after antigen receptor stimulation are the activation of tyrosine kinases. Following this, adaptor proteins are modified, recruiting phospholipases and lipid kinases to the activated receptor complexes. The next level of signaling amplifies these earlier stages by activating multiple small GTPases, serine/threonine kinases, and protein phosphatases. Together, these lead to transcription factor activation, cytoskeletal changes, and increases in cellular adhesion and metabolism, all of which contribute to T- and B-cell activation.

multiple time points after activation and from cells at multiple developmental stages. These proteomic data are then combined with known physical protein–protein interaction data extracted from the research literature to develop a more comprehensive picture of the composition and dynamics of large multiprotein signaling modules.

Summary.

The antigen receptors on the surface of lymphocytes are multiprotein complexes in which the antigen-binding chains interact with additional proteins that are responsible for signaling from the receptor. These protein chains carry tyrosine-containing signaling motifs known as ITAMs. Signaling chains containing ITAMs are widely used by activating receptors in many immune cell types in addition to lymphocytes. In lymphocytes, activation of the receptors by antigen results in a series of biochemical events that are broadly outlined in **Fig. 7.30**. This signaling cascade is initiated by the phosphorylation of the ITAMs by Src family kinases. The phosphorylated ITAM then recruits another tyrosine kinase, ZAP-70 in T cells and Syk in B cells. Activation of ZAP-70 or Syk results in the phosphorylation of adaptors called LAT and SLP-76 in T cells and SLP-65 in B cells, and in the activation of PI 3-kinase. Multiple signaling proteins are recruited and activated by these phosphorylated scaffolds, including phospholipase C-γ, ADAP, and Vav, whereas Akt is recruited and activated by the action of PI 3-kinase generating PIP$_3$ at the plasma membrane. PLC-γ generates inositol 1,4,5-trisphosphate (IP$_3$) and diacylglycerol (DAG). IP$_3$ has an important role in inducing changes in intracellular calcium concentrations, and DAG is involved in activating protein kinase C-θ and the small G protein Ras. In T cells, these pathways ultimately result in the activation of three transcription factors, namely, AP-1, NFAT, and NFκB; together, these transcription factors induce transcription of the cytokine IL-2, which is essential for the proliferation and further differentiation of the activated lymphocyte. In addition to transcription factor activation, antigen receptor signaling in both T cells and B cells leads to enhanced cell survival, metabolic activity, adhesiveness, and cytoskeletal reorganization. Signaling by antigen receptors is facilitated by co-receptors that become engaged as a result of receptor–antigen binding. These co-receptors are the MHC-binding CD4 and CD8 transmembrane proteins in T cells and the complement-binding B-cell co-receptor complex containing CD19 in B cells.

Co-stimulatory and inhibitory receptors modulate antigen receptor signaling in T and B lymphocytes.

Signals initiated by the T-cell and B-cell antigen receptors are essential for lymphocyte activation and determine the specificity of the adaptive immune response that is initiated. However, signaling from the antigen receptor is not on its own sufficient to activate a naive T cell or B cell. These naive lymphocytes require additional signals to achieve full activation. Receptors on T cells and B cells that can provide this necessary second signal are called **co-stimulatory receptors** and are members of either the CD28 family of proteins or of the TNF receptor superfamily. While naive T cells primarily utilize CD28 as the co-stimulatory receptor, naive B cells use the TNF receptor family member CD40. The overall function of signaling through these co-stimulatory receptors is to enhance the antigen receptor signals that induce transcription factor activation and PI 3-kinase activation, thereby ensuring activation of the T cell or B cell. In contrast to these activating co-stimulatory receptor signals, other cell-surface receptors on T cells and B cells function to down-regulate activation signals. These inhibitory receptors are important in preventing excessive immune responses that can lead to destructive inflammatory or autoimmune conditions, particularly in the case of chronic infections that are inefficiently controlled by the immune system.

7-22   The cell-surface protein CD28 is a required co-stimulatory signaling receptor for naive T-cell activation.

The signaling through the T-cell receptor complex described in the second part of the chapter is not by itself sufficient to activate a naive T cell. As noted in Chapter 1, antigen-presenting cells that can activate naive T cells bear cell-surface proteins known as co-stimulatory molecules or co-stimulatory ligands. These interact with cell-surface receptors, known as co-stimulatory receptors, on the naive T cell to transmit a signal that is required, along with antigen stimulation, for T-cell activation—this signal is sometimes called 'signal 2'. We discuss the immunological consequences of this requirement for co-stimulation in detail in Chapter 9.

The best understood of these co-stimulatory receptors is the cell-surface protein **CD28**. CD28 is present on the surface of all naive T cells and binds the co-stimulatory ligands **B7.1 (CD80) and B7.2 (CD86)**, which are expressed mainly on specialized antigen-presenting cells such as dendritic cells, once the antigen-presenting cells have had stimulation via their pattern recognition receptors. To become activated, the naive lymphocyte must engage both antigen and a co-stimulatory ligand on the same antigen-presenting cell. CD28 signaling aids antigen-dependent T-cell activation mainly by promoting T-cell proliferation, cytokine production, and cell survival. All these effects are mediated by signaling motifs present in the cytoplasmic domain of CD28.

After engagement by B7 molecules, CD28 becomes tyrosine phosphorylated by Lck in its cytoplasmic domain on tyrosine residues in a YXN motif that can recruit the adaptor protein Grb2 and in a non-ITAM motif YMNM, which binds to the regulatory subunit of PI 3-kinase. The cytoplasmic tail of CD28 also carries two proline-rich motifs (PXXP) that bind the SH3 domains of Lck and Itk. This association of CD28 with tyrosine kinases, Lck in particular, serves to amplify the activation of T-cell receptor signaling, as all downstream pathways are dependent on the initial recruitment and activity of Lck. Another effect of CD28 phosphorylation is to activate PI 3-kinase to generate PIP_3 (**Fig. 7.31**). By this mechanism, the co-stimulatory signal induced by CD28 cooperates with the T-cell receptor signal to ensure maximal activation of three of the four T-cell receptor signaling modules described in the second part of the chapter. Specifically, a high concentration of PIP_3 recruits Itk to the membrane, where Lck can phosphorylate it, thereby enhancing PLC-γ activation. PIP_3 also functions to recruit and activate Akt, which promotes cell survival and increased cellular metabolism (see Section 7.17). Finally, PIP_3 recruits Vav, leading to cytoskeletal reorganization (see Section 7.19). Thus, co-stimulatory signaling through CD28 functions to amplify most of the downstream responses to T-cell receptor stimulation (see Fig. 7.31).

 ANIMATION 7.3

Fig. 7.31 The T-cell co-stimulatory protein CD28 transduces signals that enhance antigen receptor signaling pathways. Upper panel: The amino acid sequence of the CD28 cytoplasmic tail is illustrated, along with the binding sites of several signaling proteins. Red text indicates an SH2 domain binding motif and blue text indicates SH3 domain binding motifs. Proteins known to bind to those motifs are indicated by arrows. Lower panel: The ligands for CD28, namely B7.1 and B7.2, are expressed only on specialized antigen-presenting cells (APCs), such as dendritic cells. Engagement of CD28 together with TCR binding to peptide:MHC leads to CD28 recruitment to the immune synapse, where it functions to enhance TCR signaling by binding to Lck, Grb2, and Itk. CD28 also becomes tyrosine phosphorylated, leading to the binding and activation of PI 3-kinase (PI3K), with subsequent production of PIP₃, which recruits several enzymes via their PH domains, thus bringing them together with their substrates in the membrane. The protein kinase Akt, which becomes phosphorylated by phosphoinositide-dependent protein kinase-1 (PDK1), is activated and enhances cell survival and up-regulates cell metabolism (see Fig. 7.24). Recruitment of the kinase Itk to the membrane is critical for the full activation of PLC-γ (see Fig. 7.17). PIP₃ also recruits Vav, leading to Cdc42 activation and inducing actin polymerization (see Fig. 7.26). All of these pathways are enhanced by CD28 binding to Lck.

7-23 Maximal activation of PLC-γ, which is important for transcription factor activation, requires a co-stimulatory signal induced by CD28.

One important function of co-stimulatory signaling through CD28 is to promote the maximal activation of PLC-γ via the local production of PIP₃. This recruits Itk by its PH domain, enhancing Itk phosphorylation by Lck. Activated Itk is then recruited to the phosphorylated LAT:Gads:SLP-76 complex by its SH2 and SH3 domains binding to SLP-76, where it phosphorylates and activates PLC-γ (see Fig. 7.17). PLC-γ also binds to PIP₃ generated at the membrane, further amplifying its local activation. Activated PLC-γ cleaves PIP₂ to produce the two second messengers DAG and IP₃, ultimately leading to the activation of transcription factors NFAT, AP-1, and NFκB. Thus, the full activation of PLC-γ leading to transcription factor activation requires signals emanating from both the T-cell receptor and CD28.

In T cells, one of the major functions of NFAT, AP-1, and NFκB is to act together to stimulate expression of the gene for the cytokine IL-2, which is essential for promoting T-cell proliferation, survival, and differentiation into effector cells. The promoter for the IL-2 gene contains multiple regulatory elements that must be bound by transcription factors to initiate *IL2* expression. Some control sites are already bound by transcription factors, such as Oct1, that are produced constitutively in lymphocytes, but this is not sufficient to switch on *IL2*. Only when AP-1, NFAT, and NFκB are all activated and are bound to their control sites in the *IL2* promoter is the gene expressed. NFAT and AP-1 bind to the promoter cooperatively and with higher affinity by forming a heterotrimer of NFAT, Jun, and Fos. In addition, CD28 co-stimulation further enhances transcription of *IL2* by increasing NFκB activation. Thus, the *IL2* promoter integrates signals from both the T-cell receptor and CD28 signaling pathways to ensure that IL-2 is produced only in appropriate circumstances (**Fig. 7.32**). CD28 co-stimulation also induces the phosphorylation of NF-90, an mRNA-binding protein that stabilizes the IL-2 mRNA. Together, the CD28-induced increase in

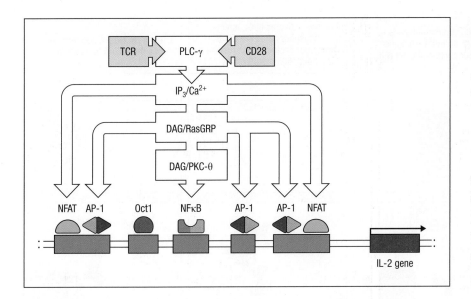

Fig. 7.32 Simplified scheme depicting multiple signaling pathways that converge on the *IL2* promoter. AP-1, NFAT, and NFκB binding to the promoter of the IL-2 gene integrate multiple signaling pathways emanating from the T-cell receptor (TCR) and CD28 into a single output, the production of the cytokine IL-2. The MAPK pathway activates AP-1; calcium activates NFAT; and protein kinase C activates NFκB. All three pathways are required to stimulate transcription of *IL2*. Activation of the gene requires both the binding of NFAT and AP-1 to a specific promoter element, and the additional binding of AP-1 on its own to another site. Oct1 is a transcription factor that is required for transcription of *IL2*. Unlike the other transcription factors, it is constitutively bound to the promoter and is therefore not regulated by T-cell receptor or CD28 signaling.

IL-2 gene transcription plus the increase in IL-2 mRNA stability lead to substantially increased production of IL-2 by activated T cells, in addition to the general amplification of T-cell receptor signals by CD28 co-stimulation.

7-24 TNF receptor superfamily members augment T-cell and B-cell activation.

While naive T- and B-cell activation requires signaling through the antigen receptors on these cells, T-cell receptor and B-cell receptor signaling is not sufficient to activate the cells. For naive T cells, an additional co-stimulatory signal is required and, as discussed earlier (see Sections 7-22 and 7-23), is frequently provided by the CD28 receptor. For naive B cells, the additional activation signal can be contributed by direct interactions between the pathogen and an innate pattern-recognition receptor (PRR), such as a TLR, on the B cell. An alternative second signal for B-cell activation can be provided by interactions between the B cell and a CD4 T follicular helper cell. These two forms of second signals for B-cell activation do not produce equivalent outcomes, however. More effective B-cell activation, leading to the production of all classes of antibodies and to the formation of memory B cells, requires B-cell activation signals that are contributed by CD4 T cells. One component of this mechanism is the production of T-cell cytokines, which bind to and stimulate their receptors on the B-cell surface (see Chapter 10). The second and more essential component provided by the CD4 T cells is the stimulation of CD40 on the B cell by the CD40 ligand expressed on the T cell. The importance of the CD40–CD40-ligand interaction for B-cell responses to protein antigens is highlighted by the discovery that a severe immunodeficiency disease resulting from impaired antibody responses is caused by the absence of CD40 ligand expression on an individual's CD4 T cells. Because of the presence of the CD40L gene on the X chromosome, this disease is generally observed in boys.

 CD40 Ligand Deficiency

CD40 is a member of the large TNF receptor superfamily, which consists of more than 20 members. While some members of this family, such as Fas (see Chapter 11), are specialized to induce cell death, the majority of TNF receptor superfamily members, including CD40, primarily activate the NFκB pathway after receptor stimulation, leading to enhanced cell survival (**Fig. 7.33**). TNF receptor superfamily members signal by a mechanism distinct from that of antigen receptors, as it does not involve the activation of tyrosine kinases. Instead, stimulation of TNF receptors recruits adaptor proteins known as TRAFs (TNF receptor–associated factors). In addition to serving as simple

| Prior to stimulation, TRAF ubiquitin ligases bind cIAP and NIK leading to ubiquitination and degradation of NIK | CD40L stimulation leads to TRAF ubiquitination and degradation, releasing NIK | NIK activates IKKα, which phosphorylates the NFκB precursor protein, p100, resulting in p100 ubiquitination | p100 is cleaved to p52, forming an active NFκB heterodimer |

Fig. 7.33 The TNF receptor superfamily member CD40 is an important co-stimulatory molecule on B cells. Several members of the TNF receptor superfamily are expressed on T cells and B cells. A key function of these receptors is the activation of NFκB, which occurs by a pathway distinct from the one initiated by antigen receptor stimulation and is often referred to as the non-canonical NFκB pathway. TNF receptor superfamily members also activate PI 3-kinase signaling pathways (not shown). One important TNF receptor superfamily member on B cells is CD40. Prior to stimulation, TRAF molecules, which are ubiquitin ligases, are associated in a complex with cIAP (another ubiquitin ligase) and the NFκB-inducing kinase (NIK). Under these steady-state conditions, TRAF binding promotes ubiquitination and degradation of NIK. When CD40 is stimulated by binding to CD40L, the aforementioned complex is recruited to the intracellular domain of CD40. TRAF2 catalyzes K63-linked ubiquitination of cIAP, leading to cIAP-mediated K48-linked ubiquitination of TRAF3. This leads to TRAF3 degradation, releasing NIK, and allowing NIK to phosphorylate and activate IκB kinase α (IKKα). IKKα phosphorylates the NFκB precursor protein p100, inducing its cleavage to form the active p52 subunit, which remains bound to relB to form the active NFκB transcription factor.

adaptors that promote the assembly of multiprotein complexes, five of the six known TRAFs also function as E3 ubiquitin ligases. This activity contributes to the ability of most TNF receptor superfamily members to activate the NFκB pathway, using a pathway distinct from the one initiated by antigen receptor stimulation and often referred to as the **non-canonical NFκB pathway** (see Fig. 7.33).

CD40 is constitutively expressed on B cells and functions during B-cell activation in response to antigen recognition by the B-cell receptor. Additional TNF receptor superfamily members are also expressed on B cells, and each of them is important in B-cell survival at a particular stage of B-cell maturation, including B cells that have differentiated into antibody-secreting cells or memory cells. Similarly, TNF receptor superfamily members are expressed on T cells, many of which are up-regulated after T-cell activation. These molecules, such as OX40, 4-1BB, CD30, and CD27, contribute important survival signals and function to enhance cellular metabolism at later stages of the T-cell response to infection (see Chapter 11).

7-25 Inhibitory receptors on lymphocytes down-regulate immune responses by interfering with co-stimulatory signaling pathways.

CD28 belongs to a family of structurally related receptors that are expressed by lymphocytes and bind B7 family ligands. Some, such as the receptor ICOS, which is discussed in Chapter 9, act as activating receptors, but others inhibit signaling by the antigen receptors, can stimulate apoptosis, and are important in regulating the immune response. Inhibitory receptors related to CD28 and expressed by T cells include **CTLA-4** (CD152) and **PD-1 (programmed death-1)**, while the **B and T lymphocyte attenuator (BTLA)** is expressed by both T cells and B cells. Of these, CTLA-4 seems to be the most important: mice lacking CTLA-4 die at a young age from an uncontrolled proliferation of T cells in multiple organs, whereas loss of PD-1 or BTLA causes less marked changes that alter the magnitude of responses after lymphocyte activation, rather than causing widespread spontaneous lymphoproliferation. Both CTLA-4 and PD-1 have been targeted for the development of protein-based therapeutics

Fig. 7.34 CTLA-4 has a higher affinity for B7 than does CD28 and engages it in a multivalent orientation. CD28 and CTLA-4 are both expressed as dimers on the cell surface and both bind to two ligands of B7.1, which is a dimer, and B7.2, which is not. However, the orientations of the B7 binding of CD28 and of CTLA-4 differ in a way that contributes to the inhibitory action of CTLA-4. One dimer of CD28 engages just one dimer of B7.1. But one dimer of CTLA-4 binds in such a way that two different dimers of B7.1 are engaged at once, allowing these molecules to cluster into complexes of high avidity. This, together with the higher affinity of CTLA-4 for B7 molecules, may give CTLA-4 an advantage in competing for available B7 molecules on an antigen-presenting cell, providing one mechanism by which it could block the co-stimulation of T cells.

that block the activities of these receptors. The goal of these therapeutics is to enhance T-cell responses by inhibiting these inhibitory receptors, a therapeutic strategy referred to as **checkpoint blockade** (see Chapter 16). Recent clinical data demonstrate that both CTLA-4 and PD-1 blockade have efficacy in the treatment of some cancers by enhancing the patient's own antitumor T-cell responses.

CTLA-4 is induced on activated T cells and binds to the same co-stimulatory ligands (B7.1 and B7.2) as CD28, but CTLA-4 engagement inhibits T-cell activation rather than enhancing it (**Fig. 7.34**). The function of CTLA-4 is controlled largely by regulation of its surface expression. Initially, CTLA-4 resides on intracellular membranes but moves to the cell surface after T-cell receptor signaling. The surface expression of CTLA-4 is controlled by phosphorylation of the tyrosine-based motif GVYVKM in its cytoplasmic tail. When this motif is not phosphorylated, it is able to bind to the clathrin adaptor molecule AP-2, which removes CTLA-4 from the surface. When it is phosphorylated, this motif cannot bind AP-2, and CTLA-4 remains in the membrane, where it can bind B7 molecules on antigen-presenting cells.

CTLA-4 has a higher affinity for its B7 ligands than does CD28, and, apparently of importance for its inhibitory function, it engages B7 molecules in a different orientation. CD28, CTLA-4, and B7.1 are all expressed as homodimers. A CD28 dimer engages one B7.1 dimer in a direct one-to-one correspondence, but a CTLA-4 dimer engages two different B7.1 dimers in a configuration that allows for extended cross-linkages that confer high avidity to the interaction (see Fig. 7.34). The precise mechanism of CTLA-4–mediated inhibition of T cells is still unclear. Initial evidence favored a role for inhibitory phosphatases recruited to the CTLA-4 cytoplasmic tail, a mechanism used by other inhibitory receptors described in the next section. Additional evidence also indicates that inhibition mediated by CTLA-4 may, in part, result from blocking the binding of CD28 to B7 or, in some cases, by stripping B7 molecules from the antigen-presenting cell membrane, thereby reducing CD28-dependent co-stimulation.

7-26 Inhibitory receptors on lymphocytes down-regulate immune responses by recruiting protein or lipid phosphatases.

Some other receptors that can inhibit lymphocyte activation possess motifs in their cytoplasmic regions that are known as the **immunoreceptor tyrosine-based inhibition motif** (**ITIM**; consensus sequence $[I/V]XYXX[L/I]$, where X is any amino acid) (**Fig. 7.35**) or the related **immunoreceptor tyrosine-based switch motif** (**ITSM**; consensus sequence $TXYXX[V/I]$). When the tyrosine in an ITIM or ITSM is phosphorylated, it can recruit inhibitory phosphatases, **SHP (SH2-containing phosphatase)** and **SHIP (SH2-containing**

B cells, T cells, and NK cells express receptors that contain immunoreceptor tyrosine-based inhibition motifs

PIR-B   FcγRIIB   CD22   BTLA, PD-1   KIR2DL   KIR3DL

Fig. 7.35 Some lymphocyte cell-surface receptors contain motifs involved in down-regulating activation. Several receptors that transduce signals inhibiting lymphocyte or NK-cell activation contain one or more ITIMs (immunoreceptor tyrosine-based inhibition motifs) in their cytoplasmic tails (red rectangles). ITIMs bind to various phosphatases that, when activated, inhibit signals derived from ITAM-containing receptors.

inositol phosphatase), via their SH2 domains. SHP is a protein tyrosine phosphatase that removes phosphate groups added by tyrosine kinases to a variety of proteins. SHIP is an inositol phosphatase that removes the phosphate from PIP_3 to generate PIP_2, thus reversing the recruitment of proteins such as Tec kinases, PLC-γ, and Akt to the cell membrane and inhibiting signaling.

One ITIM-containing receptor is PD-1 (see Fig. 7.35), which is induced transiently on activated T cells, B cells, and myeloid cells. It can bind to the B7 family ligands **PD-L1 (programmed death ligand-1; B7-H1)** and **PD-L2 (programmed death ligand-2; B7-DC)**. Despite their names, we now understand that these proteins function as ligands for the inhibitory receptor PD-1, rather than acting directly in cell death. PD-L1 is constitutively expressed by a wide variety of cells, whereas PD-L2 expression is induced on antigen-presenting cells during inflammation. Because PD-L1 is expressed constitutively, regulation of PD-1 expression could have a critical role in controlling T-cell responses. For example, signaling by pro-inflammatory cytokines can repress PD-1, a mechanism that might contribute to enhancing the T-cell response. Mice lacking PD-1 gradually develop autoimmunity, presumably because of an inability to regulate T-cell activation. In chronic infections, the widespread expression of PD-1 reduces the effector activity of T cells; this helps to limit potential damage to bystander cells, but at the expense of pathogen clearance. Protein-based therapeutics that inhibit PD-1 binding to its ligands have also provided clinical benefit in checkpoint blockade strategies used for treating some cancers (see Section 16-17). Although it is not known whether PD-1 blockade is acting to directly enhance T-cell recognition of infected cells and tumor cells in all disease models, recent evidence indicates that antiviral or antitumor T cells that respond in individuals treated with PD-1 blockade require CD28. A potential function of PD-1 on T cells in inhibiting CD28 co-stimulatory signaling is also supported by direct biochemical evidence that PD-1 recruits the tyrosine phosphatase SHP2 and that this phosphatase acts to efficiently dephosphorylate the cytoplasmic tail of CD28, thereby curtailing the overall activation signal.

BTLA contains an ITIM and an ITSM and is expressed on activated T cells and B cells, as well as on some cells of the innate immune system. Unlike other CD28 family members, however, BTLA does not interact with B7 ligands but binds a member of the TNF receptor family called the **herpes virus entry molecule (HVEM)**; this receptor is highly expressed on resting T cells and immature dendritic cells. When BTLA and HVEM are coexpressed on the same cell, BTLA utilizes a second mechanism that further inhibits lymphocyte activation. In this configuration, BLTA binds to HVEM and prevents HVEM from binding to alternative partners that would stimulate NFκB-dependent pro-survival signaling pathways downstream of HVEM. Alternatively, when BTLA and HVEM are expressed on different cells, the interaction of these two receptors functions to stimulate the positive pro-survival signal in the HVEM-expressing cell.

Other receptors on B cells and T cells also contain ITIMs and can inhibit cell activation when ligated along with the antigen receptors. One example is the receptor **FcγRIIB** on B cells, which binds the Fc region of IgG antibodies and is the only Fc receptor expressed on B cells. As a result, antigens present as immune complexes containing IgG antibodies are poor at activating naive B cells because of the co-engagement of the B-cell receptor with this inhibitory Fc receptor. This mechanism provides B cells with a means of monitoring the levels of antigen-specific antibodies in their environment. The inhibitory signal transduced by FcγRIIB results from phosphorylation of the ITIM in the receptor cytoplasmic tail, leading to recruitment of SHIP into a complex with the B-cell receptor to block the actions of PI 3-kinase (**Fig. 7.36**). The importance of this pathway is illustrated by the fact that FcγRIIB deficiencies are associated with B-cell hyperreactivity in humans with and mouse models of autoimmunity, such as systemic lupus erythematosus. Another inhibitory receptor on

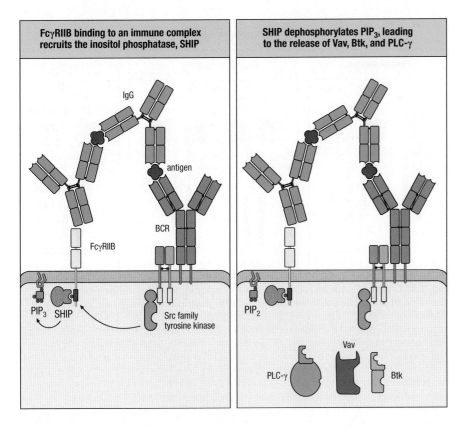

Fig. 7.36 The ITIM-containing Fc receptor inhibits B-cell receptor signaling by recruiting the inositol phosphatase SHIP. When the B-cell receptor binds an antigen that is already present in immune complexes with IgG, the ITIM-containing Fc receptor FcγRIIB is engaged at the same time as the B-cell receptor. The Src family kinase present at the B-cell receptor (BCR) phosphorylates the ITIM motif of FcγRIIB, which then recruits the SH2-containing inositol phosphatase, SHIP. SHIP dephosphorylates PIP$_3$ in the plasma membrane, generating PIP$_2$. PH domain–containing enzymes, such as Vav, Btk, and PLC-γ, depend on their PH domain binding to PIP$_3$ for their stable recruitment to the activated B-cell receptor complex. The loss of PIP$_3$ terminates the recruitment of these enzymes and inhibits B-cell receptor signaling.

B cells is **CD22**, a transmembrane protein that recognizes sialic acid–modified glycoproteins commonly found on mammalian cells but rarely on microbial pathogen surfaces. CD22 contains an ITIM that interacts with SHP, a phosphatase that can dephosphorylate adaptors such as SLP-65 that associate with CD22, thereby inhibiting signaling from the B-cell receptor.

The ITIM motif is also an important motif in signaling by receptors on NK cells that inhibit the killer activity of these cells (see Section 3-26). These inhibitory receptors recognize MHC class I molecules and inhibit the release of the NK cell's cytotoxic granules when the NK cell recognizes a healthy uninfected cell. In NK cells, ITIM-containing receptors play an important role in setting the threshold for NK-cell activation by balancing positive signals from ITAM-containing receptors.

7-27 Knowledge of lymphocyte receptor signaling pathways can be exploited to engineer chimeric antigen receptors.

In 1991, a seminal paper reported that a chimeric receptor formed by fusing the extracellular and transmembrane portions of the CD8 protein with the cytoplasmic tail of the T-cell receptor ζ chain was sufficient to transduce activation signals that mimicked those of the intact T-cell receptor complex (**Fig. 7.37**). More than 20 years later, in 2014, the US Food and Drug Administration licensed the first use of this concept, now called chimeric antigen receptor (CAR) T-cell therapy (CAR-T therapy), for the treatment of patients with B-cell lymphomas. This treatment is implemented by isolating and expanding the patient's T cells in culture and transducing them with a gene encoding the chimeric receptor, as discussed further in Chapter 16. For patients with B-cell lymphoma, the chimeric antigen receptor is composed of an antibody fragment that binds to CD19, a surface receptor expressed on the lymphoma tumor cells. This anti-CD19 antibody domain forms the extracellular portion of the chimeric receptor, and it is fused to a transmembrane domain and cytoplasmic tail containing multiple signaling domains. The patient's

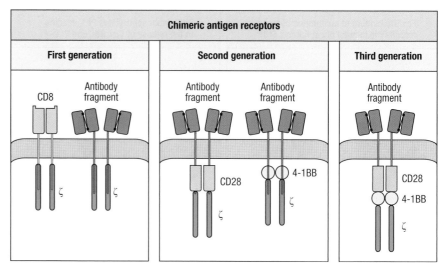

Fig. 7.37 Chimeric antigen receptors (CARs) link extracellular antigen-binding domains of antibodies to intracellular T-cell signaling domains. Initial studies from A. Weiss demonstrated that a simple chimeric antigen receptor, composed of the extracellular domain of CD8 and the intracellular domain of TCRζ, was sufficient to activate T cells when aggregated into multimers by anti-CD8 antibodies. This study led to the development of a chimeric receptor in which the extracellular CD8 domain was replaced by an antibody fragment. These chimeric receptors are often referred to as first-generation CAR. The next phase of this approach (second-generation CAR) included signaling domains from a co-stimulatory receptor, such as CD28 or 4-1BB. Third-generation CAR includes all three signaling domains: one from TCRζ, one from a CD28 family member, and one from a TNF receptor family member.

T cells, now expressing the chimeric antigen receptor, are then infused back into the patient. The CD19 antibody domain directs the CAR-T cells to bind to the tumor cells, and this interaction triggers signaling via the attached signaling domains. When expressed in cytotoxic T cells, CD19 recognition by the chimeric receptor leads to killing of the tumor cells. For other tumor types, the extracellular domain consists of an antibody fragment that recognizes a surface antigen on the relevant tumor cells.

Several generations of chimeric antigen receptors have been developed and tested in patients. Initial versions included sequences from the T-cell receptor ζ chain as the sole intracellular signaling domain. CAR-T cells expressing this chimeric receptor showed little clinical benefit, predominantly because of the failure of the infused CAR-T cells to expand and persist in patients. Improved efficacy was observed with second-generation chimeric receptors that included two signaling domains in the intracellular tail, one derived from the T-cell receptor ζ chain and a second derived from a co-stimulatory receptor, such as CD28 or the TNF receptor family member 4-1BB. These second-generation approaches provided substantial clinical benefit in a subset of patients. Third-generation chimeric receptors provide even better clinical effects. These receptors include three signaling domains, one derived from the T-cell receptor ζ chain, one from a CD28 family receptor (CD28 or ICOS), and one from a TNF receptor family member, most commonly 4-1BB (see Fig. 7.37). These recent advances in cancer therapy, using patients' T cells and modifying them to target tumor cells for killing, highlight the importance of studies aimed at understanding lymphocyte receptor signaling pathways.

Summary.

Signaling through the antigen receptors on T cells and B cells is essential for the activation of these cells. However, for naive T and B cells, the signal through the T-cell receptor or B-cell receptor is not sufficient to initiate a response. In addition to the antigen receptor signals, these cells require signals through accessory receptors that serve to monitor the environment of the cell to ensure the presence of an infection. An important secondary signaling system in naive T cells is provided by the CD28 family of co-stimulatory proteins, which bind members of the B7 family of proteins. Activating members of the CD28 family provide co-stimulatory signals that amplify the signal from the T-cell receptor and are important in ensuring the activation of naive T cells by the appropriate target cell. In B cells, these secondary signals are provided by members of the TNF receptor superfamily, such as CD40. Inhibitory members of the CD28 and other receptor families function to attenuate or completely block signaling by activating receptors. The regulated expression of activating and inhibitory receptors and their ligands generates a sophisticated level of control of immune responses that is an ongoing area of active investigation.

Summary to Chapter 7.

Signaling by cell-surface receptors of many different sorts is crucial to the ability of the immune system to respond appropriately to foreign pathogens. The importance of these signaling pathways is demonstrated by the many diseases that are due to aberrant signaling, including both immunodeficiency diseases and autoimmune diseases. Common features of many signaling pathways are the generation of second messengers such as calcium and phosphoinositides and the activation of both serine/threonine and tyrosine kinases. An important concept in the initiation of signaling pathways by receptor proteins is the recruitment of signaling proteins to the plasma membrane and the assembly of multiprotein signaling complexes. In many cases, signal transduction leads to the activation of transcription factors that lead directly or indirectly to the proliferation, differentiation, and effector function of activated lymphocytes. Signal transduction also serves to mediate changes in the cytoskeleton that are important for cell functions such as migration and shape changes. These steps of the T-cell and B-cell receptor signaling pathways are summarized in Fig. 7.30.

While we are beginning to understand the basic circuitry of signal transduction pathways, it is important to keep in mind that we do not yet understand why these pathways are so complex. One reason might be that the signaling pathways have roles in properties such as amplification, robustness, diversity, and efficiency of signaling responses. An important goal for the future will be to understand how the design of each signaling pathway contributes to the particular quality and sensitivity needed for specific signaling responses. The application of this knowledge to designing immune-based therapies for diseases such as cancer highlights the importance of these investigations.

Discussion Questions

7.1 Explain the function of adaptor proteins in signaling pathways, and name two protein domains often found in adaptor proteins.

7.2 Describe two mechanisms by which protein phosphorylation can alter the function of an enzyme important in a signaling pathway.

7.3 Because antigen receptors are present at the lymphocyte plasma membrane, a key step in antigen receptor signaling is the recruitment of signaling proteins to the membrane. List three mechanisms by which signaling proteins can be recruited to the plasma membrane.

7.4 There are two major mechanisms for terminating signaling pathways. Describe these two mechanisms, and indicate the most important difference between these two mechanisms.

7.5 Studies have shown that the ITAM sequences in the T-cell receptor signaling chains (for example, the T-cell receptor ζ chain) are constitutively phosphorylated and have ZAP-70 bound in nonstimulated T cells. Yet this does not lead to the constitutive activation of downstream signaling pathways. Explain why constitutive ITAM phosphorylation and ZAP-70 binding does not result in constitutive T-cell receptor signaling activation.

7.6 T-cell activation can be initiated by treatment of T cells with two pharmacological agents: phorbol myristate acetate (PMA) and ionomycin. Which natural products generated by T-cell receptor signaling are these pharmacological agents mimicking? Name three T-cell proteins that would be dispensable for T-cell activation when cells are treated with PMA and ionomycin.

7.7 Many T-cell receptor–stimulated signaling events involve the phosphorylation of enzymes, adaptor proteins, or transcription factors in T cells. Name an example of a protein that is activated by protein dephosphorylation. Also, name an example of a protein for which T-cell receptor stimulation induces phosphorylation of that protein, leading to inactivation of the protein.

7.8 The PI 3-kinase pathway activates enzymes that control many metabolic and biosynthetic pathways in activated lymphocytes. A number of these PI 3-kinase–dependent responses can be inhibited by the immunosuppressive drug rapamycin. List three fundamental features of cells (for example, total nuclear DNA content, total RNA content, number of mitochondria) that would be altered by treating activated T or B cells with rapamycin.

7.9 The immune synapse is an organized site of interaction between T cells and antigen-presenting cells or target cells. The formation of the immune synapse requires T-cell receptor signaling. Would inhibitors of RNA synthesis block the formation of the immune synapse after T-cell receptor stimulation? Would inhibitors of protein tyrosine kinases block this process? How does the activation of a Rho family GTPase contribute to the formation of the immune synapse?

7.10 How is B-cell activation mediated by B-cell receptor signaling enhanced by the innate immune response; for example, when the antigen recognized by the B-cell receptor is on the surface of a bacterium?

7.11 CD28 is known as a co-stimulatory receptor. When engaged by CD80 or CD86, CD28 functions to amplify most of the downstream responses to T-cell receptor stimulation. Yet, stimulation of CD28 in the absence of T-cell receptor stimulation is unable to activate a T cell. Which key step(s) in T-cell receptor signaling is CD28 unable to mediate on its own?

7.12 CD40 is an important receptor on B cells and contributes signals that are essential for B-cell activation leading to the production of all classes of antibodies and to the formation of memory B cells. Unlike many signaling receptors on B cells and T cells, CD40 signaling does not require the activation of protein tyrosine kinases. How does CD40 signaling lead to the activation of the transcription factor NFκB?

7.13 In addition to co-stimulatory receptors, lymphocytes express a variety of inhibitory receptors. Why might the immune system have evolved to include inhibitory receptors, and what might occur if these receptors did not exist?

General references.

Alberts, B., Heald, R., Johnson, A., Morgan, D., Raff, M., Roberts, K., and Walter, P.: *Molecular Biology of the Cell*, 7th ed. New York: W. W. Norton, 2022.

Gomperts, B., Kramer, I., and Tatham, P.: *Signal Transduction*. San Diego: Elsevier, 2002.

Marks, F., Klingmüller, U., and Müller-Decker, K.: *Cellular Signal Processing*. New York: Garland Science, 2009.

Samelson, L., and Shaw, A. (eds.): *Immunoreceptor Signaling*. Cold Spring Harbor, NY: Cold Spring Harbor Laboratory Press, 2010.

Section references.

7-1 Transmembrane receptors convert extracellular signals into intracellular biochemical events.

Lin, J., and Weiss, A.: T cell receptor signaling. *J. Cell Sci.* 2001, **114**:243–244.

Smith-Garvin, J.E., Koretzky, G.A., and Jordan, M.S.: T cell activation. *Annu. Rev. Immunol.* 2009, **27**:591–619.

7-2 Intracellular signal propagation is mediated by large multiprotein signaling complexes.

Balagopalan, L., Coussens, N.P., Sherman, E., Samelson, L.E., and Sommers, C.L.: The LAT story: a tale of cooperativity, coordination, and choreography. *Cold Spring Harb. Perspect. Biol.* 2010, **2**:a005512.

Jordan, M.S., and Koretzky, G.A.: Coordination of receptor signaling in multiple hematopoietic cell lineages by the adaptor protein SLP-76. *Cold Spring Harb. Perspect. Biol.* 2010, **2**:a002501.

Lim, W.A., and Pawson, T.: Phosphotyrosine signaling: evolving a new cellular communication system. *Cell* 2010, **142**:661–667.

Scott, J.D., and Pawson, T.: Cell signaling in space and time: where proteins come together and when they're apart. *Science* 2009, **326**:1220–1224.

7-3 Small G proteins act as molecular switches in many different signaling pathways.

Etienne-Manneville, S., and Hall, A.: Rho GTPases in cell biology. *Nature* 2002, **420**:629–635.

Mitin, N., Rossman, K.L., and Der, C.J.: Signaling interplay in Ras superfamily function. *Curr. Biol.* 2005, **15**:R563–R574.

7-4 Signaling proteins are recruited to the membrane by a variety of mechanisms.

Buday, L.: Membrane-targeting of signaling molecules by SH2/SH3 domain-containing adaptor proteins. *Biochim. Biophys. Acta* 1999, **1422**:187–204.

Fruman, D.A., and Cantley, L.C.: Phosphoinositide 3-kinase in immunological systems. *Sem. Immunol.* 2002, **14**:7–18.

Lemmon, M.A.: Membrane recognition by phospholipid-binding domains. *Nat. Rev. Mol. Cell Biol.* 2008, **9**:99–111.

7-5 Post-translational modifications of proteins can both activate and inhibit signaling responses.

Ciechanover, A.: Proteolysis: from the lysosome to ubiquitin and the proteasome. *Nat. Rev. Mol. Cell Biol.* 2005, **6**:79–87.

Hurley, J.H., Lee, S., and Prag, G.: Ubiquitin-binding domains. *Biochem. J.* 2006, **399**:361–372.

Liu, Y.C., Penninger, J., and Karin, M.: Immunity by ubiquitylation: a reversible process of modification. *Nat. Rev. Immunol.* 2005, **5**:941–952.

Wertz, I.E., and Dixit, V.M.: Signaling to NFκB: regulation by ubiquitination. *Cold Spring Harb. Perspect. Biol.* 2010, **2**:a003350.

7-6 The activation of many receptors generates small-molecule second messengers.

Kresge, N., Simoni, R.D., and Hill, R.L.: Earl W. Sutherland's discovery of cyclic adenine monophosphate and the second messenger system. *J. Biol. Chem.* 2005, **280**:39–40.

Rall, T.W., and Sutherland, E.W.: Formation of a cyclic adenine ribonucleotide by tissue particles. *J. Biol. Chem.* 1958, **232**:1065–1076.

7-7 Antigen receptors consist of variable antigen-binding chains associated with invariant chains that carry out the signaling function of the receptor.

Brenner, M.B., Trowbridge, I.S., and Strominger, J.L.: Cross-linking of human T cell receptor proteins: association between the T cell idiotype beta subunit and the T3 glycoprotein heavy subunit. *Cell* 1985, **40**:183–190.

Call, M.E., Pyrdol, J., Wiedmann, M., and Wucherpfennig, K.W.: The organizing principle in the formation of the T cell receptor-CD3 complex. *Cell* 2002, **111**:967–979.

Kuhns, M.S., and Davis, M.M.: TCR signaling emerges from the sum of many parts. *Front. Immunol.* 2012, **3**:159.

Reth, M.: Antigen receptors on B lymphocytes. *Annu. Rev. Immunol.* 1992, **10**:97–121.

Samelson, L.E., Harford, J.B., and Klausner, R.D.: Identification of the components of the murine T cell antigen receptor complex. *Cell* 1985, **43**:223–231.

Tolar, P., Sohn, H.W., Liu, W., and Pierce, S.K.: The molecular assembly and organization of signaling active B-cell receptor oligomers. *Immunol. Rev.* 2009, **232**:34–41.

7-8 Antigen recognition by the T-cell receptor and its co-receptors transduces a signal across the plasma membrane to initiate signaling.

Klausner, R.D., and Samelson, L.E.: T cell antigen receptor activation pathways: the tyrosine kinase connection. *Cell* 1991, **64**:875–878.

Liu, B., Chen, W., Evavold, B.D., and Zhu, C.: Accumulation of dynamic catch bonds between TCR and agonist peptide-MHC triggers T cell signalling. *Cell* 2014, **157**:357–368.

Weiss, A., and Littman, D.R.: Signal transduction by lymphocyte antigen receptors. *Cell* 1994, **76**:263–274.

7-9 Antigen recognition by the T-cell receptor and its co-receptors leads to phosphorylation of ITAMs by Src family kinases, generating the first intracellular signal in a signaling cascade.

Au-Yeung, B.B., Deindl, S., Hsu, L.-Y., Palacios, E.H., Levin, S.E., Kuriyan, J., and Weiss, A.: The structure, regulation, and function of ZAP-70. *Immunol. Rev.* 2009, **228**:41–57.

Bartelt, R.R., and Houtman, J.C.D.: The adaptor protein LAT serves as an integration node for signaling pathways that drive T cell activation. *Wiley Interdiscip. Rev. Syst. Biol. Med.* 2013, **5**:101–110.

Chan, A.C., Iwashima, M., Turck, C.W., and Weiss, A.: ZAP-70: a 70 Kd protein-tyrosine kinase that associates with the TCR zeta chain. *Cell* 1992, **71**:649–662.

Iwashima, M., Irving, B.A., van Oers, N.S., Chan, A.C., and Weiss, A.: Sequential interactions of the TCR with two distinct cytoplasmic tyrosine kinases. *Science* 1994, **263**:1136–1139.

Okkenhaug, K., and Vanhaesebroeck, B.: PI3K in lymphocyte development, differentiation and activation. *Nat. Rev. Immunol.* 2003, **3**:317–330.

Zhang, W., Sloan-Lancaster, J., Kitchen, J., Trible, R.P., and Samelson, L.E.: LAT: the ZAP-70 tyrosine kinase substrate that links T cell receptor to cellular activation. *Cell* 1998, **92**:83–92.

7-10 Phosphorylated ITAMs recruit and activate the tyrosine kinase ZAP-70.

Au-Yeung, B.B., Shah, N.H., Shen, L., and Weiss, A.: ZAP-70 in signalling, biology, and disease. *Annu. Rev. Immunol.* 2018, **36**:127–153.

Yan, Q., Barros, T., Visperas, P.R., Deindl, S., Kadlecek, T.A., Weiss, A., and Kuriyan, J.: Structural basis for activation of ZAP-70 by phosphorylation of the SH2-kinase linker. *Mol. Cell. Biol.* 2013, **33**:2188–2201.

7-11 ITAMs are also found in other receptors on leukocytes that signal for cell activation.

Lanier, L.L.: Up on the tightrope: natural killer cell activation and inhibition. *Nat. Immunol.* 2008, **9**:495–502.

7-12 Activated ZAP-70 phosphorylates adaptor proteins and promotes PI 3-kinase activation.

Zhang, W., Sloan-Lancaster, J., Kitchen, J., Trible, R.P., and Samelson, L.E.: LAT: the ZAP-70 tyrosine kinase substrate that links T cell receptor to cellular activation. *Cell* 1998, **92**:83–92.

7-13 Activated PLC-γ generates the second messengers diacylglycerol and inositol trisphosphate that lead to transcription factor activation.

Berg, L.J., Finkelstein, L.D., Lucas, J.A., and Schwartzberg, P.L.: Tec family kinases in T lymphocyte development and function. *Annu. Rev. Immunol.* 2005, **23**:549–600.

Yang, Y.R., Choi, J.H., Chang, J.-S., Kwon, H.M., Jang, H.-J., Ryu, S.H., and Suh, P.-G.: Diverse cellular and physiological roles of phospholipase C-γ1. *Adv. Biol. Regul.* 2012, **52**:138–151.

7-14 Ca²⁺ entry activates the transcription factor NFAT.

Hogan, P.G., Chen, L., Nardone, J., and Rao, A.: Transcriptional regulation by calcium, calcineurin, and NFAT. *Genes Dev.* 2003, **17**:2205–2232.

Hogan, P.G., Lewis, R.S., and Rao, A.: Molecular basis of calcium signaling in lymphocytes: STIM and ORAI. *Annu. Rev. Immunol.* 2010, **28**:491–533.

Picard, C., McCarl, C.A., Papolos, A., Khalil, S., Lüthy, K., Hivroz, C., LeDeist, F., Rieux-Laucat, F., Rechavi, G., Rao, A., *et al.* STIM1 mutation associated with a syndrome of immunodeficiency and autoimmunity. *N. Engl. J. Med.* 2009, **360**:1971–1980.

Prakriya, M., Feske, S., Gwack, Y., Srikanth, S., Rao, A., and Hogan, P.G.: Orai1 is an essential pore subunit of the CRAC channel. *Nature* 2006, **443**:230–233.

7-15 Ras activation stimulates the mitogen-activated protein kinase (MAPK) relay and induces expression of the transcription factor AP-1.

Das, J., Ho, M., Zikherman, J., Govern, C., Yang, M., Weiss, A., Chakraborty, A.K., and Roose, J.P.: Digital and hysteresis characterize Ras activation in lymphoid cells. *Cell* 2009, **136**:337–351.

Downward, J., Graves, J.D., Warne, P.H., Rayter, S., and Cantrell, D.A.: Stimulation of P21ras upon T-cell activation. *Nature* 1990, **346**:719–723.

Leevers, S.J., and Marshall, C.J.: Activation of extracellular signal-regulated kinase, ERK2, by P21ras oncoprotein. *EMBO J.* 1992, **11**:569–574.

Roskoski, R.: ERK1/2 MAP kinases: structure, function, and regulation. *Pharmacol. Res.* 2012, **66**:105–143.

Shaw, A.S., and Filbert, E.L.: Scaffold proteins and immune-cell signalling. *Nat. Rev. Immunol.* 2009, **9**:47–56.

7-16 Protein kinase C activates the transcription factors NFκB and AP-1.

Blonska, M., and Lin, X.: CARMA1-mediated NFκB and JNK activation in lymphocytes. *Immunol. Rev.* 2009, **228**:199–211.

Matsumoto, R., Wang, D., Blonska, M., Li, H., Kobayashi, M., Pappu, B., Chen, Y., Wang, D., and Lin, X.: Phosphorylation of CARMA1 plays a critical role in T cell receptor-mediated NFκB activation. *Immunity* 2005, **23**:575–585.

Qiao, Q., Yang, C., Zheng, C., Fontan, L., David, L., Yu, X., Bracken, C., Rosen, M., Melnick, A., Egelman, E.H., and Wu, H.: Structural architecture of the CARMA1/Bcl10/MALT1 signalosome: nucleation-induced filamentous assembly. *Mol. Cell* 2013, **51**:766–779.

Rueda, D., and Thome, M.: Phosphorylation of CARMA1: the link(Er) to NFκB activation. *Immunity* 2005, **23**:551–553.

Sommer, K., Guo, B., Pomerantz, J.L., Bandaranayake, A.D., Moreno-García, M.E., Ovechkina, Y.L., and Rawlings, D.J.: Phosphorylation of the CARMA1 linker controls NFκB activation. *Immunity* 2005, **23**:561–574.

Thome, M., and Weil, R.: Post-translational modifications regulate distinct functions of CARMA1 and BCL10. *Trends Immunol.* 2007, **28**:281–288.

7-17 PI 3-kinase activation up-regulates cellular metabolic pathways via the serine/threonine kinase Akt.

Gamper, C.J., and Powell, J.D.: All PI3Kinase signaling is not mTOR: dissecting mTOR-dependent and independent signaling pathways in T cells. *Front. Immunol.* 2012, 3:312.

Kane, L.P., and Weiss, A.: The PI-3 kinase/Akt pathway and T cell activation: pleiotropic pathways downstream of PIP3. *Immunol. Rev.* 2003, 192:7–20.

Pearce, E.L.: Metabolism in T cell activation and differentiation. *Curr. Opin. Immunol.* 2010, 22:314–320.

7-18 T-cell receptor signaling leads to enhanced integrin-mediated cell adhesion.

Bezman, N., and Koretzky, G.A.: Compartmentalization of ITAM and integrin signaling by adapter molecules. *Immunol. Rev.* 2007, 218:9–28.

Dimitrov, S., Gouttefangeas, C., Besedovsky, L., Jensen, A.T.R., Chandran, P.A., Rusch, E., Businger, R., Schindler, M., Lange, T., Born, J., *et al.:* Activated integrins identify functional antigen-specific CD8+ T cells within minutes after antigen stimulation. *Proc. Natl. Acad. Sci. USA* 2018, 115:E5536-E5545. doi: 10.1073/pnas.1720714115.

Mor, A., Dustin, M.L., and Philips, M.R.: Small GTPases and LFA-1 reciprocally modulate adhesion and signaling. *Immunol. Rev.* 2007, 218:114–125.

Stinchcombe, J.C., Bossi, G., Booth, S., and Griffiths, G.M. The immunological synapse of CTL contains a secretory domain and membrane bridges. *Immunity* 2001, 15:751–761.

7-19 T-cell receptor signaling induces cytoskeletal reorganization by activating the small GTPase Cdc42.

Burkhardt, J.K., Carrizosa, E., and Shaffer, M.H.: The actin cytoskeleton in T cell activation. *Annu. Rev. Immunol.* 2008, 26:233–259.

Moulding, D.A., Record, J., Malinova, D., and Thrasher, A.J.: Actin cytoskeletal defects in immunodeficiency. *Immunol. Rev.* 2013 256:282–299.

Tybulewicz, V.L.J., and Henderson, R.B.: Rho family GTPases and their regulators in lymphocytes. *Nat. Rev. Immunol.* 2009, 9:630–644.

7-20 The logic of B-cell receptor signaling is similar to that of T-cell receptor signaling, but some of the signaling components are specific to B cells.

Cambier, J.C., Pleiman, C.M., and Clark, M.R.: Signal transduction by the B cell antigen receptor and its coreceptors. *Annu. Rev. Immunol.* 1994, 12:457–486.

DeFranco, A.L., Richards, J.D., Blum, J.H., Stevens, T.L., Law, D.A., Chan, V.W., Datta, S.K., Foy, S.P., Hourihane, S.L., and Gold, M.R.: Signal transduction by the B-cell antigen receptor. *Ann. N.Y. Acad. Sci.* 1995, 766:195–201.

Harwood, N.E., and Batista, F.D.: New insights into the early molecular events underlying B cell activation. *Immunity* 2008, 28:609–619.

Harwood, N.E., and Batista, F.D.: Early events in B cell activation. *Annu. Rev. Immunol.* 2010, 28:185–210.

Koretzky, G.A., Abtahian, F., and Silverman, M.A.: SLP76 and SLP65: complex regulation of signalling in lymphocytes and beyond. *Nat. Rev. Immunol.* 2006, 6:67–78.

Kurosaki, T., and Hikida, M.: Tyrosine kinases and their substrates in B lymphocytes. *Immunol. Rev.* 2009, 228:132–148.

7-21 Antigen receptor signaling is a dynamic process that evolves over time.

Caron, E., Roncagalli, R., Hase, T., Wolski, W.E., Choi, M., Monoita, M.G., Durand, S., Garcia-Blesa, A., Fierro-Monti, I., Sajic, T., *et al.:* Precise temporal profiling of complexes in primary cells using SWATH mass spectrometry. *Cell Rep.* 2017, 18:3219–3226.

Su, X., Ditlev, J.A., Hui, E., Xing, W., Banjade, S., Okrut, J., King, D.S., Taunton, J., Rosen, M.K., and Vale, R.D.: Phase separation of molecules promotes T cell receptor signal transduction. *Science* 2016, 352:595–599.

7-22 The cell-surface protein CD28 is a required co-stimulatory signaling receptor for naive T cell activation.

Acuto, O., and Michel, F.: CD28-mediated co-stimulation: a quantitative support for TCR signalling. *Nat. Rev. Immunol.* 2003, 3:939–951.

Frauwirth, K.A., Riley, J.L., Harris, M.H., Parry, R.V., Rathmell, J.C., Plas, D.R., Elstrom, R.L., June, C.H., and Thompson, C.B.: The CD28 signaling pathway regulates glucose metabolism. *Immunity* 2002, 16:769–777.

Sharpe, A.H.: Mechanisms of costimulation. *Immunol. Rev.* 2009, 229:5–11.

7-23 Maximal activation of PLC-γ, which is important for transcription factor activation, requires a co-stimulatory signal induced by CD28.

Chen, L., and Flies, D.B.: Molecular mechanisms of T cell co-stimulation and co-inhibition. *Nat. Rev. Immunol.* 2013, 13:227–242.

7-24 TNF receptor superfamily members augment T-cell and B-cell activation.

Chen, L., and Flies, D.B.: Molecular mechanisms of T cell co-stimulation and co-inhibition. *Nat. Rev. Immunol.* 2013, 13:227–242.

Rickert, R.C., Jellusova, J., and Miletic, A.V.: Signaling by the tumor necrosis factor receptor superfamily in B-cell biology and disease. *Immunol. Rev.* 2011, 244:115–133.

7-25 Inhibitory receptors on lymphocytes down-regulate immune responses by interfering with co-stimulatory signaling pathways.

Qureshi, O.S., Zheng, Y., Nakamura, K., Attridge, K., Manzotti, C., Schmidt, E.M., Baker, J., Jeffery, L.E., Kaur, S., Briggs, Z., *et al.:* Trans-endocytosis of CD80 and CD86: a molecular basis for the cell-extrinsic function of CTLA-4. *Science* 2011, 332:600–603.

Rudd, C.E., Taylor, A., and Schneider, H.: CD28 and CTLA-4 coreceptor expression and signal transduction. *Immunol. Rev.* 2009, 229:12–26.

7-26 Inhibitory receptors on lymphocytes down-regulate immune responses by recruiting protein or lipid phosphatases.

Acuto, O., Di Bartolo, V., and Michel, F.: Tailoring T-cell receptor signals by proximal negative feedback mechanisms. *Nat. Rev. Immunol.* 2008, 8:699–712.

Chen, L., and Flies, D.B.: Molecular mechanisms of T cell co-stimulation and co-inhibition. *Nat. Rev. Immunol.* 2013, 13:227–242.

7-27 Knowledge of lymphocyte receptor signaling pathways can be exploited to engineer chimeric antigen receptors.

Guedan, S., Posey Jr., A.D., Shaw, C., Wing, A., Da, T., Patel, P.R., McGettigan, S.E., Casado-Medrano, V., Kawalekar, O.U., Uribe-Herranz, M., *et al.:* Enhancing CAR T cell persistence through ICOS and 4-1BB costimulation. *JCI Insight* 3:1–17.

Irving, B.A., and Weiss, A.: The cytoplasmic domain of the T cell receptor zeta chain is sufficient to couple receptor-associated signal transduction pathways. *Cell* 1991, 64:891–901.

Pang, Y., Hou, X., Yang, C., Liu, Y., and Jiang, G.: Advances on chimeric antigen receptor-modified T-cell therapy for oncotherapy. *Mol. Cancer* 2018, 17:91–100.

The Development of B and T Lymphocytes

8

After birth, the production of new lymphocytes, or **lymphopoiesis**, takes place in specialized lymphoid tissues—the **central (or primary) lymphoid tissues**—which are the bone marrow for most B cells and the thymus for most T cells. Precursors for both populations originate in the bone marrow, but whereas B cells complete most of their development there, the precursors of most T cells migrate to the thymus, where they develop into mature T cells. A major goal of lymphopoiesis is to generate a diverse repertoire of B-cell receptors and T-cell receptors on circulating B and T cells, respectively, thereby enabling an individual to make adaptive immune responses against the wide range of pathogens encountered during a lifetime. In the fetus and the juvenile, the central lymphoid tissues are the sources of large numbers of new lymphocytes, which migrate to populate the **peripheral (or secondary) lymphoid tissues** such as lymph nodes, spleen, and mucosal lymphoid tissue, a process that generally slows with age. This chapter will focus on the development of T cells and B cells from their uncommitted progenitors, with an emphasis on the major populations of CD4$^+$ and CD8$^+$ T cells and B cells. The development of additional subsets of T cells and B cells, such as invariant NKT (iNKT) cells, T_{reg} cells, $\gamma\delta$ TCR$^+$ T cells, B-1 B cells, and marginal zone B cells, will be briefly discussed.

The structure of the antigen receptor genes expressed by B cells and T cells, and the mechanisms by which a complete antigen receptor is assembled, were described in Chapters 4 and 5. Once an antigen receptor has been formed, rigorous testing is required to select lymphocytes that carry useful antigen receptors; that is, antigen receptors that can recognize a wide spectrum of pathogens and yet will not react against an individual's own cells. Given the incredible diversity of receptors the rearrangement process can generate, it is important that those lymphocytes that mature are likely to be useful in recognizing and responding to foreign antigens, especially as an individual can express only a small fraction of the total possible receptor repertoire in his or her lifetime. We describe how the specificity and affinity of the receptor for self ligands are tested to determine whether the immature lymphocyte will either survive and join the mature repertoire or die. In general, it seems that developing lymphocytes whose receptors interact weakly with self antigens or that bind self antigens in a particular way receive a signal that enables them to survive. This process, known as **positive selection**, is particularly critical in the development of $\alpha\beta$ T cells (which recognize composite antigens consisting of peptides bound to MHC molecules) because it ensures that an individual's T cells will be able to respond to peptides bound to one's own MHC molecules.

In contrast, lymphocytes with strongly self-reactive receptors must be eliminated to prevent autoimmune reactions; this process of **negative selection** is one of the ways in which the immune system is made self-tolerant. The default fate of developing lymphocytes, in the absence of any signal being received from the receptor, is death by apoptosis, and as we will see, the vast majority of developing lymphocytes die before emerging from the central lymphoid organs or before completing maturation in the peripheral lymphoid organs.

IN THIS CHAPTER

Development of B lymphocytes.

Development of T lymphocytes.

Positive and negative selection of T cells.

In this chapter we describe the different stages of the development of B cells and T cells in mice and humans from the uncommitted stem cell in the bone marrow up to the mature, functionally specialized lymphocyte with a unique antigen receptor ready to respond to a foreign antigen. The final stages in the life history of a mature lymphocyte, in which an encounter with its antigen activates it to become an effector or memory lymphocyte, are discussed in Chapters 9–11. We now know that the B-and T-cell development that predominates during late fetal life and after birth is distinct from waves of lymphocyte development that take place earlier in fetal ontogeny. These earlier waves originate from stem cells found in the fetal liver and in even more primitive hematopoietic tissues in the developing embryo. Unlike the lymphocytes that develop from bone marrow stem cells, B and T cells that develop from these early fetal progenitors generally populate mucosal and epithelial tissues and function in innate immune responses. In the adult, these subsets of lymphocytes are minority populations in peripheral lymphoid tissues.

This chapter will focus on B and T cells that develop from bone marrow stem cells and that compose the cells of the adaptive immune response (see Figs 1.7 and 1.20). These lymphocyte subsets, along with innate lymphoid cells (ILCs), are derived from lymphoid progenitor cells, which themselves derive from the multipotent **hematopoietic stem cells (HSCs)** that give rise to all blood cells (see Fig. 1.3). Development from precursors into cells that are committed to becoming B cells or T cells occurs over several stages of differentiation, as cells gradually acquire lineage-specific properties and lose properties of immature cells. In the case of lymphocyte development, cells become committed first to the lymphoid lineage, as opposed to the myeloid, and then to either the B-cell or the T-cell lineage (**Fig. 8.1**).

Fig. 8.1 A multipotent hematopoietic stem cell generates all the cells of the immune system. In the bone marrow or other hematopoietic sites, the multipotent stem cell gives rise to cells with progressively more limited potential. A simplified progression is shown here. The lymphoid–myeloid primed multipotent progenitor (LMPP), for example, has lost its stem-cell properties. The first differentiated branch leads to cells with myeloid and erythroid potential (common myeloid progenitors, CMPs; and megakaryocyte–erythroid progenitors, MEPs), and the other differentiated branches lead to several lymphoid progenitors, including early innate lymphoid progenitors (EILPs), common lymphoid progenitors (CLPs), and early thymic progenitors (ETPs). The myeloid–erythroid branch gives rise to all nonlymphoid cellular blood elements, including circulating monocytes and granulocytes, as well as the macrophages and dendritic cells that reside in tissues and peripheral lymphoid organs (not shown). The branches of lymphoid progenitors are heterogeneous, and each progenitor is biased to give rise to different subsets of lymphoid cells after successive stages of differentiation in either the bone marrow or thymus. EILPs generally produce innate lymphoid cells, including NK cells, innate lymphoid cells (groups 1–3 ILCs), and lymphoid tissue inducer (LTi) cells. CLPs are biased toward producing B cells, and ETPs migrate to the thymus and preferentially produce T cells. There is considerable plasticity in these pathways, in that in certain circumstances progenitor cells may switch their commitment.

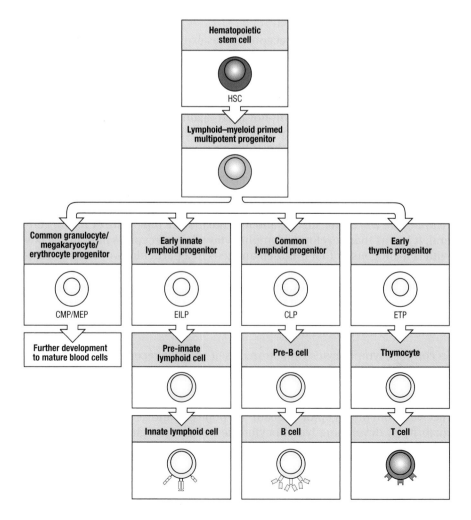

Development of B lymphocytes.

The main phases of a B lymphocyte's life history are shown in **Fig. 8.2**. The stages of both B-cell and T-cell development are defined mainly by the successive steps in the assembly and expression of functional antigen-receptor genes. At each step of lymphocyte development, the progress of gene rearrangement is monitored; the major recurring theme is that successful gene rearrangement leads to the production of a protein chain that serves as a signal for the cell to progress to the next stage. We will see that a developing B cell is presented with opportunities for multiple rearrangements that increase the likelihood of expressing a functional antigen receptor, but there are also checkpoints that reinforce the requirement that each B cell express just one receptor specificity. We will start by looking at how the earliest recognizable cells of the B-cell lineage develop from the multipotent hematopoietic stem cells in the bone marrow, and at what point the B-cell and T-cell lineages diverge.

8-1 Lymphocytes derive from hematopoietic stem cells in the bone marrow.

The specialized microenvironment of the bone marrow provides signals both for the development of lymphocyte progenitors from hematopoietic stem cells and for the subsequent differentiation of B cells. Such signals act on the developing lymphocytes to switch-on key genes that direct the developmental program and are produced by the network of specialized nonlymphoid connective tissue **stromal cells** that are in intimate contact with the developing lymphocytes (**Fig. 8.3**). The contribution of the stromal cells is twofold. First, they form specific adhesive contacts with the developing lymphocytes by interactions between cell-adhesion molecules and their ligands. Second, they provide soluble and membrane-bound cytokines and chemokines that control lymphocyte differentiation and proliferation.

Fig. 8.2 B cells develop in the bone marrow and migrate to peripheral lymphoid organs, where they can be activated by antigens. In the first phase of development, progenitor B cells in the bone marrow rearrange their immunoglobulin genes. This phase is independent of antigen but is dependent on interactions with bone marrow stromal cells (first panels). It ends in an immature B cell that carries an antigen receptor in the form of cell-surface IgM (second panels), and in the second phase the immature B cell can now interact with antigens in its environment. Immature B cells that are strongly stimulated by antigen at this stage are removed from the repertoire by receptor editing or by apoptosis, thus removing many self-reactive B cells from the repertoire. In the third phase of development, the surviving immature B cells emerge into the periphery and mature to express IgD as well as IgM. They can now be activated by encounter with their specific foreign antigen in a peripheral lymphoid organ (third panels). Activated B cells proliferate and differentiate into antibody-secreting plasma cells and long-lived memory cells (fourth panels).

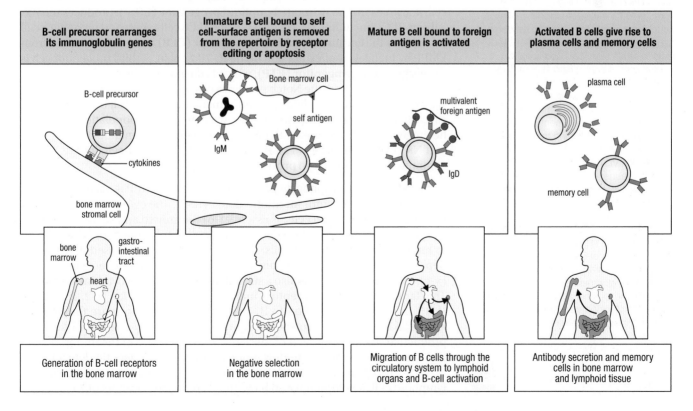

B-cell precursor rearranges its immunoglobulin genes	Immature B cell bound to self cell-surface antigen is removed from the repertoire by receptor editing or apoptosis	Mature B cell bound to foreign antigen is activated	Activated B cells give rise to plasma cells and memory cells
Generation of B-cell receptors in the bone marrow	Negative selection in the bone marrow	Migration of B cells through the circulatory system to lymphoid organs and B-cell activation	Antibody secretion and memory cells in bone marrow and lymphoid tissue

	Lymphoid–myeloid primed multipotent progenitor	Common lymphoid progenitor	Early pro-B cell	Late pro-B cell	Pre-B cell	Immature B cell
Ikaros, PU.1						
E2A						
FOXO1, EBF						
PAX5/BSAP						

Fig. 8.3 The early stages of B-cell development are dependent on bone marrow stromal cells. Interaction of B-cell progenitors with bone marrow stromal cells is required for development to the immature B-cell stage. The designations pro-B cell and pre-B cell refer to defined phases of B-cell development, as described in Fig. 8.4. Lymphoid–myeloid primed multipotent progenitor cells express the receptor tyrosine kinase FLT3, which binds to its ligand on stromal cells. Signaling through FLT3 is required for differentiation to the next stage, the common lymphoid progenitor. The chemokine CXCL12 (SDF-1) acts to retain stem cells and lymphoid progenitors at appropriate stromal cells in the bone marrow. The receptor for interleukin-7 (IL-7) is present at this stage, and IL-7 produced by stromal cells is required for the development of B-lineage cells. Progenitor cells bind to the adhesion molecule VCAM-1 on stromal cells through the integrin VLA-4 and also interact through other cell-adhesion molecules (CAMs). The adhesive interactions promote the binding of the receptor tyrosine kinase Kit (CD117) on the surface of the pro-B cell to stem-cell factor (SCF) on the stromal cell, which activates the kinase and induces the proliferation of B-cell progenitors. The actions of the listed transcription factors in B-cell development are discussed in the text. The pink horizontal bands denote the expression of particular proteins at the indicated stages of development.

 X-linked Severe Combined Immune Deficiency

The hematopoietic stem cells first differentiate into **lymphoid–myeloid primed multipotent progenitors (LMPPs)**, which can produce both lymphoid and myeloid cells but are no longer self-renewing stem cells. LMPPs express a cell-surface receptor tyrosine kinase known as FLT3, which binds the membrane-bound FLT3 ligand on stromal cells. Additionally, LMPPs express transcription factors and receptors that are required for the development of multiple hematopoietic lineages, such as the transcription factors PU.1 and Ikaros, and the receptor tyrosine kinase Kit. In the next stage, LMPPs produce three major subsets of progenitor cells that give rise to all the lymphocyte lineages (see Fig. 8.1). One progenitor cell, known as the **early innate lymphoid progenitor (EILP)**, produces the ILC subsets, ILC1 (including NK cells), ILC2, and ILC3 cells. A second progenitor cell is known as the **common lymphoid progenitor (CLP)** and is distinguished from LMPP by high levels of expression of the IL-7Rα chain. A third progenitor cell is the **early thymic progenitor (ETP)**, which is the major subset of T-cell progenitors; these cells express the Notch protein, a cell-surface receptor that transduces signals essential for T-cell lineage commitment. Progenitor cell transfer and lineage repopulation experiments have shown that the CLP population is actually heterogeneous; while some CLPs have broad potential to generate B cells, T cells, and NK cells, the majority of CLPs are biased toward the B-cell lineage. B cell–committed CLPs give rise to **pro-B cells** (see Fig. 8.3).

The production of lymphocyte progenitors from the LMPP is accompanied by expression of the receptor for interleukin-7 (IL-7). The cytokine IL-7, secreted by bone marrow stromal cells, is essential for the growth and survival of innate lymphoid cells, the majority of developing T cells, and in mice (but possibly not in humans) of developing B cells. The IL-7 receptor is composed of two polypeptides, the IL-7 receptor α chain and the common cytokine receptor γ chain (γ-c), so called because it is also a subunit of five additional cytokine receptors. This family of cytokine receptors includes the receptors for IL-2, IL-4, IL-9, IL-15, and IL-21, in addition to IL-7. These receptors also share the tyrosine kinase Jak3, a signaling protein that binds exclusively to γ-c and is required for productive signaling by each of these receptors. Because of the importance of IL-7 for murine lymphocyte development, mice with a genetic deficiency in IL-7, IL-7 receptor α, γ-c, or Jak3 all exhibit a severe block in B-cell and innate lymphoid cell development and have greatly reduced numbers of T cells.

8-2 Commitment to B cell, T cell, or innate lymphoid cell lineages is regulated by distinct networks of transcription factors.

B-cell development is initiated by the activation of the helix–loop–helix transcription factor E2A (see Fig. 8.3). In CLPs, E2A induces the expression of a second transcription factor FOXO1, which together with E2A promotes the expression of the early B-cell factor (EBF). EBF and FOXO1 then act in a positive amplification pathway that orchestrates the B lineage–specific programs of gene expression that include the up-regulation of PAX5. After these changes, the CLP cells transition to become pro-B cells, which receive proliferation and survival signals from IL-7.

As B-lineage cells mature, they migrate within the marrow, remaining in contact with the stromal cells. The earliest stem cells lie in a region called the **endosteum**, which lines the inner cavity of the long bones such as the femur and tibia. Developing B-lineage cells make contact with reticular stromal cells in the trabecular spaces, and as they mature they move toward the central sinus of the marrow cavity. The final stages of development of immature B cells into mature B cells occur in peripheral lymphoid organs, such as the spleen, which we describe in Sections 8-8 and 8-9 of this chapter.

Innate lymphoid cells also develop in the bone marrow. A key aspect of innate lymphoid cell development is the expression of a transcriptional regulator, Id2. This protein acts as a competitive inhibitor of E2A and prevents the E2A proteins from promoting B-cell development. Additional transcription factors, such as NFIL3 and TOX, are essential for innate lymphoid cell development. In contrast to B cells and innate lymphoid cells, T cells develop in the thymus rather than in the bone marrow. Once in the thymus, the ETP receives signals through the Notch receptor, a key step in driving T-cell commitment, a process that will be discussed in more detail in Section 8-14.

8-3 B-cell development begins by rearrangement of the heavy-chain locus.

The stages of B-cell development are, in the order they occur, **early pro-B cell**, **late pro-B cell**, **large pre-B cell**, **small pre-B cell**, **immature B cell**, and **mature B cell** (Fig. 8.4). Rearrangement of the heavy-chain locus is initiated in the pro-B cell when E2A and EBF induce the expression of several key proteins that enable gene rearrangement to occur, including the RAG-1 and RAG-2 components of the V(D)J recombinase (see Chapter 5). Only one gene locus is rearranged at a time, in a fixed sequence. The first rearrangement to take place is the joining of a D gene segment to a J segment at the immunoglobulin heavy-chain locus (*Igh*). D to J_H rearrangement takes place mostly in the early pro-B-cell stage but can be seen as early as the common lymphoid progenitor. In the absence of E2A or EBF, this initial rearrangement event fails to occur. Another key protein induced by E2A and EBF is the transcription factor PAX5, one isoform of which is known as the B-cell activator protein (BSAP) (see Fig. 8.3). Among the targets of PAX5 are the gene for the B-cell co-receptor component CD19 and the gene for Igα, a signaling component of both the pre-B-cell receptor and the B-cell receptor (see Section 7-7). In the absence of PAX5, pro-B cells fail to develop further down the B-cell pathway but can be induced to give rise to T cells and myeloid cell types, indicating that PAX5 is required for commitment of the pro-B cell to the B-cell lineage. PAX5 also induces the expression of the B-cell linker protein (BLNK), an SH2-containing scaffold protein that is required for further development of the pro-B cell and for signaling from the mature B-cell antigen receptor (see Section 7-20). The temporal expressions of some of the transcription factors, surface proteins, and receptors required for B-cell development are listed in Fig. 8.3 and Fig. 8.4.

		Stem cell	Early pro-B cell	Late pro-B cell	Large pre-B cell	Small pre-B cell	Immature B cell	Mature B cell
H-chain genes		Germline	D–J rearranging	V–DJ rearranging	VDJ rearranged	VDJ rearranged	VDJ rearranged	VDJ rearranged
L-chain genes		Germline	Germline	Germline	Germline	V–J rearranging	VJ rearranged	VJ rearranged
Surface Ig		Absent	Absent	Absent	μ chain transiently at surface as part of pre-B-cell receptor. Mainly intracellular	Intracellular μ chain	IgM expressed on cell surface	IgD and IgM made from alternatively spliced H-chain transcripts

Protein	**Function**							
RAG-1	Lymphoid-specific recombinase							
RAG-2								
TdT	N-nucleotide addition							
λ5	Surrogate light-chain components							
VpreB								
Igα	Signal transduction							
Igβ								
CD45R								
Btk								
CD19								
Kit	Growth factor receptor							
IL-7R								
CD43	Unknown							
CD24								
BP-1	Amino-peptidase							

Fig. 8.4 The development of a B-lineage cell proceeds through several stages marked by the rearrangement and expression of the immunoglobulin genes. The stem cell has not yet begun to rearrange its immunoglobulin (Ig) gene segments; they are in the germline configuration found in all nonlymphoid cells. The heavy-chain (H-chain) locus rearranges first. Rearrangement of a D gene segment to a J_H gene segment starts in the common lymphoid progenitor and occurs mostly in early pro-B cells, generating late pro-B cells in which V_H to DJ_H rearrangement occurs. A successful VDJ_H rearrangement leads to the expression of a complete immunoglobulin heavy chain as part of the pre-B-cell receptor, which signals via Igα, Igβ, and Btk (see Fig 7.28). Once this occurs, the cell is stimulated to become a large pre-B cell, which proliferates to become small resting pre-B cells; at this point the cells cease expression of the surrogate light chains (λ5 and VpreB) and express the μ heavy chain alone as an intracellular protein. Small pre-B cells reexpress the RAG proteins and start to rearrange the light-chain (L-chain) genes. Upon successfully assembling a light-chain gene, a cell becomes an immature B cell that expresses a complete IgM molecule at the cell surface, which also signals via Igα and Igβ. Mature B cells produce a δ heavy chain as well as a μ heavy chain, by a mechanism of alternative mRNA splicing (see Fig. 5.12), and are marked by the additional appearance of IgD on the cell surface. All stages through the development of immature B cells take place in the bone marrow; the final maturation to IgM^+IgD^+ mature B cells occurs in the spleen. The earliest B-lineage surface markers are CD19 and CD45R (B220 in the mouse), which are expressed throughout B-cell development. A pro-B cell is also distinguished by the expression of CD43 (a marker of unknown function), Kit (CD117), and the IL-7 receptor. A late pro-B cell starts to express CD24 (a marker of unknown function). A pre-B cell is phenotypically distinguished by the expression of the enzyme BP-1, whereas Kit is no longer expressed.

Although the V(D)J recombinase system operates in both B- and T-lineage cells and uses the same core enzymes, rearrangements of T-cell receptor genes do not occur in B-lineage cells, nor do complete rearrangements of immunoglobulin genes occur in T cells. The ordered rearrangement events that do occur are associated with lineage-specific low-level transcription of the gene segments about to be joined.

The initial D to J_H rearrangements in the immunoglobulin heavy-chain locus (**Fig. 8.5**) typically occur on both alleles, at which point the cell becomes a late pro-B cell. Most D to J_H joins in humans are potentially useful, because most human D gene segments can be translated in all three reading frames without encountering a stop codon. Thus, there is no need for a special mechanism to distinguish successful D to J_H joints, and at this early stage there is also no need to ensure that only one allele undergoes rearrangement. Indeed, given the likely rate of failure at later stages, starting off with two successfully rearranged D–J_H sequences may be an advantage.

To produce a complete immunoglobulin heavy chain, the late pro-B cell now proceeds with a rearrangement of a V_H gene segment to a DJ_H sequence. In

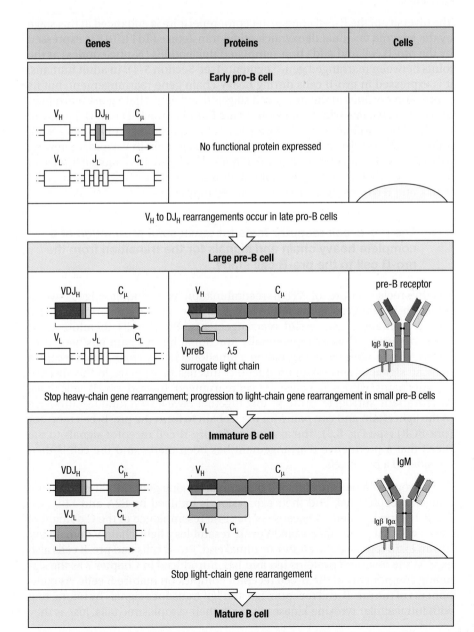

Fig. 8.5 A productively rearranged immunoglobulin gene is immediately expressed as a protein by the developing B cell. In early pro-B cells, heavy-chain gene rearrangement is initiated with D to J_H rearrangements. As shown in the top panels, no functional μ protein is expressed, although transcription occurs (red arrow). In late pro-B cells, V_H to DJ_H rearrangement occurs on one chromosome first. If no functional H-chain is produced, V_H to DJ_H rearrangement occurs on the second chromosome. As soon as a productive heavy-chain gene rearrangement takes place, μ chains are expressed by the cell in a complex with two other chains, λ5 and VpreB, which together make up a surrogate light chain. The whole immunoglobulin-like complex is known as the pre-B-cell receptor (center panels). It is associated with two other protein chains, Igα and Igβ, which signal the B cell to halt heavy-chain gene rearrangement; this drives the transition to the large pre-B-cell stage by inducing proliferation. Failure to produce a functional H-chain leading to a pre-B-cell receptor signal leads to cell death. The progeny of large pre-B cells stop dividing and become small pre-B cells, in which light-chain gene rearrangements commence. $V_κ$–$J_κ$ rearrangement (see Section 5-2) occurs first, and if unsuccessful, $V_λ$ to $J_λ$ rearrangement occurs next. Successful light-chain gene rearrangement results in the production of a light chain that binds the μ chain to form a complete IgM molecule, which is expressed together with Igα and Igβ at the cell surface, as shown in the bottom panels. Signaling via this surface receptor complex is thought to trigger the cessation of light-chain gene rearrangement. Failure to produce a functional L chain leads to cell death.

contrast to D to J_H rearrangement, V_H to DJ_H rearrangement occurs first on only one chromosome. A successful rearrangement leads to the production of intact μ heavy chains, after which V_H to DJ_H rearrangement ceases and the cell becomes a pre-B cell. Pro-B cells that do not produce a μ chain are eliminated, as they fail to receive an important survival signal mediated by the **pre-B-cell receptor** (see Section 8-3). At least 45% of pro-B cells are lost at this stage. In at least two out of three cases, the first V_H to DJ_H rearrangement is nonproductive. Because each amino acid is encoded by a triplet of nucleotides, only one out of three rearrangements produces an in-frame junction. When this initial rearrangement is out of frame, rearrangement then occurs on the other chromosome, again with a theoretical two in three chance of failure. A rough estimate of the chance of generating a pre-B cell is thus 55% [1-(2/3 × 2/3)]. The actual frequency is somewhat lower, because the V gene segment repertoire contains pseudogenes that can rearrange yet have major defects that prevent the expression of a functional protein. An initial nonproductive rearrangement does not automatically lead to pro-B-cell elimination, as it is possible for most loci to undergo successive rearrangements on the same chromosome, and where that fails, the locus on the other chromosome will rearrange.

The diversity of the B-cell antigen-receptor repertoire is enhanced at this stage by the enzyme terminal deoxynucleotidyl transferase (TdT). TdT is expressed by the pro-B cell and adds non-templated nucleotides (N-nucleotides) at the joints between rearranged gene segments (see Section 5-4). In adult humans, it is expressed in pro-B cells during heavy-chain gene rearrangement, but its expression declines at the pre-B-cell stage during light-chain gene rearrangement. This explains why N-nucleotides are found in the V–D and D–J joints of nearly all heavy-chain genes but only in about a quarter of human light-chain joints. N-nucleotides are rarely found in mouse light-chain V–J joints, showing that TdT is switched off slightly earlier in the development of mouse B cells. In fetal development, when the peripheral immune system is first being supplied with T and B lymphocytes, TdT is expressed only at low levels, if at all.

8-4 The pre-B-cell receptor tests for successful production of a complete heavy chain and signals for the transition from the pro-B cell to the pre-B cell stage.

The imprecise nature of V(D)J recombination is a double-edged sword. Although it produces increased diversity in the antibody repertoire, it also results in many unsuccessful rearrangements. Pro-B cells therefore need a way of testing whether a potentially functional heavy chain has been produced. They do this by incorporating a functional heavy chain into a receptor that can signal its successful production. This test takes place in the absence of light chains, whose loci have not yet rearranged. Instead, pro-B cells make two invariant 'surrogate' proteins that together have a structural resemblance to the light chain and can pair with the μ chain to form the pre-B-cell receptor (pre-BCR) (see Fig. 8.5). The assembly of a pre-B-cell receptor signals to the B cell that a productive rearrangement has been made, and the cell is then considered a pre-B cell.

The surrogate chains are encoded by nonrearranging genes separate from the antigen receptor loci, and their expression is induced by E2A and EBF (see Fig. 8.4). One is called **λ5** because of its close resemblance to the C domain of the λ light chain; the other, called **VpreB**, resembles a light-chain V domain but has an extra region at the amino-terminal end. Pro-B cells and pre-B cells also express the invariant proteins Igα and Igβ, introduced in Chapter 7 as the signaling components of the B-cell receptor complex on mature B cells. As components of the pre-B-cell receptor, Igα and Igβ transduce signals by interacting with intracellular tyrosine kinases through their cytoplasmic tails, just as they function to transduce signals through the antigen receptor on mature B cells (see Section 7-7).

Formation of the pre-B-cell receptor and signaling through this receptor provide an important checkpoint that mediates the transition between the pro-B cell and the pre-B cell. In mice that either lack λ5 or have mutant heavy-chain genes that cannot form the pre-B-cell receptor, B-cell development is blocked after heavy-chain gene rearrangement. In normal B-cell development, the pre-B-cell receptor complex is expressed transiently, perhaps because the production of λ5 mRNA stops as soon as pre-B-cell receptors begin to be formed. Although present at only low levels on the cell surface, the pre-B-cell receptor generates signals required for the transition from pro-B cell to pre-B cell. No antigen or other external ligand seems to be involved in signaling by the receptor. Instead, pre-B-cell receptors are thought to interact with each other, forming dimers or oligomers that generate signals as described in Section 7-8. Dimerization involves 'unique' regions in the amino termini of λ5 and VpreB proteins that are not present in other immunoglobulin-like domains and which mediate the cross-linking of adjacent pre-B-cell receptors on the cell surface (**Fig. 8.6**). Pre-B-cell receptor signaling requires the scaffold protein BLNK and Bruton's tyrosine kinase (Btk), an intracellular Tec-family tyrosine kinase (see Section 7-20). In humans and mice, deficiency of BLNK leads to a block in B-cell development at the pro-B-cell stage. In humans, mutations in the BTK gene cause a profound B lineage–specific immune deficiency, **Bruton's X-linked agammaglobulinemia (XLA)**, in which no mature B cells are produced. The block in B-cell development caused by mutations in *BTK*

X-linked
Agammaglobulinemia

Amino-terminal tails on VpreB and λ5 in adjacent pre-B-cell receptor molecules bind each other and cross-link the receptors, inducing clustering and signaling

Fig. 8.6 **The pre-B-cell receptor initiates signaling through spontaneous dimerization induced by the unique regions of VpreB and λ5.** Two surrogate protein chains, VpreB (orange) and λ5 (green), substitute for a light chain and bind to a heavy chain, thus allowing its surface expression. VpreB substitutes for the light-chain V region in this surrogate interaction, while λ5 takes the part of the light-chain constant region. Both VpreB and λ5 contain 'unique' amino-terminal regions that are not present in other immunoglobulin-like domains, shown here as unstructured tails extending out from the globular domains. These amino-terminal regions associated with one pre-B-cell receptor can interact with the corresponding regions on the adjacent pre-B-cell receptor, promoting the spontaneous formation of pre-B-cell receptor dimers on the cell surface. Dimerization generates signaling from the pre-B-cell receptor that is dependent on the presence of the ITAM-containing signaling chains Igα and Igβ. The signals cause the inhibition of RAG-1 and RAG-2 expression and the proliferation of the large pre-B cell.

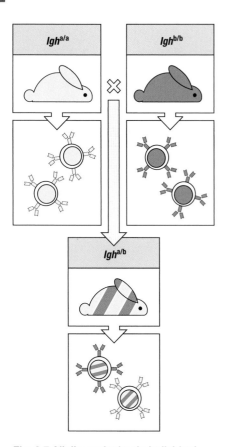

Fig. 8.7 Allelic exclusion in individual B cells. Most species have genetic polymorphisms of the constant regions of their immunoglobulin heavy-chain and light-chain genes; these polymorphisms lead to amino acid differences between the encoded proteins. These variants of heavy-chain or light-chain proteins expressed by different individuals in a species are known as allotypes. In rabbits, for example, all of the B cells in an individual homozygous for the *a* allele of the immunoglobulin heavy-chain locus (*Igh*$^{a/a}$) will express immunoglobulin of allotype a, whereas in an individual homozygous for the *b* allele (*Igh*$^{b/b}$) all the B cells make immunoglobulin of allotype b. In a heterozygous animal (*Igh*$^{a/b}$), which carries the *a* allele at one of the Igh loci and the *b* allele at the other, individual B cells can be shown to express surface immunoglobulin of either the a-allotype or the b-allotype, but not both (bottom panel). This allelic exclusion reflects the productive rearrangement of only one of the two *Igh* alleles in the B cell, because the production of a successfully rearranged immunoglobulin heavy chain forms a pre-B-cell receptor, which signals the cessation of further heavy-chain gene rearrangement.

is almost total, interrupting the transition from pre-B cell to immature B cell. A similar but less severe defect called **X-linked immunodeficiency, or xid**, arises from mutations in the Btk gene in mice.

8-5   Pre-B-cell receptor signaling inhibits further heavy-chain locus rearrangement and enforces allelic exclusion.

The signaling generated by pre-B-cell receptor clustering halts further rearrangement of the heavy-chain locus. Successful rearrangements at both heavy-chain alleles could result in a B cell producing two receptors of different antigen specificities. To prevent this, signaling by the pre-B-cell receptor enforces **allelic exclusion**, the state in which only one of the two alleles of a gene is expressed in a diploid cell. Allelic exclusion, which occurs at both the heavy-chain locus and the light-chain loci, was discovered in the 1960s and provided one of the original pieces of experimental support for the theory that one lymphocyte expresses one type of antigen receptor (**Fig. 8.7**).

Signaling from the pre-B-cell receptor promotes heavy-chain allelic exclusion in three ways. First, it reduces V(D)J recombinase activity by directly reducing the expression of the RAG1 and RAG2 genes. Second, it further reduces levels of RAG-2 by indirectly causing this protein to be targeted for degradation, which occurs when RAG-2 is phosphorylated in response to the entry of the pro-B cell into S phase (the DNA synthesis phase) of the cell cycle. Finally, pre-B-cell receptor signaling reduces access of the heavy-chain locus to the recombinase machinery, although the precise details of this process are not clear. At a later stage of B-cell development, RAG proteins will again be expressed in order to carry out light-chain locus rearrangement, but at that point the heavy-chain locus does not undergo further rearrangement. In the absence of pre-B-cell receptor signaling, allelic exclusion of the heavy-chain locus does not occur.

A second important role of pre-B-cell receptor signaling is to stimulate proliferative expansion of B-cell precursors with a successful heavy-chain rearrangement, initiating their transition into the large pre-B-cell stage. In response to IL-7, the cells undergo several rounds of cell division, expanding the population by about 30- to 60-fold. Thus, a deficiency in pre-B-cell receptor signaling causes a profound reduction in the numbers of pre-B cells and mature B cells that develop.

8-6   Pre-B cells rearrange the light-chain locus and express cell-surface immunoglobulin.

After several rounds of cell division, large pre-B cells transition to become resting small pre-B cells. RAG proteins are produced again in the small pre-B cells, and rearrangement of the light-chain locus begins. Each of these cells can make a different rearranged light-chain gene, and so cells with many different antigen specificities are generated from a single pre-B cell, a process that makes an important contribution to overall B-cell receptor diversity.

Light-chain rearrangement also exhibits allelic exclusion. Rearrangements at the light-chain locus generally take place at only one allele at a time, a process regulated by a mechanism not currently understood. The light-chain loci lack D segments, and rearrangement occurs by V to J joining, and if a particular VJ rearrangement fails to produce a functional light chain, repeated rearrangements of unused V and J gene segments at the same allele can occur (**Fig. 8.8**). Several attempts at productive rearrangement of a light-chain gene can therefore be made on one chromosome before initiating any rearrangements on the second chromosome. This greatly

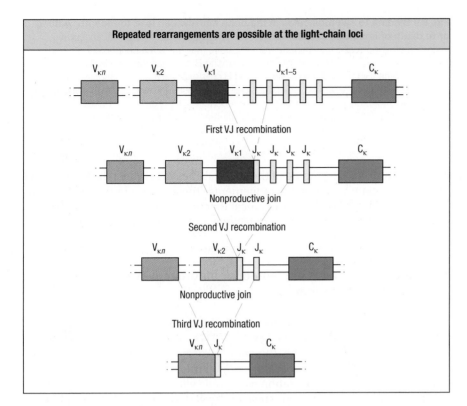

Repeated rearrangements are possible at the light-chain loci

First VJ recombination

Nonproductive join

Second VJ recombination

Nonproductive join

Third VJ recombination

Fig. 8.8 Nonproductive light-chain gene rearrangements can be rescued by further rearrangement. The organization of the light-chain loci in mice and humans offers many opportunities for the rescue of pre-B cells that initially make an out-of-frame rearrangement. Light-chain rescue is illustrated here at the human κ locus. If the first rearrangement is nonproductive, a 5' V_κ gene segment can recombine with a 3' J_κ gene segment to remove the out-of-frame join located between them and to replace it with a new rearrangement. In principle, this can happen up to five times on each chromosome, because there are five functional J_κ gene segments in humans. If all rearrangements of κ-chain genes fail to yield a productive light-chain join, λ-chain gene rearrangement may succeed (not shown).

increases the chances of eventually generating an intact light chain, especially as there are two different light-chain loci. As a result, many cells that reach the pre-B-cell stage succeed in generating progeny that bear intact IgM molecules and can be classified as immature B cells. Figure 8.4 lists some of the proteins involved in V(D)J recombination and shows how their expression is regulated throughout B-cell development. Figure 8.5 summarizes the stages of B-cell development up to the point of assembly of a complete surface immunoglobulin. Developing B cells that fail to assemble a complete surface immunoglobulin undergo apoptosis in the bone marrow and are eliminated from the B-cell pool.

As well as allelic exclusion, light chains also display **isotypic exclusion**; that is, the expression of only one type of light chain—κ or λ—by an individual B cell. Again, the mechanism regulating this process is not known. In mice and humans, the κ light-chain locus tends to rearrange before the λ locus. This was deduced from the observation that myeloma cells secreting λ light chains generally have both their κ and λ light-chain genes rearranged, whereas in myelomas secreting κ light chains, generally only the κ genes are rearranged. This order is occasionally reversed, however, and λ gene rearrangement does not absolutely require the previous rearrangement of the κ genes. The ratios of κ-expressing versus λ-expressing mature B cells vary from one extreme to the other in different species. In mice and rats it is 95% κ to 5% λ, in humans it is typically 65%:35%, and in cats it is 5%:95%, the opposite of that in mice. These ratios correlate most strongly with the number of functional V_κ and V_λ

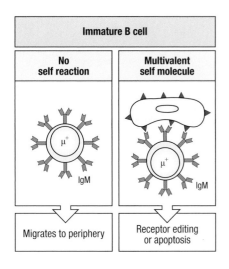

Immature B cell

No self reaction	Multivalent self molecule

IgM	IgM

Migrates to periphery	Receptor editing or apoptosis

Fig. 8.9 Binding to self molecules in the bone marrow can lead to receptor editing or to death of immature B cells. Left panel: Immature B cells that do not encounter antigen mature normally; they migrate from the bone marrow to the peripheral lymphoid tissues, where they may become mature recirculating B cells bearing both IgM and IgD on their surface. Right panel: When developing B cells express receptors that recognize multivalent ligands, for example, ubiquitous cell-surface self molecules such as those of the MHC, these receptors are eliminated from the repertoire. The B cells either undergo receptor editing (see Fig. 8.10), thereby eliminating the self-reactive receptor, or undergo programmed cell death (apoptosis), resulting in clonal deletion.

gene segments in the genome of the species. They also reflect the kinetics and efficiency of gene segment rearrangements. The κ:λ ratio in the mature lymphocyte population is useful in clinical diagnostics, because an aberrant κ:λ ratio indicates the dominance of one clone and the presence of a lymphoproliferative disorder.

8-7   Immature B cells are tested for autoreactivity before they leave the bone marrow.

Once a rearranged light chain has paired with a μ chain, IgM can be expressed on the cell surface (as a surface IgM, or sIgM) and the pre-B cell becomes an immature B cell. At this stage, the antigen receptor is first tested for reactivity to self antigens, or autoreactivity. The elimination of autoreactive B cells ensures that the B-cell population as a whole will be tolerant of self antigens. The **tolerance** produced at this stage of B-cell development is known as **central tolerance** because it arises in a central lymphoid organ, the bone marrow. However, B cells leaving the bone marrow are not fully mature and require additional maturation steps that take place in peripheral lymphoid organs (see Sections 8-8 and 8-9). As we shall see later in the chapter and in Chapter 15, self-reactive B cells that escape central tolerance may still be removed from the repertoire after they have left the bone marrow, a process that takes place during the final peripheral stages of B-cell maturation and is referred to as peripheral tolerance, described in Section 8-8.

sIgM associates with Igα and Igβ to form a functional B-cell receptor complex, and the fate of an immature B cell in the bone marrow depends on signals delivered from this receptor complex when it interacts with ligands in the environment. Igα signaling is particularly important in dictating the emigration of B cells from the bone marrow and/or their survival in the periphery: mice that express Igα with a truncated cytoplasmic domain that cannot signal show a fourfold reduction in the number of immature B cells in the marrow and a hundredfold reduction in the number of peripheral B cells. The release of immature B cells from the bone marrow into the circulation is also dependent on their expression of **S1PR1**, a G protein–coupled receptor that binds to the lipid ligand S1P and promotes cell migration toward the high concentrations of S1P that exist in the blood (see Section 8-28).

Immature B cells that have no strong reactivity to self antigens continue to mature (**Fig. 8.9**). They leave the marrow via sinusoids that enter the central sinus, enter the circulation, and are carried by the venous blood supply to the spleen. If, however, the newly expressed receptor encounters a strongly cross-linking antigen in the bone marrow—that is, if the B cell is strongly self-reactive—development is arrested at this stage, and the cell undergoes further gene rearrangements in an attempt to replace the autoreactive receptor with a new receptor that is not self-reactive. This mechanism is termed **receptor editing**.

Receptor editing is the predominant mechanism of central tolerance for B cells in the bone marrow (**Fig. 8.10**). When an immature B cell first produces sIgM, RAG proteins are still being made. If the receptor is not self-reactive, the

Fig. 8.10 Replacement of light chains by receptor editing can rescue some self-reactive B cells by changing their antigen specificity. When a developing B cell expresses antigen receptors that are strongly cross-linked by multivalent self antigens such as MHC molecules on cell surfaces (top panel), its development is arrested. The cell decreases surface expression of IgM and does not turn off the RAG genes (second panel). Continued synthesis of RAG proteins allows the cell to continue light-chain gene rearrangement. This usually leads to a new productive rearrangement and the expression of a new light chain, which combines with the previous heavy chain to form a new receptor; the process is called receptor editing (third panel). If this new receptor is not self-reactive, the cell is 'rescued' and continues normal development, much like a cell that had never reacted with self antigen (bottom left panel). If the cell remains self-reactive, it may be rescued by another cycle of rearrangement; however, if it continues to react strongly with self antigen, it will undergo apoptosis, resulting in clonal deletion of the self-reactive cell from the repertoire of B cells (bottom right panel).

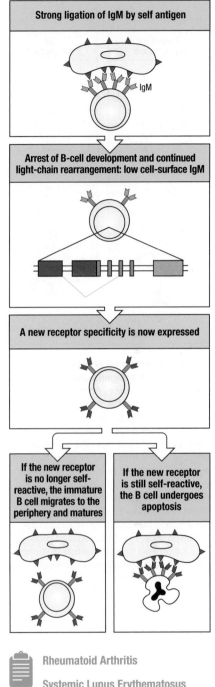

absence of sIgM cross-linking allows gene rearrangement to cease, and B-cell development continues, with RAG proteins eventually disappearing. For an autoreactive receptor, however, an encounter with the self antigen results in strong cross-linking of sIgM; RAG expression continues, and light-chain gene rearrangement can continue, as described in Fig. 8.8. These secondary rearrangements can rescue immature self-reactive B cells by deleting the self-reactive light-chain gene and replacing it with another sequence. If the new light chain is not autoreactive, the B cell continues normal development. If the receptor remains autoreactive, rearrangement continues until a non-autoreactive receptor is produced or until no additional light-chain V and J gene segments are available for recombination, at which time the immature B cell undergoes apoptosis, a process known as **clonal deletion**. The importance of receptor editing as a mechanism of tolerance is well established, as defects in this process contribute to the human autoimmune diseases systemic lupus erythematosus and rheumatoid arthritis, two diseases characterized by high levels of autoreactive antibodies (see Chapter 15).

It was originally thought that the successful production of a heavy chain and a light chain caused the almost instantaneous shutdown of light-chain locus rearrangement and that this ensured both allelic and isotypic exclusion. The unexpected ability of self-reactive B cells to continue to rearrange their light-chain genes, even after having made a productive rearrangement, suggests an alternative mechanism of allelic exclusion, in which the fall in the level of RAG proteins that follows a successful non-autoreactive rearrangement could be the principal means by which light-chain rearrangement is terminated. It is now apparent that allelic exclusion is not absolute, as there are rare B cells that express two different light chains.

The fact that central tolerance is not perfect and some self-reactive B cells are allowed to mature reflects the balance that the immune system strikes between purging all self-reactivity and maintaining the ability to respond to pathogens. If the elimination of self-reactive cells were too efficient, the receptor repertoire might become too limited and thus unable to recognize a wide variety of pathogens. Some autoimmune disease is the price of this balance: we shall see in Chapter 15 that weakly self-reactive lymphocytes can be activated and cause disease under conditions such as inflammation or when the self antigen becomes available or reaches an unusually high concentration because of tissue damage.

Rheumatoid Arthritis

Systemic Lupus Erythematosus

8-8 Lymphocytes that encounter sufficient quantities of self antigens in the periphery are eliminated.

While large numbers of self-reactive B cells are purged from the population of new lymphocytes in the bone marrow, only lymphocytes specific for self antigens that are expressed in or can reach this organ are affected. Some antigens, like the thyroid product thyroglobulin, are highly tissue specific or are

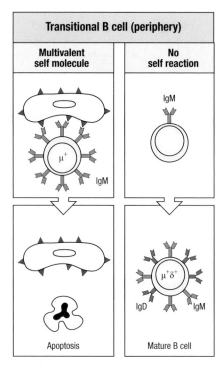

Fig. 8.11 Transitional B cells that recognize self antigens undergo peripheral tolerance. After emigrating from the bone marrow and entering the circulation, B cells are known as transitional B cells. Not yet fully mature, these cells are still subject to tolerance in the spleen after engagement of their sIgM receptor by a self antigen. Transitional B cells that encounter a multivalent self antigen receive a strong B-cell receptor signal and undergo cell death. Transitional B cells with no strong self reaction continue their maturation into mature B cells. The final stages of B-cell maturation lead to up-regulation of surface IgD (sIgD) and take place in the B-cell follicles in the spleen.

compartmentalized so that little if any is available in the circulation. Therefore, newly emigrated self-reactive B cells that encounter their specific self antigen in the periphery must also be eliminated (**Fig. 8.11**). This tolerance mechanism, which acts on newly emigrated B cells that are not yet functionally mature, is known as **peripheral tolerance**.

In the absence of an infection, newly emigrated B cells that encounter a strongly cross-linking antigen in the periphery will undergo clonal deletion. This was elegantly shown in studies of B cells expressing B-cell receptors specific for H-2K^b MHC class I molecules. These B cells are deleted even when, in transgenic animals, the expression of the H-2K^b molecule is restricted to the liver by the use of a liver-specific gene promoter. There is no receptor editing: B cells that encounter multivalent self-antigens in the periphery undergo apoptosis directly, unlike their counterparts in the bone marrow, which attempt further receptor rearrangements. This difference may be due to the fact that the B cells in the periphery are somewhat more mature and can no longer rearrange their light-chain loci.

8-9 Newly formed B cells arriving in the spleen turn over rapidly and require cytokines and positive signals through the B-cell receptor for maturation and long-term survival.

When B cells emerge from the bone marrow into the periphery, they are not yet functionally mature and are referred to as **transitional B cells**. As discussed above, their final maturation in the periphery provides an opportunity for these B cells to encounter peripheral self antigens and to undergo tolerance. Transitional B cells express high levels of sIgM but little surface IgD (sIgD), whereas mature B cells express low levels of IgM and high levels of IgD; while the changes in expression of sIgM and sIgD as B cells mature is well documented, the function of sIgD on mature B cells is not known.

Most B cells leaving the bone marrow will not survive to become fully mature B cells. **Figure 8.12** shows the possible fates of newly produced B cells that enter the periphery. The daily output of new B cells from the bone marrow is roughly 5–10% of the total B-lymphocyte population in the steady-state peripheral pool. In unimmunized animals, the size of this pool seems to remain constant, due to homeostasis, which means that the stream of new B cells needs to be balanced by the removal of an equal number of peripheral B cells. However, the majority of peripheral mature B cells are long-lived, and only 1–2% of these die each day. Thus, most of the B cells that die are in the rapidly turning-over peripheral population of transitional B-cells, of which more than 50% die every 3 days. The failure of most newly formed B cells to survive for more than a few days in the periphery seems to be due to competition between peripheral B cells for access to the follicles in the spleen. If newly produced transitional B cells do not enter a follicle, their passage through the periphery is halted and they eventually die. The limited number of lymphoid follicles cannot accommodate all of the B cells generated each day, and so there is continual competition for entry.

The follicle provides signals necessary for B-cell survival. In particular, the TNF family member **BAFF** (for B-cell activating factor belonging to the TNF family) is made by several cell types but is produced abundantly by the follicular dendritic cells (FDCs). FDCs are non-hematopoietic cells resident in the B-cell follicles that are specialized to capture antigens for recognition by B-cell antigen receptors (see Section 9-1). B cells express three different receptors for BAFF; namely, BAFF-R, BCMA, and TACI. BAFF-R is the most important for follicular B-cell survival, because mutant mice lacking BAFF-R have mainly transitional B cells and few long-lived peripheral B cells. BCMA and TACI also bind the related TNF family cytokine APRIL, which is not required for the survival of transitional B cells but is important for IgA antibody production, as we shall see in Chapter 10.

Fig. 8.12 Transitional B cells complete their maturation in B-cell follicles in the spleen. The micrograph in the top panel shows a cross-sectional view of a mouse spleen indicating the distribution of B cells (anti-B220; brown) and T cells (anti-CD3; blue) composing the white pulp. Surrounding the B cell–rich follicles (intense brown staining) are the marginal zones (also brown due to presence of B220⁺ B cells). The white pulp cords sit within the red pulp, which is rich in myeloid cells (mostly macrophages), plasma cells, and passing red blood cells. Transitional B cells that have left the bone marrow must complete their maturation in the B-cell follicles of the spleen, where they receive necessary maturation and survival signals (middle panel). One essential component is a low level of signaling through the B-cell receptor. A second essential factor is the expression of BAFF, a TNF family member, on follicular dendritic cells (FDCs). BAFF stimulates the receptor BAFF-R on transitional B cells, promoting B-cell survival. Newly emigrated transitional B cells (T1) exhibit high levels of surface IgM, little surface IgD, and the BAFF-R. In the B-cell follicles, these cells up-regulate CD21 to become transitional stage 2 B cells (T2). Finally, the cells up-regulate surface IgD and become long-lived mature B cells. The majority of long-lived B cells are recirculating B cells, known as follicular B cells. A second, less numerous subset is the marginal zone B-cell population. Marginal zone B cells are thought to be weakly self-reactive and express very high levels of the complement receptor CD21. These cells migrate to the marginal zones of the splenic white pulp, an area at the white pulp–red pulp junctions. In this location, marginal zone B cells are poised to make rapid responses to blood-borne antigens or pathogens. Transitional T1 B cells that are excluded from the follicles fail to receive maturation and survival signals and will die within 2–3 days of leaving the bone marrow (bottom panel).

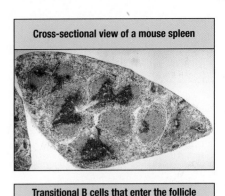

Cross-sectional view of a mouse spleen

Transitional B cells that enter the follicle receive maturation and survival signals and differentiate into follicular B cells or marginal zone B cells

Blood

B-cell follicle
transitional B cell (T1)
transitional B cell (T2)
follicular B cell
IgM
BAFF-R
BAFF
CD21
IgD
follicular dendritic cell
marginal zone B cell
Marginal zone

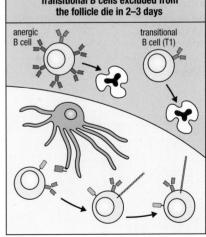

Transitional B cells excluded from the follicle die in 2–3 days

anergic B cell
transitional B cell (T1)

Transitional B cells in the spleen proceed through two distinct **transitional stages**, called T1 and T2, defined by the absence or presence of the B-cell co-receptor component CD21 (complement receptor 2) (see Section 2-13 and Section 7-20). In mice lacking BAFF, newly arising B cells progress to the T1 stage in the spleen but fail to express CD21, and the mice lack mature B cells. Signaling through the B-cell receptor is also required for transitional B cells in the spleen to progress through the T1 and T2 stages and enter the long-lived peripheral B-cell pool. In this case, the B-cell receptor signals do not arise from high-affinity interactions between the sIgM of the B-cell receptor and an antigen, which would induce strong signals; instead, these B-cell receptor signals are thought to be weak signals that are potentially generated by low-affinity recognition of self antigens, although the precise mechanism responsible for this signaling is not known. These weak B-cell receptor signals together with the BAFF-R signals are essential to promote the final stages of B-cell maturation in the periphery. Dysregulation of the appropriate balance between B-cell receptor and BAFF-R signaling occurs in individuals who overexpress BAFF and has been linked to the development of autoimmune diseases that result from a failure to purge autoreactive B cells, such as Sjögren's syndrome.

The majority of peripheral B cells that reside in the spleen and other peripheral lymphoid organs are known as **follicular B cells**, sometimes referred to as B-2 B cells. A second, minor population of B cells found in the spleen consists of **marginal zone B cells**, named for their predominance at the marginal zones that lie at the white pulp–red pulp junctions (see Fig. 8.12). Follicular and marginal zone B cells both derive from a common lineage that develops in the bone marrow and bifurcates during the final stage of B-cell maturation in the splenic follicles. Experiments reconstituting the signals promoting peripheral B-cell maturation in cell culture, starting from immature B-cell precursors, indicate that follicular versus marginal zone B-cell lineages diverge at the transitional T2 stage, as cells transition to the fully mature stage. Like follicular B cells, marginal zone B cells are dependent on BAFF signals and are missing in mice lacking BAFF expression. Marginal zone B cells can be identified by their expression of very high levels of the complement receptor CD21. Studies using rearranged immunoglobulin gene knock-in mice that express a single B-cell receptor specificity on all developing B cells have demonstrated that some B-cell receptors predominantly generate follicular B cells, whereas others generate marginal zone B cells. These findings indicate that the specificity of the B-cell receptor is a major factor in determining the final commitment of transitional B cells to the follicular versus the marginal zone lineage; however, the details of this process are still not fully understood. Because of their location, marginal zone B cells are poised to make rapid responses to antigens or pathogens filtered from the blood. Therefore, it is thought that marginal zone B cells represent an early line of defense for blood-borne pathogens.

Peripheral B cells also include memory B cells, which are generated in addition to antibody-producing plasma cells from mature B cells after their first encounter with antigen; we will return to B-cell memory in Chapter 11. Competition for follicular entry favors mature B cells that are already established in the relatively long-lived and stable peripheral B-cell pool. Mature B cells have undergone phenotypic changes that might make their access to the follicles easier; for example, they express CXCR5, the receptor for CXCL13, which is expressed by FDCs (see Section 10-3). They also have increased expression of CD21 compared with immature newly developed B cells, which enhances the signaling capacity of the B cell.

The B-cell receptor plays a positive role in the maturation and continued recirculation of peripheral B cells. Mice that lack the tyrosine kinase Syk, which is involved in signaling from the B-cell receptor (see Section 7-20), have transitional B cells but fail to develop mature B cells. Thus, a Syk-transduced signal may be required for final B-cell maturation or for the survival of mature B cells. Furthermore, continual expression of the B-cell receptor is required for B-cell survival, as is evident from the loss of all B cells in mice whose B-cell receptor is conditionally deleted specifically in mature B cells. Although each B-cell receptor has a unique specificity, antigen-specific interactions may not induce the signals used for final B-cell maturation and survival; the receptor could, for example, be responsible for 'tonic' signaling, in which a weak but important signal is generated by the assembly of the receptor complex and infrequently triggers some or all of the downstream signaling events.

8-10 B-1 B cells are an innate lymphocyte subset that arises early in development.

Thus far, this chapter has focused on the development of the majority populations of B cells that reside in peripheral lymphoid organs, such as follicular B cells and marginal zone B cells. These two populations compose the B-cell arm of the adaptive immune response. A third important subset of B cells, called **B-1 B cells**, is part of the innate immune system. These cells are present only in low numbers in peripheral lymphoid organs but are found in large numbers in the peritoneal and pleural cavities. B-1 B cells are the major source of 'natural' antibodies, which are constitutively produced circulating antibodies that are secreted by these B cells prior to any infections. Most antibodies made by B-1 B cells recognize capsular polysaccharide antigens, and B-1 B cells are important in controlling infections of pathogenic viruses and bacteria.

One important feature of B-1 B cells is that they can produce antibodies of the IgM class without 'help' from T cells. Although this response can be enhanced by T-cell cooperation, the antibodies first appear within 48 hours of exposure to antigen, when T cells cannot be involved. The lack of an antigen-specific interaction with helper T cells might explain why immunological memory is not generated as a result of B-1 cell responses: repeated exposures to the same antigen elicit similar or decreased responses with each exposure. While the precise functions of B-1 B cells are still not clear, mice deficient in B-1 B cells are more susceptible to infection with *Streptococcus pneumoniae* because they fail to produce an anti-phosphocholine antibody that provides protection against this bacterium. Because a significant fraction of the B-1 B cells can make antibodies of this specificity, and because no antigen-specific T-cell help is required, a potent response can be produced early in infection with this pathogen. Whether human B-1 B cells have the same role is not certain.

Property	B-1 B cells	Follicular B cells	Marginal zone B cells
When first produced	Fetus	After birth	After birth
N-regions in VDJ junctions	Few	Extensive	Yes
V-region repertoire	Restricted	Diverse	Partly restricted
Primary location	Body cavities (peritoneal, pleural)	Peripheral lymphoid organs	Spleen
Dependence on BAFF	No	Yes	Yes
Dependence on IL-7	No	Yes	Yes
Mode of renewal	Self-renewing	Replaced from bone marrow	Long-lived
Spontaneous production of immunoglobulin	High	Low	Low
Isotypes secreted	IgM >> IgG	IgG > IgM	IgM > IgG
Response to carbohydrate antigen	Yes	Maybe	Yes
Response to protein antigen	Maybe	Yes	Yes
Requirement for T-cell help	No	Yes	Sometimes
Somatic hypermutation	Low to none	High	?
Memory development	Little or none	Yes	?

Fig. 8.13 A comparison of the properties of B-1 B cells, follicular B cells, and marginal zone B cells. In addition to developing in the liver, B-1 B cells can develop in unusual sites in the mouse fetus, such as the omentum. B-1 B cells predominate in the young animal, although they probably can be produced throughout life. Being produced mainly during fetal and neonatal life, their rearranged variable-region sequences contain few N-nucleotides. In contrast, marginal zone B cells accumulate after birth and do not reach peak levels in the mouse until 8 weeks of age. Follicular B cells and marginal zone B cells share a common precursor population, the transitional T2 B cells in the spleen; as a consequence, both subsets are dependent on IL-7 and BAFF signals for their development in the mouse. In contrast, B-1 B cell development does not require IL-7 or BAFF. B-1 B cells are best thought of as a partly activated self-renewing pool of lymphocytes that are selected by ubiquitous self and foreign antigens. Because of this selection, and possibly because the cells are produced early in life, the B-1 B cells have a restricted repertoire of variable regions and antigen-binding specificities. Marginal zone B cells also have a restricted repertoire of V-region specificities that may be selected by a set of antigens similar to those that select B-1 B cells. B-1 B cells seem to be the major population of B cells in certain body cavities, most likely because of exposure at these sites to antigens that drive B-1 B cell proliferation. Marginal zone B cells remain in the marginal zone of the spleen and are not thought to recirculate. Partial activation of B-1 B cells leads to the secretion of mainly IgM antibody; B-1 B cells contribute much of the IgM that circulates in the blood. The limited diversity of both the B-1 and marginal zone B-cell repertoire and the propensity of these cells to react with common bacterial carbohydrate antigens suggest that they carry out a more primitive, less adaptive immune response than follicular B cells. In this regard they are comparable to γδ T cells.

Unlike follicular and marginal zone B cells that develop from bone marrow stem cells, the majority of B-1 B cells are generated from progenitor cells found in the fetal liver (**Fig. 8.13**). During late fetal and early neonatal stages in mice, B-1 B cells are produced in large numbers. After birth, the development of follicular and marginal zone B cells predominates, and few B-1 B cells are made. Current evidence indicates that the progenitor cells giving rise to B-1 B cells are committed to this lineage and are distinct from those producing follicular and marginal zone B cells. Whereas follicular and marginal zone B cells are absent in mice lacking BAFF or the BAFF-R, these deficiencies have no effect on the development or survival of B-1 B cells. Additionally, the weak B-cell receptor signals that promote the final stages of follicular and marginal zone B-cell maturation in the spleen require the non-canonical NFκB activation pathway (see Section 7-24), a signaling pathway that is dispensable for B-1 B-cell development. Cytokine requirements also differ between these developmental pathways. B-1 B cells develop normally in mice lacking IL-7 or IL-7R signaling components, defects that prevent the development of follicular and marginal zone B cells. Finally, follicular and marginal zone B-cell development also requires the transcription factor PU.1, which is not needed for the development of B-1 B cells.

Summary.

In this section, we have followed B-cell development from the earliest progenitors in the bone marrow to the long-lived mature peripheral B-cell pool (**Fig. 8.14**). The heavy-chain locus is rearranged first and, if this is successful, a μ heavy chain is produced that combines with surrogate light chains to form the pre-B-cell receptor; this is the first checkpoint in B-cell development.

	B cells	Heavy-chain genes	Light-chain genes	Intracellular proteins	Surface marker proteins	
ANTIGEN INDEPENDENT	Common lymphoid progenitor	Germline	Germline	RAG-1 RAG-2 TdT λ5, VpreB	CD34, CD45, CD93	**BONE MARROW**
	Early pro-B cell	D–J rearranged	Germline	TdT λ5, VpreB	CD34, CD45R, CD93, IL-7R, MHC class II, CD10, CD19, CD38	
	Late pro-B cell	V–DJ rearranged	Germline	λ5, VpreB	CD45R, CD93, IL-7R, MHC class II, CD10, CD19, CD38, CD20	
	Large pre-B cell	VDJ rearranged	Germline	μ RAG-1 RAG-2	CD45R, CD93, IL-7R, MHC class II, pre-BCR, CD19, CD38, CD20	
	Small pre-B cell	VDJ rearranged	V–J rearrangement		CD45R, CD93, MHC class II, CD19, CD38, CD20	
	Immature B cell	VDJ rearranged. μ heavy chain produced in membrane form	VJ rearranged		CD45R, MHC class II, IgM, CD19, CD20, CD24, CD93, CD21, CD38, CD23⁻/⁺	
ANTIGEN DEPENDENT	Transitional B cell				CD45R, MHC class II, IgM, CD19, CD20, CD24, CD93, CD21, CD38, CD23⁻/⁺	**PERIPHERY**
	Marginal zone B cell	VDJ rearranged. Alternative splicing yields μ + δ mRNA that encodes IgM and IgD. IgM predominates			CD45R, MHC class II, IgMhi, IgDlo, CD19, CD20, CD1, CD9, CD21, CD22, CD35	
	Mature follicular B cell	VDJ rearranged. Alternative splicing yields μ + δ mRNA that encodes IgM and IgD. IgD predominates			CD45R, CD93, MHC class II, IgMlo, IgDhi, CD19, CD20, CD21, CD22, CD23, CD24, CD38	
	Lymphoblast	Alternative splicing yields secreted μ chains		Ig	CD45R, MHC class II, CD19, CD20, CD21	
	Memory B cell	Often isotype switched to Cγ, Cα, or Cε. Somatic hypermutation	Somatic hypermutation		CD45R, MHC class II, IgM, IgG, IgA, IgDneg, CD19, CD20, CD38, CD80	
TERMINAL DIFFERENTIATION	Plasmablast and plasma cell	Alternative splicing yields both membrane and secreted Ig. In plasma cells, Ig is predominantly secreted	VJ rearranged	Ig	CD138, plasma cell antigen-1, CD38	

Fig. 8.14 A summary of the development of B-lineage cells. The state of the immunoglobulin genes, the expression of some essential intracellular proteins, and the expression of some cell-surface molecules are shown for successive stages of conventional B-cell development. During antigen-driven B-cell differentiation, the immunoglobulin genes undergo further changes, such as class switching and somatic hypermutation (see Chapter 10), which are evident in the immunoglobulins produced by memory cells and plasma cells.

Production of the pre-B-cell receptor signals successful heavy-chain gene rearrangement and causes cessation of this rearrangement, thus enforcing allelic exclusion. It also initiates pre-B-cell proliferation, generating numerous progeny in which subsequent light-chain rearrangement can be attempted. If the initial light-chain gene rearrangement is productive, a complete immuno-globulin B-cell receptor is formed, gene rearrangement again ceases, and the B cell continues its development. If the first light-chain gene rearrangement is unsuccessful, rearrangement continues until either a productive rearrange-ment is made or all available J regions are used up. If no productive rearrange-ment is made, the developing B cell dies. Once a complete immunoglobulin receptor is expressed on the surface of the cell, immature B cells undergo tolerance to self antigens. This process begins in the bone marrow and con-tinues for a short time after immature B cells emigrate to the periphery. For the majority of B cells, the final stages of maturation occur in the B-cell folli-cles of the spleen and require the TNF family member BAFF as well as signals through the B-cell receptor.

Development of T lymphocytes.

Like B cells, T lymphocytes derive from the multipotent hematopoietic stem cells in the bone marrow. However, T-cell progenitors migrate from the bone marrow via the blood to the thymus, where they mature (**Fig. 8.15**); this is the reason for the name thymus-dependent (T) lymphocytes, or T cells. T-cell development parallels that of B cells in many ways, including the orderly and stepwise rearrangement of antigen receptor genes, the sequential testing for successful gene rearrangement, and the eventual assembly of a heterodi-meric antigen receptor. Nevertheless, T-cell development in the thymus has some features not seen for B cells, such as the generation of two distinct lin-eages of T cells expressing antigen receptors encoded by distinct genes, the

Fig. 8.15 T cells undergo development in the thymus and migrate to the peripheral lymphoid organs, where they are activated by foreign antigens. T-cell precursors migrate from the bone marrow to the thymus, where they commit to the T-cell lineage after Notch receptor signaling. In the thymus, T-cell receptor genes are rearranged (top first panel); αβ T-cell receptors that are compatible with self MHC molecules transmit a survival signal on interacting with thymic epithelium, leading to positive selection of the cells that bear them. Self-reactive receptors transmit a signal that leads to cell death, and cells bearing them are removed from the repertoire in a process of negative selection (top second panel). T cells that survive selection mature and leave the thymus to circulate in the periphery; they repeatedly leave the blood to migrate through the peripheral lymphoid organs, where they may encounter their specific foreign antigen and become activated (top third panel). Activation leads to clonal expansion and differentiation into effector T cells. Some of these are attracted to sites of infection, where they can kill infected cells or activate macrophages and other innate immune cells not pictured (top fourth panel); others are attracted into B-cell areas, where they help to activate an antibody response (not shown).

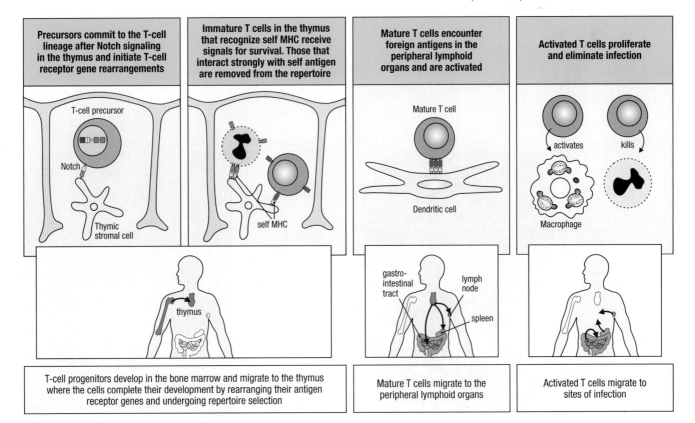

Precursors commit to the T-cell lineage after Notch signaling in the thymus and initiate T-cell receptor gene rearrangements

Immature T cells in the thymus that recognize self MHC receive signals for survival. Those that interact strongly with self antigen are removed from the repertoire

Mature T cells encounter foreign antigens in the peripheral lymphoid organs and are activated

Activated T cells proliferate and eliminate infection

T-cell precursor

Notch

Thymic stromal cell

self MHC

Mature T cell

Dendritic cell

activates

kills

Macrophage

thymus

gastro-intestinal tract

lymph node

spleen

T-cell progenitors develop in the bone marrow and migrate to the thymus where the cells complete their development by rearranging their antigen receptor genes and undergoing repertoire selection

Mature T cells migrate to the peripheral lymphoid organs

Activated T cells migrate to sites of infection

γδ lineage and the αβ lineage. Developing T cells, which are known generally as **thymocytes**, also undergo rigorous selection that depends on interactions with thymic cells and that shapes the mature repertoire of T cells to ensure self MHC restriction as well as self-tolerance. We begin with a general overview of the stages of thymocyte development and its relationship to thymic anatomy before considering gene rearrangement and the mechanisms of selection.

8-11 T-cell progenitors originate in the bone marrow, but all the important events in T-cell development occur in the thymus.

The thymus is situated in the upper anterior thorax, just above the heart. It consists of numerous lobules, each clearly differentiated into an outer cortical region—the **thymic cortex**—and an inner **medulla** (**Fig. 8.16**). In young individuals, the thymus contains large numbers of developing T-cell precursors embedded in a network of epithelia known as the **thymic stroma**. This provides a unique microenvironment for T-cell development analogous to that provided for B cells by the stromal cells of the bone marrow.

The thymic epithelium arises early in embryonic development from endoderm-derived structures known as the third pharyngeal pouches. These epithelial tissues form a rudimentary thymus, or **thymic anlage**. The thymic anlage is colonized by cells of hematopoietic origin that give rise to large numbers of thymocytes, which are committed to the T-cell lineage, and to **intrathymic dendritic cells**. Thymocytes are not simply passengers within the thymus: they influence the arrangement of the thymic epithelial cells on which they depend for survival, inducing the formation of a reticular epithelial structure that surrounds the developing thymocytes.

The cellular architecture of the human thymus is illustrated in Fig. 8.16. Bone marrow–derived cells are differentially distributed between the thymic cortex and medulla. The cortex contains only immature thymocytes and scattered

Fig. 8.16 The cellular organization of the human thymus. The thymus, which lies in the midline of the body, above the heart, is made up of several lobules, each of which contains discrete cortical (outer) and medullary (central) regions. As shown in the diagram on the left, the cortex consists of immature thymocytes (dark blue); branched cortical epithelial cells (pale blue), with which the immature cortical thymocytes are closely associated; and scattered macrophages (yellow), which are involved in clearing apoptotic thymocytes. The medulla consists of mature thymocytes (dark blue) and medullary epithelial cells (orange), along with macrophages (yellow) and dendritic cells (yellow) of bone marrow origin. Hassall's corpuscles are probably also sites of cell degradation. The thymocytes in the outer cortical cell layer are proliferating immature cells, whereas the deeper cortical thymocytes are mainly immature T cells undergoing thymic selection. The photograph shows the equivalent section of a human thymus, stained with hematoxylin and eosin. The cortex is darkly stained, whereas the medulla is lightly stained.

macrophages, whereas more mature thymocytes, along with dendritic cells, macrophages, and some B cells, are found in the medulla. As will be discussed later, this organization reflects the different developmental events that occur in these two compartments.

The importance of the thymus in immunity was first discovered through experiments on mice; indeed, most of our knowledge of T-cell development in the thymus comes from the mouse. It was found that surgical removal of the thymus (**thymectomy**) at birth resulted in immunodeficient mice, focusing interest on this organ at a time when the difference between T and B lymphocytes in mammals had not yet been defined. Much evidence, including observations in immunodeficient children, has since confirmed the importance of the thymus in T-cell development. In **DiGeorge syndrome** in humans and in mice with the *nude* mutation, the thymus does not form, and the affected individual produces B lymphocytes but few T lymphocytes. DiGeorge syndrome is a complex combination of cardiac, facial, endocrine, and immune defects associated with deletions of chromosome 22q11. The *nude* mutation in mice is due to a defect in the gene for Foxn1, a transcription factor required for terminal epithelial-cell differentiation; the name *nude* was given to this mutation because it also causes hairlessness. Rare cases of a defect in the human FOXN1 gene (which is on chromosome 17) have been associated with T-cell immunodeficiency, absence of a thymus, congenital alopecia, and nail dystrophy.

In mice, the thymus continues to develop for 3–4 weeks after birth, whereas in humans it is fully developed at birth. The rate of T-cell production by the thymus is greatest before puberty. After puberty, the thymus begins to shrink, and the production of new T cells in adults is reduced, although it does continue throughout life. In both mice and humans, removal of the thymus after puberty is not accompanied by any notable loss of T-cell function or numbers. Thus, it seems that once the T-cell repertoire is established, immunity can be sustained without the production of significant numbers of new T cells; the pool of peripheral T cells is instead maintained by long-lived T cells and also by division of some mature T cells.

8-12 T-cell precursors proliferate extensively in the thymus, but most die there.

T-cell precursors arriving in the thymus from the bone marrow spend up to a week differentiating there before they enter a phase of intense proliferation. In a young adult mouse the thymus contains about 10^8 to 2×10^8 thymocytes. About 5×10^7 new cells are generated each day; however, only about 10^6 to 2×10^6 (roughly 2–4%) of these leave the thymus each day as mature T cells. Despite the disparity between the number of T cells generated in the thymus and the number leaving, the thymus does not continue to grow in size or cell number. This is because about 98% of the thymocytes developing in the thymus die by apoptosis (see Section 1-13). Cells undergoing apoptosis are recognized and ingested by macrophages, and apoptotic bodies, which are the residual condensed chromatin of apoptotic cells, are seen inside macrophages throughout the thymic cortex (**Fig. 8.17**). This apparently profligate waste of thymocytes is a crucial part of T-cell development because it reflects the intensive screening that each thymocyte undergoes for the ability to recognize self peptide:self MHC complexes and for self-tolerance.

8-13 Successive stages in the development of thymocytes are marked by changes in cell-surface molecules.

Like developing B cells, developing thymocytes pass through a series of distinct stages. These are marked by changes in the status of the T-cell receptor genes and in the expression of the T-cell receptor, and by changes in the

DiGeorge Syndrome

Fig. 8.17 Developing T cells that undergo apoptosis are ingested by macrophages in the thymic cortex. The left panel shows a section through the thymic cortex and part of the medulla in which cells have been stained for apoptosis using a red dye. The thymic cortex is to the right in the photograph. Apoptotic cells are scattered throughout the cortex but are rare in the medulla likely due to the lower density of thymocytes in the medulla. The right panel shows at higher magnification a section of thymic cortex that has been stained red for apoptotic cells and blue for macrophages. The apoptotic cells can be seen within macrophages. Magnifications: left panel, ×45; right panel, ×164.

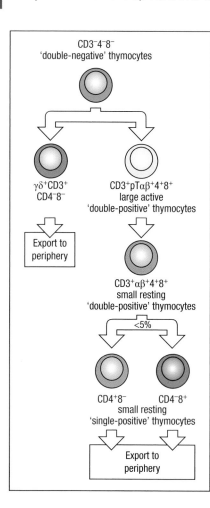

CD3⁻4⁻8⁻
'double-negative' thymocytes

γδ⁺CD3⁺
CD4⁻8⁻

CD3⁺pTαβ⁺4⁺8⁺
large active
'double-positive' thymocytes

Export to
periphery

CD3⁺αβ⁺4⁺8⁺
small resting
'double-positive' thymocytes

<5%

CD4⁺8⁻   CD4⁻8⁺
small resting
'single-positive' thymocytes

Export to
periphery

Fig. 8.18 Distinct lineages of thymocytes are produced in the thymus. CD4, CD8, and T-cell receptor complex molecules (CD3, and the T-cell receptor α and β chains) are important cell-surface molecules for identifying thymocyte subpopulations. The earliest cell population in the thymus does not express any of these proteins, and because these cells do not express CD4 or CD8, they are called 'double-negative' thymocytes. These cells include precursors that give rise to two T-cell lineages: the minority population of γδ T cells (which lack CD4 or CD8 even when mature), and the majority αβ T-cell lineage. The development of prospective αβ T cells proceeds through stages in which both CD4 and CD8 are expressed by the same cell; these are known as 'double-positive' thymocytes. Early on, these cells are large proliferating cells. Later, they become small resting double-positive cells that express low levels of the T-cell receptor. Most thymocytes die within the thymus after becoming small double-positive cells, but those cells whose receptors can interact with self peptide:self MHC molecular complexes lose expression of either CD4 or CD8 and increase the level of expression of the T-cell receptor. The outcome of this process is the 'single-positive' thymocytes, which, after maturation, are exported from the thymus as mature single-positive CD4 or CD8 T cells.

expression of cell-surface proteins such as the CD3 complex (see Section 7-7) and the co-receptor proteins CD4 and CD8 (see Section 4-21). These surface changes reflect the state of functional maturation of the cell, and particular combinations of cell-surface proteins are used as markers for T cells at different stages of differentiation. Two distinct lineages of T cells—αβ and γδ, which have different types of T-cell receptor chains—are produced early in T-cell development. Later, αβ T cells develop into two distinct functional subsets—CD4 T cells and CD8 T cells.

When progenitor cells first enter the thymus from the bone marrow, they lack most of the surface molecules characteristic of mature T cells, and their receptor genes are not rearranged. These cells are often referred to as 'double-negative' thymocytes, as they lack expression of both CD4 and CD8. Double-negative thymocytes give rise to the major population of αβ T cells and the minor population of γδ T cells (**Fig. 8.18**). If injected into the peripheral circulation, these lymphoid progenitors can even give rise to B cells and NK cells, although it is uncertain whether individual thymic progenitor cells retain this multipotency or whether the progenitor-cell population consists of a mixture of cells, only some of which are fully committed to the αβ or γδ T-cell lineage.

In the postnatal thymus, only ~60% of the double-negative thymocytes are immature T cells. The double-negative thymocyte pool (about 5% of all thymocytes) also includes two populations of more mature T cells that belong to minority lineages, including T cells expressing γδ T-cell receptors (Fig. 8.18) and T cells bearing αβ T-cell receptors of very limited diversity (iNKT cells; see Section 6-18). Here and in subsequent discussions, we reserve the term 'double-negative thymocytes' for the immature thymocytes that do not yet express a complete T-cell receptor molecule. These double-negative thymocytes give rise to both γδ and αβ T cells (see Fig. 8.18), although most of them develop along the αβ pathway. Mature γδ T cells remain double-negative and are exported to the periphery to populate various tissue sites (see Section 8-17). αβ T cells progress through several additional stages before leaving the thymus. First the double-negative thymocytes progress to a stage known as 'double-positive,' where thymocytes co-express both CD4 and CD8 receptors. Lastly, thymocyte development generates two different subsets: one subset expressing CD4 but not CD8 (CD4⁺8⁻) and a second subset expressing CD8 but not CD4 (CD4⁻8⁺), both of which are exported from the thymus into the periphery (Fig. 8.18).

8-14 Commitment to the T-cell lineage occurs in the thymus after Notch signaling.

T lymphocytes develop from a lymphoid progenitor in the bone marrow that also gives rise to B lymphocytes. Some of these progenitors leave the bone marrow and migrate to the thymus. In the thymus, these progenitor cells are known as early thymic progenitors (ETPs). ETPs receive a signal from thymic epithelial cells that is transduced through a receptor called Notch to switch-on specific genes. Notch signaling is widely used in animal development to specify tissue differentiation; in lymphocyte development, the Notch signal instructs the precursor to commit to the T-cell lineage rather than the B-cell lineage. Notch signaling is required throughout T-cell development and is also thought to help regulate other T-cell lineage choices, including the αβ versus γδ choice.

Notch signaling in thymic progenitor cells is essential to initiate the T cell–specific gene expression program and commitment to the T-cell lineage (**Fig. 8.19**). Notch signaling induces the expression of two transcription factors, T-cell factor-1 (TCF1) and GATA3, both of which are required for T-cell development. Together, TCF1 and GATA3 initiate expression of several T lineage–specific genes, such as those encoding components of the CD3 complex, as well as *RAG1*, a gene required for T-cell receptor and B-cell receptor gene rearrangements. However, TCF1 and GATA3 are not sufficient to induce the entire program of T cell–specific gene expression. A third transcription factor, Bcl11b, is required to induce T-lineage commitment by restricting progenitor cells from adopting alternative fates; this final phase of T-cell commitment is a necessary prerequisite for activating the complete T-cell gene expression program.

Notch signaling also induces the expression of the IL-7 receptor α chain. IL-7 is an important cytokine that is produced by the thymic stroma, and IL-7 receptor signaling is essential for maintaining the survival of thymic progenitor cells. The receptor for IL-7 is composed of the IL-7 receptor α chain and a receptor subunit called γ-c that is shared with several other cytokine receptors (see Sections 3-15 and 3-16). All of the cytokine receptors that use γ-c as a subunit activate the tyrosine kinase Jak3, which is essential for receptor signaling. In the absence of IL-7, IL-7 receptor α, γ-c, or Jak3, a severe block in T-cell development occurs in both mice and humans. In fact, the human primary immunodeficiency disease characterized by a lack of T cells and NK cells, X-linked severe combined immune deficiency (X-linked SCID) disease, is caused by a genetic deficiency leading to the absence of γ-c protein expression.

X-linked Severe Combined Immune Deficiency

Interactions with the thymic stroma trigger an initial phase of differentiation along the T-cell lineage pathway, followed by cell proliferation and the expression of the first cell-surface molecules specific for T cells; for example, CD2 and (in mice) Thy-1. At the end of this phase, which can last about a week, the thymocytes bear distinctive markers of the T-cell lineage but do not express any of the three cell-surface markers that define mature T cells. These are the CD3:T-cell receptor complex and the co-receptors CD4 or CD8. Because of the absence of CD4 and CD8, such cells are called **double-negative thymocytes** (see Fig. 8.18).

The αβ pathway is shown in more detail in Fig. 8.19. The double-negative stage can be further subdivided into four stages on the basis of the state of differentiation. The earliest stage of thymocyte development is the early thymic progenitor (ETP), sometimes referred to as **DN1** cells. ETPs express Kit, the receptor for stem-cell factor (SCF) (see Figure 8.3); in these cells, the genes encoding both chains of the T-cell receptor are in the germline configuration, and the cells retain the potential to develop into T cells, B cells, NK cells, and some myeloid cells. As thymocytes mature, they begin to express CD25 (the α chain of the IL-2 receptor) along with Kit on their surface and gradually lose the potential to develop into non-T-cell lineages; these cells are called **pro-T cells**, sometimes referred to as **DN2** cells. Kit expression is lost at the next stage of thymocyte maturation; these cells are **pre-T cells**, or **DN3** cells, and are fully committed to develop into T cells, having lost the potential to develop into any other hematopoietic lineages.

Fig. 8.19 The stages of αβ T-cell development in the mouse thymus correlate with the program of gene rearrangement and the expression of cell-surface proteins, signaling proteins, and transcription factors.
Early thymic progenitors (ETPs) are triggered to proliferate and become thymocytes committed to the T-cell lineage through interactions with Notch ligands expressed on the thymic stroma. T-cell commitment requires Notch signaling to induce the expression of TCF1 and GATA3, which in turn induce the expression of Bcl11b. This gene expression program begins in the ETP [also known as double-negative (DN1)] cells that express CD44 and Kit. Cells become irreversibly committed to the T-cell lineage at the subsequent (pro-T; DN2) stage, which is marked by expression of CD25, the α chain of the IL-2 receptor. Then the pro-T (CD44+CD25+) cells begin to rearrange the β-chain locus, becoming CD44low and Kitlow, and they become pre-T (DN3) cells. The small pre-T cells are arrested in the CD44lowCD25+ stage until they productively rearrange the β-chain locus; the in-frame β chain then pairs with a surrogate chain called pTα to form the pre-T-cell receptor (pre-TCR), which is expressed on the cell surface and triggers entry into the cell cycle. Expression of small amounts of pTα:β on the cell surface in association with CD3 signals the cessation of β-chain gene rearrangement and triggers rapid cell proliferation, which causes the loss of CD25. The cells are then known as large pre-T (DN4) cells. CD4 and CD8 expression is initiated, and the CD4+CD8+ double-positive cells cease to proliferate. These nonproliferating small CD4+CD8+ double-positive cells begin efficient rearrangement at the α-chain locus. The cells then express low levels of an αβ T-cell receptor and the associated CD3 complex and are ready for selection. Most cells die by failing to be positively selected or as a consequence of negative selection, but some are selected to mature into CD4 or CD8 single-positive cells and eventually to leave the thymus. Maturation of CD4+CD8+ double-positive cells into CD4 or CD8 single-positive cells is regulated by transcription factors ThPOK and Runx3, respectively. KLF2 is first expressed at the single-positive stage; if it is absent, thymocytes exhibit a defect in emigrating to peripheral lymphoid tissues, due in part to their failure to express receptors involved in trafficking, such as the sphingosine 1-phosphate (S1P) receptor, S1PR1 (see Fig. 8.32). The individual contributions to T-cell development of the other proteins are discussed in the text.

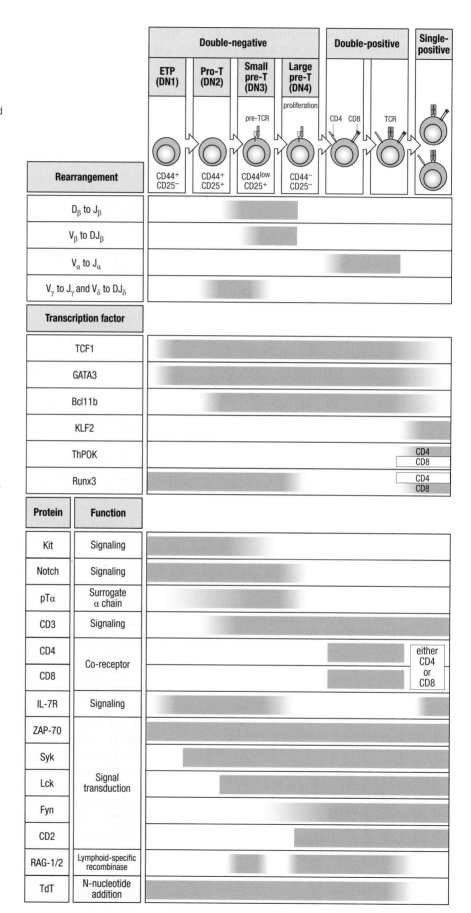

8-15   After T-cell commitment, thymocyte development is regulated by T-cell receptor rearrangement, expression, and signaling.

Rearrangement of the T-cell receptor β-chain locus begins in pro-T cells with some D_β to J_β rearrangements and continues in pre-T cells with V_β to DJ_β rearrangement. Cells that fail to make a successful rearrangement of the β-chain locus remain at the pre-T stage and soon die, whereas cells that make productive β-chain gene rearrangements and express the β-chain protein progress to a large pre-T cell stage, often called the **DN4** stage. These cells undergo proliferation, leading to the loss of CD25 expression. In spite of its usefulness in identifying these thymocyte subsets, the functional significance of the transient expression of CD25 is unclear: conventional CD4 and CD8 T cells develop normally in mice in which the IL-2 gene has been deleted by gene knockout (see Appendix I, Section A-36). By contrast, Kit is quite important for the development of the earliest double-negative thymocytes, in that mice lacking Kit have a much smaller number of double-negative T cells. In addition, continual Notch signaling is important for progression through each stage of T-cell development.

In thymocytes at the pre-T cell stage (see Fig. 8.19), the expressed β chains pair with a surrogate pre-T-cell receptor α chain called **pTα** (pre-T-cell **α**), which allows the assembly of a complete **pre-T-cell receptor** (pre-TCR) that is analogous in structure and function to the pre-B-cell receptor. The pre-TCR is expressed on the cell surface in a complex with the CD3 molecules that provide the signaling components of T-cell receptors (see Section 7-7). As with the pre-B-cell receptor, the assembly of the CD3:pre-T-cell receptor complex causes constitutive signaling that does not require interaction with a ligand. Recent structural evidence shows that the pre-TCR forms dimers in a manner similar to pre-BCR dimerization. The pTα Ig domain makes two important contacts. It associates with the constant-region Ig domain of the V_β subunit to form the pre-TCR itself. A distinct surface of the pTα then binds to a V_β domain from another pre-TCR molecule, forming a bridge between two different pre-TCRs. The region of contact with the V_β involves residues that are highly conserved across many V_β families. In this way, expression of the pre-TCR induces ligand-independent dimerization, which leads to cell proliferation, the arrest of further β-chain gene rearrangement, and the expression of both CD8 and CD4.

Double-positive thymocytes make up the vast majority of thymocytes. Once the large double-positive thymocytes have ceased to proliferate and have become small double-positive cells, the α-chain locus begins to rearrange. As we will see later in this chapter, the structure of the α locus (see Section 5-10) allows multiple successive attempts at rearrangement, so that it is successfully rearranged in most developing thymocytes. Thus, most double-positive cells produce an αβ T-cell receptor during their relatively short life span. Small double-positive thymocytes initially express low levels of the T-cell receptor. Not all double-positive thymocytes continue the developmental process to become mature T cells. On the basis of selection processes that depend on T-cell receptor signaling, a small subset of double-positive cells down-regulates one of the two co-receptor molecules, becoming either CD4 or CD8 **single-positive thymocytes** (see Fig. 8.18 and Fig. 8.19). Single-positive thymocytes continue to undergo selection processes that shape the T-cell repertoire and promote the development of multiple T-cell lineages, including conventional CD4 and CD8 T cells, T_{reg} cells, NK-T cells, MAIT cells, and others (see Section 8-27). Thus, of the original pool of double-positive thymocytes, only about 2% survive and are exported from the thymus to form the peripheral T-cell repertoire. Overall, the time between the entry of a T-cell progenitor into the thymus and the export of its mature progeny is estimated to be about 3 weeks in the mouse.

ANIMATION 8.1

8-16 Thymocytes at different developmental stages are found in distinct parts of the thymus.

The thymus is divided into two main regions, a peripheral cortex and a central medulla (see Fig. 8.16). Most T-cell development takes place in the cortex; only mature single-positive thymocytes are seen in the medulla. Initially, progenitors from the bone marrow enter the thymus from the blood at the cortico-medullary junction and migrate to the outer cortex (**Fig. 8.20**). At the outer edge of the cortex, in the subcapsular region of the thymus, large immature double-negative thymocytes proliferate vigorously; these cells are thought to represent committed thymocyte progenitors and their immediate progeny and will give rise to all subsequent thymocyte populations. Deeper in the cortex, most of the thymocytes are small double-positive cells. The cortical stroma is composed of epithelial cells with long branching processes that express both MHC class II and MHC class I molecules on their surface. The thymic cortex is densely packed with thymocytes, and the branching processes of the thymic cortical epithelial cells make contact with almost all cortical thymocytes. Contact between the MHC molecules on thymic cortical epithelial cells and the receptors of developing T cells has a crucial role in positive selection, as we will see later in this chapter.

After positive selection, developing T cells migrate from the cortex to the medulla. The medulla contains fewer lymphocytes, and those present are predominantly the newly matured single-positive T cells that will eventually leave the thymus. The medulla plays a role in negative selection. The antigen-presenting cells in this environment include dendritic cells that express co-stimulatory molecules, which are generally absent from the cortex. In addition, specialized medullary epithelial cells present peripheral antigens for the negative selection of T cells reactive for these self antigens.

8-17 T cells with αβ or γδ receptors arise from a common progenitor.

T cells bearing γδ receptors differ from αβ T cells in that they are found primarily in epithelial and mucosal sites and lack expression of the CD4 and CD8 co-receptors; in comparison with αβ T cells, relatively little is known about the ligands recognized by the γδ T-cell receptors, which are thought not to be MHC restricted (see Section 4-23). Recall from Section 5-10 that different genetic loci are used to make these two types of T-cell receptors. The γ and δ loci are

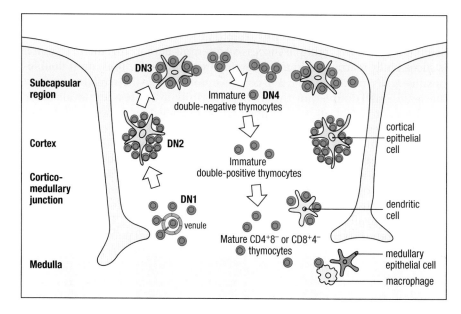

Fig. 8.20 Thymocytes at different developmental stages are found in distinct parts of the thymus. The earliest precursor thymocytes enter the thymus from the bloodstream via venules near the cortico-medullary junction. Ligands that interact with the receptor Notch are expressed in the thymus and act on the immigrant cells to commit them to the T-cell lineage. As these cells differentiate through the early CD4−CD8− double-negative (DN) stages described in the text, they migrate from the cortico-medullary junction to the outer cortex. DN3 cells reside near the subcapsular region, where they undergo proliferation. As the progenitor matures further to the CD4+CD8+ double-positive stage, it migrates back through the cortex. Finally, the medulla contains mature single-positive T cells, which eventually leave the thymus.

the first to undergo rearrangement, followed shortly thereafter by the β locus. In addition, the δ locus is contained within the α locus, so rearrangements at the α locus eliminate the δ coding sequences on the chromosome. While the mechanism regulating commitment of individual precursor cells to the αβ versus the γδ lineage is still not understood, there is some plasticity in this process. This can be deduced from the pattern of gene rearrangements found in thymocytes and in mature γδ and αβ T cells. Mature γδ T cells can contain rearranged β-chain genes, although 80% of these are nonproductive, and mature αβ T cells often contain rearranged, but mostly out-of-frame, γ-chain genes.

8-18   T cells expressing γδ T-cell receptors arise in two distinct phases during development.

Although γδ T cells arise from the same progenitors as αβ T cells, most mature γδ T cells are components of the innate rather than the adaptive immune system. When their maturation in the thymus is complete, the cells have acquired a defined effector function that can be rapidly elicited after their activation. After emigration from the thymus, most γδ T cells home to mucosal and epithelial sites in the body and take up stable residence in these locations.

In mice, the majority of γδ T cells in the body arise during embryonic development and the early neonatal period. In the fetal thymus, the first T cells to develop are γδ T cells that all express T-cell receptors assembled from the same V_γ and V_δ regions (**Fig 8.21**). These cells populate the epidermis; the T cells become wedged among the keratinocytes and adopt a dendritic-like form that has given them the name of **dendritic epidermal T cells (DETCs)** (Fig. 8.22). The DETCs provide surveillance of the skin and respond to infection and injury by producing cytokines and chemokines. These factors induce inflammation to enhance pathogen clearance, and they promote wound healing to repair lesions in the skin. In steady-state conditions, DETCs also produce growth factors that help maintain epidermal growth and survival.

After the development of DETC cells, a second subset of γδ T cells develops in the fetal thymus. These cells home to mucosal epithelia of tissues such as the reproductive tract and the lung, and also to the dermis of the skin. This subset is programmed to produce inflammatory cytokines such as IL-17 when stimulated and is thought to play a role in responses to infection and injury. Like the DETCs, these IL-17–producing γδ T ($T_{\gamma\delta}$-17) cells express T-cell receptors that are essentially invariant, being composed of a single V_γ–V_δ combination. However, the two subsets, DETCs and the fetal $T_{\gamma\delta}$-17 cells, express T-cell receptors that use distinct V_γ gene segments—$V_{\gamma 5}$ in the DETCs and $V_{\gamma 6}$ in the $T_{\gamma\delta}$-17 cells. As fetal thymocytes do not express the enzyme TdT, there are no N-nucleotides contributing additional diversity at the junctions between V, D, and J gene segments of the T-cell receptors in these two fetally derived subsets of γδ T cells. Why certain V, D, and J gene segments are selected for rearrangement at particular times during embryonic development remains incompletely understood.

DETCs and the $V_{\gamma 6}$-positive $T_{\gamma\delta}$-17 cells develop exclusively from the early wave of hematopoietic stem cells derived from the fetal liver (see Fig. 8.21). Consequently, these two γδ T-cell subsets arise only for a brief period of time in the fetal thymus, and then never again. A second phase of γδ T-cell development is initiated in the fetal thymus just before birth. This phase persists at a low level in the adult thymus throughout life and produces several subsets of cells, each with distinct effector functions and tissue-homing properties. Like the DETCs and fetal $T_{\gamma\delta}$-17 cells, these later-developing γδ T cells can be generally classified by their usage of distinct V_γ–V_δ regions in their T-cell receptors (see Fig. 8.21), although the receptor sequences within each population are more diverse because of the presence of N-region nucleotides added by TdT.

Fig. 8.21 The rearrangement of T-cell receptor γ and δ genes in the mouse proceeds in waves of cells expressing different Vγ and Vδ gene segments. At about 2 weeks of gestation in the mouse, the $C_{\gamma 1}$ locus is expressed with its closest V gene ($V_{\gamma 5}$). After a few days, $V_{\gamma 5}$-bearing cells decline in number in the thymus (first row of panels) and are replaced by cells expressing the next most proximal gene, $V_{\gamma 6}$. Both these rearranged γ chains are expressed with the same rearranged δ-chain gene, as shown in the lower panels, and there is little junctional diversity in either the V_{γ} or the V_{δ} chain. As a consequence, most of the γδ T cells produced in each of these early waves share the same specificity, although the antigen recognized in each case is not known. The $V_{\gamma 5}$-bearing cells become established selectively in the epidermis; they are programmed to secrete keratinocyte growth factor and inflammatory cytokines and chemokines. In contrast, $V_{\gamma 6}$-bearing cells become established in the lung, the dermis of the skin, and the epithelium of the reproductive tract and are programmed to secrete IL-17. The next wave of γδ development begins on day 17 of gestation and produces two different populations. One population rearranges and expresses the $V_{\gamma 4}$ chain, which pairs with heterogeneous delta chains. These $V_{\gamma 4}$-bearing cells are the second subset of $T_{\gamma \delta}$-17 (IL-17–secreting) cells and home to lymph nodes, spleen, lung, and the dermis of the skin. The second population in this wave expresses $V_{\gamma 1}$ and homes to lymph nodes, spleen, and liver. Some of these cells are paired with $V_{\delta 6}$ chains and are programmed to secrete IL-4 and IFN-γ, and represent γδ NKT cells. Finally, the last wave of γδ T-cell development begins late during fetal development and persists into adulthood. This last wave includes a heterogeneous population of cells bearing $V_{\gamma 1}$, $V_{\gamma 2}$, and $V_{\gamma 4}$ chains paired with many different delta chains. These cells home to lymphoid organs and are programmed to secrete IFN-γ. The other population in this last wave are cells bearing the $V_{\gamma 7}$ chain paired with heterogeneous delta chains. These γδ cells home to the intestinal epithelium and are programmed to secrete IFN-γ as well as antimicrobial compounds. Although γδ T cells continue to be produced after birth, at this stage the αβ T-cell lineage becomes the dominant population developing in the thymus.

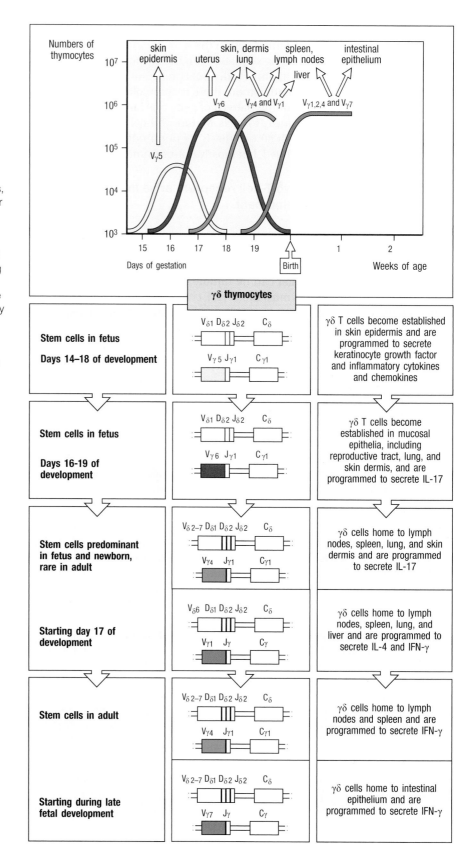

One population of these later-developing γδ T cells is programmed to secrete IL-17 when activated; these represent a second subset of $T_{\gamma\delta}$-17 cells that express a different V_{γ} region than do the fetal $T_{\gamma\delta}$-17 cells. Specifically, these later-developing $T_{\gamma\delta}$-17 cells express T-cell receptors using the $V_{\gamma4}$ region. This $T_{\gamma\delta}$-17 subset is found in all lymphoid organs, as well as in the skin dermis and the intestinal epithelium, where the cells provide rapid inflammatory signals in response to bacterial and parasitic infections. In addition, γδ T cells using the $V_{\gamma7}$ region in their T-cell receptors also develop in this second phase. The $V_{\gamma7}$-positive γδ T cells home specifically to the intestinal epithelium. In that location, the cells are poised to respond to gut microbes that breach the epithelial barrier and are important producers of antibacterial compounds as well as IFN-γ.

In contrast to the γδ T-cell subsets that reside in barrier tissues such as the skin and intestinal epithelium, γδ T cells are also found in lymphoid organs. The majority of the lymphoid-resident γδ T cells arise during the late fetal–early neonatal period as well as thereafter, and represent a more diverse population expressing the $V_{\gamma1}$ region. $V_{\gamma1}$-positive T cells are composed of two major groups—an IFN-γ– plus IL-4–producing subset that homes to the liver as well as several lymphoid organs, and an IFN-γ–producing subset that homes to all lymphoid organs. The former population of cells, which can be identified by their expression of a unique TCRδ chain ($V_{\delta6}$) that is paired to a $V_{\gamma1}$ chain, is remarkably similar to the αβ T-cell receptor–expressing subset of iNKT cells, and the cells are therefore often referred to as γδ NKT cells. Unlike the mucosal and epithelial resident γδ T-cell populations, whose importance in tissue homeostasis, repair, and innate defense against infections has been well established, the functions of γδ T cells within secondary lymphoid organs are still not well understood.

8-19 Successful synthesis of a rearranged β chain allows the production of a pre-T-cell receptor that triggers cell proliferation and blocks further β-chain gene rearrangement.

We now return to the development of αβ T cells. The rearrangement of the β- and α-chain loci closely parallels the rearrangement of immunoglobulin heavy-chain and light-chain loci during B-cell development (see Sections 8-3 through 8-6). As shown in **Fig. 8.23**, the β-chain gene segments rearrange first, with the D_{β} gene segments rearranging to J_{β} gene segments, and this is followed by V_{β} to DJ_{β} rearrangement. If no functional β chain can be synthesized from this rearrangement, the cell will not be able to produce a pre-T-cell receptor and will die. However, unlike B cells with nonproductive heavy-chain gene rearrangements, thymocytes with nonproductive β-chain VDJ rearrangements can be rescued by further rearrangement, which is possible because of the two clusters of D_{β} and J_{β} gene segments upstream of two C_{β} genes (see Fig. 5.14). The likelihood of a productive VDJ join at the β locus is therefore somewhat higher than the 55% chance for a productive immunoglobulin heavy-chain gene arrangement.

Once a productive β-chain gene rearrangement has occurred, the β chain is expressed together with the invariant pTα and the CD3 molecules (see Fig. 8.23) and is transported in this complex to the cell surface. The pTα:β complex is a functional pre-T-cell receptor analogous to the µ:VpreB:λ5 pre-B-cell receptor complex in B-cell development (see Section 8-4). Expression of the pre-T-cell receptor at the small pre-T cell (DN3) stage of thymocyte development induces signals that cause the phosphorylation and degradation of RAG-2, thus halting β-chain gene rearrangement and ensuring allelic exclusion at the β locus. These signals also induce the large pre-T cell (DN4) stage, in which rapid cell proliferation occurs, and eventually the co-receptor proteins CD4 and CD8 are expressed. The pre-T-cell receptor signals constitutively via the

Fig. 8.22 Dendritic epidermal T cells reside within the epithelial layer, forming an interdigitating network with Langerhans cells. This face-on view of a murine epidermal sheet shows Langerhans cells (green) and dendritic epidermal T cells (DETCs; red) forming an interdigitating network within the layers of the epidermis. The epidermal epithelial cells are not visible in this fluorescence image. The branching dendritic-like form of these γδ T cells is the source of their name. Although the ligands for all γδ T-cell receptors are not known, some γδ T cells recognize nonclassical MHC molecules (see Sections 6-16, 6-17, and 6-20), which can be induced in epithelia by stresses such as UV damage or pathogens. Thus, DETCs may serve as sentinels of such damage, producing cytokines that activate the innate immune response and, in turn, adaptive immunity.

Fig. 8.23 The stages of gene rearrangement in αβ T cells. The sequence of gene rearrangements is shown, together with an indication of the stage at which the events take place and the nature of the cell-surface receptor molecules expressed at each stage. The β-chain locus rearranges first, in CD4⁻CD8⁻ double-negative thymocytes expressing CD25 and low levels of CD44. As with immunoglobulin heavy-chain genes, D to J gene segments rearrange before V gene segments rearrange to DJ (second and third panels). It is possible to make up to four attempts to generate a productive rearrangement at the β-chain locus, because there are four D gene segments with two sets of J gene segments associated with each TCRβ-chain locus (not shown). The productively rearranged gene is expressed initially within the cell and then at low levels on the cell surface. It associates with pTα, a surrogate 33-kDa α chain that is equivalent to λ5 in B-cell development, and this pTα:β heterodimer forms a complex with the CD3 chains (fourth panel). The expression of the pre-T-cell receptor signals the developing thymocytes to halt b-chain gene rearrangement and to undergo multiple cycles of division. At the end of this proliferative burst, the CD4 and CD8 molecules are expressed, the cell ceases cycling, and the α chain is now able to undergo rearrangement. The first α-chain gene rearrangement deletes all δ D, J, and C gene segments on the chromosome, although these are retained as a circular DNA, indicating that these are nondividing cells (bottom panel). This permanently inactivates the δ-chain gene. Rearrangements at the α-chain locus can proceed through several cycles, because of the large number of Vα and Jα gene segments, so that productive rearrangements almost always occur. When a functional α chain is produced that pairs efficiently with the b chain, the CD3lowCD4⁺CD8⁺ thymocyte is ready to undergo selection for its ability to recognize self peptides in association with self MHC molecules.

cytoplasmic protein kinase Lck, an Src family tyrosine kinase (see Fig. 7.12), but seems not to require a ligand on the thymic epithelium. Lck subsequently associates with the co-receptor proteins. In mice genetically deficient in Lck, T-cell development is arrested before the CD4⁺CD8⁺ double-positive stage, and no α-chain gene rearrangements can be made.

The role of the expressed β chain in suppressing further β-locus rearrangement can be demonstrated in mice containing a rearranged TCRβ transgene: these mice express the transgenic β chain on virtually 100% of their T cells, and rearrangement of their endogenous β-chain genes is strongly suppressed. The importance of pTα has been shown in mice deficient in pTα, in which there is a hundredfold decrease in αβ T cells and an absence of allelic exclusion at the β locus.

During the proliferation of large pre-T cells triggered by expression of the pre-T-cell receptor, the RAG1 and RAG2 genes are repressed (see Fig. 8.19). Hence, no rearrangement of the α-chain locus occurs until the proliferative phase ends, at which time *RAG1* and *RAG2* are transcribed again, and the functional RAG-1:RAG-2 complex accumulates. This ensures that each cell in which a β-chain gene has been successfully rearranged gives rise to many CD4$^+$CD8$^+$ thymocytes. Once the cells stop dividing, each of them can independently rearrange its α-chain genes, so that a single functional β chain can be associated with many different α chains in the progeny cells. During the period of α-chain gene rearrangement, αβ T-cell receptors are first expressed, and selection by self peptide:self MHC complexes on the thymus cells can begin.

The progression of thymocytes from the double-negative to the double-positive and finally to the single-positive stage is accompanied by a distinct pattern of expression of proteins involved in DNA rearrangement, signaling, and T cell–specific gene expression (see Fig. 8.19). Postnatal thymocytes continually express TdT, the enzyme responsible for the insertion of N-nucleotides, and consequently, N-nucleotides are found at the junctions of all rearranged α and β genes. T-cell receptor signaling proteins, such as the tyrosine kinases Lck and ZAP-70, are expressed from an early stage in thymocyte development. Lck is important in signaling from the pre-T-cell receptor, thereby playing a role in αβ T-cell development; Lck is also important for γδ T-cell development. In contrast, gene knockout studies (see Appendix I, Section A-36) show that ZAP-70, although expressed from the double-negative stage onward, is not essential for pre-T-cell receptor signaling, as double-negative thymocytes also express the related Syk kinase, which is capable of fulfilling this role. ZAP-70 is required later, to promote the development of single-positive thymocytes from double-positive thymocytes, as Syk is no longer expressed at this stage. Fyn, a Src family kinase similar to Lck, is expressed at increasing levels from the double-positive stage onward. It is not essential for the development of αβ thymocytes as long as Lck is present but is required for the development of iNKT cells (see Section 8-27).

8-20   T-cell α-chain genes undergo successive rearrangements until positive selection or cell death intervenes.

The T-cell receptor α-chain genes are comparable to the immunoglobulin κ and λ light-chain genes in that they do not have D gene segments and are rearranged only after their partner receptor chain has been expressed. As with the light-chain genes, repeated attempts at α-chain gene rearrangement are possible, as illustrated in **Fig. 8.24**. The presence of multiple V$_α$ gene segments, and about 60 J$_α$ gene segments spread over some 80 kilobases of DNA, allows many successive V$_α$ to J$_α$ rearrangements to take place at both α-chain alleles. This means T cells with an initial nonproductive α-gene rearrangement are much more likely to be rescued by a subsequent rearrangement than are B cells with a nonproductive light-chain gene rearrangement.

One key difference between B and T cells is that the final assembly of an immunoglobulin leads to the cessation of gene rearrangement and initiates the further differentiation of the B cell, whereas rearrangement of the V$_α$ gene segments continues in T cells unless there is signaling by a self peptide:self MHC complex that positively selects the receptor (see Section 8-22). This means many T cells have in-frame rearrangements on both chromosomes and so can produce two types of α chains. This is possible because expression of the T-cell receptor is not in itself sufficient to shut off gene rearrangement.

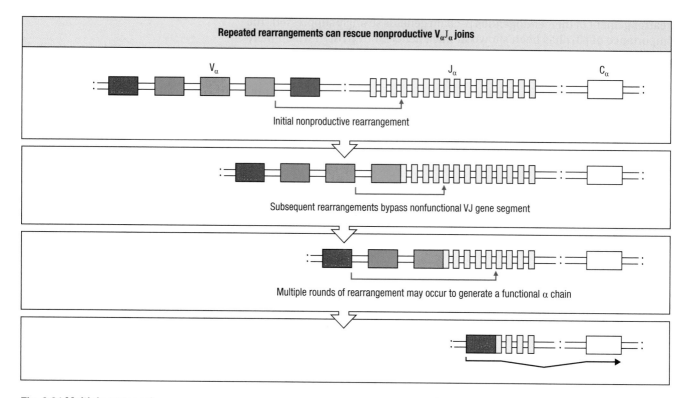

Repeated rearrangements can rescue nonproductive V$_\alpha$J$_\alpha$ joins

Initial nonproductive rearrangement

Subsequent rearrangements bypass nonfunctional VJ gene segment

Multiple rounds of rearrangement may occur to generate a functional α chain

Fig. 8.24 Multiple successive rearrangement events can rescue nonproductive T-cell receptor α-chain gene rearrangements. The multiplicity of V and J gene segments at the α-chain locus allows successive rearrangement events to 'leapfrog' over previously rearranged VJ segments, deleting any intervening gene segments. The α-chain rescue pathway resembles that of the immunoglobulin κ light-chain genes (see Section 8-6), but the number of possible successive rearrangements is greater. α-chain gene rearrangement continues until either a productive rearrangement leads to positive selection or the cell dies.

Continued rearrangements on both chromosomes can allow several different α chains to be produced successively as well as simultaneously in each developing T cell and to be tested for self peptide:self MHC recognition in partnership with the same β chain. This phase of gene rearrangement lasts for 3 or 4 days in the mouse and ceases only when positive selection occurs as a consequence of receptor engagement or when the cell dies. One can predict that if the frequency of positive selection is sufficiently low, roughly one in three mature T cells will express two productively rearranged α chains at the cell surface. This has been confirmed for both human and mouse T cells. Thus, in the strict sense, T-cell receptor α-chain genes are not subject to allelic exclusion.

T cells with dual specificity might be expected to give rise to inappropriate immune responses if the cell is activated through one receptor yet can act upon target cells recognized by the second receptor. However, only one of the two receptors is likely to be able to recognize peptide presented by a self MHC molecule expressed in that individual, and so each T cell will still have only a single T-cell receptor that can function in antigen recognition. This is because once a thymocyte has been positively selected by self peptide:self MHC recognition, α-chain gene rearrangement ceases. Thus, the existence of cells with two α-chain genes productively rearranged and two α chains expressed at the cell surface does not truly challenge the idea that a single functional specificity is expressed by each cell.

Summary.

The thymus provides a specialized and architecturally organized microenvironment for the development of mature T cells. Precursors of T cells migrate from the bone marrow to the thymus, where they interact with environmental cues, such as ligands for the Notch receptor, that drive commitment to the T lineage. Developing thymocytes develop along one of several T-cell lineages: the most prominent subsets in the thymus are γδ T cells, conventional αβ T cells, and αβ T cells with receptors of very limited diversity, such as iNKT cells.

T-cell progenitors develop along the γδ or the αβ T-cell lineages. Early in ontogeny, the production of γδ T cells predominates over production of αβ T cells, and these cells populate several peripheral tissues, including the skin, the intestine, and other mucosal and epithelial surfaces. These subsets predominantly develop from fetal liver (rather than bone marrow) stem cells. Later, more than 90% of thymocytes express αβ T-cell receptors. In developing thymocytes, the γ, δ, and β genes are the first to rearrange. Cells of the αβ lineage that rearrange a functional β chain form a pre-T-cell receptor that signals thymocyte proliferation, α-chain gene rearrangement, and CD4 and CD8 expression. Most steps in T-cell development take place in the thymic cortex, whereas the medulla contains mainly mature T cells.

Positive and negative selection of T cells.

Up to the stage at which an αβ receptor is produced, T-cell development is independent of MHC proteins or antigen. From this point onward, developmental decisions in the αβ T-cell lineage depend on the interaction of the receptor with peptide:MHC ligands it encounters in the thymus. Here we consider this phase of T-cell development.

8-21 Overview of positive and negative selection of αβ lineage T cells.

T-cell precursors committed to the αβ lineage at the pre-T (DN3) stage undergo vigorous proliferation in the subcapsular region and progress to the large pre-T (DN4) transitional stage. These cells then rapidly transit through an immature CD4 or CD8 single-positive stage and become double-positive cells that express low levels of the T-cell receptor and both the CD4 and CD8 co-receptors as they move deeper into the thymic cortex. These double-positive cells have a life span of only about 3–4 days unless they are rescued by engagement of their T-cell receptor. The rescue of double-positive cells from programmed cell death and their maturation into CD4 or CD8 single-positive cells is the process known as positive selection. Only about 10–30% of the T-cell receptors generated by gene rearrangement will be able to recognize self peptide:self MHC complexes and thus function in self MHC–restricted responses to foreign antigens (see Chapter 4); those that have this capability are initially selected for survival in the thymus.

After this initial selection, thymocytes undergo additional selection events on the basis of their T-cell receptor recognition properties (**Fig. 8.25**). Some very strongly self-reactive thymocytes undergo negative selection as double-positive cells while still in the thymic cortex; these cells die by

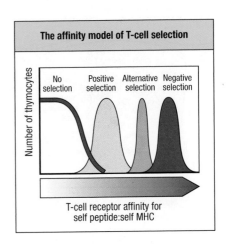

Fig. 8.25 The affinity model of T-cell positive and negative selection. Random TCRα- and TCRβ-chain gene rearrangements generate a large pool of immature thymocytes expressing a varied repertoire of specificities. The T-cell receptors on many of these cells fail to have sufficient binding strength to the self peptide:self MHC complexes on thymic epithelium and so receive no signals. These cells, labeled 'No selection,' die by neglect. Another fraction of immature thymocytes is positively selected because their T-cell receptors bind with sufficient strength to the self peptide:self MHC complexes on thymic epithelium to generate T-cell receptor–dependent survival signals ('Positive selection'). From this cohort of positively selected thymocytes, negative selection removes those thymocytes whose receptors have excessively strong reactivity to self peptides complexed with self MHC molecules (resulting in clonal deletion), thereby establishing self-tolerance of the mature T-cell population ('Negative selection'). A small subset of positively selected cells receiving signals slightly weaker than those inducing negative selection is induced into alternative lineages, such as regulatory T cells (T_reg cells), NK-T cells, intraepithelial lymphocytes (IELs) or MAIT cell subsets ('Alternative selection'). Maturation of thymocytes into these alternative lineages often involves specific cytokine signals or recognition of MHC class Ib molecules.

apoptosis. The remaining surviving thymocytes begin their maturation into CD4 or CD8 single-positive cells and move into the thymic medulla. The unique environment of the thymic medulla includes a variety of cell types that interact with maturing thymocytes. If the maturing thymocyte has strong reactivity to a self antigen found in the medulla, negative selection will occur. Cells with weaker levels of self-reactivity can be induced to differentiate into alternative T-cell lineages. One alternative lineage is regulatory T cells, a population of T cells (primarily CD4 T cells) that is important in preventing onset of autoimmune disease (see Chapter 15). Additional subsets of T cells whose T-cell receptors recognize MHC class Ib molecules (see Chapter 6) are also selected in the thymic medulla after recognition of their self MHC molecules. These less abundant alternative T-cell lineages include invariant NKT (iNKT) cells and mucosal-associated invariant T (MAIT) cells, which recognize CD1d and MR-1 MHC class Ib molecules, respectively.

8-22 Only thymocytes whose receptors interact with self peptide:self MHC complexes can survive and mature.

Early experiments using bone marrow chimeras (see Appendix I, Section A-33) and thymic grafting provided evidence that MHC molecules in the thymus influence the MHC-restricted T-cell repertoire. However, mice transgenic for rearranged T-cell receptor genes provided the first conclusive evidence that the interaction of the T cell with self peptide:self MHC complexes is necessary for the survival of immature T cells and their maturation into naive CD4 or CD8 T cells. For these experiments, the rearranged α- and β-chain genes were cloned from a T-cell clone (see Appendix I, Section A-21) whose origin, antigen specificity, and MHC restriction were known. When such genes are introduced into the mouse genome, they are expressed early during thymocyte development. As a consequence of expressing functional transgene-encoded TCRα- and TCRβ-chain proteins in developing T cells, the rearrangement of endogenous T-cell receptor genes is inhibited, albeit to different degrees. In general, endogenous β-chain gene rearrangement is inhibited completely, but that of α-chain genes is inhibited only incompletely, because the mechanism for terminating α-chain rearrangements requires T-cell receptor signaling as well as the expression of an α-chain protein (see Section 8-20). The result is that most of the developing thymocytes in TCR transgenic mouse lines express the T-cell receptor encoded by the transgenes. Studies using T-cell receptor αβ transgenic mice showed that thymocytes bearing a particular T-cell receptor could develop to the double-positive stage independently of the MHC class I or class II proteins expressed in that thymus. In contrast, the transgenic thymocytes developed into mature CD4 or CD8 single-positive thymocytes only if the thymus expressed the same self MHC molecule as that on which the original T-cell

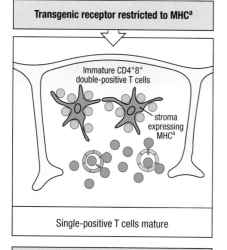

Transgenic receptor restricted to MHCᵃ

Immature CD4⁺8⁺ double-positive T cells

stroma expressing MHCᵃ

Single-positive T cells mature

Transgenic receptor restricted to MHCᵃ

Immature CD4⁺8⁺ double-positive T cells

stroma expressing MHCᵇ

No single-positive T cells mature

Fig. 8.26 Positive selection is demonstrated by the development of T cells expressing rearranged T-cell receptor transgenes. In mice transgenic for rearranged αβ T-cell receptor genes, the maturation of T cells depends on the MHC allele expressed in the thymus. If the transgenic mice express the same MHC allele in their thymic stromal cells as that of the mouse from which the rearranged TCRα-chain and TCRβ-chain genes originally developed (both MHCᵃ; top panel), then the T cells expressing the transgenic T-cell receptor will develop from the double-positive stage (pale green) into mature single-positive T cells (dark green). If the MHCᵃ-restricted TCR transgenes are genetically crossed into a different MHC background (MHCᵇ; yellow, bottom panel), then developing T cells expressing the transgenic receptor will progress to the double-positive stage but will fail to mature further. This failure is due to the absence of an interaction between the transgenic T-cell receptor and MHC molecules on the thymic cortex, and thus no signal for positive selection is delivered, leading to apoptotic death by neglect.

clone was selected (**Fig. 8.26**). Additional experimental strategies have confirmed that thymocytes require TCR interactions with self peptide:self MHC for positive selection. One striking example is the finding that mice lacking all MHC class I and class II expression show a complete arrest of thymocyte maturation at the CD4⁺CD8⁺ stage.

8-23 Positive selection coordinates the expression of CD4 or CD8 with the specificity of the T-cell receptor and the potential effector functions of the T cell.

At the time of positive selection, the thymocyte expresses both CD4 and CD8 co-receptor molecules. By the end of thymic selection, mature αβ T cells ready for export to the periphery have stopped expressing one of these co-receptors. The majority of these cells belong to the conventional CD4 or CD8 T-cell lineages. Less abundant subsets, such as iNKT cells (discussed further in Section 8-27) and a subset of regulatory T cells expressing CD4 and high levels of CD25 (the IL-2 receptor α chain), also develop in the thymus from CD4⁺CD8⁺ cells. Moreover, almost all mature T cells that express CD4 have receptors that recognize peptides bound to self MHC class II molecules and are programmed to become cytokine-secreting helper T cells. In contrast, most of the cells that express CD8 have receptors that recognize peptides bound to self MHC class I molecules and are programmed to become cytotoxic effector cells. Thus, positive selection also determines the cell-surface phenotype and functional potential of the mature T cell, selecting the appropriate co-receptor for efficient antigen recognition and the appropriate program for the T cell's eventual functional differentiation in an immune response.

The importance of MHC molecules in this selection is illustrated by the human immunodeficiency diseases caused by mutations that lead to an absence of MHC molecules on lymphocytes and thymic epithelial cells. People who lack MHC class II molecules have CD8 T cells, but only a few, highly abnormal CD4 T cells; a similar result has been obtained in mice in which MHC class II expression has been eliminated by targeted gene disruption (**Fig. 8.27**) (see Appendix I, Section A-36). Likewise, mice and humans that lack MHC class I molecules have few CD8 T cells. Thus, MHC class II molecules are predominantly required for CD4 T-cell development, whereas MHC class I molecules are predominantly required for CD8 T-cell development.

In mature T cells, the co-receptor functions of CD8 and CD4 depend on their respective abilities to bind invariant sites on MHC class I and MHC class II

Fig. 8.27 Thymic cortical epithelial cells mediate positive selection. In the thymus of normal mice (first panels), which express MHC class II molecules on epithelial cells in the thymic cortex (blue) as well as on medullary epithelial cells (orange) and bone marrow–derived cells (yellow), both CD4 (blue) and CD8 (red) T cells mature. Double-positive thymocytes are shown as half red and half blue. The second panels represent mutant mice in which MHC class II expression has been eliminated by targeted gene disruption; in these mice, few CD4 T cells develop, although CD8 T cells develop normally. In MHC class II–negative mice containing an MHC class II transgene engineered so that it is expressed only on the epithelial cells of the thymic cortex (third panels), normal numbers of CD4 T cells mature. In contrast, if a mutant MHC class II molecule with a defective CD4-binding site is expressed (fourth panel), positive selection of CD4 T cells does not take place. This indicates that the cortical epithelial cells are the critical cell type mediating positive selection and that the MHC class II molecule needs to be able to interact with the CD4 protein.

Normal MHC class II expression	MHC class II–negative mutant	Mutant with MHC class II transgene expressed in cortical thymic epithelium	Mutant with MHC class II transgene expressed that cannot interact with CD4
Both CD8 and CD4 T cells mature	CD8 T cells mature	Both CD8 and CD4 T cells mature	CD8 T cells mature

Fig. 8.28 Positive-selection signaling requires cooperation between the T-cell receptor and the CD4 or CD8 co-receptor. In double-positive thymocytes with T-cell receptors recognizing peptide:MHC class II complexes, the CD4 co-receptor recruits the Lck tyrosine kinase to the receptor to initiate signaling, leading to the maturation of CD4+ T cells (left panel). In contrast, double-positive thymocytes with T-cell receptors recognizing peptide:MHC class I complexes have cooperative recognition of peptide:MHC by the T-cell receptor plus the CD8 co-receptor. This also recruits Lck to the receptor to initiate signaling, leading to the maturation of CD8+ T cells (right panel). This cooperation between the T-cell receptor and the co-receptor is required for efficient positive selection of double-positive thymocytes.

MHC Class II Deficiency

MHC Class I Deficiency

Fig. 8.29 The MHC molecules that induce positive selection determine CD4 versus CD8 lineage development and transcriptional programming. Double-positive thymocytes with T-cell receptors recognizing peptide:MHC class II complexes receive strong and persistent signaling, leading to the up-regulation of the transcription factor ThPOK. ThPOK induces the maturation of CD4+ T cells and promotes the expression of 'helper' T-cell genes (left panel). In contrast, double-positive thymocytes with T-cell receptors recognizing peptide:MHC class I complexes receive curtailed signaling. This weaker signaling together with cytokines induces the expression of the transcription factor Runx3 and the maturation of CD8+ T cells. Runx3 promotes the expression of 'cytotoxic' T-cell genes (right panel). This mechanism ensures that mature CD4+ and CD8+ T cells acquire the functional properties of cytokine production and target-cell killing, respectively, that match their T-cell receptor specificity for peptides bound to MHC class II versus MHC class I molecules.

molecules (see Section 4-21). Co-receptor binding to an MHC molecule is also required for normal positive selection. In thymocytes, nearly all of the Lck is associated with CD4 and CD8 co-receptors, providing a mechanism to ensure that signaling is initiated only in thymocytes bearing T-cell receptors that bind to MHC molecules. Thus, positive selection depends on engagement of both the antigen receptor and co-receptor by an MHC molecule, and this signal determines the survival of single-positive cells that express the appropriate co-receptor (**Fig. 8.28**).

T-cell receptor signaling regulates this choice of the CD4 versus the CD8 lineage by controlling the expression of two transcription factors, ThPOK and Runx3 (**Fig. 8.29**). The role of ThPOK was identified through a naturally occurring loss-of-function mutation in mice that lacked CD4 T-cell development. In mice lacking ThPOK, MHC class II–restricted thymocytes are redirected toward the CD8 lineage. ThPOK is up-regulated in preselection

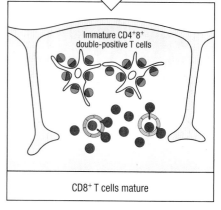

double-positive thymocytes by strong and persistent T-cell receptor signaling, where it reinforces its own expression and represses expression of Runx3; together, the expression of ThPOK and absence of Runx3 lead to CD4 commitment and the ability to express cytokine genes typical of CD4 cells. If T-cell signaling is of insufficient strength or duration, however, ThPOK is not induced; instead, this T-cell receptor signal, together with intrathymic cytokines, induces Runx3 up-regulation. Runx3 functions to silence CD4 expression, maintain CD8 expression, and promote the expression of genes typical of CD8 T cells; namely, genes that encode proteins involved in target-cell killing.

While the majority of double-positive thymocytes that undergo positive selection develop into either CD4 or CD8 single-positive T cells, the thymus also generates less numerous populations of other T-cell subsets with specialized functions; these will be discussed further in Section 8-27.

8-24   Thymic cortical epithelial cells mediate positive selection of developing thymocytes.

Thymus transplantation studies indicate that stromal cells are important for positive selection. These cells form a web of cell processes that make close contacts with the double-positive T cells undergoing positive selection. Direct evidence that thymic cortical epithelial cells mediate positive selection comes from an ingenious manipulation of mice whose MHC class II genes have been eliminated by targeted gene disruption (see Fig. 8.27). Mutant mice that lack MHC class II molecules do not normally produce CD4 T cells. To test the role of the thymic epithelium in positive selection, an MHC class II gene was placed under the control of a promoter that restricted the gene's expression to thymic cortical epithelial cells. This was then introduced as a transgene into the MHC class II–mutant mice, and CD4 T-cell development was restored. A variant of this experiment showed that, to promote the development of CD4 T cells, the MHC class II molecule on the thymic cortical epithelium must be able to interact effectively with CD4. Thus, when the MHC class II transgene expressed in the thymus contains a mutation that prevents binding of the MHC to CD4, very few CD4 T cells develop. Equivalent studies of CD8 interaction with MHC class I molecules showed that co-receptor binding is also necessary for the positive selection of CD8 cells.

The critical role of the thymic cortical epithelium in positive selection raises the question whether there is anything distinctive about the antigen-presenting properties of these cells. The thymic stromal cells may simply be in closest proximity to the developing thymocytes, as there are very few macrophages and dendritic cells in the cortex to perform the antigen presentation. In addition, however, thymic epithelium differs from other tissues in the expression of key proteases that are involved in MHC class I and class II antigen processing (see Chapter 6). Cortical epithelial cells express cathepsin L as opposed to the more widely expressed cathepsin S, and mice deficient in cathepsin L have severely impaired CD4 T-cell development. Thymic epithelial cells from mice lacking cathepsin L exhibit a relatively high proportion of MHC class II molecules on their surface that retain the class II–associated invariant chain peptide (CLIP) (see Fig. 6.11). Cortical epithelial cells also express a unique proteasome subunit, β5T, whereas other cells express β5 or β5i. Mice deficient in β5T have severely impaired CD8 T-cell development. Because mice that lack either cathepsin L or β5T still have normal levels of MHC on the surface of their thymic cortical cells, it would seem that it is the peptide repertoire displayed by the MHC molecules on cortical epithelial cells that is responsible for altering T-cell development, although the mechanism is still unclear.

8-25   T cells that react strongly with self antigens are deleted in the thymus.

When the T-cell receptor of a mature naive T cell is strongly ligated by a peptide:MHC complex displayed on a specialized antigen-presenting cell in a peripheral lymphoid organ, the T cell is activated to proliferate and produce effector T cells. In contrast, when the T-cell receptor of a developing thymocyte is similarly ligated by a self peptide:self MHC complex in the thymus, it dies by apoptosis. The response of immature T cells to stimulation by antigen is the basis of negative selection. Elimination of immature T cells in the thymus prevents their potentially harmful activation later, should they encounter the same self peptide:self MHC complexes when they are mature T cells.

Negative selection has been demonstrated using TCR-transgenic mice expressing T-cell receptors specific for self peptides derived from proteins encoded on the Y chromosome, and thus expressed only in male mice. Thymocytes bearing these receptors disappear from the developing T-cell population in male mice at the double-positive stage of development, and no single-positive cells bearing the transgenic receptors mature. By contrast, in female mice, which lack the male-specific peptide, T cells bearing the transgenic receptors mature normally. Negative selection to male-specific peptides has also been demonstrated in nontransgenic mice and also occurs by deletion of T cells.

TCR-transgenic mice were very useful for the classic experiments above, but they express a functional T-cell receptor earlier during development than normal mice and have a very high frequency of cells reactive to any particular peptide. A more realistic system for evaluating negative selection involves the transgenic expression of only the β chain of a T-cell receptor reactive to a given peptide antigen. In such mice, the β chain pairs with endogenous α chains, yet the frequency of peptide-reactive T cells is sufficient for detection using peptide:MHC tetramers (see Appendix I, Section A-24). These and other more physiologic approaches showed that clonal deletion can occur at either the double-positive or the single-positive stage, presumably depending on where the T cell encounters the antigen that causes deletion. Thus, negative selection of developing T cells can take place in the thymic cortex to self antigens presented on bone marrow–derived antigen-presenting cells, as well as in the thymic medulla, as discussed below.

The experiments outlined above illustrate the principle that self peptide:self MHC complexes encountered in the thymus purge the mature T-cell repertoire of cells bearing self-reactive receptors. One obvious problem with this scheme is that many tissue-specific proteins, such as pancreatic insulin, would not be expected to be expressed in the thymus. However, it is now clear that many such 'tissue-specific' proteins are expressed by certain stromal cells in the thymic medulla, providing a mechanism for intrathymic negative selection to proteins that are otherwise restricted to tissues outside the thymus. Another important function of the intrathymic expression of tissue-specific proteins is to promote the development of CD4 regulatory T cells, a subset of self-reactive T cells (see Fig. 8.26) with an important role in maintaining self-tolerance (discussed further in Section 8-27 and Chapter 15). The expression of some, but not all, tissue-specific proteins in the thymic medulla is controlled by a gene called **_AIRE_ (autoimmune regulator)**. AIRE is expressed in medullary stromal cells (**Fig. 8.30**), interacts with many proteins involved in transcription, and seems to lengthen transcripts that would otherwise terminate earlier. Mutations in _AIRE_ give rise to the human autoimmune disease known as **autoimmune polyendocrinopathy–candidiasis–ectodermal dystrophy (APECED) or autoimmune polyglandular syndrome type I**, highlighting the important role of intrathymic expression of tissue-specific proteins in maintaining tolerance to self. Together, negative selection and the development of self-reactive regulatory T cells provide two major mechanisms of

AIRE expression in the thymus

Fig. 8.30 AIRE is expressed in the medulla of the thymus and promotes the expression of proteins normally expressed in peripheral tissues. Expression of AIRE by thymic medullary cells is limited to the medullary region of the thymus, where it is expressed in a subset of epithelial-like cells. The expression of the thymic medullary epithelial marker MTS10 is shown in red. AIRE expression is shown in green by immunofluorescence and is present in only a fraction of the medullary epithelial cells.

self-tolerance. There are, however, additional mechanisms operating in the periphery that can prevent mature T cells from responding to tissue-specific self antigens; these are discussed in Chapter 15, when we consider the problem of autoimmune responses and their avoidance.

As negative selection occurs throughout thymocyte development, both in the thymic cortex and in the medulla, it is likely to be mediated by antigen presentation by several different cell types. Bone marrow–derived dendritic cells present self antigens expressed by the cells or acquired by uptake from their environment or by handoff from medullary epithelial cells. In addition, medullary epithelial cells expressing AIRE, and thus presenting a wide range of self antigens, can directly induce thymocyte negative selection.

Autoimmune Polyendocrinopathy–Candidiasis–Ectodermal Dystrophy (APECED)

8-26 The specificity and/or the strength of signals for negative and positive selection must differ.

T cells undergo both positive selection for self MHC restriction and negative selection for self-tolerance by interacting with self peptide:self MHC complexes expressed on stromal cells in the thymus. An unresolved issue is how the interaction of the T-cell receptor with self peptide:self MHC complexes distinguishes between these opposite outcomes. First, more receptor specificities must be positively selected than are negatively selected. Otherwise, all the cells that were positively selected in the thymic cortex would be eliminated by negative selection, and no T cells would ever be produced. Second, the consequences of the interactions that lead to positive and negative selection must differ: cells that recognize self peptide:self MHC complexes on cortical epithelial cells are induced to mature, whereas those whose receptors might confer strong and potentially damaging autoreactivity are induced to die.

Currently, the choice between positive and negative selection is thought to hinge on the strength of self peptide:self MHC binding by the T-cell receptor, an idea known as the **affinity hypothesis** (see Fig. 8.26). Low-affinity interactions rescue the cell from death by neglect, leading to positive selection; high-affinity interactions induce apoptosis and thus negative selection. Because more complexes are likely to bind weakly than strongly, this model explains the positive selection of a larger repertoire of cells than are negatively selected. How this quantitative difference in receptor affinity translates into a qualitatively distinct cell fate is still an area of active investigation. Many of the biochemical signals induced by low-affinity interactions are weaker or of shorter duration than those from high-affinity interactions. However, low-affinity interactions lead to sustained activation of the protein kinase Erk, whereas high-affinity interactions lead to only transient activation of Erk, suggesting that differential activation of this or other MAPKs might determine the outcome of thymic selection. Indeed, experiments showed that developing T cells need to engage low-affinity ligands for more than 24 hours for positive selection to occur.

8-27 αβ T cells diverge into multiple lineages at the CD4+ and CD8+ single-positive stage in the thymic medulla.

Positive and negative selection of conventional CD4+ and CD8+ αβ T cells are not the only processes that occur during the late stages of thymocyte maturation. Once CD4+ and CD8+ single-positive cells arise and migrate into the thymic medulla, additional T-cell receptor and cytokine signals can divert thymocytes into one of several alternative cell lineages (see Fig. 8.26). As discussed earlier (see Section 8-25), thymocytes with strong reactivity to self-peptide:MHC complexes on medullary dendritic cells or AIRE-expressing epithelial cells can undergo negative selection; the remaining CD4+ and CD8+ single-positive thymocytes continue their maturation into conventional CD4

Fig. 8.31 The selection of CD4⁺ T_reg cells in the thymic medulla requires moderately high affinity for self peptide:self MHC. Thymocytes from mice expressing a fluorescent reporter that monitors T-cell receptor signal strength were analyzed by flow cytometry. CD4⁺ T_reg cells, identified by their expression of the transcription factor FoxP3 (not shown), were compared with conventional CD4⁺ single-positive thymocytes. The increased fluorescence seen in the T_reg subset indicates that these cells are receiving stronger T-cell receptor stimulation in the thymus than that received by the conventional CD4⁺ cells undergoing maturation. For comparison, the fluorescent signal from thymocytes that do not carry the fluorescent reporter gene are shown ('Reporter-negative').

and CD8 T cells, T_reg cells, iNKT cells (see Section 6-18), or CD8⁺ intraepithelial lymphocytes (IELs). Additional lineages of T cells also develop at this stage, but as these are not as well understood, they will not be discussed further.

One important subset that develops in the thymic medulla is the thymically derived T_reg cell subset, a population of CD4⁺ T cells that function to maintain self-tolerance. T_reg cells develop from CD4⁺ single-positive thymocytes whose T-cell receptors have moderately high affinity for self peptide:self MHC complexes (see Fig. 8.26), as indicated by studies using mice expressing a fluorescent reporter that monitors T-cell receptor signal strength. Examination of thymocytes from these mice showed that T_reg cells express high levels of the fluorescent reporter, indicating that they likely express T-cell receptors with high affinity for self (**Fig. 8.31**). During their maturation, T_reg cells up-regulate the transcription factor FoxP3 and express high levels of CD25, the IL-2 receptor α chain. Furthermore, T_reg cell development depends on IL-2 receptor signaling, a cytokine signal that is not required for the development of conventional T cells.

A second specialized subset of T cells that develops in the thymic medulla is a lineage known as **invariant NKT cells (iNKT cells)** based on their use of a restricted T-cell receptor repertoire and their expression of the NK1.1 receptor commonly found on NK cells. iNKT cells are activated as part of the early response to many infections; they differ from the major lineage of αβ T cells in recognizing CD1 molecules rather than MHC class I or MHC class II molecules (see Section 6-18). Unlike other T cells, iNKT cells require for their development a T-cell receptor interaction with CD1 molecules expressed on thymocytes and a signal through the adaptor protein SAP. iNKT cells, like γδ T cells, acquire a defined effector program during their development in the thymus. Therefore, these cells exhibit a memory-cell phenotype when they leave the thymus and migrate to peripheral lymphoid tissues and mucosal surfaces. iNKT cells have been suggested to develop in response to 'agonist' signaling. Recent studies have revealed that CD1-binding lipid antigens produced by the commensal microbes in the gut are an important source of these agonist ligands, and that the composition of the gut microbiome regulates the development of iNKT cells early in life. Because agonist stimulation of immature T cells is also known to cause clonal deletion, it is not yet clear which activating interactions lead to clonal deletion in the thymus and which lead to selection of T_reg cells or the nonconventional iNKT cells.

A third important subset of specialized αβ T-cell receptor–expressing T cells are CD8⁺ intraepithelial lymphocytes (IELs). Unlike conventional CD8⁺ T cells, IELs express a homodimer of the CD8α chain, rather than the CD8αβ heterodimer found on conventional T cells. Mature CD8αα IELs are found in the intestinal epithelium, interdigitated between epithelial cells. Although these cells appear capable of self-renewal in the intestinal tissue, current evidence indicates that they develop from thymic progenitor cells, which then migrate to the intestine and become resident IELs. In the intestinal tissue, these cells function to protect the mucosal barrier against infection or injury caused by gut microbes, especially at the time of gut colonization immediately after birth. Like thymically derived T_reg cells and iNKT cells, T-cell receptor αβ IELs require strong T-cell receptor signaling for their development.

8-28 Thymic emigration is controlled by signaling through a G protein–coupled receptor.

After completing their maturation in the thymic medulla, a process that takes 1–2 weeks, surviving thymocytes emigrate from the thymus and enter the bloodstream (**Fig. 8.32**). Emigration requires recognition of the lipid molecule sphingosine 1-phosphate (S1P) by the G protein–coupled receptor S1PR1, which is expressed by thymocytes during their final maturation. S1P is present in high concentration in blood and lymph, and mature thymocytes are drawn toward it. Mature thymocytes also express CD62L (L-selectin), a lymph node–homing receptor that facilitates the localization of mature naive T cells to peripheral lymphoid organs after their emigration from the thymus.

8-29 T cells that encounter sufficient quantities of self antigens for the first time in the periphery are eliminated or inactivated.

Many autoreactive T cells are purged during their development in the thymus. As discussed in Section 8-25, this negative selection process is facilitated by the AIRE protein, which promotes the expression of many tissue-specific antigens in thymic medullary epithelial cells. Nonetheless, not all self antigens are expressed in the thymus, and some autoreactive T cells complete their maturation and migrate to the periphery. Our understanding of the fates of autoreactive T cells in the periphery comes mainly from the study of mice transgenic for self-reactive T-cell receptors. In some cases, T cells reacting to self antigens in the periphery are eliminated. This usually follows a brief period of activation and cell division and so is known as **activation-induced cell death**.

The question immediately arises: If the encounter of a mature naive lymphocyte and a self antigen leads to cell death, why does this not also happen to a mature lymphocyte that recognizes a pathogen-derived antigen? The answer is that infection sets up inflammation, which induces the expression of co-stimulatory molecules on the antigen-presenting dendritic cells and the production of cytokines promoting lymphocyte activation. The outcome of an encounter with antigen in these conditions is the activation, proliferation, and differentiation of the lymphocyte to effector-cell status. In the absence of infection or inflammation, dendritic cells still process and present self antigens, but in the absence of co-stimulatory and other signals, any interaction of a mature lymphocyte with its specific antigen seems to result in a tolerance-inducing (**tolerogenic**) signal from the antigen receptor.

Summary.

The stages of thymocyte development up to the expression of the pre-T-cell receptor—including the decision between commitment to either the αβ or the γδ lineage—are all independent of interactions with peptide:MHC antigens. With the successful rearrangement of α-chain genes and expression of the T-cell receptor, αβ thymocytes undergo further development that is determined by the interactions of their T-cell receptors with self peptides presented by the MHC molecules on the thymic stroma. CD4+CD8+ double-positive thymocytes whose receptors interact with self peptide:self MHC complexes on thymic cortical epithelial cells are positively selected and will eventually mature into CD4 or CD8 single-positive cells. T cells that react too strongly with self antigens are deleted in the thymus, a process driven by bone marrow–derived antigen-presenting cells and AIRE-expressing epithelial cells in the medullary region of the thymus. The outcome of positive and negative selection is the generation of a mature conventional T-cell repertoire that is both MHC-restricted and self-tolerant. Some nonconventional T-cell lineages undergo 'agonist' selection after strong T-cell receptor signaling. Precisely how the recognition of self peptide:self MHC ligands by the T-cell receptor leads to either positive or negative selection remains an unsolved problem.

Summary to Chapter 8.

B-cell and T-cell lineages form from an uncommitted hematopoietic stem cell. The somatic gene rearrangements that generate the highly diverse repertoire of antigen receptors—immunoglobulin for B cells, and the T-cell receptor for

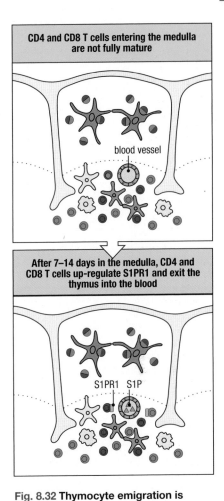

CD4 and CD8 T cells entering the medulla are not fully mature

blood vessel

After 7–14 days in the medulla, CD4 and CD8 T cells up-regulate S1PR1 and exit the thymus into the blood

S1PR1 S1P

Fig. 8.32 Thymocyte emigration is induced by signaling through the sphingosine 1-phosphate receptor, S1PR1. CD4 and CD8 single-positive thymocytes that have successfully survived positive and negative selection are found in the medulla but are not yet fully mature. At the termination of the maturation process, which takes 7–14 days, the CD4 and CD8 single-positive thymocytes up-regulate the sphingosine 1-phosphate (S1P) receptor, known as S1PR1. S1PR1 is a G protein–coupled receptor that promotes chemotaxis of the cells toward the ligand S1P. Because of the high levels of S1P in the blood, single-positive thymocytes are induced to leave the thymus by entering the blood, where they become part of the recirculating naive T-cell population.

T cells—occur in the early stages of the development of T cells and B cells from a common bone marrow–derived lymphoid progenitor. Mammalian B-cell development takes place in fetal liver and, after birth, in the bone marrow; T cells also originate from stem cells in the fetal liver or in the bone marrow but undergo most of their development in the thymus. Much of the somatic recombination machinery, including the RAG proteins that are an essential part of the V(D)J recombinase, is common to both B and T cells. In both B and T cells, gene rearrangements begin with the loci that contain D gene segments and proceed successively at each locus. The first step in B-cell development is the rearrangement of the locus for the immunoglobulin heavy chain, and for T cells it is the β chain. In each case, the developing cell is allowed to proceed to the next stage of development only if the rearrangement has produced an in-frame sequence that can be translated into a protein expressed on the cell surface: either the pre-B-cell receptor or the pre-T-cell receptor. Cells that do not generate successful rearrangements for both receptor chains die by apoptosis.

Once a functional antigen receptor has appeared on the cell surface, the lymphocyte is tested in two ways. Positive selection tests for the potential usefulness of the antigen receptor, whereas negative selection removes self-reactive cells from the lymphocyte repertoire, rendering it tolerant to the antigens of the body. Positive selection is particularly important for T cells, because it ensures that only cells bearing T-cell receptors that can recognize antigen in combination with self MHC molecules will continue to mature. Positive selection also coordinates the choice of co-receptor expression. CD4 becomes expressed by T cells harboring MHC class II–restricted receptors, and CD8 becomes expressed by cells harboring MHC class I–restricted receptors. This ensures the optimal use of these receptors in responses to pathogens. For B cells, positive selection seems to occur at the final transition from immature to mature B cells, which occurs in peripheral lymphoid tissues. Tolerance to self antigens is enforced by negative selection at different stages throughout the development of both B and T cells, and positive selection likewise seems to represent a continual process.

Discussion Questions

8.1 Hematopoietic progenitor cells found in the adult bone marrow, such as lymphoid–myeloid primed multipotent progenitor cells, are the precursors to several lineages of more committed progenitors. On the basis of your knowledge of these more committed progenitors, such as the common lymphoid progenitor or the common granulocyte/megakaryocyte/erythrocyte progenitor, what might be the advantage of having progenitors that are not committed to generating only a single lineage of mature hematopoietic cells?

8.2 Multiple checkpoints are in place during B-cell development in the bone marrow, to ensure the most efficient generation of mature B cells expressing a functional immunoglobulin protein. What is the first of these checkpoints, and how is this checkpoint enforced?

8.3 When recombination processes are impaired during B-cell development, such as occurs when RAG-1 or RAG-2 is defective, the number of pre-B cells in the bone marrow is profoundly reduced. What is the explanation for this observed reduction in pre-B cells?

8.4 Why might individuals with defects in receptor editing in the bone marrow have increased susceptibility to autoimmune diseases such as systemic lupus erythematosus or rheumatoid arthritis?

8.5 In a healthy individual, the number of circulating B cells remains relatively constant over time. As a consequence, large variations in the number of circulating B cells in an individual are used as a diagnostic indicator of disease, such as an infection or a malignancy. What process during B-cell maturation ensures that an individual maintains a relatively constant number of circulating B cells?

8.6 The bone marrow progenitor cells that enter the thymus and develop into T cells have the potential to generate other lineages of lymphocytes (for example, B cells). What key signaling pathway is required for these progenitor cells to commit to the T-cell lineage, and how is this accomplished?

8.7 As for B cells, antigen receptor gene rearrangements in developing T cells occur in an ordered series of steps. For T cells developing in the αβ T-cell lineage, which rearrangements occur first, and what are the consequences of success versus failure in generating a productive antigen receptor chain protein at this step?

8.8 Positive selection of αβ T cells in the thymus is coordinated with commitment to the CD4 or CD8 T-cell lineage. Why is it important that these two processes are coordinately regulated?

8.9 The immunomodulatory drug FTY720 causes rapid and profound reductions in the number of circulating T cells. This drug is an inhibitor of a G protein–coupled receptor expressed on medullary thymocytes and circulating naive T cells. What is the likely target of FTY720, and why does it cause rapid reduction in the number of T cells in the blood?

General references.

Melchers, F.: Checkpoints that control B cell development. *J. Clin. Invest.* 2015, **125**:2203–2210. doi: 10.1172/JCI78083.

Shah, D.K., and Zuniga-Pflucker, J.C.: An overview of the intrathymic intricacies of T cell development. *J. Immunol.* 2014, **192**:4017–4023. doi: 10.4049/jimmunol.1302259.

Section references.

8-1   Lymphocytes derive from hematopoietic stem cells in the bone marrow.

Funk, P.E., Kincade, P.W., and Witte, P.L.: Native associations of early hematopoietic stem-cells and stromal cells isolated in bone-marrow cell aggregates. *Blood* 1994, **83**:361–369.

Harly, C., Cam, M., Kaye, J., and Bhandoola, A.: Development and differentiation of early innate lymphoid progenitors. *J. Exp. Med.* 2018, **215**:249–262. doi: 10.1084/jem.20170832.

8-2   Commitment to B cell, T cell, or innate lymphoid cell lineages is regulated by distinct networks of transcription factors.

Boller, S., and Grosschedl, R.: The regulatory network of B-cell differentiation: a focused view of early B-cell factor 1 function. *Immunol. Rev.* 2014, **261**: 102–115. doi: 10.1111/imr.12206.

8-3   B-cell development begins by rearrangement of the heavy-chain locus.

Allman, D., Li, J., and Hardy, R.R.: Commitment to the B lymphoid lineage occurs before DH-JH recombination. *J. Exp. Med.* 1999, **189**:735–740.

Hardy, R.R., Carmack, C.E., Shinton, S.A., Kemp, J.D., and Hayakawa, K.: Resolution and characterization of pro-B and pre-pro-B cell stages in normal mouse bone marrow. *J. Exp. Med.* 1991, **173**:1213–1225.

Medvedovic, J, Ebert, A., Tagoh, H., and Busslinger, M.: Pax5: a master regulator of B cell development and leukemogenesis. *Adv. Immunol.* 2011, **111**:179–206. doi: 10.1016/B978-0-12-385991-4.00005-2.

8-4   The pre-B-cell receptor tests for successful production of a complete heavy chain and signals for the transition from the pro-B cell to the pre-B cell stage.

Bankovich, A.J., Raunser, S., Juo, Z.S., Walz, T., Davis, M.M., and Garcia, K.C.: Structural insight into pre-B cell receptor function. *Science* 2007, **316**:291–294.

Grawunder, U., Leu, T.M.J., Schatz, D.G., Werner, A., Rolink, A.G., Melchers, F., and Winkler, T.H.: Down-regulation of Rag1 and Rag2 gene expression in pre-B cells after functional immunoglobulin heavy-chain rearrangement. *Immunity* 1995, **3**:601–608.

Monroe, J.G.: ITAM-mediated tonic signalling through pre-BCR and BCR complexes. *Nat. Rev. Immunol.* 2006, **6**:283–294.

8-5   Pre-B-cell receptor signaling inhibits further heavy-chain locus rearrangement and enforces allelic exclusion.

Loffert, D., Ehlich, A., Muller, W., and Rajewsky, K.: Surrogate light-chain expression is required to establish immunoglobulin heavy-chain allelic exclusion during early B-cell development. *Immunity* 1996, **4**:133–144.

Melchers, F., ten Boekel, E., Yamagami, T., Andersson, J., and Rolink, A.: The roles of preB and B cell receptors in the stepwise allelic exclusion of mouse IgH and L chain gene loci. *Semin. Immunol.* 1999, **11**:307–317.

Ochiai, K., Maienschein-Cline, M., Mandal, M., Triggs, J.R., Bertolino, E., Sciammas, R., Dinner, A.R., Clark, M.R., and Singh, H.: A self-reinforcing regulatory network triggered by limiting IL-7 activates pre-BCR signalling and differentiation. *Nat. Immunol.* 2012, **13**:300–307. doi: 10.1038/ni.2210.

8-6   Pre-B cells rearrange the light-chain locus and express cell-surface immunoglobulin.

Gorman, J.R., van der Stoep, N., Monroe, R., Cogne, M., Davidson, L., and Alt, F.W.: The Igκ 3′ enhancer influences the ratio of Igκ versus IgλB lymphocytes. *Immunity* 1996, **5**:241–252.

Sleckman, B.P., Gorman, J.R., and Alt, F.W.: Accessibility control of antigen receptor variable region gene assembly—role of *cis*-acting elements. *Annu. Rev. Immunol.* 1996, **14**:459–481.

8-7   Immature B cells are tested for autoreactivity before they leave the bone marrow.

Casellas, R., Shih, T.A., Kleinewietfeld, M., Rakonjac, J., Nemazee, D., Rajewsky, K., and Nussenzweig, M.C.: Contribution of receptor editing to the antibody repertoire. *Science* 2001, **291**:1541–1544.

Nemazee, D.: Receptor editing in lymphocyte development and central tolerance. *Nat. Rev. Immunol.* 2006, **6**:728–740.

Prak, E.L., and Weigert, M.: Light-chain replacement—a new model for antibody gene rearrangement. *J. Exp. Med.* 1995, **182**:541–548.

8-8   Lymphocytes that encounter sufficient quantities of self antigens in the periphery are eliminated.

Goodnow, C.C., Crosbie, J., Jorgensen, H., Brink, R.A., and Basten, A.: Induction of self-tolerance in mature peripheral B lymphocytes. *Nature* 1989, **342**:385–391.

Russell, D.M., Dembic, Z., Morahan, G., Miller, J.F.A.P., Burki, K., and Nemazee, D.: Peripheral deletion of self-reactive B cells. *Nature* 1991, **354**:308–311.

8-9   Newly formed B cells arriving in the spleen turn over rapidly and require cytokines and positive signals through the B-cell receptor for maturation and long-term survival.

Lam, K.P., Kuhn, R., and Rajewsky, K.: *In vivo* ablation of surface immunoglobulin on mature B cells by inducible gene targeting results in rapid cell death. *Cell* 1997, **90**:1073–1083.

Levine, M.H., Haberman, A.M., Sant'Angelo, D.B., Hannum, L.G., Cancro, M.P., Janeway, C.A., Jr., and Shlomchik, M.J.: A B-cell receptor-specific selection step governs immature to mature B cell differentiation. *Proc. Natl. Acad. Sci. USA* 2000, **97**:2743–2748.

Loder, F., Mutschler, B., Ray, R.J., Paige, C.J., Sideras, P., Torres, R., Lamers, M.C., and Carsetti, R.: B cell development in the spleen takes place in discrete steps and is determined by the quality of B cell receptor-derived signals. *J. Exp. Med.* 1999, **190**:75–89.

Schiemann, B., Gommerman, J.L., Vora, K., Cachero, T.G., Shulga-Morskaya, S., Dobles, M., Frew, E., and Scott, M.L.: An essential role for BAFF in the normal development of B cells through a BCMA-independent pathway. *Science* 2001, **293**:2111–2114.

Wen, L., Brill-Dashoff, J., Shinton, S.A., Asano, M., Hardy, R.R., and Hayakawa, K.: Evidence of marginal-zone B cell-positive selection in spleen. *Immunity* 2005, 23:297–308.

8-10 B-1 B cells are an innate lymphocyte subset that arises early in development.

Montecino-Rodriguez, E., and Dorshkind, K.: B-1 B cell development in the fetus and adult. *Immunity* 2012, 36:13–21.

8-11 T-cell progenitors originate in the bone marrow, but all the important events in T-cell development occur in the thymus.

Carlyle, J.R., and Zúñiga-Pflücker, J.C.: Requirement for the thymus in α:β T lymphocyte lineage commitment. *Immunity* 1998, 9:187–197.
Takahama, Y., Ohigashi, I., Baik, S., and Anderson, G.: Generation of diversity in thymic epithelial cells. *Nat. Rev. Immunol.* 2017, 17:295–305. doi: 10.1038/nri.2017.12.

8-12 T-cell precursors proliferate extensively in the thymus, but most die there.

Shortman, K., Egerton, M., Spangrude, G.J., and Scollay, R.: The generation and fate of thymocytes. *Semin. Immunol.* 1990, 2:3–12.
Surh, C.D., and Sprent, J.: T-cell apoptosis detected *in situ* during positive and negative selection in the thymus. *Nature* 1994, 372:100–103.

8-13 Successive stages in the development of thymocytes are marked by changes in cell-surface molecules.

Borowski, C., Martin, C., Gounari, F., Haughn, L., Aifantis, I., Grassi, F., and von Boehmer, H.: On the brink of becoming a T cell. *Curr. Opin. Immunol.* 2002, 14:200–206.

8-14 Commitment to the T-cell lineage occurs in the thymus after Notch signaling.

Hosokawa, H., and Rothenberg, E.V.: Cytokines, transcription factors, and the initiation of T-cell development. *Cold Spring Harb. Perspect. Biol.* 2018, 10:a028621. doi: 10.1101/schperspect.a028621.
Pui, J.C., Allman, D., Xu, L., DeRocco, S., Karnell, F.G., Bakkour, S., Lee, J.Y., Kadesch, T., Hardy, R.R., Aster, J.C., *et al.*: Notch1 expression in early lymphopoiesis influences B versus T lineage determination. *Immunity* 1999, 11:299–308.
Radtke, F., Wilson, A., Stark, G., Bauer, M., van Meerwijk, J., MacDonald, H.R., and Aguet, M.: Deficient T cell fate specification in mice with an induced inactivation of Notch1. *Immunity* 1999, 10:547–558.

8-15 After T-cell commitment, thymocyte development is regulated by T-cell receptor rearrangement, expression, and signaling.

Borowski, C., Li, X., Aifantis, I., Gounari, F., and von Boehmer, H.: Pre-TCRα and TCRα are not interchangeable partners of TCRβ during T lymphocyte development. *J. Exp. Med.* 2004, 199:607–615.
Dudley, E.C., Petrie, H.T., Shah, L.M., Owen, M.J., and Hayday, A.C.: T-cell receptor β chain gene rearrangement and selection during thymocyte development in adult mice. *Immunity* 1994, 1:83–93.
Philpott, K.I., Viney, J.L., Kay, G., Rastan, S., Gardiner, E.M., Chae, S., Hayday, A.C., and Owen, M.J.: Lymphoid development in mice congenitally lacking T cell receptor αβ-expressing cells. *Science* 1992, 256:1448–1453.
von Boehmer, H., Aifantis, I., Azogui, O., Feinberg, J., Saint-Ruf, C., Zober, C., Garcia, C., and Buer, J.: Crucial function of the pre-T-cell receptor (TCR) in TCRβ selection, TCRβ allelic exclusion and α:β versus γ:δ lineage commitment. *Immunol. Rev.* 1998, 165:111–119.

8-16 Thymocytes at different developmental stages are found in distinct parts of the thymus.

Ladi, E., Yin, X., Chtanova, T., and Robey, E.A.: Thymic microenvironments for T cell differentiation and selection. *Nat. Immunol.* 2006, 7:338–343. doi: 10.1038/ni1323.

8-17 T cells with αβ or γδ receptors arise from a common progenitor.

Kang, J., and Raulet, D.H.: Events that regulate differentiation of αβ TCR+ and γδ TCR+ T cells from a common precursor. *Semin. Immunol.* 1997, 9:171–179.
Kreslavsky, T., Garbe, A.I., Krueger, A., and von Boehmer, H.: T cell receptor-instructed αβ versus γδ lineage commitment revealed by single-cell analysis. *J. Exp. Med.* 2008, 205:1173–1186.

8-18 T cells expressing γδ T-cell receptors arise in two distinct phases during development.

Dunon, D., Courtois, D., Vainio, O., Six, A., Chen, C.H., Cooper, M.D., Dangy, J.P., and Imhof, B.A.: Ontogeny of the immune system: γ:δ and α:β T cells migrate from thymus to the periphery in alternating waves. *J. Exp. Med.* 1997, 186:977–988.
Narayan, K., Sylvia, K.E., Malhotra, N., Yin, C.C., Martens, G., Vallerskog, T., Kornfeld, H., Xiong, N., Cohen, N.R., Brenner, M.B., *et al.*: Intrathymic programming of effector fates in three molecularly distinct gamma:delta T cell subtypes. *Nat. Immunol.* 2012, 13:511–518.
Xiong, N., and Raulet, D.H.: Development and selection of γδ T cells. *Immunol. Rev.* 2007, 215:15–31.

8-19 Successful synthesis of a rearranged β chain allows the production of a pre-T-cell receptor that triggers cell proliferation and blocks further β-chain gene rearrangement.

Pang, S.S., Berry, R., Chen, Z., Kjer-Nielsen, L., Perugini, M.A., King, G.F., Wang, C., Chew, S.H., La Gruta, N.L., Williams, N.K., *et al.*: The structural basis for autonomous dimerization of the pre-T-cell antigen receptor. *Nature* 2010, 467:844–848.
von Boehmer, H., Aifantis, I., Azogui, O., Feinberg, J., Saint-Ruf, C., Zober, C., Garcia, C., and Buer, J.: Crucial function of the pre-T-cell receptor (TCR) in TCRβ selection, TCRβ allelic exclusion and α:β versus γ:δ lineage commitment. *Immunol. Rev.* 1998, 165:111–119.

8-20 T-cell α-chain genes undergo successive rearrangements until positive selection or cell death intervenes.

Marrack, P., and Kappler, J.: Positive selection of thymocytes bearing α:β T cell receptors. *Curr. Opin. Immunol.* 1997, 9:250–255.
Padovan, E., Casorati, G., Dellabona, P., Meyer, S., Brockhaus, M., and Lanzavecchia, A.: Expression of two T-cell receptor α chains: dual receptor T cells. *Science* 1993, 262:422–424.
Petrie, H.T., Livak, F., Schatz, D.G., Strasser, A., Crispe, I.N., and Shortman, K.: Multiple rearrangements in T-cell receptor α-chain genes maximize the production of useful thymocytes. *J. Exp. Med.* 1993, 178:615–622.

8-21 Overview of positive and negative selection of αβ lineage T cells.

Gascoigne, N.R.J., Rybakin, V., Acuto, O., and Brzostek, J.: TCR signal strength and T cell development. *Annu. Rev. Cell Dev. Biol.* 2016, 32:327–348. doi: 10.1146/annurev-cellbio-111315-125324.

8-22 Only thymocytes whose receptors interact with self peptide:self MHC complexes can survive and mature.

Hogquist, K.A., Tomlinson, A.J., Kieper, W.C., McGargill, M.A., Hart, M.C., Naylor, S., and Jameson, S.C.: Identification of a naturally occurring ligand for thymic positive selection. *Immunity* 1997, 6:389–399.

Kisielow, P., Teh, H.S., Blüthmann, H., and von Boehmer, H.: **Positive selection of antigen-specific T cells in thymus by restricting MHC molecules.** *Nature* 1988, 335:730–733.

8-23 Positive selection coordinates the expression of CD4 or CD8 with the specificity of the T-cell receptor and the potential effector functions of the T cell.

Egawa, T., and Littman, D.R.: ThPOK acts late in specification of the helper T cell lineage and suppresses Runx-mediated commitment to the cytotoxic T cell lineage. *Nat. Immunol.* 2008, 9:1131–1139.

Etzensperger, R., Kadakia, T., Tai, X., Alag, A., Guinter, T.I., Egawa, T., Erman, B., and Singer, A.: Identification of lineage-specifying cytokines that signal all CD8[+] cytotoxic lineage fate decisions in the thymus. *Nat. Immunol.* 2017, 18:1218–1227. doi: 10.1038/ni.3847.

He, X., Xi, H., Dave, V.P., Zhang, Y., Hua, X., Nicolas, E., Xu, W., Roe, B.A., and Kappes, D.J.: The zinc finger transcription factor Th-POK regulates CD4 versus CD8 T-cell lineage commitment. *Nature* 2005, 433:826–833.

8-24 Thymic cortical epithelial cells mediate positive selection of developing thymocytes.

Cosgrove, D., Chan, S.H., Waltzinger, C., Benoist, C., and Mathis, D.: The thymic compartment responsible for positive selection of CD4[+] T cells. *Int. Immunol.* 1992, 4:707–710.

Murata, S., Sasaki, K., Kishimoto, T., Niwa, S.-I., Hayashi, H., Takahama, Y., and Tanaka, K.: Regulation of CD8[+] T cell development by thymus-specific proteasomes. *Science* 2007, 316:1349–1353.

Nakagawa, T., Roth, W., Wong, P., Nelson, A., Farr, A., Deussing, J., Villadangos, J.A., Ploegh, H., Peters, C., and Rudensky, A.Y.: Cathepsin L: critical role in Ii degradation and CD4 T cell selection in the thymus. *Science* 1998, 280:450–453.

8-25 T cells that react strongly with self antigens are deleted in the thymus.

Anderson, M.S., and Su, M.A.: Aire and T cell development. *Curr. Opin. Immunol.* 2011, 23:198–206.

Anderson, M.S., Venanzi, E.S., Klein, L., Chen, Z., Berzins, S.P., Turley, S.J., von Boehmer, H., Bronson, R., Dierich, A., Benoist, C., *et al.*: Projection of an immunological self shadow within the thymus by the aire protein. *Science* 2002, 298:1395–1401.

Kishimoto, H., and Sprent, J.: Negative selection in the thymus includes semimature T cells. *J. Exp. Med.* 1997, 185:263–271.

McCaughtry, T.M., Baldwin, T.A., Wilken, M.S., and Hogquist, K.A.: Clonal deletion of thymocytes can occur in the cortex with no involvement of the medulla. *J. Exp. Med.* 2008, 205:2575–2584.

8-26 The specificity and/or the strength of signals for negative and positive selection must differ.

Alberola-Ila, J., Hogquist, K.A., Swan, K.A., Bevan, M.J., and Perlmutter, R.M.: Positive and negative selection invoke distinct signaling pathways. *J. Exp. Med.* 1996, 184:9–18.

Ashton-Rickardt, P.G., Bandeira, A., Delaney, J.R., Van Kaer, L., Pircher, H.P., Zinkernagel, R.M., and Tonegawa, S.: **Evidence for a differential avidity model of T-cell selection in the thymus.** *Cell* 1994, 76:651–663.

Bommhardt, U., Scheuring, Y., Bickel, C., Zamoyska, R., and Hunig, T.: **MEK activity regulates negative selection of immature CD4[+]CD8[+] thymocytes.** *J. Immunol.* 2000, 164:2326–2337.

Hogquist, K.A., Jameson, S.C., Heath, W.R., Howard, J.L., Bevan, M.J., and Carbone, F.R.: **T-cell receptor antagonist peptides induce positive selection.** *Cell* 1994, 76:17–27.

8-27 αβ T cells diverge into multiple lineages at the CD4[+] and CD8[+] single-positive stage in the thymic medulla.

Jordan, M.S., Boesteanu, A., Reed, A.J., Petrone, A.L., Holenbeck, A.E., Lerman, M.A., Naji, A., and Caton, A.J.: Thymic selection of CD4[+]CD25[+] regulatory T cells induced by an agonist self-peptide. *Nat. Immunol.* 2001, 2:301–306.

Moran, A.E., and Hogquist, K.A.: T-cell receptor affinity in thymic development. *Immunology* 2012, 135:261–267.

Moran, A.E., Hozapfel, K.L., Xing, Y., Cunningham, N.R., Maltzman, J.S., Punt, J., and Hogquist, K.A.: T cell receptor signal strength in Treg and iNKT cell development demonstrated by a novel fluorescent reporter mouse. *J. Exp. Med.* 2011, 208:1279–1289. doi: 10.1084/jem.20110308.

8-28 Thymic emigration is controlled by signaling through a G protein–coupled receptor.

Matloubian, M., Lo, C.G., Cinamon, G., Lesneski, M.J., Xu, Y., Brinkmann, V., Allende, M.L., Proia, R.L., and Cyster, J.G.: Lymphocyte egress from thymus and peripheral lymphoid organs is dependent on S1P receptor 1. *Nature* 2004, 427:355–360.

Zachariah, M.A., and Cyster, J.G.: Neural crest-derived pericytes promote egress of mature thymocytes at the corticomedullary junction. *Science* 2010, 328:1129–1135.

8-29 T cells that encounter sufficient quantities of self antigens for the first time in the periphery are eliminated or inactivated.

Fink, P.J., and Hendricks, D.W.: Post-thymic maturation: young T cells assert their individuality. *Nat. Rev. Immunol.* 2011, 11:544–549.

Steinman, R.M., and Nussenzweig, M.C.: Avoiding horror autotoxicus: the importance of dendritic cells in peripheral T cell tolerance. *Proc. Natl. Acad. Sci. USA* 2002, 99:351–358.

Xing, Y., and Hogquist, K.A.: T-cell tolerance: central and peripheral. *Cold Spring Harb. Perspect. Biol.* 2012, 4:a006957.

T Cell–Mediated Immunity

9

An adaptive immune response is initiated when a pathogen overwhelms innate defense mechanisms. As the pathogen replicates and antigen accumulates, sensor cells of the innate immune system become activated to trigger the adaptive immune response. While some infections may be dealt with solely by innate immunity, as discussed in Chapters 2 and 3, host defense against most pathogens, almost by definition, requires recruitment of adaptive immunity; that is, T and B lymphocytes. This is borne out by immunodeficiency syndromes that are associated with failure of particular parts of the adaptive immune response, to be discussed in Chapter 13.

In the next three chapters, we will learn how the adaptive immune response involving antigen-specific T cells and B cells is initiated and deployed. T-cell responses that lead to cellular immunity will be considered first, in this chapter. B-cell responses that lead to antibody-mediated, or humoral, immunity will be considered in Chapter 10. In Chapter 11, we will consider the dynamics of T-cell and B-cell responses in the context of their integration with innate immunity and how this culminates in one of the most important features of adaptive immunity—immunological memory.

Once T cells have completed their primary development in the thymus, they are released into circulation. On reaching a secondary (or peripheral) lymphoid organ—whether a lymph node, the spleen, or mucosal lymphoid tissue—they leave the blood to migrate through the lymphoid tissue in search of their cognate antigen. Circulating T cells that have not yet encountered their specific antigens are known as **naive T cells**. A naive T cell has very limited functional activity, and if it fails to detect its antigen as it migrates through a secondary lymphoid tissue, it soon exits and returns to the circulation with the same limited functionality. If, however, the naive T cell does encounter its antigen—presented as a peptide:MHC complex on the surface of a conventional dendritic cell—it typically becomes activated and is induced to proliferate and differentiate over several days within

IN THIS CHAPTER

Development and function of secondary lymphoid organs—sites for the initiation of adaptive immune responses.

Naive T-cell activation, clonal expansion, and differentiation into effector and memory T cells.

General properties of effector T cells and their cytokines.

T cell–mediated cytotoxicity.

that lymphoid tissue to generate many progeny (termed **clonal expansion**) possessing new activities that contribute to removal of the source of antigen. These clonal progeny are called **effector T cells**, and, unlike naive T cells, they perform their acquired functions as soon as they encounter their specific antigen on other cells—generally without requirement for further differentiation. Effector T cells also change their pattern of recirculation, such that many are directed to sites of pathogen entry in nonlymphoid tissues, while others are directed to interact with B cells within the lymphoid tissue to provide 'help' for the production of pathogen-specific antibodies. The initial antigenic response of naive T cells is often referred to as **priming**, and the more general initial antigenic response is referred to as a **primary immune response**, to distinguish it from a subsequent reencounter with the same pathogen in a **secondary (or recall) immune response**.

As we will see, there are several functional classes of effector T cells that can be generated in a primary response, each specialized for the clearance of different types of pathogens. Because of their requirement to recognize peptide antigens presented by MHC molecules, all effector T cells act on other host cells—not on the pathogen itself—to bring about eradication of the pathogen. CD8 T cells recognize pathogen peptides presented by MHC class I molecules, and naive CD8 T cells differentiate into cytotoxic T cells, or **cytotoxic T lymphocytes (CTLs)**, that recognize and kill cells infected by intracellular pathogens such as viruses, which can replicate within host cells. Because MHC class I is expressed on all nucleated cells, CTLs can kill infected cells anywhere in the body. CD4 T cells recognize pathogen peptides presented by MHC class II molecules and have a more flexible repertoire of effector activities. Naive CD4 T cells can differentiate down distinct pathways that generate effector subsets with different immunological functions. The main CD4 effector-cell subsets are T helper 1 (T_H1), T_H2, T_H17, and T follicular helper (T_{FH}), which activate MHC class II–bearing target cells, such as macrophages, mucosal epithelial cells, and B cells, to enhance those cells' activity against the pathogen. Naive CD4 T cells can also differentiate into **regulatory T cells, or T_{reg} cells**, which inhibit the initiation and extent of immune activation. Because the range of host cells that express MHC class II is much more restricted than that of MHC class I, the cellular targets of effector CD4 T cells are also more restricted. The interactions of both CD8 and CD4 effector T cells with target cells is mediated both by direct contact between the T cell and the target cell and by the release of cytokines, which can act locally on target cells or on other cells at a distance to orchestrate the clearance of antigen.

Unlike innate immune cells, which respond to pathogens within minutes to hours, the activation, proliferation, and differentiation of naive T cells into effector T cells takes several days, resulting in a substantial period of delay during which the innate immune system must restrain the pathogen prior to the participation of effector T cells and the antibodies they have helped induce. Once the adaptive immune response is fully developed, the pathogen is typically cleared, resulting in elimination of the antigens that have driven the adaptive response. In the wake of antigen clearance and resolution of the inflammatory response provoked by a pathogen, most of the effector T cells that were generated to combat the infection die off. However, a fraction remains as long-lived **memory T cells**, which can retain effector functions and persist for months to years at substantially higher numbers than their naive clonal precursors to accelerate pathogen clearance should future challenges arise.

In this chapter, we will first consider how the structure of secondary lymphoid tissues enables the interaction of rare clones of circulating T cells with dendritic cells that may bear the antigens they recognize. We will then consider how naive T cells become activated to differentiate into effector T cells that help other immune cells to clear pathogens. Some of the effector functions of T cells will be considered in this chapter; others will be discussed in the context of T-cell help for B-cell production of antibodies in Chapter 10 and the actions of effector cells to heighten the activation of the innate immune system in Chapter 11.

Development and function of secondary lymphoid organs—sites for the initiation of adaptive immune responses.

As discussed in Chapters 1 and 8, the primary lymphoid organs—the thymus and bone marrow—are the tissue sites for selection of antigenic receptor repertoires of T and B cells, respectively. Adaptive immune responses are initiated in the secondary lymphoid organs—lymph nodes, spleen, and the mucosa-associated lymphoid tissue (MALT), such as the Peyer's patches in the gut. The architecture of these tissues is similar throughout the body and is structured to provide a crossroads for the interaction of rare clonal precursors of recirculating T and B cells with their cognate antigens—whether presented by dendritic cells in the case of T cells or recognized as free antigens in the case of B cells. In view of the rarity of naive T cells that recognize a specific peptide:MHC complex—roughly 100 cells in the entire immune repertoire of approximately 100 million T cells in the mouse (~1 in every million T cells)—and the large area over which an infectious agent can invade, the antigens derived from the pathogen (or in some instances the pathogen itself) must be transported from sites of pathogen entry to secondary lymphoid tissues to facilitate recognition of the antigen by lymphocytes. As we will see, these tissues are structured for the efficient delivery of naive T and B cells and their antigens into a small volume in secondary lymphoid organs to enable the adaptive immune system to overcome the daunting task of effective surveillance of the entire body for pathogens despite the rarity of naive clonal precursors. Moreover, when naive lymphocytes do recognize antigen, the secondary lymphoid tissues serve as the site for rapid clonal expansion as antigen-activated T and B cells divide rapidly and differentiate for several days prior to their release back into the circulation where they can redistribute to sites of infection. Thus, secondary lymphoid tissues are sites of both initiation and amplification of the nascent adaptive response. In this part of the chapter we will first consider the development and structure of secondary lymphoid organs that enable these interactions. We will then discuss how naive T cells are directed to exit the blood and enter secondary lymphoid organs, then exit these tissues to recirculate back to blood. This will be followed by consideration of how dendritic cells pick up antigen and travel to local lymphoid organs, where they can both present antigen to T cells and activate them.

9-1 Secondary lymphoid structures are specialized to facilitate the interaction of circulating T and B lymphocytes with antigen.

The various secondary lymphoid organs are organized roughly along the same lines (see Chapter 1), having distinct areas in which B cells and T cells are concentrated—the B-cell and T-cell zones. They also contain macrophages, dendritic cells, and nonleukocyte stromal cells that are critical to the structural organization and function of these tissues. In the case of the spleen, which is specialized for the capture of antigens that enter the bloodstream,

Spleen

Red pulp

dendritic cell

marginal sinus

B-cell zone

central arteriole

B-cell follicle

T-cell zone (PALS)

B cell   T cell

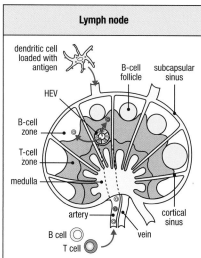

Lymph node

dendritic cell loaded with antigen

B-cell follicle   subcapsular sinus

HEV

B-cell zone

T-cell zone

medulla

artery

cortical sinus

B cell

T cell   vein

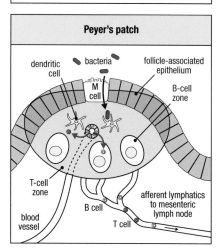

Peyer's patch

dendritic cell   bacteria   follicle-associated epithelium

M cell   B-cell zone

T-cell zone

blood vessel

B cell   afferent lymphatics to mesenteric lymph node

T cell

Fig. 9.1 Secondary lymphoid tissues serve as anatomic crossroads for interactions of antigens and lymphocytes. Secondary lymphoid tissues are specialized to facilitate interactions between lymphocytes and antigens. In the spleen (upper panel), antigen (denoted by red dots) is delivered via arterioles that branch from the central arteriole to the marginal sinus, which is the boundary between the white pulp and red pulp. In the marginal sinus, antigen can be taken up by marginal zone B cells, macrophages, or dendritic cells, the last of which can transport antigen into the T-cell zones of the periarteriolar lymphoid sheath, or PALS. T and B cells enter the spleen via the same route as antigen and leave the marginal sinus to travel to either the PALS or the B-cell follicles. In lymph nodes (middle panel), antigen is delivered in lymph either free or as cargo of dendritic cells that have taken up the antigen in the tissues drained by the lymph node. The antigen is conducted via afferent lymphatics to the subcapsular sinus, from which it is delivered to T-cell zones, where T cells can recognize it on the surface of dendritic cells; or, in the case of B cells, it is detected as an intact antigen, often on the surface of macrophages at the border of B-cell follicles. T and B cells enter the lymph node via high endothelial venules (HEVs) in T-cell zones, and then diverge into T-cell and B-cell zones. In the intestines (lower panel), antigens are transported from the lumen via the microfold cells (M cells)—specialized epithelial cells that overlay Peyer's patches and other lymphoid follicles—to dendritic cells that reside immediately beneath the epithelium. Antigen-loaded dendritic cells are then surveyed by T cells in T-cell zones, and if the antigens they bear are not recognized by T cells locally, the dendritic cells can migrate to mesenteric lymph nodes to be further surveyed. As in the lymph nodes, T and B cells enter the Peyer's patches via HEVs in the T-cell zones.

the lymphoid tissue component is called the **white pulp** (**Fig. 9.1**). The white pulp is demarcated from the **red pulp**—which is specialized for the removal of damaged or senescent red blood cells—by a **marginal sinus**, a vascular network that is formed from branches of a small arterial vessel (the central arteriole) around which the white pulp is organized. Circulating T and B cells are initially delivered to the marginal sinus, which is a highly organized region of cells that is specialized for the capture of blood-borne antigens or intact microbes, such as viruses and bacteria. It is rich in specialized populations of macrophages and dendritic cells and contains a unique population of B cells, the **marginal zone B cells**, which do not recirculate. Pathogens reaching the bloodstream are efficiently trapped in the marginal sinus by dendritic cells and macrophages, which can then deliver pathogen-derived antigen into the white pulp, and by marginal zone B cells, which appear adapted to provide rapid responses to pathogens that enter the marginal zone—particularly the production of IgM antibodies directed against certain pathogens.

From the marginal sinus, incoming T and B cells migrate centrally along marginal zone bridging channels toward the central arteriole, where they bifurcate into T-cell zones that are clustered around the central arteriole—the so-called **periarteriolar lymphoid sheath (PALS)**—and B-cell zones, or follicles, that are located more peripherally between the PALS and the marginal sinus. Some follicles may contain **germinal centers**, in which B cells involved in an adaptive immune response are proliferating and undergoing somatic hypermutation (see Section 1-16 and Chapter 8). The antigen-driven production of germinal centers will be described in detail when we consider B-cell responses in Chapter 10.

Other types of cells are found within the B-cell and T-cell areas and are important for the structural and functional organization of secondary lymphoid organs. In the spleen, T-cell zones and the marginal zone bridging channels contain a network of **fibroblast reticular cells (FRCs)**, which are stromal cells that produce an extracellular scaffold of reticular fibers connecting the marginal sinus to the PALS and produce chemokines that attract T cells to enter from the marginal sinus. This network serves as a 'highway system' along which T cells migrate as they move from the marginal sinus into the PALS. A similar network is present in lymph nodes and will be discussed in more detail in Section 9-4.

The B-cell zone contains a network of **follicular dendritic cells (FDCs)**, which are concentrated mainly in the area of the follicle most distant from the central arteriole. Despite their name, FDCs are not of bone-marrow origin. Instead, they resemble FRCs and are specialized stromal cells that are limited to

B-cell zones, where they produce the chemokine CXCL13, which acts on the chemokine receptor CXCR5 on B cells to attract them to B-cell follicles. FDCs form a network through which B cells move into and within B-cell follicles. FDCs are also specialized for the capture of antigen in the form of immune complexes—complexes of antigen, antibody, and complement. The immune complexes are not internalized but remain intact on the surface of the FDC for prolonged periods of time, where the antigen can be recognized by B cells to drive germinal center responses, to be discussed in Chapter 10.

As in the spleen, the T cells and B cells in lymph nodes are organized into discrete T-cell and B-cell areas (see Fig. 9.1). B-cell follicles in the lymph nodes have a structure and composition similar to those of B-cell follicles in the spleen and are located just under the outer capsule of the lymph node in the cortex. T-cell zones surround the follicles in the paracortical areas. Unlike the spleen, lymph nodes have connections to both the blood system and the lymphatic system. Lymph conducted to lymph nodes by afferent lymphatic vessels enters into the **subcapsular sinus**, into which antigen and antigen-bearing dendritic cells are initially delivered from the tissues. T and B cells enter the lymph node via small blood vessels called **high endothelial venules (HEVs)**, which are found in T-cell zones and are so named because of their unusually thick endothelial-cell lining that is specialized for the recruitment of circulating lymphocytes into lymph nodes and mucosal lymphoid tissues.

The **mucosa-associated lymphoid tissue (MALT)** is associated with the body's mucosal epithelial surfaces, which provide physical barriers against infection. **Peyer's patches** are one example and are lymph node–like structures interspersed at intervals just beneath the gut epithelium in the distal portion of the small intestine, where they sample antigens from the intestinal lumen. Like the spleen and lymph nodes, these structures are organized into B-cell follicles and T-cell zones (see Fig. 9.1). The epithelium overlying them contains specialized **M cells** that are adapted to channel antigens and pathogens directly from the gut lumen to the underlying lymphoid tissue (see Section 1-17 and Chapter 12). Peyer's patches and similar tissue present in other mucosal tissues (for example, tonsils) provide specialized sites where B cells become preferentially committed to the synthesis of IgA. These lymphoid tissues will be discussed in more detail in the context of the mucosal immune system in Chapter 12.

9-2 The development of secondary lymphoid tissues is initiated by lymphoid tissue inducer cells and cytokines of the tumor necrosis factor family.

Before considering how secondary lymphoid organs contribute to adaptive immunity, we will briefly look at how these organs develop in the first place. Lymphatic vessels are formed during embryonic development from endothelial cells that originate from blood vessels. Some endothelial cells in the early venous system begin to express Prox1, a member of the homeobox family of transcription factors. These cells bud from veins, migrate away, and reassociate to form a parallel network of lymphatic vessels. Mice lacking Prox1 have normal arteries and veins but fail to form a lymphatic system, showing this factor to be critical to development of the lymphatic endothelium.

At sites destined to become lymphoid organs, **retinoic acid**, a signaling molecule derived from vitamin A that is probably produced by local nerve endings, stimulates mesenchymal cells to produce the chemokine **CXCL13**, which acts to recruit circulating hematopoietic cells called **lymphoid tissue inducer (LTi) cells** that express the receptor for CXCL13, **CXCR5**. LTi cells are a subtype of type 3 innate lymphoid cells (ILC3 cells; see Section 3-23) that initiate the formation of lymph nodes and Peyer's patches by producing TNF family proteins known as **lymphotoxins (LTs)**. LTs activate differentiation of the mesenchymal cells into **stromal organizer cells**, which are precursors of fibroblast

Retinoic acid signals mesenchymal cells to produce CXCL13, which attracts circulating LTi cells that express CXCR5	Production of LT by LTi cells induces differentiation of mesenchymal cells into stromal organizer cells, which produce additional chemokines	The recruitment of more LTi cells by CXCL13 and the recruitment of dendritic cell precursors by CCL21 and CCL19 forms the nascent lymphoid tissue	The development of HEVs results in the recruitment of T and B cells in response to chemokines produced by stromal organizer cells and the HEV endothelium	LT-β and TNF-α produced by B cells induces differentiation of follicular dendritic cells, which produce CXCL13 to establish B-cell follicles

Fig. 9.2 The development of secondary lymphoid organs is orchestrated by the interplay of lymphoid tissue inducer (LTi) cells and stromal cells. During embryonic development, LTi cells arise in the fetal liver and are recruited to sites of future lymphoid organs by CXCL13, which is produced by mesenchymal cells under the influence of retinoic acid and binds CXCR5 expressed on the circulating LTi cells (first panel). The source of retinoic acid is not clear, but it appears to be produced by nerves, at least in some sites. Once recruited from the blood into the tissue, LTi cells express lymphotoxin (LT), which acts on LT-β receptors expressed on mesenchymal cells to induce their differentiation into stromal organizer cells (second panel). The cellular organization of developing lymphoid organs is initiated when, in addition to the further recruitment of LTi cells by

CXCL13, stromal organizer cells begin to secrete the chemokines CCL21 and CCL19, which recruit dendritic-cell precursors that express CCR7, the receptor for CCL21 and CCL19 (third panel). Stromal organizer cells also stimulate the development of high endothelial venules (HEVs), which also produce CCL21 and facilitate the recruitment of CCR7-expressing B cells and T cells immediately after birth (fourth panel). Incoming B cells produce LT-β and TNF-α, both of which are needed to induce the differentiation of follicular dendritic cells (FDCs), which then become the dominant source of CXCL13. The production of CXCL13 drives the organization of B cells into discrete B-cell areas (follicles) around the FDCs and contributes to the further recruitment of B cells from the circulation into the lymph node (fifth panel). LTβR, LT-β receptor.

ANIMATION 9.1

reticular cells (FRCs) and follicular dendritic cells (FDCs) that induce the development of high endothelial venules (HEVs) and produce new chemokines (**CCL21** and **CCL19**) that recruit additional LTi cells as well as dendritic-cell precursors and lymphocytes to these sites (**Fig. 9.2**). Completion of lymphoid tissue development follows the recruitment of B cells, which provide both LTs and TNF-α required for the differentiation of FDCs, which in turn promote the development of B-cell follicles (**Fig. 9.3**). The normal development of the white pulp of the spleen also depends on lymphotoxins and TNF-α.

A critical signal for the differentiation of stromal organizer cells in all developing secondary lymphoid tissues, including lymph nodes, the splenic white pulp, and Peyer's patches, is delivered to mesenchymal cells by the LT-β receptor (see Fig. 9.3). Although this receptor can bind two different ligands—a membrane-bound heterotrimer consisting of one soluble molecule of LT-α that is anchored by two membrane-bound molecules of LT-β (that is, LT-$\alpha_1\beta_2$) and LIGHT—for most lymphoid tissues LT-$\alpha_1\beta_2$ is nonredundant. Accordingly, mice deficient for LT-β receptor, LT-α, or LT-β fail to develop most lymph nodes. An exception is the lymph nodes that drain mucosal tissues—cervical and mesenteric lymph nodes, and possibly lumbar and sacral lymph nodes (see Chapter 12), development of which is absent in both LT-β receptor–deficient mice and LT-α–deficient mice, but not LT-β–deficient mice, suggesting that an alternative ligand for LT-β receptor (possibly LIGHT) can compensate in the face of LT-β deficiency. In addition to lymphotoxins, TNF-α is required for the normal development of lymphoid tissues because of its co-requirement for the development of FDCs that are required to organize B-cell zones; FDCs are lacking in mice deficient for either TNF-α or its receptor TNFR-I (see Fig. 9.3). These mice do have lymph nodes and Peyer's patches, because they express LTs, but these structures lack FDCs and thus B-cell follicles.

		Effects seen in receptor- or ligand-knockout mice				
Receptor	Ligands	Spleen	Peripheral lymph node	Mesenteric lymph node	Peyer's patch	Follicular dendritic cells
LT-β receptor	LT-α₁β₂ LIGHT	Distorted architecture No marginal zones	Absent in LT-β receptor and LT-β KO Present in LIGHT KO	Absent in LT-β receptor KO Present in LT-β KO	Absent	Absent
TNFR-I	TNF-α LT-α₃	Distorted architecture	Absent in LT-α KO Present in TNF-α and TNFR-I KO	Absent in LT-α KO Present in TNF-α and TNFR-I KO	Absent in LT-α KO Reduced in TNF-α and TNFR-I KO	Absent

Fig. 9.3 The role of TNF family members in the development of secondary lymphoid organs. The role of TNF family members in the development of secondary lymphoid organs has been deduced mainly from the study of knockout (KO) mice deficient in certain TNF family receptors or their ligands. The defects are organized here with respect to the two main receptors, TNFR-I and the LT-β receptor, and selected members of their ligands, TNF-α and the lymphotoxins (LTs). Note that each of these receptors can bind multiple ligands, but the loss of distinct ligands can lead to different phenotypes, as indicated in the figure. This is due to the ability of the different ligands to bind different sets of receptors (not shown). The LT-α protein chain contributes to two distinct ligands, the LT-α₃ trimer and the LT-α₁β₂ heterotrimer, each of which acts through a distinct receptor. In general, signaling through the LT-β receptor is required for lymph-node and follicular dendritic cell (FDC) development and for normal splenic architecture, whereas signaling through TNFR-I is also required for FDCs and normal splenic architecture but not for lymph-node development.

Because LT-β is also required for FDC development, mice deficient for LT-β or the LT-β receptor lack normal FDCs in the spleen and any residual lymph nodes. Administration of the appropriate LT to adult mice deficient in these molecules does not restore development of lymph nodes or Peyer's patches, indicating that there are critical developmental periods during which these cytokines act to induce the development of these lymphoid tissues.

9-3 T-cell entry into lymphoid tissues occurs across specialized small blood vessels and is mediated by the sequential actions of adhesion molecules and chemokine receptors.

Circulating T and B cells enter developing and mature secondary lymphoid tissues from the blood by a common route but are then directed into their respective compartments under the control of distinct chemokines that are produced by stromal cells resident in the T- and B-cell zones. Entry of all lymphocytes into lymph nodes and mucosal lymphoid tissues from blood occurs across high endothelial venules (HEVs), through cell–cell interactions that are not antigen-specific but are governed by cell-adhesion molecules. The spleen is the exception, as entry into the white pulp is via the marginal sinus, not HEVs (see Fig. 9.1). Here we will discuss lymphocyte entry of T cells into lymph nodes and mucosal lymphoid tissues. The dynamics of B-cell trafficking will be discussed further in Chapter 10.

The process of T-cell entry into lymphoid tissues from blood is highly efficient and is orchestrated in a manner similar to the recruitment of circulating leukocytes to inflamed tissues (see Section 3-19 and Fig. 3.30): initial tethering and rolling along the endothelial surface of HEVs via selectin–addressin interactions; activation of integrins by chemokines that decorate the endothelial-cell surface; firm adhesion of the T cell to the endothelial surface; and transmigration, or diapedesis, across the endothelial layer into the paracortical areas, or T-cell zones (**Fig. 9.4**).

The selectins are important for guiding lymphocytes to particular tissues, a phenomenon known as **homing**. In the case of naive T cells, this process is mediated by **L-selectin (CD62L)**, which serves as an important marker for these cells and others that circulate through T-cell zones of

Leukocyte Adhesion Deficiency

ANIMATION 9.2

| Circulating lymphocyte enters a high endothelial venule in the lymph node | Binding of L-selectin to GlyCAM-1 and CD34 allows rolling interaction | LFA-1 is activated by CCR7 signaling in response to CCL21 or CCL19 bound to endothelial surface | Activated LFA-1 binds tightly to ICAM-1 | Lymphocyte crosses the endothelium and enters the lymph node via diapedesis |

Fig. 9.4 Lymphocytes in circulation in blood enter lymph nodes by crossing the walls of high endothelial venules in stages that involve the activity of adhesion molecules, chemokines, and chemokine receptors. T cells and B cells enter lymph nodes via sequential interactions with specialized endothelium of high endothelial venules (HEVs). Shown here is entry of a naive T cell. The first step is the binding of L-selectin on the T cell to sulfated carbohydrates (sulfated sialyl-Lewis^X) of GlyCAM-1 and CD34, vascular addressins that are expressed on the endothelium of the HEV. This induces rolling of the T cell on endothelial-cell surfaces. Chemokines produced by fibroblast reticular cells (FRCs) in the T-cell zones of the lymphoid tissue (CCL21 and CCL19) or by the endothelial cells themselves (CCL21) are bound to a proteoglycan matrix on the HEV surface and are recognized by chemokine receptors on the rolling T cell, leading to activation of LFA-1. This induces both increased affinity of LFA-1 and its clustering on the T-cell surface to increase overall avidity, causing the T cell to bind tightly to ICAM-1 and arrest on the endothelial cell, which is followed by migration across the endothelium between adjacent endothelial cells, or diapedesis. As in the case of neutrophil migration (see Fig. 3.30), matrix metalloproteinases on the lymphocyte surface (not shown) enable the lymphocyte to penetrate the basement membrane under the endothelium so it can crawl into the surrounding T-cell zone in the paracortex of the lymph node along the chemokine gradient.

secondary lymphoid organs (**Fig. 9.5**). As we will discuss later, L-selectin is also expressed by regulatory T cells, as well as a subset of memory T cells such that they retain a recirculatory pattern similar to that of naive T cells. The exit of naive lymphocytes from the blood is initiated by weak attachment to the wall of the HEV that results in the rolling of the cell along the endothelial surface (see Fig. 9.4). Selectins are cell-surface molecules with a common core structure and are distinguished by the presence of different lectin-like domains in their extracellular portion. The lectin domains bind particular sugar groups, and each selectin binds to a specific cell-surface carbohydrate structure. L-selectin binds to the carbohydrate moiety— sulfated sialyl-Lewis^X—of mucin-like molecules called vascular addressins, which are expressed on the surface of the endothelial cells of the specialized venules in lymphoid organs. Two of these addressins, CD34 and GlyCAM-1 (see Fig. 9.5, upper left panel), are expressed on high endothelial venules in lymph nodes. A third addressin, mucosal addressin cell-adhesion molecule-1 (**MadCAM-1**), is expressed on endothelium in mucosae and the marginal sinus of the spleen and guides lymphocyte entry into mucosal lymphoid tissue, such as the Peyer's patches in the gut, and the white pulp of the spleen (see Fig. 9.5, upper right panel).

Through the process of rolling on the luminal surface of the HEV endothelium, the T cell is able to survey the surface of endothelial cells for chemokines that attract them into T-cell zones of lymphoid tissues (see Fig. 9.4). The chemokines CCL19, produced by FRCs, and CCL21, produced by both FRCs and HEV cells, are unique in directing migration into T-cell zones. Both chemokines are ligands for the chemokine receptor **CCR7**, which is expressed by naive T cells; mice that lack CCR7 do not form normal T-cell zones and have impaired primary immune responses. Like L-selectin, CCR7 is also expressed by regulatory T cells and a subset of memory T cells that recirculate through T-cell zones of secondary lymphoid organs. As with leukocyte migration to other tissue sites (see Section 3-18), recognition of chemokines on the endothelial surface of the HEV by CCR7 induces signaling that activates the integrin **LFA-1** (see Section 3-2 and Fig. 7.25), increasing affinity for its two ligands, ICAM-2 and ICAM-1 (Fig. 9.5 and **Fig. 9.6**). At homeostasis, ICAM-1 is expressed only on endothelial cells of the HEV in secondary lymphoid tissues, whereas ICAM-2 is constitutively expressed on all endothelial cells. The organization of LFA-1 molecules in the lymphocyte membrane is also altered by chemokine stimulation, such that they become

Fig. 9.5 Different selectins and integrins are used by lymphocytes to enter different lymphoid tissues. L-selectin is expressed on naive T cells and recognizes carbohydrate motifs. Its binds to sulfated sialyl-Lewis^X moieties on the vascular addressins CD34 and GlyCAM-1, which are expressed on the luminal surface of HEV endothelial cells (top left panel). CD34 is expressed in appropriately glycosylated form only on HEV cells, although it is found in other forms on other endothelial cells; GlyCAM-1 is expressed only on HEV cells. The addressin MAdCAM-1 is expressed on mucosal endothelium and guides lymphocytes to mucosal lymphoid tissue (top right panel). The configuration shown represents mouse MAdCAM-1, which contains an IgA-like domain closest to the cell membrane; human MAdCAM-1 has an elongated mucin-like domain and lacks the IgA-like domain. Integrins are heterodimeric proteins containing a β chain, which defines the class of integrin, and an α chain, which defines the different integrins within a class. The α chain is larger than the β chain and contains binding sites for divalent cations that may be important in signaling. LFA-1 (integrin $\alpha_L\beta_2$) is expressed on all leukocytes (bottom left panel). It binds ICAMs and is important in cell migration into lymph nodes. Integrin $\alpha_4\beta_7$ (also known as lymphocyte Peyer's patch adhesion molecule, or LPAM-1) is expressed by a subset of naive T cells and contributes to lymphocyte entry into mucosal lymphoid tissues and the white pulp of the spleen by supporting adhesive interactions with the vascular addressin MAdCAM-1 (bottom right panel).

Fig. 9.6 Activation of LFA-1 by chemokine signaling on naive T cells occurs via G-protein signaling. As a naive T cell rolls on HEV endothelium, CCR7 expressed on the T cell detects the chemokines CCL21 and CCL19 that are bound to proteoglycans on the surface of endothelial cells. Binding of CCL21 or CCL19 by CCR7 induces its association with the G-protein complex (left panel), inducing exchange of GDP for GTP and leading to its dissociation into the G_α and $G_\beta G_\gamma$ subunits, the latter of which leads to activation of the small GTPase Rap1 (middle panel). GTP-bound Rap1 leads to a conformational change in LFA-1, inducing its transition from a low-affinity state to a high-affinity state and its clustering on the T-cell surface (right panel), which combine to greatly increase the avidity of LFA-1 for the ICAM ligands that are displayed on the HEV surface.

concentrated into microclusters in areas of cell–cell contact on the rolling lymphocyte (see Fig. 9.6). Together with the affinity change in LFA-1, this produces higher avidity, and thus stronger binding, of LFA-1 to ICAM-1 or ICAM-2, which arrests the T cell on the endothelial surface and enables it to cross the HEV and enter the lymphoid tissue. In the mucosal lymphoid tissues and spleen, some naive and effector T cells use another integrin heterodimer, $\alpha_4\beta_7$, for adhesion to MadCAM-1 and arrest of the rolling T cell on the vascular endothelium.

9-4 T cells are highly motile within T-cell zones as they survey dendritic cells for cognate antigen.

Once naive T cells have entered the T-cell zone across HEVs, CCR7 directs their continued locomotion as they migrate along the three-dimensional network created by the same fibroblast reticular cells (FRCs) that produce CCL19 and CCL21 (**Fig. 9.7**). These chemokines bind to proteoglycans in the extracellular matrix of channels formed and lined by FRCs, through which the T cells crawl as they search for cognate antigen. As we will see in Section 9-6, because dendritic cells activated in the tissues by antigen uptake also express CCR7, they co-localize to the same channels within the FRC network in T-cell zones, thereby facilitating interactions with T cells that are transmigrating there.

Compared to T cells, the dendritic cells (DCs) that migrate into T-cell zones are relatively immobile. Yet, because they project long dendrites, they provide tremendous surface area for contact with T cells as the T cells scan their surfaces for specific peptide:MHC complexes. In view of the high motility of T cells (about two cell diameters per minute), their high density within the FRC network, and the extensive projections of DCs, it is estimated that a given T cell contacts ~100 DCs per hour. With a dwell time of up to 24 hours within a given lymphoid tissue, it is therefore possible for a given T cell to survey thousands of DCs per day—essentially every DC that might bear the T cell's cognate antigen during its transit of a T-cell zone. Moreover, by some estimates the T-cell

Fig. 9.7 Fibroblast reticular cells form a network in the T-cell zones of lymphoid tissues that facilitates interactions of naive T cells and dendritic cells. Fibroblast reticular cells (FRCs) within the T-cell zones of secondary lymphoid organs produce an extracellular matrix containing reticulin and collagen fibrils that form a meshwork, referred to as lymphoid conduits, that is invested by a continuous layer of FRCs. The conduits extend from the floor of the subcapsular sinus throughout the paracortex of lymph nodes and serve as a scaffold for the network of FRCs as well as a conduction system to deliver free antigens that enter the lymph node via afferent lymphatics to dendritic cells in T-cell zones. The surfaces of the sinusoid-like spaces created by the FRC networks are decorated with CCL21 and CCL19 produced by the FRCs and serve as a 'highway system' along which CCR7-bearing T cells navigate in search of cognate antigen on dendritic cells, which are also attracted to these sites by the same chemokines. A similar network (not shown) is formed by follicular dendritic cells (FDCs) in B-cell follicles and is decorated with the B-cell chemoattractant, CXCL13.

Fig. 9.8 Naive T cells encounter antigen during their recirculation through secondary lymphoid organs. Naive T cells recirculate through secondary lymphoid organs, such as a lymph node (shown here), entering from the arterial blood via the specialized vascular endothelium of high endothelial venules (HEVs). Entry into the lymph node is regulated by chemokines (not shown) that direct the T cells' migration through the HEV wall and into the paracortical areas, where the T cells encounter mature dendritic cells (top panel). Those T cells shown in green do not encounter their specific antigen; they receive a survival signal through their interaction with self peptide:self MHC complexes and IL-7, and leave the lymph node through the lymphatics to return to the circulation (second panel). T cells shown in blue encounter their specific antigen on the surface of mature dendritic cells; they lose their ability to exit from the node and become activated to proliferate and to differentiate into effector T cells (third panel). After several days, these antigen-specific effector T cells regain the expression of receptors needed to exit from the node, leave via the efferent lymphatics, and enter the circulation in greatly increased numbers (bottom panel).

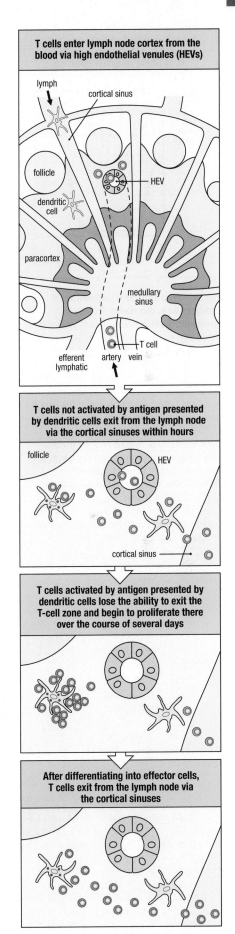

receptor can be activated by recognition of just a single antigenic peptide:MHC complex. In view of their high rates of recirculation to, and concentration in, T-cell zones along with incoming dendritic cells, and the high efficiency with which T cells can scan DCs for their cognate peptide:MHC complex, each T cell has a high probability of encountering antigen derived from a pathogen that has set up an infection anywhere in the body.

If naive T cells do not encounter their specific antigen during their transit through a T-cell zone, they exit from the lymphoid organ and reenter the bloodstream, where they continue to recirculate—returning to the blood via the efferent lymphatics in the case of lymph nodes or MALT or directly back to blood in the spleen, which has no lymphatics (**Fig. 9.8**; see also Fig. 9.1). If, however, a naive T cell recognizes its specific antigen on the surface of an activated dendritic cell, its locomotion is arrested, and it is retained much longer in the T-cell zone where it proliferates for several days, undergoing a remarkable number of cell divisions that gives rise to effector T cells and memory cells of identical antigenic specificity that vastly outnumber their naive precursors, as we will discuss further in Section 9-9. At the end of this period, most effector T cells exit the lymphoid organ and reenter the blood-stream, through which they migrate to the sites of infection to coordinate pathogen clearance with innate immune cells (see Chapter 11), whereas others interact with B cells and migrate instead to B-cell zones, where they participate in the germinal center response to support antibody production (see Chapter 10).

As indicated above, the efficiency with which T cells screen antigen-presenting cells in lymph nodes is very high, as can be seen by the rapid trapping of antigen-specific T cells in a single lymph node containing antigen; within 48 hours of antigen delivery, nearly all antigen-specific T cells in the body can be trapped in the lymph node draining a site of infection (**Fig. 9.9**). In addition to the high efficiency of T-cell surveillance of the T-cell zone for antigen, local inflammation that accompanies pathogen penetration of innate defenses stimulates a marked increase in the influx, and a decrease in efflux, of lymphocytes into and out of the involved lymph node. This is the basis for local lymph node swelling that typically accompanies infection. Such efficiency is crucial for the initiation of an adaptive immune response, as only one naive T cell out of ~10^6, or ~100 of each clonal precursor per animal (in mice), is likely to be specific for a particular antigenic epitope, and adaptive immunity depends on the activation, differentiation, and expansion of these rare cells to adequately deal with an infection.

9-5 The exit of T cells from T-cell zones of lymphoid tissues is controlled by a chemotactic lipid.

T cells exit from a lymph node via the cortical sinuses, which lead into the medullary sinus and then the efferent lymphatic vessel. The egress of T cells from secondary lymphoid organs involves the phospholipid molecule

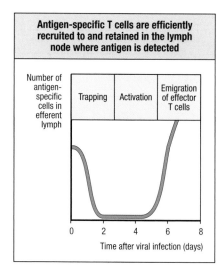

Antigen-specific T cells are efficiently recruited to and retained in the lymph node where antigen is detected

Fig. 9.9 Trapping and activation of antigen-specific naive T cells in lymphoid tissue. Naive T cells entering the lymph node from the blood encounter antigen-presenting dendritic cells in T-cell zones. T cells that recognize their specific antigen bind stably to the dendritic cells and are activated through their T-cell receptors, resulting in their retention within the lymph node as they develop into effector T cells. By 3–6 days after their activation and differentiation, activated effector T cells begin leaving the lymph node in large numbers via the efferent lymphatics. Lymphocyte recirculation and recognition are so effective that all the naive T cells in the peripheral circulation specific for a particular antigen can be trapped by that antigen in one node within 2 days.

sphingosine 1-phosphate (S1P) (**Fig. 9.10**). S1P has chemotactic activity and signaling properties similar to those of chemokines, in that the receptors for S1P are G protein–coupled receptors (GPCRs). S1P is constitutively produced by endothelial cells lining lymphatic vessels and the cortical and medullary sinuses of lymph nodes and is actively degraded by an enzyme, S1P lyase, that is produced in the lymphoid tissue. A concentration gradient of S1P is therefore established between the T-cell zones and the lymph.

Naive T cells recently arrived from the blood express low levels of the S1P receptor, **S1PR1**, due to its internalization and down-regulation by S1P present in blood. During the hours required for reexpression of the receptor, naive T cells are able to migrate within T-cell zones without sensing the S1P gradient. The up-regulation of S1PR1 by naive T cells that fail to recognize antigen activates their migration to the cortical and medullary sinuses and out the efferent lymphatic vessel, ultimately returning them to the blood via the thoracic duct (see Section 1–16).

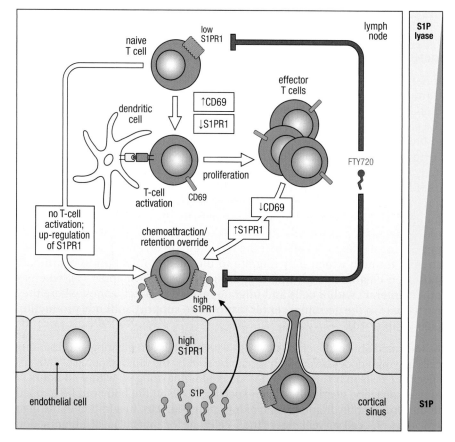

Fig. 9.10 The egress of lymphocytes from lymphoid tissue is mediated by a sphingosine 1-phosphate gradient. The level of sphingosine 1-phosphate (S1P) within lymphoid tissue is low compared with that in blood and lymph, due to the production by stromal cells within T-cell zones of the enzyme S1P lyase, which degrades S1P. This creates an S1P gradient (indicated by shading), such that S1P levels are low in T-cell zones and high in cortical sinuses and efferent lymphatics. The sphingosine 1-phosphate receptor 1 (S1PR1), which is expressed by naive T cells, is present at low levels on the surface of naive T cells that have recently entered T-cell zones, because the high levels of S1P in blood down-regulate the receptor. In the absence of antigen recognition, S1PR1 surface expression on the naive T-cell surface increases, allowing the cell to sense the S1P gradient, which directs its egress from the T-cell zones into a cortical sinus and thus into the efferent lymphatic vessel. T cells activated by an antigen-expressing dendritic cell up-regulate CD69, which acts to internalize S1PR1 expression and cause retention in the T-cell zone. Antigen-activated T cells eventually reexpress S1PR1 as CD69 expression decreases and egress from the lymph node along the S1P gradient. FTY720, an immunomodulatory molecule that cannot be inactivated by S1P lyase, inhibits T-cell egression by down-modulating expression of S1PR1 by ligand-induced internalization within the lymph node. FTY720 may also activate S1PR1-mediated closure of egress ports on the sinusoidal endothelium by enhancing junctional contacts (not shown).

T cells activated by antigen in lymphoid organs undergo more sustained down-regulation of S1PR1 that persists for several days, during clonal expansion and effector T-cell differentiation. This is due to actions of **CD69**, a surface protein induced within a few hours of T-cell receptor signaling that acts to internalize S1PR1. During this period, activated T cells cannot respond to the S1P gradient and do not exit the lymphoid organ. After several days of proliferation and effector T-cell differentiation, as T-cell activation wanes, CD69 expression decreases and S1PR1 reappears on the surface of effector T cells, allowing the effector T cells to migrate out of the lymphoid tissue in response to the S1P gradient.

Regulation of the exit of both naive and effector lymphocytes from secondary lymphoid organs by S1P is the basis for a new kind of potential immunosuppressive drug, FTY720 (fingolimod). FTY720 inhibits immune responses by preventing lymphocytes from returning to the circulation, thereby sequestering them in lymphoid tissues and causing rapid onset of lymphopenia (a lack of lymphocytes in the blood). *In vivo*, FTY720 becomes phosphorylated and mimics S1P and acts as an agonist for S1P receptors. Phosphorylated FTY720 is not degraded by S1P lyase and therefore causes chronic inactivation and down-regulation of S1P receptors, leading to trapping of T cells in secondary lymphoid organs. FTY720 may also inhibit lymphocyte exit by effects on lymphatic endothelial cells that increase tight junction formation and close exit portals normally used by T cells.

ANIMATION 9.3

9-6 Activation of conventional dendritic cells stimulates their maturation and migration to T-cell zones to induce naive T-cell activation.

Dendritic cells (DCs) are central players that bridge innate and adaptive immunity; DCs are sentinel cells that sense pathogens as part of the innate immune system and activate naive T-cell responses to initiate adaptive immunity. Like DCs, macrophages and B cells express MHC class II molecules and can process and present antigen to T cells—hence they are referred to collectively as 'professional' antigen-presenting cells (APCs) (**Fig. 9.11**).

	Dendritic cells	**Macrophages**	**B cells**
Antigen uptake	+++ Macropinocytosis and phagocytosis by tissue dendritic cells	+++ Macropinocytosis +++ Phagocytosis	Antigen-specific receptor (Ig) ++++
MHC expression	Low on immature dendritic cells High on dendritic cells in lymphoid tissues	Inducible by bacteria and cytokines – to +++	Constitutive Increases on activation +++ to ++++
Co-stimulation delivery	Constitutive by mature, nonphagocytic lymphoid dendritic cells ++++	Inducible – to +++	Inducible – to +++
Location	Ubiquitous throughout the body	Lymphoid tissue Connective tissue Body cavities	Lymphoid tissue Peripheral blood
Effect	Results in activation of naive T cells	Results in activation of macrophages by effector and memory T cells	Results in delivery of help to B cell by T$_{FH}$ cells

Fig. 9.11 The properties of the various antigen-presenting cells (APCs). Dendritic cells, macrophages, and B cells are the main cell types involved in the presentation of foreign antigens to T cells. These cells vary in their means of antigen uptake, MHC class II expression, co-stimulator expression, the type of antigen they present effectively, their locations in the body, and their surface adhesion molecules (not shown). Antigen presentation by dendritic cells is primarily involved in activating naive T cells for expansion and differentiation. Macrophages present antigen primarily to receive help from effector and memory T cells in the form of cytokines or surface molecules that enhance their killing of phagocytosed microbes, whereas B cells present antigen to TFH cells to recruit their help for germinal center responses that produce class-switched, high-affinity antibodies. The degree of activity for each of the indicated functions is indicated on an arbitrary scale from '–' (no activity) to '++++' (highest activity).

Immature conventional dendritic cells resident in tissues encounter pathogens and are activated by MAMPs

TLR signaling induces expression of CCR7 and enhances processing of pathogen-derived antigens and down-regulation of non-CCR7 chemokine receptors and antigen-uptake receptors

CCR7 directs migration of dendritic cells into the lymph node. This is associated with reduced synthesis of new MHC molecules and expression of co-stimulatory molecules

Activated dendritic cell in T-cell zone primes naive T cells

Fig. 9.12 Conventional dendritic cells in nonlymphoid tissues undergo sequential steps of antigen uptake, migration, and maturation to deliver antigens to T cells in lymphoid tissues. See text for details.

However, DCs appear to be unique in their activation of naive T cells. The delivery of antigen from a site of infection to lymphoid tissue is actively aided by the innate immune response. Following the sensing of a breach of innate barrier defenses by a pathogen, antigen is delivered to secondary lymphoid tissues by two mechanisms: as free antigen carried via draining lymph or by blood; or as cell-associated antigen, carried primarily by DCs that have taken up antigen in tissue sites. One effect of innate immunity is an inflammatory reaction that increases the rate of entry of blood plasma into an infected tissue and thus increases the drainage of extracellular fluid into the lymph, taking with it free, or soluble, antigen that is carried to lymphoid tissues. Even more important for initiation of the adaptive response is the activation of dendritic cells that have taken up particulate and soluble antigens at the site of infection (**Fig. 9.12**).

Although there are two major classes of dendritic cells—**conventional (or classical) dendritic cells (cDCs)** and **plasmacytoid dendritic cells (pDCs)** (**Fig. 9.13**; see also Section 3-1)—the principal antigen-presenting cells tasked with naive T-cell activation are conventional dendritic cells. The major function of cDCs is to ingest and degrade protein antigens and present them as peptides bound to MHC class I or MHC class II molecules (see Chapter 6). There are two major subsets of conventional dendritic cells, **cDC1** and **cDC2**, which are specialized for the presentation of antigens derived from different classes of pathogen, as will be discussed in detail in the next section. Both subsets of cDCs are most abundant in non-lymphoid tissues, particularly at barrier tissue sites, such as the intestines, lung, and skin, where they are strategically positioned in close contact with surface epithelia through which most pathogens enter. They are also present in solid organs such as the heart and kidneys. Conventional dendritic cells that reside in these sites at steady state are often referred to as **nonlymphoid tissue (NLT)-resident (or migratory) cDCs**; because naive T cells do not circulate to nonlymphoid tissues, these cDCs must migrate to T-cell zones to activate them. Conventional dendritic cells also populate secondary lymphoid organs, where they can handle antigens that are delivered directly to the lymphoid tissue, whether introduced across the epithelial barrier to mucosa-associated lymphoid tissue, via the lymph to

Fig. 9.13 Conventional and plasmacytoid dendritic cells have different roles in the immune response. Mature conventional dendritic cells (left panel) are primarily concerned with the activation of naive T cells. There are several subsets of conventional dendritic cells, but these all process antigen efficiently, and when they are mature they express MHC proteins and co-stimulatory molecules for priming naive T cells. Immature dendritic cells lack many of the cell-surface molecules shown here but have numerous surface receptors that recognize pathogen molecules, including most of the Toll-like receptors (TLRs) and receptors that facilitate antigen uptake. Plasmacytoid dendritic cells (right panel) are sentinels primarily for viral infections and secrete large amounts of type I interferons. This category of dendritic cell is thought to play a minimal role in priming naive T cells, but they express the intracellular receptors TLR-7 and TLR-9 for sensing viral infections.

lymph nodes, or via the bloodstream to the spleen. These **lymphoid tissue (LT)-resident cDCs** are also able to receive antigen from migratory cDCs in some settings.

In accord with their primacy as APCs for naive T-cell activation, all cDCs are highly active at the uptake and processing of antigen, both by receptor-mediated phagocytosis and by macropinocytosis (see Sections 3-1 and 6-1). However, cDCs at all tissue sites express only low levels of co-stimulatory molecules at steady state and are often referred to as **immature cDCs**, reflecting their inability to activate naive T cells. It is only after their recognition of microbial-associated molecular patterns or damage-associated molecular patterns (MAMPs or DAMPs) that immature cDCs are activated to become **mature cDCs** and express the high levels of co-stimulatory molecules required to activate naive T cells (Fig. 9.13 and **Fig. 9.14**). DC maturation can be enhanced, but not replaced, by stimulation with inflammatory cytokines, such as TNF and IL-1. Activated cDCs alter their integrin and

Dendritic cells in peripheral tissues

Dendritic cells in the lymphatic circulation

Dendritic cells in lymphoid tissues

Fig. 9.14 Dendritic cells in different stages of activation and migration. The panels show fluorescence micrographs of dendritic cells stained for MHC class II molecules in green and for a lysosomal protein in red. Unactivated dendritic cells (top panel) have many long processes, or dendrites, from which the cells get their name. The cell bodies are difficult to distinguish in this low-power image, but the cells contain many endocytic vesicles that stain both for MHC class II molecules and for the lysosomal protein; when these two colors overlap they give rise to a yellow fluorescence, as shown here. Activated dendritic cells leave the tissues to migrate through the lymphatics to secondary lymphoid tissues. During this migration their morphology changes. The dendritic cells stop phagocytosing antigen, and staining for the lysosomal protein is beginning to be distinct from that for MHC class II molecules (center panel). The dendritic cell now has many folds of membrane, which gave these cells their original name of 'veil' cells. Finally, in the lymph nodes, dendritic cells express high levels of peptide:MHC complexes and co-stimulatory molecules and are very good at stimulating naive CD4 and naive CD8 T cells. At this stage, the activated dendritic cells do not phagocytose, and the red staining of the lysosomal protein is quite distinct from the green-stained MHC class II molecules displayed at high density on many dendritic processes (bottom panel).

chemokine receptor expression to enable them to leave their initial tissue of residence to traffic to T-cell zones of secondary lymphoid tissues. A remarkable diversity of receptors expressed by immature DCs underlies their recognition of a broad range of extracellular and intracellular signals that induce their activation and maturation and help to define distinct functions of cDC subsets (see Sections 3-1 and 6-5).

Between them, immature cDC1 and cDC2 cells express all members of the TLR family except for TLR-8, which is functionally redundant with TLR-7 (see Fig. 3.10). Thus, cDCs can be activated effectively by any TLR ligand and, therefore, by nearly any pathogen. In addition to TLRs, several other pattern-recognition receptors (PRRs) that are used by dendritic cells to take up pathogens also provide maturation signals. This includes an array of members of the C-type lectin family of receptors, which recognize a diversity of carbohydrates on microbes to facilitate their uptake. Examples include the lectin **DC-SIGN**, which binds mannose and fucose residues present on a wide range of pathogens; DEC 205; and **Dectin-1**, which recognizes β-(1,3)-linked glucans found in fungal cell walls (see Section 3-1). Other receptors that enhance pathogen binding, such as receptors for complement or phagocytic receptors such as the mannose receptor, may also contribute to dendritic-cell activation, in addition to augmenting phagocytosis. Other extracellular antigens are taken up nonspecifically by the process of **macropinocytosis**, in which large volumes of surrounding fluid are engulfed. In this way, microbes that have evolved strategies to escape recognition by phagocytic receptors, such as bacteria with thick polysaccharide capsules, can be ingested. The versatility in pathways for antigen uptake enables dendritic cells to present antigens from virtually any type of microbe, including fungi, parasites, viruses, and bacteria (**Fig. 9.15**).

A critical result of PRR and inflammatory cytokine signaling is significant alteration in the chemokine receptors and integrins expressed by dendritic cells that induces their mobilization from sites of antigen capture to T-cell zones—whether within the lymphoid tissue in which they reside in

Routes of antigen processing and presentation by dendritic cells				
Receptor-mediated phagocytosis	**Macropinocytosis**	**Viral infection**	**Cross-presentation after phagocytic or macropinocytic uptake**	**Transfer from incoming dendritic cell to resident dendritic cell**
Type of pathogen presented: Extracellular bacteria, fungi	Extracellular bacteria, soluble antigens, virus particles	Viruses	Viruses	Viruses
MHC molecules loaded: MHC class II	MHC class II	MHC class I	MHC class I	MHC class I, MHC class II
Type of naive T cell activated: CD4 T cells	CD4 T cells	CD8 T cells	CD8 T cells	CD8 T cells, CD4 T cells

Fig. 9.15 The different routes by which dendritic cells can take up, process, and present protein antigens. Uptake of antigens into the endocytic system, either by receptor-mediated phagocytosis or by macropinocytosis, is considered the major route for delivering peptides to MHC class II molecules for presentation to CD4 T cells (first two panels). Production of antigens in the cytosol, for example, as a result of viral infection, is thought to be the major route for delivering peptides to MHC class I molecules for presentation to CD8 T cells (third panel). It is possible, however, for exogenous antigens taken into the endocytic pathway to be delivered into the cytosol for eventual delivery to MHC class I molecules for presentation to CD8 T cells, a process called cross-presentation (fourth panel). Finally, antigens can be transmitted from one APC to another, whether for presentation to CD8 or CD4 T cells (fifth panel).

the case of LT-resident cDCs or within a draining lymph node in the case of migratory cDCs. PRR signaling induces expression of CCR7, which is required for activated cDCs to sense and migrate along gradients of CCL19 and CCL21—the same chemokines used by naive T cells to home to T-cell zones. CCL19 and CCL21 immobilized on the lymphatic endothelium allow migratory cDCs to enter the afferent lymphatics and navigate through the lymphatics to T-cell zones. Whereas T cells must cross the wall of high endothelial venules to leave the blood and reach the T-cell zones, dendritic cells entering via the afferent lymphatics migrate into T-cell zones via the floor of the subcapsular sinus. In addition to the *de novo* expression of CCR7, activated cDCs must down-modulate their expression of chemokine receptors that act to retain them in their tissue of residence. Although details of how this occurs are not fully understood, desensitization of these receptors by enhanced local expression of the chemokines they bind may play a role.

Signaling through CCR7 not only induces the migration of cDCs into T-cell zones, but, together with other activating signals such as type I interferons, TNF, and IL-1, it may also contribute to their enhanced antigen-presenting function (see Fig. 9.13). By the time activated dendritic cells arrive within T-cell zones, they are no longer able to engulf antigens by phagocytosis or macropinocytosis. They also express high levels of the two main co-stimulatory molecules: the structurally related transmembrane glycoproteins B7.1 (CD80) and B7.2 (CD86), which deliver co-stimulatory signals by interacting with CD28 expressed on naive T cells (see Section 7-22). Moreover, as discussed in Section 6-9, activated cDCs enhance the surface expression of pathogenic peptide:MHC class II complexes by increasing the longevity of newly loaded MHC class II molecules coincident with activation-induced down-regulation of MARCH-1 E3 ligase, which otherwise promotes the internalization and degradation of surface peptide:MHC class II complexes (see Section 6-9). DC activation also shuts off the transcriptional regulator CIITA, thereby preventing new expression of MHC class II molecules. In combination, these actions enable mature cDCs to present peptide:MHC class II complexes loaded at the time of pathogen uptake for very extended periods of time. Loss of the MARCH-1 E3 ligase similarly extends the life span of surface-expressed CD86 (B7.2). Activated dendritic cells also secrete the chemokine CCL19 and express high levels of adhesion molecules, which may enhance their recruitment of, and binding to, naive T cells. Together, these properties of mature cDCs markedly increase the opportunity for pathogen-derived antigens to be recognized by incoming naive T cells.

Despite their enhanced presentation of pathogen-derived peptide antigens, activated dendritic cells also present self peptides. Although the presence of self-peptide:MHC complexes could present a problem for the maintenance of self-tolerance, several mechanisms normally prevent these self peptides from inducing an immune response. First, the T-cell receptor repertoire has largely been purged of receptors that recognize self peptides during thymic development (see Chapter 8), so that T-cell responses against most ubiquitous self antigens are avoided. This is referred to as **central tolerance**. In addition, dendritic cells in the lymphoid tissues that have not been activated by infection will bear self-peptide:MHC complexes on their surface, derived from the breakdown of their own proteins and tissue proteins present in the extracellular fluid. Because these cells do not express the appropriate co-stimulatory molecules, however, they do not have the same capacity to activate naive T cells as do activated dendritic cells. Although the details remain unclear, the presentation of self peptides by LT-resident, immature dendritic cells may induce an alternative program of activation in naive T cells that favors immune regulation and T-cell deletion rather than immune activation (see also Section 9-17).

The induction of co-stimulatory activity in antigen-presenting cells by common microbial constituents is believed to allow the immune system to distinguish antigens borne by infectious agents from antigens associated with innocuous proteins, including self proteins. Indeed, many foreign proteins do not induce an immune response when injected on their own because they fail to induce co-stimulatory activity in antigen-presenting cells. When such protein antigens are mixed with bacteria, however, they become immunogenic, because the bacteria induce the essential co-stimulatory activity in cells that ingest the protein. Bacteria or bacterial components used in this way are known as **adjuvants** (see Appendix I, Section A-1). We will see in Chapter 15 how self proteins mixed with bacterial adjuvants can induce autoimmune disease, illustrating the crucial importance of the regulation of co-stimulatory activity in the discrimination of self from nonself.

9-7 Subsets of conventional dendritic cells are specialized for different modes of antigen presentation.

Conventional dendritic cells are composed of two major subsets—cDC1 and cDC2—that are present in all tissues and share the same general properties discussed in the past section. However, cDC1 and cDC2 cells have distinct ontogeny and distinct roles for priming different types of naive T cells in response to different types of pathogens, hence the subdivision (**Fig. 9.16**). Although specifics of the functions of cDC subsets are still being defined, it is now apparent that cDC1 cells are specialized for the activation of naive CD8 T cells, which recognize intracellular pathogens that introduce antigens into the cytosol and are processed and loaded onto MHC class I molecules. cDC1 cells are primarily responsible for **cross-priming**; that is, the activation of naive CD8 T cells by **cross-presentation** (see Section 9-13; see also Sections 6-1 and 6-5). For this reason, they are also critical for antitumor immune surveillance, to be discussed further in Chapter 16.

Feature	Conventional DC subset	
	cDC1	**cDC2**
Common surface markers	CD11c MHC class II	CD11c MHC class II
Unique surface markers	XCR1 BDCA-3 CLEC9A	CD11b BDCA-1 Dectin-1
Nonlymphoid tissues (migratory DCs)	CD103 CD24	CD11b CD24 SIRPα CD103*
Lymphoid tissues (LT-resident DCs)	CD8αα CD24	CD4 SIRPα
Key transcription factors	BATF3 IRF8	Notch2 IRF4
TLRs	TLR-3+, various	TLR-3-, various
Cytokines produced	IL-12	IL-23, IL-6, TGF-β
Major functions	Antigen presentation to naive CD8 T cells Cross-presentation	Antigen presentation to naive CD4 T cells
Pathogens	Intracellular	Extracellular

Fig. 9.16 Phenotypic and functional features of type 1 and type 2 conventional dendritic cells. This chart highlights the characteristics of conventional dendritic cell 1 (cDC1) and conventional dendritic cell 2 (cDC2). *CD103 is expressed by a subset of cDC2 cells.

In contrast to cDC1 cells, cDC2 cells appear to be specialized for the presentation of extracellular pathogens whose antigens are delivered via vesicular compartments to be loaded onto MHC class II, and thus activate naive CD4 T cells. However, while details are unclear, some CD4 T cells—particularly those that respond to some intracellular pathogens—may receive their activating signals not on cDC2 cells but on cDC1 cells (see Section 9-13). Both subsets encompass migratory and LT-resident cDCs; both cDC1 and cDC2 cells are arrayed at nearly all of the portals of antigen entry in the body, whether in nonlymphoid or lymphoid tissues. Although there are some differences in the cell-surface markers that distinguish them across species, these subsets appear to be analogous in mice and humans.

While all cDCs express the α integrin **CD11c**, as well as MHC class II and **CD24**, the cDC1 subset is defined by the unique expression of the chemokine receptor **XCR1**, the ligand for which is **XCL1** (lymphotactin), which is produced by activated CD8 T cells and NK cells (see Fig. 9.16). Other cDC1-specific markers include CLEC9A, a member of the C-type lectin receptor family that facilitates uptake of necrotic cells (see Section 6-5), and blood dendritic cell antigen 3 (BDCA-3), the function of which is unclear. cDC1s are also distinguished from cDC2s by their expression of **TLR-3**, the endosomal TLR that recognizes double-stranded RNA (dsRNA). Because dsRNA is an intermediate in the replication of many viruses—including those with DNA or single-stranded RNA (ssRNA) genomes—TLR-3 is an important sensor for products of viral replication in host cells that are damaged by viral infection or killed by cytolytic cells; that is, PAMPs that are linked to pathogens best handled by cross-presentation to CD8 T cells. Type 1 cDCs are also the principal producers of IL-12, which, as we will discuss later, is important for the differentiation of both CD8 T cells and the T_H1 subset of CD4 T cells. cDC1 cells can be further divided by the expression of **CD8αα** and **CD103** (the latter being the $α_E$ component of $α_Eβ_7$ integrin), which generally distinguish cDC1 cells resident in lymphoid tissues and nonlymphoid tissues, respectively.

Cells of the cDC2 subset are the most numerous in secondary lymphoid tissues and are defined by expression of the integrin component **CD11b**, which is also expressed on some macrophages, and BDCA-1. In contrast to cDC1 cells, cDC2 cells lack expression of TLR-3 and produce less IL-12, but appear to be the principal producers of IL-23 and IL-6, which are important for the induction of T_H17 responses, as we will discuss. Type 2 cDCs also appear to be dominant in the induction of T_H2 and T_{FH} cells, albeit by undefined mechanisms. Markers for discriminating LT-resident and migratory cDC2 cells that are comparable to CD8αα and CD103 for cDC1 cells have yet to be defined. Although differences in methods of antigen uptake, phagolysosomal processing, and relative expression of MHC class I and MHC class II have been considered, the mechanistic basis for the subdivision of labor between cDC1 and cDC2 cells remains to be completely defined.

Not all cell-bound antigen delivered to lymphoid tissues arrives via migratory cDCs. Although migratory cDCs are typically the dominant source, antigens taken up by **monocyte-derived DCs (MoDCs)** may also contribute in the response to some pathogens. As their name implies, MoDCs are derived from circulating monocytes that are recruited into inflamed tissues, where they take up antigen that is then delivered to T-cell zones of lymphoid tissues. Although they are poor stimulators of naive T cells, MoDCs are able to transfer antigens to LT-resident cDCs, which in turn activate naive T cells. Moreover, in some cases, such as infections with herpes simplex or influenza viruses, the dendritic cells that migrate to the lymph nodes from peripheral tissues may not be the same cells that finally present antigen to naive T cells. In a herpes simplex infection, for example, dendritic cells residing in the dermis of skin capture antigen and transport it to the draining lymph nodes. There, some antigen is transferred to

Fig. 9.17 Langerhans cells take up antigen in the skin and migrate to the regional lymph nodes, where they can transfer antigen to cDC1 cells to prime CD8 T cells or directly prime CD4 T cells. Langerhans cells (LCs; yellow) are a type of nonlymphoid tissue–resident macrophage with dendritic morphology that resides in the epidermis of the skin. LCs ingest antigen in various ways, including uptake from infected keratinocytes, which are the principal epithelial cells that make up the epidermis (not shown; first panel). After antigen uptake locally, LCs then migrate to the lymph nodes (second panel). There they can transfer their antigen to cDC1 cells (orange; third panel), which, in turn, prime naive CD8 cells, or they can prime CD4 T cells directly (fourth panel).

CD8αα-positive, LT-resident cDCs, which in turn activate naive CD8 T cells. This type of transfer means that antigens from viruses that rapidly kill the dendritic cells they infect can still be presented by uninfected dendritic cells that have been activated via their TLRs to take up the dying dendritic cells and cross-present this material. This may also provide a mechanism to amplify antigen presentation by allowing multiple LT-resident cDCs to present antigen carried by a single migratory DC.

Finally, in rare microenvironments, cDCs are absent. Perhaps the best example is the epidermis of the skin, which normally lacks both cDC1 and cDC2 cells. Here, the initiation of CD8 T-cell responses is dependent on a specialized tissue-resident macrophage, the **Langerhans cell**, for initial uptake and transport of antigen to draining lymph nodes, where it can be transferred to CD8αα-positive, LT-resident cDC1 cells (**Fig. 9.17**). Thus, cross-presentation by LT-resident cDC1 cells is critical for the responses to many antigens imported by Langerhans cells, which are themselves less efficient at CD8 T-cell priming. In contrast, Langerhans cells appear to be the principal APCs for initiation of some CD4 T-cell responses, particularly those of T_H17 cells (see Section 12-24).

Summary.

An adaptive immune response is generated when naive T cells contact activated antigen-presenting cells in the secondary lymphoid organs. These tissues have a specialized architecture that facilitates efficient interaction between circulating lymphocytes and their target antigens. The formation and organization of the secondary lymphoid organs are controlled by proteins of the TNF family and their receptors (TNFRs). Lymphoid tissue inducer (LTi) cells expressing lymphotoxin-α_1b_2 (LT-$\alpha_1\beta_2$) interact with stromal cells expressing the LT-β receptor in the developing embryo to induce chemokine production, which in turn initiates formation of the lymph nodes and Peyer's patches. Similar interactions between lymphotoxin-expressing B cells and TNFR-I–expressing follicular dendritic cells (FDCs) establish the normal architecture of the spleen and lymph nodes. B and T cells are partitioned into distinct areas within lymphoid tissue by specific chemokines.

To ensure that rare antigen-specific T cells survey the body effectively for pathogen-bearing antigen-presenting cells, T cells continually recirculate through T-cell zones of all secondary lymphoid organs where they are brought into contact with antigen-presenting cells from many different tissue sites. The migration of naive T cells into lymphoid organs is guided by the chemokine receptor CCR7, which binds CCL19 or CCL21 produced by stromal cells in the T-cell zones of secondary lymphoid tissues and displayed on the specialized endothelium of high endothelial venules (HEVs). L-selectin expressed by naive T cells initiates their rolling along the specialized surfaces of HEVs, where contact with these chemokines induces a switch in the integrin LFA-1 expressed by T cells to a configuration with affinity for the ICAM-1 expressed on the HEV endothelium. This initiates strong adhesion, diapedesis, and migration of the T cells into the T-cell zone. There, naive T cells meet antigen-bearing dendritic cells, of which there are two main populations: type 1 and type 2 conventional dendritic cells (cDC1 and cDC2). Conventional dendritic cells continually survey nonlymphoid tissues for invading pathogens and are the dendritic cells responsible for activating naive T cells. Contact with pathogens delivers signals to dendritic cells via TLRs and other pattern-recognition receptors (PRRs) that accelerate antigen processing and the production of foreign-peptide:self-MHC complexes. TLR signaling also induces expression of CCR7 by dendritic cells, which directs their migration to T-cell zones of secondary lymphoid organs, where they encounter and activate naive T cells.

Naive T-cell activation, clonal expansion, and differentiation into effector and memory T cells.

As we learned in the previous section, the perpetual recirculation of naive T cells from blood to T-cell zones of secondary lymphoid tissues and back to blood is contingent on absence of activation by cognate antigen. For an individual T cell, this pattern of recirculation can persist for years. Because the migration of a T cell to any particular secondary lymphoid tissue is random, and because a single naive T cell can survey about one lymph organ per day, even a clonal population of 100 naive T cells can theoretically survey up to 100 different lymphoid tissues per day. Thus, despite the fact that the diversity of antigen receptors on naive T cells is great and the number of cells in any clonal population is small, the chances that any given T cell within the repertoire will engage its antigen after infection is high. Still, for a clonal population to eradicate an invading pathogen, which in the case of viruses or bacteria can involve an inoculum of thousands to millions of microorganisms that can rapidly amplify their numbers exponentially, T cells must expand their own numbers and functional capabilities to succeed in defending the host.

We now consider the generation of effector and memory T cells from naive T cells. The activation and differentiation of naive T cells, often called priming, is distinct from the later responses of effector T cells to antigen on their target cells and from the responses of memory T cells to subsequent encounters with the same antigen. Priming of naive CD8 T cells by antigen presented on cDC1 cells

Fig. 9.18 Adhesion molecules involved in APC–T-cell interactions. Adhesion molecules of the immunoglobulin superfamily bind to adhesion molecules of various types, including integrins (LFA-1 and VLA-4) and other immunoglobulin superfamily members [the CD2–CD58 (LFA-2–LFA-3) interaction] to mediate cell–cell contact between APCs and T cells.

ANIMATION 9.4 ▶

generates cytotoxic T cells capable of directly killing pathogen-infected cells. Naive CD4 T cells activated by antigen presented on cDC2 cells—and in some cases, cDC1 cells—develop into a diverse array of effector cell types depending on the nature of the signals they receive during priming. CD4 effector activity can also include cytotoxicity, but more frequently it involves the secretion of a set of cytokines that direct target cells toward a more pathogen-specific response.

As we will learn, the activation of naive T cells is contingent on at least three signals. The primary signal is T-cell receptor (TCR) recognition of antigenic peptide:MHC on the surface of activated conventional dendritic cells. Activation of the naive T cell also requires co-recognition of co-stimulatory molecules displayed by the same cDC, often referred to as the second signal. Finally, cytokines that control differentiation into different types of effector cells, the so-called third signal, are often delivered to the activated naive T cell by the antigen-presenting DC itself, but they may also be produced by other innate immune cells. All these events are set in motion by earlier signals that arise from the initial detection of the pathogens by the innate immune system and the delivery of antigen to regional lymphoid tissues. The result is a tremendous increase in the number of pathogen-specific T cells—termed clonal expansion—and their acquisition, via effector-cell differentiation, of enhanced functional properties tailored for the eradication of the pathogen that incited their response.

9-8 Conventional dendritic cells deliver multiple signals for the activation of naive T cells.

As naive T cells migrate through FRC channels in the T-cell zones of lymphoid tissues, they bind transiently to each dendritic cell they encounter. Binding is mediated by interactions between LFA-1 or CD2 on the T cell and ICAM-1/ICAM-2 or CD58, respectively, on the dendritic cell (**Fig. 9.18**). The transient binding provides time for a T cell to scan the large number of MHC molecules displayed on the surface of cDCs for its cognate peptide. Most encounters of naive T cells with DCs do not, however, result in the recognition of an antigen, and the T cell must disengage the DC so that it can continue its migration. How naive T cells disengage from their antigen-negative targets is not known, although evidence suggests that, at least in the case of CD4 T cells, binding to MHC class II molecules without engagement of the T-cell receptor provides a signal for the cell to detach. In those rare cases in which a naive T-cell's TCR recognizes its peptide:MHC ligand, signaling through the T-cell receptor induces a conformational change in LFA-1 that greatly increases its affinity for ICAM-1 and ICAM-2 (see Section 7-19)—like that induced by signaling through CCR7 as the naive T cell enters the lymphoid tissue across HEVs (see Section 9-3). The change in LFA-1 stabilizes the association between the antigen-specific T cell and the antigen-presenting cell (**Fig. 9.19**). The association can persist

Fig. 9.19 Transient adhesive interactions between T cells and antigen-presenting cells are stabilized by specific antigen recognition. When a T cell binds to its specific ligand on an antigen-presenting cell, intracellular signaling through the T-cell receptor (TCR) induces a conformational change in LFA-1 that causes it to bind with higher affinity to ICAMs on the antigen-presenting cell. Not shown, but also contributory, is activation-induced clustering of LFA-1 molecules on the T cell that increases binding avidity for ICAM on the APC. The T cell shown here is a CD4 T cell.

Fig. 9.20 Three kinds of signals are involved in the activation of naive T cells by antigen-presenting cells. Binding of the foreign-peptide:self-MHC complex by the T-cell receptor and, in this example, a CD4 co-receptor transmits a signal to the T cell that antigen has been encountered. Effective activation of naive T cells requires a second signal, the co-stimulatory signal, to be delivered by the same antigen-presenting cell (APC). CD28 on the T cell encounters B7 molecules on the antigen-presenting cell and delivers the second signal, whose net effect is the increased proliferation and survival of the T cell that has received the first (TCR) signal. For CD4 T cells in particular, different pathways of differentiation produce subsets of effector T cells that carry out different effector responses, depending on the nature of a third signal delivered by the antigen-presenting cell. Cytokines commonly, but not exclusively, represent the third signal involved in directing this differentiation.

ANIMATION 9.5

for several days, during which time the naive T cell proliferates, and its progeny, which can also adhere to the same DC, differentiate into effector T cells.

At least three types of signals are produced by the activating cDC over the time the T cell engages it (**Fig. 9.20**). The first is generated from the interaction of a specific peptide:MHC complex with the T-cell receptor. Engagement of the T-cell receptor with its specific peptide antigen is essential for activating a naive T cell and engages several key signaling pathways (see Chapter 7). However, even if the co-receptor—CD4 or CD8—is also ligated, this does not, on its own, activate a naive T cell to proliferate and differentiate into effector T cells. Expansion and differentiation of naive T cells involve at least two additional signals: co-stimulatory signals that promote the activation and expansion of the T cells, and cytokines that direct T-cell differentiation into one of the different subsets of effector T cells. Additional signals, such as Notch ligands, can contribute to the effector differentiation of naive T cells, although these signals appear to be of less importance than those of lineage-specifying cytokines (discussed in Section 9-14).

As discussed in Section 7-22, the co-stimulatory molecules required for initial T-cell activation are the B7 family molecules, **B7.1** (CD80) and **B7.2** (CD86). These homodimeric members of the immunoglobulin superfamily are found exclusively on APCs and, in the case of naive T cells are co-expressed by the same cDC on which activating peptide:MHC complexes are engaged. The receptor for B7 molecules on the T cell is **CD28**, a member of the immunoglobulin superfamily (see Section 7-22). Signaling through CD28 that is induced by B7 molecules enhances activation of PLC-γ and other signals transduced through the TCR that are required for activation of transcription factors and PI 3-kinase, which initiate the processes of T-cell division and differentiation (see Section 7-22); targeted deficiency of B7 molecules or experimental blockade of the binding of B7 molecules to CD28 inhibits naive T-cell activation.

9-9   T-cell activation induces metabolic changes that prepare the T cell for rapid clonal expansion and differentiation.

Naive T cells have condensed chromatin and little cytoplasm and are generally arrested in the G0 stage of the cell cycle (**Fig. 9.21**); that is, at any given time most are not progressing through the cell cycle—they have low metabolic activity and synthesize little RNA or protein. Their primary fuel is glucose, which is converted by glycolysis to pyruvate that feeds the TCA cycle in mitochondria, where **oxidative phosphorylation (OXPHOS)** efficiently generates ATP. Within hours of activation, signals generated by antigen recognition induce the cells to undergo a metabolic shift to accommodate an increased demand for macromolecular biosynthesis and energy production in preparation for entry into the cell cycle (**Fig. 9.22**). The resultant increase in cell size and change in morphology that accompanies the cell's preparation for cell division is referred to as **blast transformation** (see Fig. 9.21).

Fig. 9.21 Antigen-induced activation of naive T cells initiates changes in morphology, metabolic activity, and progression into the cell cycle.
In the initial minutes to hours after TCR recognition of antigen on a cDC, signals emanating from the TCR and CD28 activate transcription factors such as NFAT, AP-1, and NFκB that induce the transcription of genes whose products are required for retention of the activated T cell within the lymphoid tissue (for example, CD69) and for its proliferation and differentiation into an effector T cell (for example, IL-2 and IL-2Rα). Activation of Akt–mTOR signaling shifts the energy metabolism of the T cell to ramp up aerobic glycolysis to increase macromolecule synthesis in preparation for rapid cell growth (blast transformation; upper panels and middle panels) prior to cell division. The activated T cell leaves the quiescent, G0 phase and enters the cell cycle (lower panels), first transitioning to the first gap phase (G1), during which the cell grows larger and copies organelles. This is followed by the synthesis phase, or S phase, during which the genome is duplicated. A second gap phase follows (G2), during which the cell grows further, increasing the synthesis of macromolecules and organelles prior to mitosis (M), where the cell divides and apportions a complete genome to each of the two daughter cells generated. Antigen-activated T cells typically begin to divide the first of many cell divisions within 2–3 days, initiating the process of clonal expansion that rapidly increases the number of clonal progeny that can participate in the adaptive immune response.

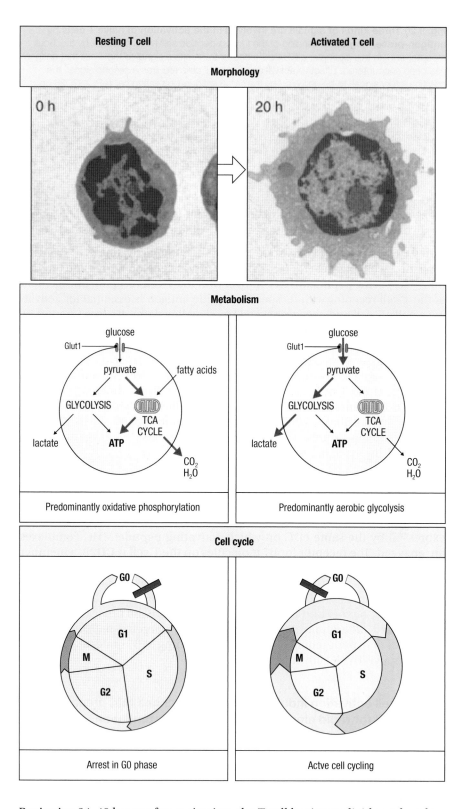

Beginning 24–48 hours after activation, the T cell begins to divide and undergoes remarkably rapid cell division to produce large numbers of progeny (clonal expansion) as it differentiates (**Fig. 9.23**). Activation of Akt downstream of TCR and CD28 signaling stimulates the mTOR pathway to increase the activated T cell's metabolic and biosynthetic capabilities as it transitions from G0 to G1 and enters the cell cycle. Activation of Akt–mTOR signaling stimulates **aerobic glycolysis** and increases the uptake of glucose to fuel this pathway—while also increasing the OXPHOS pathway to meet energy demands. Although

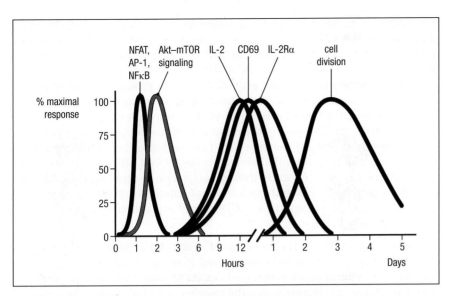

Fig. 9.22 Naive T-cell activation induced by TCR- and CD28-mediated signaling leads to sequential waves of signaling protein activation, gene expression, and cell-cycle progression that lead to rapid cell division and clonal expansion. Shown is a time-course of signaling that leads to new gene expression and entry into the cell cycle that occurs minutes to days after T-cell activation. A number of key transcription factors, including NFAT, AP-1, and NFκB, rapidly undergo changes in expression and/or post-translational modifications by signaling kinases upon activation by TCR and CD28 signaling. These factors then bind regulatory elements in many genes to activate their expression, including the genes encoding IL-2, CD69, and IL-2Rα. Activation of the Akt–mTOR signaling cascade induces metabolic changes in the activated T cell to prepare it for transition from G0 to G1 as it enters the cell cycle.

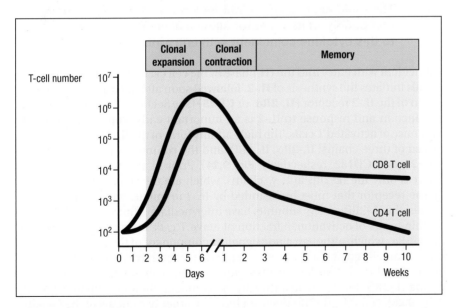

Fig. 9.23 The initial T-cell response to antigen results in rapid clonal expansion that is followed by clonal contraction as the immune response wanes. Because naive T cells of a given antigenic specificity are present in such low numbers (for most clones in mice, approximately 100 cells), they must undergo a remarkable amplification in cell numbers after initial activation in order to adequately cope with an infection. Naive T cells begin to enter the cell cycle within ~48 hours after activation and begin dividing very rapidly. In the case of CD4 T cells, clonal expansion can lead to an ~1000-fold increase in number compared to the initial clone size. For CD8 T cells, clonal expansion can increase the starting T-cell number as much as ~50,000-fold. After antigen clearance, the large majority of clonal progeny produced undergo programmed cell death to reduce the clonal pool size as homeostasis is restored—a process referred to as clonal contraction. The increased number of clonal members that persist long-term after clonal contraction are termed memory T cells.

a less efficient pathway for ATP generation than OXPHOS, aerobic glycolysis supports anabolic metabolism that is required for rapid cell division, including the up-regulation of a number of biosynthetic pathways—mitochondrial biogenesis, protein synthesis, nucleotide synthesis, and lipid biosynthesis—while also repressing catabolic activities, such as protein degradation. The resultant shift in cellular energetics and metabolism supports the ability of T cells to divide once every 4–6 hours, which can result in an approximately 1,000- to 10,000-fold increase in the number of clonal progeny over a period of several days (see Fig. 9.23). Because CD8 T cells exercise their effector function through direct interaction with their targets (target-cell killing) and CD4 T cells generally exercise their function through activation of other immune effector cells (for example, B cells and granulocytes) that themselves undergo proliferative increases, the magnitude of CD8 clonal expansion is typically greater than that of CD4 T cells.

As the inciting pathogen is cleared, most of the clonal progeny generated to eradicate the pathogen must be eliminated to restore homeostasis, a process referred to as **clonal contraction** (see Fig. 9.23), which will be considered in detail in Chapter 11. Nevertheless, the number of clonal progeny that survive clonal contraction and are retained as memory T cells exceeds that of the number of clonal precursors, such that their number is typically increased at least 1–2 orders of magnitude. Memory T cells have enhanced responsiveness to recall challenges with antigen and, like naive T cells, can persist for years without requirement for recognition of their cognate antigen. The persistence of memory T cells is accompanied by a shift in their metabolism back to a maintenance program and a G0 ground state. We will discuss the properties of memory T cells further in Chapter 11.

9-10 The rapid expression of interleukin-2 and the high-affinity component of its receptor allow activated T cells to respond to this cytokine coincident with entry into the cell cycle.

Coincident with entry into the G1 phase of the cell cycle, a fraction of activated T cells initiates the synthesis of **IL-2**, followed soon after by expression of the α chain of the IL-2 receptor (**IL-2Rα**, or **CD25**) (see Sections 7-21 and 7-22). The production and response to IL-2 is an important early step in the antigenic response of activated T cells. The high-affinity form of the IL-2 receptor is composed of three chains: IL-2Rα, IL-2Rβ, and the common γ (γ$_c$) chain (CD25, CD122, and CD132, respectively; **Fig. 9.24**). Prior to activation, naive T cells express only the IL-2Rβ and γ$_c$ chains, which are the signaling components of the receptor that must be liganded by IL-2 to initiate signaling. By themselves, the IL-2Rβ and γ$_c$ subunits have intermediate affinity for IL-2 binding. Within hours of activation, a fraction of naive T cells up-regulates expression of IL-2Rα, which, although a nonsignaling component of the receptor, confers a substantially greater affinity of the trimeric receptor by capturing and tethering IL-2 to the T-cell surface in an orientation that facilitates the binding of IL-2 to the IL-2Rβ and γ$_c$ chains, thereby cross-linking them to initiate signaling (**Fig. 9.25**). Notably, IL-2Rα does not bind the other two chains of the receptor once the quaternary complex with IL-2 is formed. Rather, the initial binding of IL-2 by IL-2Rα facilitates its 'presentation' of IL-2 to the IL-2Rβ and γ$_c$ subunits to form the signaling complex. Thus, the expression of IL-2Rα allows the T cell to respond to very low concentrations of IL-2.

Unlike naive T cells, regulatory T cells (T$_{reg}$ cells) constitutively and uniformly express IL-2Rα, and thus can rapidly form the high-affinity signaling complex upon binding IL-2 (see Figs. 9.24 and 9.25). As will be discussed later (see Section 9-17), by expressing the high-affinity IL-2 receptor, T$_{reg}$ cells can outcompete T cells that do not express IL-2Rα for binding of the limited quantities of IL-2 that are available early in the response to antigen. In this way, T$_{reg}$

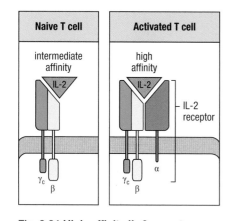

Fig. 9.24 High-affinity IL-2 receptors are three-chain structures that are present only on activated T cells. On resting T cells, the IL-2 receptor β chain (IL-2Rβ; CD122) and common γ chain (γ$_c$; CD132) are expressed constitutively. They bind IL-2 with intermediate affinity. Activation of T cells induces the synthesis of the IL-2 receptor α chain (IL-2Rα; CD25), which captures IL-2 and presents it to the IL-2Rβ and γ$_c$ chains to form the high-affinity heterotrimeric receptor that signals into the T cell. The IL-2Rβ and γ$_c$ chains show similarities in amino acid sequence to that of cell-surface receptors for other growth hormones that regulate cell growth and differentiation.

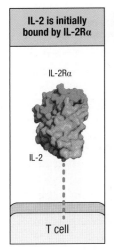

IL-2 is initially bound by IL-2Rα

IL-2Rα

IL-2

T cell

IL-2 bound by IL-2Rα is presented to the IL-2Rβ and γc chains to dimerize them and initiate signaling

IL-2Rβ

IL-2Rγc

T cell

Fig. 9.25 Structural features of the IL-2 receptor. Shown are the structures of the IL-2 receptor in complex with IL-2. In the first panel, the initial complex of IL-2 with IL-2Rα (CD25) is shown. IL-2Rα–bound IL-2 then binds IL-2Rβ and γc to form the signaling trimeric IL-2 receptor (second panel, front and lateral views). Note that while IL-2Rα contacts IL-2, it does not contact the IL-2Rβ and γc chains in the quaternary complex, whereas IL-2 contacts both the IL-2Rβ and γc chains to bring them into close apposition to induce signaling.

cells act as a 'sink' for IL-2 to limit its availability to other cells. However, once activated, naive T cells up-regulate IL-2Rα to effectively compete with T_{reg} cells for binding of IL-2. The binding of IL-2 by these developing T cells triggers signaling that supports their activation and differentiation and may also enhance their proliferation and survival (**Fig. 9.26**).

On the basis of *in vitro* studies, IL-2 was long thought to be required for the proliferation of naive T cells. However, *in vivo* studies indicate that while IL-2 can augment T-cell proliferation and survival, other functions of IL-2 might be more important. Thus, as we will learn, while IL-2 favors the development of some subsets of effector T cells after initial activation—and is essential for the maintenance of regulatory T cells, which cannot produce their own IL-2—it also represses the development of other subsets of CD4 T cells despite their robust clonal expansion after antigenic priming. This suggests IL-2 is dispensable for the proliferation of at least some developing T cells. Indeed, mice deficient for IL-2 or IL-2Rα receptor develop uncontrolled T-cell proliferation and multiorgan autoimmunity because of the absence of regulatory T cells, indicating an indispensable role for IL-2 in T_{reg} cell maintenance but not for the clonal expansion of at least some non-T_{reg} cells. As will be discussed further in Section 9-15, this points to a complex and important role for IL-2 in regulating the developmental fate of effector T cells early in their differentiation and suggests other roles for IL-2 in the adaptive immune response.

9-11 Additional co-stimulatory and inhibitory receptors are engaged after initial T-cell activation to control clonal expansion and contraction.

Once a naive T cell has been activated, it expresses additional surface molecules that act either to amplify and sustain clonal expansion or to restrain it. These molecules include receptors that belong to both the CD28 and the TNF receptor families. Here we consider those family members that facilitate or impede the initial clonal expansion of T cells after priming; members of the CD28 and the TNF receptor families that play other important roles in the interactions between APCs and T cells will be considered in later sections.

Fig. 9.26 Activated T cells either secrete or respond to IL-2. Unlike effector T cells, which can produce a diversity of cytokines depending on the mature effector phenotype, naive T cells primarily produce IL-2 when activated by antigen. However, secretion of IL-2 or expression of the high-affinity component of its receptor, IL-2Rα, typically appears to be differentially induced on activated T cells. Thus, IL-2 produced by one T cell binds to the high-affinity IL-2 receptor of a different T cell, so-called paracrine signaling, which induces enhanced T-cell growth and altered differentiation of the cell receiving the IL-2 signal.

Resting T cells express only a moderate-affinity IL-2 receptor (IL-2Rβ and γc chains only)

moderate-affinity IL-2 receptor

T cell

IL-2

IL-2Rα

Some activated T cells express a high-affinity IL-2 receptor (IL-2Rα, IL-2Rβ and γc chains), and some secrete IL-2

Binding of IL-2 to its receptor promotes enhanced proliferation and can modulate T-cell differentiation

Fig. 9.27 CTLA-4 is an inhibitory receptor for B7 molecules. Naive T cells express CD28, which delivers a co-stimulatory signal on binding B7 molecules (see Fig. 9.20), thereby driving the survival and expansion of the T cells. Activated T cells express increased levels of CTLA-4 (CD152), which attenuate TCR signaling through three mechanisms. First, because CTLA-4 has a higher affinity than CD28 for B7 molecules and can simultaneously bind two B7 molecules (compared to only one for CD28), it outcompetes CD28 for B7 binding (left panel). CTLA-4 can also remove B7 molecules from the dendritic-cell surface, thereby depleting the co-stimulatory function of the DC (middle panel). Finally, CTLA-4 may deliver negative signals that repress the activating signals generated through the TCR (right panel). Thus, expression of CTLA-4 by the activated T cell serves to attenuate the proliferative phase of the T-cell response.

In addition to CD28, B7 molecules can be engaged by **CTLA-4** (CD152), which, although related in sequence to CD28, acts to restrain, rather than promote, T-cell activation and clonal expansion (**Fig. 9.27**; see also Section 7-25). Unlike CD28, which binds a single B7 homodimer, CTLA-4 can bind a pair of B7 homodimers and has an affinity for B7 that is about 20 times higher than that of CD28. It is clear that one mechanism by which CTLA-4 inhibits T-cell activation is by outcompeting CD28 for interaction with B7 molecules expressed by antigen-presenting cells. Moreover, it has been shown that CTLA-4 can physically remove B7 molecules from the surface of activated APCs, effectively stripping them of their co-stimulatory capability. Finally, although CTLA-4 does not contain an immunoreceptor tyrosine-based inhibition motif (ITIM), some data indicate that it can also generate negative signals that repress T-cell activation.

Unlike CD28, which is constitutively expressed by naive T cells, surface expression of CTLA-4 is induced only after activation of naive T cells, making activated T cells less sensitive than naive T cells to stimulation by the antigen-presenting cell and also restricting IL-2 production. Thus, binding of CTLA-4 to B7 molecules plays a central role in limiting the response of activated T cells to antigen and B7. This has been confirmed in mice with a disrupted CTLA-4 gene; such mice develop a fatal disorder characterized by a massive overgrowth of lymphocytes. As will be discussed in Section 9-17, unlike naive T cells, regulatory T cells constitutively express CTLA-4 on the cell surface, where it acts to limit the co-stimulatory activity of APCs that bear antigens recognized by the T_{reg} cell TCR.

Programmed death protein-1 (PD-1) is another member of the CD28 family that acts to restrain T-cell responses after their initiation, albeit by a different mechanism. PD-1 is induced by TCR signaling on nearly all activated T cells and recognizes one of two ligands: PD-L1, which is expressed by many cell types, and PD-L2, which is expressed on APCs at sites of inflammation. Unlike CTLA-4, the cytoplasmic domain of PD-1 does contain an ITIM, which acts to repress signaling through CD28 (see Section 7-26). Antibodies that block PD-1 or CTLA-4 signaling, so-called **checkpoint inhibitors**, are the basis for immunotherapies that are now employed for treatment of certain malignancies that impair the antitumor function of T cells, to be discussed in greater detail in Chapter 16.

Several members of the TNF and TNFR families (for example, OX40L and OX40) can deliver co-stimulatory signals that sustain T-cell survival and may

Fig. 9.28 Multiple members of the TNF–TNFR superfamily can activate the non-canonical NFκB pathway to enhance and sustain T-cell responses. See text for details.

amplify clonal expansion after the initial priming event (**Fig. 9.28**). These pathways all seem to function by activating NFκB through a TRAF-dependent, non-canonical NFκB pathway (see Section 7-24), although other signaling pathways (for example, PI 3-kinase–Akt) appear to be activated by at least some of the family members. While much remains to be learned about the orchestration of this family of co-stimulators and their functions, signals activating these pathways appear to be preferentially delivered by monocyte-derived DCs (MoDCs) rather than cDCs, and may act at sites of T-cell activation in lymphoid tissues as well as in nonlymphoid tissues to which recently activated T cells are recruited. Thus, the actions of these co-stimulators take place with delayed kinetics relative to initial priming by cDCs and are induced by a different APC.

Another TNF family ligand, CD40L, which is expressed on the surface of the T cell soon after initial activation, signals via its CD40 receptor on cDCs and other APCs to up-regulate expression of B7 molecules, thereby providing an amplifying feed-forward signal loop that enhances T-cell clonal expansion. The role of the CD40–CD40L pair in amplifying a T-cell response is demonstrated in mice lacking CD40L; when these mice are immunized, the clonal expansion of responding T cells is curtailed at an early stage. As we will see in subsequent sections in this chapter and the next, CD40L also plays critical roles in activating naive B cells and in signaling cDCs and macrophages to enhance their expression of cytokines, such as IL-12. Thus, deleterious mutations of *CD40L* in humans cause a form of severe immunodeficiency (see Chapter 13).

CD40 Ligand Deficiency

9-12 Proliferating T cells differentiate into effector T cells that are programmed for altered tissue homing and loss of a requirement for co-stimulation to act.

During the period of rapid cell division that follows their activation, naive T cells differentiate into effector T cells that acquire the ability to produce a range of effector molecules required for specialized helper or cytotoxic functions when they reencounter antigen. Effector T cells undergo additional changes that distinguish them from naive T cells. One of the most important is in their activation requirements: once a T cell has differentiated into an effector cell,

| Stimulation of naive T cell | Proliferating T cell | Active effector T cells kill virus-infected target cells |

RECOGNITION   PROLIFERATION   DIFFERENTIATION   EFFECTOR FUNCTION

Fig. 9.29 Effector T cells can respond to their target cells without co-stimulation. Naive T cells that recognize antigen on the surface of an antigen-presenting cell and receive the required signals (left panel) become activated and can secrete and respond to IL-2. IL-2 signaling enhances clonal expansion and contributes to the differentiation of the T cells to effector-cell status (central panel). Once the cells have differentiated into effector T cells, encounters with target cells bearing specific antigen can trigger their effector actions without the need for co-stimulation. Thus, as illustrated here (right panel), cytotoxic T cells can kill any virus-infected target cell, including those that do not express co-stimulatory molecules.

an encounter with its specific antigen results in an immune attack without the need for co-stimulation. This distinction is particularly easy to understand for cytotoxic CD8 T cells, which must be able to act on any cell infected with a virus, whether or not the infected cell can express co-stimulatory molecules (**Fig. 9.29**). However, this feature is also important for the effector function of CD4 cells, as effector CD4 T cells must be able to activate B cells and macrophages that have taken up antigen irrespective of whether or not those cells initially express co-stimulatory molecules.

Changes are also seen in the cell-adhesion molecules and receptors expressed by effector T cells. As we will discuss in more detail in Chapter 11, effector T cells lose cell-surface L-selectin and therefore cease to recirculate through lymph nodes. Instead, they express glycans that serve as ligands for P- and E-selectins (for example, **P-selectin glycoprotein ligand-1,** or **PSGL-1**), which are up-regulated on inflamed vascular endothelial cells and allow effector T cells to roll on the blood vessels at sites of inflammation. They also express higher levels of LFA-1 and CD2 than do naive T cells, as well as the integrin $\alpha_4\beta_1$ (**VLA-4**), which allows them to bind to vascular endothelium bearing the adhesion molecule **VCAM-1**, which is also expressed on the inflamed endothelium. As we will see, effector T cells that develop in mucosal tissues or the lymph nodes draining them are also induced to express the $\alpha_4\beta_7$ integrin heterodimer, which acts as a 'homing receptor' for the mucosal addressin, MadCAM-1. This altered deployment of cell-adhesion molecules and receptors by effector T cells allows them to exit the bloodstream and enter sites of infection, where they orchestrate the local immune responses. These changes in the T-cell surface are summarized in **Fig. 9.30** and will be discussed further in Chapter 11.

9-13   CD8 T cells can be activated in different ways to become cytotoxic effector cells.

Naive T cells fall into two broad classes, one of which expresses the co-receptor CD8 on its surface, and the other expresses the co-receptor CD4. The CD8 co-receptor recognizes MHC class I molecules, hence CD8 T cells are MHC class I–restricted for recognition of their cognate antigen. Naive CD8 T cells typically differentiate into cytotoxic T cells (often called cytotoxic

						Cell-surface molecules						
T cell	T-cell receptor	L-selectin	CCR7	LFA-1	CD45RA	CD45RO	CD2	S1PR1	$\alpha_4\beta_7$	VLA-4	PSGL-1	CD44
Naive	+	++	++	+	+	−	+	+	+/−	−	−	+
Effector	+	−	−	++	−	+	++	−	++/−	+	+	++

Fig. 9.30 Activation of T cells changes the expression of several cell-surface molecules. The example here is a CD4 T cell. Resting naive T cells express L-selectin, through which they home to lymph nodes, but express relatively low levels of other adhesion molecules such as CD2, LFA-1, and $\alpha_4\beta_7$. Upon activation, expression of L-selectin ceases and, instead, expression of ligands for P- and E-selectins is induced (for example, PSGL-1), which allow the activated T cells to roll on P- and E-selectins expressed on endothelium at sites of inflammation. Increased amounts of the integrin LFA-1 are also produced, which is activated to bind its ligands, ICAM-1 and ICAM-2. A newly expressed integrin called VLA-4, which allows T cells to arrest on inflamed vascular endothelium, ensures that activated T cells can enter nonlymphoid tissues at sites where they are likely to encounter infection. On T cells activated in mucosal lymphoid tissues, there is up-regulation of $\alpha_4\beta_7$ integrin, which similarly serves to direct these cells to nonlymphoid mucosal sites where they reencounter antigen. Activated T cells also have on their surface a higher density of the adhesion molecule CD2, increasing the avidity of their interaction with potential target cells, as well as a higher density of the adhesion molecule CD44. Alternative splicing of the RNA transcript of the CD45 gene induced by antigenic activation causes a change in the isoform of CD45 that is expressed on human T cells: naive T cells preferentially express the CD45RA isoform, while effector and memory T cells express the CD45RO isoform. In mice, there is a similar change from high expression of the CD45RB isoform on naive T cells to low expression of CD45RB in previously activated T cells (not shown). CD45RO associates with the T-cell receptor and CD4 more efficiently to make previously activated T cells more sensitive to stimulation by low concentrations of peptide:MHC complexes. Finally, the sphingosine 1-phosphate receptor 1 (S1PR1) is expressed by naive T cells, allowing cells that do not become activated to egress from lymphoid tissues (see Fig. 9.10). Down-regulation of S1PR1 for several days after activation prevents T-cell egress during the period of proliferation and differentiation. After several days, it is expressed again, allowing effector cells to exit from the lymphoid tissues.

T lymphocytes, or CTLs), which are specialized for killing target cells bearing their cognate antigen (**Fig. 9.31**). CTLs are important in defense against intracellular pathogens, especially viruses and some intracellular bacteria. Effector CD8 T cells are also central to antitumor immunity. Because all nucleated cells in the body express MHC class I molecules and can process cytosolic antigens to load them, essentially any cell in the body can be targeted for killing by CTLs.

Naive CD8 T cells recognize peptide antigens processed and loaded onto MHC class I of cDC1 cells from two cytosolic sources: antigens of pathogens that can infect the cytosol of cDC1 cells directly and those derived via cross-presentation. Like other cells, dendritic cells are directly susceptible to infection by some viruses, which enter the cytoplasm by binding to cell-surface molecules that act as entry receptors. Viral proteins synthesized in the cytoplasm of dendritic cells are processed in the proteasome and presented on the cell surface as peptides loaded onto MHC class I molecules after transport into the endoplasmic reticulum, as in any other type of virus-infected cell (see Chapter 6). Similarly, bacteria that have evolved mechanisms to escape the phagosome after uptake by phagocytes, such as *Listeria monocytogenes*, shed antigens in the cytosol that can be loaded onto MHC class I molecules and recognized by CD8 T cells.

Uptake of extracellular virus particles or virus-infected cells into the endocytic pathway by macropinocytosis or phagocytosis can also result in the presentation of viral peptides on MHC class I molecules. This phenomenon, known as

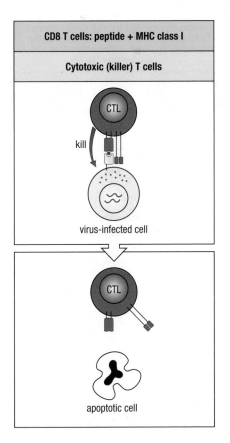

CD8 T cells: peptide + MHC class I

Cytotoxic (killer) T cells

CTL

kill

virus-infected cell

CTL

apoptotic cell

Fig. 9.31 Cytotoxic CD8 T cells are specialized to kill cells infected with intracellular pathogens. Cytotoxic CD8 T cells (cytotoxic T lymphocytes; CTLs) kill target cells that display at their cell surface the peptide fragments of cytosolic pathogens (most notably viruses) that are bound to MHC class I molecules.

Antigens taken up by cDC1 during cross-presentation may activate both naive CD8 and CD4 T cells

APC stimulates effector CD4 T cell to induce the expression of CD40L and IL-2

Stimulation of APC through CD40 increases B7 and CD70, which both co-stimulate the naive CD8 T cell, and also increases APC production of IL-12

Fig. 9.32 CD8 T-cell responses can be enhanced by CD4 T cells. CD8 T cells that recognize antigen on weakly co-stimulatory cells may become activated only in the presence of CD4 T cells interacting with the same antigen-presenting cell (APC). CD40 ligand (CD40L) expressed by the activated CD4 T cells can signal via CD40 on the dendritic cell to up-regulate its expression of B7 molecules to enhance CD8 activation and may also induce increased levels of other co-stimulatory activity on the dendritic cell (for example, CD70, which is recognized by CD27 expressed by the CD8 T cell), a process known as licensing of the dendritic cell. CD40 signaling also can enhance DC expression of IL-12, which enhances differentiation of CD8 T cells. Finally, the CD4 T cell may also produce abundant IL-2, which helps drive CD8 T-cell proliferation and differentiation.

cross-presentation, is an alternative to the usual cytosolic pathway for MHC class I antigen processing (see Section 6-5 and Section 9-7). In this case, viral antigens that enter dendritic cells via endocytic or phagocytic vesicles may be diverted to the cytosol for proteasomal degradation and transferred to the endoplasmic reticulum for loading onto MHC class I molecules. The result is that viruses that do not directly infect dendritic cells can nevertheless stimulate the activation of naive CD8 T cells. Cross-presentation is typically mediated by cDC1 cells, which are specialized for stimulating T-cell responses to intracellular pathogens and are the principal APC for CD8 T-cell priming (see Section 6-5 and Section 9-7). Any viral infection can therefore lead to the generation of cytotoxic effector CD8 T cells, whether or not the virus can directly infect dendritic cells.

In addition to priming CD8 T cells, some antigens taken up in the process of cross-presentation can be presented by MHC class II molecules on type 1 cDCs to co-activate naive CD4 T cells. CD4 T cells that recognize antigens presented by the same cDC1 cell may amplify the activation of naive CD8 T cells by further activating the antigen-presenting cell, so-called **licensing** of the dendritic cell, by directly recruiting CD4 T-cell help (**Fig. 9.32**). The production by the CD4 T cell of CD40L can induce the cDC1 cell to express heightened levels of B7 and CD70, which bind CD28 and CD27, respectively, on the CD8 T cell to amplify its response. Naive CD4 T cells activated on the same DC as a naive CD8 T cell may also provide IL-2 to the activated CD8 cell, which can enhance CD8 T-cell memory through mechanisms not yet understood. Finally, heightened IL-12 production by antigen-presenting cDC1 cells is also induced by CD40 signaling. In addition to enhancing the differentiation of CTLs, IL-12 may also promote the development of T_H1 cells from the activated CD4 T cell, as we will discuss shortly. Therefore, cooperativity between naive CD8 and CD4 T cells in the context of cross-presentation of antigens derived from intracellular pathogens may induce concomitant CTL and T_H1 responses that later act together in tissue sites of infection, as we will discuss further in Chapter 11.

Although plasmacytoid dendritic cells (pDCs) do not play a direct role in antigen presentation to naive CD8 T cells, like CD4 T cells they also contribute signals to cDC1 cells for CD8 T-cell effector differentiation. This is mediated principally through their abundant production of type I interferons. Specialized for the detection of viral infections by their unique pattern of nucleic acid–sensing TLRs, activated pDCs produce high levels of IFN-α and IFN-β that act on cDC1 cells to increase their production of IL-12. This may also enhance T_H1 responses activated by type 1 cDCs.

9-14   CD4 T cells differentiate into several functionally distinct subsets.

In contrast to CD8 T cells, naive CD4 T cells can differentiate into several types of helper or regulatory T effector cells that orchestrate different immune functions. The main helper subsets are T helper 1 (T_H1), T_H2, T_H17, T follicular helper (T_{FH}), and regulatory T (T_{reg}) cells. The T_H1, T_H2, and T_H17 subsets are elicited by different classes of pathogens and are defined on the basis of the

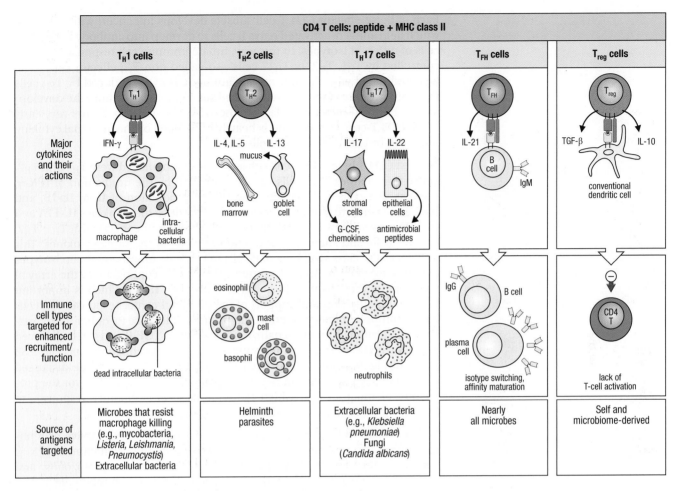

Fig. 9.33 Subsets of effector CD4 T cells are specialized to help different target cells eradicate different classes of pathogens. Unlike CD8 T cells, which act directly on infected target cells to eliminate pathogens, CD4 T cells typically enhance the effector functions of other cells that eradicate pathogens—whether cells of the innate immune system or, in the case of T_{FH} cells, antigen-specific B cells. T_H1 cells (first panels) produce cytokines, such as IFN-γ, which activate macrophages, enabling them to destroy intracellular microorganisms more efficiently. T_H2 cells (second panels) produce cytokines that recruit and activate eosinophils (IL-5) as well as mast cells and basophils (IL-4) and promote enhanced barrier immunity at mucosal surfaces (IL-13) to eradicate helminths. T_H17 cells (third panels) secrete IL-17 family cytokines that induce local epithelial and stromal cells to produce chemokines that recruit neutrophils to sites of

infection. T_H17 cells also produce IL-22, which along with IL-17 can activate epithelial cells at barrier sites to enhance barrier integrity and repair, and produce antimicrobial peptides that kill bacteria. T_{FH} cells (fourth panels) form cognate interactions with naive B cells through linked recognition of antigen and traffic to B-cell follicles, where they promote the germinal center response. T_{FH} cells can produce cytokines characteristic of other subsets that participate in type 1, 2, and 3 immune responses to influence isotype class-switching, but they primarily produce IL-21, which is important for optimal production of high-affinity, class-switched antibodies. Regulatory T cells (right panels) generally suppress naive T-cell responses and can produce immune regulatory cytokines, such as IL-10 and TGF-β, which regulate the response of effector T cells directly or via repression of pro-inflammatory cytokines.

different combinations of cytokines that they secrete (**Fig. 9.33**). These subsets cooperate with different innate effector cells of the myelomonocytic series (granulocytes and monocyte/macrophages) and with innate lymphoid cells (ILCs) to form integrated 'immune modules' specialized for the clearance of the different classes of pathogens (see Fig. 3.36 and also Chapter 11). One of these subsets will typically become predominant as an immune response progresses, especially in persistent infections, autoimmunity, or allergies. As we will discuss further in Chapter 11, the functional features of these T-cell subsets parallel in many ways those of ILCs, which, although lacking antigenic receptors, produce many of the same patterns of effector cytokines or cytotoxins. Alternatively, naive CD4 T cells can differentiate into T_{reg} cells, which respond to self antigens or nonpathogenic microbes that are components of the commensal microbiota that is normally resident at barrier tissues, such as the intestines, as we will discuss in Chapter 12.

Each of these effector CD4 T-cell subsets develops in concert with T_{FH} cells, which help antigen-activated naive B cells to develop into antibody-producing cells of different isotypes. In this way, innate immune cell responses that are controlled by T_H1, T_H2, or T_H17 cells—so-called non-T_{FH} effector cells—will be coordinated with the appropriate antibody isotypes induced by T_{FH} cells that enhance their function. As we shall see in the next section, the developmental bifurcation between T_{FH} and non-T_{FH} effector cells occurs very early in the CD4 T-cell response and is heavily influenced by the principal cytokine produced by activated naive T cells—IL-2.

The first CD4 T helper (T_H) cell subsets to be distinguished were T_H1 and T_H2, hence their names. T_H1 cells are characterized by the production of **IFN-γ**, whereas T_H2 cells are characterized by the production of **IL-4**, **IL-13**, and **IL-5**. T_H17 cells are so named because they produce the cytokines **IL-17A** and **IL-17F**; they also produce **IL-22**. T_{FH} cells develop in concert with T_H1, T_H2, or T_H17 cells and share the production of some of the same cytokines. This influences the class switching of B cells to generate immunoglobulin isotypes that bind to different innate immune effector cells contingent on the array of Fc receptors they display. T_{FH} cells also produce **IL-21**, which is important for B-cell maturation and support of the germinal center response. T_{reg} cells have immunoregulatory function and promote tolerance to, rather than clearance of, the antigens they recognize. They produce **TGF-β** and can be induced to produce **IL-10** upon further antigen-driven differentiation (see Fig. 9.33 and also Fig. 9.34 later in text; see also Section 9-17). As will be discussed in Chapter 12, T_{FH} cells that develop in concert with T_{reg} cells favor the production of mucosal IgA, which reinforces anti-inflammatory responses to nonpathogenic constituents of the healthy microbiome.

T_H1 cells help to eradicate infections by microbes that can survive or replicate within macrophages and are characterized by the production of IFN-γ. Pathogens targeted by T_H1 cells include certain viruses, protozoans, and intracellular bacteria, such as the mycobacteria that cause tuberculosis and leprosy. These bacteria are phagocytosed by macrophages in the usual way, but they can evade the intracellular killing mechanisms described in Chapter 3. If a T_H1 cell recognizes microbial antigens displayed on the surface of an infected macrophage, it will activate the macrophage further by releasing IFN-γ, which enhances the macrophage's microbicidal activity. T_{FH} cells that develop in concert with T_H1 cells can promote B-cell class switching that favors production of opsonizing IgG antibodies, such as IgG2a in mouse and IgG3 in humans. We will describe the macrophage-activating functions of T_H1 cells and the enhancement of the function of other innate effector cells by T_H2 and T_H17 cells in more detail in Chapter 11.

T_H2 cells help to control infections by multicellular parasites, particularly helminths, by promoting responses mediated by eosinophils, basophils, mast cells, as well as mucus-producing cells in mucosal epithelia. T_H2 cells also play an important role in the repair of tissue damage that results from infection. T_{FH} cells that develop in concert with T_H2 cells promote class switching of B cells to produce IgE, the primary role of which is to arm eosinophils, basophils, and mast cells to fight infections by helminths. IgE is also the antibody responsible for allergies and asthma, making T_H2 differentiation and type 2 immune responses of considerable medical interest.

T_H17 cells are typically induced in response to extracellular bacteria and fungi and amplify neutrophilic and monocytic responses that help to clear such pathogens (see Fig. 9.33). In addition to stimulating increased production and recruitment of neutrophils from the bone marrow, the effector cytokines produced by T_H17 cells are important in activating barrier epithelial cells in the gastrointestinal, respiratory, and urogenital tracts and in the skin to produce antimicrobial peptides that resist microbial invasion. T_{FH} cells that develop together with T_H17 cells also promote B-cell class switching to opsonizing IgG2 and IgG3 antibodies, which arm neutrophils and monocytes for enhanced phagocytosis.

As noted earlier, T_{FH} cells contribute to the eradication of most classes of pathogens through their unique role in providing help to B cells to promote germinal center responses—irrespective of the pattern of immune response with which they are associated. Thus, T_{FH} cells are elicited in the context of type 1, type 2, or type 3 immune responses, where they play a central role in the development of distinct patterns of class-switched antibodies. T_{FH} cells are identified primarily by their expression of the chemokine receptor CXCR5 after antigenic priming, which directs their mobilization toward B-cell follicles where CXCL13 is constitutively produced by stromal cells.

Prior to the discovery of T_{FH} cells, a point of controversy had been the role of CD4 T-effector subsets in providing B-cell help. Although historically it was thought B-cell help was a primary function of T_H2 cells, it is now clear that the T_{FH} cell, rather than T_H1, T_H2, or T_H17 cells, is the effector T cell that provides help to B-cells for high-affinity antibody production. Nevertheless, T_{FH} cells develop as a component of type 1, 2, or 3 immune responses and share production of some of the same lineage-defining cytokines as T_H1, T_H2, and T_H17 cells to drive the differentiation of naive B cells to alternative patterns of isotype switching. This explains how, in the course of an infection, B cells can receive help to switch to IgE through the presence of 'T_H2' cytokines or switch to other isotypes such as IgG2a through the presence of 'T_H1' cytokines. We will return to the helper functions of T_{FH} cells in more detail in Chapters 10 and 11.

All the effector T cells described above are involved in activating target cells that bear their antigens to enhance responses that help clear pathogens from the body. Another major branch of CD4 T cells has a different function. These are called regulatory T cells, or T_{reg} cells, because their function is to promote immune tolerance to the antigens they recognize. T_{reg} cells achieve this, at least in part, by preventing or limiting other T cell–driven immune responses, including those that might otherwise cause immune-mediated disease, such as autoimmunity. Two pathways of regulatory T cell development are currently recognized. One occurs during positive selection by self antigens in the thymus and produces natural T_{reg} cells or thymically derived T_{reg} cells (nT_{reg} cells or tT_{reg} cells, respectively; see Section 8-27). The other occurs in T-cell zones of secondary (peripheral) lymphoid organs, where naive CD4 T cells develop into T_{reg} cells under the influence of particular environmental cues, as we discuss in Section 9-17. This group is known as induced or peripheral T_{reg} cells (iT_{reg} or pT_{reg} cells, respectively) to distinguish them from those that develop in the thymus. In addition to self antigens, pT_{reg} cells can be induced in response to microbial antigens derived from microbes that normally live as commensal organisms in different host tissues, such as the gut, respiratory tract, and skin. This will be discussed further in Section 9-17 and in Chapter 12.

9-15 Cytokines play a central role in guiding the differentiation of CD4 T cells down distinct pathways.

Having briefly described the types and functions of CD4 T-cell subsets, we will now consider how they are derived from naive T cells. The fate of the progeny of a naive CD4 T cell is largely defined during the initial priming period and is regulated by signals provided by the local environment, whether by the priming antigen-presenting cell, other innate immune cells that have been activated by a pathogen, or by activated CD4 T cells themselves. As noted previously, the principal determinants of the developmental fate of naive CD4 T cells are the combination and balance of lineage-specifying cytokines, which are integrated with TCR and co-stimulatory signaling during priming. The five main subsets into which naive CD4 T cells may develop—T_H1, T_H2, T_H17, T_{FH},

Fig. 9.34 Cytokines are the principal determinants of alternative programs of CD4 T-cell effector differentiation.
Antigen-presenting cells, principally dendritic cells, as well as other innate immune cells can provide various cytokines that induce the development of naive CD4 T cells into distinct subsets. The environmental conditions, such as the exposure to various pathogens, determine which cytokines the innate sensor cells will produce. T_H1 cells differentiate in response to sequential IFN-γ and IL-12 signaling, whereas T_H2 cells differentiate in response to IL-4. IL-6 produced by dendritic cells acts with transforming growth factor-β (TGF-β) to induce differentiation of T_H17 cells, which up-regulate expression of the IL-23 receptor and become responsive to IL-23. Mouse T_{FH} cells also require IL-6 for their development, although it does not appear that human T_{FH} cells do, and it is not currently understood what additional signals might induce their differentiation from naive precursors in either species. When pathogens are absent, the presence of TGF-β and IL-2, and the lack of IL-6, favor the development of peripheral T_{reg} (pT_{reg}) cells.

Fate-specifying cytokines

IFN-γ IL-12	IL-4	TGF-β IL-6 IL-23	IL-6?	TGF-β IL-2
IFN-γ	IL-4, IL-5, IL-13	IL-17, IL-22	IL-21	TGF-β, IL-10
T_H1 cells	T_H2 cells	T_H17 cells	T_{FH} cells	pT_{reg} cells

and peripheral regulatory T cells (pT_{reg} cells)—are associated with distinct signals that induce their formation, different transcription factors that drive their differentiation, and unique cytokines and surface markers that define their identity (**Fig. 9.34**; see also Fig. 9.33).

T_H1 development is induced when there is a predominance of interferons (for example, IFN-γ) and IL-12 during the early stages of naive T-cell activation. As described in Section 3-16, many key cytokines, including the interferons and IL-12, stimulate a JAK–STAT intracellular signaling pathway that results in the activation of specific gene networks. Different members of the JAK and STAT families are activated by different cytokines. Each of the effector pathways is dependent on a distinct pattern of STAT activation downstream of the lineage-specifying cytokines to program a unique transcription factor network that defines the gene-expression profile of mature effector T cells (**Fig. 9.35**). For T_H1 development, **STAT1** and **STAT4** are critical and are sequentially activated by interferons (type I, IFN-α and IFN-β; or type II, IFN-γ) and IL-12, respectively, which are produced by innate immune cells early during infection. Activated group 1 ILCs, or NK cells, may also be an important source of IFN-γ, whereas activated plasmacytoid DCs produce abundant type I interferons. Finally, T_H1 cells themselves may provide IFN-γ, thus reinforcing the signal for the differentiation of more T_H1 cells through a positive feedback loop. The activation of STAT1 by interferons also induces the expression of another transcription factor, **Tbet**, which switches on the genes for IFN-γ and the inducible component of the IL-12 receptor, IL-12Rβ2 (the other component of the receptor, IL-12Rβ1, is already expressed on naive T cells). These T cells are now committed to becoming T_H1 cells and can be further activated by IL-12 produced by dendritic cells and macrophages to induce STAT4 signaling. STAT4 further up-regulates Tbet expression and completes T_H1 programming. Because of its central role in programming T_H1 development, Tbet is sometimes referred to as a 'master regulator' of T_H1 cell differentiation.

Fig. 9.35 Different members of the STAT family of transcription factors are coupled to cytokine receptors that specify CD4 T-cell subset development.
With the exception of TGF-β, which participates in both T_H17 and pT_{reg} development, the cytokines that specify the development of distinct effector cells typically activate different members of the STAT family of transcription factors. T_H1 cell differentiation is dependent on sequential activation of STAT1 and STAT4 by binding of IFN-γ and IL-12 to their respective receptors on antigen-activated naive CD4 T cells. Both of these STAT factors promote the expression of Tbet, which in turn cooperates with STAT1 and STAT4 to program T_H1 differentiation. T_H2 cell differentiation is dependent on STAT6 activation downstream of IL-4 receptor signaling. STAT6 acts to increase GATA3 expression, which cooperates with STAT6 to program T_H2 differentiation. IL-6 activates STAT3, which, in concert with TGF-β, participates in the induction of RORγt expression and T_H17 differentiation. IL-23, which acts later in T_H17 differentiation, also activates STAT3 to sustain and amplify the T_H17 program. The programming of T_{FH} cell differentiation by STAT factors is not fully understood, although STAT3 actions upstream of Bcl-6 expression are essential for T_{FH} development in mice. Activation of STAT5 by IL-2 is important in pT_{reg} differentiation and acts upstream of FoxP3 expression.

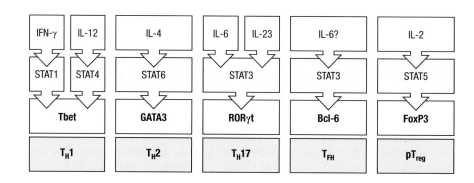

IFN-γ	IL-12	IL-4	IL-6	IL-23	IL-6?	IL-2
STAT1	STAT4	STAT6	STAT3		STAT3	STAT5
Tbet		GATA3	RORγt		Bcl-6	FoxP3
T_H1		T_H2	T_H17		T_{FH}	pT_{reg}

T_H2 development requires IL-4. When an antigen-activated naive T cell encounters IL-4, its receptor activates **STAT6**, which promotes expression of the transcription factor **GATA3**. GATA3 is a powerful activator of the genes encoding several cytokines produced by T_H2 cells, such as IL-4 and IL-13. GATA3 also induces its own expression, thereby stabilizing T_H2 differentiation via a cell-intrinsic positive feedback loop. The initial source of IL-4 that triggers a T_H2 response has long been debated. Eosinophils, basophils, and mast cells are each attractive possibilities because they can produce abundant IL-4 when activated by chitin, a polysaccharide present in helminth parasites, as well as in insects and crustaceans, which induces T_H2 responses. In mice treated with chitin, eosinophils and basophils are recruited into tissues and are activated to produce IL-4. In humans, group 2 ILCs can also produce IL-4, suggesting that these cells might contribute to T_H2 differentiation, although this is unproven. Clearly, there are several innate immune cells that might contribute IL-4 for T_H2 development, and the cellular source might differ, contingent on the inciting antigen. Similar to the positive feedback for T_H1 cell development provided by IFN-γ produced by activated T_H1 cells, IL-4 produced by activated T_H2 cells may amplify T_H2 development from naive T-cell precursors.

T_H17 cells arise when the cytokines IL-6 and TGF-β predominate during naive CD4 T-cell activation (see Figs. 9.33 and 9.34). Development of T_H17 cells requires the actions of **STAT3**, which is activated by IL-6 signaling. The signature transcription factor, or master regulator, of T_H17 cell differentiation is **RORγt**, a nuclear hormone receptor that is central to stabilizing the development of T_H17 cells. Developing T_H17 cells express the receptor for the cytokine IL-23, rather than the IL-12 receptor typical of T_H1 cells, and the expansion and further development of T_H17 effector activity seem to require IL-23, similar to the requirement for IL-12 in effective T_H1 responses (see Figs. 9.33 and 9.34). IL-21, which can be produced by T_H17 cells early in their development, has been proposed as an autocrine factor for T_H17 cell development and growth, although mice deficient for IL-21 or its receptor show no obvious impairment in T_H17 responses to infection. Notably, recent studies indicate that ongoing IL-6 signaling is required for the maintenance of T_H17 cells, indicating a nonredundant role for this cytokine both in the induction and maintenance of the T_H17 program. The initial source of IL-6 and TGF-β required for T_H17 cell differentiation appears to be cDC2 cells, although other innate immune cells activated by microbial products can also produce these cytokines. Unlike T_H1 or T_H2 cells, T_H17 cells do not appear to directly induce further T_H17 cell development from naive CD4 T cells via positive feedback, as they do not produce IL-6. However, IL-17 produced by T_H17 cells appears to enhance IL-6 production by innate immune cells and provides an indirect mechanism for reinforcing T_H17 differentiation from naive precursors.

It remains to be determined what cytokine signals—if any—are required for the initial commitment of activated CD4 T cells into T_{FH} cells. Unlike the other helper subsets, the requirements for T_{FH} differentiation are not yet clearly established and may differ between mice and humans. IL-6 seems to be important for T_{FH} development in mice but may be dispensable for development of this subset in humans. However, both species share a requirement for the transcription factor **Bcl-6** for T_{FH} development. Induction of Bcl-6 is required for the expression of CXCR5, the chemokine receptor for CXCL13, which is produced by the follicular dendritic cells and other stromal cells of the B-cell follicle. CXCR5 is essential for T_{FH} localization in follicles and is not expressed by other effector T-cell subsets. T_{FH} cells also express ICOS, the ligand for which (ICOSL) is expressed abundantly by B cells. ICOS, a member of the CD28 family, is crucial for the helper activity of T_{FH} cells, as we will see in Chapter 10. In addition to production of low amounts of cytokines characteristic of the effector T-cell subsets with which they develop in parallel (for example, IFN-γ, IL-4, or IL-17) and which promote different patterns of B-cell class switching,

Fig. 9.36 CD4 T cells differentially express IL-2 and IL-2Rα after initial activation contingent on strength of TCR signaling, leading to alternative developmental programming. See text for details.

| Stronger TCR signaling induces naive CD4 T cells to produce IL-2; less strong signaling induces IL-2Rα and response to IL-2 via paracrine signaling | More highly activated T cell up-regulates ICOS, Bcl-6, and CXCR5; less activated T cell up-regulates BLIMP-1 and S1PR1 | T_FH cell migrates to border of B-cell follicle and engages B cell; non-T_FH effector cell migrates to cortical sinus and exits lymphoid tissue |

T_FH cells produce high amounts of IL-21, a cytokine that supports the proliferation and differentiation of B cells into antibody-producing plasma cells.

One cytokine that appears to be important in T_FH development is IL-2—not by its presence, but rather by its absence (**Fig. 9.36**). Unlike effector T cells, which produce an array of 'effector' cytokines when reactivated by antigen, naive T cells are limited to production of primarily IL-2 when initially activated—and then by only a fraction of antigen-activated cells. Although still an area of active study, it now appears that differential expression of IL-2 by activated naive CD4 T cells is linked to their developmental fate, such that IL-2 producers preferentially become T_FH cells whereas IL-2 nonproducers preferentially become non-T_FH effector cells (for example, T_H1, T_H2). This would appear to be counterintuitive, as IL-2 activates STAT5, which induces the expression of the transcription factor **BLIMP-1**, which in turn represses the transcriptional actions of the central T_FH transcription factor, Bcl-6. Thus, IL-2 is a potent inhibitor of T_FH differentiation, yet cells destined for a T_FH fate are the producers of IL-2.

However, because expression of IL-2 and IL-2Rα appear to be reciprocal, the fraction of cells producing IL-2—those fated to develop into T_FH cells—are resistant to its signaling, whereas cells that do not express IL-2, but instead express IL-2Rα, become activated by IL-2—despite their lack of its production. This suggests IL-2 signaling in nascent T-cell responses is primarily paracrine, not autocrine. The basis for this is likely related to the directional secretion of some cytokines, as we will discuss in Section 9-18. Thus, IL-2 and IL-2Rα appear to be differentially expressed by activated T cells fated to become T_FH and non-T_FH effectors, respectively. The outlier would appear to be T_H17 cells, the development of which, like T_FH cells, is also inhibited by IL-2. How divergence of T_FH and T_H17 development occurs despite their shared repression by IL-2 is currently unknown. Also, mechanisms that control the differential expression of IL-2 and IL-2Rα following activation of naive T cells are not yet understood. However, the strength of TCR and CD28 co-signaling appears to be contributory: stronger activation favors IL-2 expression and T_FH cell development, whereas weaker activation favors IL-2Rα expression and non-T_FH cell development.

Peripheral regulatory T (pT_reg) cells differ from thymic regulatory T (tT_reg) cells in that they develop upon antigen recognition in secondary lymphoid tissues, not the thymus. However, like tT$_{reg}$ cells, pT$_{reg}$ cells are distinguished by expression of the transcription factor **FoxP3**, and they appear to be functionally equivalent to tT$_{reg}$ cells. Peripheral T$_{reg}$ cells develop when naive T cells are activated in the presence of the cytokines TGF-β and IL-2 in the absence of IL-6 and other pro-inflammatory cytokines. Another factor that is critical to pT$_{reg}$ cell development is all-*trans*-retinoic acid (at-RA, or simply RA), a derivative of vitamin A that binds the nuclear retinoic acid receptor (RAR). As we will discuss in Chapter 12, both TGF-β and RA are abundant in the mucosa of the gut, where the antigens derived from commensal microbes stimulate the development of pT$_{reg}$ cells to maintain tolerance to the intestinal microbiome.

Importantly, the shared requirement for TGF-β in the development of pT$_{reg}$ and T$_H$17 cells is a basis for the overlapping programming of these two subsets, such that the presence or absence of IL-6 and RA is central in determining whether TGF-β co-signaling leads to the development of immunosuppressive pT$_{reg}$ cells or pro-inflammatory T$_H$17 cells (**Fig. 9.37**). The generation of IL-6 by innate immune cells, particularly cDC2 cells, is regulated by the detection of pathogen signatures by innate sensor cells. In the absence of pathogens, IL-6 production is low, favoring differentiation of the immunosuppressive pT$_{reg}$ cells and so preventing unwanted immune responses. Both pT$_{reg}$ and tT$_{reg}$ cells can also produce TGF-β, which in certain contexts can act in an inhibitory manner to suppress immune responses and inflammation and may act to support further pT$_{reg}$ differentiation. Both types of T$_{reg}$ cells can also undergo further differentiation to produce the immunoregulatory cytokine IL-10, as we will consider further in Section 9-17, as well as in Chapters 11 and 12.

9-16 CD4 T-cell subsets can cross-regulate each other's differentiation through the cytokines they produce.

The various subsets of helper CD4 T cells have quite different immune functions. For the immune response to efficiently control different types of pathogens, it must orchestrate a coordinated effector response that is dominated by one of these subsets. A principal means of achieving this is through the distinct ensemble of cytokines that are produced by the different subsets. Importantly, some of these same cytokines also participate in positive and negative feedback loops that control the differentiation of helper T cells from naive precursors, thereby providing a mechanism to promote one pattern of effector response while suppressing others. For example, TGF-β produced by T$_{reg}$ cells inhibits the development of both T$_H$1 and T$_H$2 cells. And both IFN-γ (produced by T$_H$1 cells) and IL-4 (produced by T$_H$2 cells) potently inhibit T$_H$17 development, promoting T$_H$1 or T$_H$2 development, respectively (**Fig. 9.38**). Similarly, there is cross-regulation between T$_H$1 and T$_H$2 cells. IL-4 produced by T$_H$2 cells potently inhibits T$_H$1 development. Conversely, IFN-γ, a product of T$_H$1 cells, can inhibit the proliferation of T$_H$2 cells. As these cytokines are produced only after effector-cell development, their actions would appear to be limited to the later stages of an ongoing primary antigenic response or in a secondary, recall response. In this way, cytokines produced by effector T cells likely reinforce the differentiation of their own kind from naive precursor cells.

The adverse consequences of inappropriate cross-regulation of effector T-cell responses by cytokines have been demonstrated in a number of infectious models in mice. Such studies reinforce the notion that induction of the appropriate effector CD4 T-cell subset is crucial for pathogen clearance and show that subtle differences in CD4 T-cell responses can have a significant impact on the outcome of infection. One example is the murine model of infection by the protozoan parasite *Leishmania major*, which requires a T$_H$1 response and activation of macrophages for clearance. C57BL/6 mice

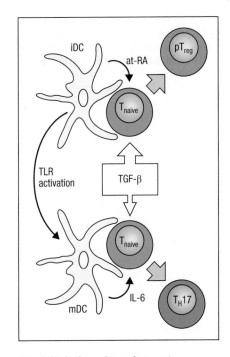

Fig. 9.37 A shared requirement for TGF-β in the differentiation of pT$_{reg}$ and T$_H$17 cells provides a developmental link that reflects their complementary roles in promoting mutualism with the microbiota. A major site for the deployment of pT$_{reg}$ and T$_H$17 cells is mucosal tissues, particularly the intestines, where the immune system must cope with an extraordinarily high density of microbial organisms that compose the microbiota. While the microbiota provides its host with important metabolic functions, it also represents a potential threat as some of its constituents are opportunistic pathogens that can cause serious infections if they breach the mucosal barrier. As an adaptation to restrain untoward inflammation directed against the microbiota while retaining the capacity to mount a host-protective immune response should barrier breach occur, the developmental balance between pT$_{reg}$ cells, which suppress inflammatory responses against the microbiota, and T$_H$17 cells, which promote host-protective inflammatory responses, is determined by the balance between production of the vitamin A metabolite all-*trans*-retinoic acid (at-RA) and production of the pro-inflammatory cytokine IL-6 by mucosal dendritic cells. At homeostasis, antigens derived from the microbiota are presented by a specialized subset of resident dendritic cells that produce high amounts of at-RA, but little IL-6 (so-called immature DC, or iDC). However, when antigens are recognized in the context of TLR-stimulating signals, at-RA production is suppressed in favor of IL-6, resulting in a 'mature' DC (mDC) that favors the development of T$_H$17 effector cells.

Fig. 9.38 The subsets of CD4 T cells each produce cytokines that can negatively regulate the development or effector activity of other subsets. Under homeostatic conditions, TGF-β produced by T_{reg} cells represses T_H1 and T_H2 responses in order to promote T_{reg} development. Under inflammatory conditions that favor IL-6 production, TGF-β production by T_{reg} cells similarly inhibits the activation of T_H1 or T_H2 responses (upper panels) in order to facilitate the development of T_H17 cells, which otherwise would be potently inhibited by IFN-γ or IL-4. Conversely, if signals are present to induce T_H1 or T_H2 cells, the cytokines IFN-γ or IL-4 produced by them can override the effect of IL-6 and inhibit T_H17 development (lower center panel). IFN-γ produced by T_H1 cells blocks the growth of T_H2 cells (right panels). On the other hand, IL-4 produced by TH2 cells dominantly prevents T_H1 cell development in favor of T_H2 (left panels). Although not shown, all T-cell subsets can produce IL-10 under conditions of chronic antigen stimulation, which inhibits the production of IL-12, IL-4, and IL-23 by dendritic cells and macrophages, thereby suppressing the development and/or maintenance of T_H1, T_H2, and T_H17 cells.

produce T_H1 cells that protect the animal by activating infected macrophages to kill *L. major*. In BALB/c mice infected with *L. major*, however, CD4 T cells fail to differentiate into T_H1 cells; instead, they become T_H2 cells, which are unable to activate macrophages to inhibit *Leishmania* growth. This difference seems to result from a population of memory T cells that are specific for gut-derived antigens but cross-react with an antigen, LACK (*Leishmania* analog of the receptors of activated C kinase), expressed by the *Leishmania* parasite. These memory cells are present in both strains of mice, but for unknown reasons they produce IL-4 in BALB/c mice but not in C57BL/6 mice. In BALB/c mice, the small amount of IL-4 secreted by these memory cells during *Leishmania* infection drives new *Leishmania*-specific CD4 T cells to become T_H2 cells instead of T_H1 cells, leading to failure of pathogen elimination and death. The preferential development of T_H2 rather than T_H1 cells in BALB/c mice can be reversed if IL-4 is blocked early during infection by anti-IL-4 antibody, but this treatment is ineffective if delayed after a week or so of infection, demonstrating the crucial importance of cytokines early in developmental decisions made by naive T cells (**Fig. 9.39**).

9-17 Regulatory T cells are a subset of CD4 T cells that restrains immune responses to maintain self-tolerance.

Regulatory T cells play a central role in preventing autoreactive immune responses and fall into different groups that are defined by their different developmental origins and functions. Thymic regulatory T (tT_{reg}) cells develop during positive selection in the thymus (see Section 8-27) and are characterized by constitutive expression of IL-2Rα, high levels of L-selectin (CD62L) and CCR7, as well as CTLA-4. As their name implies, peripheral regulatory T (pT_{reg}) cells arise in the periphery from naive CD4 T cells (see Section 9-14) and also express IL-2Rα, CD62L, CCR7, and CTLA-4. Collectively, T_{reg} cells represent about 5–10% of the CD4 T cells in circulation. A hallmark of both thymic and peripheral T_{reg} cells is their expression of the transcription factor FoxP3, which, among other actions, interferes with the interaction between

AP-1 and NFAT at the IL-2 gene promoter, preventing transcriptional activation of the gene and production of IL-2. Accordingly, although T_{reg} cells are highly dependent on IL-2 for their development and survival, they are unable to produce it. They are thus dependent on other immune cells for the IL-2 that sustains them.

Thymic T_{reg} cells develop from potentially self-reactive T cells that express conventional $\alpha\beta$ T-cell receptors and are selected in the thymus by high-affinity binding to MHC molecules containing self-peptides (see Section 8-27). They exert their regulatory function after export to secondary lymphoid tissues, where—like naive CD4 and CD8 T cells, so-called conventional T cells—they continually recirculate between blood and T-cell zones, where they survey resident and migratory cDCs for antigen. It is not currently known whether tT_{reg} cells are activated to express their regulatory function in the periphery by the same self antigens that selected them in the thymus or by other self or nonself antigens, but antigen recognition on APCs is required for their actions to inhibit the activation of conventional T cells. The critical role for tT_{reg} cells in maintaining immune tolerance to self antigens is demonstrated in humans and mice that are defective in, or deficient for, FoxP3, which results in fatal multi-organ autoimmunity (described further in Chapter 15). In essence, release of the T_{reg} cell 'brake' on naive T-cell priming by autoantigens releases uncontrolled effector T-cell differentiation that can target self antigens.

Multiple mechanisms appear to contribute to the ability of T_{reg} cells to inhibit the priming of conventional T cells by cDCs, but principal among these are interactions that interfere with the capacity of these antigen-presenting cells to provide activating signals. The expression of high levels of CTLA-4 on the surface of T_{reg} cells is thought to permit them to compete for B7 expressed by antigen-presenting cells, thereby preventing adequate co-stimulation of naive T cells. CTLA-4 is an inhibitory receptor for B7 that has a higher affinity for its ligand than that of its activating family member, CD28, and therefore can outcompete CD28 for their shared ligand. Moreover, it has been shown that CTLA-4 expressed on T_{reg} cells can physically remove B7 molecules from the surface of antigen-presenting cells, thereby depleting them of co-stimulatory activity. Similarly, by constitutively expressing the high-affinity α chain of the IL-2 receptor (IL-2Rα, and lacking the ability to produce IL-2 themselves, T_{reg} cells appear to sequester IL-2 from naive T cells, which lack IL-2Rα expression until activated. Finally, T_{reg} cells can produce TGF-β, which can inhibit the development and function of T_H1 and T_H2 cells.

Other functions of T_{reg} cells are not as well understood but are acquired only after they undergo further differentiation after antigen activation in secondary lymphoid tissues. These T_{reg} cells, called **effector regulatory T (eT_{reg}) cells**, resemble other effector CD4 T cells in that they alter their movement to sites of pathogen entry or inflammation in nonlymphoid tissues, where they act to restrain antigenic responses by T_H1, T_H2, or T_H17 cells (see Chapter 11). A key cytokine produced by eT_{reg} cells is IL-10, which inhibits the expression of MHC molecules and co-stimulatory molecules by antigen-presenting cells as a means of limiting the responses of other effector T cells. IL-10 also inhibits the production of pro-inflammatory cytokines by antigen-presenting cells. For example, IL-10 potently inhibits the production of IL-12 and IL-23 by APCs and thus impairs their ability to promote the differentiation and maintenance of T_H1 and T_H17 cells, respectively.

Although they differentiate in secondary lymphoid tissues after export from the thymus, peripheral T_{reg} cells also express FoxP3 and share most of the phenotypic and functional features of thymic T_{reg} cells. A major function of pT_{reg} cells is the prevention of inflammatory immune responses to antigens of the commensal microbiota, particularly bacteria and fungi that are residents

Fig. 9.39 The development of CD4 T-cell subsets can be manipulated by altering the cytokines acting during the early stages of infection. Elimination of infection with the intracellular protozoan parasite *Leishmania major* requires a T_H1 response, because IFN-γ is needed to activate the macrophages that provide protection. BALB/c mice are normally susceptible to *L. major* because they generate a T_H2 response to the pathogen. This is because they produce IL-4 early during infection, and this induces naive T cells to develop into the T_H2 lineage (see the text). Treatment of BALB/c mice with neutralizing anti-IL-4 antibodies at the beginning of infection inhibits this IL-4 and prevents the diversion of naive T cells toward the T_H2 lineage; these mice develop a protective T_H1 response.

in mucosal tissues and skin, and to dietary antigens to which the host must maintain tolerance. Here, pT_{reg} cells appear to be the dominant source of IL-10, deficiency of which causes inflammatory bowel disease, an immune-mediated disease of the intestines characterized by chronic reactivity against antigens of the intestinal microbiota (see also Section 15-17). As discussed in Section 9-15 and considered in more detail in Chapter 12, the differentiation of pT_{reg} cells in the intestines is favored by the presence of antigen-presenting cells that produce retinoic acid (RA). RA produced by intestinal cDCs acts with TGF-β to induce pT_{reg} cell differentiation while suppressing the differentiation of T_H17 cells (see Fig. 9.37). The antagonistic balance of RA and IL-6 therefore controls the differentiation of pT_{reg} cells and T_H17 cells, respectively, in the intestinal lymphoid tissues.

CD4 T cells that lack FoxP3 expression but produce immunosuppressive cytokines characteristic of T_{reg} cells have also been described. One such population, referred to as **type 1 regulatory (T_R1) cells**, has been defined largely by their production of IL-10 but absence of FoxP3 expression. However, we now recognize that many different cells, including T_H1, T_H2, T_H17, and B cells, can produce IL-10 under certain circumstances, such as during chronic responses to persistent antigen. Therefore, it is uncertain whether T_R1 cells represent a distinct subset of T cells, and if so, whether they have unique functions in immune regulation.

Summary.

The initiation of adaptive immunity is one of the most compelling narratives in immunology. The crucial first step in adaptive immunity is the activation, or priming, of naive antigen-specific T cells by antigen-presenting cells within the lymphoid tissues through which they constantly circulate. The most distinctive feature of antigen-presenting cells is the expression of cell-surface co-stimulatory molecules, of which the B7 molecules are the most important. Naive T cells will respond to antigen only when the antigen-presenting cell presents both a specific antigen to the T-cell receptor and a B7 molecule to CD28 on the T cell. This dual requirement for both receptor ligation and co-stimulation by the same antigen-presenting cell helps to prevent naive T cells from responding to self antigens on tissue cells, which lack co-stimulatory activity.

Activation of naive T cells leads to their proliferation and differentiation into effector T cells, the critical event in most adaptive immune responses. Various combinations of cytokines regulate the type of effector T cell that develops in response to antigen. In turn, the cytokines present during primary T-cell activation are influenced by the innate immune system. Once an expanded clone of T cells acquires effector function, its progeny can act on any target cell that displays antigen on its surface. Effector T cells have a variety of functions. CD8 cytotoxic T cells recognize virus-infected cells and kill them. T_H1 effector cells promote the activation of macrophages to enhance their killing of intracellular pathogens. T_H2 cells promote mucosal barrier immunity against helminth pathogens by amplifying the effector activities of innate effector cells such as eosinophils, basophils, and mast cells, which ultimately eliminate the worms. The elimination of certain types of bacteria and fungi is orchestrated by T_H17 cells, particularly at barrier sites, where they recruit neutrophils to sites of infection and promote the production of antimicrobial peptides by epithelial cells. T_{FH} cells are specialized for interactions with B cells and localization to the B-cell follicle and germinal centers, where they provide help for antibody production and isotype switching. Regulatory CD4 T-cell subsets restrain the immune response by preventing the activation of self-reactive naive T cells by antigen-presenting cells and by producing inhibitory cytokines that limit the effector responses of other T-cell subsets.

General properties of effector T cells and their cytokines.

Once a T cell has been primed and has undergone differentiation in the T-cell zones of a lymphoid tissue, it migrates out of the T-cell zone to perform its function. As we will learn further in Chapter 10, T_{FH} cells act on their B-cell targets without leaving the lymphoid tissue in which they were primed; they migrate to the border between T-cell and B-cell zones, where they are reactivated by an antigen-presenting B cell that has taken up the T cell's cognate antigen via its B-cell receptor (membrane-associated IgM). Most other effector T cells emigrate from their site of activation in lymphoid tissues and enter the blood, either directly if primed by antigen in the spleen or via the efferent lymphatics and thoracic duct if primed in lymph nodes. Because of the cell-surface changes that have occurred during their differentiation, effector T cells can now migrate into tissues, particularly at sites of infection. They are guided to these sites by changes in the adhesion molecules expressed on the endothelium of the local blood vessels as a result of infection, and by local chemotactic factors, as will be discussed further in Chapter 11.

Effector proteins expressed by the T cell, whether cell-associated (for example, CD40L) or secreted (for example, cytokines), are often focused on the target by mechanisms that are activated by antigen recognition. This focusing mechanism is common to all types of effector T cells and is an important mechanism controlling the efficiency and selectivity of immune effector responses, irrespective of the target cell engaged. The initial binding of an effector T cell to its target, like that of a naive T cell to an antigen-presenting cell, is an antigen-nonspecific interaction mediated by LFA-1 and CD2. The levels of LFA-1 and of CD2 are twofold to fourfold higher on effector T cells than on naive T cells, such that effector T cells can bind efficiently to target cells that have less ICAM and CD58, respectively, on their surface than do activated conventional DCs. As for naive T cells that engage cDCs, this interaction is transient unless recognition of antigen on the target cell by the T-cell receptor triggers an increase in the affinity of the T-cell's LFA-1 for its ligands. The T cell then binds more tightly to its target and remains bound long enough to release its effector molecules. Because effector CD4 T cells have to switch on new genes and synthesize new proteins to carry out their effector actions, they must maintain contact with their targets for relatively long periods (hours). Cytotoxic T cells, by contrast, can be observed under the microscope attaching to and dissociating from successive targets relatively rapidly as they kill them, as we shall see later. Killing of the target or some local change in the T cell allows the effector T cell to detach and address new targets.

9-18   An immunological synapse can form between effector T cells and their targets to direct the release of effector molecules.

As we learned in Chapter 7, when binding to cells that express their specific antigenic peptide:self MHC complexes on target cells, the T cell sometimes forms a specialized structure at the site of cell–cell contact that facilitates focused secretion of its effector molecules onto the target; this structure is called the supramolecular activation complex (SMAC), or immune (immunological) synapse (see Section 7-19). Other cell-surface molecules also cluster here. For example, the tight binding of LFA-1 to ICAM-1 induced by ligation of the T-cell receptor creates a molecular seal that surrounds the T-cell receptor and its co-receptor (**Fig. 9.40**; see also Fig. 7.5). In some cases, the contact surface organizes into two zones: a central zone known as the central supramolecular activation complex (cSMAC) and an outer zone known as the peripheral supramolecular activation complex (pSMAC). The cSMAC contains most of the signaling proteins known to be important in T-cell activation.

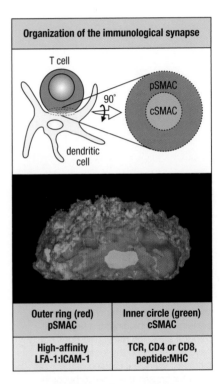

Organization of the immunological synapse

Outer ring (red) pSMAC	Inner circle (green) cSMAC
High-affinity LFA-1:ICAM-1	TCR, CD4 or CD8, peptide:MHC

Fig. 9.40 The area of contact between an effector T cell and another cell forms an immunological synapse. Proteins in the contact area between the T cell and the APC form a structure called the immunological synapse, also known as the supramolecular activation complex (SMAC), which is organized into two distinct regions: the outer, or peripheral SMAC (pSMAC), indicated by the red ring; and the inner, or central SMAC (cSMAC), indicated in bright green. The cSMAC is enriched in the T-cell receptor (TCR), CD4 or CD8, and peptide:MHC complexes. The pSMAC is enriched in the integrin LFA-1 and ICAM-1. A confocal fluorescence micrograph of the area of contact between a CD4 T cell and an APC (as viewed through one of the cells) is shown below the schematic.

ANIMATION 9.6

The pSMAC is notable mainly for the presence of the LFA-1 and the cytoskeletal protein talin, which connects LFA-1 to the actin cytoskeleton (see Section 3-18). The immunological synapse is not a static structure, as may be inferred from Fig. 9.40, but is quite dynamic. TCRs move from the periphery into the cSMAC, where they undergo endocytosis through ubiquitin-mediated degradation involving the E3 ligase Cbl (see Section 7-5). Because TCRs are being degraded in the cSMAC, signaling is actually weaker there than in the peripheral contact areas, where microclusters of TCRs are being formed and are highly active (see Section 7-8).

ANIMATION 9.7

Wiscott-Aldrich Syndrome

Clustering of TCRs signals a reorientation of the cytoskeleton that polarizes the effector cell and focuses the release of effector molecules at the site of contact with the target cell. This is illustrated for a cytotoxic T cell in **Fig. 9.41**. An important intermediary in reorganization of the cytoskeleton downstream of T-cell receptor signaling is the Wiskott–Aldrich syndrome protein (WASp), defects in which result in the inability of T cells to become polarized, among other effects, and cause an immune deficiency syndrome for which the protein is named (see Section 7-19 and Section 13-5). Activation and recruitment of WASp by TCR signaling is mediated by the adaptor protein Vav (see Section 7-19). Polarization starts with the local reorganization of the cortical actin cytoskeleton at the site of contact; this in turn leads to the reorientation of the microtubule-organizing center (MTOC)—the structure from which the microtubule cytoskeleton is produced—and reorientation of the Golgi apparatus, through which most proteins destined for secretion travel. In the cytotoxic T cell, the cytoskeletal reorientation focuses exocytosis of the preformed cytotoxic granules at the site of T-cell contact with its target cell. In CD4 effector T cells, cytoskeletal polarization also focuses the secretion of newly synthesized effector molecules induced by ligation of the T-cell receptor. For example,

Fig. 9.41 The cellular polarization of T cells during specific antigen recognition allows effector molecules to be focused on the antigen-bearing target cell. The example illustrated here is a CD8 cytotoxic T cell. Cytotoxic T cells contain specialized lysosomes called cytotoxic granules (shown in red in the left panels), which contain cytotoxic proteins. Initial binding to a target cell through adhesion molecules does not have any effect on the location of the cytotoxic granules. Binding of the T-cell receptor causes the T cell to become polarized: reorganization within the cortical actin cytoskeleton at the site of contact aligns the microtubule-organizing center (MTOC), which in turn aligns the secretory apparatus, including the Golgi apparatus (GA), toward the target cell. Proteins stored in cytotoxic granules derived from the Golgi are then directed specifically onto the target cell. The photomicrograph in panel a shows an unbound, isolated cytotoxic T cell. The microtubule cytoskeleton is stained in green and the cytotoxic granules in red. Note how the granules are dispersed throughout the T cell. Panel b depicts a cytotoxic T cell bound to a (larger) target cell. The granules are now clustered in the bound T cell at the site of cell–cell contact. The electron micrograph in panel c shows the release of granules from a cytotoxic T cell.

IFN-γ and IL-4 produced by T_H1 and T_H2 cells, respectively, may be confined and concentrated at the site of contact with the target cell.

Thus, the T-cell receptor controls the delivery of effector molecules to target cells in three ways: it induces tight binding of effector cells to their target cells to create a narrow space in which effector molecules can be concentrated; it focuses delivery of effector molecules at the site of contact by inducing a reorientation of the secretory apparatus of the effector cell; and it triggers the synthesis and/or release of the effector molecules. All these mechanisms contribute to targeting actions of effector molecules onto the cell bearing specific antigen. Effector T-cell activity is thus highly selective for appropriate target cells, even though effector molecules themselves are not antigen-specific.

9-19　The effector functions of T cells are determined by the array of effector molecules they produce, which can act locally or at a distance.

The effector molecules produced by effector T cells fall into two broad classes: cytotoxins, which are stored in specialized cytotoxic granules and released by CD8 cytotoxic T cells, and cytokines or membrane-associated proteins, which are synthesized *de novo* by all effector T cells. Cytotoxins are the principal effector molecules of cytotoxic T cells (discussed later in Section 9-22). Their release must be tightly regulated because they are not specific; they can penetrate the lipid bilayer and trigger apoptosis in any cell. By contrast, effector CD4 T cells act mainly through the production of cytokines and membrane-associated proteins, and their actions are largely restricted to cells bearing MHC class II molecules that express receptors for these proteins. Secreted cytokines and membrane-associated molecules often act in concert to mediate their effects. Although cytokines can act on the secreting T cell itself (autocrine actions), it often directs its effector functions onto other cells (paracrine actions). The main effector molecules produced by CD8 and CD4 effector T cells are summarized in **Fig. 9.42**; the major effector T-cell cytokines and their effects on different target cells are summarized in **Fig. 9.43** (see also a more comprehensive list of cytokines of immunological interest in Appendix III).

In many cases the formation of an immunological synapse ensures the polarized release of cytokines so that they are concentrated at the site of contact with the target cell (see Section 9-18). Moreover, the actions of many cytokines synergize with those of membrane-bound effector molecules. The effect, therefore, is combinatorial, and because the membrane-bound effectors can bind only to receptors on an interacting cell, this is another mechanism by which selective effects of cytokines are focused on the target cell. The effects of some cytokines are further restricted to target cells by tight regulation of their synthesis downstream of TCR signaling: the synthesis of IL-2, IL-4, and IFN-γ, for example, is controlled by mRNA instability, so that their secretion by T cells does not continue after the antigen engagement on the target cell has ended.

In other instances, cytokines have distant effects. For example, IL-3 and GM-CSF are released by T_H1, T_H2, and T_H17 cells and act on bone marrow cells to stimulate increased production of macrophages and granulocytes, which are important innate effector cells in both antibody-mediated and T cell–mediated immunity. IL-17A and IL-17F produced by T_H17 cells act both on barrier epithelium, such as in the intestinal and respiratory tracts, and on stromal cells, activating them to produce G-CSF, which enhances production of neutrophils by the bone marrow. The production by T_H2 cells of IL-5 stimulates bone marrow production of eosinophils. Whether a given cytokine effect is local or more distant is likely to reflect the amounts released, the degree to which this release is focused on the target cell, and the stability of the cytokine *in vivo*.

CD8 T cells: peptide + MHC class I		CD4 T cells: peptide + MHC class II							
Cytotoxic (killer) T cells		T_H1 cells		T_H2 cells		T_H17 cells		T_{FH} cells	
Cytotoxic effector molecules	Others	Macrophage-activating effector molecules	Others	Barrier immunity–activating effector molecules	Others	Barrier immunity–activating effector molecules, neutrophil recruitment	Others	B-cell help	Others
Perforin Granzymes Granulysin Fas ligand	IFN-γ LT-α TNF-α	IFN-γ GM-CSF TNF-α CD40 ligand Fas ligand	IL-3 LT-α CXCL2 (GROβ)	IL-4 IL-5 IL-13 CD40 ligand	IL-3 GM-CSF IL-10 TGF-β CCL11 (eotaxin) CCL17 (TARC)	IL-17A IL-17F IL-22 CD40 ligand	IL-3 TNF-α GM-CSF CCL20	IL-21 IL-4 CD40 ligand	TNF-α LT-α CXCL13

Fig. 9.42 The different types of effector T-cell subsets produce different effector molecules. CD8 T cells are predominantly killer T cells that recognize peptide:MHC class I complexes. They release perforin (which helps deliver granzymes into the target cell) and granzymes (which are pro-proteases that are activated intracellularly to trigger apoptosis in the target cell), and often also produce the cytokine IFN-γ. They also carry the membrane-bound effector molecule Fas ligand (CD178). When this binds to Fas (CD95) on a target cell, it activates apoptosis in the Fas-bearing cell. The various functional subsets of CD4 T cells recognize peptide:MHC class II complexes. T_H1 cells are specialized to activate macrophages that are infected by or have ingested pathogens; they secrete IFN-γ to activate the infected cell, as well as other effector molecules. They can express membrane-bound CD40 ligand and/or Fas ligand. CD40 ligand triggers activation of the target cell, whereas Fas ligand triggers the death of Fas-bearing targets, and so which molecule is expressed strongly influences T_H1 function. T_H1 cells also produce chemokines (for example, CXCL2) that enhance the recruitment of monocytes to enhance type 1 immune responses.

T_H2 cells are specialized for promoting immune responses to the multicellular parasites—helminths. They provide cytokines (IL-4, IL-5, and IL-13) that enhance helminth clearance through their actions to enhance eosinophil, mast cell, basophil, and barrier epithelial cell activities. They can also produce CD40 ligand and chemokines that preferentially recruit innate effector cells that enhance type 2 immune responses, as well as cytokines that promote tissue repair/healing. T_H17 cells produce members of the IL-17 family and IL-22 that both can activate barrier epithelial cell activities and can promote acute inflammation by helping to recruit neutrophils to sites of infection. They also produce CCL20, a chemokine that assists in coordination of type 3 immune responses. T_{FH} cells produce the cytokine IL-21, which is important in helping B cells mature into class-switched antibody-producers, as well as some cytokines that participate in class switching characteristic of type 1, 2, or 3 immune responses (for example, IL-4). Importantly, CD40 ligand expressed by T_{FH} cells is critical to the activation and differentiation of antigen-bearing B cells with which they interact.

9-20　Effector T cells express several TNF family cytokines.

Most effector T cells express members of the TNF family as membrane-associated proteins on the cell surface. These include TNF-α, the lymphotoxins (LTs), Fas ligand (CD178), and CD40 ligand, the last two always being cell-surface associated. TNF-α is made by T cells in soluble and membrane-associated forms and assembles into a homotrimer. Secreted LT-α is a homotrimer, but LT-α can also heterotrimerize with the transmembrane member of this family called LT-β (see Section 9-2). The receptors for TNF-α and LT-α (TNFR-I and TNFR-II) form homotrimers when bound to their ligands. The trimeric structure is characteristic of nearly all members of the TNF family (see Fig. 9.28), and the ligand-induced trimerization of their receptors is critical in initiating signaling.

Fas ligand (FasL) and CD40 ligand (CD40L) bind respectively to the transmembrane proteins Fas (CD95) and CD40 on target cells. Fas contains a 'death' domain in its cytoplasmic tail, and binding of Fas by FasL induces death by apoptosis in the Fas-bearing cell (see Fig. 9.45). Other TNFR family members, including TNFR-I, are also associated with death domains and can also induce apoptosis under some circumstances. Thus, TNF-α and LT-α can induce apoptosis by binding to TNFR-I.

CD40 Ligand Deficiency

CD40L is particularly important for CD4 T-cell effector function; its expression is induced on T_H1, T_H2, T_H17, and T_{FH} cells, and it delivers activating signals to B cells and innate immune cells through CD40. As we have seen, CD40L also plays an important role in licensing type 1 cDCs for heightened

Cytokine	T-cell source	Effects on					Effect of gene knockout
		B cells	T cells	Macrophages	Hematopoietic cells	Other tissue cells	
Interleukin-2 (IL-2)	Naive, T_H1, some CD8	Stimulates growth and J-chain synthesis	Growth and differentiation	–	–	–	↓T-cell responses IBD
Interferon-γ (IFN-γ)	T_H1, T_{FH}, CTL	Differentiation IgG2a synthesis (mouse)	Inhibits T_H2 and T_H17 cell differentiation	Activation, ↑MHC class I and class II	Activates NK cells	Antiviral ↑MHC class I and class II	Susceptible to mycobacteria, some viruses
Lymphotoxin-α (LT-α, TNF-β)	T_H1, some CTL	Inhibits	Kills	Activates, induces NO production	Activates neutrophils	Kills fibroblasts and tumor cells	Absence of lymph nodes Disorganized spleen
Interleukin-4 (IL-4)	T_H2, T_{FH}	Activation, growth IgG1, IgE ↑MHC class II induction	Growth, survival	Promotes marginal zone macrophage activation	↑Growth of mast cells	–	No T_H2
Interleukin-5 (IL-5)	T_H2	Mouse: Differentiation IgA synthesis	–	–	↑Eosinophil growth and differentiation	–	Reduced eosinophilia
Interleukin-13 (IL-13)	T_H2	IgG1, IgE class switch	–	Promotes marginal zone macrophage	–	↑Production of mucus (goblet cell)	Impaired helminth expulsion
Interleukin-17 (IL-17)	T_H17, T_{FH}	Promotes IgG2a, IgG2b, IgG3 (mouse)	–	–	Stimulates neutrophil recruitment	Stimulates fibroblasts and epithelial cells to secrete chemokines	Impaired antibacterial defense
Interleukin-22 (IL-22)	T_H17	–	–	–	–	Stimulates mucosal epithelium and skin to produce antimicrobial peptides	Impaired antibacterial defense
Interleukin-21 (IL-21)	T_{FH}, some T_H1, T_H17, CTL	Stimulates B-cell growth, germinal center formation, IgG class switching	Promotes CTL memory	–	–	–	Deficient antibody responses
Transforming growth factor-β (TGF-β)	T_{reg}, T_{FH}	Inhibits growth IgA switch factor	T_H17 and iT_{reg} differentiation, inhibits T_H1 and T_H2	Inhibits activation	Activates neutrophils	Inhibits/ stimulates cell growth	Death at ~10 weeks
Interleukin-10 (IL-10)	T_{reg}, some T_H1, T_H2, T_H17, CTL	↑MHC class II	Inhibits T_H1	Inhibits cytokine release	Co-stimulates mast cell growth	–	IBD
Interleukin-3 (IL-3)	T_H1, T_H2, T_H17, some CTL	–	–	–	Growth factor for progenitor hematopoietic cells (multi-CSF)	–	–
Tumor necrosis factor-α (TNF-α)	T_H1, T_H17, some T_H2, some CTL	–	–	Activates, induces NO production	–	Activates microvascular endothelium	Susceptibility to Gram + sepsis
Granulocyte–macrophage colony-stimulating factor (GM-CSF)	T_H1, T_H17, some T_H2, some CTL	Differentiation	Inhibits growth?	Activation Differentiation to dendritic cells	↑Production of granulocytes and macrophages (myelopoiesis) and dendritic cells	–	–

Fig. 9.43 The nomenclature and functions of well-defined T-cell cytokines. Each cytokine has multiple activities on different cell types and is typically produced only after T-cell activation by antigen. Major activities of effector cytokines are highlighted in red. The mixture of cytokines secreted by a given cell type produces many effects through what is called a 'cytokine network.' ↑, increase; ↓, decrease; CTL, cytotoxic T lymphocyte; NK cells, natural killer cells; CSF, colony-stimulating factor; Gram +, Gram positive; IBD, inflammatory bowel disease; NO, nitric oxide.

activation of naive CD8 T cells. The cytoplasmic tail of CD40 lacks a death domain; instead, it is linked downstream to proteins called TRAFs (TNF receptor–associated factors). CD40 is involved in the activation of B cells and macrophages; the ligation of CD40 on B cells promotes growth and iso-type switching, whereas CD40 ligation on macrophages induces them to secrete higher amounts of pro-inflammatory cytokines (for example, TNF-α) and become receptive to much lower concentrations of IFN-γ. Deficiency in CD40 ligand expression is associated with immunodeficiency, as we will learn in Chapter 13.

Summary.

Interactions between effector T cells and their targets are initiated by transient antigen-nonspecific adhesion. T-cell effector functions are elicited only when peptide:MHC complexes on the surface of the target cell are recognized by the receptor on an effector T cell. This recognition event triggers the effector T cell to adhere more strongly to the antigen-bearing target cell and to release its effector molecules directly at the target cell, leading to the activation or death of the target. The immunological consequences of antigen recognition by an effector T cell are determined largely by the set of effector molecules that the T cell produces on binding a specific target cell. CD8 cytotoxic T cells store preformed cytotoxins in specialized cytotoxic granules whose release is tightly focused at the site of contact with the infected target cell, thus killing it without killing any uninfected cells nearby. Cytokines and members of the TNF family of membrane-associated effector proteins are synthesized *de novo* by most effector T cells. Membrane-associated effector molecules can deliver signals only to an interacting cell bearing the appropriate receptor, whereas soluble cytokines can act on cytokine receptors expressed locally on the target cell or on other cells at a distance. The actions of cytokines and membrane-associated effector molecules through their specific receptors, together with the effects of the cytotoxins released by CD8 cells, account for most of the effector functions of T cells.

T cell–mediated cytotoxicity.

All viruses and some bacteria and single-cell protozoans multiply in the cyto-plasm of infected cells; indeed, a virus is a highly sophisticated parasite that has no biosynthetic or metabolic apparatus of its own and, in consequence, can replicate only inside cells. Although susceptible to antibody-mediated clearance before they enter cells, once they enter cells these pathogens are not accessible to antibodies and can be eliminated only by the destruction or mod-ification of the infected cells in which they replicate. This role in host defense is largely filled by cytotoxic CD8 T cells, although T_H1 cells may also acquire cytotoxic capacities. The crucial role of cytotoxic T cells in limiting such infec-tions is seen in the increased susceptibility of animals artificially depleted of these T cells or of mice or humans that lack the MHC class I molecules that present antigen to CD8 T cells. The elimination of infected cells without the destruction of healthy tissue requires the cytotoxic mechanisms of CD8 T cells to be both powerful and accurately targeted.

9-21 Cytotoxic T cells induce target cells to undergo programmed cell death via extrinsic or intrinsic pathways of apoptosis.

To deprive intracellular pathogens of their cellular host, cytotoxic T cells target the infected host cells for death. Cytotoxic T cells kill by inducing their targets to

| CTL recognizes and binds virus-infected cell | CTL programs target for death, inducing DNA fragmentation | CTL migrates to new target | Target cells die by apoptosis; neighboring uninfected cell is not killed |

Fig. 9.44 Cytotoxic CD8 T cells can induce apoptosis in infected target cells while sparing neighboring uninfected cells. Specific recognition of peptide:MHC complexes on an infected target cell by a cytotoxic CD8 T cell (CTL) leads to the death of the target cell by apoptosis. CTLs can recycle to kill multiple targets, so called 'serial killing.' Each killing requires the same series of steps, including receptor binding and the directed release of cytotoxic proteins stored in granules. Although all the cells in a tissue are susceptible to killing by the cytotoxic proteins of CTLs, the polarized release of the cytotoxic granules onto infected cells by specific antigen recognition ensures that neighboring cells are spared.

undergo **apoptosis** (**Fig. 9.44**; see also Fig. 9.31). Apoptosis is a regulated process that is induced either by specific extracellular signals or by the lack of signals required for survival. It proceeds by a series of cellular events that include plasma-membrane blebbing, changes in the distribution of membrane lipids, and enzymatic fragmentation of chromosomal DNA. A hallmark of apoptosis is the fragmentation of nuclear DNA into pieces 200 base pairs long through the activation of nucleases that cleave genomic DNA between nucleosomes. Two general pathways are involved in the induction of apoptotic cell death (**Fig. 9.45**). One, called the **extrinsic pathway of apoptosis**, is mediated by the activation of so-called death receptors by extracellular ligands. Engagement of ligand stimulates apoptosis in receptor-bearing cells. The other pathway is known as the **intrinsic** (or **mitochondrial**) **pathway of apoptosis** and is typically induced in response to noxious stimuli (for example, ultraviolet irradiation or chemotherapeutic drugs) or lack of the growth factors required for survival. Common to both pathways is the activation of specialized proteases called aspartic acid–specific cysteine proteases, or caspases, which were introduced in Chapter 3 for their role in processing the cytokines IL-1 and IL-18 to their mature forms.

Like many other proteases, caspases are synthesized as inactive pro-enzymes, in this case, pro-caspases, in which the catalytic domain is inhibited by an adjacent pro-domain. Pro-caspases are activated by other caspases that cleave the protein to release the inhibitory pro-domain. There are two classes of caspases involved in the apoptotic pathway: **initiator caspases** promote apoptosis by cleaving and activating other caspases; **effector caspases** initiate the cellular changes associated with apoptosis. The extrinsic pathway uses two related initiator caspases, caspase 8 and caspase 10, whereas the intrinsic pathway uses caspase 9. Both pathways use caspases 3, 6, and 7 as effector caspases. The effector caspases cleave a variety of proteins that are critical for cellular integrity and also activate enzymes that promote the death of the cell. For example, they cleave and degrade nuclear proteins that are required for the structural integrity of the nucleus and activate the endonucleases that fragment the chromosomal DNA.

Cytotoxic T cells can induce target-cell death by either the extrinsic or the intrinsic apoptotic pathway. The extrinsic pathway is mediated by expression of FasL and TNF-α or LT-α, receptors for which [Fas (CD95) and TNFR-I, respectively] are expressed by other cells of the immune system, as well as non-immune-system cells. Activation of the extrinsic pathway (or death receptor pathway) leads to the formation of the **death-inducing signaling complex (DISC)** (see Fig. 9.45, upper panel). The first step in Fas-mediated

 ANIMATION 9.8

 ANIMATION 9.9

Extrinsic pathway

| Trimeric Fas ligand (FasL) binds to and trimerizes Fas | Clustering of the death domains (DDs) in the Fas cytoplasmic domains allows Fas to recruit FADD via its death domain | The clustered death effector domains (DEDs) of FADD recruit and activate pro-caspase 8 via similar DEDs in the pro-caspase | Activated caspase 8 cleaves pro-caspase 3, which then cleaves I-CAD, releasing CAD to enter the nucleus and cleave DNA |

FasL

Fas

death domain (DD)

FADD — death domain (DD), death effector domain (DED)

DISC — pro-caspase 8

pro-caspase 3 cleavage

cleaved I-CAD

CAD

| In a normal cell, cytochrome *c* is present only in mitochondria | When programmed cell death is induced, the mitochondria release cytochrome *c*, which binds to and induces a conformational change in Apaf-1 | Apaf-1:cytochrome *c* complex self-assembles into an apoptosome, which recruits and activates multiple copies of pro-caspase 9, which in turn activates pro-caspase 3 | Caspase 3 cleaves I-CAD, releasing CAD to enter the nucleus and cleave DNA |

CAD I-CAD

cytochrome *c*

pro-caspase 9

Apaf-1

CARD domain

pro-caspase 3

Apaf-1

pro-caspase 3 cleavage

caspase 3

CAD

cleaved I-CAD

Intrinsic pathway

Fig. 9.45 Apoptosis of target cells can be induced by the extrinsic or intrinsic pathway. Induction of apoptosis can occur by either the extrinsic pathway (upper panels) or the intrinsic pathway (lower panels). Apoptosis induced by the extrinsic pathway is typically mediated via signaling through one of several 'death' receptors of the TNF receptor superfamily, such as Fas, which contain a so-called death domain (DD) in their cytoplasmic tails. When Fas ligand (FasL) binds Fas, this trimerizes the receptor (upper first panel). The adaptor protein FADD (also known as MORT-1) also contains a death domain and can bind to the clustered death domains of Fas (upper second panel). FADD also contains a domain called a death effector domain (DED), which allows it to recruit pro-caspase 8 (or pro-caspase 10, not shown), which also contains a DED (upper third panel). Clustered pro-caspase 8 cleaves itself to form an active enzyme that is released from the death-inducing signaling complex, or DISC, allowing active caspase 8 to then cleave executioner caspases, such as pro-caspase 3; this results in the activation of enzymes such as I-CAD, which can cleave DNA (upper fourth panel). Induction of apoptosis by the intrinsic pathway (lower panels) is mediated by the mitochondrial release of cytochrome *c*, which induces formation of the apoptosome, which in turn activates pro-caspase 9 to initiate programmed cell death. In normal cells, cytochrome *c* is confined to the mitochondria (lower first panel). However, after stimulation of the intrinsic pathway, there is mitochondrial outer membrane permeabilization (MOMP)—typically induced by activation of members of the Bcl-2 family that can form pore complexes (for example, Bax and Bak; see Fig. 9.46)—allowing cytochrome *c* to leak out into the cytosol (lower second panel), where it is bound by Apaf-1. The conformational change that ensues in Apaf-1 induces self-assembly of the multimeric apoptosome, which recruits pro-caspase 9 (lower third panel). Clustering of pro-caspase 9 by the apoptosome activates it, allowing it to cleave downstream caspases, such as pro-caspase 3, resulting in the activation of proteases and nucleases, such as I-CAD (lower fourth panel).

formation of the DISC is binding of the homotrimeric FasL, which results in the trimerization of Fas. This causes the death domains of Fas to bind to the death domain of FADD (Fas-associated via death domain), an adaptor protein that is recruited to the activated death domains of a number of TNF receptor superfamily members. In addition to its death domain, FADD contains an additional domain called a death effector domain (DED) that can bind to DEDs present in other proteins. When FADD is recruited to Fas, the DED of FADD then recruits the initiator caspase pro-caspase 8 (and/or pro-caspase 10) via interaction with a DED in the pro-caspase. The high local concentration of these caspases in association with activated receptors allows the caspases to cleave themselves, resulting in their activation. Once activated, caspases 8 and 10 are released from the receptor complex and can activate the downstream effector caspases that induce apoptosis. Loss-of-function mutations in Fas leads to the increased survival of lymphocytes and is one cause of the disease **autoimmune lymphoproliferative syndrome (ALPS)**. This disease can also be due to mutations in FasL and in caspase 10.

Because the distribution of these receptors is somewhat restricted, cytotoxic T cells have acquired a more universal mechanism for inducing cell death in antigen-specific targets: the directional release of cytotoxic granules that activate the intrinsic pathway of apoptosis (see Section 9.22). When cytotoxic T cells engage target cells that express cognate antigen, they can induce target-cell death within 5 minutes, although death can take hours to become fully evident (see Fig. 9.44). The rapidity of this response reflects the release of preformed effector molecules that are delivered to the target cell. In addition to killing the host cell, the apoptotic mechanism may also act directly on cytosolic pathogens. For example, the nucleases that are activated in apoptosis to destroy cellular DNA can also degrade viral DNA. This prevents the assembly of virions and the release of infectious virus, which could otherwise infect nearby cells. Other enzymes activated in the course of apoptosis may destroy nonviral cytosolic pathogens. Apoptosis is therefore preferable to necrosis as a means of killing infected cells; in cells dying by necrosis, intact pathogens are released from the dead cell, and these can continue to infect healthy cells or parasitize the macrophages that ingest them.

Apoptosis by the intrinsic pathway is triggered by the release of **cytochrome c** from mitochondria, which triggers the activation of caspases. Once released into the cytoplasm, cytochrome c binds Apaf-1 (apoptotic protease activating factor-1), stimulating its oligomerization to form the **apoptosome**. The apoptosome then recruits an initiator caspase, pro-caspase 9, aggregation of which promotes its self-cleavage and frees its catalytic domain to activate effector caspases (see Fig. 9.45, lower panel).

The release of cytochrome c is controlled by interactions between members of the **Bcl-2 family** of proteins. The Bcl-2 family of proteins is defined by the presence of one or more Bcl-2 homology (BH) domains and can be divided into two general groups: members that promote apoptosis, and members that inhibit apoptosis (**Fig. 9.46**). Pro-apoptotic Bcl-2 family members, such as Bax, Bak, and Bok (referred to as 'executioners'), bind to mitochondrial membranes and can directly cause cytochrome c release. How they do this is still not known, but they may form pores in the mitochondrial membranes.

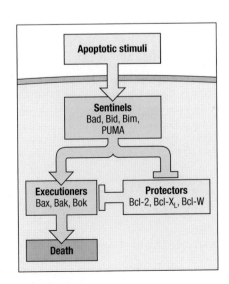

Fig. 9.46 General scheme of intrinsic pathway regulation by the Bcl-2 family of proteins. Extracellular apoptotic stimuli activate a group of pro-apoptotic (sentinel) proteins. Sentinel proteins can function either to block the protection provided by pro-survival, protector proteins or to directly activate pro-apoptotic, executioner proteins. In mammalian cells, apoptosis is mediated by the executioner proteins Bax, Bak, and Bok. In normal cells, these proteins are prevented from acting by the protector proteins (Bcl-2, Bcl-X$_L$, and Bcl-W). The release of activated executioner proteins causes the release of cytochrome c and subsequent cell death, as shown in Fig. 9.45.

Protein in granules of cytotoxic T cells	Actions on target cells
Perforin	Aids in delivering contents of granules into the cytoplasm of target cell
Granzymes	Serine proteases, which activate apoptosis once in the cytoplasm of the target cell
Granulysin	Has antimicrobial actions and can induce apoptosis

Fig. 9.47 **Cytotoxic effector proteins released by cytotoxic T cells.**

The anti-apoptotic Bcl-2 family members are induced by stimuli that promote cell survival. The best known of the anti-apoptotic proteins is Bcl-2 itself. The gene *Bcl2* was first identified as an oncogene in a B-cell lymphoma, and its overexpression in tumors makes the cells more resistant to apoptotic stimuli and thus more likely to progress to an invasive cancer. Other members of the inhibitory family include Bcl-X_L and Bcl-W. Anti-apoptotic proteins function by binding to the mitochondrial membrane to block the release of cytochrome *c*. The precise mechanism of inhibition is not clear, but they may function by directly blocking the function of the pro-apoptotic family members.

In addition to the executioners, another set of pro-apoptotic Bcl-2 family members, termed 'sentinels,' promotes apoptosis through dual actions: once activated by apoptotic stimuli, these proteins, which include Bad, Bid, Bim, and PUMA, can both block the activity of the anti-apoptotic proteins and act directly to promote the activity of the executioner pro-apoptotic proteins.

9-22 Cytotoxic effector proteins that trigger apoptosis are contained in the granules of cytotoxic CD8 T cells.

The principal mechanism of cytotoxic T-cell action is the calcium-dependent release of specialized cytotoxic granules upon recognition of antigen on the surface of a target cell. Cytotoxic granules are modified lysosomes containing at least three distinct classes of cytotoxic effector proteins that are expressed specifically in cytotoxic T cells: perforin, granzymes, and granulysin (**Fig. 9.47**). These proteins are stored in cytotoxic granules in an active form, but conditions within the granules prevent their actions until after release. **Perforin** acts by forming pores in, or perforating, the target-cell plasma membrane, which both causes direct damage to the target cell and forms a conduit through which other contents of cytotoxic granules are delivered into the cytosol of the target cell. **Granzymes**, of which there are 5 in humans and 10 in the mouse, activate apoptosis once delivered to the target-cell cytosol via pores formed by perforin. **Granulysin**, which is expressed in humans but not in mice, has antimicrobial activity and, at high concentrations, is also able to induce apoptosis in target cells. Cytotoxic granules also contain the proteoglycan **serglycin**, which acts as a scaffold, forming a complex with perforin and the granzymes. Both perforin and granzymes are required for effective target-cell killing. In cytotoxic cells that lack granzymes, the presence of perforin alone can kill target cells, but large numbers of cytotoxic cells are needed because the killing is very inefficient. In contrast, cytotoxic T cells from mice lacking perforin are unable to kill other cells because of the lack of a mechanism to form pores that deliver granzymes into the target cell.

Granzymes trigger apoptosis in the target cell both by directly activating caspases and by inducing mitochondrial release of cytochrome *c*, which also activates caspases (**Fig. 9.48**). The two most abundant granzymes are granzymes A and B. Granzyme A triggers cell death by caspase-independent mitochondrial damage, through mechanisms that are not completely understood. Granzyme B, like the caspases, cleaves proteins after aspartic acid residues and directly activates caspase 3, thereby activating a caspase proteolytic cascade, which eventually activates caspase-activated deoxyribonuclease (CAD) by cleaving an inhibitory protein (I-CAD) that binds to and inactivates CAD. This nuclease is believed to be the enzyme that degrades DNA in target cells. Granzyme B also targets mitochondria to activate the intrinsic apoptotic pathway; it cleaves the protein Bid (BH3-interacting domain death agonist protein), either directly or indirectly by activated caspase 3, causing disruption of the mitochondrial outer membrane and the release from the mitochondrial intermembrane space of pro-apoptotic molecules such as cytochrome *c*. As discussed in Section 9-21, cytochrome *c* is central to amplification of the intrinsic apoptotic cascade, as it initiates assembly of the apoptosome with

Fig. 9.48 Perforin, granzymes, and serglycin are released from cytotoxic granules and deliver granzymes into the cytosol of target cells to induce apoptosis. Recognition of its antigen on a virus-infected cell by a cytotoxic CD8 T cell induces the T cell to release the contents of its cytotoxic granules in a directed fashion. Perforin and granzymes, in a complex with the proteoglycan serglycin, are delivered to the membrane of the target cell (top panel). Perforin permeabilizes the target-cell membrane to allow the entry of the granule contents into the cytosol of the target cell, and the introduced granzymes then act on specific intracellular targets such as the proteins Bid and pro-caspase 3 (second panel). Either directly or indirectly, the granzymes cause the cleavage of Bid into truncated Bid (tBid) and the cleavage of pro-caspase 3 into an active caspase (third panel). tBid displaces the protective Bcl-2 family member, Bcl-X$_L$, from its interaction with the executioner Bcl-2 family member, Bax, resulting in Bax multimerization to form a pore to induce mitochondrial outer membrane permeabilization (MOMP). This results in mitochondrial release of cytochrome c into the cytosol, which promotes apoptosis by inducing the formation of the apoptosome that activates pro-caspase 9, which in turn further amplifies caspase 3 activation (see lower panels of Fig. 9.45). Activated caspase 3 targets I-CAD to release caspase-activated deoxyribonuclease (CAD), which fragments the DNA (bottom panel).

Apaf-1, which in turn activates the initiator caspase 9 (see Fig. 9.45, lower panels). Thus, granzyme B acts directly to activate the effector caspase 3 and indirectly to activate the initiator caspase 9.

Cells undergoing programmed cell death are rapidly ingested by phagocytic cells, which recognize a change in the cell membrane: phosphatidylserine, which is normally found only in the inner leaflet of the membrane, replaces phosphatidylcholine as the predominant phospholipid in the outer leaflet. The ingested cell is broken down and completely digested by the phagocyte without the induction of co-stimulatory proteins. Thus, apoptosis is normally an immunologically 'quiet' process; that is, apoptotic cells do not normally contribute to or stimulate immune responses.

9-23 Cytotoxic T cells are selective serial killers of targets expressing a specific antigen.

When cytotoxic T cells are offered a mixture of equal amounts of two target cells, one bearing a specific antigen and the other not, they kill only the target cell bearing the specific antigen. The 'innocent bystander' cells and the cytotoxic T cells themselves are not killed. The cytotoxic T cells are probably not killed because release of the cytotoxic effector molecules is highly polarized via an immune synapse. As we saw in Fig. 9.41, cytotoxic T cells orient their Golgi apparatus and microtubule-organizing center to focus secretion on the point of contact with a target cell (**Fig. 9.49**). Cytotoxic T cells attached to several different target cells reorient their secretory apparatus toward each cell in turn and kill them one by one, strongly suggesting that the mechanism whereby cytotoxic mediators are released allows attack at only one point of contact at any one time. The narrowly focused action of cytotoxic CD8 T cells allows them to kill single infected cells in a tissue without creating widespread tissue damage (see Fig. 9.44) and is of crucial importance in tissues where cell regeneration does not occur, as with the neurons of the central nervous system, or is very limited, as in the pancreatic islets.

Cytotoxic T cells (cytotoxic T lymphocytes; CTLs) can kill their targets rapidly because during effector differentiation from naive precursors, developing CTLs synthesize and store preformed cytotoxic proteins that are maintained in an inactive state in the cytotoxic granule by serglycin. Reactivation of the CTL by ligation of its T-cell receptor not only stimulates rapid release of preformed cytotoxins but also induces *de novo* synthesis of perforin and granzymes, so that the supply of cytotoxic granules is replenished as serial killing of targets proceeds. This makes it possible for a single CD8 T cell to kill a series of targets in rapid succession.

ANIMATION 9.10

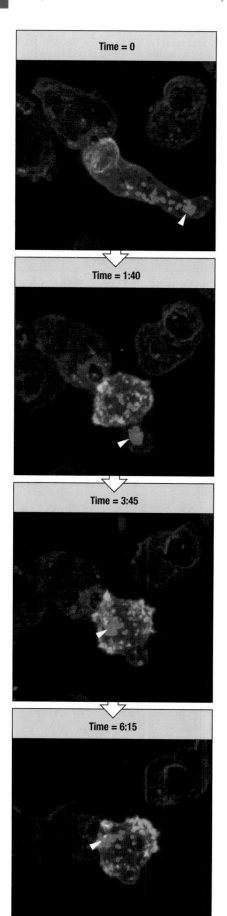

Fig. 9.49 Effector molecules are released from cytotoxic granules of a CTL in a highly polar fashion. The granules and centrosome of cytotoxic T cells (cytotoxic T lymphocytes; CTLs) can be labeled with fluorescent proteins, allowing their movements to be followed by time-lapse microscopy. Here is shown a series of pictures taken during the interaction of a CTL (green cell) with a target cell (red cell), which is eventually killed. In the top panel, at time 0, the CTL has just made contact with a target cell. At this time, the cytotoxic granules of the T cell (red dots) and the centrosome (small blue dots; arrowhead) trail the main body of the T cell and are distant from the point of contact. In the second panel, after 1 minute and 40 seconds have elapsed, the granules and centrosome have begun to move toward the target cell, a move that has nearly been completed in the fourth panel (time 6:15). After the granule contents have been released into the space between the T cell and the target, the target cell will undergo apoptosis (not shown). The T cell will then disengage from the target cell, whereupon it can go on to recognize and kill other targets.

9-24 Cytotoxic T cells also act by releasing cytokines.

Inducing apoptosis in target cells is the main way in which cytotoxic CD8 T cells eliminate infection. However, most cytotoxic CD8 T cells also release the cytokines IFN-γ, TNF-α, and LT-α, which contribute to host defense in other ways. IFN-γ inhibits viral replication directly and induces the increased expression of MHC class I molecules and other proteins that are involved in peptide loading of these newly synthesized MHC class I molecules in infected cells. This increases the chance that infected cells will be recognized as target cells for cytotoxic attack. IFN-γ also activates macrophages, which serve as both innate effector cells and as antigen-presenting cells, and stimulates the production of chemokines (for example, CXCL9, CXCL10, and CXCL11) that recruit additional macrophages and CD8 T cells to sites of infection. Finally, TNF-α and LT-α can induce apoptosis in target cells that express TNFR-I via the extrinsic pathway (see Sections 9-20 and 9-21), providing an alternative mechanism for killing of cells infected with pathogens that have the capability to subvert the perforin/granzyme mode of killing (see Chapter 13). Thus, cytotoxic effector CD8 T cells act in a variety of ways to limit the spread of cytosolic pathogens.

Summary.

Cytotoxic effector CD8 T cells are essential in host defense against many intracellular pathogens, most commonly, viruses. CTLs can kill any cell harboring such pathogens by recognizing foreign peptides that are transported to the cell surface bound to MHC class I molecules. Cytotoxic CD8 T cells perform their killing function by releasing three types of preformed cytotoxic proteins: granzymes, which use multiple mechanisms to induce apoptosis in any type of target cell; perforin, which acts in the delivery of granzymes into the target cell; and granulysin, which has antimicrobial activity and is pro-apoptotic. These properties allow the cytotoxic T cell to attack and destroy virtually any cell infected with a cytosolic pathogen. TNF family molecules, such as Fas and TNF-α, may also induce apoptosis on some target cells that express their receptors. However, this pathway is less important in most infections than that mediated by cytotoxic granules. Cytotoxic CD8 T cells also produce IFN-γ, which inhibits viral replication and is an important inducer of MHC class I molecule expression and macrophage activation. Cytotoxic T cells kill infected targets with remarkable precision, sparing adjacent normal cells. This precision is crucial in minimizing tissue damage while allowing the eradication of infected cells.

Summary to Chapter 9.

An adaptive immune response is initiated when naive T cells encounter specific antigen on the surface of an antigen-presenting cell in T-cell zones of secondary lymphoid tissues. In most cases, the antigen-presenting cells responsible for activating naive T cells, and inducing their clonal expansion, are conventional dendritic cells that express the co-stimulatory molecules B7.1 and B7.2. Conventional dendritic cells not only reside in lymphoid tissues but also survey the periphery, where they encounter pathogens, take up antigen at sites of infection, become activated through innate recognition, and migrate to local lymphoid tissue. The dendritic cell may become a potent direct activator of naive T cells or it may transfer antigen to dendritic cells resident in secondary lymphoid organs that prime T cells. Plasmacytoid dendritic cells contribute to rapid responses against viruses by producing type I interferons. Activated T cells produce IL-2, which is important in modulating early proliferation and differentiation of T cells; various other signals drive the differentiation of several types of effector T cells, which primarily act by releasing mediators directly onto their target cells. This triggering of effector T cells by peptide:MHC complexes occurs independently of co-stimulation, so that any infected target cell can be activated or destroyed by an effector T cell. Cytotoxic CD8 T cells kill target cells infected with cytosolic pathogens, thus removing sites of pathogen replication. CD4 T cells can become specialized effectors that in turn promote distinct arms of the immune response by targeting different innate and adaptive immune cells for enhanced effector function: macrophages (T_H1); eosinophils, basophils, and mast cells (T_H2); neutrophils (T_H17); or B cells (T_{FH}). Thus, effector T cells control virtually all known effector mechanisms of the adaptive and innate immune responses. In addition, subsets of CD4 regulatory T cells help control and limit immune responses by suppressing T-cell activity.

Discussion Questions

9.1 Secondary lymphoid organs are specialized for the induction of adaptive immune responses. What cells and molecules are important for the development of lymph nodes? Describe the structural features of lymph nodes and the processes of recruitment and migration of T cells through this tissue.

9.2 Dendritic cells that reside in nonlymphoid tissues are key sentinel cells that bridge innate and adaptive immunity. Describe the different types of dendritic cells, their roles in the immune response, and how they become activated to initiate an immune response in lymphoid tissues.

9.3 Activation of a naive T cell requires interaction with a conventional dendritic cell (cDC). Which molecules on T cells are involved in this process, and which molecules do they interact with on the dendritic cell? What consequences would you expect if these molecules were deficient in an individual?

9.4 CD4 T cells can develop into several subsets of effector cells. Describe the known CD4 subsets and define their major immunological functions. Describe the role of dendritic cells and different types of pathogens in generating each subset. What are the key transcription factors that contribute to the development of each CD4 subset? What are the principal cytokines produced by each subset?

9.5 T_{FH} cells are uniquely specialized to provide help to B cells for T-dependent antibody responses. Describe the features of T_{FH} cells that equip them for this function.

9.6 Effector CD8 T cells (CTLs) kill infected targets via cell–cell contact. Describe the process by which CTLs induce target-cell death, including common and unique features of the induction of apoptotic cell death by the extrinsic versus intrinsic pathways. How do CTLs kill infected target cells but spare uninfected neighboring cells?

General references.

Coffman, R.L.: Origins of the T_H1-T_H2 model: a personal perspective. *Nat. Immunol.* 2006, 7:539–541.

Heath, W.R., and Carbone, F.R.: Dendritic cell subsets in primary and secondary T cell responses at body surfaces. *Nat. Immunol.* 2009, 10:1237–1244.

Jenkins, M.K., Chu, H.H., McLachlan, J.B., and Moon, J.J.: On the composition of the preimmune repertoire of T cells specific for peptide-major histocompatibility complex ligands. *Annu. Rev. Immunol.* 2010, 28:275–294.

Springer, T.A.: Traffic signals for lymphocyte recirculation and leukocyte emigration: the multistep paradigm. *Cell* 1994, 76:301–314.

Weaver, C.T.: One road to the T_H17 pathway: how TH1 led to TH17 (and vice versa), and first came last. *Nat. Immunol.* 2020, 21:819–821.

Zhu, J., Yamane, H., and Paul, W.E.: Differentiation of effector CD4 T cell populations. *Annu. Rev. Immunol.* 2010 28:445–489.

Section references.

9-1 Secondary lymphoid structures are specialized to facilitate the interaction of circulating T and B lymphocytes with antigen.

Liu, Y.J.: Sites of B lymphocyte selection, activation, and tolerance in spleen. *J. Exp. Med.* 1997, **186**:625–629.

Loder, F., Mutschler, B., Ray, R.J., Paige, C.J., Sideras, P., Torres, R., Lamers, M.C., and Carsetti, R.: B cell development in the spleen takes place in discrete steps and is determined by the quality of B cell receptor-derived signals. *J. Exp. Med.* 1999, **190**:75–89.

Mebius, R.E.: Organogenesis of lymphoid tissues. *Nat. Rev. Immunol.* 2003, **3**:292–303.

9-2 The development of secondary lymphoid tissues is initiated by lymphoid tissue inducer cells and cytokines of the tumor necrosis factor family.

Cyster, J.G.: Blown away: the unexpected role of lymphotoxin in lymphoid organ development. *J. Immunol.* 2014, **192**:2007–2009.

Douni, E., Akassoglou, K., Alexopoulou, L., Georgopoulos, S., Haralambous, S., Hill, S., Kassiotis, G., Kontoyiannis, D., Pasparakis, M., Plows, D., *et al.*: Transgenic and knockout analysis of the role of TNF in immune regulation and disease pathogenesis. *J. Inflamm.* 1996, **47**:27–38.

Fu, Y.X., and Chaplin, D.D.: Development and maturation of secondary lymphoid tissues. *Annu. Rev. Immunol.* 1999, **17**:399–433.

Mariathasan, S., Matsumoto, M., Baranyay, F., Nahm, M.H., Kanagawa, O., and Chaplin, D.D.: Absence of lymph nodes in lymphotoxin-α (LTα)-deficient mice is due to abnormal organ development, not defective lymphocyte migration. *J. Inflamm.* 1995, **45**:72–78.

Mebius, R.E., and Kraal, G.: Structure and function of the spleen. *Nat. Rev. Immunol.* 2005, **5**:606–616.

Roozendaal, R., and Mebius, R.E.: Stromal-immune cell interactions. *Annu. Rev. Immunol.* 2011, **29**:23–43.

Wigle, J.T., and Oliver, G.: Prox1 function is required for the development of the murine lymphatic system. *Cell* 1999, **98**:769–778.

9-3 T-cell entry into lymphoid tissues occurs across specialized small blood vessels and is mediated by the sequential actions of adhesion molecules and chemokine receptors.

Cyster, J.G.: Chemokines and cell migration in secondary lymphoid organs. *Science* 1999, **286**:2098–2102.

Cyster, J.G.: Chemokines, sphingosine-1-phosphate, and cell migration in secondary lymphoid organs. *Annu. Rev. Immunol.* 2005, **23**:127–159.

Hogg, N., Henderson, R., Leitinger, B., McDowall, A., Porter, J., and Stanley, P.: Mechanisms contributing to the activity of integrins on leukocytes. *Immunol. Rev.* 2002, **186**:164–171.

Kunkel, E.J., Campbell, D.J., and Butcher, E.C.: Chemokines in lymphocyte trafficking and intestinal immunity. *Microcirculation* 2003, **10**:313–323.

Laudanna, C., Kim, J.Y., Constantin, G., and Butcher, E.: Rapid leukocyte integrin activation by chemokines. *Immunol. Rev.* 2002, **186**:37–46.

Lo, C.G., Lu, T.T., and Cyster, J.G.: Integrin-dependence of lymphocyte entry into the splenic white pulp. *J. Exp. Med.* 2003, **197**:353–361.

Luo, B.H., Carman, C.V., and Springer, T.A.: Structural basis of integrin regulation and signaling. *Annu. Rev. Immunol.* 2007, **25**:619–647.

Rosen, S.D.: Ligands for L-selectin: homing, inflammation, and beyond. *Annu. Rev. Immunol.* 2004, **22**:129–156.

Rosen, H., and Goetzl, E.J.: Sphingosine 1-phosphate and its receptors: an autocrine and paracrine network. *Nat. Rev. Immunol.* 2005, **5**:560–570.

von Andrian, U.H., and Mempel, T.R.: Homing and cellular traffic in lymph nodes. *Nat. Rev. Immunol.* 2003, **3**:867–878.

9-4 T cells are highly motile within T-cell zones as they survey dendritic cells for cognate antigen.

Caux, C., Ait-Yahia, S., Chemin, K., de Bouteiller, O., Dieu-Nosjean, M.C., Homey, B., Massacrier, C., Vanbervliet, B., Zlotnik, A., and Vicari, A.: Dendritic cell biology

and regulation of dendritic cell trafficking by chemokines. *Springer Semin. Immunopathol.* 2000, **22**:345–369.

Gretz, J.E., Anderson, A.O., and Shaw, S.: Cords, channels, corridors and conduits: critical architectural elements facilitating cell interactions in the lymph node cortex. *Immunol. Rev.* 1997, **156**:11–24.

Itano, A.A., and Jenkins, M.K.: Antigen presentation to naïve CD4 T cells in the lymph node. *Nat. Immunol.* 2003, **4**:733–739.

Miller, M.J., Wei, S.H., Parker, I., and Cahalan, M.D.: Two-photon imaging of lymphocyte motility and antigen response in intact lymph node. *Science* 2002, **296**:1869–1873.

Picker, L.J., and Butcher, E.C.: Physiological and molecular mechanisms of lymphocyte homing. *Annu. Rev. Immunol.* 1993, **10**:561–591.

Qi, H., Kastenmuller, W., and Germain, R.N.: Spatiotemporal basis of innate and adaptive immunity in secondary lymphoid tissue. *Annu. Rev. Cell Dev. Biol.* 2014, **30**:141–167.

Steptoe, R.J., Li, W., Fu, F., O'Connell, P.J., and Thomson, A.W.: Trafficking of APC from liver allografts of Flt3L-treated donors: augmentation of potent allostimulatory cells in recipient lymphoid tissue is associated with a switch from tolerance to rejection. *Transpl. Immunol.* 1999, **7**:51–57.

Stoll, S., Delon, J., Brotz, T.M., and Germain, R.N.: Dynamic imaging of T cell-dendritic cell interactions in lymph nodes. *Science* 200, **296**: 1873–1876.

9-5 The exit of T cells from T-cell zones of lymphoid tissues is controlled by a chemotactic lipid.

Cyster, J.G., and Schwab, S.R.: Sphingosine-1-phosphate and lymphocyte egress from lymphoid organs. *Annu. Rev. Immunol.* 2012, **30**:69–94.

9-6 Activation of conventional dendritic cells stimulates their maturation and migration to T-cell zones to induce naive T-cell activation.

Allan, R.S., Waithman, J., Bedoui, S., Jones, C.M., Villadangos, J.A., Zhan, Y., Lew, A.M., Shortman, K., Heath, W.R., and Carbone, F.R.: Migratory dendritic cells transfer antigen to a lymph node-resident dendritic cell population for efficient CTL priming. *Immunity* 2006, **25**:153–162.

Blander, J.M., and Medzhitov, R.: Toll-dependent selection of microbial antigens for presentation by dendritic cells. *Nature* 2006, **440**:808–812.

Germain, R.N., Miller, M.J., Dustin, M.L., and Nussenzweig, M.C.: Dynamic imaging of the immune system: progress, pitfalls and promise. *Nat. Rev. Immunol.* 2006, **6**:497–507.

Iwasaki, A., and Medzhitov, R.: Toll-like receptor control of adaptive immune responses. *Nat. Immunol.* 2004, **10**:988–995.

Miller, M.J., Wei, S.H., Cahalan, M.D., and Parker, I.: Autonomous T cell trafficking examined *in vivo* with intravital two-photon microscopy. *Proc. Natl. Acad. Sci. USA* 2003, **100**:2604–2609.

Murphy, T.L., and Murphy, K.M.: Transcriptional control of dendritic cell development. *Annu. Rev. Immunol.* 2016, **34**:93–119.

Reis e Sousa, C.: Toll-like receptors and dendritic cells: for whom the bug tolls. *Semin. Immunol.* 2004, **16**:27–34.

9-7 Subsets of conventional dendritic cells are specialized for different modes of antigen presentation.

Anderson, D.A., Dutertre, C.-A., Ginhoux, F., and Murphy, K.M.: Genetic models of human and mouse dendritic cell development and function. *Nat. Rev. Immunol.* 2021, **21**:101–115.

Asselin-Paturel, C., and Trinchieri, G.: Production of type I interferons: plasmacytoid dendritic cells and beyond. *J. Exp. Med.* 2005, **202**:461–465.

Belz, G.T., Carbone, F.R., and Heath, W.R.: Cross-presentation of antigens by dendritic cells. *Crit. Rev. Immunol.* 2002, **22**:439–448.

Eisenbarth, S.C.: Dendritic cell subsets in T cell programming: location dictates function. *Nat. Rev. Immunol.* 2019, **19**:89–103.

Ferris, S.T., Durai, V., Wu, R., Theisen, D.J., Ward, J.P., Bern, M.D., Davidson, J.T., Bagadia, P., Liu, T., Briseño, C.G., *et al.*: cDC1 prime and are licensed by CD4+ T cells to induce anti-tumour immunity. *Nature* 2020, **584**:624–629.

Guermonprez, P., Valladeau, J., Zitvogel, L., Thery, C., and Amigorena, S.: **Antigen presentation and T cell stimulation by dendritic cells.** *Annu. Rev. Immunol.* 2002, **20**:621–667.

Shortman, K., and Heath, W.R.: **The CD8+ dendritic cell subset.** *Immunol. Rev.* 2010, **234**:18–31.

Shortman, K., and Naik, S.H.: **Steady-state and inflammatory dendritic-cell development.** *Nat. Rev. Immunol.* 2007, **7**:19–30.

Swiecki, M., and Colonna, M.: **Unraveling the functions of plasmacytoid dendritic cells during viral infections, autoimmunity, and tolerance.** *Immunol. Rev.* 2010, **234**:142–162.

9-8　Conventional dendritic cells deliver multiple signals for the activation of naive T cells.

Bour-Jordan, H., and Bluestone, J.A.: **CD28 function: a balance of costimulatory and regulatory signals.** *J. Clin. Immunol.* 2002, **22**:1–7.

Chen, L., and Flies, D.B.: **Molecular mechanisms of T cell co-stimulation and co-inhibition.** *Nat. Rev. Immunol.* 2013, **13**:227–242.

Greenwald, R.J., Freeman, G.J., and Sharpe, A.H.: **The B7 family revisited.** *Annu. Rev. Immunol.* 2005, **23**:515–548.

Kapsenberg, M.L.: **Dendritic-cell control of pathogen-driven T-cell polarization.** *Nat. Rev. Immunol.* 2003, **3**:984–993.

9-9　T-cell activation induces metabolic changes that prepare the T cell for rapid clonal expansion and differentiation.

Geltink, R.I.K., Kyle, R.L., and Pearce, E.L.: **Unraveling the complex interplay between T cell metabolism and function.** *Annu. Rev. Immunol.* 2018, **36**:461–488.

MacIver, N.J., Michalek, R.D., and Rathmell, J.C.: **Metabolic regulation of T lymphocytes.** *Annu. Rev. Immunol.* 2013 **31**:259–283.

9-10　The rapid expression of interleukin-2 and the high-affinity component of its receptor allow activated T cells to respond to this cytokine coincident with entry into cell cycle.

Acuto, O., and Michel, F.: **CD28-mediated co-stimulation: a quantitative support for TCR signalling.** *Nat. Rev. Immunol.* 2003, **3**:939–951.

Gaffen, S.L.: **Signaling domains of the interleukin 2 receptor.** *Cytokine* 2001, **14**:63–77.

Seko, Y., Cole, S., Kasprzak, W., Shapiro, B.A., and Ragheb, J.A.: **The role of cytokine mRNA stability in the pathogenesis of autoimmune disease.** *Autoimmun. Rev.* 2006, **5**:299–305.

Wang, X., Rickert, M., and Garcia, K.C.: **Structure of the quaternary complex of interleukin-2 with its α, β, and γc receptors.** *Science* 2005, **310**:1159–1163.

Zhou, X.Y., Yashiro-Ohtani, Y., Nakahira, M., Park, W.R., Abe, R., Hamaoka, T., Naramura, M., Gu, H., and Fujiwara, H.: **Molecular mechanisms underlying differential contribution of CD28 versus non-CD28 costimulatory molecules to IL-2 promoter activation.** *J. Immunol.* 2002, **168**:3847–3854.

9-11　Additional co-stimulatory and inhibitory receptors are engaged after initial T-cell activation to control clonal expansion and contraction.

Croft, M.: **The role of TNF superfamily members in T-cell function and diseases.** *Nat. Rev. Immunol.* 2009, **9**:271–285.

Greenwald, R.J., Freeman, G.J., and Sharpe, A.H.: **The B7 family revisited.** *Annu. Rev. Immunol.* 2005, **23**:515–548.

Watts, T.H.: **TNF/TNFR family members in costimulation of T cell responses.** *Annu. Rev. Immunol.* 2005, **23**:23–68.

9-12　Proliferating T cells differentiate into effector T cells that are programmed for altered tissue homing and loss of a requirement for co-stimulation to act.

Gudmundsdottir, H., Wells, A.D., and Turka, L.A.: **Dynamics and requirements of T cell clonal expansion *in vivo* at the single-cell level: effector function is linked to proliferative capacity.** *J. Immunol.* 1999, **162**:5212–5223.

London, C.A., Lodge, M.P., and Abbas, A.K.: **Functional responses and costimulator dependence of memory CD4+ T cells.** *J. Immunol.* 2000, **164**:265–272.

Schweitzer, A.N., and Sharpe, A.H.: **Studies using antigen-presenting cells lacking expression of both B7-1 (CD80) and B7-2 (CD86) show distinct requirements for B7 molecules during priming versus restimulation of Th2 but not Th1 cytokine production.** *J. Immunol.* 1998, **161**:2762–2771.

9-13　CD8 T cells can be activated in different ways to become cytotoxic effector cells.

Andreasen, S.O., Christensen, J.E., Marker, O., and Thomsen, A.R.: **Role of CD40 ligand and CD28 in induction and maintenance of antiviral CD8+ effector T cell responses.** *J. Immunol.* 2000, **164**:3689–3697.

Blazevic, V., Trubey, C.M., and Shearer, G.M.: **Analysis of the costimulatory requirements for generating human virus-specific *in vitro* T helper and effector responses.** *J. Clin. Immunol.* 2001, **21**:293–302.

Seder, R.A., and Ahmed, R.: **Similarities and differences in CD4+ and CD8+ effector and memory T cell generation.** *Nat. Immunol.* 2003, **4**:835–842.

Weninger, W., Manjunath, N., and von Andrian, U.H.: **Migration and differentiation of CD8+ T cells.** *Immunol. Rev.* 2002, **186**:221–233.

9-14　CD4 T cells differentiate into several functionally distinct subsets.

Basu, R., Hatton, R.D., and Weaver, C.T.: **The Th17 family: flexibility follows function.** *Immunol. Rev.* 2013, **252**:89–103.

Bluestone, J.A., and Abbas, A.K.: **Natural versus adaptive regulatory T cells.** *Nat. Rev. Immunol.* 2003, **3**:253–257.

Crotty, S.: **Follicular helper T cells (T_FH).** *Annu. Rev. Immunol.* 2011, **29**:621–663.

Littman, D.R., and Rudensky, A.Y.: **Th17 and regulatory T cells in mediating and restraining inflammation.** *Cell* 2010, **140**:845–858.

Murphy, K.M., and Reiner, S.L.: **The lineage decisions of helper T cells.** *Nat. Rev. Immunol.* 2002, **2**:933–944.

9-15　Cytokines play a central role in guiding the differentiation of CD4 T cells down distinct pathways.

DiToro, D., Winstead, C.J., Pham, D., Witte, S., Andargachew, R., Singer, J.R., Wilson, C.G., Zindl, C.L., Luther, R.J., Silberger, D.J., *et al.*: **Differential IL-2 expression defines developmental fates of follicular versus nonfollicular helper T cells.** *Science* 2018, **361**:eaao2933.

O'Shea, J.J., and Paul, W.E.: **Mechanisms underlying lineage commitment and plasticity of helper CD4+ T cells.** *Science* 2010, **327**:1098–1102.

Reese, T.A., Liang, H.E., Tager, A.M., Luster, A.D., Van Rooijen, N., Voehringer, D., and Locksley, R.M.: **Chitin induces the accumulation in tissue of innate immune cells associated with allergy.** *Nature* 2007, **447**:92–96.

Szabo, S.J., Sullivan, B.M., Peng, S.L., and Glimcher, L.H.: **Molecular mechanisms regulating Th1 immune responses.** *Annu. Rev. Immunol.* 2003, **21**:713–758.

Weaver, C.T., Harrington, L.E., Mangan, P.R., Gavrieli, M., and Murphy, K.M.: **Th17: an effector CD4 lineage with regulatory T cell ties.** *Immunity* 2006, **24**:677–688.

9-16　CD4 T-cell subsets can cross-regulate each other's differentiation through the cytokines they produce.

Croft, M., Carter, L., Swain, S.L., and Dutton, R.W.: **Generation of polarized antigen-specific CD8 effector populations: reciprocal action of interleukin-4 and IL-12 in promoting type 2 versus type 1 cytokine profiles.** *J. Exp. Med.* 1994, **180**:1715–1728.

Harrington, L.E., Hatton, R.D., Mangan, P.R., Turner, H., Murphy, T.L., Murphy, K.M., and Weaver, C.T.: **Interleukin 17-producing CD4+ effector T cells develop via a lineage distinct from the T helper type 1 and 2 lineages.** *Nat. Immunol.* 2005, **6**:1123–1132.

Nakamura, T., Kamogawa, Y., Bottomly, K., and Flavell, R.A.: **Polarization of IL-4- and IFN-γ-producing CD4+ T cells following activation of naïve CD4+ T cells.** *J. Immunol.* 1997, **158**:1085–1094.

Seder, R.A., and Paul, W.E.: **Acquisition of lymphokine producing phenotype by CD4+ T cells.** *Annu. Rev. Immunol.* 1994, **12**:635–673.

Szabo, S.J., Dighe, A.S., Gubler, U., and Murphy, K.M.: Regulation of the interleukin (IL)-12R beta 2 subunit expression in developing T helper 1 (Th1) and Th2 cells. *J. Exp. Med.* 1997, **185**:817–824.

9-17 Regulatory T cells are a subset of CD4 T cells that restrains immune responses to maintain self-tolerance.

Fontenot, J.D., and Rudensky, A.Y.: A well adapted regulatory contrivance: regulatory T cell development and the forkhead family transcription factor Foxp3. *Nat. Immunol.* 2005, **6**:331–337.
Roncarolo, M.G., Bacchetta, R., Bordignon, C., Narula, S., and Levings, M.K.: Type 1 T regulatory cells. *Immunol. Rev.* 2001, **182**:68–79.
Sakaguchi, S.: Naturally arising Foxp3-expressing CD25⁺CD4⁺ regulatory T cells in immunological tolerance to self and non-self. *Nat. Immunol.* 2005, **6**:345–352.
Sakaguchi, S., Yamaguchi, T., Nomura, T., and Ono, M.: Regulatory T cells and immune tolerance. *Cell* 2008, **133**:775–787.
Saraiva, M., and O'Garra, A.: The regulation of IL-10 production by immune cells. *Nat. Rev. Immunol.* 2010, **10**:170–181.

9-18 An immunological synapse can form between effector T cells and their targets to direct the release of effector molecules.

Bossi, G., Trambas, C., Booth, S., Clark, R., Stinchcombe, J., and Griffiths, G.M.: The secretory synapse: the secrets of a serial killer. *Immunol. Rev.* 2002, **189**:152–160.
Montoya, M.C., Sancho, D., Vicente-Manzanares, M., and Sanchez-Madrid, F.: Cell adhesion and polarity during immune interactions. *Immunol. Rev.* 2002, **186**:68–82.
Trambas, C.M., and Griffiths, G.M.: Delivering the kiss of death. *Nat. Immunol.* 2003, **4**:399–403.

9-19 The effector functions of T cells are determined by the array of effector molecules they produce, which can act locally or at a distance.

Basler, C.F., and Garcia-Sastre, A.: Viruses and the type I interferon antiviral system: induction and evasion. *Int. Rev. Immunol.* 2002, **21**:305–337.
Boulay, J.L., O'Shea, J.J., and Paul, W.E.: Molecular phylogeny within type I cytokines and their cognate receptors. *Immunity* 2003, **19**:159–163.
Guidotti, L.G., and Chisari, F.V.: Cytokine-mediated control of viral infections. *Virology* 2000, **273**:221–227.
Harty, J.T., Tvinnereim, A.R., and White, D.W.: CD8⁺ T cell effector mechanisms in resistance to infection. *Annu. Rev. Immunol.* 2000, **18**:275–308.
Proudfoot, A.E.: Chemokine receptors: multifaceted therapeutic targets. *Nat. Rev. Immunol.* 2002, **2**:106–115.

9-20 Effector T cells express several TNF family cytokines.

Hehlgans, T., and Mannel, D.N.: The TNF–TNF receptor system. *Biol. Chem.* 2002, **383**:1581–1585.
Ware, C.F.: Network communications: lymphotoxins, LIGHT, and TNF. *Annu. Rev. Immunol.* 2005, **23**:787–819.

9-21 Cytotoxic T cells induce target cells to undergo programmed cell death via extrinsic or intrinsic pathways of apoptosis.

Aggarwal, B.B.: Signalling pathways of the TNF superfamily: a double-edged sword. *Nat. Rev. Immunol.* 2003, **3**:745–756.
Ashton-Rickardt, P.G.: The granule pathway of programmed cell death. *Crit. Rev. Immunol.* 2005, **25**:161–182.
Borner, C.: The Bcl-2 protein family: sensors and checkpoints for life-or-death decisions. *Mol. Immunol.* 2003, **39**:615–647.
Bratton, S.B., and Salvesen, G.S.: Regulation of the Apaf-1-caspase-9 apoptosome. *J. Cell Sci.* 2010, **123**:3209–3214.
Chowdhury, D., and Lieberman, J.: Death by a thousand cuts: granzyme pathways of programmed cell death. *Annu. Rev. Immunol.* 2008, **26**:389–420.
Green, D.R., Droin, N., and Pinkoski, M.: Activation-induced cell death in T cells. *Immunol. Rev.* 2003, **193**:70–81.
Siegel, R.M.: Caspases at the crossroads of immune-cell life and death. *Nat. Rev. Immunol.* 2006, **6**:308–317.
Strasser, A.: The role of BH3-only proteins in the immune system. *Nat. Rev. Immunol.* 2005, **5**:189–200.

9-22 Cytotoxic effector proteins that trigger apoptosis are contained in the granules of cytotoxic CD8 T cells.

Barry, M., Heibein, J.A., Pinkoski, M.J., Lee, S.F., Moyer, R.W., Green, D.R., and Bleackley, R.C.: Granzyme B short-circuits the need for caspase 8 activity during granule-mediated cytotoxic T-lymphocyte killing by directly cleaving Bid. *Mol. Cell Biol.* 2000, **20**:3781–3794.
Grossman, W.J., Revell, P.A., Lu, Z.H., Johnson, H., Bredemeyer, A.J., and Ley, T.J.: The orphan granzymes of humans and mice. *Curr. Opin. Immunol.* 2003, **15**:544–552.
Lieberman, J.: The ABCs of granule-mediated cytotoxicity: new weapons in the arsenal. *Nat. Rev. Immunol.* 2003, **3**:361–370.
Pipkin, M.E., and Lieberman, J.: Delivering the kiss of death: progress on understanding how perforin works. *Curr. Opin. Immunol.* 2007, **19**:301–308.

9-23 Cytotoxic T cells are selective serial killers of targets expressing a specific antigen.

Jenkins, M.R., and Griffiths, G.M.: The synapse and cytolytic machinery of cytotoxic T cells. *Curr. Opin. Immunol.* 2010, **22**:308–313.
Stinchcombe, J.C., and Griffiths, G.M.: Secretory mechanisms in cell-mediated cytotoxicity. *Annu. Rev. Cell Dev. Biol.* 2007, **23**:495–517.
Veugelers, K., Motyka, B., Frantz, C., Shostak, I., Sawchuk, T., and Bleackley, R.C.: The granzyme B-serglycin complex from cytotoxic granules requires dynamin for endocytosis. *Blood* 2004, **103**:3845–3853.

9-24 Cytotoxic T cells also act by releasing cytokines.

Kristensen, N.N., Madsen, A.N., Thomsen, A.R., and Christensen, J.P.: Cytokine production by virus-specific CD8⁺ T cells varies with activation state and localization, but not with TCR avidity. *J. Gen. Virol.* 2004, **85**:1703–1712.

The Humoral Immune Response

Many pathogens multiply in the body's extracellular spaces, and even intracellular pathogens can spread by moving through the extracellular fluids. The extracellular spaces are protected by the adaptive **humoral immune response**, in which antibodies produced by B cells act to destroy extracellular microorganisms and their products and prevent the spread of intracellular infections. As we introduced in Section 1-20, antibodies contribute to immunity in three main ways: **neutralization**, **opsonization**, and **complement activation** (**Fig. 10.1**). Antibodies can bind to pathogens and prevent their entry into cells and therefore are said to neutralize the pathogen; antibodies may also bind bacterial toxins, preventing their action or ability to enter cells. Recall that there are different forms of antibodies, known as antibody **classes** or **isotypes**, which differ in their constant regions (C regions). Antibodies of some classes can facilitate the uptake of pathogens by phagocytes by binding to certain Fc receptors through their C regions. Other Fc receptors interact with the C regions of other antibody isotypes to mediate different effector functions, such as mast-cell degranulation. Finally, antibodies bound to pathogens can activate proteins of the classical pathway of the complement system, as we described in Chapter 2. This can opsonize the pathogen by placing other complement proteins onto the pathogen's surface, helping to recruit phagocytic cells to the site of infection and activating the membrane-attack complex, which can directly lyse certain microorganisms by forming pores in their membranes. The choice of which effector mechanisms are used is influenced by the heavy-chain isotype of the antibodies produced, which determines their class (see Section 4-6).

In the first part of this chapter, we describe the interactions of naive B cells with antigen and helper T cells that lead to the activation of B cells and antibody production. Some microbial antigens can provoke antibody production without T-cell help, but activation of naive B cells by antigens usually involves help from activated CD4 T cells, especially from T follicular helper (T_{FH}) cells (see Section 9-14). Some activated B cells then differentiate into antibody-secreting **plasma cells** and memory B cells. Most antibody responses undergo a process called affinity maturation, in which antibodies of greater affinity for their target antigen are produced by the somatic hypermutation of antibody variable-region (V-region) genes. We examine the molecular mechanism of somatic hypermutation and its immunological consequences, as well as class switching—a process that generates the different classes of antibodies that confer functional diversity on the antibody response. Both affinity maturation and class switching occur only in B cells and require T-cell help. In the second part of the chapter, we introduce the distributions and functions of various classes of antibody, in particular those secreted into mucosal sites. In the

IN THIS CHAPTER

B-cell activation by antigen and helper T cells.

The distributions and functions of immunoglobulin classes.

The destruction of antibody-coated pathogens via Fc receptors.

Fig. 10.1 Antibodies mediate the humoral immune response through neutralization, opsonization, and complement activation. After being secreted by plasma cells, antibodies protect the host from infection in three main ways. They can inhibit the toxic effects or infectivity of pathogens or their products by binding to them, a process called neutralization (top panel). When bound to pathogens, the antibody's Fc region can bind to Fc receptors on accessory cells, such as macrophages and neutrophils, helping these cells to ingest and kill the pathogen. This process is called opsonization (middle panel). Antibodies can trigger complement by activating C1, the first step in the classical complement pathway. Deposition of complement proteins enhances opsonization and can also directly kill certain bacterial cells by activating the membrane-attack complex (bottom panel).

third part of the chapter, we discuss in detail how the Fc region of the antibody engages various effector mechanisms to contain and eliminate infections. Like the T-cell response, the humoral immune response produces immunological memory, which is discussed in Chapter 11.

B-cell activation by antigen and helper T cells.

The surface immunoglobulin that serves as the **B-cell antigen receptor (BCR)** plays two roles in B-cell activation in response to pathogens. Like the antigen receptor on T cells, the BCR initiates a signaling cascade upon binding antigens derived from the microbe. In addition, the BCR can deliver the antigen to intracellular sites for antigen processing, generating antigenic peptides bound to MHC class II molecules that are returned to the B-cell surface. These peptide:MHC class II complexes are recognized by antigen-specific helper T cells that have already differentiated in response to the same pathogen. The effector T cells express surface molecules and cytokines that help the B cell to proliferate and to differentiate into antibody-secreting cells and into memory B cells. A structure called the germinal center (see Section 10-6) is formed during an intermediate phase of the antibody response, before the emergence of long-term plasma cells that generate antibody or of memory B cells.

Some microbial antigens can activate B cells directly in the absence of T-cell help, and the ability of B cells to respond directly to these antigens provides a rapid response to many important pathogens. However, the fine-tuning of antibody responses to increase the affinity of the antibody for the antigen and the switching to most immunoglobulin classes other than IgM depend on the interaction of antigen-stimulated B cells with helper T cells and other cells in the secondary (or peripheral) lymphoid organs. Thus, antibodies induced by microbial antigens alone tend to have lower affinity and to be less functionally versatile than those induced with T-cell help.

10-1   Activation of B cells by antigen involves signals from the B-cell receptor and either helper T cells or microbial antigens.

As we learned in Chapter 8, activation of naive T cells requires signals derived from the T-cell receptor as well as co-stimulatory signals provided by professional antigen-presenting cells. Similarly, in addition to signals derived from the B-cell receptor, naive B cells also require accessory signals that can arise either from a helper T cell or, in some cases, directly from microbial constituents (**Fig. 10.2**).

Protein antigens alone are unable to induce antibody responses in animals or humans who lack T cells, and they are therefore known as **thymus-dependent (TD) antigens** and typically require antigen-specific T-cell help. The T cells involved are CD4 T cells that reside in the lymphoid tissues and are not fully differentiated T_H1, T_H2, or T_H17 effector cells, can become T_{FH} cells (see Section 9-14), and can enter B-cell follicular regions and induce B cells to proliferate and secrete antibody in response to protein antigens. To receive T-cell help, the B cell must display antigen on its surface in a form that a T cell can recognize. This occurs when antigen bound by surface immunoglobulin on the B cell is internalized and degraded within the B cell and peptides derived from it are returned to the cell surface in a complex with MHC class II molecules (see Fig. 10.2, first panel). When the CD4 T cell recognizes these peptide:MHC complexes, it provides the B cell with signals that favor survival and induce proliferation. These signals include the activation of **CD40** on B cells by the T-cell–expressed ligand, **CD40L** (CD154),

Fig. 10.2 A second signal is required for B-cell activation by either thymus-dependent or thymus-independent antigens. The first signal (indicated as '1') required for B-cell activation is delivered through its antigen receptor (BCR) and activates several pathways as described in Chapter 7. Signaling by the BCR is enhanced by the co-receptors CD21 and CD19, which interact with C3b on opsonized microbial surfaces. For thymus-dependent antigens (first panel), a second signal (indicated as '2') is delivered by a helper T cell (T_H) that recognizes degraded fragments of the antigen as peptides bound to MHC class II molecules on the B-cell surface. CD40L on the helper T cell binds to CD40 on the B cell, activating both the canonical NFκB signaling via IKK and the non-canonical NFκB signaling pathway via NFκB-inducing kinase (NIK). This induces expression of pro-survival genes such as *Mcl1* (myeloid cell leukemia-1). For thymus-independent antigens (second panel), a second signal can be delivered through Toll-like receptors that recognize antigen-associated TLR ligands, such as bacterial lipopolysaccharide (LPS) or bacterial DNA, as described in Chapter 3.

and production of various cytokines by T cells, including **IL-21** (Fig. 10.3). CD40 signaling can activate both the **canonical NFκB pathway** and the **non-canonical NFκB pathway** (see Section 7-24) and enhances B-cell survival by inducing the expression of anti-apoptotic molecules such as Mcl-1 (myeloid cell leukemia-1), a protein related to the Bcl-2 family, and B-cell

Fig. 10.3 CD4 T cells provide several signals that activate B cells and control their subsequent differentiation. After antigen binding to the B-cell receptor delivers the first signal for B-cell activation (not shown), the T_FH cell delivers additional signals when it recognizes a peptide:MHC class II complex on the B-cell surface (first panel). Besides expression of CD40 ligand, the T_FH cell secretes several important cytokines, including IL-21, which activates the transcription factor STAT3 to enhance B-cell proliferation and survival. T cells can also produce cytokines that will regulate isotype switching (see Section 10-12). After receiving these signals, activated B cells begin to proliferate (second panel), enter the germinal center, and eventually become plasma cells or memory B cells (third panel).

differentiation by inducing metabolic programs and transcription factors such as BLIMP that promote antibody secretion. IL-21 signaling activates STAT3 and enhances cellular proliferation and differentiation into plasma cells and memory B cells. Other cytokines produced by T cells include IL-6, TGF-β, IFN-γ, and IL-4, which provide signals that can regulate the type of antibody produced, as we will see in Section 10-12.

While B-cell responses to protein antigens rely on help from T cells, some microbial constituents can induce antibody production in the absence of helper T cells. These microbial antigens are known as **thymus-independent (TI) antigens** because they can induce antibody responses in individuals who have no T lymphocytes. Such antigens typically contain highly repetitive epitopes, such as the polysaccharides of bacterial cell walls, and can activate signaling by the BCR on B cells. In such cases, a second signal can be derived from direct recognition of a common microbial constituent, such as lipopolysaccharide (LPS), which can activate TLR signaling in the B cell (see Fig. 10.2, second panel), activating the NFκB pathway, as described in Chapter 3. Thymus-independent antibody responses provide some early protection against extracellular bacteria, and we will return to them later.

10-2 Linked recognition of antigen by T cells and B cells promotes robust antibody responses.

B-cell activation by antigens on microbial surfaces can be greatly stimulated by the concurrent deposition of complement on these pathogens. The **B-cell co-receptor complex** contains the cell-surface proteins CD19, CD21, and CD81 (see Fig. 7.29). When **CD21**, or complement receptor 2 (CR2), binds to the complement fragments C3d and C3dg that are deposited on microbial surfaces (see Section 2-13), it is brought near to the activated B-cell receptor bound to the same surface. CD21 and CD19 are associated with each other, and CD19 becomes phosphorylated by a complex of proteins associated with the activated B-cell receptor. This recruits phosphatidylinositol 3-kinase (PI 3-kinase), which cooperates with the BCR to stimulate several downstream pathways, enhancing proliferation, differentiation, and antibody production (see Fig. 10.2, arrow 1). This effect is shown when mice are immunized with the experimental antigen hen egg-white lysozyme coupled to three linked molecules of C3dg. In this case, less C3dg-modified lysozyme is more effective in inducing antibody in the absence of added adjuvant than is unmodified lysozyme.

For T-dependent antibody responses, the T cells involved are activated by fragments of the same antigen as is recognized by the B cells; this is called **linked recognition**. However, the peptide recognized by the helper T cell is likely to differ from the protein epitope recognized by the B cell's antigen receptor. Natural antigens, such as viruses and bacteria, contain multiple proteins and carry both protein and carbohydrate epitopes. For linked recognition to occur, the peptide recognized by the T cell must be physically associated with the antigen recognized by the B cell's receptor, so that the B cell can take up and present the appropriate peptide to the T cell. For example, a B cell that recognizes an epitope on a viral coat protein will internalize the complete virus particle. The B cell can degrade multiple viral proteins into peptides for display on MHC class II molecules on the B-cell surface. CD4 T cells specific for such viral peptides may have been activated by dendritic cells earlier in the infection. Some of these can become T$_{FH}$ cells and express CXCR5, which allows them to enter the same regions where B cells reside (discussed later). When these activated T$_{FH}$ cells encounter their cognate peptide presented on B cells, the T cells in turn provide specific signals that help B cells to generate antibodies against the viral coat protein (**Fig. 10.4**).

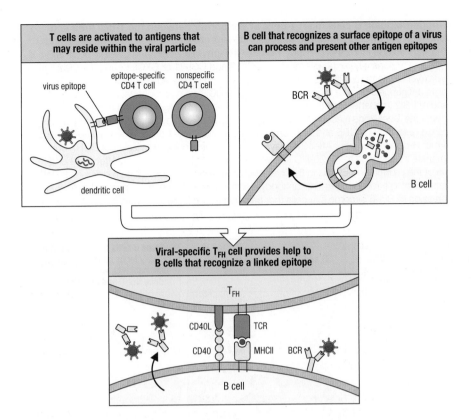

Fig. 10.4 T cells and B cells that recognize antigens contained within the same molecular complex can engage productively. In this example, an internal viral protein harbors a peptide epitope (shown as red) that is presented by MHC class II molecules and is recognized by a CD4 T cell. The virus also harbors a native epitope on an external viral coat protein (shown as blue) that is recognized by the surface immunoglobulin on a B cell. If the virus is captured and presented by a dendritic cell, a peptide-specific CD4 T cell (blue) becomes activated (top left panel), whereas nonspecific T cells (green) remain inactive. If the virus is recognized by a specific B cell (top right panel), peptides derived from internal viral proteins are processed and presented by MHC class II molecules. When the activated T cell recognizes its peptide on this B cell (bottom panel), the T cell will deliver various accessory signals to the B cell that promote antibody production against the coat protein. This process is known as linked recognition.

Linked recognition relies on the concentration of the appropriate peptide for presentation by MHC class II molecules on the B-cell surface. B cells whose B-cell receptor binds a particular antigen are 10,000 times more efficient at displaying peptide fragments of that antigen on their MHC class II molecules than are B cells that have B-cell receptors of irrelevant specificities. Linked recognition was originally discovered through studies of the production of antibodies against haptens, which are small chemical groups that cannot elicit antibody responses on their own (see Appendix I, Section A-1). But haptens that are coupled to a carrier protein become immunogenic—known as the **hapten carrier effect**—for two reasons. The protein can carry multiple hapten groups, allowing it to cross-link B-cell receptors. T cells that are activated against peptides of the carrier protein and which became T_{FH} cells have also taken part in the germinal center reaction to strengthen the antibody response to the hapten. Accidental coupling of a hapten to a protein is responsible for the allergic responses shown by many people to the antibiotic penicillin, which reacts with host proteins to form a coupled hapten that can stimulate an antibody response, as we will learn in Chapter 14. Vaccine design can take advantage of linked recognition, as in the vaccine used to immunize infants against *Haemophilus influenzae* type b (see Section 16-7).

10-3 B cells that encounter their antigens migrate toward the boundaries between B-cell and T-cell areas in secondary lymphoid tissues.

The frequency of naive B cells specific for most protein antigens is extremely low (less than 1 in 10,000). The frequency can be higher for some conserved carbohydrate or phospholipid antigens, such as galactose-α-1,3-galactose (α-Gal), which may react with up to 0.2% of all peripheral B cells in humans. Nonetheless, the chance of a random encounter between a T and a B cell with the same antigen specificity should be less than 1 in 10^8, making it remarkable that B cells ever interact with T_H cells with similar antigen specificity. For these reasons, linked recognition requires a precise regulation of the migration

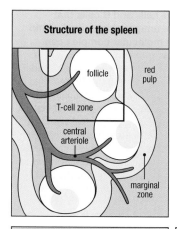

Structure of the spleen

follicle

red pulp

T-cell zone

central arteriole

marginal zone

Fig. 10.5 Antigen-binding B cells meet T cells at the border between the T-cell area and a B-cell follicle in secondary lymphoid tissues. Antigens enter the spleen from the blood and collect in T-cell zones and follicles (top panel). Naive CCR7-positive T cells and CXCR5-positive B cells migrate to distinct regions where the chemokines CCL19 and CCL21 or CXCL13 and the EBI2 ligand 7α,25-dihydroxycholesterol (7α,25-HC), respectively, are being produced (first lower panel). If a B cell encounters its antigen, either on a follicular dendritic cell (FDC) or a macrophage, it induces expression of CCR7 and of EBI2 (the latter increasing its responsiveness to EBI2 ligands) and migrates toward the border with the T-cell zone (second lower panel). T cells activated by antigen-presenting dendritic cells induce expression of CXCR5 and EBI2 and migrate to this same border, where linked recognition induces further B-cell proliferation. After 2–3 days, some B cells reduce expression of CCR7 but retain EBI2 and migrate in response to 7α,25-HC to the outer follicle (third lower panel). After another day or so, some of the proliferating B cells in the interfollicular regions near the red pulp differentiate into plasmablasts, forming a focus of terminal antibody-secreting cells (fourth lower panel). T cells that induce expression of Bcl-6 become T_{FH} cells that participate with B cells there to form a germinal center reaction.

| Before activation, resting B cells express CXCR5 and reside in follicles and T cells express CCR7 and reside in T-cell zones | Activated B cells induce CCR7 and EBI2, and T cells induce CXCR5, and both cells migrate to follicular and interfollicular regions | B and T cells aggregate at the periphery of follicles | Some B cells migrate to form a primary focus and differentiate into plasmablasts, while some T cells induce Bcl-6 and become T_{FH} cells |

resting B cells

resting T cells

CXCL13

FDC

CCL21

7α, 25HC

interfollicular zone

dendritic cell

activated B cells

activated T cells

T_{FH}

primary focus

of activated B and T cells—orchestrated by several sets of ligands and receptors—into specific locations within the lymphoid tissues, which serves to increase the chances of a productive interaction (**Fig. 10.5**).

Naive T cells and B cells express the **sphingosine 1-phosphate receptor 1 (S1PR1)**, which they use to egress from the secondary lymphoid tissues (see Section 9-5). However, before they exit, they initially occupy and are retained in two distinct zones, the **T-cell areas** and the **primary lymphoid follicles** (or B-cell areas or B-cell zones), respectively. These zones are established by different patterns of chemokine receptor expression and chemokine production. Naive T cells express the chemokine receptor **CCR7** and localize to zones where its ligands, **CCL19** and **CCL21**, are highly expressed by stromal cells and dendritic cells (see Section 9-3). Circulating naive B cells express **CXCR5**, and when they migrate into lymphoid tissues, they enter the primary lymphoid follicles, where the chemokine **CXCL13** is abundant. Within the follicle, stromal cells and a specialized cell type, the **follicular dendritic cell (FDC)**, secrete CXCL13. The FDC is a nonphagocytic cell of non-hematopoietic origin that bears numerous long processes; it functions by trapping antigen using Fc receptors and complement receptors on its cell surface for access by B cells in the follicle.

Once in the follicle, naive B cells encounter the soluble TNF-family cytokine **BAFF** (see Section 8-9), which is secreted by FDCs, stromal cells, dendritic cells, monocytes, and T_{FH} cells and which acts as a survival factor for B cells. BAFF can act through three receptors, but its major actions in promoting survival are through **BAFF-R** (**Fig. 10.6**). BAFF-R signals through **TRAF3** (see Section 3-7) to activate the non-canonical NFκB pathway and induces expression of Bcl-X_L, an anti-apoptotic member of the Bcl-2 family. Two other receptors for BAFF are **TACI** and **BCMA**, which signal through TRAF2, TRAF5, and TRAF6 to induce signaling pathways

Fig. 10.6 BAFF and APRIL promote B-cell survival and regulate differentiation.
BAFF (B-cell activating factor, also called B-lymphocyte stimulator, or BLyS) and APRIL (a proliferation-inducing ligand) are both members of the TNF superfamily of cytokines. They are initially produced as membrane-bound trimers by several cell types. BAFF is produced by FDCs and other cells in the B-cell follicle, where it supports B-cell survival. Its main receptor, BAFF-R, signals through TRAF3 and NIK to activate the non-canonical NFκB pathway, leading to the RelB:p52 transcription factor and inducing expression of Bcl-X$_L$, a protein similar in function to Bcl-2 described in Section 9-21. BAFF also binds to the receptors TACI (transmembrane activator and calcium modulator and cyclophilin ligand interactor) and BCMA (B-cell maturation antigen), although its affinity for BCMA is relatively weak. Naive and recently activated B cells express only BAFF-R and TACI, while BCMA is expressed by plasma cells. These receptors also activate the non-canonical NFκB pathway.

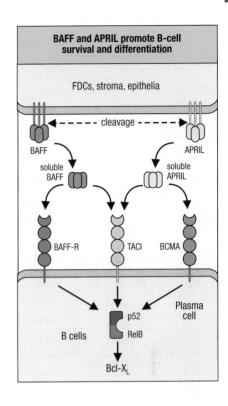

involved in B-cell activation. TACI is highly expressed on follicular and germinal center B cells, but BCMA is expressed by plasma cells and has a relatively low affinity for BAFF. TACI and BCMA also bind the related cytokine **APRIL**, a survival factor for plasma cells.

Antigens derived from microorganisms and viruses are transported into lymph nodes via the afferent lymph and into the spleen via the blood. Opsonized antigens bearing C3b or C3dg accumulate in the B-cell follicles because they are trapped by complement receptors CR1 and CR2 expressed on the surface of FDCs. While small soluble antigens may diffuse directly into the follicle, opsonized particulate antigens can also be taken up by specialized macrophages residing in the **subcapsular sinus** (SCS) of lymph nodes and the **marginal sinus** of the spleen, regions that are both adjacent to the B-cell follicles (**Fig. 10.7**). These macrophages seem to retain the antigen on their surface rather than ingesting and degrading it. These antigens can then be sampled and carried by antigen-specific follicular B cells. B cells of any antigen specificity could also acquire antigen from these macrophages via their complement receptors and transport it within the follicle. In the spleen, marginal zone B cells shuttle between that site and the follicle, carrying antigen trapped in the marginal zone for deposition on FDCs. SCS macrophages can also actively function to restrict the dissemination of infection. For example, in mice, infection of these macrophages in lymph nodes by vesicular stomatitis virus (VSV), a relative of rabies virus, triggers the cells to produce interferon and to recruit

Fig. 10.7 Opsonized antigens are captured and preserved by subcapsular sinus macrophages. Macrophages residing in the lymph node subcapsular sinus (SCS) express complement receptors 1 and 2 (CR1 and CR2, respectively), are poorly endocytic, and have reduced levels of lysosomal enzymes compared with macrophages in the medulla. Opsonized antigen arriving from the afferent lymphatics binds to CR1 and CR2 on the surface of SCS macrophages. Instead of being completely degraded by these macrophages, some antigen is retained on the cell surface, where it can be presented and transferred to the surface of follicular B cells. B cells are then able to transport the antigen into the follicle, where it can be trapped on the surfaces of follicular dendritic cells.

Fig. 10.8 Induction of SAP in T$_{FH}$ cells allows SLAM family receptors to mediate sustained contact with B cells. The SLAM receptor family members SLAM, Ly108, and CD84 are expressed on T cells and B cells and mediate homotypic interactions that lead to adhesion between cells. SLAM can also enhance signaling by the T-cell receptor to augment production of cytokines such as IL-21 that help B cells. The SLAM-associated molecule SAP is a signaling adaptor that is required for one SLAM receptor to sustain binding with another. T cells initially express SAP at low levels that are insufficient for sustained adhesion between T and B cells. Fully differentiated T$_{FH}$ cells express high levels of the transcription factor Bcl-6, which increases SAP expression to a level sufficient to sustain cell–cell interactions and allow for the delivery of CD40L and cytokine signals to B cells.

plasmacytoid dendritic cells (pDCs). Type I interferon produced by pDCs restricts further viral spread, which would otherwise eventually pass on to the central nervous system.

After a naive follicular B cell first encounters specific antigen, either soluble antigen or displayed by FDCs or macrophages, within a few hours it will become positioned in the outer follicles of lymphoid tissue close to the sites where antigen enters the lymph node or spleen. This positioning is orchestrated by the B cell's expression of a chemoattractant receptor, **EBI2** (GPR183), whose ligands are oxysterols such as 7α,25-dihydroxycholesterol. Non-hematopoietic reticular cells in the outer follicular and interfollicular regions are the primary sources of these ligands. After sampling antigens there for 6 hours to 1 day, the B cell induces expression of CCR7, which functions together with EBI2 to distribute activated B cells along the interface between the B-cell follicle and the T-cell zone, where CCL21 is expressed.

During an immune response, T cells are activated within the T-cell zones by dendritic cells. When naive T cells are activated, some will proliferate, differentiate into effector cells, up-regulate expression of S1PR1, and exit the lymphoid tissue. However, others will up-regulate CXCR5 and migrate to the border with the B-cell follicle. There, T cells can encounter B cells activated during the same response, increasing the chance that they might recognize linked antigens presented by activated B cells that have recently moved to this location (see Fig. 10.5).

10-4   T cells express surface molecules and cytokines that activate B cells, which in turn promote T$_{FH}$ cell development.

When a CD4 T cell encounters an activating peptide presented by B cells, it responds by expressing receptors and cytokines that in turn activate B cells. As mentioned earlier, the CD40L expressed by CD4 T cells activates CD40 on B cells to increase B-cell survival and also induces B-cell expression of co-stimulatory molecules, especially those of the B7 family. CD40L expressed by CD4 T cells provides a general help for B cells, and in human CD40L deficiency, there is loss of all switched Ig isotypes. T cells also secrete several cytokines that regulate B-cell proliferation and antibody production. Primary among these is IL-21, which is produced early in immune responses and which activates the transcription factor **STAT3** in B cells to support proliferation and differentiation. IL-21 exerts similar autocrine effects on CD4 T cells, including T$_{FH}$ cells. Later in the antibody response, the T cells will produce other cytokines, such as IL-4 and IFN-γ, that are characteristic of the other T helper subsets (described in Chapter 9). These will impact B-cell differentiation, particularly class switching, as we discuss later.

This first interaction between T and B cells not only provides important help to B cells but also influences T-cell differentiation by means of signals provided by the B cell. The co-stimulatory molecule B7.2 (CD86) is up-regulated during B-cell activation and stimulates T cells by ligation of CD28. Activated B cells also express **ICOSL**, another member of the B7 family and a ligand for **ICOS** (inducible co-stimulatory protein), which is expressed by T cells. This T- and B-cell interaction, provided by linked recognition, activates ICOS signaling in T cells and is important for the completion of T$_{FH}$ differentiation (see Section 9-15), leading to induction of the transcription factors **Bcl-6** and **c-Maf**.

The ability of T$_{FH}$ cells to successfully deliver these signals to B cells depends on intimate contact between these cells. Specific adhesion molecules, including several Ig superfamily receptors of the **SLAM (signaling lymphocyte activation molecule)** family, help to prolong and stabilize cell–cell contact. T$_{FH}$ cells and B cells both express SLAM (CD150), **CD84**, and **Ly108**, which promote cell adhesion through homotypic binding interactions (**Fig. 10.8**).

The cytoplasmic regions of these SLAM family receptors all interact with an adaptor protein, **SAP (SLAM-associated protein)**, which becomes highly expressed by T_{FH} cells and which is necessary for prolonging cell–cell contact mediated by these receptors. The transcription factors Bcl-6 and c-Maf characteristic of T_{FH} cells are also required for SAP expression and so help sustain the contact between B and T_{FH} cells. The SAP gene is inactivated in **X-linked lymphoproliferative (XLP) syndrome**, which is associated with a T-cell and NK-cell lymphoproliferative disorder and with a defect in antibody production due to failed interactions between T_{FH} cells and B cells in the germinal center, discussed later. In contrast to CD40L deficiency, in XLP syndrome there is often hypergammaglobulinemia and hyper-IgE.

X-linked Lymphoproliferative Syndrome

The regulated migration of activated B cells and T_{FH} cells to the same location in the secondary lymphoid organ increases the chance that linked recognition will occur and deliver appropriate help for B-cell differentiation. B cells stimulated chronically with antigen that fail to interact with a T_{FH} cell within 1–2 days will become anergic and exhibit a shorter life span (~5 days) compared with naive B cells (~40 days). B cells that are transiently exposed to antigen can return to the naive state in the absence of T cell help.

10-5 Some activated B cells differentiate into antibody-secreting plasmablasts and plasma cells.

After their initial activation by antigen, B cells migrate to the boundary of the follicle where they interact with helper T cells. B cells that have received T-cell help migrate from the follicle border to continue to proliferate and differentiate. Two to three days after activation, B cells begin to decrease expression of CCR7 and retain expression of EBI2 (see Fig. 10.5). Decreased expression of CCR7 causes B cells to move away from the boundary with the T-cell zone: EBI2 directs their migration back to the interfollicular regions and the subcapsular sinus in the lymph nodes, or, in the spleen, to the splenic bridging channels, a region between the T-cell area and the red pulp. Here, some B cells will form an emerging aggregate of differentiating B cells, which in lymph nodes is located in the medullary cords, where lymph drains out of the node. In the spleen, this can be seen as extrafollicular foci in the splenic red pulp, which are called **primary foci**. Primary foci are apparent by about 5 days after an infection or immunization with an antigen not previously encountered.

B cells proliferate for several days, and this constitutes the first phase of the primary humoral immune response. Some of these proliferating B cells differentiate into antibody-synthesizing **plasmablasts** in the primary focus. Not all B cells activated by the initial interaction with CD4 T_H cells will move into the primary focus. Some will migrate into the lymphoid follicle as described later. Plasmablasts are cells that have begun to secrete antibody, yet are still dividing and express many of the characteristics of activated B cells that allow their interaction with T cells. After a few more days, the plasmablasts in the primary focus stop dividing and may eventually die. Subsequently, plasmablasts or B cells arising from the germinal centers can migrate to the bone marrow and become long-lived plasma cells, where they continue antibody production. Many long-lived plasma cells are generated long after the primary focus has dissipated, suggesting that they arise from B cells that entered the germinal center reaction.

The properties of resting B cells, plasmablasts, and plasma cells are compared in **Fig. 10.9**. The differentiation of a B cell into a plasma cell is accompanied by many morphological changes reflecting the commitment of a plasma cell to the secretion of large amounts of antibody (several thousand antibody molecules per second), which can constitute up to 20% of all the protein synthesized by a plasma cell. Plasmablasts and plasma cells have a prominent perinuclear Golgi apparatus and an extensive rough endoplasmic reticulum that is

B-lineage cell	Intrinsic properties			Inducible by antigen stimulation		
	Surface Ig	Surface MHC class II	High-rate Ig secretion	Growth	Somatic hyper-mutation	Class switch
Resting B cell	High	Yes	No	Yes	Yes	Yes
Plasmablast	High	Yes	Yes	Yes	Unknown	Yes
Plasma cell	IgA, IgE: High / IgG: Low	Yes	Yes	No	No	No

Fig. 10.9 Plasma cells secrete antibody at a high rate but can no longer respond to antigen. Resting naive B cells have membrane-bound immunoglobulin (usually IgM and IgD) and MHC class II molecules on their surface. Although their V genes do not carry somatic mutations, B cells can take up antigen and present it to helper T cells. The T cells in return induce the B cells to proliferate and to undergo isotype switching and somatic hypermutation, but B cells do not secrete significant amounts of antibody during this period. Plasmablasts have an intermediate phenotype. They secrete antibody but retain substantial surface immunoglobulin and MHC class II molecules and so can continue to take up and present antigen to T cells. Plasmablasts early in the immune response and those activated by T-independent antigens have usually not undergone somatic hypermutation and class switching, and therefore secrete IgM. Plasma cells are terminally differentiated cells that secrete antibodies. Plasma cells have low levels of surface immunoglobulin but can express MHC class II molecules and may suppress T_{FH} activity in a negative feedback pathway while differentiating. Early in the immune response, they differentiate from unswitched activated B cells and secrete IgM; later in the response, they derive from activated B cells that entered the germinal center reaction and underwent class switching and somatic hypermutation. Plasma cells have lost the ability to change the class of their antibody or undergo further somatic hypermutation.

rich in immunoglobulin molecules that are being synthesized and exported into the lumen of the endoplasmic reticulum for secretion. Plasmablasts still express B7 co-stimulatory molecules B7.1 and B7.2 and MHC class II molecules; by contrast, plasma cells will eventually turn down the expression of MHC class II molecules. Nevertheless, T cells still provide important signals for plasma-cell differentiation and survival, such as IL-6 and CD40 ligand. While some plasma cells survive for only days to a few weeks after their final differentiation, others are very long lived and account for the persistence of antibody responses.

10-6 The second phase of a primary B-cell immune response occurs when activated B cells migrate into follicles and proliferate to form germinal centers.

Some activated B cells move into a primary lymphoid follicle together with their associated T_{FH} cells (**Fig. 10.10**), where they continue to proliferate and ultimately form a **germinal center**; follicles with germinal centers are also called **secondary lymphoid follicles**. Down-regulating EBI2 by B cells appears to favor germinal center formation. In mice lacking EBI2 expression in B cells, antigen-activated B cells failed to move to the border with the T-cell zone and remained near the follicular center. These mice were able to form germinal centers but generated fewer plasmablasts.

Germinal centers are composed mainly of proliferating B cells, but antigen-specific T cells make up about 10% of germinal center lymphocytes and

Fig. 10.10 Activated B cells form germinal centers in lymphoid follicles. Activation of B cells in a lymph node is shown here. Top panel: Naive circulating B cells enter lymph nodes from the blood via high endothelial venules (HEVs) and are attracted by chemokines into the primary lymphoid follicle; if these B cells do not encounter antigen in the follicle, they leave via the efferent lymphatic vessel. Second panel: B cells that have bound antigen move to the border with the T-cell area, where they may encounter activated helper T cells specific for the same antigen; these T cells interact with the B cells and activate them to begin proliferating and encourage some of them to differentiate into plasmablasts. Some B cells activated at the T-cell–B-cell border migrate as antibody-secreting plasmablasts to form extrafollicular foci in the red pulp (spleen) or an initial aggregate in the medullary cords (lymph nodes). Other B cells move back into the interior of the follicle, where they continue to proliferate and form a germinal center. Germinal centers are sites of sustained B-cell proliferation and differentiation and affinity maturation. Follicles in which germinal centers have formed are known as secondary follicles. Within the germinal center, B cells begin their differentiation into either long-lived plasma cells or memory B cells. Third and fourth panels: Plasma cells leave the germinal center and migrate to the medullary cords, where they are short-lived and persist for only a few days, or leave the lymph node altogether via the efferent lymphatics and migrate to the bone marrow, where they can persist for many months to years.

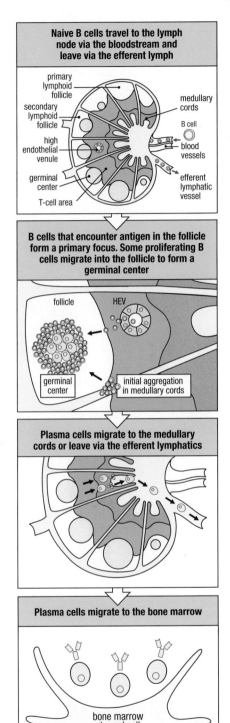

provide indispensable help to the B cells. The germinal center is an area of active cell division that forms within a surrounding region of resting B cells in the primary follicle. Proliferating germinal center B cells displace the resting B cells toward the periphery of the follicle, forming a **mantle zone** of resting cells around the two distinguishable areas of activated B cells, called the **light zone** and the **dark zone** (**Fig. 10.11**, left panel). The germinal center grows in size as the immune response proceeds, and then shrinks and finally disappears when the infection is cleared. Germinal centers are present for about 3–4 weeks after initial antigen exposure to proteins, and often for much longer when induced by live infections such as influenza viruses.

The primary focus and the germinal center reaction differ in the quality of antibody that they produce. Plasmablasts, germinal center B cells, and early memory B cells begin to emerge during the first 4–5 days of an immune response. Plasmablasts in primary foci primarily can secrete antibodies of

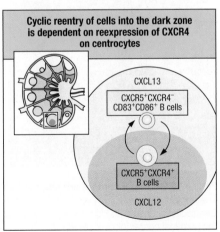

Fig. 10.11 The structure of a germinal center. The germinal center is a specialized microenvironment in which B-cell proliferation, somatic hypermutation, and selection for strength of antigen binding all occur. Closely packed centroblasts, which express CD83, CD86, CXCR4, and CXCR5, form the dark zone of the germinal center; the less densely packed light zone contains centrocytes, which express only CXCR5. Stromal cells in the dark zone produce CXCL12, which attracts the CXCR4-expressing centroblasts. Cyclic reentry describes the process by which B cells can lose and gain expression of CXCR4 and thus move from the light zone to the dark zone and back again.

the IgM isotype but can also undergo class switching to produce other isotypes independently of the germinal center reaction, which may offer some immediate protection. Recent evidence suggests that most class switching occurs before entry of B cells into the germinal center reaction. In contrast, B cells in the germinal center reaction undergo several processes that produce antibodies that are more effective in eliminating infections facilitated by their higher levels of Bcl-6 expression. These processes include **somatic hypermutation**, which alters the V regions of immunoglobulin genes (discussed shortly) and enables a process called **affinity maturation**, which selects for the survival of mutated B cells that have a high affinity for the antigen. In addition, class switching allows the selected B cells to produce antibodies with a variety of effector functions. These B cells will differentiate either into plasma cells that secrete higher-affinity and class-switched antibody in the latter part of the primary immune response or into memory B cells as described in Chapter 11. We will discuss mechanisms of class switching after a description of the germinal center reaction, even though Ig class switching can occur outside the germinal center and may occur even in TI responses.

B cells in the germinal center divide rapidly, every 6–8 hours. Initially, these rapidly proliferating B cells, called **centroblasts**, express the chemokine receptors CXCR4 and CXCR5 but markedly reduce their expression of surface immunoglobulin, particularly of IgD. Centroblasts proliferate primarily in the dark zone of the germinal center, named for its densely packed appearance in hematoxylin and eosin (H&E)-stained microscopic tissue sections (**Fig. 10.12**). Stromal cells in the dark zone produce **CXCL12 (SDF-1)**, a ligand for CXCR4 that acts to retain centroblasts in this region. As time goes on, some centroblasts reduce their rate of cell division, reduce CXCR4 expression, and begin

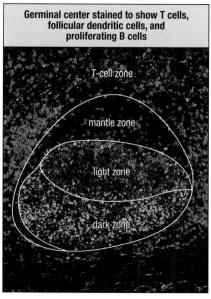

| Light micrograph of germinal center (high power) | Germinal center stained to show T cells, follicular dendritic cells, and proliferating B cells |

T-cell zone

mantle zone

light zone

dark zone

Fig. 10.12 Germinal centers are sites of intense cell proliferation and cell death. The photomicrograph (first panel) shows a section through a human tonsillar germinal center. Centroblasts, seen in the lower part of this photomicrograph, form the so-called dark zone of the germinal center. Above this region is the light zone, which appears lighter in H&E-stained micrographs in part due to the presence of the highly networked dendritic extensions of FDCs. The second panel shows immunofluorescent staining of a germinal center. B cells are found in the dark zone, light zone, and mantle zone. Proliferating cells are stained green for Ki67, an antigen expressed in nuclei of dividing cells, revealing the rapidly proliferating centroblasts in the dark zone. The dense network of follicular dendritic cells, stained red, mainly occupies the light zone. Centrocytes in the light zone proliferate to a lesser degree than centroblasts. Small recirculating B cells occupy the mantle zone at the edge of the B-cell follicle. Large masses of CD4 T cells, stained blue, can be seen in the T-cell zones, which separate the follicles. There are also significant numbers of T cells in the light zone of the germinal center.

to produce higher levels of surface immunoglobulin. These B cells are termed **centrocytes**. The loss of CXCR4 allows centrocytes to move into the light zone, containing abundant FDCs that produce the chemokine CXCL13 (BLC), a ligand for CXCR5 (see Fig. 10.11, right panel).

10-7   Germinal center B cells undergo V-region somatic hypermutation, and cells with mutations that improve affinity for antigen are selected.

Somatic hypermutation introduces mutations that change anywhere from one to a few amino acids in the immunoglobulin, producing closely related B-cell clones that differ in their affinity for antigen (**Fig. 10.13**). These mutations in the V genes are initiated by an enzyme called **activation-induced cytidine deaminase,** or **AID**, which is expressed by B cells in the extrafollicular foci and germinal centers. Before describing the enzymatic mechanisms initiated by AID, we first present a general overview of this process in which random mutations can improve antibody affinity.

The immunoglobulin V-region genes accumulate mutations at a rate of about one base pair change per 10^3 base pairs per cell division, while the rate of mutations in the rest of the cell's DNA is much lower: around one base pair change per 10^{10} base pairs per cell division. Somatic hypermutation also affects some DNA flanking the rearranged V gene but does not generally extend into the C-region exons. Because each V region (for both the heavy and light chain) is encoded by about 360 base pairs and about three out of every four base changes will alter the amino acid encoded, there is about a 50% chance during each B-cell division that a mutation will occur to the receptor.

The point mutations accumulate in a stepwise manner as the descendants of each B cell proliferate in the germinal center to form B-cell clones (**Fig. 10.14**). An altered receptor can affect the ability of a B cell to bind antigen and thus will affect the fate of the B cell in the germinal center. Most mutations have a negative impact on the ability of the B-cell receptor to bind the original antigen by preventing the correct folding of the immunoglobulin molecule or by blocking the complementarity-determining regions from binding antigen. Detrimental

Fig. 10.13 The primary antibody repertoire is diversified by processes that modify the rearranged immunoglobulin gene. First panel: The primary antibody repertoire is initially composed of IgM-containing variable regions (red) produced by V(D)J recombination and constant regions (blue) from the μ gene segment. The range of reactivity of this primary repertoire can be further modified by somatic hypermutation, by class switch recombination at the immunoglobulin loci, and in some species by gene conversion (not shown). Second panel: Somatic hypermutation results in mutations (shown as blue lines) being introduced into the heavy-chain and light-chain V regions (red), altering the affinity of the antibody for its antigen. Third panel: In class switch recombination, the initial μ heavy-chain C regions (blue in first two panels) are replaced by heavy-chain regions of another isotype (shown as yellow), modifying the effector activity of the antibody but not its antigen specificity.

	Heavy-chain V region			Light-chain V region			
	CDR1	CDR2	CDR3	CDR1	CDR2	CDR3	
Day 7 Primary response							
Day 14 Secondary response							
Day 21 Tertiary response							Increasing antibody affinity

B cells mutate their antibody genes in the dark zone of the germinal center

TFH — antigen — B cells — Light zone — Dark zone

B cells with high affinity for antigen can capture and process it for presentation by MHC class II molecules

TFH — TCR — High-affinity antibody — MHCII — low-affinity antibody

B cells that can present antigens to T$_{FH}$ cells will receive survival and mitogenic signals via CD40 and cytokines

TFH — CD40 — CD40L — low affinity antibody

B cells that receive help from T$_{FH}$ cell can reenter the dark zone to undergo additional mutations

Dark zone

Fig. 10.14 Somatic hypermutation introduces mutations into the rearranged immunoglobulin variable (V) regions that improve antigen binding. The process of somatic hypermutation can be tracked by sequencing immunoglobulin V regions from hybridomas (clones of antibody-producing cells; see Appendix I, Section A-8) established at different time points after the experimental immunization of mice. The result of one experiment is depicted here. Each V region sequenced is represented by a horizontal line. The complementarity-determining regions CDR1, CDR2, and CDR3 are shown by pink shading. Mutations that change the amino acid sequence are represented by red bars. Within a few days of immunization, the V regions within a particular clone of responding B cells begin to acquire mutations, and over the course of the next week more mutations accumulate (top panels). B cells whose V regions have accumulated deleterious mutations and can no longer bind antigen die. B cells whose V regions have acquired mutations that improve the affinity of the B-cell receptor for antigen are able to compete more effectively for antigen and receive signals that drive their proliferation and expansion. The antibodies they produce also have this improved affinity. This process of mutation and selection can continue in the lymph node germinal center through multiple cycles in response to secondary and tertiary immune responses elicited by further immunization with the same antigen (center and bottom panels). In this way, the antigen-binding efficiency of the antibody response is improved over time.

mutations may alter conserved framework regions (see Fig. 4.9) and disrupt basic immunoglobulin structure. Cells that harbor such detrimental mutations are eliminated by apoptosis either because they can no longer make a functional B-cell receptor or because they cannot take up antigen as well as sibling B cells (**Fig. 10.15**). Germinal centers are filled with apoptotic B cells that are quickly engulfed by macrophages, giving rise to the characteristic **tingible body macrophages**. These contain dark-staining nuclear debris in their cytoplasm. This process of elimination is implied by the relative scarcity of amino acid replacements

Fig. 10.15 Selection for high-affinity mutants in the germinal center relies on help provided by T$_{FH}$ cells. After activated B cells interact with T$_{FH}$ cells at the follicle border, they migrate to germinal centers (GCs), where the following events depicted here occur. In the dark zone of the GC, somatic hypermutation alters the immunoglobulin V regions (first panel). In some B cells (yellow), the mutated B-cell receptor (BCR) will have low or no affinity for the antigen, while in other B cells (orange), the mutated BCR affinity may be higher. After exiting the dark zone, the B cells with higher-affinity BCRs will capture antigen (red) trapped on follicular dendritic cells (FDCs) and then process and present it on MHC class II molecules (second panel). B cells with low-affinity BCRs will fail to capture and present antigen. B cells that present linked antigen epitopes to T$_{FH}$ cells (dark blue) will receive help through CD40L and IL-21, which promote survival and proliferation. B cells that lack antigen on MHC class II molecules receive no help and will eventually die (third panel). T cells that do not recognize the antigen presented by B cells (light blue) will not participate. Some of the proliferating B cells undergo repeated cycles of entry to the dark zone, mutation, and selection (fourth panel), and other progeny B cells undergo differentiation to either memory B cells or plasma cells (not shown).

in the framework regions, reflecting the loss of cells that had mutated any one of the many residues that are critical for immunoglobulin V-region folding. This process prevents rapidly dividing B cells from expanding to numbers that would overwhelm the lymphoid tissues. Less frequently, mutations may improve the affinity of a B-cell receptor for antigen, and these mutations will be selectively expanded (see Fig. 10.15) because the cells expressing receptors with such mutations will have an increased survival rate compared with that of low-affinity cells. Positive selection is evident in the accumulation of numerous amino acid replacements in the complementarity-determining regions (CDRs), which determine antibody specificity and affinity (see Fig. 10.14), a process we discuss in the next section. The result of selection for enhanced binding to antigen is that the nucleotide changes that alter amino acid sequences, and thus protein structure, tend to be clustered in the CDRs of the immunoglobulin V-region genes, whereas silent, or neutral, mutations that preserve amino acid sequence and do not alter protein structure are scattered throughout the V region.

▶ **ANIMATION 10.1**

10-8   Positive selection of germinal center B cells involves contact with T_FH cells and CD40 signaling.

Selection of B cells with improved affinity for antigen occurs in increments. It was originally discovered *in vitro* that resting B cells could be kept alive by simultaneously cross-linking their B-cell receptors and ligating their cell-surface CD40. *In vivo* these signals are delivered by antigen and by T_FH cells, respectively. The details of selection in the germinal center have become more clear recently from studies based on *in vivo* two-photon laser-scanning microscopy (see Appendix I, Section A-10). They show that positive selection of a B cell depends on the B cell's ability to take up antigen and to receive signals delivered by T_FH cells. It is thought that somatic hypermutation occurs in the centroblasts in the dark zone; when a centroblast reduces its rate of proliferation and becomes a centrocyte, it increases the number of B-cell receptors on its surface and moves to the light zone, where there are abundant FDCs. Antigen can be trapped and stored for long periods in the form of immune complexes on FDCs (**Fig. 10.16** and **Fig. 10.17**). The centrocyte's ability to bind antigen determines its relative ability to acquire antigen, in competition with the other clonally related centrocytes harboring different mutations. Centrocytes whose receptors bind antigen better will capture and present more peptides on their

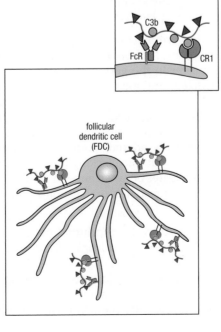

Fig. 10.16 Antigens are trapped in immune complexes that bind to the surface of follicular dendritic cells. Radiolabeled antigen localizes to, and persists in, lymphoid follicles of draining lymph nodes [see the light micrograph and the schematic representation (left panels), showing a germinal center in a lymph node]. The intense dark staining shows the localization in the germinal center of radiolabeled antigen that had been injected 3 days previously. The antigen is in the form of antigen:antibody:complement complexes bound to Fc receptors and to complement receptors CR1 or CR2 on the surface of the FDC, as depicted in the right panel and inset. These complexes may also be internalized and recycled by a nondegradative endocytic pathway (not shown). FcR, Fc receptor.

Fig. 10.17 Immune complexes bound to FDCs form iccosomes, which are released and can be taken up by B cells in the germinal center. FDCs have a prominent cell body and many dendritic processes. Immune complexes, bound to complement receptors and Fc receptors on the FDC surface, become clustered, forming prominent bead-like structures along the dendrites (a). An intermediate form of FDC is shown, which has both straight filiform dendrites and others that are becoming beaded. These beads are shed from the cell as *iccosomes* (immune complex–coated bodies), which can bind to a B cell in the germinal center (b) and be taken up by it (c). In panels b and c, the iccosome has been formed with immune complexes containing horseradish peroxidase, which is used to form electron-dense material that appears dark in the transmission electron micrographs.

surface MHC class II molecules. T_FH cells in the germinal center recognize these peptides and, as before, are activated to deliver to the B-cell signals that promote survival. Centrocytes whose mutations reduce antigen-binding affinity will take up less antigen, and so will receive weaker survival signals from T_FH cells. Successful B cells will reexpress CXCR4 and return to the dark zone, where they will undergo additional rounds of division, in effect becoming centroblasts again. Germinal center B cells that fail to acquire sufficient antigen from FDCs to engage T_FH cells will become apoptotic and disappear. This process of B-cell migration within the germinal center is known as the **cyclic reentry model** (see Fig. 10.11, right panel). In this way, the affinities of B cells are continually refined during the germinal center response (see Section 10-6). The selection process can be quite stringent. The germinal center may begin with perhaps a few hundred different clones. Competition among these various clones is based not only on their affinity for antigen but also on which epitope of which antigens they recognize. Although some clones may leave few progeny as antigen-producing B cells, they may leave progeny in the form of memory B cells.

In the germinal center, T_FH cells and B cells interact to deliver signals that are important for both cells (see Section 10-4). Mice that lack ICOS or SAP are deficient in the germinal center reaction and have severely reduced class-switched antibody responses because of defective T_FH cell function. CD40 signaling in B cells is activated by CD40L on T_FH cells and increases expression of the survival molecule Mcl-1, a relative of Bcl-2. These interactions between T_FH cells and B cells are enhanced by signals from SLAM family receptors through the adaptor protein SAP. Intravital laser-scanning microscopy has revealed that mice lacking the SLAM receptor CD84 have reduced numbers of conjugates between antigen-specific T cells and B cells, and these mice also have a reduced humoral response to antigen.

10-9 Activation-induced cytidine deaminase introduces mutations into genes transcribed in B cells.

Activation-Induced Cytidine Deaminase Deficiency

Now that we have discussed the cellular processes involved in somatic hypermutation and affinity maturation, we will delve into the details of the mutation process itself. The enzyme activation-induced cytidine deaminase (AID) is important for both somatic hypermutation and class switch recombination, as mice lacking AID have defects in both processes. People with mutations in the AID gene that inactivate the enzyme—that is, who have **activation-induced cytidine deaminase deficiency, or AID deficiency**—also lack both somatic hypermutation and class switching. This condition leads to the production of predominantly IgM antibodies and the absence of affinity maturation, a syndrome known as **hyper IgM type 2 immunodeficiency** (discussed in Section 13-9).

AID is related to enzymes that deaminate cytosine to uracil in making nucleotide precursors for RNA and DNA synthesis. Its closest homolog, **APOBEC1 (apolipoprotein B mRNA editing catalytic polypeptide 1)**, is an RNA-editing enzyme that deaminates cytosine in the context of RNA. However, AID fulfills its activity in antibody gene diversification by acting on cytosine in the DNA of the immunoglobulin locus. When AID deaminates cytidine residues in the immunoglobulin V regions, somatic hypermutation is initiated; when cytidine residues in switch regions are deaminated, class switch recombination is initiated.

AID can deaminate cytidine residues in single-stranded DNA but not double-stranded DNA (**Fig. 10.18**). AID typically acts when its target genes are being transcribed, so that the DNA double helix is temporarily unwound. Because AID is expressed primarily in germinal center B cells, but is also expressed in activated B cells, AID primarily targets the actively transcribed, rearranged V regions of the immunoglobulin genes. This process is thought to rely in part on the highly active transcription of the rearranged V regions in these B cells, where RNA polymerase may generate transient single-strand regions. Somatic hypermutation does not occur in loci that are not being actively transcribed. Rearranged V_H and V_L genes are mutated even if they are 'nonproductive' rearrangements and are not being expressed as protein, as long as they are being transcribed. Some actively transcribed genes in B cells besides those for immunoglobulins can also be affected by the somatic mutation process, but at a much lower rate. AID is also expressed in human and mouse B-cell progenitors, where it may play a role in promoting self-tolerance in developing B cells, and in non-Peyer's-patch lamina propria B cells, where it may be involved in T-independent IgA class switch and somatic mutation.

10-10   Mismatch and base-excision repair pathways contribute to somatic hypermutation after initiation by AID.

The uridine produced by AID represents a dual lesion in DNA: it is foreign to normal DNA, and it is a mismatch with the guanosine nucleoside on the opposite DNA strand. The presence of uridine in DNA can trigger several types of DNA repair—including the **mismatch repair** and the **base-excision repair** pathways—which further alter the DNA sequence. The various repair processes lead to different mutational outcomes (**Fig. 10.19**). In the mismatch repair pathway, the presence of uridine is detected by the mismatch repair proteins **MSH2** and **MSH6** (MSH2/6). They recruit nucleases that remove the complete uridine nucleotide along with several adjacent nucleotides from the damaged DNA strand. This removal is followed by a fill-in 'patch repair' by a DNA polymerase; but unlike the repair process in other cells, in B cells this DNA synthesis is error-prone and tends to introduce mutations at nearby A-T base pairs. Two error-prone polymerases that may be involved are and Polη and Polθ.

The initial steps in the base-excision repair pathway are shown in **Fig. 10.20**. In this pathway, the enzyme **uracil-DNA glycosylase (UNG)** removes the uracil base from the uridine to create an abasic site in the DNA. If no further modification is made, at the next round of DNA replication this will result in the random insertion of a nucleotide opposite the abasic site by DNA polymerase, leading to mutation. The action of UNG may, however, be followed by the

Fig. 10.18 Activation-induced cytidine deaminase (AID) is the initiator of mutations in somatic hypermutation, gene conversion, and class switching. The activity of AID, which is expressed only in B cells, requires access to the cytidine side chain of a single-strand DNA molecule (first panel), which is normally prevented by the hydrogen bonding in double-stranded DNA. AID initiates a nucleophilic attack on the exposed cytosine ring (second panel), which is resolved by the deamination of the cytidine to form uridine (third panel).

DNA in variable region or in switch region

Transcription produces local single-stranded DNA

In B cells, AID attacks cytidine in single-stranded DNA to produce uridine

AID

Uracil-DNA glycosylase (UNG) removes uracil to form apyrimidinic residue

UNG

Apurinic/apyrimidinic endonuclease-1 (APE1) cuts the backbone next to the abasic site to form a single-strand nick

APE1

Single-strand nick in DNA

Fig. 10.19 AID initiates DNA lesions whose repair leads to somatic hypermutation, class switch recombination, or gene conversion. When AID converts a cytidine (C) to uridine (U) in the DNA of an immunoglobulin gene, the final mutation produced depends on which repair pathways are used. Somatic hypermutation can result from either the mismatch repair (MSH2/6) pathway combined with an error-prone polymerase activity or from the base-excision repair (UNG) pathway. Acting together, these pathways can generate point mutations at and around the site of the original C-G pair. REV1 is a DNA repair enzyme that can synthesize DNA, or recruit other enzymes that can synthesize DNA, over the abasic sites in damaged DNA. REV1 itself will insert only C opposite the abasic site, but it can help recruit other polymerases that can also insert A, G, and T. The end result is insertion of a random nucleotide at the C-G residues where AID initially acted. Both class switch recombination and gene conversion require the formation of a single-strand break in the DNA. A single-strand break is formed when apurinic/apyrimidinic endonuclease-1 (APE1) removes a damaged residue from the DNA as part of the repair process (see Fig. 10.20, bottom two panels). In class switch recombination, single-strand breaks made in two of the so-called switch regions upstream of the C-region genes are converted to double-strand breaks. The cell's machinery for repairing double-strand breaks, which is very similar to the later stages of V(D)J recombination, then rejoins the DNA ends in a way that leads to a recombination event in which a different C-region gene is brought adjacent to the rearranged V region. Gene conversion results from the broken DNA strand using homologous sequences flanking the immunoglobulin gene as a template for repair DNA synthesis, thus replacing part of the gene with new sequences.

action of another enzyme, **apurinic/apyrimidinic endonuclease-1 (APE1)**, which excises the abasic residue to create a single-strand discontinuity (known as a single-strand nick) in the DNA at the site of the original cytidine. Repair of the single-strand nick proceeding through double-strand breaks may result in gene conversion. Gene conversion is not used in the diversification of immunoglobulin genes in humans and mice, but is of importance in some other mammals and in birds.

Somatic hypermutation involves both mutation at the original cytidines targeted by AID and mutation at nearby non-cytidine nucleotides. If the original

Fig. 10.20 The base-excision repair pathway produces single-strand nicks in DNA by the sequential actions of AID, uracil-DNA glycosylase (UNG), and apurinic/apyrimidinic endonuclease-1 (APE1). Double-stranded DNA (first panel) can be made accessible to AID by transcription that unwinds the DNA helix locally (second panel). AID, which is specifically expressed in activated B cells, converts cytidine residues to uridine residues (third panel). The ubiquitous base-excision repair enzyme UNG can then remove the uracil ring from uridine, creating an abasic site (fourth panel). The repair endonuclease APE1 then cuts the sugar–phosphate DNA backbone next to the abasic residue (fifth panel), thereby forming a single-strand nick in the DNA (sixth panel). APE1 does not excise the deoxyribose to form a single-strand nick in DNA, but rather cuts the DNA backbone to yield a 5′-deoxyribose phosphate terminus that is then removed by, for example, DNA polymerase b.

U-G mismatch is recognized by UNG, then an abasic site will be generated in the DNA (see Fig. 10.19). If no further modification is made to this site, it can be replicated without instructive base pairing from the template strand by a class of **error-prone 'translesion' DNA polymerases** that normally repair gross damage to DNA, such as that caused by ultraviolet (UV) radiation. These polymerases can incorporate any nucleotide into the new DNA strand opposite the abasic site, and after a further round of DNA replication this can result in a stable mutation at the site of the original C-G base pair.

In the mismatch repair pathway in B cells, but not in other cell types, the DNA lesion is repaired by error-prone DNA polymerases rather than by more accurate polymerases that faithfully copy the undamaged template strand. Individuals with a defect in the translesion polymerase **Polη** have relatively fewer mutations than usual at A-T, but not at C-G, in their hypermutated immunoglobulin V regions. This fact suggests that Polη is the repair polymerase involved in this pathway of somatic hypermutation. These individuals also have a form of **xeroderma pigmentosum**, a condition resulting from the inability of their cells to repair DNA damage caused by UV radiation.

10-11   AID initiates class switching to allow the same assembled V_H exon to be associated with different C_H genes in the course of an immune response.

All the progeny of a particular B cell activated in an immune response will express the same V_H gene that was generated during its development in the bone marrow, although the gene may be modified by somatic hypermutation. In contrast, that B cell's progeny may express several different C-region isotypes as the cells mature and proliferate during the immune response. The first antigen receptors expressed by B cells are IgM and IgD, and the first antibody produced in an immune response is always IgM. Later in the immune response, the same assembled V region may be expressed in IgG, IgA, or IgE antibodies. This change is known as **class switching** (or **isotype switching**), and, unlike the expression of IgD, it involves irreversible DNA recombination. It is stimulated in the course of an immune response by external signals such as cytokines released by T_H cells.

Switching from IgM to the other immunoglobulin classes occurs only after B cells have been stimulated by antigen. It is achieved through **class switch recombination**, which is a type of nonhomologous DNA recombination that is guided by stretches of repetitive DNA known as **switch regions**. Switch regions lie in the intron between the J_H gene segments and the C_μ gene, and at equivalent sites upstream of the genes for each of the other heavy-chain isotypes, with the exception of the C_δ gene, which does not require DNA rearrangement for its expression (**Fig. 10.21**, first panel). When a B cell switches from the coexpression of IgM and IgD to the expression of another subtype, DNA recombination occurs between S_μ and the S region immediately upstream of the newly chosen constant-region gene. In such a recombination event, the C_μ coding regions and the entire intervening DNA between C_μ and the S region undergoing rearrangement are deleted. Figure 10.21 illustrates switching from C_μ to C_ε in the mouse. All switch recombination events produce genes that can encode a functional protein, because the switch sequences are located in the intron between the assembled V_H exon and C exons, so that changes there cannot cause frameshift mutations.

 ANIMATION 10.2

The enzyme AID initiates class switch recombination and acts only on regions of DNA being transcribed. Certain properties of the switch region sequences promote the accessibility to AID when they are being transcribed. Each switch region consists of many repeats of a G-rich sequence element on the non-template strand. For example, S_μ consists of about 150 repeats of the sequence (GAGCT)n(GGGGGT), where n is usually 3 but can be as many as 7.

Fig. 10.21 Class switching involves recombination between specific switch signals. The top panel shows the organization of a rearranged immunoglobulin heavy-chain locus before class switching. Second panel: This figure illustrates switching between the μ and ε isotypes in the mouse heavy-chain locus. Switch regions (S) are repetitive DNA sequences that guide class switching and are found upstream of each of the immunoglobulin C-region genes, with the exception of the C_δ gene. Switching is guided by the initiation of transcription by RNA polymerase (shaded circle) through these regions from promoters (shown as arrows) located upstream of each S. Because of the repetitive sequences, RNA polymerase can stall within the S regions, allowing these regions to serve as substrates for AID, and subsequently for UNG and APE1. Third panel: These enzymes introduce a high density of single-strand nicks into the non-template DNA strand and the template strand. Staggered nicks are converted to double-strand breaks by a mechanism that is not yet understood. Fourth panel: These breaks are then recognized by the cell's double-strand break repair machinery, which involves DNA-PKcs, Ku proteins, and other repair proteins. Bottom two panels: The two switch regions, in this case S_μ and S_ε, are brought together by the repair proteins, and class switching is completed by excision of the intervening region of DNA (including C_μ and C_δ) and ligation of the S_μ and S_ε regions.

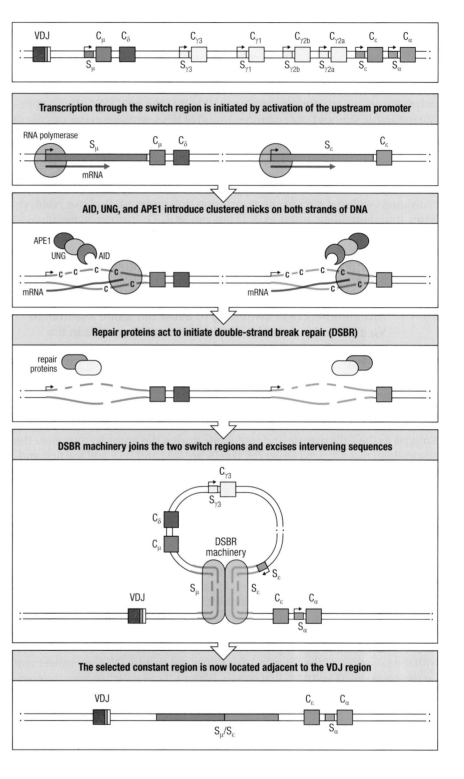

The sequences of the other switch regions ($S\gamma$, $S\alpha$, and S_ε) differ in exact sequence, but all contain repeats of the GAGCT and GGGGGT sequences. It appears that movement of RNA polymerase through this highly repetitive region is occasionally halted—called **polymerase stalling**. This may be caused by bubble-like structures, called **R-loops**, that form when the transcribed RNA displaces the non-template strand of the DNA double helix (see Fig. 10.21, third panel) due to the RNA having many G residues in tandem on one strand.

Polymerase stalling seems closely connected with the recruitment of AID to specific switch regions being transcribed. A multi-subunit RNA processing/

Fig. 10.22 RNA processed from switch region introns interacts with AID and guides its activity. Top panel: Promoters upstream of each switch region initiate transcription by RNA polymerase upstream of a rearranged V_H gene, as in the case of C_μ, shown here, or a noncoding exon for all other constant regions. In all cases, the switch region itself lies within an intron upstream of the exons encoding the constant regions. This intronic switch region RNA is removed from the primary RNA transcript by splicing at specific splice acceptor and donor sites. Middle panel: After splicing, the switch region RNA is further processed, and its repetitive elements allow the formation of putative G-quadruplex structures. Evidence indicates that these RNAs are able to bind AID, as implied in the diagram. Bottom panel: The RNA acts as a guide to bring AID to the switch region by the ability of the G-quadruplex to hybridize with the original DNA template strand from which it was transcribed.

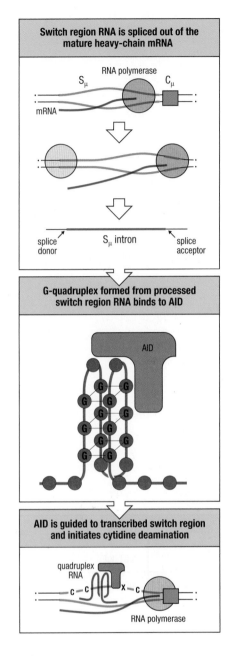

degradation complex, the **RNA exosome**, associates with AID and accumulates on transcribed switch regions, and the protein **Spt5** associates with the stalled polymerase; both are necessary for AID to generate double-strand breaks. Recent evidence indicates that AID is selectively guided to the transcribed switch by an additional mechanism that bears some similarities to the mechanism that operates in the CRISPR/Cas9 genome editing system (see Appendix I, Section A-36). After an RNA polymerase has completed transcription of one RNA template, the intron RNA harboring the switch region is spliced out. Recall that the RNA derived from the switch region contains many repeated copies of the sequences described above, with each switch region having a slightly different repeat sequence. This intronic RNA is then processed to generate many copies of an RNA structure, called a **G-quadruplex**, that is based on the G-rich repetitive element of the switch region (**Fig. 10.22**). This G-quadruplex serves a dual purpose, both binding to AID and, on the basis of sequence complementarity, associating with the switch region from which it was transcribed. Thus the G-quadruplex guides AID to the appropriate switch region, where particular palindromic sequences, such as AGCT, act as good substrates to allow its cytidine deaminase activity to act on both strands concurrently. In this way, the G-quadruplex functions in a manner similar to the synthetic guide RNAs that deliver the Cas9 endonuclease to specific genomic regions, as described in Appendix I, Section A-36). In addition, transcribed switch region DNA may also form G-quadruplex structures and recruit AID directly, providing multiple mechanisms by which the deaminase could access the DNA during class switch recombination.

After the generation of double-strand breaks in switch regions, general cellular mechanisms for repairing these breaks lead to the nonhomologous recombination between switch regions that results in class switching (see Fig. 10.21, fourth and fifth panels). The ends to be joined are brought together by the alignment of repetitive sequences common to the different switch regions, and rejoining of the DNA ends then leads to excision of all DNA between the two switch regions and the formation of a chimeric region at the junction. Loss of AID completely blocks class switching, but deficiency of UNG in both mice and humans severely impairs class switching, suggesting sequential actions of AID and UNG in generating DNA breaks. Joining of DNA ends is probably mediated by classic nonhomologous end joining [as in V(D)J recombination] as well as by a poorly understood alternative end-joining pathway. Class switching is sometimes impaired in the disease **ataxia telangiectasia**, which is caused by mutations in the DNA-PKcs family kinase **ATM**, a known DNA repair protein. The role of ATM in class switching is not yet entirely clear, however.

Ataxia Telangiectasia

10-12 Cytokines made by T_H cells direct the choice of isotype for class switching in T-dependent antibody responses.

We are now ready to explain how a particular heavy chain is selected during an immune response. It is this choice of antibody isotype that ultimately determines the effector function of antibodies, and we will see that it is largely controlled by the cytokines that are produced by T_{FH} cells in the germinal center reaction. As discussed earlier, interactions between germinal center B cells and T_H cells are essential for class switching. CD40 ligand expressed by activated helper T cells activates signaling by CD40 on B cells. Genetic deficiency of CD40 ligand greatly reduces class switching and causes abnormally high levels of plasma IgM, a condition known as **hyper IgM syndrome**. People with this defect lack antibodies of classes other than IgM and exhibit severe humoral immunodeficiency, manifested as repeated infections with common bacterial pathogens. Much of the IgM in hyper IgM syndrome may be induced by thymus-independent antigens on the pathogens that chronically infect these individuals. Nevertheless, people with CD40 ligand deficiency can make IgM antibodies in response to thymus-dependent antigens, which indicates that in the B-cell response, CD40L–CD40 interactions are most important in sustaining a response in the germinal center that leads to class switching and affinity maturation, rather than in the initial activation of B cells.

The selection of a particular C region for class switch recombination is not random but is regulated by the cytokines produced by T_H cells and other cells during the immune response. Different cytokines preferentially induce switching to different isotypes (**Fig. 10.23**). Cytokines induce class switching in part by inducing the production of RNA transcripts through the switch regions that lie 5′ to each heavy-chain C gene segment. When activated B cells are exposed to the cytokine IL-4, for example, transcription from promoters that lie upstream of the switch regions of $C_{\gamma 1}$ and C_ε can be detected a day or two before switching occurs. This will make it possible for switching to occur to either of these two heavy-chain C genes, but in any particular germinal center B cell, recombination will occur in only one. In the example of class switching shown in Fig. 10.21, transcription through the S_ε regions caused the rearrangement between the S_μ and S_ε regions, making the IgE isotype antibody. This results because IL-4 signaling activates the transcription factor **STAT6**, which initiates transcription of the Iε promoter upstream of the S_ε region. I regions are sequences immediately upstream of the switch regions. These sequences contain promoters that initiate transcription across the switch regions and are named according to the switch region they transcribe. Other cytokines activate other promoters upstream of other I-region promoters upstream of other switch regions to produce other antibody classes. T_H cells also produce IL-21, which promotes switching to IgG1 and IgG3. Transforming growth factor-β (TGF-β) induces switching to IgG2b ($C_{\gamma 2b}$) and IgA (C_α). Interferon-γ (IFN-γ) induces switching to IgG2a and IgG3. IL-5 promotes the maturation of IgA-producing B cells and can induce switching to IgG1. While it is clear that the transcription across switch regions influences their selection in undergoing class switch recombination, the basis on which cytokines are produced by T_{FH} cells and their precise impact on S-region transcription are still an active area of research.

CD40 Ligand Deficiency

Cytokines	Isotype
IL-4	IgG1, IgE
IFN-γ	IgG3, IgG2a
TGF-β	IgG2b, IgA
IL-21	IgG3, IgG1, IgA
IL-5	IgG1, IgA

Fig. 10.23 Different cytokines induce switching to different antibody classes. Cytokines induce the production of certain antibody classes by promoting transcription of mRNA from promoters upstream of the various switch regions for the different classes of antibodies. The properties of the switch region promoters determine the cytokine to which it will respond. These 'sterile' transcripts initially encode only for the C region, and not for the entire antibody. Both the process of transcription across the switch regions and the RNA derived from it contribute to allowing AID to induce the DNA rearrangement that will join the V region with a new C region for the selected isotype.

10-13 B cells that survive the germinal center reaction eventually differentiate into either plasma cells or memory cells.

When B cells have undergone affinity maturation and class switching, some eventually exit from the germinal center as developing plasma cells that produce large amounts of antibody. Germinal centers produce many more B cells than eventually are exported as memory B cells or plasma cells, indicating that entry into the memory-cell or plasma-cell compartment is tightly regulated. In B cells, the transcription factors Pax5 and Bcl-6 inhibit the expression of transcription factors required for plasma-cell differentiation, and both Pax5 and Bcl-6 are down-regulated when the B cell starts differentiating. The transcription factor IRF4 then induces the expression of **BLIMP-1**, a transcriptional repressor that switches off genes required for B-cell proliferation, class switching, and affinity maturation. B cells in which BLIMP-1 is induced become plasma cells; they cease proliferating, increase the synthesis and secretion of immunoglobulins, and change their cell-surface properties. Plasma cells down-regulate CXCR5 and up-regulate S1PR1, CXCR4, and $\alpha_4\beta_1$ integrins so that they can leave the germinal centers and home to peripheral tissues.

Some plasma cells deriving from germinal centers in lymph nodes or spleen migrate to the bone marrow, where a subset live for a long period, whereas others migrate to the medullary cords in lymph nodes or to the splenic red pulp. In general, plasma cells formed from early primary foci and germinal centers live for only a few days and are localized to the lymph node medullary cords or splenic red pulp. Plasma cells formed later in germinal centers migrate to the bone marrow and can persist for months, years, and even decades depending on the vaccine or infection. The persistence of plasma cells is the major determinant of the duration of humoral immunity. B cells that have been activated in germinal centers in mucosal tissues, and which are predominantly switched to IgA production, stay within the mucosal system. A splice variant of **XBP1 (X-box binding protein 1)** is expressed in plasma cells and helps to regulate their secretory capacity. Plasma cells in the bone marrow are the source of long-lasting, high-affinity class-switched antibody.

Other germinal center B cells differentiate into **memory B cells**. Memory B cells are long-lived descendants of cells that were once stimulated by antigen. Although some can form early in an immune response before the formation of germinal centers, most long-lived memory B cells have proliferated in the germinal center. They divide very slowly if at all; they express surface immunoglobulin but secrete no antibody or do so only at a low rate. Because the precursors of some memory B cells arise from the germinal center reaction, memory B cells can inherit the genetic changes that occur there, including somatic hypermutation and the gene rearrangements that result in a class switch. The signals that control which path of differentiation a B cell takes are still being investigated. We will briefly return to memory B cells in Chapter 11.

10-14 Some antigens do not require T-cell help to induce antibody responses.

Humans and mice with T-cell deficiencies are able to produce antibodies against thymus-independent (TI) antigens, which we introduced in Section 10-1. These antigens include certain bacterial polysaccharides, polymeric proteins, and lipopolysaccharides, which are able to stimulate naive B cells in the absence of T-cell help. These nonprotein bacterial products cannot elicit classical T-cell responses, yet they induce antibody responses in normal individuals. In addition, there are TI antigens that are not derived from bacteria; these include plant-derived mitogens and lectins, viral antigens, and superantigens, and some parasite-derived antigens.

Thymus-independent antigens fall into two classes, TI-1 and TI-2, which activate B cells by two different mechanisms. **TI-1 antigens** rely on activity that can directly induce B-cell division without T-cell help. We now understand that TI-1 antigens contain molecules that cause the proliferation and differentiation of most B cells regardless of their antigen specificity; this is known as **polyclonal activation** (Fig. 10.24, top panel). TI-1 antigens are therefore often called **B-cell mitogens**, a mitogen being a substance that induces cells to undergo

High concentration of TI-1 antigen

Polyclonal B-cell activation; nonspecific antibody response

Low concentration of TI-1 antigen

TI-1 antigen-specific antibody response

Fig. 10.24 TI-1 antigens induce polyclonal B-cell responses at high concentrations and antigen-specific antibody responses at low concentrations. At high antigen concentration, the signal delivered by the B cell–activating moiety of TI-1 antigens is sufficient to induce B-cell proliferation and antibody secretion in the absence of specific antigen binding to surface immunoglobulin. Thus, all B cells respond (top panel). At low antigen concentration, only B cells specific for the TI-1 antigen bind enough of it to focus its B cell–activating properties onto the B cell; this gives a specific antibody response to epitopes on the TI-1 antigen (bottom panel).

mitosis. For example, LPS and bacterial DNA are both TI-1 antigens because they activate TLRs expressed by B cells (see Section 3-5) and can act as mitogens. Naive murine B cells constitutively express many of the TLRs, but naive human B cells do not express high levels of most TLRs until they receive stimulation through the B-cell receptor. So by the time a B cell has been stimulated by antigen through its B-cell receptor, it is likely to express several TLRs and be responsive to stimulation by TLR ligands that accompany the antigens. Thus, when B cells are exposed to concentrations of TI-1 antigens that are 10^3–10^5 times lower than those used for polyclonal activation, only those B cells whose B-cell receptors specifically bind the TI-1 antigen become activated. At these low concentrations, amounts of TI-1 antigen sufficient for B-cell activation can be concentrated on the B-cell surface only with the aid of this specific binding (Fig. 10.24, bottom panel). B-cell responses to TI-1 antigens in the early stages of an infection may be important in defense against several extracellular pathogens, but they do not lead to affinity maturation or memory B cells, both of which require antigen-specific T-cell help.

The second class of thymus-independent antigens—**TI-2 antigens**—consists of molecules that have highly repetitive structures, such as bacterial capsular polysaccharides. These contain no intrinsic B cell–stimulating activity. Whereas TI-1 antigens can activate both immature and mature B cells, TI-2 antigens can activate only mature B cells; immature B cells, as we saw in Section 8-7, are inactivated by encounter with repetitive epitopes. Infants and young children up to about 5 years of age do not make fully effective antibody responses against polysaccharide antigens, and this might be because most of their B cells are immature, and because their spleen and lymphoid structures (for example, marginal zone) and dendritic cells are not fully developed.

Responses to several TI-2 antigens are prominently made by marginal zone B cells, a subset of non-recirculating B cells that line the border of the splenic white pulp, and by **B-1 B cells** (see Section 8-10). Marginal zone B cells are rare at birth and accumulate with age; they might therefore be responsible for most physiological TI-2 responses, which increase in efficiency with age. TI-2 antigens probably act by simultaneously cross-linking a critical number of B-cell receptors on the surface of antigen-specific mature B cells (**Fig. 10.25**, left

Fig. 10.25 B-cell activation by TI-2 antigens requires, or is greatly enhanced by, cytokines. Multiple cross-linking of the B-cell receptor by TI-2 antigens can lead to IgM antibody production (left panels), but there is evidence that, in addition, cytokines greatly augment these responses and also lead to isotype switching (right panels). It is not clear where such cytokines originate, but one possibility is that dendritic cells, which may be able to bind the antigen through innate immune system receptors on their surface and so present it to the B cells, secrete a soluble TNF family cytokine called BAFF, which can activate class switching by the B cell.

TI-2 antigens alone can signal B cells to produce IgM antibody

Activated dendritic cells release a cytokine, BAFF, that augments production of antibody against TI-2 antigens and induces class switching panels). Dendritic cells and macrophages can provide co-stimulatory signals for activation of B cells by TI-2 antigens. One of these co-stimulatory signals is BAFF, which can be secreted by dendritic cells and interacts with the receptor TACI on the B cell (Fig. 10.25, right panels). The density of TI-2 antigen epitopes is critical; excessive cross-linking of B-cell receptors renders mature B cells unresponsive or anergic, as in immature B cells, while too low a density may be insufficient for activation.

An important class of TI-2 antigens arises during infection by **capsulated bacteria**. Many common extracellular bacterial pathogens are surrounded by a polysaccharide capsule that enables them to resist ingestion by phagocytes. The bacteria not only escape direct destruction by phagocytes but also avoid stimulating T-cell responses against bacterial peptides presented by macrophages. IgM antibodies rapidly produced against the capsular polysaccharide independent of peptide-specific T-cell help will coat the bacteria, promoting their ingestion and destruction by phagocytes early in the infection.

Not all antibodies against bacterial polysaccharides are produced strictly through this TI-2 mechanism. We mentioned earlier the importance of antibodies against the capsular polysaccharide of *Haemophilus influenzae* type b in protective immunity to this bacterium. The immunodeficiency disease **Wiskott–Aldrich syndrome** is caused by defects in T cells that impair their interaction with B cells (see Chapter 13). Individuals with Wiskott–Aldrich syndrome respond poorly to protein antigens, but, unexpectedly, also fail to make IgM and IgG antibody against polysaccharide antigens and are highly susceptible to infection with encapsulated bacteria such as *H. influenzae*. The failure to make IgM seems to be due in part to greatly reduced development of the marginal zone of the spleen, which contains B cells responsible for making much of the 'natural' IgM antibody against ubiquitous carbohydrate antigens. In addition, early studies indicate that TI-2 responses are helped by IL-2 produced by T cells. Thus, IgM and IgG antibodies induced by TI-2 antigens are likely to be an important part of the humoral immune response in many bacterial infections, and in humans at least, the production of class-switched antibodies to TI-2 antigens might normally rely on some degree of T-cell help.

Wiskott–Aldrich Syndrome

As well as producing IgM, TI responses can include switching to certain other antibody classes, such as IgG3 in the mouse. This is probably the result of help from dendritic cells (see Fig. 10.25, right panels), which provide secreted cytokines, such as BAFF, and membrane-bound signals to proliferating plasmablasts as they respond to TI antigens. The distinguishing features of thymus-dependent (TD), TI-1, and TI-2 antibody responses are summarized in **Fig. 10.26**.

Summary.

B-cell activation by many antigens requires both binding of the antigen by the B-cell surface immunoglobulin—the B-cell receptor—and interaction of the B cell with antigen-specific helper T cells. Helper T cells recognize peptide fragments derived from the antigen internalized by the B cells and displayed by the B cells as peptide:MHC class II complexes. Helper T cells stimulate B cells by conjugation in germinal centers, with binding of CD40 ligand on the T cell to CD40 on the B cell, and by their release of various cytokines, such as IL-21. Activated B cells also express molecules, such as B7.2 and ICOSL, that can stimulate T cells. The initial interaction between B and T cells occurs at the border of the T-cell and B-cell areas of secondary lymphoid tissue, to which antigen-activated helper T cells and B cells migrate in response to chemokines. Further interactions between T_{FH} cells and B cells continue after migration into the follicle and the formation of a germinal center.

Fig. 10.26 Properties of different classes of antigen that elicit antibody responses. Some data indicate a minor role for T cells in antibody responses to TI-2 antigens; robust responses to TI-2 antigens can be observed in T cell–deficient mice.

	TD antigen	TI-1 antigen	TI-2 antigen
Antibody response in infants	Yes	Yes	No
Antibody production in congenitally athymic individual	No	Yes	Yes
Antibody response in absence of all T cells	No	Yes	Yes
Primes T cells	Yes	No	No
Polyclonal B-cell activation	No	Yes	No
Requires repeating epitopes	No	No	Yes
Examples of antigen	Diphtheria toxin Viral hemagglutinin Purified protein derivative (PPD) of *Mycobacterium tuberculosis*	Bacterial lipopoly-saccharide *Brucella abortus*	Pneumococcal polysaccharide *Salmonella* polymerized flagellin Dextran Hapten-conjugated Ficoll (polysucrose)

T cells induce a phase of vigorous B-cell proliferation in the germinal center reaction and direct the differentiation of clonally expanded B cells into either antibody-secreting plasma cells or memory B cells. Immunoglobulin genes expressed in B cells are diversified in the germinal center reaction by somatic hypermutation and class switching, initiated by activation-induced cytidine deaminase (AID). Unlike V(D)J recombination, these processes occur only in B cells. Somatic hypermutation diversifies the V region through the introduction of mutations that are selected for providing greater affinity for the antigen as the immune response proceeds. Class switching does not affect the V region but increases the functional diversity of immunoglobulins by replacing the C_μ region in the original immunoglobulin heavy-chain locus with another heavy-chain C region that will produce IgG, IgA, or IgE antibodies. Class switching provides antibodies with the same antigen specificity but distinct effector capacities. The switching to different antibody isotypes is regulated by cytokines released from helper T cells. Some nonprotein antigens stimulate B cells in the absence of linked recognition by peptide-specific helper T cells. Responses to these thymus-independent antigens are accompanied by only limited class switching and do not induce memory B cells. However, such responses have a crucial role in host defense against pathogens whose surface antigens cannot elicit peptide-specific T-cell responses. By contrast, evidence for memory in the TI-2 response is the permanent expansion of antigen-specific nonswitched memory B cells.

The distributions and functions of immunoglobulin classes.

Extracellular pathogens can invade most sites within the body, and so antibodies must be equally widely distributed to combat them. Most classes of antibodies are distributed by diffusion from their site of synthesis, but specialized transport mechanisms are required to deliver antibodies across the epithelial surfaces lining the mucosa of organs such as the lungs and intestine.

The particular heavy-chain isotype of the antibody can either limit antibody diffusion or engage specific transporters that deliver the antibody across epithelia. This part of the chapter describes these mechanisms and the antibody classes that use them to enter compartments of the body where their particular effector functions are appropriate. Here we restrict our discussion to the protective functions of antibodies that result solely from their binding to pathogens, and in the next part of the chapter, we discuss the effector cells and molecules that are specifically engaged by different antibody classes.

10-15 Antibodies of different classes operate in distinct places and have distinct effector functions.

The different classes of antibodies (see Fig. 4.6) are adapted to function in different compartments of the body. The functional activities and distributions for human antibodies are listed in **Fig. 10.27**. Because a given V region can become associated with any C region through class switching, the clonal progeny of a single B cell can produce antibodies that share the same specificity yet provide all of the protective functions appropriate for each body compartment. All naive B cells express cell-surface IgM and IgD. IgM is the first antibody secreted by activated B cells but is less than 10% of the immunoglobulin found in plasma. Little IgD antibody is produced at any time, while IgE contributes a small but biologically important part of the immune response. IgG and IgA are the predominant antibody classes. The overall predominance of IgG is also due in part to its longer lifetime in the plasma (see Fig. 4.7).

IgM antibodies are produced first in a humoral immune response and tend to be of low affinity. However, IgM molecules form pentamers that are stabilized by a single J-chain molecule (see Fig. 4.8) and have 10 antigen-binding sites, conferring higher overall avidity when binding to multivalent antigens such as bacterial capsular polysaccharides. This higher avidity of the pentamer compensates for the low affinity of the individual antigen-binding site within the IgM monomers. Because of the large size of the pentamers, IgM is found mainly in the bloodstream and, to a lesser extent, in the lymph, rather than in intercellular spaces within tissues. The pentameric structure of IgM makes it especially effective in activating the complement system, as we will see in

Functional activity	IgM	IgD	IgG1	IgG2	IgG3	IgG4	IgA	IgE
Neutralization	+	–	++	++	++	++	++	–
Opsonization	+	–	++	*	++	+	+	–
Sensitization for killing by NK cells	–	–	++	–	++	–	–	–
Sensitization of mast cells	–	–	+	–	+	–	–	+++
Activates complement system	+++	–	++	+	+++	–	+	–

Distribution	IgM	IgD	IgG1	IgG2	IgG3	IgG4	IgA	IgE
Transport across epithelium	+	–	–	–	–	–	+++ (dimer)	–
Transport across placenta	–	–	+++	+	++	+/–	–	–
Diffusion into extravascular sites	+/–	–	+++	+++	+++	+++	++ (monomer)	+
Mean serum level (mg ml^{-1})	1.5	0.04	9	3	1	0.5	2.1	3×10^{-5}

Fig. 10.27 Each human immunoglobulin class has specialized functions and a unique distribution. The major effector functions of each class (+++) are shaded in dark red, whereas lesser functions (++) are shown in dark pink, and very minor functions (+) in pale pink. The distributions are marked similarly, with actual average levels in serum being shown in the bottom row. IgA has two subclasses, IgA1 and IgA2. The IgA column refers to both. *IgG2 can act as an opsonin in the presence of an Fc receptor of the appropriate allotype, found in about 50% of people of Caucasian descent. The correspondence between human and mouse isotypes is as follows: human IgG1 = mouse IgG2a; human IgG2 = mouse IgG3; human IgG3 = mouse IgG2b; human IgG4 = mouse IgG1; human IgA1/2 = mouse IgA.

Section 10-19. In the absence of a J chain, IgM hexamers can also form, and these fix complement more efficiently than do pentamers, possibly because C1q is also a hexamer. However, the *in vivo* role of IgM hexamers in protecting against infections has not been fully established.

Infection of the bloodstream has serious consequences unless it is controlled quickly, and the rapid production of IgM and its efficient activation of the complement system are important in controlling such infections. These adaptive IgM responses are often dependent on T-cell help. Some IgM is produced by conventional B cells that have not undergone class switching, but most is produced by B-1 B cells. In mice, activated B-1 B cells residing in the peritoneal cavity and pleural spaces migrate to the spleen or intestinal lymphoid tissues, where they will mature into plasma cells. These cells secrete antibodies against commonly encountered carbohydrate antigens, including those of bacteria, and do not require T-cell help; they therefore provide a preformed repertoire of IgM antibodies in blood and body cavities that can recognize invading pathogens (see Section 8-10).

Antibodies of the other classes—IgG, IgA, and IgE—are smaller and diffuse easily out of the blood into the tissues. IgA can form dimers (see Fig. 4.8), but IgG and IgE are always monomeric. The affinity of the individual antigen-binding sites for their antigen is therefore critical for the effectiveness of these antibodies, and most of the B cells expressing these classes have been selected in the germinal centers for their increased affinity for antigen after somatic hypermutation.

IgG is the principal class of antibody in human blood and extracellular fluid, whereas IgA is the principal class in secretions, the most important being those from the epithelia lining the intestinal and respiratory tracts. IgG efficiently opsonizes pathogens for engulfment by phagocytes and activates the complement system, but IgA is a less potent opsonin and a weak activator of complement. IgG operates mainly in the tissues, where accessory cells and molecules are available, whereas dimeric IgA operates mainly on epithelial surfaces, where complement and phagocytes are not normally present; therefore, IgA functions chiefly as a neutralizing antibody. Monomeric IgA can be produced by plasma cells that differentiate from class-switched B cells in lymph nodes and spleen, and it acts as a neutralizing antibody in extracellular spaces and in the blood. This monomeric IgA is predominantly of the subclass IgA1; the ratio of IgA1 to IgA2 in the blood is 10:1. The IgA antibodies produced by plasma cells in the gut are dimeric and predominantly of subclass IgA2; the ratio of IgA2 to IgA1 in the gut is 3:2.

Finally, IgE antibody is present only at very low levels in blood or extracellular fluid, but it is bound avidly by receptors on **mast cells** that are found just beneath the skin and mucosa and along blood vessels in connective tissue. Antigen binding to this cell-associated IgE triggers mast cells to release powerful chemical mediators that induce reactions such as coughing, sneezing, and vomiting, which in turn can expel infectious agents, as discussed later in this chapter.

10-16 Polymeric immunoglobulin receptor binds to the Fc regions of IgA and IgM and transports them across epithelial barriers.

In the mucosal immune system, IgA-secreting plasma cells are found predominantly in the lamina propria, which lies immediately below the basement membrane of many surface epithelia. From there the IgA antibodies can be transported across the epithelium to its external surface, for example to the lumen of the gut or of the bronchi (**Fig. 10.28**). IgA antibody synthesized in the lamina propria is secreted as a dimeric IgA molecule associated with a single

| Dimeric IgA is transported into the gut lumen through epithelial cells at the base of the crypts | Dimeric IgA binds to the layer of mucus overlying the gut epithelium | IgA in the gut neutralizes pathogens and their toxins |

Fig. 10.28 Dimeric IgA is the major class of antibody present in the lumen of the gut. IgA is synthesized by plasma cells in the lamina propria and transported into the lumen of the gut through epithelial cells at the base of the crypts. pIgR is used to transport IgA across the epithelial cells. Dimeric IgA binds to the layer of mucus overlying the gut epithelium and acts as an antigen-specific barrier to pathogens and toxins in the gut lumen.

J chain. This polymeric form of IgA binds specifically to a receptor called the **polymeric immunoglobulin receptor (pIgR)**, which is present on the basolateral surfaces of the overlying epithelial cells. When the pIgR has bound a molecule of dimeric IgA, the complex is internalized and carried in a transport vesicle through the cytoplasm of the epithelial cell to its luminal surface. This process is called transcytosis. IgM also binds to the pIgR and can be secreted into the gut by the same mechanism. Upon reaching the luminal surface of the enterocyte, the antibody is released into the mucus layer covering the gut lining by proteolytic cleavage of the extracellular domain of the pIgR. The cleaved extracellular domain of the pIgR is known as **secretory component** (frequently abbreviated to **SC**) and remains associated with the antibody. Secretory component is bound to the part of the Fc region of IgA that contains the binding site for the Fcα receptor I, which is why secretory IgA does not bind to this receptor. Secretory component serves several physiological roles. It binds to mucins in mucus, acting as 'glue' to bind secreted IgA to the mucus layer on the luminal surface of the gut epithelium, where the antibody binds and neutralizes gut pathogens and their toxins (see Fig. 10.28). Secretory component also protects the antibodies against cleavage by gut enzymes.

The principal sites of IgA synthesis and secretion are the gut, the respiratory epithelium, the lactating breast, and various other exocrine glands such as the salivary and tear glands. It is believed that the primary functional role of IgA antibodies is to protect epithelial surfaces from infectious agents, just as IgG antibodies protect the extracellular spaces inside tissues. By binding bacteria, including commensal organisms, virus particles, and toxins, IgA antibodies prevent the attachment of bacteria and viruses to epithelial cells and the uptake of toxins. This action provides a first line of defense against a wide variety of pathogens. IgA is also thought to have an additional role in the gut, that of regulating the gut microbiota (see Chapter 12). The alveolar spaces in the lower respiratory tract lack the thicker mucosal layer characteristic of the upper respiratory tract, because efficient gas diffusion would be impeded by a mucus layer covering the alveolar epithelium. IgG can rapidly transudate into these spaces and is the major isotype responsible for protection there.

10-17 The neonatal Fc receptor carries IgG across the placenta and prevents IgG excretion from the body.

Newborn infants are especially vulnerable to infection, having had no previous exposure to the microbes in the environment they enter at birth. IgA antibodies are secreted in breast milk and are transferred to the gut of the newborn infant, where they provide protection from newly encountered bacteria until

Fig. 10.29 The neonatal Fc receptor (FcRn) binds to the Fc portion of IgG. The structure of a molecule of FcRn (blue) is shown bound to one chain of the Fc portion of IgG (red), at the interface of the $C_{\gamma}2$ and $C_{\gamma}3$ domains, with the $C_{\gamma}2$ region at the top. The b_2-microglobulin component of the FcRn is green. The dark-blue structure attached to the Fc portion of IgG is a carbohydrate chain, reflecting glycosylation. FcRn transports IgG molecules across the placenta in humans and also across the gut in rats and mice. It also has a role in maintaining the levels of IgG in adults. Although only one molecule of FcRn is shown binding to the Fc portion, it is thought that it takes two molecules of FcRn to capture one molecule of IgG.

the infant can synthesize its own protective antibody. IgA is not the only protective antibody that a mother passes on to her baby. Maternal IgG is transported across the placenta directly into the bloodstream of the fetus during intrauterine life; at birth, human babies have levels of plasma IgG as high as those of their mothers, and with the same range of antigen specificities. The selective transport of IgG from mother to fetus is due to an IgG transport protein in the placenta, **FcRn** (**neonatal Fc receptor**), which is closely related in structure to MHC class I molecules. Despite this similarity, FcRn binds IgG quite differently from the binding of peptide to MHC class I molecules, because its peptide-binding groove is occluded. It binds to the Fc portion of IgG molecules (**Fig. 10.29**). Two molecules of FcRn bind one molecule of IgG, bearing it across the placenta. Maternal IgG is ingested by the newborn from its mother's milk and colostrum, the protein-rich fluid secreted by the early postnatal mammary gland. In this case, FcRn transports the IgG from the lumen of the neonatal gut into the blood and tissues. Considerations of the factors that affect antibody binding to FcRn are also important in approaching maternal vaccination as a means of protecting fetuses before birth. FcRn is also found in adults in the gut, liver, endothelial cells, and on podocytes of the kidney glomeruli. Its function in adults is to maintain the levels of IgG in plasma, which it does by binding antibody, endocytosing it, and recycling it to the blood, thus preventing its excretion from the body. In the kidney, expression on podocytes is thought to aid in clearance of IgG from the glomerular basement membrane.

By means of these specialized transport systems, mammals are supplied from birth with antibodies against pathogens common in their environments. As they mature and make their own antibodies of all isotypes, these are distributed selectively to different sites in the body (**Fig. 10.30**). Thus, throughout life, class switching and the distribution of antibody classes throughout the body provide effective protection against infection in extracellular spaces.

10-18 High-affinity IgG and IgA antibodies can neutralize toxins and block the infectivity of viruses and bacteria.

Pathogens can cause damage to a host by producing toxins or by infecting cells directly, and antibodies can protect by blocking both of these actions. Many bacteria cause disease by secreting toxins that damage or disrupt the function of the host's cells (**Fig. 10.31**). Many toxins consist of separate domains for exerting toxicity and for binding to specific cell-surface receptors by which they enter cells. Antibodies that bind a toxin's receptor-binding site can prevent cell entry and protect cells from attack (**Fig. 10.32**). Antibodies that act in this way to neutralize toxins are referred to as **neutralizing antibodies**. Most toxins are active at nanomolar concentrations: a single molecule of diphtheria toxin can kill a cell. To neutralize toxins, therefore, antibodies must be able to diffuse into the tissues and bind the toxin rapidly and with high affinity. The ability of IgG antibodies to diffuse easily throughout the extracellular fluid, and their high affinity for antigen once affinity maturation has taken place, make them the principal antibodies that neutralize toxins in tissues. High-affinity IgA antibodies similarly neutralize toxins at the mucosal surfaces of the body.

Diphtheria and tetanus toxins are two bacterial toxins in which the toxic and receptor-binding functions are on separate protein chains. It is therefore possible to immunize individuals, usually as infants, with modified toxin molecules

Fig. 10.30 Immunoglobulin classes are selectively distributed in the body. IgG and IgM predominate in blood (shown here for simplicity by IgM and IgG in the heart), whereas IgG and monomeric IgA are the major antibodies in extracellular fluid within the body. Dimeric IgA predominates in secretions across epithelia, including breast milk. The fetus receives IgG from the mother by transplacental transport. IgE is found mainly associated with mast cells just beneath epithelial surfaces (especially of the respiratory tract, gastrointestinal tract, and skin). The brain is normally devoid of immunoglobulin.

| IgG | IgM | Dimeric IgA | IgE |

Disease	Organism	Toxin	Effects *in vivo*
Tetanus	*Clostridium tetani*	Tetanus toxin	Blocks inhibitory neuron action, leading to chronic muscle contraction
Diphtheria	*Corynebacterium diphtheriae*	Diphtheria toxin	Inhibits protein synthesis, leading to epithelial cell damage and myocarditis
Gas gangrene	*Clostridium perfringens*	Clostridial toxin	Phospholipase activation, leading to cell death
Cholera	*Vibrio cholerae*	Cholera toxin	Activates adenylate cyclase, elevates cAMP in cells, leading to changes in intestinal epithelial cells that result in loss of water and electrolytes
Anthrax	*Bacillus anthracis*	Anthrax toxic complex	Increases vascular permeability, leading to edema, hemorrhage, and circulatory collapse
Botulism	*Clostridium botulinum*	Botulinum toxin	Blocks release of acetylcholine, leading to paralysis
Whooping cough	*Bordetella pertussis*	Pertussis toxin	ADP-ribosylation of G proteins, leading to lymphoproliferation
		Tracheal cytotoxin	Inhibits cilia and causes epithelial cell loss
Scarlet fever	*Streptococcus pyogenes*	Erythrogenic toxin	Vasodilation, leading to scarlet fever rash
		Leukocidin Streptolysins	Kill phagocytes, allowing bacterial survival
Food poisoning	*Staphylococcus aureus*	Staphylococcal enterotoxin	Acts on intestinal neurons to induce vomiting. Also a potent T-cell mitogen (SE superantigen)
Toxic-shock syndrome	*Staphylococcus aureus*	Toxic-shock syndrome toxin	Causes hypotension and skin loss. Also a potent T-cell mitogen (TSST-1 superantigen)

Fig. 10.31 Many common diseases are caused by bacterial toxins. The toxins shown here are all exotoxins—proteins secreted by the bacteria. High-affinity IgG and IgA antibodies protect against these toxins. Bacteria also have nonsecreted endotoxins, such as lipopolysaccharide, which are released when the bacterium dies and may also mediate pathogenesis of disease.

in which the toxic chain has been denatured. These modified toxins, called **toxoids**, lack toxic activity but retain the receptor-binding site. Thus, immunization with the toxoid induces neutralizing antibodies that protect against the native toxin.

Some insect or animal venoms are so toxic that a single exposure can cause severe tissue damage or death. For these toxins, the adaptive immune

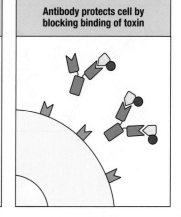

Toxin binds to cellular receptors	Endocytosis of toxin:receptor complexes	Dissociation of toxin releases its active chain, which poisons cell	Antibody protects cell by blocking binding of toxin

Fig. 10.32 Neutralization of toxins by IgG antibodies protects cells from damage. The damaging effects of many bacteria are due to the toxins they produce (see Fig. 10.31). These toxins are usually composed of several distinct moieties. One part of the toxin molecule binds a cell-surface receptor, which enables the molecule to be internalized. Another part of the toxin molecule then enters the cytoplasm and poisons the cell. Antibodies that inhibit toxin binding can prevent, or neutralize, these effects.

| **Virus binds to receptors on cell surface** |

| **Receptor-mediated endocytosis of virus** |

| **Acidification of endosome after endocytosis triggers fusion of virus with cell and entry of viral DNA** |

| **Antibody blocks binding to virus receptor and can also block fusion event** |

Fig. 10.33 Viral infection of cells can be blocked by neutralizing antibodies. For a virus to multiply within a cell, it must introduce its genes into the cell. The first step in entry is usually the binding of the virus to a receptor on the cell surface. For enveloped viruses, as shown in the figure, entry into the cytoplasm requires fusion of the viral envelope and the cell membrane. For some viruses this fusion event takes place on the cell surface (not shown); for others it can occur only within the more acidic environment of endosomes, as shown here. Non-enveloped viruses must also bind to receptors on cell surfaces, but they enter the cytoplasm by disrupting endosomes. Antibodies bound to viral surface proteins neutralize the virus, inhibiting either its initial binding to the cell or its subsequent entry.

response is too slow to be protective. Exposure to these venoms is a rare event, and protective vaccines have not been developed for use in humans. Instead, neutralizing antibodies are generated by immunizing other species, such as horses, with insect and snake venoms to produce anti-venom antibodies, or **antivenins**. The antivenins are injected into exposed individuals to protect them against the toxic effects of the venom. Transfer of antibodies in this way is known as **passive immunization** (see Appendix I, Section A-30).

Animal viruses infect cells by binding to a particular cell-surface receptor. These are often cell-type-specific proteins that determine which cells a virus can infect, or its **tropism**. Many antibodies that neutralize viruses do so by directly blocking the binding of virus to surface receptors (**Fig. 10.33**). The **hemagglutinin** of influenza virus, for example, binds to terminal sialic acid residues on the carbohydrates of glycoproteins present on epithelial cells of the respiratory tract. It is known as hemagglutinin because it recognizes and binds to similar sialic acid residues on chicken red blood cells and agglutinates these red blood cells. Antibodies against the hemagglutinin can prevent infection by the influenza virus. Such antibodies are called **virus-neutralizing antibodies**, and, as with the neutralization of toxins, high-affinity IgA and IgG antibodies are particularly important. In the case of HIV and influenza, so called **broadly neutralizing antibodies** block infection by multiple strains of the virus (see Section 13-35). However, antibodies can also neutralize viruses by interfering with the fusion mechanisms used to enter the cell's cytoplasm after binding to surface receptors.

Many bacteria have cell-surface molecules called **adhesins** that enable them to bind to the surface of host cells. This adherence is crucial to the ability of these bacteria to cause disease, whether they subsequently enter the cell, as do *Salmonella* species, or remain attached to the cell surface as extracellular pathogens (**Fig. 10.34**). *Neisseria gonorrhoeae*, the causative agent of the sexually transmitted disease gonorrhea, has a cell-surface protein known as **pilin** that enables the bacterium to adhere to the epithelial cells of the urinary and reproductive tracts and is essential to its infectivity. Antibodies against pilin can inhibit this adhesive reaction and prevent infection.

IgA antibodies secreted onto the mucosal surfaces of the intestinal, respiratory, and reproductive tracts are particularly important in inhibiting the colonization of these surfaces by pathogens and in preventing infection of the epithelial cells. Adhesion of bacteria to cells within tissues can also contribute to pathogenesis, and IgG antibodies against adhesins protect tissues from damage in much the same way as IgA antibodies protect mucosal surfaces.

10-19 Antigen:antibody complexes activate the classical pathway of complement by binding to C1q.

Chapter 2 introduced the complement system as an essential component of innate immunity. Complement activation can proceed in the absence of antibody via the **lectin pathway** through the actions of mannose-binding lectin (MBL) and ficolins. But complement is also an important effector of antibody

Fig. 10.34 Antibodies can prevent the attachment of bacteria to cell surfaces. Many bacterial infections require an interaction between the bacterium and a cell-surface receptor. This is particularly true for infections of mucosal surfaces. The attachment process involves very specific molecular interactions between bacterial adhesins and their receptors on host cells; antibodies against bacterial adhesins can block such infections.

responses via the **classical pathway**. The different pathways of complement activation converge to coat pathogen surfaces or antigen:antibody complexes with covalently attached complement fragment C3b, which acts as an opsonin to promote uptake and removal by phagocytes. In addition, the terminal complement components can form a membrane-attack complex that damages some bacteria.

In the classical pathway, complement activation is triggered by C1, a complex of C1q and the serine proteases C1r and C1s (see Section 2-7). Complement activation is initiated when antibodies that are attached to the surface of a pathogen then bind to C1 via C1q (**Fig. 10.35**). C1q can be bound by either IgM or IgG antibodies, but, because of the structural requirements of binding to C1q, neither of these antibody classes can activate complement in solution; the complement reactions are initiated only when the antibodies are already bound to multiple sites on a cell surface, normally that of a pathogen.

Each globular head of a C1q molecule can bind to one Fc region, and binding of two or more heads activates the C1 complex. In plasma, the **pentameric**

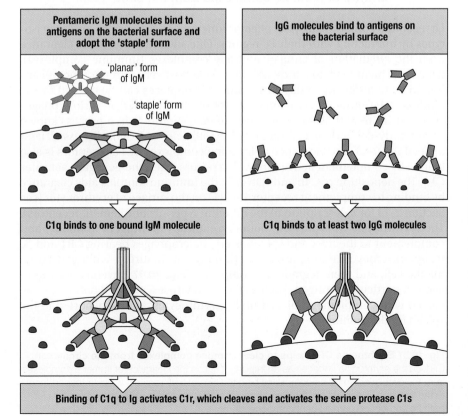

Fig. 10.35 The classical pathway of complement activation is initiated by the binding of C1q to antibody on a pathogen surface. When a molecule of IgM binds several identical epitopes on a pathogen surface, it is bent into the 'staple' conformation, which allows the globular heads of C1q to bind to the Fc regions of IgM (left panels). Multiple molecules of IgG bound on the surface of a pathogen allow the binding of a single molecule of C1q to two or more Fc regions (right panels). In both cases, the binding of C1q to the Fc regions induces a conformational change that activates the associated C1r, which becomes an active enzyme that cleaves the pro-enzyme C1s, generating a serine protease that initiates the classical complement cascade (see Chapter 2).

Fig. 10.36 **The two conformations of IgM.** The left panel shows the 'planar' conformation of soluble IgM; the right panel shows the 'staple' conformation of IgM bound to a bacterial flagellum. Magnification ×760,000.

IgM 'planar' conformation

IgM 'staple' conformation

Small antigen:antibody complexes form in the circulation

antigen

antibody

Activation of complement leads to the deposition of many molecules of C3b on the immune complex

C3b

C3 convertase

C1q

Complement receptor CR1 on erythrocytes binds the immune complexes via bound C3b

CR1

In the spleen and liver, phagocytic cells remove the immune complexes from the erythrocyte surface

FcR

IgM molecule has a planar conformation that does not bind C1q (**Fig. 10.36**, left panel); however, binding to the surface of a pathogen deforms the IgM pentamer so that it looks like a staple (Fig. 10.36, right panel), and this distortion exposes binding sites for the C1q heads. Although C1q binds with low affinity to some subclasses of IgG in solution, the binding energy required for C1q activation is achieved only when a single molecule of C1q can bind two or more IgG molecules that are held within 30–40 nm of each other as a result of binding antigen. This requires that multiple molecules of IgG be bound to a single pathogen or to an antigen in solution. For this reason, IgM is much more efficient than IgG in activating complement. The binding of C1q to a single bound IgM molecule or to two or more bound IgG molecules (see Fig. 10.35) leads to activation of the protease activity of C1r, triggering the complement cascade.

10-20 Complement receptors and Fc receptors both contribute to removal of immune complexes from the circulation.

Fc receptors confer the distinct effector functions to the various antibody isotypes by interacting with their Fc regions. One such function is the clearance from the circulation of antigen:antibody complexes (immune complexes), which can include toxins or debris from dead host cells and microorganisms bound by neutralizing antibodies. Immune complexes can be cleared by the binding of the antibody's Fc region to Fc receptors expressed on various phagocytic cells in tissues. Another function of Fc receptors is in a process known as antibody-dependent cell-mediated cytotoxicity (ADCC), discussed later in Section 10-23. The clearance of immune complexes by Fc receptors is also helped by complement activation, which occurs when the Fc region activates C1q. The deposition of C4b and C3b onto the immune complex aids clearance by binding to complement receptor 1 (CR1) on the surface of erythrocytes (see Section 2-13 for a description of the different types of complement receptors). The erythrocytes transport the bound complexes of antigen, antibody, and complement to the liver and spleen. Here, macrophages bearing CR1 and Fc receptors remove the complexes from the erythrocyte surface without destroying the cell, and then degrade the complexes (**Fig. 10.37**). Even larger aggregates of particulate antigen, such as bacteria, viruses, and cell debris, can be coated with complement, picked up by erythrocytes, and transported to the spleen for destruction.

Fig. 10.37 **Erythrocyte CR1 helps to clear immune complexes from the circulation.** CR1 on the erythrocyte surface has an important role in the clearance of immune complexes from the circulation. Immune complexes bind to CR1 on erythrocytes, which transport them to the liver and spleen, where they are removed by macrophages expressing receptors for both Fc and bound complement components.

Complement-coated immune complexes that are not removed from the circulation tend to deposit in the basement membranes of small blood vessels, most notably those of the renal glomerulus, where the blood is filtered to form urine. Immune complexes that pass through the basement membrane of the glomerulus bind to CR1 present on the renal podocytes, which are cells that lie beneath the basement membrane. The functional significance of these receptors in the kidney is unknown; however, they have an important role in the pathology of some autoimmune diseases. In the autoimmune disease **systemic lupus erythematosus (SLE)** (see Section 15-12), excessive levels of circulating immune complexes lead to their deposition in large amounts on the podocytes, damaging the glomerulus; kidney failure is the principal danger in this disease. In mice, the experimental mouse strain known as MRL/lpr develops a disease similar to SLE in humans. In these mice, inhibition of the alternative pathway of complement using a soluble form of **CRIg (complement receptor of the immunoglobulin superfamily)** leads to reduced severity of skin and renal disease. In humans, the strongest genetic risk factor for SLE is C1q deficiency, although this is very rare. Mutations in complement receptors 2 and 3 and the Fc receptor FcγRII-A are also associated with increased susceptibility to develop lupus, implying the involvement of both complement receptors and Fc receptor pathways in clearing immune complexes.

Systemic Lupus Erythematosus

Antigen:antibody complexes can also be a cause of pathology in individuals with deficiencies in the early components of complement (C1, C2, and C4). These deficiencies result in the classical complement pathway not being activated properly and immune complexes not being cleared effectively because they do not become tagged with complement. These individuals also suffer tissue damage as a result of immune-complex deposition, especially in the kidneys.

Summary.

The T cell–dependent antibody response begins with IgM secretion but quickly progresses to the production of additional antibody classes. Each class of antibody is specialized both in its localization in the body and in the functions it can perform. IgM antibodies are found mainly in blood; they are pentameric in structure. IgM is specialized to activate complement efficiently upon binding antigen and to compensate for the low affinity of a typical IgM antigen-binding site. IgG antibodies are usually of higher affinity and are found in blood and in extracellular fluid, where they can neutralize toxins, viruses, and bacteria, opsonize them for phagocytosis, and activate the complement system. IgA antibodies are synthesized as monomers, which enter blood and extracellular fluids, or they are secreted as dimeric molecules by plasma cells in the lamina propria of various mucosal tissues. IgA dimers are selectively secreted into breast milk for delivery to the newborn or transported across the epithelial layer into sites such as the lumen of the gut, where they neutralize toxins and viruses and block the entry of bacteria across the intestinal epithelium. Most IgE antibody is bound to the surface of mast cells that reside mainly just below the body surface; antigen binding to this IgE triggers local defense reactions. Antibodies can defend the body against extracellular pathogens and their toxic products in several ways. The simplest is by direct interactions with pathogens or their products; for example, by binding to the active sites of toxins and neutralizing them or by blocking their ability to bind to host cells through specific receptors. When antibodies of the appropriate isotype bind to antigens, they can activate the classical pathway of complement, which leads to the elimination of the pathogen by the various mechanisms described in Chapter 2. Soluble immune complexes of antigen and antibody also fix complement and are cleared from the circulation via complement receptors on red blood cells.

The destruction of antibody-coated pathogens via Fc receptors.

The neutralization of toxins, viruses, or bacteria by high-affinity antibodies can protect against infection but does not, on its own, solve the problem of how to remove the pathogens and their products from the body. Moreover, many pathogens cannot be neutralized by antibody and must be destroyed by other means. Many pathogen-specific antibodies do not bind to neutralizing targets on pathogen surfaces and thus need to be linked to other effector mechanisms to play their part in host defense. We have already seen how the binding of antibody to antigen can activate complement. Another important defense mechanism is the activation of a variety of **accessory effector cells** bearing Fc receptors, which are specific for the Fc portion of antibodies. These receptors facilitate the phagocytosis of antibody-bound extracellular pathogens by macrophages, dendritic cells, and neutrophils. Other, nonphagocytic cells of the immune system—NK cells, eosinophils, basophils, and mast cells (see Fig. 1.8)—are triggered to secrete stored mediators when their Fc receptors are engaged by antibody-coated pathogens. These mechanisms maximize the effectiveness of all antibodies regardless of where they bind.

10-21 The Fc receptors of accessory cells are signaling receptors specific for immunoglobulins of different classes.

The **Fc receptors** are a family of cell-surface molecules that bind the Fc portion of immunoglobulins. Each member of the Fc family recognizes immunoglobulin of one or a few closely related heavy-chain isotypes through a recognition domain on the α chain of the Fc receptor. Most Fc receptors are themselves members of the immunoglobulin gene superfamily. Different cell types bear different sets of Fc receptors, and the isotype of the antibody thus determines which types of cells will be engaged in a given response. In addition to the isotype, glycosylation of the constant regions can influence how tightly Fc receptors are engaged. The different Fc receptors, the cells that express them, and their specificities for different antibody classes are shown in **Fig. 10.38**.

Most Fc receptors function as part of a multi-subunit complex. Only the α chain is required for antibody recognition; the other chains are required for transport of the receptor to the cell surface and for signal transduction when an Fc region is bound. Some Fcγ receptors, the Fcα receptor I, and the high-affinity receptor for IgE (FcϵRI) all use a γ chain for signaling. This chain, which is closely related to the ζ chain of the T-cell receptor complex (see Section 7-7), associates noncovalently with the Fc-binding α chain. The human FcγRII-A is a single-chain receptor in which the cytoplasmic domain of the α chain replaces the function of the γ chain. These Fc receptors all transduce activating signals by virtue of their immunoreceptor tyrosine-based activation motifs, which become tyrosine phosphorylated upon receptor aggregation and recruit Src and Syk/ZAP-70 family tyrosine kinases. These tyrosine kinases propagate signals downstream. FcγRII-B1 and FcγRII-B2 are also single-chain receptors but function as inhibitory receptors because they contain an immunoreceptor tyrosine-based inhibition motif (ITIM) that engages the inositol 5'-phosphatase SHIP (see Section 7-26). The most prominent function of Fc receptors is the activation of accessory cells to attack pathogens, but they also contribute in other ways to immune responses. For example, FcγRII-B receptors negatively regulate the activities of B cells, mast cells, macrophages, and neutrophils by adjusting the threshold at which immune complexes will activate these cells. Fc receptors expressed by dendritic cells enable them to ingest antigen:antibody complexes efficiently and thus process these antigens and present their peptides to T cells.

Receptor	FcγRI (CD64)	FcγRII-A (CD32)	FcγRII-B2 (CD32)	FcγRII-B1 (CD32)	FcγRIII (CD16)	FcεRI	FcεRII (CD23)	FcαRI (CD89)	Fcα/μR
Structure	α 72 kDa; γ	α 40 kDa; γ-like domain	ITIM	ITIM	α 50–70 kDa; γ or ζ	α 45 kDa; β 33 kDa; γ 9 kDa	lectin domain trimer; N	α 55–75 kDa; γ 9 kDa	α 70 kDa
Binding	IgG1	IgG1	IgG1	IgG1	IgG1	IgE	IgE	IgA1, IgA2	IgA, IgM
	$10^8\,\mathrm{M^{-1}}$	$2 \times 10^6\,\mathrm{M^{-1}}$	$2 \times 10^6\,\mathrm{M^{-1}}$	$2 \times 10^6\,\mathrm{M^{-1}}$	$5 \times 10^5\,\mathrm{M^{-1}}$	$10^{10}\,\mathrm{M^{-1}}$	2–$7 \times 10^7\,\mathrm{M^{-1}}$ (trimer)	$10^7\,\mathrm{M^{-1}}$	$3 \times 10^9\,\mathrm{M^{-1}}$
Order of affinity	1) IgG1=IgG3 2) IgG4 3) IgG2	1) IgG1 2) IgG3=IgG2* 3) IgG4	1) IgG1=IgG3 2) IgG4 3) IgG2	1) IgG1=IgG3 2) IgG4 3) IgG2	IgG1=IgG3		2–$7 \times 10^6\,\mathrm{M^{-1}}$ (monomer)		1) IgM 2) IgA
								IgA1=IgA2	
Cell type	Macrophages Neutrophils Eosinophils	Macrophages Neutrophils Eosinophils Platelets Langerhans cells	Macrophages Neutrophils Eosinophils	B cells Mast cells	NK cells Eosinophils Macrophages Neutrophils Mast cells	Mast cells Basophils	Eosinophils B cells	Macrophages Eosinophils† Neutrophils	Macrophages B cells
Effect of ligation	Uptake Stimulation Activation of respiratory burst Induction of killing	Uptake Granule release (eosinophils)	Uptake Inhibition of stimulation	No uptake Inhibition of stimulation	Induction of killing (NK cells)	Secretion of granules	Degranulation	Uptake Induction of killing	Uptake

Fig. 10.38 Distinct receptors for the Fc region of the different immunoglobulin classes are expressed on different accessory cells. The subunit structure and binding properties of these receptors and the cell types expressing them are shown. All are immunoglobulin superfamily members except FcεRII, which is a lectin and can form trimers. The exact chain composition of any receptor can vary from one cell type to another. For example, FcγRIII in neutrophils is expressed as a molecule with a glycosylphosphatidylinositol membrane anchor without γ chains, whereas in NK cells it is a transmembrane molecule associated with γ chains. The FcγRII-B1 differs from the FcγRII-B2 by the presence of an additional exon in the intracellular region (indicated by yellow triangle). This exon prevents the FcγRII-B1 from being internalized after cross-linking. The binding affinities are taken from data on human receptors. *Only some allotypes of FcγRII-A bind IgG2. †In eosinophils, the molecular mass of the CD89α chain is 70–100 kDa.

Antibody-coated viruses that enter the cytoplasm are cleared by a system that employs a novel class of Fc receptor called **TRIM21 (tripartite motif-containing 21)**, which is expressed by a variety of immune and nonimmune cell types. TRIM21 is a cytosolic IgG receptor that has a higher affinity for IgG than that of any other Fc receptor, and it also has **E3 ligase** activity. When a virus that has bound IgG enters the cytoplasm, TRIM21 attaches to the antibody and uses its E3 ligase activity to ubiquitinate itself. This leads to the delivery of the virus-antibody complex to the proteasome, causing proteasomal degradation of virions in the cytosol before translation of virally encoded genes can occur.

10-22 Fc receptors on phagocytes are activated by antibodies bound to the surface of pathogens and enable the phagocytes to ingest and destroy pathogens.

Macrophages and neutrophils are important Fc-bearing cells in humoral immune responses. Many bacteria that are not pathogenic in normal individuals are directly recognized, ingested, and destroyed by these phagocytic cells. However, some bacterial pathogens have a **polysaccharide capsule**, a large structure that lies outside the bacterial cell membrane and resists direct engulfment by phagocytes. Such pathogens become susceptible to phagocytosis only when they are coated with antibodies and complement, which engage the Fcγ or Fcα receptors and the complement receptor CR1 on phagocytic cells, triggering bacterial uptake (**Fig. 10.39**). The stimulation of phagocytosis by complement-coated antigens binding to complement receptors is particularly important early in the immune response, before isotype-switched antibodies have been made. Capsular

| Bacterium is coated with complement and IgG antibody | When C3b binds to CR1 and antibody binds to Fc receptor, bacterium is phagocytosed | Macrophage membranes fuse, creating a membrane-enclosed vesicle, the phagosome | Lysosomes fuse with these vesicles, delivering enzymes that degrade the bacterium |

Fig. 10.39 Fc and complement receptors on phagocytes trigger the uptake and degradation of antibody-coated bacteria. Many bacteria resist phagocytosis by macrophages and neutrophils. Antibodies bound to these bacteria, however, enable the bacteria to be ingested and degraded through the interaction of the multiple Fc domains arrayed on the bacterial surface with Fc receptors on the phagocyte surface. Antibody coating also induces activation of the complement system and the binding of complement components to the bacterial surface. These can interact with complement receptors (for example, CR1) on the phagocyte. Fc receptors and complement receptors synergize in inducing phagocytosis. Bacteria coated with IgG antibody and complement are therefore more readily ingested than those coated with IgG alone. Binding of Fc and complement receptors signals the phagocyte to increase the rate of phagocytosis, to fuse lysosomes with phagosomes, and to increase its bactericidal activity.

polysaccharides belong to the TI-2 class of thymus-independent antigens and can therefore stimulate the early production of IgM antibodies, which are very effective at activating the complement system. IgM binding to encapsulated bacteria thus triggers the opsonization of these bacteria by complement and their prompt ingestion and destruction by phagocytes bearing complement receptors. Recently, Fcα/μR was discovered as a receptor that binds both IgA and IgM. Fcα/μR is expressed primarily on macrophages and B cells in the lamina propria of the intestine and in germinal centers. It is thought to have a role in the endocytosis of IgM antibody complexed with bacteria such as *Staphylococcus aureus*.

Phagocyte activation can initiate an inflammatory response that causes tissue damage. It is important that Fc receptors on phagocytes be able to distinguish antibody molecules that are bound to a pathogen from the free antibody molecules that are not bound to anything. This distinction is made possible by the aggregation of antibodies that occurs when they bind to multimeric antigens or to multivalent particulate antigens such as viruses and bacteria. Individual Fc receptors on a cell surface bind monomers of free antibody with low affinity, but when presented with an antibody-coated particle, the simultaneous binding by multiple Fc receptors results in binding of high avidity, and this is the principal mechanism by which bound antibodies are distinguished from free immunoglobulin (**Fig. 10.40**). The result is that Fc receptors enable cells to detect pathogens via the antibody molecules bound to them. Fc receptors therefore give phagocytic cells that lack intrinsic specificity the ability to identify and remove specific pathogens and their products from the extracellular spaces.

Phagocytosis is greatly enhanced by interactions between the molecules coating an opsonized microorganism and receptors on the phagocyte surface. When an antibody-coated pathogen binds to Fcγ receptors, for example,

| Free immunoglobulin does not cross-link Fc receptors |

No activation of macrophage, no destruction of bacterium

| Aggregation of immunoglobulin on bacterial surface allows cross-linking of Fc receptors |

Activation of macrophage, leading to phagocytosis and destruction of bacterium

Fig. 10.40 Bound antibody is distinguishable from free immunoglobulin by its state of aggregation. Free immunoglobulin molecules bind most Fc receptors with very low affinity and cannot cross-link Fc receptors. Antigen-bound immunoglobulin, however, binds to Fc receptors with high avidity because several antibody molecules that are bound to the same surface bind to multiple Fc receptors on the surface of the accessory cell. This Fc receptor cross-linking sends a signal to activate the cell bearing it. With Fc receptors that have ITIMs, the result is inhibition.

Fig. 10.41 Eosinophil attack on a schistosome parasite is facilitated by specific antibody binding to parasite surface antigens. This electron micrograph is of eosinophils that were obtained from the blood of a healthy donor and incubated with schistosome larvae (SL) and IgG antibodies specific for surface antigens of the larvae. Shown is one larva. In the incubation, antibodies first bind to the larval antigens, which allows numerous eosinophils (E) to bind to the Fc part of the antibodies using their Fcγ receptors. Electron micrograph courtesy of A. Butterworth.

the cell surface of the phagocyte extends around the surface of the pathogen through successive binding of the Fcγ receptors to the antibody Fc regions bound to the pathogen. This is an active process that is triggered by the stimulation of the Fcγ receptors. Phagocytosis leads to enclosure of the pathogen (or particle) in an acidified cytoplasmic vesicle—the phagosome. This then fuses with one or more lysosomes to generate a phagolysosome; lysosomal enzymes are released into the vesicle interior, where they destroy the bacterium (see Fig. 10.39). The process of intracellular killing by phagocytes was described in more detail in Chapter 3.

Some particles are too large for a phagocyte to ingest; parasitic worms are one example. In this case, the phagocyte attaches to the surface of the antibody-coated parasite via its Fcγ, Fcα, or Fcε receptors, and the contents of the secretory granules or lysosomes of the phagocyte are released by exocytosis. The contents are discharged directly onto the surface of the parasite and damage it. Thus, stimulation of Fcγ and Fcα receptors can trigger either the internalization of external particles by phagocytosis or the externalization of internal vesicles by exocytosis. The principal leukocytes involved in the destruction of bacteria are macrophages and neutrophils, whereas large parasites such as helminths are usually attacked by eosinophils (**Fig. 10.41**), nonphagocytic cells that can bind antibody-coated parasites via several different Fc receptors, including the low-affinity Fcε receptor for IgE, CD23 (see Fig. 10.38). Cross-linking of these receptors by antibody-coated surfaces activates the eosinophil to release its granule contents, which include proteins toxic to parasites (see Fig. 14.10). Cross-linking by antigen of IgE bound to the high-affinity FcεRI on mast cells and basophils also results in exocytosis of their granule contents, as we describe later.

10-23 Fc receptors activate NK cells to destroy antibody-coated targets.

Virus-infected cells are usually destroyed by T cells that recognize virus-derived peptides bound to cell-surface MHC molecules. But in addition, cells infected by some viruses can signal the presence of infection by their expression of viral envelope proteins on their cell surface. Such proteins can be recognized by antibodies originally produced against the virus particle. Host cells with such antibodies bound to them can be killed by NK cells, which we described in Chapter 3. Recall that NK cells express a limited repertoire of invariant receptors recognizing a range of ligands that are induced on abnormal cells, such as those infected with viruses. On recognition of a ligand, NK cells kill the target cells directly without the need for antibody.

As well as this innate function, NK cells can recognize and destroy antibody-coated target cells in a process called **antibody-dependent cell-mediated cytotoxicity (ADCC)**. This is triggered when antibody bound to the surface of a cell interacts with Fc receptors on the NK cell (**Fig. 10.42**). NK cells express the receptor FcγRIII (CD16), which recognizes the IgG1 and IgG3 subclasses. The killing mechanism is analogous to that of cytotoxic T cells, involving the release of cytoplasmic granules containing perforin and granzymes (see Section 9-22). ADCC has been shown to have a role in the defense against infection by viruses and represents another mechanism by which antibodies can direct an antigen-specific attack by an effector cell that itself lacks

| Antibody binds antigens on the surface of target cells | Fc receptors on NK cells recognize bound antibody | Cross-linking of Fc receptors signals the NK cell to kill the target cell | Target cell dies by apoptosis |

Fig. 10.42 Antibody-coated target cells can be killed by NK cells in antibody-dependent cell-mediated cytotoxicity (ADCC). NK cells (see Chapter 3) are large granular non-T, non-B lymphoid cells that have FcγRIII (CD16) on their surface. When these cells encounter cells coated with IgG antibody, they rapidly kill the target cell. ADCC is only one way in which NK cells can contribute to host defense.

specificity for antigen. ADCC carried out by NK cells is being considered as a potential immunotherapeutic approach in treating cancer by directing their lytic activity to cells expressing tumor-specific antigens.

10-24 Mast cells and basophils bind IgE antibody via the high-affinity Fcε receptor.

When pathogens breach an epithelial barrier, one important host defense relies on the activation of mast cells. These cells are found in particularly high concentrations in vascularized connective tissues just beneath epithelial surfaces, including the submucosal tissues of the gastrointestinal and respiratory tracts and the dermis of the skin. These large cells (see Fig. 1.8) have distinctive cytoplasmic granules that contain a mixture of chemical mediators, including histamine, that act rapidly to make local blood vessels more permeable. Mast cells have Fc receptors specific for IgE (FcεRI) and IgG (FcγRIII) and can be activated to release their granules and to secrete lipid inflammatory mediators and cytokines via antibody bound to these receptors. Most Fc receptors bind stably to the Fc regions of antibodies only when the antibodies have themselves bound antigen, and cross-linking of multiple Fc receptors is needed for strong binding. In contrast, FcεRI binds IgE antibody monomers with a very high affinity—approximately 10^{10} M^{-1}. Thus, even at the low levels of circulating IgE present in normal individuals, a substantial portion of the total IgE is bound to the FcεRI that is expressed on mast cells in tissues and on circulating basophils.

Mast cells are not directly activated by the binding of IgE to their FcεRI or by the binding of monomeric antigen to this IgE. Mast-cell activation occurs only when the bound IgE is cross-linked by multivalent antigens. This signal activates the mast cell to release the contents of its granules, which occurs in seconds (**Fig. 10.43**), to synthesize and release lipid mediators such as prostaglandin D2 and leukotriene C4, and to secrete cytokines such as TNF-α, thereby initiating a local inflammatory response. The release of stored histamine increases local blood flow and vascular permeability, which quickly leads to an accumulation of fluid and blood proteins, including antibodies, in the surrounding tissue. Shortly afterward there is an influx of blood-borne cells such as neutrophils and, later, monocytes, eosinophils, and effector lymphocytes. This influx can last from a few minutes to a few hours and produces an inflammatory response at the site of infection. Beyond their role as a front-line host defense against pathogens at epithelial barriers, mast cells are also

Fig. 10.43 IgE antibody cross-linking on mast-cell surfaces leads to a rapid release of inflammatory mediators. Mast cells are large cells found in connective tissue and can be distinguished by their secretory granules, which contain many inflammatory mediators. They bind stably to monomeric IgE antibodies through the very high-affinity receptor FcεRI. Antigen cross-linking of the bound IgE antibody molecules triggers rapid degranulation, releasing inflammatory mediators into the surrounding tissue. These mediators trigger local inflammation, which recruits cells and proteins required for host defense to sites of infection. These cells are also triggered during allergic reactions when allergens bind to IgE on mast cells.

of medical importance because of their involvement in IgE-mediated allergic responses, discussed in Chapter 14. In allergic responses, mast cells are activated by exposure to normally innocuous antigens (allergens), such as pollen, to which the individual has previously mounted a sensitizing immune response that produces allergen-specific IgE.

10-25 IgE-mediated activation of accessory cells has an important role in resistance to parasite infection.

Mast cells are thought to serve at least three important functions in host defense. First, their location near body surfaces allows them to recruit both pathogen-specific elements, such as antigen-specific lymphocytes, and nonspecific effector elements, such as neutrophils, macrophages, basophils, and eosinophils, to sites where infectious agents are most likely to enter the internal milieu. Second, the inflammation they cause increases the flow of lymph from sites of antigen deposition to the regional lymph nodes, where naive lymphocytes are first activated. Third, the ability of mast-cell products to trigger muscular contraction can contribute to the physical expulsion of pathogens from the lungs or the gut. Mast cells respond rapidly to the binding of antigen to surface-bound IgE antibodies, and their activation leads to the initiation of an inflammatory response and the recruitment and activation of basophils and eosinophils, which contribute further to the inflammatory response (see Chapter 14). IgE-mediated responses are important in the defense against parasite infestation.

A role for mast cells in the clearance of parasites is suggested by the accumulation of mast cells in the intestine, known as **mastocytosis**, that accompanies helminth infection, and by observations in W/W^V mutant mice, which have a profound mast-cell deficiency caused by a mutation in the gene c-*kit*. These mutant mice show impaired clearance of the intestinal nematodes *Trichinella spiralis* and *Strongyloides* species. Clearance of *Strongyloides* is even more impaired in W/W^V mice that lack IL-3 and so also fail to produce basophils. Thus, both mast cells and basophils seem to contribute to defense against these helminth parasites.

Other evidence points to the importance of IgE antibodies and eosinophils in the defense against parasites. Infection with certain types of multicellular parasites, particularly helminths, is strongly associated with the production of IgE antibodies and the presence of abnormally large numbers of eosinophils (eosinophilia) in blood and tissues. Furthermore, experiments in mice show that depletion of eosinophils by polyclonal anti-eosinophil antisera increases the severity of infection with the parasitic helminth *Schistosoma mansoni*. Eosinophils seem to be directly responsible for helminth destruction; examination of infected tissues shows degranulated eosinophils adhering to helminths, and experiments *in vitro* have shown that eosinophils can kill *S. mansoni* in the presence of anti-schistosome IgG or IgA antibodies (see Fig. 10.41).

The role of IgE, mast cells, basophils, and eosinophils can also be seen in resistance to the feeding of blood-sucking ixodid ticks. Skin at the site of a tick bite has degranulated mast cells and an accumulation of degranulated basophils and eosinophils, an indicator of recent activation. Subsequent resistance to feeding by these ticks develops after the first exposure, suggesting a specific immunological mechanism. Mice deficient in mast cells show no such acquired resistance to ticks, and in guinea pigs the depletion of either basophils or eosinophils by specific polyclonal antibodies also reduces resistance to tick feeding. Finally, experiments in mice showed that resistance to ticks is mediated by specific IgE antibody. Thus, many clinical studies and experiments support a role for this system of IgE bound to the high-affinity FcεRI in host resistance to pathogens that enter across epithelia or exoparasites such as ticks that breach it.

Summary.

Antibody-coated pathogens are recognized by effector cells through Fc receptors that bind to various antibody C regions. Binding activates the cell and triggers destruction of the pathogen, through either phagocytosis, granule release, or both. Fc receptors compose a family of proteins, each of which recognizes particular antibody classes, or isotypes. Fc receptors on macrophages and neutrophils recognize the constant regions of IgG or IgA antibodies bound to a pathogen and trigger the engulfment and destruction of such bacteria. Binding to the Fc receptor also induces the production of microbicidal agents in the intracellular vesicles of the phagocyte. Eosinophils are important in the elimination of parasites too large to be engulfed; they bear Fc receptors specific for the constant region of IgG, as well as receptors for IgE; aggregation of these receptors triggers the release of toxic substances onto the surface of the parasite. NK cells, tissue mast cells, and blood basophils also release their granule contents when their Fc receptors are engaged. The high-affinity receptor for IgE is expressed constitutively by mast cells and basophils and can bind free monomeric antibody. When IgE bound to a mast cell is cross-linked by multivalent antigens, it triggers the release of histamine and other mediators that increase the blood flow to sites of infection, thus enabling an immediate response to pathogens at their site of first entry. Mast cells are found principally below epithelial surfaces of the skin and beneath the basement membrane of the digestive and respiratory tracts.

Summary to Chapter 10.

The humoral immune response to infection involves the production of antibody by plasma cells derived from B lymphocytes, the binding of this antibody to the pathogen, and the elimination of the pathogen by phagocytic cells and molecules of the humoral immune system. The production of antibody typically involves help from CD4 T cells that are reactive to a peptide fragment of the antigen recognized by the B cell, a phenomenon called linked recognition. An activated B cell first moves to the T-zone–B-zone boundary in secondary lymphoid tissues, where it may encounter its cognate T cell and begin to proliferate. Some B cells become plasmablasts, while others move to the germinal center, where somatic hypermutation and class switch recombination can take place. B cells that bind antigen with the highest affinity are selected for survival and further differentiation, leading to affinity maturation of the antibody response. Cytokines made by helper T cells direct class switching, leading to the production of antibody of various classes that can be distributed to various body compartments.

IgM antibodies are produced early in an infection by conventional B cells and are also made in the absence of infection by subsets of nonconventional B cells in particular locations (as natural antibodies). IgM has a major role in protecting against infection in the bloodstream, whereas isotypes secreted later in an adaptive immune response, such as IgG, diffuse into the tissues. Antigens that have highly repeating antigenic determinants and which contain mitogens—called TI antigens—can elicit IgM and some IgG independently of T-cell help, and this provides an early protective immune response. Multimeric IgA is produced in the lamina propria and is transported across epithelial surfaces, whereas IgE is made in small amounts and binds avidly to receptors on the surface of basophils and mast cells.

Antibodies that bind with high affinity to critical sites on toxins, viruses, and bacteria can neutralize them. However, pathogens and their products are destroyed and removed from the body largely through uptake into phagocytes and degradation inside these cells. Antibodies that coat pathogens bind to Fc receptors on phagocytes, which are thereby triggered to engulf and destroy the pathogen. Binding of antibody C regions to Fc receptors on other cells leads to the exocytosis of stored mediators; this is particularly important in parasite infections, in which Fcε-expressing mast cells are triggered by the binding of antigen to IgE antibody to release inflammatory mediators directly onto parasite surfaces. Antibodies can also initiate the destruction of pathogens by activating the complement system. Complement components can opsonize pathogens for uptake by phagocytes and recruit phagocytes to sites of infection. Receptors for complement components and Fc receptors often synergize in activating the uptake and destruction of pathogens and immune complexes. Thus, the humoral immune response is targeted to the infecting pathogen through the production of specific antibody; however, the effector actions of that antibody are determined by its heavy-chain isotype.

Discussion Questions

10.1 Describe the differences between thymus-dependent (TD) and thymus-independent (TI) antigens. What kind of T cells provide help for activation of naive B cells in response to TD antigens, and by what mechanism?

10.2 What is meant by linked recognition regarding T-cell help for B-cell responses? In what way is this process a 'coincidence detector,' and what advantages does this process provide?

10.3 What part of the antibody molecule determines its particular effector function? Compare and contrast the properties of the IgM and the various IgG isotypes.

10.4 The locations of T and B cells change during a TD antibody response. Describe the mechanisms that regulate their movement at the various stages of a response.

10.5 Describe the processes that regulate the cyclic reentry of centroblasts and centrocytes between the light and dark zones of the germinal center reaction.

10.6 Somatic hypermutation induced by AID in activated B cells is converted into affinity maturation by selective processes in the germinal center. Describe these processes and explain how they lead to enhanced antibody affinity for antigen.

10.7 Which class of antibody is responsible for activation of mast cells, and how does this process occur? What type of pathogens is this class of antibody directed against, and what undesirable reactions can these antibodies cause?

10.8 Describe the interaction between antibodies and the complement system, and explain how this interaction aids in the elimination of pathogens.

10.9 What classes of maternal antibodies are found in breast milk, and how are they transported to the newborn? Birds possess this class of antibody and secrete it into the crop milk they feed to their offspring. What does this fact indicate about mammalian evolution?

General references.

Bournazos, S., Wang, T.T., Dahan, R., Maamary, J., and Ravetch, J.V.: **Signaling by antibodies: recent progress.** *Annu. Rev. Immunol.* 2017, **35**:285–311.

Cyster, J.G., and Allen, C.D.C.: **B cell responses: cell interaction dynamics and decisions.** *Cell* 2019, **177**:524–540.

Mesin, L., Ersching, J., and Victora, G.D. **Germinal center B cell dynamics.** *Immunity* 2016, **45**:471–482.

Section references.

10-1 Activation of B cells by antigen involves signals from the B-cell receptor and either helper T cells or microbial antigens.

Maglione, P.J., Simchoni, N., Black, S., Radigan, L., Overbey, J.R., Bagiella, E., Bussel, J.B., Bossuyt, X., Casanova, J.L., Meyts, I., *et al.*: **IRAK-4- and MyD88 deficiencies impair IgM responses against T-independent bacterial antigens.** *Blood* 2014, **124**:3561–3571.

Opferman, J.T., Letai, A., Beard, C., Sorcinelli, M.D., Ong, C.C., and Korsmeyer, S.J.: **Development and maintenance of B and T lymphocytes requires antiapoptotic MCL-1.** *Nature* 2003, **426**:671–676.

Pasare, C., and Medzhitov, R.: **Control of B-cell responses by Toll-like receptors.** *Nature* 2005, **438**:364–368.

Vikstrom, I., Carotta, S., Lüthje, K., Peperzak, V., Jost, P.J., Glaser, S., Busslinger, M., Bouillet, P., Strasser, A., Nutt, S.L., and Tarlinton, D.M.: **Mcl-1 is essential for germinal center formation and B cell memory.** *Science* 2010, **330**:1095–1099.

10-2 Linked recognition of antigen by T cells and B cells promotes robust antibody responses.

Barrington, R.A., Zhang, M., Zhong, X., Jonsson, H., Holodick, N., Cherukuri, A., Pierce, S.K., Rothstein, T.L., and Carroll, M.C.: **CD21/CD19 coreceptor signaling promotes B cell survival during primary immune responses.** *J. Immunol.* 2005, **175**:2859–2867.

Eskola, J., Peltola, H., Takala, A.K., Kayhty, H., Hakulinen, M., Karanko, V., Kela, E., Rekola, P., Ronnberg, P.R., Samuelson, J.S., *et al.*: **Efficacy of *Haemophilus influenzae* type b polysaccharide-diphtheria toxoid conjugate vaccine in infancy.** *N. Engl. J. Med.* 1987, **317**:717–722.

MacLennan, I.C.M., Gulbranson-Judge, A., Toellner, K.M., Casamayor-Palleja, M., Chan, E., Sze, D.M.Y., Luther, S.A., and Orbea, H.A.: **The changing preference of T and B cells for partners as T-dependent antibody responses develop.** *Immunol. Rev.* 1997, **156**:53–66.

McHeyzer-Williams, L.J., Malherbe, L.P., and McHeyzer-Williams, M.G.: **Helper T cell-regulated B cell immunity.** *Curr. Top. Microbiol. Immunol.* 2006, **311**:59–83.

Nitschke, L.: **The role of CD22 and other inhibitory co-receptors in B-cell activation.** *Curr. Opin. Immunol.* 2005, **17**:290–297.

Rickert, R.C.: **Regulation of B lymphocyte activation by complement C3 and the B cell coreceptor complex.** *Curr. Opin. Immunol.* 2005, **17**:237–243.

10-3 B cells that encounter their antigens migrate toward the boundaries between B-cell and T-cell areas in secondary lymphoid tissues.

Cinamon, G., Zachariah, M.A., Lam, O.M., Foss, F.W., Jr., and Cyster, J.G.: **Follicular shuttling of marginal zone B cells facilitates antigen transport.** *Nat. Immunol.* 2008, **9**:54–62.

Heesters, B.A., Myers, R.C., and Carroll, M.C.: **Follicular dendritic cells: dynamic antigen libraries.** *Nat. Rev. Immunol.* 2014, **14**:495–504.

Iannacone, M., Moseman, E.A., Tonti, E., Bosurgi, L., Junt, T., Henrickson, S.E., Whelan, S.P., Guidotti, L.G., and von Andrian, U.H.: **Subcapsular sinus macrophages prevent CNS invasion on peripheral infection with a neurotropic virus.** *Nature* 2010, **465**:1079–1083.

Kalled, S.L.: **Impact of the BAFF/BR3 axis on B cell survival, germinal center maintenance and antibody production.** *Semin. Immunol.* 2006, **18**:290–296.

Lu, E., and Cyster, J.G.: **G-protein coupled receptors and ligands that organize humoral immune responses.** *Immunol. Rev.* 2019, **289**:158–172.

Okada, T., and Cyster, J.G.: **B cell migration and interactions in the early phase of antibody responses.** *Curr. Opin. Immunol.* 2006, **18**:278–285.

Vincent, F.B., Saulep-Easton, D., Figgett, W.A., Fairfax, K.A., and Mackay, F.: **The BAFF/APRIL system: emerging functions beyond B cell biology and autoimmunity.** *Cytokine Growth Factor Rev.* 2013, **24**:203–215.

10-4 T cells express surface molecules and cytokines that activate B cells, which in turn promote T$_{FH}$ cell development.

Choi, Y.S., Kageyama, R., Eto, D., Escobar, T.C., Johnston, R.J., Monticelli, L., Lao, C., and Crotty, S.: **ICOS receptor instructs T follicular helper cell versus effector cell differentiation via induction of the transcriptional repressor Bcl6.** *Immunity* 2011, **34**:932–946.

Crotty, S.: **T follicular helper cell biology: a decade of discovery and diseases.** *Immunity* 2019, **50**:1132–1148.

Hatzi, K., Nancem J.P., Kroenke, M.A., Bothwell, M., Haddad, E.K., Melnick, A., and Crotty, S.: **BCL6 orchestrates Tfh cell differentiation via multiple distinct mechanisms.** *J. Exp. Med.* 2015, **212**:539–553.

Turner, J.S., Ke, F., and Grigorova, I.L.: **B cell receptor crosslinking augments germinal center B cell selection when T cell help is limiting.** *Cell Rep.* 2018, **25**:1395–1403.

Yoshinaga, S.K., Whoriskey, J.S., Khare, S.D., Sarmiento, U., Guo, J., Horan, T., Shih, G., Zhang, M., Coccia, M.A., Kohno, T., *et al.*: **T-cell co-stimulation through B7RP-1 and ICOS.** *Nature* 1999, **402**:827–832.

10-5 Some activated B cells differentiate into antibody-secreting plasmablasts and plasma cells.

Gatto, D., Wood, K., and Brink, R.: **EBI2 operates independently of but in cooperation with CXCR5 and CCR7 to direct B cell migration and organization in follicles and the germinal center.** *J. Immunol.* 2011, **187**:4621–4628.

Horst, A., Hunzelmann, N., Arce, S., Herber, M., Manz, R.A., Radbruch, A., Nischt, R., Schmitz, J., and Assenmacher, M.: **Detection and characterization of plasma cells in peripheral blood: correlation of IgE+ plasma cell frequency with IgE serum titre.** *Clin. Exp. Immunol.* 2002, **130**:370–378.

Moser, K., Tokoyoda, K., Radbruch, A., MacLennan, I., and Manz, R.A.: **Stromal niches, plasma cell differentiation and survival.** *Curr. Opin. Immunol.* 2006, **18**:265–270.

Radbruch, A., Muehlinghaus, G., Luger, E.O., Inamine, A., Smith, K.G., Dorner, T., and Hiepe, F.: **Competence and competition: the challenge of becoming a long-lived plasma cell.** *Nat. Rev. Immunol.* 2006, **6**:741–750.

Tellier, J., and Nutt, S.L. **Plasma cells: the programming of an antibody-secreting machine.** *Eur. J. Immunol.* 2019, **49**:30–37.

10-6 The second phase of a primary B-cell immune response occurs when activated B cells migrate into follicles and proliferate to form germinal centers.

Allen, C.D., Okada, T., and Cyster, J.G.: **Germinal-center organization and cellular dynamics.** *Immunity* 2007, **27**:190–202.

Cozine, C.L., Wolniak, K.L., and Waldschmidt, T.J.: **The primary germinal center response in mice.** *Curr. Opin. Immunol.* 2005, **17**:298–302.

Kerfoot, S.M., Yaari, G., Patel, J.R., Johnson, K.L., Gonzalez, D.G., Kleinstein, S.H., and Haberman, A.M.: **Germinal center B cell and T follicular helper cell development initiates in the interfollicular zone.** *Immunity* 2011, **34**:947–960.

Krzyzak, L., Seitz, C., Urbat, A., Hutzler, S., Ostalecki, C., Gläsner, J., Hiergeist, A., Gessner, A., Winkler, T.H., Steinkasserer, A., and Nitschke, L.: **CD83 modulates B cell activation and germinal center responses.** *J. Immunol.* 2016, **196**:3581–3594.

Kunkel, E.J., and Butcher, E.C.: **Plasma-cell homing.** *Nat. Rev. Immunol.* 2003, **3**:822–829.

Roco, J.A., Mesin, L., Binder, S.C., Nefzger, C., Gonzalez-Figueroa, P., Canete, P.F., Ellyard, J., Shen, Q., Robert, P.A., Cappello, J., *et al.*: **Class-switch recombination occurs infrequently in germinal centers.** *Immunity* 2019, **51**:337–350.

Victora, G.D., Dominguez-Sola, D., Holmes, A.B., Deroubaix, S., Dalla-Favera, R., and Nussenzweig, M.C.: **Identification of human germinal center light and dark zone cells and their relationship to human B-cell lymphomas.** *Blood* 2012, **120**:2240–2248.

10-7 Germinal center B cells undergo V-region somatic hypermutation, and cells with mutations that improve affinity for antigen are selected.

Anderson, S.M., Khalil, A., Uduman, M., Hershberg, U., Louzoun, Y., Haberman, A.M., Kleinstein, S.H., and Shlomchik, M.J.: **Taking advantage: high-affinity B cells in the germinal center have lower death rates, but similar rates of division, compared to low-affinity cells.** *J. Immunol.* 2009, **183**:7314–7325.

Bannard, O., and Cyster, J.G.: **Germinal centers: programmed for affinity maturation and antibody diversification.** *Curr. Opin. Immunol.* 2017, **45**:21–30.

Gitlin, A.D., Shulman, Z., and Nussenzweig, M.C.: **Clonal selection in the germinal centre by regulated proliferation and hypermutation.** *Nature* 2014, **509**:637–640.

Li, Z., Woo, C.J., Iglesias-Ussel, M.D., Ronai, D., and Scharff, M.D.: **The generation of antibody diversity through somatic hypermutation and class switch recombination.** *Genes Dev.* 2004, **18**:1–11.

Victora, G.D., and Mesin, L.: **Clonal and cellular dynamics in germinal centers.** *Curr. Opin. Immunol.* 2014, **28**:90–96.

10-8 Positive selection of germinal center B cells involves contact with T_{FH} cells and CD40 signaling.

Bannard, O., Horton, R.M., Allen, C.D., An, J., Nagasawa, T., and Cyster, J.G.: **Germinal center centroblasts transition to a centrocyte phenotype according to a timed program and depend on the dark zone for effective selection.** *Immunity* 2013, **39**:912–924.

Cannons, J.L., Qi, H., Lu, K.T., Dutta, M., Gomez-Rodriguez, J., Cheng, J., Wakeland, E.K., Germain, R.N., and Schwartzberg, P.L.: **Optimal germinal center responses require a multistage T cell:B cell adhesion process involving integrins, SLAM-associated protein, and CD84.** *Immunity* 2010, **32**:253–265.

Heesters, B.A., Chatterjee, P., Kim, Y.A., Gonzalez, S.F., Kuligowski, M.P., Kirchhausen, T., and Carroll, M.C.: **Endocytosis and recycling of immune complexes by follicular dendritic cells enhances B cell antigen binding and activation.** *Immunity* 2013, **38**:1164–1175.

Shulman, Z., Gitlin, A.D., Weinstein, J.S., Lainez, B., Esplugues, E., Flavell, R.A., Craft, J.E., and Nussenzweig, M.C.: **Dynamic signaling by T follicular helper cells during germinal center B cell selection.** *Science* 2014, **345**:1058–1062.

Tas, J.M., Mesin, L., Pasqual, G, Targ, S., Jacobsen, J.T., Mano, Y.M., Chen, C.S., Weill, J.C., Reynaud, C.A., Browne, E.P., *et al.*: **Visualizing antibody affinity maturation in germinal centers.** *Science* 2016, **351**:1048–1054.

Victora, G.D., Schwickert, T.A., Fooksman, D.R., Kamphorst, A.O., Meyer-Hermann, M., Dustin, M.L., and Nussenzweig, M.C.: **Germinal center dynamics revealed by multiphoton microscopy with a photoactivatable fluorescent reporter.** *Cell* 2010, **143**:592–605.

Wang, Z., Karras, J.G., Howard, R.G., and Rothstein, T.L.: **Induction of bcl-x by CD40 engagement rescues sIg-induced apoptosis in murine B cells.** *J. Immunol.* 1995, **155**:3722–3725.

10-9 Activation-induced cytidine deaminase introduces mutations into genes transcribed in B cells.

Bransteitter, R., Pham, P., Scharff, M.D., and Goodman, M.F.: **Activation-induced cytidine deaminase deaminates deoxycytidine on single-stranded DNA but requires the action of RNase.** *Proc. Natl. Acad. Sci. USA* 2003, **100**:4102–4107.

Cantaert, T., Schickel, J.N., Bannock, J.M., Ng, Y.S., Massad, C., Oe, T., Wu, R., Lavoie, A., Walter, J.E., Notarangelo, L.D., *et al.*: **Activation-induced cytidine deaminase expression in human B cell precursors is essential for central B cell tolerance.** *Immunity* 2015, **43**:884–895.

Muramatsu, M., Kinoshita, K., Fagarasan, S., Yamada, S., Shinkai, Y., and Honjo, T.: **Class switch recombination and hypermutation require activation-induced cytidine deaminase (AID), a potential RNA editing enzyme.** *Cell* 2000, **102**:553–563.

Petersen-Mahrt, S.K., Harris, R.S., and Neuberger, M.S.: **AID mutates *E. coli* suggesting a DNA deamination mechanism for antibody diversification.** *Nature* 2002, **418**:99–103.

Pham, P., Bransteitter, R., Petruska, J., and Goodman, M.F.: **Processive AID-catalyzed cytosine deamination on single-stranded DNA stimulates somatic hypermutation.** *Nature* 2003, **424**:103–107.

Suzuki, K., Meek, B., Doi, Y., Honjo, T., and Fagarasan, S.: **Two distinctive pathways for recruitment of naive and primed IgM+ B cells to the gut lamina propria.** *Proc. Natl. Acad. Sci. USA.* 2005, **102**:2482–2486.

Yu, K., Huang, F.T., and Lieber, M.R.: **DNA substrate length and surrounding sequence affect the activation-induced deaminase activity at cytidine.** *J. Biol. Chem.* 2004, **279**:6496–6500.

10-10 Mismatch and base-excision repair pathways contribute to somatic hypermutation after initiation by AID.

Basu, U., Chaudhuri, J., Alpert, C., Dutt, S., Ranganath, S., Li, G., Schrum, J.P., Manis, J.P., and Alt, F.W.: **The AID antibody diversification enzyme is regulated by protein kinase A phosphorylation.** *Nature* 2005, **438**:508–511.

Chaudhuri, J., Khuong, C., and Alt, F.W.: **Replication protein A interacts with AID to promote deamination of somatic hypermutation targets.** *Nature* 2004, **430**:992–998.

Delbos, F., Aoufouchi, S., Faili, A., Weill, J.C., and Reynaud, C.A.: **DNA polymerase eta is the sole contributor of A/T modifications during immunoglobulin gene hypermutation in the mouse.** *J. Exp. Med.* 2007, **204**:17–23.

Di Noia, J.M., and Neuberger, M.S.: **Molecular mechanisms of antibody somatic hypermutation.** *Annu. Rev. Biochem.* 2007, **76**:1–22.

Neuberger, M.S.: **Antibody diversification by somatic mutation: from Burnet onwards.** *Immunol. Cell Biol.* 2008, **86**:124–132.

Schenten, D., Kracker, S., Esposito, G., Franco, S., Klein, U., Murphy, M., Alt, F.W., and Rajewsky, K.: **Pol zeta ablation in B cells impairs the germinal center reaction, class switch recombination, DNA break repair, and genome stability.** *J. Exp. Med.* 2009, **206**:477–490.

Zan, H., Shima, N., Xu, Z., Al-Qahtani, A., Evinger III, A.J., Zhong, Y., Schimenti, J.C., and Casali, P.: **The translesion DNA polymerase theta plays a dominant role in immunoglobulin gene somatic hypermutation.** *EMBO J.* 2005, **24**:3757–3769.

10-11 AID initiates class switching to allow the same assembled V_H exon to be associated with different C_H genes in the course of an immune response.

Basu, U., Meng, F.L., Keim, C., Grinstein, V., Pefanis, E., Eccleston, J., Zhang, T., Myers, D., Wasserman, C.R., Wesemann, D.R., *et al.*: **The RNA exosome targets the AID cytidine deaminase to both strands of transcribed duplex DNA substrates.** *Cell* 2011, **144**:353–363.

Boboila, C., Yan, C., Wesemann, D.R., Jankovic, M., Wang, J.H., Manis, J., Nussenzweig, A., Nussenzweig, M., and Alt, F.W.: **Alternative end-joining catalyzes class switch recombination in the absence of both Ku70 and DNA ligase 4.** *J. Exp. Med.* 2010, **207**:417–427.

Pavri, R., Gazumyan, A., Jankovic, M., DiVirgilio, M., Klein, I., Ansarah-Sobrinho, C., Resch, W., Yamane, A., Reina San-Martin, B., Barreto, V., et al.: **Activation-induced cytidine deaminase targets DNA at sites of RNA polymerase II stalling by interaction with Spt5.** *Cell* 2010, **143**:122–133.

Qiao, Q., Wang, L., Meng, F.L., Hwang, J.K., Alt, F.W., and Wu, H.: **AID recognizes structured DNA for class switch recombination.** *Mol. Cell* 2017, **67**:361–373.

Revy, P., Muto, T., Levy, Y., Geissmann, F., Plebani, A., Sanal, O., Catalan, N., Forveille, M., Dufourcq-Lagelouse, R., Gennery, A., et al.: **Activation-induced cytidine deaminase (AID) deficiency causes the autosomal recessive form of the hyper-IgM syndrome (HIGM2).** *Cell* 2000, **102**:565–575.

Shinkura, R., Tian, M., Smith, M., Chua, K., Fujiwara, Y., and Alt, F.W.: **The influence of transcriptional orientation on endogenous switch region function.** *Nat. Immunol.* 2003, **4**:435–441.

Yewdell, W.T., Kim, Y., Chowdhury, P., Lau, C.M., Smolkin, R.M., Belcheva, K.T., Fernandez, K.C., Cols, M., Yen, W.F., Vaidyanathan, B., et al.: **A hyper-IgM syndrome mutation in activation-induced cytidine deaminase disrupts G-quadruplex binding and genome-wide chromatin localization.** *Immunity.* 2020, **53**:952–970.

Yu, K., Chedin, F., Hsieh, C.-L., Wilson, T.E., and Lieber, M.R.: **R-loops at immunoglobulin class switch regions in the chromosomes of stimulated B cells.** *Nat. Immunol.* 2003, **4**:442–451.

Zheng, S., Vuong, B.Q., Vaidyanathan, B., Lin, J.Y., Huang, F.T., and Chaudhuri, J.: **Non-coding RNA generated following lariat debranching mediates targeting of AID to DNA.** *Cell* 2015, **161**:762–773.

10-12 Cytokines made by T$_H$ cells direct the choice of isotype for class switching in T-dependent antibody responses.

Avery, D.T., Bryant, V.L., Ma, C.S., de Waal Malefyt, R., and Tangye, S.G.: **IL-21-induced isotype switching to IgG and IgA by human naive B cells is differentially regulated by IL-4.** *J. Immunol.* 2008, **181**:1767–1779.

Collins, J.T., and Dunnickm, W.A.: **Cutting edge: IFN-gamma regulated germline transcripts are expressed from gamma2a transgenes independently of the heavy chain 3′ enhancers.** *J. Immunol.* 1999, **163**:5758–5762.

Francke, U., and Ochs, H.D.: **The CD40 ligand, gp39, is defective in activated T cells from patients with X-linked hyper-IgM syndrome.** *Cell* 1993, **72**:291–300.

Matsumoto, R., Matsumoto, M., Mita, S., Hitoshi, Y., Ando, M., Araki, S., Yamaguchi, N., Tominaga, A., and Takatsu, K.: **Interleukin-5 induces maturation but not class switching of surface IgA-positive B cells into IgA-secreting cells.** *Immunology* 1989, **66**:32–38.

Messner, B., Stütz, A.M., Albrecht, B., Peiritsch, S., and Woisetschläger, M.: **Cooperation of binding sites for STAT6 and NF kappa B/rel in the IL-4-induced up-regulation of the human IgE germline promoter.** *J. Immunol.* 1997, **159**:3330–3337.

Mizoguchi, C., Uehara, S., Akira, S., and Takatsu, K.: **IL-5 induces IgG1 isotype switch recombination in mouse CD38-activated sIgD-positive B lymphocytes.** *J. Immunol.* 1999, **162**:2812–2829.

Park, S.R., Seo, G.Y., Choi, A.J., Stavnezer, J., and Kim, P.H.: **Analysis of transforming growth factor-beta1-induced Ig germ-line gamma2b transcription and its implication for IgA isotype switching.** *Eur. J. Immunol.* 2005, **35**:946–956.

Seo, G.Y., Park, S.R., and Kim, P.H.: **Analyses of TGF-beta1-inducible Ig germ-line gamma2b promoter activity: involvement of Smads and NF-kappaB.** *Eur. J. Immunol.* 2009, **39**:1157–1166.

10-13 B cells that survive the germinal center reaction eventually differentiate into either plasma cells or memory cells.

Martins, G., and Calame, K.: **Regulation and functions of Blimp-1 in T and B lymphocytes.** *Annu. Rev. Immunol.* 2008, **26**:133–169.

Nera, K.P., and Lassila, O.: **Pax5—a critical inhibitor of plasma cell fate.** *Scand. J. Immunol.* 2006, **64**:190–199.

Omori, S.A., Cato, M.H., Anzelon-Mills, A., Puri, K.D., Shapiro-Shelef, M., Calame, K., and Rickert, R.C.: **Regulation of class-switch recombination and plasma cell differentiation by phosphatidylinositol 3-kinase signaling.** *Immunity* 2006, **25**:545–557.

Radbruch, A., Muehlinghaus, G., Luger, E.O., Inamine, A., Smith, K.G., Dorner, T., and Hiepe, F.: **Competence and competition: the challenge of becoming a long-lived plasma cell.** *Nat. Rev. Immunol.* 2006, **6**:741–750.

Shapiro-Shelef, M., Lin, K.I., McHeyzer-Williams, L.J., Liao, J., McHeyzer-Williams, M.G., and Calame, K.: **Blimp-1 is required for the formation of immunoglobulin secreting plasma cells and pre-plasma memory B cells.** *Immunity* 2003, **19**:607–620.

10-14 Some antigens do not require T-cell help to induce antibody responses.

Balazs, M., Martin, F., Zhou, T., and Kearney, J.: **Blood dendritic cells interact with splenic marginal zone B cells to initiate T-independent immune responses.** *Immunity* 2002, **17**:341–352.

Bekeredjian-Ding, I., and Jego, G.: **Toll-like receptors—sentries in the B-cell response.** *Immunology* 2009, **128**:311–323.

Craxton, A., Magaletti, D., Ryan, E.J., and Clark, E.A.: **Macrophage- and dendritic cell-dependent regulation of human B-cell proliferation requires the TNF family ligand BAFF.** *Blood* 2003, **101**:4464–4471.

Fagarasan, S., and Honjo, T.: **T-independent immune response: new aspects of B cell biology.** *Science* 2000, **290**:89–92.

Garcia De Vinuesa, C., Gulbranson-Judge, A., Khan, M., O'Leary, P., Cascalho, M., Wabl, M., Klaus, G.G., Owen, M.J., and MacLennan, I.C.: **Dendritic cells associated with plasmablast survival.** *Eur. J. Immunol.* 1999, **29**:3712–3721.

MacLennan, I., and Vinuesa, C.: **Dendritic cells, BAFF, and APRIL: innate players in adaptive antibody responses.** *Immunity* 2002, **17**:341–352.

Mond, J.J., Lees, A., and Snapper, C.M.: **T cell-independent antigens type 2.** *Annu. Rev. Immunol.* 1995, **13**:655–692.

Ruprecht, C.R., and Lanzavecchia, A.: **Toll-like receptor stimulation as a third signal required for activation of human naive B cells.** *Eur. J. Immunol.* 2006, **36**:810–816.

Snapper, C.M., Shen, Y., Khan, A.Q., Colino, J., Zelazowski, P., Mond, J.J., Gause, W.C., and Wu, Z.Q.: **Distinct types of T-cell help for the induction of a humoral immune response to *Streptococcus pneumoniae*.** *Trends Immunol.* 2001, **22**:308–311.

Yanaba, K., Bouaziz, J.D., Matsushita, T., Tsubata, T., and Tedder, T.F.: **The development and function of regulatory B cells expressing IL-10 (B10 cells) requires antigen receptor diversity and TLR signals.** *J. Immunol.* 2009, **182**:7459–7472.

10-15 Antibodies of different classes operate in distinct places and have distinct effector functions.

Benhnia, M.R., McCausland, M.M., Laudenslager, J., Granger, S.W., Rickert, S., Koriazova, L., Tahara, T., Kubo, R.T., Kato, S., Crotty, S., et al.: **Hybrid IgG4/IgG4 Fc antibodies form upon 'Fab-arm' exchange as demonstrated by SDS-PAGE or size-exclusion chromatography.** *Mol. Immunol.* 2010, **47**:1592–1594.

Suzuki, K., Meek, B., Doi, Y., Muramatsu, M., Chiba, T., Honjo, T., and Fagarasan, S.: **Aberrant expansion of segmented filamentous bacteria in IgA-deficient gut.** *Proc. Natl. Acad. Sci. USA* 2004, **101**:1981–1986.

Ward, E.S., and Ghetie, V.: **The effector functions of immunoglobulins: implications for therapy.** *Ther. Immunol.* 1995, **2**:77–94.

10-16 Polymeric immunoglobulin receptor binds to the Fc regions of IgA and IgM and transports them across epithelial barriers.

Ghetie, V., and Ward, E.S.: **Multiple roles for the major histocompatibility complex class I-related receptor FcRn.** *Annu. Rev. Immunol.* 2000, **18**:739–766.

Johansen, F.E., and Kaetzel, C.S.: **Regulation of the polymeric immunoglobulin receptor and IgA transport: new advances in environmental factors that stimulate pIgR expression and its role in mucosal immunity.** *Mucosal Immunol.* 2011, **4**:598–602.

Kaetzel, C.S.: **Cooperativity among secretory IgA, the polymeric immunoglobulin receptor, and the gut microbiota promotes host-microbial mutualism.** *Immunol. Lett.* 2014, **162**:10–21.

Mostov, K.E.: **Transepithelial transport of immunoglobulins.** *Annu. Rev. Immunol.* 1994, **12**:63–84.

Stadtmueller, B.M., Yang, Z., Huey-Tubman, K.E., Roberts-Mataric, H., Hubbell, W.L., and Bjorkman, P.J.: Biophysical and biochemical characterization of avian secretory component provides structural insights into the evolution of the polymeric Ig receptor. *J. Immunol.* 2016, **197**:1408–1414.

Turula, H., and Wobus, C.E.: The role of the polymeric immunoglobulin receptor and secretory immunoglobulins during mucosal infection and immunity. *Viruses* 2018, **10**:237–252.

10-17   The neonatal Fc receptor carries IgG across the placenta and prevents IgG excretion from the body.

Akilesh, S., Huber, T.B., Wu, H., Wang, G., Hartleben, B., Kopp, J.B., Miner, J.H., Roopenian, D.C., Unanue, E.R., and Shaw, A.S.: Podocytes use FcRn to clear IgG from the glomerular basement membrane. *Proc. Natl. Acad. Sci. USA* 2008, **105**:967–972.

Burmeister, W.P., Gastinel, L.N., Simister, N.E., Blum, M.L., and Bjorkman, P.J.: Crystal structure at 2.2 Å resolution of the MHC-related neonatal Fc receptor. *Nature* 1994, **372**:336–343.

Roopenian, D.C., and Akilesh, S.: FcRn: the neonatal Fc receptor comes of age. *Nat. Rev. Immunol.* 2007, **7**:715–725.

Wilcox, C.R., Holder, B., and Jones, C.E.: Factors affecting the FcRn-mediated transplacental transfer of antibodies and implications for vaccination in pregnancy. *Front. Immunol.* 2017, **8**:1294.

10-18   High-affinity IgG and IgA antibodies can neutralize toxins and block the infectivity of viruses and bacteria.

Brandtzaeg, P.: Role of secretory antibodies in the defence against infections. *Int. J. Med. Microbiol.* 2003, **293**:3–15.

Caskey, M., Klein, F., and Nussenzweig, M.C.: Broadly neutralizing anti-HIV-1 monoclonal antibodies in the clinic. *Nat. Med.* 2019, **25**:547–553.

Haghi, F., Peerayeh, S.N., Siadat, S.D., and Zeighami, H.: Recombinant outer membrane secretin PilQ(406-770) as a vaccine candidate for serogroup B *Neisseria meningitidis*. *Vaccine* 2012, **30**:1710–1714.

Kaufmann, B., Chipman, P.R., Holdaway, H.A., Johnson, S., Fremont, D.H., Kuhn, R.J., Diamond, M.S., and Rossmann, M.G.: Capturing a flavivirus pre-fusion intermediate. *PLoS Pathog.* 2009, **5**:e1000672.

Nybakken, G.E., Oliphant, T., Johnson, S., Burke, S., Diamond, M.S., and Fremont, D.H.: Structural basis of West Nile virus neutralization by a therapeutic antibody. *Nature* 2005, **437**:764–769.

Sougioultzis, S., Kyne, L., Drudy, D., Keates, S., Maroo, S., Pothoulakis, C., Giannasca, P.J., Lee, C.K., Warny, M., Monath, T.P., *et al.*: *Clostridium difficile* toxoid vaccine in recurrent C. difficile-associated diarrhea. *Gastroenterology* 2005, **128**:764–770.

10-19   Antigen:antibody complexes activate the classical pathway of complement by binding to C1q.

Cooper, N.R.: The classical complement pathway. Activation and regulation of the first complement component. *Adv. Immunol.* 1985, **37**:151–216.

Sörman, A., Zhang, L., Ding, Z., and Heyman, B.: How antibodies use complement to regulate antibody responses. *Mol. Immunol.* 2014, **61**:79–88.

Thielens, N.M., Tedesco, F., Bohlson, S.S., Gaboriaud, C., and Tenner, A.J.: C1q: A fresh look upon an old molecule. *Mol. Immunol.* 2017, **89**:73–83.

10-20   Complement receptors and Fc receptors both contribute to removal of immune complexes from the circulation.

Dong, C., Ptacek, T.S., Redden, D.T., Zhang, K., Brown, E.E., Edberg, J.C., McGwin, G., Jr., Alarcón, G.S., Ramsey-Goldman, R., Reveille, J.D., *et al.*: Fcγ receptor IIIa single-nucleotide polymorphisms and haplotypes affect human IgG binding and are associated with lupus nephritis in African Americans. *Arthritis Rheumatol.* 2014, **66**:1291–1299.

Leffler, J., Bengtsson, A.A., and Blom, A.M.: The complement system in systemic lupus erythematosus: an update. *Ann. Rheum. Dis.* 2014, **73**:1601–1606.

Lieberman, L.A., Mizui, M., Nalbandian, A., Bossé, R., Crispín, J.C., and Tsokos, G.C.: Complement receptor of the immunoglobulin superfamily reduces murine lupus nephritis and cutaneous disease. *Clin. Immunol.* 2015, **160**:286–291.

Nash, J.T., Taylor, P.R., Botto, M., Norsworthy, P.J., Davies, K.A., and Walport, M.J.: Immune complex processing in C1q-deficient mice. *Clin. Exp. Immunol.* 2001, **123**:196–202.

Walport, M.J., Davies, K.A., and Botto, M.: C1q and systemic lupus erythematosus. *Immunobiology* 1998, **199**:265–285.

10-21   The Fc receptors of accessory cells are signaling receptors specific for immunoglobulins of different classes.

Li, T., DiLillo, D.J., Bournazos, S., Giddens, J.P., Ravetch, J.V., and Wang, L.X.: Modulating IgG effector function by Fc glycan engineering. *Proc. Natl. Acad. Sci. USA.* 2017, **114**:3485–3490.

Mallery, D.L., McEwan, W.A., Bidgood, S.R., Towers, G.J., Johnson, C.M., and James, L.C.: Antibodies mediate intracellular immunity through tripartite motif-containing 21 (TRIM21). *Proc. Natl. Acad. Sci. USA* 2010, **107**:19985–19990.

Pincetic, A., Bournazos, S., DiLillo, D.J., Maamary, J., Wang, T.T., Dahan, R., Fiebiger, B.M., and Ravetch, J.V.: Type I and type II Fc receptors regulate innate and adaptive immunity. *Nat. Immunol.* 2014, **15**:707–716.

Shibuya, A., Sakamoto, N., Shimizu, Y., Shibuya, K., Osawa, M., Hiroyama, T., Eyre, H.J., Sutherland, G.R., Endo, Y., Fujita, T., *et al.*: Fcα/μ receptor mediates endocytosis of IgM-coated microbes. *Nat. Immunol.* 2000, **1**:441–446.

Stefanescu, R.N., Olferiev M., Liu, Y., and Pricop, L.: Inhibitory Fc gamma receptors: from gene to disease. *J. Clin. Immunol.* 2004, **24**:315–326.

10-22   Fc receptors on phagocytes are activated by antibodies bound to the surface of pathogens and enable the phagocytes to ingest and destroy pathogens.

Dierks, S.E., Bartlett, W.C., Edmeades, R.L., Gould, H.J., Rao, M., and Conrad, D.H.: The oligomeric nature of the murine Fc epsilon RII/CD23. Implications for function. *J. Immunol.* 1993, **150**:2372–2382.

Hogan, S.P., Rosenberg, H.F., Moqbel, R., Phipps, S., Foster, P.S., Lacy, P., Kay, A.B., and Rothenberg, M.E.: Eosinophils: biological properties and role in health and disease. *Clin. Exp. Allergy* 2008, **38**:709–750.

Karakawa, W.W., Sutton, A., Schneerson, R., Karpas, A., and Vann, W.F.: Capsular antibodies induce type-specific phagocytosis of capsulated *Staphylococcus aureus* by human polymorphonuclear leukocytes. *Infect. Immun.* 1986, **56**:1090–1095.

Mukai, K., Tsaim, M., Starklm, P., Marichalm, T., and Galli, S.J.: IgE and mast cells in host defense against parasites and venoms. *Semin. Immunopathol.* 2016, **38**:581–603.

10-23   Fc receptors activate NK cells to destroy antibody-coated targets.

Chung, A.W., Rollman, E., Center, R.J., Kent, S.J., and Stratov, I.: Rapid degranulation of NK cells following activation by HIV-specific antibodies. *J. Immunol.* 2009, **182**:1202–1210.

Ochoa, M.C., Minute, L., Rodriguez, I., Garasa, S., Perez-Ruiz, E., Inogés, S., Melero, I., and Berraondo, P.: Antibody-dependent cell cytotoxicity: immunotherapy strategies enhancing effector NK cells. *Immunol. Cell Biol.* 2017, **95**:347–355.

Sulica, A., Morel, P., Metes, D., and Herberman, R.B.: Ig-binding receptors on human NK cells as effector and regulatory surface molecules. *Int. Rev. Immunol.* 2001, **20**:371–414.

Takai, T.: Multiple loss of effector cell functions in FcRγ-deficient mice. *Int. Rev. Immunol.* 1996, **13**:369–381.

Wang, W., Erbe, A.K., Hank, J.A., Morris, Z.S., and Sondel, P.M.: NK cell-mediated antibody-dependent cellular cytotoxicity in cancer immunotherapy. *Front. Immunol.* 2015, **6**:368.

10-24 Mast cells and basophils bind IgE antibody via the high-affinity Fcε receptor.

Beaven, M.A., and Metzger, H.: Signal transduction by Fc receptors: the FcεRI case. *Immunol. Today* 1993, **14**:222–226.

Galli, S.J., Starkl, P., Marichal, T., and Tsai, M.: Mast cells and IgE in defense against venoms: possible "good side" of allergy? *Allergo J. Int.* 2016, **65**:3–15.

Kalesnikoff, J., Huber, M., Lam, V., Damen, J.E., Zhang, J., Siraganian, R.P., and Krystal, G.: Monomeric IgE stimulates signaling pathways in mast cells that lead to cytokine production and cell survival. *Immunity* 2001, **14**:801–811.

10-25 IgE-mediated activation of accessory cells has an important role in resistance to parasite infection.

Capron, A., Riveau, G., Capron, M., and Trottein, F.: Schistosomes: the road from host-parasite interactions to vaccines in clinical trials. *Trends Parasitol.* 2005, **21**:143–149.

Grencis, R.K.: Th2-mediated host protective immunity to intestinal nematode infections. *Philos. Trans. R. Soc. Lond. B Biol. Sci.* 1997, **352**:1377–1384.

Grencis, R.K., Else, K.J., Huntley, J.F., and Nishikawa, S.I.: The in vivo role of stem cell factor (c-kit ligand) on mastocytosis and host protective immunity to the intestinal nematode *Trichinella spiralis in mice. Parasite Immunol.* 1993, **15**:55–59.

Kasugai, T., Tei, H., Okada, M., Hirota, S., Morimoto, M., Yamada, M., Nakama, A., Arizono, N., and Kitamura, Y.: Infection with *Nippostrongylus brasiliensis* induces invasion of mast cell precursors from peripheral blood to small intestine. *Blood* 1995, **85**:1334–1340.

Ushio, H., Watanabe, N., Kiso, Y., Higuchi, S., and Matsuda, H.: Protective immunity and mast cell and eosinophil responses in mice infested with larval *Haemaphysalis longicornis* ticks. *Parasite Immunol.* 1993, **15**:209–214.

Integrated Dynamics of Innate and Adaptive Immunity

11

Throughout this book we have examined the separate ways in which the innate and the adaptive immune responses protect against invading pathogens. In this chapter, we consider how the cells and molecules of the immune system work as an integrated defense system to eliminate or control different types of infectious agents, and also how the adaptive immune system provides long-lasting protective immunity. In Chapters 2 and 3, we saw how innate immunity is brought into play in the earliest phases of an infection and is probably sufficient to prevent colonization of the body by most microorganisms encountered in the environment. We also introduced **innate lymphoid cells (ILCs)**, which, although lacking antigen-specific receptors, have many of the same functional features as effector CD4 T-cell subsets and cytotoxic CD8 T cells and act early during infection to generate distinct types of immune responses to different types of pathogens. Although present in many tissues, ILCs are most abundant in barrier tissues, such as the intestinal and respiratory mucosae, which they populate in the perinatal period and where they reside throughout life, poised to respond rapidly to pathogens to impair or eliminate their spread at these major sites of entry.

However, most pathogens have developed strategies to evade innate immune defenses and establish a focus of infection. In these circumstances, the innate immune response sets the stage for the induction of an adaptive immune response, which is orchestrated by signals that emanate from innate immune sensor cells, such as conventional dendritic cells (cDCs), and is coordinated with innate immune effector cells to bring about pathogen clearance. In the **primary immune response**, which occurs against a pathogen encountered for the first time, tissue-resident ILCs respond rapidly to cytokines that are released by innate immune sensor cells at the site of infection to bias the recruitment of circulating innate immune effector cells toward those most appropriate for limiting pathogen growth and dissemination over the first few hours to days of invasion. Concurrent with this response, clonal expansion and differentiation of naive lymphocytes into effector T cells and antibody-secreting B cells is initiated in secondary lymphoid organs. However, the adaptive response requires several days to weeks to fully mature, largely due to the rarity of antigen-specific precursor cells that must increase their numbers and functionality over the early course of infection. After their clonal expansion and initial differentiation in the secondary lymphoid tissues, effector T cells migrate to sites of infection where, along with pathogen-specific antibodies, they enhance the recruitment and functions of innate immune effector cells and, in most cases, effectively target the pathogen for elimination (**Fig. 11.1**).

During this period, specific **immunological memory** is also established by adaptive immune cells. This ensures a rapid reinduction of antigen-specific antibody and effector T cells on encounter with the same pathogen during a **secondary (or recall) immune response**, thus providing long-lasting and often lifelong protection against the pathogen. Immunological memory is discussed in the last part of this chapter. Memory responses differ in several ways from primary responses. We discuss the reasons for this, and what is known about how immunological memory is maintained.

Fig. 11.1 The course of a typical acute infection that is cleared by an adaptive immune response. 1. The infectious agent colonizes, and its numbers increase as it replicates. The innate immune response is initiated immediately after detection of the pathogen. 2. When antigens from the pathogen are presented by dendritic cells to lymphocytes, the adaptive immune response is initiated; the pathogen continues to grow, restrained by responses of the innate immune system. At this stage, immunological memory also starts to be induced. 3. After 4–7 days, effector cells and molecules of the adaptive immune response begin to contribute to the host response and act to clear the infection. 4. When the infection has been cleared and antigen becomes undetectable, the immune response ceases, but persistent antibody and memory T and B cells provide lasting protection against reinfection in most cases.

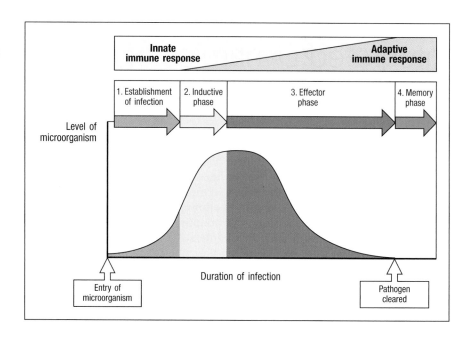

Integration of innate and adaptive immunity in response to specific types of pathogens.

The immune response is dynamic, and both its nature and intensity change over time. It begins with the antigen-independent responses of innate immunity and becomes both more focused on the pathogen and more potent as the antigen-specific adaptive immune response matures. The character of the response differs contingent on the type of pathogen encountered. Different types of pathogens (intracellular and extracellular bacteria, viruses, helminth parasites, and fungi) elicit different types of immune response (types 1, 2, 3, or cytotoxic), so that the most appropriate immune response is induced for effective elimination of the pathogen. The innate immune system not only participates in the initiation of adaptive T and B cell responses but also provides effector cells from the blood (for example, monocytes, eosinophils, and neutrophils) and reinforces pathways of the different types of immunity throughout infection. Early in the response, different subsets of innate lymphoid cells—already resident in tissues since fetal development—are activated by cytokines produced by innate sensor cells. This early activation of ILCs acts to constrain pathogen entry at the initial site of infection and prevent dissemination while the adaptive response develops. However, the more sensitive and specific actions of effector T cells and class-switched, affinity-matured antibodies are often required for the complete elimination of infection, known as **sterilizing immunity**. In this part of the chapter, we provide an overview of how the different phases of an immune response are orchestrated in space and time and then discuss how distinct cytokines from innate sensor cells activate different innate lymphoid cell subsets to restrain pathogen invasion and direct pathogen-specific defenses while the adaptive response is developing.

11-1 The course of an infection can be divided into several distinct phases.

Although some pathogen-associated molecular patterns (PAMPs) of different types of pathogens are shared, others are not. These differences contribute to the induction of four distinct patterns, or 'modules,' of innate and adaptive immunity, which can be broadly grouped into two subsets, cytotoxic or helper responses, with the latter comprising types 1, 2, and 3, as will be discussed in the next section. Irrespective of the inciting pathogen and the pattern of immune response it provokes, however, the tempo of the host response is similar and can be broken down into various stages (see Fig. 11.1, and see Fig. 3.37).

In the first stage of infection, a new host is exposed to infectious agents either shed by an infected individual or present in the environment. The numbers, route of transmission, mode of transmission, and stability of an infectious agent outside the host determine its infectivity. The first contact with a new host occurs through an epithelial surface, such as the skin or the mucosal surfaces of the respiratory, gastrointestinal, or urogenital tracts. After making contact, an infectious agent must establish a focus of infection. It must either adhere to the epithelial surface and colonize it or penetrate it to replicate in the tissues (**Fig. 11.2**). Bites by arthropods (insects and ticks) and wounds breach the epidermal barrier and help some microorganisms gain entry through the skin.

Only when a microorganism has successfully established a focus of infection in the host does disease occur (see Fig. 11.2). With few exceptions, little damage will be caused unless the pathogen spreads from the original focus or secretes toxins that spread to other parts of the body. Extracellular pathogens spread by direct extension of the infection through the lymphatics or the bloodstream. Although some pathogens have evolved mechanisms to use blood cells to ferry them to other organs, spread into the bloodstream usually occurs only after the lymphatic system has been overwhelmed. Obligate intracellular pathogens spread from cell to cell; they do so either by direct transmission from one cell to the next or by release into the extracellular fluid and reinfection of both adjacent and distant cells. Facultative intracellular pathogens can do the same

ANIMATION 11.1

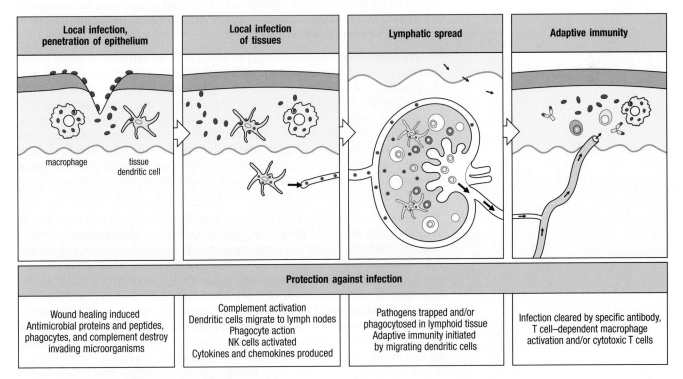

Fig. 11.2 Infections and the responses to them can be divided into a series of stages. These stages are illustrated for a pathogenic microorganism (red) entering across a wound in an epithelium. The microorganism first adheres to epithelial cells and then invades beyond the epithelium into underlying tissues (first panel). A local innate immune response helps to contain the infection and delivers antigen and antigen-loaded dendritic cells to lymphatics (second panel) and then to local lymph nodes (third panel). This leads to an adaptive immune response in the lymph node that involves the activation and differentiation of T cells and B cells with the eventual production of effector T cells and antibody, which coordinate with innate immune cells to clear the infection (fourth panel).

after a period of survival in the extracellular environment. In contrast, some of the bacteria that cause gastroenteritis exert their effects without spreading into the tissues. They establish a site of infection on the luminal surface of the epithelium lining the gut and cause pathology by damaging the epithelium or by secreting toxins that cause damage either *in situ* or after crossing the epithelial barrier and entering the circulation.

The establishment of a focus of infection in tissues and the response of the innate immune system produces changes in the immediate environment. Many microorganisms are repelled or kept in check at this stage by innate defenses, which are triggered by stimulation of the various germline-encoded pattern-recognition receptors expressed by innate sensor cells—such as epithelial cells, tissue-resident mast cells, macrophages, and dendritic cells (see Chapters 2 and 3). Cytokines and chemokines produced by pathogen-activated innate sensor cells initiate local inflammation and activate ILCs. These responses are activated within minutes to hours and are sustained for at least several days. The inflammatory response is induced through activation of the endothelium of local postcapillary venules to express selectins, integrin ligands, and chemokines recognized by circulating granulocytes and monocytes (**myelomonocytic cells**; see Fig. 3.30). This leads to the recruitment of these circulating innate effector cells, particularly neutrophils and monocytes, thereby increasing the numbers of phagocytes available for microbe clearance. As monocytes enter tissue and become activated, additional inflammatory cells are attracted into the infected tissue so that the inflammatory response is maintained and reinforced. Leakiness of the inflamed endothelium also leads to the influx of serum proteins, including complement, activation of which in a primary infection occurs mainly via the alternative and lectin pathways (see Fig. 2.15). This results in the production of the anaphylatoxins C3a and C5a, which further activate the vascular endothelium, and C3b, which opsonizes microbes for more effective clearance by recruited phagocytes. Some aspects of this early phase of the inflammatory response are nonspecific for the type of pathogen, whereas others are not.

Concordant with the production of pro-inflammatory cytokines such as TNF-α and IL-1β, which activate nonspecific inflammation, innate sensor cells produce additional cytokines that differentially activate specific subsets of ILCs within the first hours of an infection. This is due to the expression of unique PAMPs—or unique combinations of PAMPs—by different types of pathogens, which elicit different patterns of cytokines from innate sensor cells. This has important consequences in directing the type of immune response that will be mounted against the pathogen, as subsets of ILCs are differentially activated to produce their own effector cytokines and chemokines contingent on the pattern of cytokines produced by innate sensor cells (**Fig. 11.3**).

The products of activated ILCs clearly amplify and coordinate local innate responses that are better tailored to resist specific types of pathogens, and they also alter the recruitment and maturation of different myelomonocytic (granulocyte–monocyte) innate effector cells at the site of infection. It is less clear whether cytokines produced by ILCs may also guide the development of naive T cells into distinct effector subsets (for example, T_H1, T_H2, or T_H17 cells)—either directly, by acting on activated naive T cells themselves, or indirectly, by modulating the activation of conventional dendritic cells (cDCs) that migrate to regional lymphoid tissues to prime naive T cells. The lack of experimental approaches to specifically deplete ILC subsets without similarly depleting corresponding T-cell subsets with which they share specific cytokines and transcription factors has made it difficult to assess the role of ILCs in guiding the development of effector T cells. However, although ILCs are found in secondary lymphoid organs in small numbers, they are highly abundant in barrier tissues, and it seems likely that if ILCs do play a role in effector T-cell lineage specification, it may be via effects of their cytokines on modulating activation

Cytotoxic ILC	Group 1 ILCs	Group 2 ILCs	Group 3 ILCs
			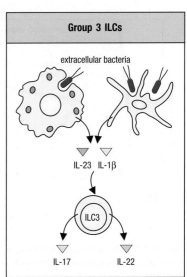

Fig. 11.3 Cytokines produced by innate sensor cells activate innate lymphoid cells (ILCs). The microbial-associated molecular patterns (MAMPs) expressed by different types of pathogens stimulate distinct cytokine responses from innate sensor cells, such as dendritic cells, macrophages, or epithelial cells—including specialized tuft cells present in mucosae that sense small molecules produced by helminths. These cells, in turn, stimulate different subsets of ILCs to produce different effector cytokines that act to coordinate and amplify the innate response.

of migratory cDCs. In any case, ILCs perform an important function during the first few days of an emerging immune response to coordinate the type of innate defense that is most effective at restraining pathogen growth while buying time for the adaptive response to occur.

Adaptive immunity is triggered when an infection eludes or overwhelms innate defenses (see Fig. 11.1). Adaptive immune responses are initiated in the local lymphoid tissue in response to antigens presented by dendritic cells activated during the course of the innate immune response (see Fig. 11.2, second and third panels). Antigen-specific effector T cells and antibody-secreting B cells are generated by clonal expansion and differentiation over several days, as innate responses orchestrated by ILCs 'buy time' for the adaptive response to mature. Within several days of infection, antigen-specific T cells and then antibodies are released into the blood and from there can enter the site of infection (see Fig. 11.2, fourth panel). Adaptive responses amplify innate defenses and confer antigen-specific targeting by innate effector mechanisms that can eliminate pathogens more precisely. For example, antibodies can activate complement to directly kill pathogens, can opsonize pathogens for enhanced phagocytosis, and can arm Fc-bearing innate effector cells for release of microbicidal factors or recruit the cytocidal actions of natural killer (NK) cells, an action called antibody-dependent cell-mediated cytotoxicity (ADCC). Effector CD8 T cells can directly kill antigen-bearing target cells via similar cytocidal cytotoxic actions, and effector CD4 T cells can directly release cytokines onto macrophages to enhance their microbicidal actions.

Resolution of the infection typically involves complete clearance of the pathogen—and thus the source of antigens—over the course of days to weeks, following which most effector lymphocytes die—a stage known as **clonal contraction** (see Section 9-9 and Section 11-16). What remains are long-lived antibody-producing plasma cells that sustain circulating antibodies for months to years and residual memory B and T cells that may also persist for years or even a lifetime, poised for an accelerated adaptive response in the event of future encounters with the same pathogen. Thus, in addition to clearing the infectious agent, an effective adaptive immune response prevents reinfection. For some infectious agents, this protection is essentially absolute, whereas for others infection is only reduced or attenuated on reexposure to the pathogen.

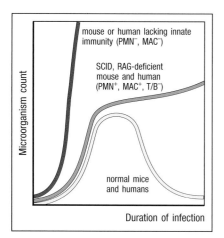

Fig. 11.4 The time course of infection in normal and immunodeficient mice and humans. The red curve shows the rapid growth of microorganisms in the absence of innate immunity, when macrophages (MAC) and polymorphonuclear leukocytes (PMN) are lacking. The green curve shows the course of infection in mice and humans that have innate immunity but have no T or B lymphocytes and so lack adaptive immunity. The yellow curve shows the normal course of an infection in immunocompetent mice and humans.

Acquired
Immune Deficiency
Syndrome (AIDS)

It is not known how many infections are dealt with solely by the nonadaptive mechanisms of innate immunity, because such infections are eliminated early and produce little in the way of symptoms or pathology. Innate immunity does, however, seem to be essential for effective host defense, as shown by the progression of infection in mice that lack components of innate immunity despite having an intact adaptive immune system; adaptive immunity is dependent on innate immunity (**Fig. 11.4**). Conversely, many infections can be curbed—but typically not cleared—in the absence of adaptive immunity. Thus, the two arms of immunity are typically interlinked and often interdependent.

Little or no residual pathology follows an effective primary adaptive immune response to many types of infection. In some cases, however, the infection itself, or the response it induces, causes significant tissue damage. In yet other cases, such as infection with cytomegalovirus or *Mycobacterium tuberculosis*, the pathogen is contained but not eliminated and can persist in a latent form. If the adaptive immune response is later weakened, as it is in acquired immune deficiency syndrome (AIDS) or in medical interventions that impair immunity (for example, organ transplantation or treatment with certain biologic agents, such as anti-TNFs), these pathogens may resurface to cause virulent systemic infections. We will focus on the strategies used by certain pathogens to evade or subvert adaptive immunity, and thereby establish a persistent, or chronic, infection, in Chapter 13.

11-2 The effector mechanisms that are recruited to clear an infection can be organized into immune modules.

Most infections ultimately engage both T cell– and B cell–mediated adaptive immunity, and in many cases, both are helpful in clearing or containing the pathogen and setting up protective immunity. However, the relative importance of the different effector mechanisms, and the classes of antibody induced, vary with different pathogens. Different types of immune responses are coordinated through activation of distinct **immune effector modules** (see Section 1-19). In each type of immune response, a specific collection of innate and adaptive mechanisms acts together to eliminate a specific type of pathogen.

Broadly speaking, there are two major subsets of immune modules—cytotoxic and helper—that are generally aligned around the eradication of intracellular pathogens that do not require phagocytes for their elimination (for example, viruses) versus the eradication of extracellular pathogens (for example, bacteria, fungi, helminths) and those intracellular pathogens that require phagocytes for their elimination (for example, intracellular bacteria and some single-cell parasites, or protozoa), respectively. Cells in the cytotoxic module (for example, NK cells and CTLs) can kill infected targets directly, whereas cells in each of the helper modules (types 1–3) act indirectly to coordinate with subsets of circulating or tissue-resident myelomonocytic cells whose microbicidal functions they recruit and/or enhance (**Fig. 11.5**). Circulating myelomonocytic cells include, in order of their decreasing abundance in circulating blood, neutrophils, monocytes (which enter inflamed tissues and differentiate into macrophages), eosinophils, and basophils. Tissue-resident mast cells, which share many functions with basophils, are also included, as mast-cell precursors can be recruited to some tissues, such as intestine, during certain types of infections. To date, ILCs that correspond with additional T-cell subsets, such as T_{FH} and T_{reg} cells, have not been definitively identified, although this is an area of active study. The absence of ILC homologs of T_{FH} and T_{reg} cells may reflect the primary role of these T-cell subsets in influencing the development and function of other adaptive immune cells rather than innate immune cells. Of course, there are exceptions to this classification, and some pathogens recruit more than one module (for example, cytotoxic and type 1 responses are often

Fig. 11.5 Integration of ILCs, T-cell subsets, and innate effector cells into immune effector modules. The major inductive and effector cytokines and transcription factors (for example, EOMES, Tbet, GATA3, RORγt, and AHR) that are associated with each effector module are shown. See text for details. Although the developmental origins of ILCs are still under investigation, it appears that all ILCs are derived from a common ILC precursor (CILCP) that develops from the common lymphoid precursor (CLP) that also gives rise to the B- and T-cell lineages in the bone marrow (not shown). CILCPs diverge into either an NK-cell precursor (NKP) or a common helper-like ILC precursor (CHILP), which gives rise to ILC1, ILC2, and ILC3. This is analogous to the divergence of the CD4 and CD8 lineages from double-positive (DP) precursors in the thymus.

recruited together, and type 3 responses can transition to type 1 responses), but as a conceptual framework this is a useful system for understanding the integration of innate immunity and adaptive immunity.

Whereas natural killer (NK) cells and cytotoxic T lymphocytes (CTLs) evolved to eradicate their target pathogens primarily via cell-mediated cytotoxicity (see Section 3-24 and Section 9-21), the three interlinked helper ILC and CD4 T-cell modules (ILC1/ILC2/ILC3 and $T_H1/T_H2/T_H17$, respectively) appear to have evolved to enhance and coordinate the functions of, and integrate adaptive immunity with, different arms of the myelomonocytic pathway for optimal eradication of their target pathogens: monocyte/macrophages are enhanced by **ILC1** cells and T_H1 cells; eosinophils, basophils, and mast cells by **ILC2** cells and T_H2 cells; and neutrophils by **ILC3** cells and T_H17 cells. The cytokines produced by each of these ILC and helper T-cell subsets also has important local actions on epithelial cells in the tissues in which they are resident or to which they are recruited. Each of the four major types of immune responses are controlled by and integrated through cytokine and chemokine networks, as discussed later.

Cytotoxic responses are characterized by the actions of NK cells and CTLs, which are specialized for killing host cells infected by intracellular pathogens, stressed or damaged host cells, and tumor cells. NK cells can also be armed by IgG antibodies for ADCC, and both NK cells and CTLs produce IFN-γ, which activates macrophages. **Type 1** responses are characterized by the actions of group 1 ILCs (ILC1), T_H1 cells, opsonizing IgG antibody isotypes (for example, IgG1 and IgG2 in mice), and macrophages in response to intracellular pathogens, including intracellular bacteria, viruses, and parasites (see Fig. 11.5). **Type 2** responses are characterized by the actions of group 2 ILCs (ILC2), T_H2 cells, IgE, and the innate effector cells eosinophils, basophils, and tissue mast cells, which are armed for function by IgE bound to surface Fcε receptors. Type 2 responses are primarily induced by, and target, multicellular parasites, or helminths, although some parasitic protozoans also provoke type 2 immunity. **Type 3** responses are characterized by the actions of group 3 ILCs (ILC3), T_H17 cells, opsonizing IgG isotypes, and neutrophils in response to extracellular bacteria and fungi. It is the activation of NK cells and different subsets of ILCs that coordinates the local innate response at the site of pathogen entry prior to the development and recruitment of polarized CTL, T_H1, T_H2, or T_H17 antigen-specific responses induced by type 1 or type 2 conventional dendritic cells (cDC1 or cDC2 cells) in secondary lymphoid tissues. Unlike the effector CD4 T cells with which they share overlapping functional features, ILCs do not require antigenic priming and differentiation in order to acquire their effector functions. Instead, they seed barrier tissues prior to birth and, in mice, expand in number and acquire their full functionality prior to weaning and stably populate their tissue of residence throughout life. Thus, ILCs are able to respond rapidly to amplify the activities of other resident and recruited innate effector cells. However, with few exceptions, ILCs are largely nonmotile; they are bound geographically within barrier tissues and, unlike T cells, must often engage the innate effector cells whose functions they enhance at a distance via the secreted factors they produce. In the next section, we will consider in more detail the induction and actions of ILC subsets, as these responses precede and are integrated with adaptive T- and B-cell responses.

11-3 Subsets of ILCs are early responders of the immune response.

As discussed in Chapter 3, NK cells and ILC1 cells are characterized by their production of IFN-γ in response to IL-12 and IL-18 produced by pathogen-activated dendritic cells and macrophages. However, NK cells differ from ILC1 cells in their developmental origins and in their expression of cytotoxic granules containing perforin and granzymes, analogous to those expressed by CTLs (see Fig. 11.5). Moreover, unlike ILC1 cells, which are abundant in barrier tissues but rare in blood and spleen, NK cells circulate in blood and constitute a substantial fraction of mononuclear cells in the spleen. NK cells are therefore mobile, whereas ILC1 cells are largely stationary in the tissue sites they populate around birth.

The rapid induction of the cytolytic activity of NK cells through the recognition of surface molecules expressed on the target cells by a range of inhibitory and activating receptors (see Section 3-25) enables NK-cell killing of a range of pathogen-infected cells—in advance of the antigen-driven development and deployment of cytolytic CD8 T cells. When armed by IgG bound to their Fc receptors, NK cells can kill targets in an antigen-specific mode despite their lack of expression of antigenic receptors like those expressed by B and T cells. Finally, NK cells play a unique role in the killing of host cells that have lost expression of MHC class I molecules because of down-regulation by certain viruses; this killing activity occurs via release of activation restraints on the NK cell by inhibitory receptors that recognize MHC class I (see Section 3-25).

In contrast to NK cells, ILC1 cells most closely mirror T_H1 cells. Like T_H1 cells, they lack the cytolytic granules that are characteristic of NK cells and CTLs and appear to participate in the clearance of intracellular pathogens primarily through their activation of infected macrophages by the release of IFN-γ. Thus, through production of IL-12 and IL-18, macrophages and dendritic cells can rapidly induce ILC1 production of IFN-γ, which acts back on macrophages to induce the heightened killing of intracellular pathogens in barrier tissues such as the gastrointestinal (GI) and respiratory tracts several days prior to the development and deployment of T_H1 cells.

ILC2 cells that reside in mucosal tissues are preferentially activated by the cytokines **thymic stromal lymphopoietin (TSLP)**—a STAT5-activating cytokine—and IL-33 and IL-25, all of which are produced in response to helminths. Activation of at least some ILC2 cells, including those in the respiratory tract, is also dependent on **leukotrienes**, which are short-lived, lipid signaling molecules derived from arachidonic acid (eicosanoids). Although details of the contributions of each of these inputs is not completely understood, activation of ILC2 cells appears to differ in different tissues. TSLP and IL-33 are produced by epithelial cells, stromal cells, and macrophages that sense molecular patterns common to helminths, such as chitin, a polysaccharide polymer of β-(1,4)-N-acetylglucosamine that is a widespread constituent of helminths and the exoskeletons of insects and of some fungi. IL-33 is an alarmin that is released by cell death, suggesting that an important inducer of the ILC2 response is tissue injury. The principal source of IL-25 is a specialized secretory epithelial cell found in mucosal tissues—the **tuft cell**—which is specialized for chemosensing of molecules produced by type 2 pathogens, including the metabolite **succinate**, as well as a range of tastants and odorants, via G protein–coupled succinate and taste receptors, respectively (see Fig. 11.3; detailed further in Chapter 12). Tuft cells can also produce TSLP and eicosanoids. Activated ILC2 cells rapidly produce large amounts of IL-13 and IL-5; IL-13 stimulates mucus production by goblet cells in the epithelium and mucosal smooth muscle contractions that facilitate worm expulsion—the so-called 'weep-and-sweep' response. IL-13 also stimulates increased differentiation of goblet cells and tuft cells, providing a feed-forward mechanism for amplifying type 2 responses (see Chapter 12). IL-5 stimulates the production and activation of eosinophils that can kill worms. Unlike T_H2 cells, with which they share many functional features, ILC2 cells appear to produce little or no IL-4 in mice, suggesting that expression of IL-4 may impart unique functions to T_H2 cells in inflamed tissues. However, eosinophils and basophils that are recruited by chemokines produced by ILC2 cells are activated to produce IL-4 in response to the IL-5 and IL-13 produced by ILC2 cells, possibly providing an indirect mechanism by which T_H2 differentiation is directed by ILC2 cells. Moreover, IL-13 produced by ILC2 cells appears to regulate the activation and migration to regional lymphoid tissues of dendritic cells that promote T_H2 differentiation, although it is unclear whether these dendritic cells can also produce IL-4.

ILC3 cells play a critical early role in defense against extracellular bacteria and fungi at barrier tissues. Similar to T_H17 cells, ILC3 cells are responsive to IL-23 and IL-1β; these cytokines elicit the production of IL-17 and IL-22, which promote early type 3 responses. IL-17 is a pro-inflammatory cytokine that acts on a variety of cells, including stromal cells, epithelial cells, and myeloid cells, to stimulate the production of other pro-inflammatory cytokines (for example, IL-6, IL-1β), hematopoietic growth factors (G-CSF and GM-CSF), and chemokines that recruit neutrophils and monocytes. IL-17 and IL-22 act on epithelial cells in mucosal tissues and skin to induce their production of antimicrobial peptides (AMPs), and IL-22 promotes enhanced barrier integrity.

As with other ILCs, the cytokines produced by ILC3 cells act indirectly via IL-6 and IL-1β in a positive feedback loop to enhance type 3 responses by increasing local production of IL-23 and IL-1β. Through induction of elevated IL-6, IL-1β, and IL-23, ILC3 cells might also promote the differentiation of T_H17 cells in mucosal lymphoid tissues, although this is unproven.

In a further parallel with effector CD4 T cells, an important feature of helper ILCs is that they activate other innate immune cells to kill or expel microbes, but they do not do so themselves. Instead, myelomonocytic cells, and even cells of barrier epithelia, are the agents of ILCs and effector CD4 T cells; they are recruited and/or activated through the pro-inflammatory cytokines and chemokines that these lymphoid cells produce in response to infection or tissue injury. As we will discuss later, because of their ability to focus effector cytokines on antigen-bearing target cells and to induce B-cell maturation and the production of class-switched antibodies, effector CD4 T cells provide an additional layer of licensing of innate effector cells that increases their lethality and ability to achieve microbial clearance.

Summary.

Integration of the innate and adaptive immune responses is required for effective protection of the host against pathogenic microorganisms. The responses of the innate immune system act early to restrain pathogens during the time required for the adaptive immune response to fully develop. Different types of pathogens cause the activation of different patterns of cytokine production by innate sensor cells. This, in turn, promotes the activation of different patterns of innate lymphoid cells (ILCs), which act locally to enhance barrier defense and recruit innate effector cells to sites of infection in advance of the arrival of antigen-specific CD4 and CD8 T cells whose functions they mirror. Coordination of the induction of different immune modules that are composed of related subsets of ILCs, innate effector cells, effector CD4 T cells, and class-switched antibodies underlies the different types of immunity directed against different types of pathogens.

Effector CD4 T cells augment the effector functions of innate immune cells.

In Chapter 9 we described how dendritic cells loaded with their antigen cargo migrate from the infected tissue to enter T-cell zones of secondary lymphoid tissues, where they initiate the adaptive immune response. We also discussed how CD8 T cells are primed to become cytotoxic effectors that are specialized for killing infected target cells that express MHC class I molecules, enabling them to eradicate intracellular infections in any nucleated cell. We also saw how transcription factor networks activated by specific cytokines direct the differentiation of naive CD4 T cells into distinct classes of effector CD4 T cells—T_H1, T_H2, and T_H17 (see Fig. 9.33). In Chapters 9 and 10 we discussed the specialized role of T_{FH} cells, which engage antigen-bearing B cells to control antibody class-switching and B-cell maturation in germinal centers in the context of type 1, type 2, and type 3 responses.

We now turn our attention to the specialized roles of subsets of these effector CD4 T cells after their differentiation in, and emigration from, secondary lymphoid tissues to orchestrate the functions of innate immune cells at sites of infection.

As discussed in Chapter 9 and in the preceding sections of this chapter, the pattern of cytokines produced by cells of the innate immune response during the early course of infection is determined by how the pathogen influences the behavior of innate sensor cells that engage it. This has a major impact on how T cells differentiate during their initial contact with dendritic cells, thus determining the subsets of effector T cells that are generated. In turn, the recruitment of effector T cells to sites of infection sustains, amplifies, and enhances innate effector cell responses initiated by ILCs through effector mechanisms that require antigen-specific recognition, whether through cell–cell contact between CD4 or CD8 T cells and cell targets bearing their cognate antigens, or via pathogen-specific antibodies that T_FH cells help promote. In this part of the chapter, we will discuss how the differentiation of effector CD4 T cells alters their expression of surface receptors to program their egress from secondary lymphoid tissues and to sites of infection. We will then consider how T_H1, T_H2, and T_H17 cells interact with innate immune cells at sites of infection to bring about the clearance of the specific pathogens that elicit their development and recruitment. Finally, we will consider how the primary effector response is terminated as the pathogen is eliminated.

11-4 Effector T cells are guided to specific tissues and sites of infection by changes in their expression of adhesion molecules and chemokine receptors.

As discussed in Chapters 9 and 10, when naive T cells differentiate into effector T cells, changes occur in the expression of specific surface molecules that redirect their trafficking from T-cell zones into B-cell zones, in the case of T_FH cells, or from lymphoid to nonlymphoid tissues, in the case of other effector T cells. This includes changes in the expression of selectins and their ligands, integrins, and chemokine receptors. As we will see, some of these changes are generic; they are common to all CD4 and CD8 effector T cells. Others are tissue-specific, facilitating the recruitment of T cells back to the tissues in which they were primed. Yet others are T-cell subset-specific, particularly in the patterns of chemokine receptor expression, which direct T_FH cells to germinal centers, where they provide help to developing B cells, or direct T_H1, T_H2, and T_H17 cells to the same tissue sites as the myelomonocytic cells whose effector functions they will coordinate.

Activated naive CD4 T cells destined to become T_FH cells acquire expression of CXCR5 and lose expression of CCR7 and S1PR1 (see Section 9-15 and Section 10-3). Loss of CCR7 results in unresponsiveness to the T cell–zone chemokines CXCL21 and CXCL19, while sustained down-regulation of S1PR1 renders these cells insensitive to the S1P gradient that would otherwise guide their egress from the lymphoid tissue back to blood (see Section 9-5). The constitutive expression of CXCL13 by follicular dendritic cells establishes a gradient that acts via CXCR5 to attract developing T_FH cells from the T-cell zone, first to the border between the T-cell zone and a B-cell follicle where they can interact with B cells that present their cognate antigen and then into the B-cell follicle where they provide help to germinal center B cells. Unlike T_FH cells, other effector CD4 and CD8 T cells must leave the lymphoid tissue in which they have developed to interact with myeloid cells that present antigen at sites of infection in nonlymphoid tissues. As for T_FH cells, the exodus of these non-T_FH effector T cells from T-cell zones requires their loss of CCR7, but unlike T_FH cells, they reexpress S1PR1 as CD69 is down-regulated to direct them out of the lymphoid tissue and back into the blood (see Section 9-5).

Most non-T_FH effector cells also shed **L-selectin (CD62L)**, which mediates rolling on the high endothelial venules of secondary lymphoid tissues such as lymph nodes, in favor of **P-selectin glycoprotein ligand-1 (PSGL-1)**, a homodimeric sialoglycoprotein that is the major ligand for tethering and rolling on the P- and E-selectin expressed by endothelial cells activated by inflammatory cytokines (for example, TNF and IL-1) at sites of inflammation (**Fig. 11.6**). In

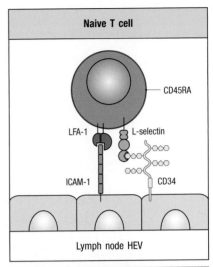

Naive T cell

CD45RA

LFA-1   L-selectin

ICAM-1   CD34

Lymph node HEV

Effector T cell

LFA-1   CD45RO

VLA-4   PSGL-1

ICAM-1   E-selectin

VCAM-1   P-selectin

Activated peripheral vascular endothelium

Fig. 11.6 Effector T cells change their surface molecules, allowing them to home to sites of infection. Naive T cells home to lymph nodes through the binding of L-selectin to sulfated carbohydrates displayed by various proteins, such as CD34 and GlyCAM-1 (not shown), on the high endothelial venule (HEV; upper panel). After encounter with antigen, many of the differentiated effector T cells lose expression of L-selectin, leave the lymph node about 4–5 days later, and now express the integrin VLA-4 and increased levels of LFA-1. These bind to VCAM-1 and ICAM-1, respectively, on peripheral vascular endothelium at sites of inflammation (lower panel). On differentiating into effector cells, T cells also alter their splicing of the mRNA encoding the cell-surface protein CD45, a receptor-type protein tyrosine phosphatase (PTP). The CD45RO isoform expressed by effector T cells lacks one or more exons that encode extracellular domains present in the CD45RA isoform expressed by naive T cells and appears to make effector T cells more sensitive to stimulation by specific antigen.

contrast to granulocytes and monocytes, which constitutively express glycosyltransferases necessary for biosynthesis of selectin ligands, T cells express these enzymes only after effector T-cell development. Effector differentiation induces expression of the glycosyltransferase **α-(1,3)-fucosyltransferase VII (FucT-VII)**, a key enzyme required for both P- and E-selectin ligand generation. Thus, although PSGL-1 is expressed by both naive and effector T cells, it is appropriately glycosylated for selectin binding only by effector T cells.

The expression of integrins that are important for the recruitment of effector T cells to inflamed tissues is also induced (see Fig. 11.6). Effector T cells retain expression of **LFA-1 ($\alpha_L\beta_2$)**, which is also expressed by naive T-cell precursors. However, they also synthesize the integrin $\alpha_4\beta_1$, or **VLA-4**, which binds to the adhesion molecule **VCAM-1**, a member of the immunoglobulin superfamily related to ICAM-1. When effector T cells are activated by chemokine signaling, VLA-4 is altered so that it can bind with high affinity to VCAM-1, similar to chemokine-induced binding of ICAM-1 by activated LFA-1 (see Section 3-18). Thus, chemokines activate VCAM-1 to bind VLA-4 on vascular endothelial cells near sites of inflammation, allowing extravasation of effector T cells. Although both VCAM-1 and ICAM-1 are expressed on activated endothelial-cell surfaces, there appears to be preferential utilization of the two adhesion pairs in some inflamed tissue vascular beds, with recruitment of effector T cells being more dependent on VLA-4 in some tissues, and more dependent on LFA-1 in others.

Expression of some adhesion molecules by effector T cells is programmed within the specific secondary lymphoid tissues in which they are primed such that they preferentially home back to the associated nonlymphoid tissues. Thus, the site of priming appears to imprint effector T cells with the ability to traffic to particular tissues. This is achieved by the expression of adhesion molecules that bind selectively to tissue-specific addressins. In this context, the adhesion molecules are often known as **homing receptors**. As an example, cDCs that prime T cells in the gut-associated lymphoid tissue (GALT) preferentially induce T-cell expression of the integrin $\alpha_4\beta_7$, which binds to the mucosal vascular addressin **MAdCAM-1** that is constitutively expressed by endothelial cells of high endothelial venules (HEVs) in GALT and in postcapillary venules within the gut mucosa (see Chapter 12). In this way, T cells primed in the GALT preferentially traffic to the gut.

T cells primed in the GALT also express specific chemokine receptors that bind chemokines produced constitutively—and specifically—by the gut epithelium. Thus, at homeostasis, CCR9 expressed on T cells primed in lymphoid tissues of the small intestine recruit those T cells back to the small intestine along a CCL25 gradient. In contrast, T cells primed in skin-draining lymph nodes preferentially home back to the skin. They are induced to express the adhesion molecule **cutaneous lymphocyte antigen (CLA)**, an isoform of PSGL-1 that differs in its pattern of glycosylation and binds to E-selectin on cutaneous vascular endothelium (**Fig. 11.7**). CLA-expressing T lymphocytes also express the chemokine receptors CCR4 and CCR10, which bind the chemokines CCL17 (TARC) and CCL27 (CTACK), respectively. These chemokines are constitutively produced by cells in the epidermis of the skin and line the endothelium of cutaneous blood vessels. Because these tissue-homing chemokines are produced at steady state, they are referred to as **homeostatic chemokines**. They are analogous to chemokines produced constitutively in lymphoid tissues at steady state, such as CCL19 and CCL21, which direct CCR7-bearing naive T cells along a gradient from the endothelium of HEVs to T-cell zones (**Fig. 11.8**). Homeostatic chemokines can be contrasted with **inflammatory chemokines**, which are elicited in the context of infection to recruit circulating immune cells to sites of inflammation.

In addition to the general and tissue-specific changes in trafficking molecules induced during effector T-cell differentiation, loss of CCR7 expression

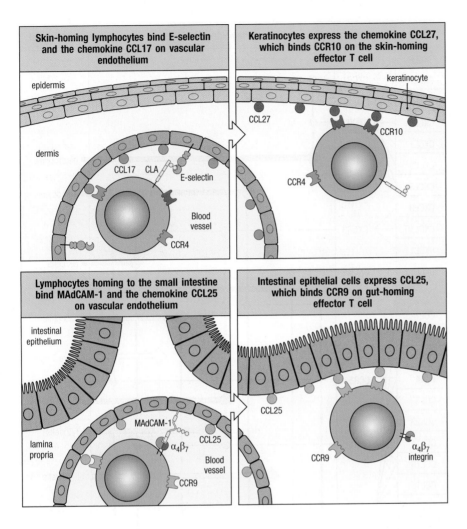

Skin-homing lymphocytes bind E-selectin and the chemokine CCL17 on vascular endothelium

epidermis

dermis

CCL17 CLA

E-selectin

Blood vessel

CCR4

Keratinocytes express the chemokine CCL27, which binds CCR10 on the skin-homing effector T cell

keratinocyte

CCL27

CCR10

CCR4

Lymphocytes homing to the small intestine bind MAdCAM-1 and the chemokine CCL25 on vascular endothelium

intestinal epithelium

lamina propria

MAdCAM-1

CCL25

$\alpha_4\beta_7$

Blood vessel

CCR9

Intestinal epithelial cells express CCL25, which binds CCR9 on gut-homing effector T cell

CCL25

CCR9

$\alpha_4\beta_7$ integrin

Fig. 11.7 Skin- and gut-homing T cells use particular combinations of integrins and chemokines to migrate specifically to their target tissues. Circulating lymphocytes primed in lymph nodes draining the skin bind to the endothelium lining a cutaneous blood vessel by interactions between cutaneous lymphocyte antigen (CLA) and constitutively expressed E-selectin on the endothelial cells (upper left panel). The adhesion is strengthened by an interaction between lymphocyte chemokine receptor CCR4 and the endothelial chemokine CCL17. Once through the endothelium, effector T lymphocytes are attracted to keratinocytes of the epidermis by the chemokine CCL27, which binds to the receptor CCR10 on lymphocytes (upper right panel). Similarly, $\alpha_4\beta_7$ expressed on circulating lymphocytes primed in gut-associated lymphoid tissue initially binds MAdCAM-1 (lower left panel), then uses CCR9 to move along a CCL25 chemokine gradient to traverse the endothelium and migrate to the intestinal epithelium (lower right panel).

is accompanied by subset-specific induction of other chemokine receptors. This results in distinct patterns of chemokine receptor expression by T_H1, T_H2, and T_H17 cells, which guides their differential recruitment to sites of inflammation contingent on the local patterns of inflammatory chemokines induced by innate immune responses to different types of pathogens (**Fig. 11.9**). For example, T_H1 cells express CCR5, which is also expressed on monocytes that mature into macrophages as they enter the inflammatory site. Thus, both T_H1 cells and the innate effector cells whose effector functions they enhance are recruited to the same tissue site by the same chemokines (see Fig. 11.8). As is the case for many other chemokine receptors, CCR5 has multiple ligands (CCL3, CCL4, CCL5, and CCL8), which may be induced by different cellular sources and by different pathogens targeted by type 1 immunity. Some of these are produced by activated macrophages themselves after their recruitment to the inflammatory site. This provides a feed-forward mechanism by which the emerging innate response is amplified and then contributes to the recruitment of T_H1 cells, which provide antigen-dependent 'help' to further activate the macrophages, as we discuss in Section 11-6. T_H1 cells also express CXCR3, which is shared by NK cells and cytotoxic CD8 T cells. In response to CXCR3 ligands—CXCL9, CXCL10, and CXCL11—these cells are recruited to the same inflammatory site to coordinate the cell-mediated killing of targets infected by intracellular pathogens, such as *Listeria monocytogenes*, which require the concerted actions of both T_H1 cells and cytotoxic effectors to clear the bacterium from macrophages and other cellular hosts.

T_H2 and T_H17 cells display different patterns of inflammatory chemokine receptors, some of which, like those expressed by T_H1 cells, are shared with

Fig. 11.8 Chemokine networks coordinate the interactions of innate and adaptive immune-cell populations. Chemokines are classified into four families on the basis of structural differences: CXCL, CCL, XCL, and CX3CL1. Chemokines (see the first column) can also be classified as pro-inflammatory (pink), homeostatic (green), and mixed function (yellow). Chemokines bind to a subfamily of seven-transmembrane G protein–coupled receptors, which are classified as CXCR, CCR, XCR, and CX3CR1 on the basis of the class of chemokines they bind. Many, but not all, of the chemokine–chemokine receptor networks that coordinate immune modules are represented here. The connection between receptors and cell types on which they are expressed is indicated by the 'circuit' representation of lines and connecting nodes. To connect chemokines and their receptors to target cells, follow a horizontal line and turn on a vertical one at each node; the rhomboids (diamond shapes) link vertical lines to the cell type. Note that most chemokine receptors can bind multiple chemokines.

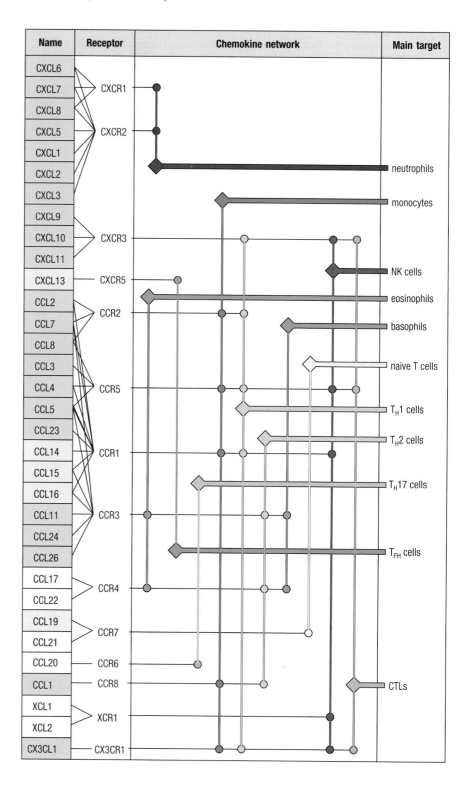

the myelomonocytic cells with which they interact in inflamed tissues (see Figs. 11.8 and 11.9). The shared expression pattern of chemokine receptors by innate and adaptive effector cells represents an important mechanism for the spatiotemporal coordination and integration of immune effector modules in response to different types of pathogen (see Fig. 11.8). Thus, the local release of cytokines and chemokines at the site of infection has far-reaching consequences. In addition to recruiting granulocytes and monocytes, which constitutively express their specific complement of chemokine receptors while in circulation, changes induced in endothelial cells lining blood vessels also enable newly generated effector T lymphocytes to enter infected tissues. Once in the tissue, recruited T cells may undergo further maturation and are activated to produce T helper cell subset–specific cytokines that further increase specific chemokine production by innate immune cells in an additional feed-forward mechanism that results in further effector T cell and innate effector cell trafficking into the tissue.

11-5 Pathogen-specific effector T cells are progressively enriched at sites of infection where they may undergo further maturation to acquire full effector function.

In the early stage of the adaptive immune response, only a minority of the effector T cells that enter infected tissues will be specific for pathogen. This is because activation of the endothelium of local blood vessels by inflammatory cytokines induces expression of selectins, integrin ligands, and chemokines that can recruit any circulating effector or memory T cell that expresses the appropriate trafficking receptors, irrespective of its antigenic specificity. This limits the potency of the antigen-specific response early. Moreover, at least for type 2 responses, T_H2 cells primed in secondary lymphoid organs require additional maturational signals in the inflamed tissue to which they are recruited to acquire full effector responses. As will be discussed in Section 11-10, the same cytokines that activate ILC2 cells—TSLP, IL-33, and IL-25—appear to be required for complete differentiation of T_H2 cells, at least in some target tissues, and this late-stage differentiation appears to be independent of signals from ILC2. Thus, sensing of module-specific innate cytokines may provide a mechanism to control the final activation of effector T cells, representing a further parallel with ILCs and a common local tissue checkpoint to regulate the effector response.

However, specificity and potency of the reaction is rapidly increased as the number and maturation state of pathogen-specific T cells increases and recognition of antigen within the inflamed tissue retains them there. Although the precise mechanisms controlling retention of antigen-activated effector T cells in the inflamed tissue are not entirely understood, it is thought that some of the same mechanisms that retain antigen-activated naive T cells within secondary lymphoid tissues during early effector T-cell development are at play. Thus, incoming T cells that are activated by antigen reexpress CD69, leading to down-regulation of S1PR1, and perhaps other members of the S1P receptor family, depriving them of the signal needed for tissue egress. Antigen-induced persistence of receptors for local chemokines may also contribute to retention of pathogen-specific T cells. Conversely, effector and memory T cells that enter tissues but do not recognize their cognate antigen are not retained there. While some may undergo apoptosis locally, most probably enter the afferent lymphatics and migrate to the draining lymph nodes and eventually return to the bloodstream. T cells in the afferent lymph that drains tissues therefore express markers of effector or memory T cells, characterized by expression of the CD45RO isoform of the cell-surface molecule CD45 and lack of L-selectin (see Fig. 11.6). Through the selective retention of pathogen-specific T cells and loss of nonspecific T cells, by the peak of an adaptive immune response, after several days of clonal expansion and differentiation, a large fraction of the T cells recruited to the inflamed tissue will be specific for the inciting pathogen and will be fully activated to eliminate it.

11-6 T_H1 cells coordinate and amplify the host response to intracellular pathogens through classical activation of macrophages.

Type 1 responses (see Fig. 11.5) are important for the eradication of pathogens that have evolved mechanisms to survive and replicate within host cells, particularly those that do so within macrophages. T_H1 cells are the principal

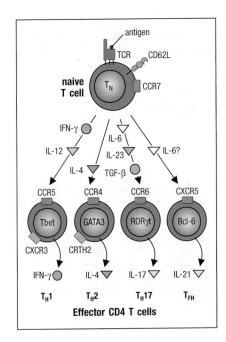

Fig. 11.9 The expression of adhesion and chemokine receptors is altered during effector T-cell differentiation. During a primary immune response, specific cytokines derived from the innate immune system (indicated along the four diverging arrows) and unique master transcription factors (Tbet, GATA3, RORγt, and Bcl-6) direct naive CD4 T cells to differentiate into T_H1, T_H2, T_H17, or T_{FH} effector cells. Effector T cells of each subset lose expression of L-selectin (CD62L) and CCR7 and express characteristic chemokine receptors.

Fig. 11.10 T$_H$1 cells activate macrophages to become highly microbicidal. When an effector T$_H$1 cell specific for a bacterial peptide contacts an infected macrophage, the T cell is induced to secrete the macrophage-activating factor IFN-γ and to express CD40 ligand and other products that may activate the macrophage. Together these newly synthesized T$_H$1 proteins activate the macrophage for heightened intracellular killing and enhanced production of pro-inflammatory cytokines.

T-cell helpers for macrophages; they enhance the ability of macrophages to destroy intracellular pathogens taken up via phagocytosis. Thus, in the case of infections by intracellular bacteria such as mycobacteria and *Salmonella* or by protozoa such as *Leishmania* and *Toxoplasma*, all of which can survive within macrophages, T$_H$1 cells activate macrophages to heighten their microbicidal function. T$_H$1 cells can also participate in viral infections, whether to provide help to infected macrophages—or other MHC class II–expressing cells, such as the inflamed intestinal epithelium—to inhibit viral replication and destroy virus particles or to coordinate with cytotoxic CD8 T cells that recognize virus-infected cells and destroy them (see Chapter 9). T$_{FH}$ cells that differentiate in the context of type 1 responses induce the production of subclasses of IgG antibodies (for example, IgG2a and IgG2c in mice; IgG2 and IgG3 in humans) that can opsonize intracellular pathogens that are released into the extracellular environment, neutralize virus particles in the blood and extracellular fluid, and arm NK cells for ADCC. Historically, overexuberant, tissue-damaging T cell–mediated immunity orchestrated by type 1 responses has been referred to as **delayed-type hypersensitivity**, to be distinguished from **immediate hypersensitivity**, such as allergic reactions and asthma, which are characterized by poorly controlled type 2 responses (see Section 11-10 and Chapters 14 and 15).

Single-cell pathogens of all types are ingested by macrophages and are often destroyed without the need for additional macrophage activation. However, in several clinically important infections, such as those caused by mycobacteria, pathogens ingested by macrophages are not killed and may even serve as hosts for chronic infection. Such microorganisms are able maintain themselves in the hostile environment of phagosomes—shielded from the effects of both antibodies and cytotoxic T cells—by inhibiting the fusion of phagosomes and lysosomes, preventing the acidification required to activate lysosomal proteases, or escaping the phagosome into the macrophage cytoplasm. Nevertheless, peptides derived from such microorganisms can be displayed by MHC class II molecules on the macrophage surface, where they are recognized by antigen-specific effector T$_H$1 cells. The T$_H$1 cell is stimulated to synthesize membrane-associated proteins and secrete cytokines that enhance the macrophage's antimicrobial defenses and enable it to either eliminate the pathogen or control its growth and spread (**Fig. 11.10**). This boost to antimicrobial mechanisms is often referred to as 'classical' macrophage activation, the result of which is the so-called **classically activated macrophage**, or **M1 macrophage** (**Fig. 11.11**). Although the range of macrophage subsets and activation states is still being defined, the M1 designation is useful in distinguishing the macrophage functions induced in the context of T$_H$1 responses from those induced by other types of immune responses, such as M2 macrophages induced in the context of T$_H$2 responses (see Section 11-10).

Macrophages require two main signals for classical activation. Both are delivered by T$_H$1 cells. One signal is the cytokine IFN-γ; the other is CD40L (see Fig. 11.10). Both signals are elicited by recognition of pathogenic peptide:MHC class II molecules on the macrophage surface by the T$_H$1 cell. Because CD40L and its receptor on the macrophage (CD40) are cell surface–associated molecules, and IFN-γ is thought to be delivered primarily across an immunological synapse that forms between the T cell and the macrophage, the T$_H$1 cell's effector actions are primarily focused on macrophages that harbor intracellular pathogens. T$_H$1 cells can also produce lymphotoxin and TNF-α, which, like CD40L, are TNF family cytokines that may contribute to M1-type macrophage activation. However, because inherited deficiency of *CD40L*, the most common cause of **X-linked hyper IgM syndrome**, results in defects in the killing of certain intracellular pathogens (for example, mycobacteria; see Section 13-8), it is likely that CD40L has a nonredundant role in macrophage activation.

CD40 Ligand Deficiency

Macrophages activated by T_H1 cells acquire potent antimicrobial effector activities, as illustrated in Fig. 11.11. This includes the induction of several key lysosomal enzymes that enhance the production of microbicidal reactive oxygen and nitrogen species after the fusion of phagosomes with lysosomes, as described in Section 3-2. In addition to inducing mechanisms for increased intracellular killing, T_H1 cells induce other changes in macrophages that enhance their recruitment of T-cell help. IFN-γ produced by T_H1 cells is a potent inducer of antigen processing and presentation; it stimulates increased synthesis of MHC class I and class II molecules and B7 molecules (CD80 and CD86) and is unique in up-regulating components of the MHC class II antigen-processing machinery (for example, invariant chain, HLA-DM; see Chapter 6), collectively making the macrophage more effective at presenting antigen to sustain T-cell help. IFN-γ also enhances expression of CD40 and TNF receptors on the M1 macrophage surface (see Figs. 11.10 and 11.11), resulting in heightened responsiveness to CD40L and TNF-α. In addition, M1 macrophages are activated by CD40L to secrete IL-12, which increases the amount of IFN-γ produced by ILC1 cells and T_H1 cells, thereby promoting a positive feedback loop that enhances macrophage activation.

Another important function of T_H1 cells is the recruitment of additional phagocytic cells to sites of infection. T_H1 cells recruit monocytes—the precursors of macrophages—by multiple mechanisms (**Fig. 11.12**). Activated T_H1 cells make the hematopoietic growth factors IL-3 and GM-CSF, which stimulate the production of new monocytes in the bone marrow and result in increased monocytes in circulation. TNF-α and LT-α secreted by T_H1 cells at sites of infection up-regulate endothelial-cell expression of selectins and integrin ligands that enhance the local recruitment of monocytes. Chemokines such as CXCL2, which is produced by T_H1 cells at inflammatory sites, direct the migration of monocytes through the vascular endothelium and into the infected tissue, where they differentiate into macrophages (see Section 3-1). Moreover, the secretion of cytokines and chemokines by M1 macrophages to enhance the recruitment of monocytes to sites of infection—including TNF-α and IL-1β—is increased by the actions of T_H1 cells. Collectively, these T_H1-mediated effects provide a positive feedback loop that amplifies and sustains type 1 responses until the pathogen is controlled or eliminated.

Certain intracellular bacteria, including some mycobacteria and *Listeria monocytogenes*, have evolved mechanisms to escape from phagocytic vesicles and enter the cytoplasm, where they are no longer susceptible to the microbicidal actions of activated macrophages. However, their presence can be detected by cytotoxic CD8 T cells. The pathogens released when macrophages are killed by these CTLs can be killed in the extracellular environment by antibody-mediated mechanisms or phagocytosed by freshly recruited macrophages. In this circumstance, the provision of T_H1-mediated 'help' for the development of CTLs, such as the provision of IL-2, may play an important role in coordinating the T_H1 and CTL responses.

11-7 Activation of macrophages by T_H1 cells must be tightly regulated to avoid tissue damage.

As discussed in Chapter 9, distinguishing features of effector T cells are their capacity for antigen-induced activation of effector functions with limited requirement for co-stimulation, and also their efficient delivery of effector molecules through polarized secretion or expression of cytokines and cell-surface molecules—often through formation of an immunological synapse with an antigen-bearing cell (see Section 9-18). After a T_H1 cell recognizes its cognate antigen expressed by a macrophage, the secretion of effector

Fig. 11.11 Macrophages activated by T_H1 cells undergo changes that increase their antimicrobial effectiveness and amplify the immune response. Activated macrophages increase their expression of CD40 and of TNF receptors, and are also stimulated to secrete TNF-α. CD40 ligand (CD40L) and TNF-α synergize with IFN-γ secreted by T_H1 cells to induce classical, or M1, macrophage activation characterized by production of nitric oxide (NO) and superoxide (O_2^-). The macrophage also up-regulates its B7 molecules in response to binding CD40L and TNF-α and increases its expression of MHC class II molecules in response to IFN-γ, thus enabling a positive feed-forward loop that enhances activation of T_H1 cells.

ANIMATION 11.2

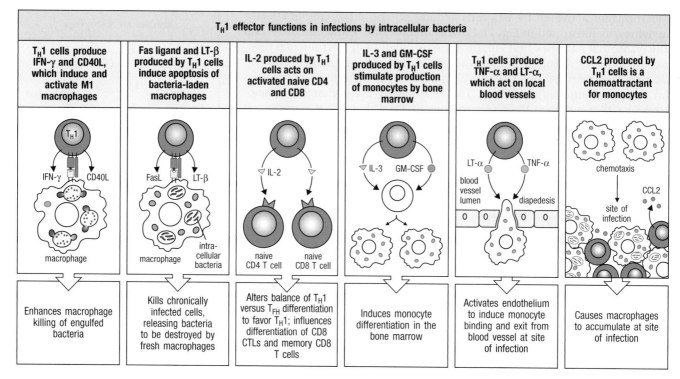

Fig. 11.12 The immune response to intracellular bacteria is coordinated by activated T$_H$1 cells. The activation of T$_H$1 cells by infected macrophages results in the synthesis of cytokines that both induce M1 macrophage activation and coordinate the immune response to intracellular pathogens. IFN-γ, CD40 ligand, and TNF-α synergize in activating the macrophage, which allows it to kill engulfed pathogens. Chronically infected macrophages lose the ability to kill intracellular bacteria, and membrane-bound Fas ligand or LT-β produced by the T$_H$1 cell can kill these macrophages, releasing the engulfed bacteria, which are taken up and killed by fresh macrophages. In this way, IFN-γ and LT-β synergize in the removal of intracellular bacteria. IL-2 produced by T$_H$1 cells augments effector T-cell differentiation and CD8 memory-cell development. IL-3 and GM-CSF stimulate the production of new monocytes by acting on hematopoietic stem cells in the bone marrow. New macrophages are recruited to the site of infection by the actions of secreted TNF-α, LT-α, and other cytokines on vascular endothelium, which signal monocytes to leave the bloodstream and enter the tissues where they become macrophages. Chemokines with monocyte chemotactic activity (for example, CCL3) signal monocytes to migrate into sites of infection and accumulate there. Thus, the T$_H$1 cell coordinates a macrophage response that is highly effective in destroying intracellular infectious agents.

molecules can take several hours. Therefore, T$_H$1 cells must adhere to their target cells longer than cytotoxic CD8 T cells, which can deliver a death signal in minutes and then detach to interact with other targets. However, similar to cytotoxic T cells, the T$_H$1 cell orients its secretory machinery toward the site of contact with the macrophage and secretes newly synthesized cytokines there (see Fig. 9.41). CD40 ligand also seems to be delivered to the same contact site. So, although all macrophages have receptors for IFN-γ and may respond to this cytokine, the infected macrophage that presents antigen to the T$_H$1 cell is more likely to become activated than nearby uninfected macrophages.

In addition to more efficiently focusing activating signals on infected macrophages, the antigen-specific induction of macrophage activation may play an important role in limiting tissue injury. By targeting only infected macrophages through peptide:MHC recognition, T$_H$1 cells minimize 'collateral damage' to normal components of the inflamed tissue that might otherwise result from oxygen radicals, NO, and proteases that are toxic to host cells as well as to the pathogen that is targeted for destruction. Thus, antigen-specific macrophage activation by T$_H$1 cells is a means to deploy this powerful defensive mechanism to maximum effect while minimizing local tissue damage. In this regard, it is notable that although ILC1 cells are also producers of IFN-γ , they lack antigen receptors that can focus the cytokine on infected macrophages for more efficient activation. It is not yet known whether ILC1 cells have other mechanisms with which to direct IFN-γ onto macrophages—analogous to the activating and inhibitory receptors deployed by NK cells—or whether they play a more limited role in macrophage activation, and whether the IFN-γ they produce downstream of activating signals is more important in indirectly modulating the local inflammatory response.

11-8 Chronic activation of macrophages by T_H1 cells mediates the formation of granulomas to contain intracellular pathogens that cannot be cleared.

Some intracellular pathogens, most notably *Mycobacterium tuberculosis*, are sufficiently resistant to the microbicidal effects of activated macrophages that they are incompletely eliminated by a type 1 response. This gives rise to chronic, low-level infection that requires an ongoing T_H1 response to prevent pathogen proliferation and spread. In this circumstance, chronic coordination between T_H1 cells and macrophages underlies the formation of the immunological reaction called the **granuloma**, in which microbes are held in check within a central area of macrophages surrounded by activated lymphocytes (**Fig. 11.13**). A characteristic feature of granulomas is the fusion of several macrophages to form **multinucleated giant cells**, which can be found at the border of the central focus of activated macrophages and the lymphocytes that surround them and which appear to have heightened antimicrobial activity. A granuloma serves to 'wall off' pathogens that resist destruction. In tuberculosis, the centers of large granulomas can become isolated and the cells there die, probably from a combination of lack of oxygen and the cytotoxic effects of activated macrophages. As the dead tissue in the center resembles cheese, this process is called 'caseous' necrosis. Thus, the chronic activation of T_H1 cells can cause significant pathology. The absence of the T_H1 response, however, leads to the more serious consequence of death from disseminated infection, which is seen frequently in individuals with AIDS and concomitant mycobacterial infection.

11-9 Defects in type 1 immunity reveal its important role in the elimination of intracellular pathogens.

In mice whose gene for IFN-γ or CD40 ligand has been deleted by gene targeting, classical macrophage activation is impaired; consequently, the animals succumb to sublethal doses of *Mycobacterium, Salmonella,* and *Leishmania* species. Classical macrophage activation is also crucial in controlling vaccinia virus. However, although IFN-γ and CD40 ligand are probably the most important effector molecules synthesized by T_H1 cells, the immune response to pathogens that proliferate in macrophage vesicles is complex, and other cytokines secreted by T_H1 cells may also be crucial (see Fig. 11.12).

The depletion of CD4 T cells in people with HIV/AIDS causes ineffective T_H1 responses that can lead to the dissemination of microbes that are normally cleared by macrophages. This is the case with the opportunist fungal pathogen *Pneumocystis jirovecii* (see also Chapter 13). The lungs of healthy people are kept clear of *P. jirovecii* by phagocytosis and intracellular killing by alveolar macrophages. Pneumonia caused by *P. jirovecii* is, however, a frequent cause of death in people with AIDS. In the absence of CD4 T cells, phagocytosis of *P. jirovecii* and intracellular killing by lung macrophages are impaired, and the pathogen colonizes the surface of the lung epithelium and invades lung tissue. The requirement for CD4 T cells seems to be due, at least in part, to a

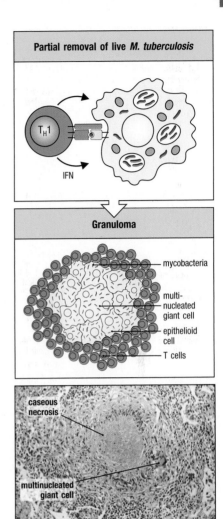

Partial removal of live *M. tuberculosis*

T_H1

IFN

Granuloma

mycobacteria

multi-nucleated giant cell

epithelioid cell

T cells

caseous necrosis

multinucleated giant cell

Fig. 11.13 Granulomas form when an intracellular pathogen or its constituents cannot be completely eliminated. When mycobacteria such as *M. tuberculosis* (red) resist the effects of macrophage activation, a characteristic localized inflammatory response called a granuloma develops. This consists of a central core of infected macrophages. The core may include multinucleated giant cells, which are fused macrophages, surrounded by large macrophages often called epithelioid cells, but in granulomas caused by mycobacteria the core usually becomes necrotic—referred to as caseous necrosis because of the cheese-like consistency of material that accumulates in the necrotic centers. Mycobacteria can persist in the cells of the granuloma. The central core is surrounded by T cells, many of which are CD4-positive. The exact mechanisms by which this balance is achieved, and how it breaks down, are not fully understood. An example of a caseating granuloma in the lung of an individual with tuberculosis is shown in the bottom panel.

requirement for the macrophage-activating cytokines IFN-γ and TNF-α produced by T_H1 cells.

11-10 T_H2 cells coordinate type 2 responses to expel intestinal helminths and repair tissue injury.

Type 2 immunity is primarily elicited in response to helminth parasites: roundworms (nematodes) and two types of flatworms—tapeworms (cestodes) and flukes (trematodes). Unlike microbial pathogens, or 'micropathogens' (bacteria, viruses, fungi, and protozoa), which replicate rapidly and can overwhelm host defenses by sheer numbers, most helminths do not replicate in their mammalian host. Moreover, helminths are multicellular; they are metazoan 'macropathogens' that are far too large—ranging in size from approximately 1 mm to more than 1 meter—to be engulfed by host phagocytic cells. Host defense against helminthic pathogens therefore requires very different strategies.

In the developing world, the intestines of virtually all humans and domestic animals are colonized by helminth parasites. Many of these infections may be cleared rapidly by the generation of an effective type 2 response, although often the host response is only successful in reducing worm burden, not in completely clearing the parasite, resulting in chronic disease. In these circumstances, the parasite persists for long periods despite the host's attempts to expel it, and it causes disease by competing with the host for nutrients or by causing local tissue injury. As noted earlier (see Section 11-6), aberrant type 2 responses can cause chronic immediate hypersensitivity diseases, typified by allergic reactions or asthma.

Irrespective of the type of helminth involved or its site of host entry, the host adaptive response is orchestrated by T_H2 cells (**Fig. 11.14**; and see Fig. 9.33). The T_H2 response is induced by the actions of worm products on a variety of different innate cells: epithelial cells, including tuft cells; mast cells; cDC2 cells; and perhaps ILC2 cells. Type 2 conventional dendritic cells required for the presentation of helminth antigens to naive CD4 T cells appear to be activated by IL-13 produced by ILC2 cells and by innate cytokines, such as epithelium-derived TSLP, which repress the development of T_H1- and T_H17-inducing dendritic cells in favor of dendritic cells that promote T_H2 cell differentiation. The initial source of the IL-4 required for T_H2 cell differentiation appears to be context-specific and redundant. Thus, although several cell types have been proposed as the source, including iNKT cells, mast cells, and basophils, none of these has been proven to be essential.

The initial development of T_H2 cells in draining lymphoid tissues is followed by their exodus to sites of helminth invasion, where they may undergo further maturation driven by the same cytokines that activate ILC2 cells—TSLP, IL-33, and IL-25. Mature T_H2 cells activated in sites of infection produce many of the same cytokines as ILC2 cells to enhance both the recruitment and function of circulating type 2 innate effector cells (eosinophils and basophils) and the activation of tissue-resident innate effectors (mast cells). Like T_H1 and T_H17 cells, T_H2 cells express a distinct complement of chemokine receptors that is shared with the circulating innate effector cells with which they interact, thus selectively guiding the T_H2 cells to sites of ongoing type 2 responses (see Figs. 11.8 and 11.9). Thus, CCR3 and CCR4 are expressed by T_H2 cells, eosinophils, and basophils. The chemokines recognized by these receptors (the CCR3-binding eotaxins CCL11, CCL24, and CCL26) are induced by the actions of IL-13 and IL-4 on multiple innate immune cells in tissue sites of helminth infection. Each of these cells also expresses CRTH2, the ligand for which—prostaglandin D2 (PGD2)—is produced in abundance by activated tissue mast cells, as

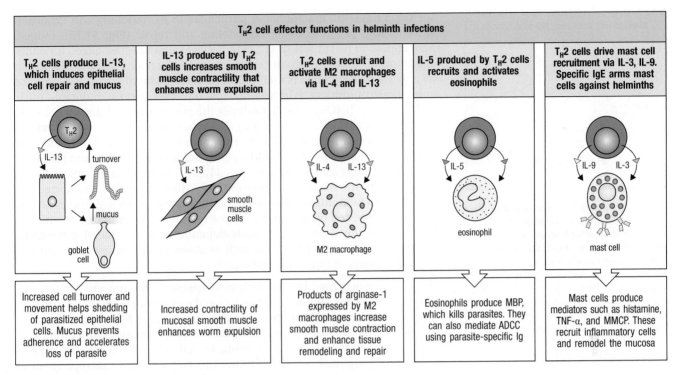

Fig. 11.14 Protective responses to intestinal helminths are mediated by T_H2 cells. Most intestinal helminths induce both protective and pathological immune responses by CD4 T cells. T_H2 responses tend to be protective, creating an unfriendly environment for the parasite and leading to its expulsion and the generation of protective immunity (see the text for details). M2 macrophage, alternatively activated macrophage; MBP, major basic protein; MMCP, mucosal mast cell protease.

well as by T$_H$2 cells themselves and possibly by tuft cells. Hence, each cell in the type 2 immune module (ILC2 cells, eosinophils, basophils, mast cells, and T$_H$2 cells) can further amplify the recruitment of circulating type 2 cells through this chemokine network.

Although the T$_H$2 effector response can coordinate the direct killing of some worms by enhancing innate effector-cell functions, a major focus of the anti-helminth response is expelling the worms and limiting the tissue damage they cause when they invade the host—functions that are mediated by type 2 cytokines. IL-13 directly enhances the production of mucus by goblet cells, activates smooth muscle cells in mucosal tissues for hypermotility, and increases the migration and turnover of epithelial cells in the mucosa (see Fig. 11.14, first panel). In the intestines, which are the most common site of worm infestation, each of these actions is a critical component of the host response, as it helps to eliminate parasites that have attached to the epithelium and decreases the surface area available for colonization.

The response to helminths generates IgE antibody, induced by IL-4–producing T$_{FH}$ cells that develop in concert with T$_H$2 cells (see Fig. 11.14). IgE binds to Fcε receptors expressed by mast cells, eosinophils, and basophils, which arms them for antigen-specific recognition and activation. Type 2 adaptive responses also promote production of IgG1, which is recognized by macrophages and engages them in the type 2 response. IL-4 produced by T$_H$2 cells and IL-13 produced by both T$_H$2 cells and ILCs can induce differentiation of **alternatively activated macrophages** (also called **M2 macrophages**). Unlike classically activated M1 macrophages, which acquire new functions after interaction with T$_H$1 cells and are potent activators of inflammation

Fig. 11.15 Macrophages activated by T$_H$2 cells undergo changes that increase their effectiveness in eradicating helminths and promote tissue repair responses. Macrophages activated by T$_H$2 cells up-regulate expression of the IL-4 and IL-13 receptors (for example, IL-4Rα) and are induced to express arginase-1, which results in the secretion of ornithine and proline. Ornithine enhances smooth muscle contractility, which can enhance worm expulsion and may be directly cytotoxic to some helminth larvae. It also promotes tissue repair. Proline is a critical amino acid for collagen synthesis, which is important for tissue remodeling and repair. M2 macrophages can also repress local tissue inflammation through their production of IL-1 receptor antagonist (IL-1RA) and a decoy IL-1 receptor (IL-1RII), both of which act to inhibit IL-1 receptor signaling. M2 macrophages also produce the anti-inflammatory cytokine IL-10 as well as TGF-β, which has pleiotropic effects in wound healing.

(see Fig. 11.11), M2 macrophages participate in worm killing and expulsion and may also promote tissue remodeling and repair (**Fig. 11.15**). Indeed, there appear to be subsets of M2 macrophages that are specialized for either anti-helminth actions or tissue repair. In any case, a major difference between M1 and M2 macrophages is their different metabolism of arginine to produce antipathogen products. Whereas M1 macrophages express inducible nitric oxide synthase (iNOS), which produces the potent intracellular microbicide nitric oxide (NO) (see Section 3-2), M2 macrophages express **arginase-1**, which produces ornithine and proline from arginine. Along with other factors, ornithine increases the contractility of mucosal smooth muscle and promotes tissue remodeling and repair (see Fig. 11.15). Through a mechanism that is unclear, ornithine has also been found to be directly toxic to IgG-coated larvae of certain helminths. Because helminths that have invaded tissues are too large to be ingested by macrophages, the targeted release of toxic mediators directly onto the worm by antibody-dependent cell-mediated cytotoxicity (ADCC) enables macrophages, as well as eosinophils (discussed shortly), to attack these large extracellular pathogens.

Macrophages activated by T$_H$2 cells also appear to be important in walling off invading worms and in repairing tissue damage caused as worms migrate through host tissues. These 'tissue repair' functions of M2 macrophages are dependent on secreted factors important in tissue remodeling and include the stimulation of collagen production, formation of which requires proline generated by arginase-1 activity. Moreover, T$_H$2-activated macrophages can also induce the formation of granulomas that entrap worm larvae in tissues. In this regard, antigen-specific macrophage activation by T$_H$2 cells has non-redundant function in type 2 responses. Although ILC2 cells and innate effector cells may promote M2 macrophage activation via IL-13, they appear to be unable to sustain this response, at least in part because they are sessile and unable to engage and directly deliver cytokines to antigen-bearing macrophages through cell–cell contacts. Thus, in several models of worm infection, anti-helminth responses are considerably impaired in Rag-deficient or T cell–depleted mice, demonstrating that sustained and optimal alternative activation of macrophages requires T$_H$2 cells.

The IL-5 produced by T$_H$2 cells and ILC2 cells recruits and activates eosinophils (see Fig. 11.14), which have direct toxic effects on worms via the release of cytotoxic molecules stored in their secretory granules, such as major basic protein (MBP). In addition to Fcε receptors that arm them for degranulation via bound IgE, eosinophils bear Fc receptors for IgG and IgA and can mediate ADCC against IgG- and IgA-coated parasites (see Fig. 10.38). They also express the Fcα receptor (CD89) and degranulate in response to stimulation by secretory IgA.

IL-3 and IL-9 produced by T$_H$2 cells in the mucosae recruit, expand, and activate a specialized population of mast cells known as **mucosal mast cells** (see Fig. 11.14). The innate cytokines IL-25 and IL-33 also activate mucosal mast cells early in a response to helminths. Mucosal mast cells differ from their counterparts in other tissues by having only small numbers of IgE receptors and producing very little histamine. When activated by cytokines or by the binding of worm antigens to receptor-bound IgE, mucosal mast cells release large amounts of preformed inflammatory mediators that are stored in secretory granules: prostaglandins, leukotrienes, and several proteases, including the mucosal mast cell protease (MMCP-1), which can degrade the epithelial tight junctions to increase epithelial permeability and enable fluid flow into the mucosal lumen. Together, the mast cell–derived mediators increase vascular and epithelial permeability, increase intestinal motility, stimulate the production of mucus by goblet cells, and induce leukocyte recruitment, all of which contribute to the 'weep-and-sweep' response that helps to expel parasites from the host.

11-11 T_H17 cells coordinate type 3 responses to enhance the clearance of extracellular bacteria and fungi.

The subset of effector T cells generated in response to infection by extracellular bacteria and fungi is T_H17, so-named because of its unique production of IL-17 among CD4 T-cell subsets. At homeostasis, T_H17 cells are deployed almost exclusively in the intestinal mucosa, where they contribute to the mutualistic relationship between the host and the intestinal microbiota—which is composed of extracellular bacteria and some fungi. However, they are also critical for defense against pathogenic extracellular bacteria and fungi that invade at barrier sites as well as components of the normal microbiota that may enter the host when epithelial barrier function is compromised, whether as the result of trauma or pathogenic infection. In these settings, a principal function of T_H17 cells is the orchestration of type 3 responses, in which neutrophils are the principal innate effector cell.

As discussed in Chapter 9, the development of T_H17 cells is guided by the combined actions of TGF-β and the pro-inflammatory cytokines IL-6, IL-1, and IL-23 (see Fig. 9.34). In the intestines of mice, these cytokines are preferentially produced by cDC2 cells that recognize PAMPs produced by extracellular bacteria, such as flagellin, which is recognized by TLR-5, or PAMPs produced by fungi, such as β-glucan polymers of glucose expressed by yeast and fungi that are recognized by Dectin-1. As for T_H1 and T_H2 cells, the egress of T_H17 cells from secondary lymphoid tissues is associated with altered chemokine expression: primarily the induction of CCR6, the ligand for which (CCL20) is produced by activated epithelial cells in mucosal tissues and skin, and by T_H17 cells themselves and ILC3 cells (**Fig. 11.16**; and see Fig. 11.5). Also like T_H1 and T_H2 cells, T_H17 cells primed in secondary lymphoid tissues may require additional maturational signals within inflamed tissues to which they are recruited for full effector function (for example, IL-23).

T_H17 effector functions in infections by extracellular bacteria				
IL-17 and IL-22 produced by T_H17 cells induce the production of antimicrobial peptides by epithelial cells	IL-22 produced by T_H17 cells increases epithelial cell turnover	IL-17 produced by T_H17 cells activates stromal cells and myeloid cells to produce G-CSF, which stimulates neutrophil production in bone marrow	IL-17 produced by T_H17 cells activates stromal cells and epithelial cells to produce chemokines that recruit neutrophils	CCL20 produced by T_H17 cells is a chemoattractant for other T_H17 cells
Direct killing or growth inhibition of bacteria attached to the epithelium	Increased epithelial cell division and shedding impairs bacterial colonization	Increases numbers of circulating neutrophils to sustain supply of short-lived innate effectors at infection site	Recruitment of neutrophils to the site of infection	Increased recruitment of T_H17 cells to site of infection

Fig. 11.16 The immune response to extracellular bacteria and some fungi is coordinated by activated T_H17 cells. T_H17 cells activated by antigen-bearing macrophages and dendritic cells in barrier tissues (for example, intestinal or respiratory mucosae, urogenital tract, and skin) produce cytokines that activate local epithelial and stromal cells to coordinate the immune response to extracellular bacteria and some types of fungi.

T$_H$17 cells are stimulated to release IL-17A and IL-17F when activated by antigen at sites of infection (see Fig. 11.16). A primary effect of these cytokines is the enhanced production and recruitment of neutrophils. The receptor for IL-17A and IL-17F is expressed widely on cells such as fibroblasts, epithelial cells, and keratinocytes. IL-17 induces these cells to secrete various cytokines, including IL-6, which may amplify and sustain the T$_H$17 response, and the hematopoietic factor granulocyte colony-stimulating factor (G-CSF), which increases the production of neutrophils by the bone marrow. IL-17 also stimulates production of the chemokines CXCL8 and CXCL2, the receptors for which (CXCR1 and CXCR2) are primarily expressed by neutrophils (see Fig. 11.8). Thus, one important action of IL-17 at sites of infection is to induce local cells to secrete cytokines and chemokines that attract neutrophils—a function shared with ILC3 cells.

T$_H$17 cells also produce IL-22, a member of the IL-10 family that acts cooperatively with IL-17 to induce the expression by epithelial cells of antimicrobial proteins (see Fig. 11.16). These include β-defensins and the C-type lectins, Reg3β and Reg3γ, all of which can directly kill bacteria (see Section 2-4). IL-22 and IL-17 can also induce epithelial cells to produce metal-binding proteins that are bacteriostatic and fungistatic. **Lipocalin-2** limits iron availability to bacterial pathogens; S100A8 and S100A9 are two antimicrobial peptides that heterodimerize to form the antimicrobial protein **calprotectin**, which sequesters zinc and manganese from microbes. Many of these antimicrobial agents are also produced by neutrophils recruited to the site of infection; calprotectin has been reported to compose up to a third of the cytosolic protein of neutrophils. IL-22 also stimulates the proliferation and shedding of epithelial cells as a mechanism to deprive bacteria and fungi of a 'foothold' for colonization at epithelial surfaces. While ILC3 cells in barrier tissues respond rapidly to pathogens to produce IL-22, pathogen-specific T$_H$17 cells have been shown to amplify and sustain the production of IL-22 at sites of infection.

As in type 1 and type 2 responses, integration of innate and adaptive effector cells in the type 3 response is mediated in large part by the production of pathogen-specific antibodies that opsonize extracellular bacteria and fungi for destruction by neutrophils, macrophages, and complement. T$_{FH}$ cells that develop coordinately with T$_H$17 cells promote the production of high-affinity IgG and IgA antibodies by plasma cells that can express CCR6 and thereby localize to sites of type 3 responses in barrier tissues, where they can arm neutrophils and macrophages 'on-site.' Antibodies are critical for the clearance of primary infections by common extracellular bacteria that elicit type 3 responses, such as *Staphylococcus aureus* and *Streptococcus pneumoniae*.

11-12 Effector T cells continue to respond to maturational and maintenance signals as they carry out their effector functions in target tissues.

The commitment of CD4 T cells to distinct lineages of effector cells occurs in secondary lymphoid tissues, such as lymph nodes. However, the effector activities of these cells are not defined simply by the signals received in the lymphoid tissues. Increasing evidence indicates that at least some activities of effector CD4 T cells—and perhaps also their maintenance in inflamed tissues—are contingent on signals they receive once they enter sites of infection. In view of the potential for each of the effector subsets to cause immune-mediated disease, about which we will learn more in Chapters 14 and 15, this requirement likely reflects the need for tissue checkpoints that provide ongoing regulation of effector T-cell functions to minimize the risk of allergy or autoimmunity.

Fig. 11.17 The cytokines IL-12 and IL-23 have a component in common, as do their receptors. The heterodimeric cytokines IL-12 and IL-23 both contain the p40 subunit, and the receptors for IL-12 and IL-23 have in common the IL-12Rβ1 subunit, which binds the p40 subunit. IL-12 signaling primarily activates the transcriptional activator STAT4, which increases IFN-γ production. IL-23 primarily activates STAT3, but also activates STAT4 weakly (not shown). Both cytokines augment the activity and/or proliferation of the CD4 subsets that express receptors for them; T_H1 cells express IL-12R, and T_H17 cells express primarily IL-23R, but can also express low levels of IL-12R (not shown). Mice deficient in p40 lack expression of both of these cytokines and manifest immune defects as a result of deficiencies in both T_H1 and T_H17 activities.

As we have seen, commitment of naive T cells to become T_H1, T_H2, or T_H17 cells is triggered by antigenic priming in the context of different inductive cytokines: IFN-α/β or IFN-γ; IL-4; or TGF-β and IL-6, respectively. These initial conditions appear insufficient, however, to generate complete or fully effective responses. To complete effector differentiation, each T-cell subset also requires stimulation by another cytokine: IL-12 in the case of T_H1 cells; IL-23 in the case of T_H17 cells; and probably TSLP in the case of T_H2 cells. Note that each of these cytokines also plays a role in activation of the corresponding ILC subset. As will be discussed in Section 11-13, each of these STAT-activating cytokines can also act in concert with a pro-inflammatory NFκB-activating cytokine (for example, IL-18 for T_H1 cells or IL-1 for T_H17 cells) to induce some functions of their target effector T cell.

In the case of T_H1 and T_H17 cells, the cytokines IL-12 and IL-23 are closely related in structure; each is a heterodimer, and they have a subunit in common (**Fig. 11.17**). IL-12 is composed of one p40 (IL-12p40) and one p35 (IL-12p35) subunit, whereas IL-23 has the p40 (IL-12p40) subunit and a unique p19 (IL-23p19) subunit. T_H1 cells express the receptor for IL-12; T_H17 cells express the receptor for IL-23. As will be discussed later (Section 11-14), T_H17 cells can also express low levels of the receptor for IL-12, which has important implications for their terminal differentiation. As for the ligands, the receptors for IL-12 and IL-23 are also related. They have a common subunit, IL-12Rβ1, which is expressed by naive T cells and binds the shared IL-12p40 subunit of IL-12 and IL-23. Upon receipt of differentiating cytokine signals, developing T_H1 cells synthesize IL-12Rβ2, the inducible component of the mature IL-12 receptor heterodimer, which binds the IL-12p35 subunit of IL-12; T_H17 cells synthesize IL-23R, the inducible component of the mature IL-23 receptor, which binds IL-23p19.

IL-12 and IL-23 play important roles in the maturation and functional activities of T_H1 and T_H17 cells, respectively. Like many other cytokines, both act through the JAK–STAT intracellular signaling pathway (see Fig. 9.35). IL-23 signaling primarily activates the intracellular transcriptional activator STAT3, but it also activates STAT4. In contrast, IL-12 strongly activates STAT4, with minimal activation of STAT3. IL-23 does not initiate the commitment of naive CD4 T cells to become T_H17 cells, but it does stimulate their expansion and contributes to their maintenance and full effector activities. Many *in vivo* responses that depend on IL-17 are diminished in the absence of IL-23. For example, mice lacking the IL-23–specific subunit p19 show decreased production of IL-17A and IL-17F in the lung after infection by *Klebsiella pneumoniae*.

While IL-12 contributes to the early development of T_H1 cells, it also appears to contribute to the effector activity of committed T_H1 cells at sites of infection. Studies of two different pathogens have shown that the initial differentiation of T_H1 cells is not sufficient for protection and that continual signals may be required. Mice deficient in IL-12p40 can resist initial infection by *Toxoplasma gondii* as long as IL-12 is administered continually. If IL-12 is administered during the first 2 weeks of infection, p40-deficient mice survive the initial infection and establish a latent chronic infection characterized by cysts containing

T$_H$1 cells from mice cured of infection with *L. major* are transferred into Rag-2– or IL-12p40–deficient mice, which are then injected with *L. major*

T$_H$1 cells protect Rag-2–deficient mice, but mice lacking the IL-12p40 subunit show progressive growth of the parasite

Fig. 11.18 Continual IL-12 is necessary for resistance to pathogens requiring T$_H$1 responses. Mice that have eliminated an infection with *Leishmania major* and have generated T$_H$1 cells specific to the pathogen were used as a source of T cells that were adoptively transferred either into Rag-2–deficient (*Rag2$^{-/-}$*) mice, which lack T cells and B cells and cannot control *L. major* infection but can produce IL-12, or into mice lacking IL-12p40 (*Il12b$^{-/-}$*), which cannot produce IL-12. On subsequent infection of the Rag-2–deficient mice, lesions did not enlarge because the transferred T$_H$1 cells conferred immunity. But despite the fact that the transferred cells were already differentiated T$_H$1 cells, they did not confer resistance to IL-12p40–deficient mice, which lacked a source of IL-12 to support T$_H$1 function.

the pathogen. When IL-12 administration is stopped, however, these mice gradually reactivate the latent cysts and the animals eventually die of toxoplasmic encephalitis. IFN-γ production by pathogen-specific T cells decreases in the absence of IL-12 but can be restored by IL-12 administration. Similarly, the adoptive transfer of differentiated T$_H$1 cells from mice cured of *Leishmania major* protects Rag-deficient mice infected by *L. major*, but it cannot protect IL-12p40–deficient mice (**Fig. 11.18**). Together, these experiments indicate that T$_H$1 cells continue to respond to signals after their initial priming and that continual IL-12 may be needed to sustain the effectiveness of differentiated T$_H$1 cells against at least some pathogens.

T$_H$2 cells also appear to receive cytokine signals that are important for their full effector function and/or maintenance in inflamed tissues. Although details of their specific roles remain to be defined, TSLP, IL-33, and IL-25 have all been implicated in the late maturation of T$_H$2 cells after their entry into sites of type 2 inflammation. It has also been shown that TSLP, the receptor for which is expressed by naive CD4 T cells, may promote the differentiation of a subset of T$_H$2 cells that express IL-15, IL-5, and IL-9 without IL-4, raising the possibility that under conditions of high production of TSLP, differentiation of T$_H$2 cells is favored at the expense of type 2 T$_{FH}$ cells.

11-13 Effector T cells can be activated to release cytokines independently of antigen recognition.

A central paradigm in adaptive immunity is the requirement for antigen recognition by the cognate receptors of naive lymphocytes to induce their differentiation into mature effector cells. However, effector T cells also acquire the ability to be activated by pairs of cytokines, independently of antigen recognition by their T-cell receptor. The cytokine pairs that mediate this 'noncognate' function of differentiated effector cells appear to be the same as those that activate the ILC subset that parallels each T-cell subset (**Fig. 11.19**). And in each case, the pair of stimulating cytokines includes one cytokine that activates a receptor that signals via a STAT factor, and one that activates a receptor that signals via NFκB—typically a member of the IL-1 receptor family. Thus, for both T$_H$1 cells and ILC1 cells, stimulation by IL-12 (STAT4) plus IL-18 induces production of IFN-γ. Similarly, stimulation of T$_H$2 and ILC2 cells by TSLP (STAT5) plus IL-25 or IL-33 produces IL-5 and IL-13. T$_H$2 cells, like ILC2 cells, also express the CRTH2 receptor for prostaglandin D2 (PGD2), and can be induced to express their effector cytokines by coordinate activation with PGD2 plus IL-33. Finally, both T$_H$17 and ILC3 cells produce IL-17 and IL-22 when stimulated by IL-23 (STAT3) plus IL-1.

In this way, mature effector CD4 T cells can acquire innate-like functional properties that allow them to amplify different types of immune responses without the requirement for antigen recognition. Note that in the case of type 1

Fig. 11.19 Effector T cells can be activated to release cytokines independently of antigen recognition. Analogous to ILCs, effector T cells can be stimulated to produce effector cytokines independently of T-cell receptor signaling via the coordinate actions of pairs of cytokines.

and type 3 cells, the IL-1 family member involved (IL-18 and IL-1, respectively) is produced by inflammasome activation in myeloid cells. Conversely, IL-33, which activates type 2 responses, is inactivated by the inflammasome, indicating another basis for counterregulation between type 2 and type 1 or type 3 immune responses and suggesting that IL-33 favors tissue repair. Although the precise role of noncognate activation of effector T cells by cytokines is not clearly defined, it may provide a mechanism to augment effector T-cell function during active tissue inflammation in primary responses. It may also be a means by which tissue-resident memory T cells that remain in nonlymphoid tissues after clearance of pathogen in a primary response could be rapidly recruited in recall, or memory, responses in an antigen-independent manner (see Section 11-20), essentially serving innate-like functions similar to ILCs.

11-14 Effector CD4 T cells demonstrate plasticity and cooperativity that enable adaptation during antipathogen responses.

Thus far we have discussed subsets of effector CD4 T cells as though they are intrinsically stable, such that their functional phenotype is unchanging after their development. Similarly, we have discussed the different types of immunity as though they are unimodal; that is, only one type of response is recruited to clear a given pathogen. Although this is often the case, it is not always so. Just as the pathogens can modify their tactics to evade destruction, so too can the elicited effector T cells adapt in order to clear these pathogens. Adaptation can occur by flexibility in the programming of individual T cells, referred to as **T-cell plasticity**, wherein effector T cells can transition into different cytokine phenotypes contingent on changes in the local inflammatory environment. It can also occur as a result of cooperation between different subsets of T cells. Plasticity applies to cells of the same clonal origin and thus identical antigenic specificity, whereas cooperation applies to cells that develop from different clonal precursors and target different antigens, typically at different stages of an infection.

Although some degree of plasticity has been experimentally demonstrated for each of the major effector CD4 subsets, it appears to be most prevalent in type 3 responses. It is common for T_H17 cells to deviate, or be 'reprogrammed,' into T_H1-type cells—a process referred to as **transdifferentiation (Fig. 11.20)**. Transdifferentiation was discovered using cytokine reporter mice, in which T_H17 cells that express IL-17F could be identified and isolated on the basis of their expression of a cell-associated reporter molecule controlled by the gene *Il17f*. When T_H17 cells isolated using the reporter were restimulated in the presence of the T_H1-polarizing cytokine IL-12, their progeny rapidly lost expression of IL-17 and acquired expression of IFN-γ. Moreover, repetitive restimulation of T_H17 cells with the T_H17 lineage cytokine IL-23 could lead to a subset of progeny that also acquired features of T_H1 cells. In both cases, transdifferentiation of T_H17 cells into T_H1 cells required expression of the T_H1-associated transcription factor Tbet and loss of the T_H17-associated transcription factor RORγt, both of which were contingent on activation of STAT4 by the IL-12 and IL-23 receptors. Thus, T_H17 cells deficient for either Tbet or STAT4 failed to transdifferentiate into T_H1 cells; that is, they lost their intrinsic 'T_H17-cell plasticity.' Recent studies have suggested that type 3 ILCs may similarly undergo an ILC3 to ILC1 transition, although this has been difficult to prove experimentally.

An example of the importance of effector T-cell plasticity and cooperativity between subsets is found in host protection against facultative intracellular bacterial pathogens, such as *Salmonella*, which, unlike obligate extracellular bacteria, have also evolved mechanisms to survive within macrophages that are not activated by IFN-γ. Early in infection, *Salmonella* can colonize the intestinal epithelium similarly to other enteric Gram-negative pathogens. During this period, a T_H17 response dominates, resulting in a robust IL-17– and

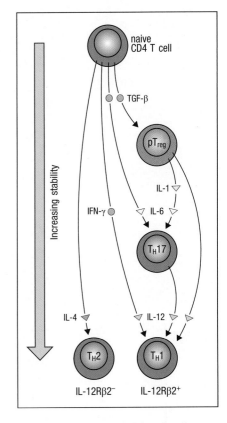

Fig. 11.20 Plasticity of CD4+ T-cell subsets. There is a hierarchy of stability of effector and regulatory CD4 T cells. Naive CD4+ T cells are multipotent, whereas T_H1 and T_H2 cells appear to be relatively stable, or at 'ground state'; that is, they are highly resistant to transitioning into other effector-cell phenotypes. Peripheral regulatory T (pT_reg) cells and T_H17 cells are less stable and can transition into other subsets, depending on prevailing cytokines. When acted on by IL-6 and IL-1, pT_reg cells can transition, or 'transdifferentiate,' into T_H17 cells, or when acted on by IL-12, they can become T_H1 cells. T_H17 cells acted on by IL-12 can transition into T_H1 cells. Notably, the transdifferentiation of pT_reg cells into T_H17 cells or of T_H17 cells into T_H1 cells appears to be unidirectional, or irreversible. Developing T_H2 cells (left) repress expression of the inducible component of the IL-12 receptor (IL-12Rβ) and are unresponsive to IL-12; pT_reg, T_H17, and T_H1 subsets (right) remain responsive to IL-12.

IL-22–induced influx of neutrophils that engulf extracellular bacteria and the release of antimicrobial proteins that restrain bacterial growth in the intestinal lumen. During this intestinal phase of infection, much of the T-cell response appears to be directed against antigenic epitopes within bacterial flagellins, which are potent activators of TLR-5. Activation of this innate sensor promotes IL-23 expression by cDC2 cells in the intestine, thereby inducing a type 3 immune response. Flagellin-specific T_H1 cells also emerge during the early intestinal phase of infection and may arise from T_H17 cell precursors as a result of plasticity. To escape destruction by macrophages activated for intracellular killing by these 'ex-T_H17' T_H1 cells, *Salmonella* simultaneously down-regulates the expression of flagellin and begins synthesizing new proteins, such as SseI and SseJ, that suppress intracellular killing within macrophages. This allows *Salmonella* to both evade detection by flagellin-specific T cells and use the host macrophage as a safe haven to shield it from extracellular killing—at least temporarily—as the infection spreads systemically.

During the systemic phase of the infection, the T-cell response shifts to become focused on those antigens that enable the intracellular lifestyle of the pathogen. Some of these newly expressed antigens appear to activate cytosolic sensors within cDC1 cells, which produce IL-12 to activate pathogen-specific T_H1 cells and a type 1 response. The pathogen can now be cleared by T_H1-induced macrophage activation directed against these newly expressed antigens. Because the antipathogen response now includes both type 3 and type 1 immunity to different sets of antigens that the bacterium requires for its extracellular and intracellular lifestyles, *Salmonella* is deprived of a niche for its survival and is cleared from the host.

11-15 Integration of cell- and antibody-mediated immunity is critical for protection against many types of pathogens.

The type of effector response required for host protection depends on the infectious strategy and lifestyle of the pathogen. Central to the integration of innate immunity and adaptive immunity in each immune module is the production of pathogen-specific, class-switched antibodies. Antibodies can function directly to neutralize pathogens and/or their toxins and can activate microbicidal actions of the complement pathway. They can also act indirectly by enhancing the uptake and destruction of pathogens by phagocytes in type 1 and type 3 responses or by arming innate immune effector cells to direct their degranulation in the context of type 2 responses (**Fig. 11.21**; and see Sections 10-22 through 10-25 and Sections 11-6 through 11-11). Although the signals that control the developmental fate of T_{FH} cells are yet to be fully characterized, there appears to be overlap with signals controlling the development of each subset of non-T_{FH} effector CD4 T cells. Accordingly, many of the same subset-specific cytokines produced by non-T_{FH} effector cells to modulate the antimicrobial actions of different innate effector cells are produced by T_{FH} cells to direct B-cell class switching to specific antibody isotypes that are targeted to the same innate effector cells. Thus, whereas IL-21 produced by most T_{FH} cells induces class switching to IgG1—a component of each of the helper immune response types (for example, types 1, 2, and 3)—IL-4 produced by T_{FH} cells in type 2 responses is required for IgE class switching, and IFN-γ produced by type 1 T_{FH} cells promotes IgG2 (mouse) or IgG3 (human) class switching while repressing IgE class switching. The coordinated differentiation of T_{FH} with non-T_{FH} effector T cells thus results in antibody isotypes that are appropriately matched to the types of innate effector cells that dominate each type of infection to enhance their functions.

As we learned in Chapter 10, the targeting of specific antibody isotypes to different innate effector cells is determined by the pattern of Fc receptors (FcRs) they express (see Fig. 11.21). In this way, different antibody isotypes

Immune module	Cytotoxic	Type 1	Type 2			Type 3
	NK cell	macrophage	eosinophil	basophil	mast cell	neutrophil
Innate effector cell and major Fc receptors expressed	FcγRIII	FcγRIII, FcγRI, FcαRI, FcγRIIA	FcγRI, FcγRIII, FcεRII, FcαRI	FcεRI	FcεRI	FcγRI, FcγRIIA, FcαRI
Principal antibody isotypes bound	IgG1, IgG3	IgG1, IgG3, IgA	IgE, IgG1, IgG3, IgA	IgE		IgG1, IgG3, IgA

Fig. 11.21 The innate effector cells of each immune module are armed by different antibody isotypes on the basis of the pattern of Fc receptors they express. See text for details.

preferentially activate different innate effector cells. The affinity of the FcR for each immunoglobulin Fc region it recognizes dictates whether the receptor binds free antibody or requires prior binding of the antibody to multivalent antigen (see Section 10-21 for more detailed discussion). For most FcRs, the binding affinity for Fc regions is such that antibody is only bound in aggregate. For high-affinity FcRs, such as FcεRI, free antibody can be bound and becomes, in essence, an antigen-specific receptor that couples antigen recognition (via antibody) to Fc-receptor signaling. Irrespective of the mode of antibody isotype binding, FcR signaling requires cross-linking by multivalent antigen and, in the case of ITAM-coupled FcRs, activates the innate effector cell.

In the case of phagocytic innate effector cells, such as macrophages or neutrophils, opsonizing IgG isotypes produced in type 1 or type 3 responses promote the phagocytosis and destruction of antibody-decorated pathogens by activating Fcγ receptors (for example, FcγRI or FcγRIIA). This enables phagocytic targeting of extracellular bacteria—or intracellular bacteria as they move from cell to cell, and may be particularly important for clearing small numbers of remaining bacteria toward the end of the antipathogen response. Opsonizing and complement-fixing antibodies are critical for clearance of many encapsulated extracellular bacteria, such as *Streptococcus pneumoniae*, *Haemophilus influenzae*, and *Neisseria meningitidis*, which evade alternative pathway activation and uptake by phagocytes.

Binding of IgG1 to the same Fc receptors on eosinophils induces the targeted release of eosinophilic granules onto IgG1-decorated parasites rather than phagocytosis. IgE, which is bound with high affinity by FcεRI expressed on basophils and mast cells or by FcεRII on eosinophils, is uniquely induced by type 2 T_{FH} cells that produce IL-4 and recognizes free- or pathogen-associated antigens to stimulate granule and lipid mediator release from these innate effector cells. Similarly, IL-5 produced by type 2 T_{FH} cells induces IgA, which binds to FcαRI on eosinophils. Thus, the antibody isotypes induced in the context of a type 2 response are critical to amplification and focusing of the anti-parasite response by nonphagocytic innate effector cells.

Specific antibody isotypes are also important in defense against many of the intracellular pathogens that provoke a cytotoxic immune response, particularly viruses. Despite the ability of CTLs to directly kill infected cells—and the inability of CD8 T cells to provide help for B cells—high-affinity, pathogen-specific IgG or IgA antibodies are typically generated in CTL responses. This is mediated by T_{FH} cells that differentiate in parallel with effector CD8 T cells. Although the generation of class-switched antibodies generally lags that of CTLs—and in some viral infections the initial infection may be cleared without an antibody response—the role of antibodies in viral clearance is critical for host defense against some viruses (for example, Ebola virus). IgG1 and IgG3 produced in the context of cytotoxic and type 1 responses also arm NK cells for ADCC via FcγRIII (CD16). In this way, pathogen-derived antigens that are expressed on the surface of infected cells can target the cells for killing by an antibody-dependent mechanism. NK cell–mediated ADCC has been shown to contribute to host defense against several viral and intracellular bacterial infections, including influenza and *Salmonella*.

11-16 Resolution of an infection is accompanied by the death of most effector T cells and persistence of a small number of long-lived memory T cells.

When a pathogen is eliminated by an immune response, so too are the pathogen-specific antigens that drive the clonal expansion and differentiation of effector T cells. In the absence of antigen, and as a consequence of its loss, most effector T cells undergo apoptotic cell death, removing themselves from the T-cell repertoire (see Fig. 9.23). In mice, greater than 90% of clonally expanded T cells die upon clearance of specific antigen. As we will discuss later, the cells that persist following this 'clonal contraction' are **memory T cells**. Although details of the mechanisms resulting in clonal contraction of effector T cells remain incompletely understood, it appears to be due, at least in part, to the loss of pro-survival signals that are produced by ongoing antigenic stimulation and/or cytokine signaling.

One signal that is contributed by T-cell receptor (TCR) stimulation is the production of IL-2, which is lost with the loss of antigen. Also, expression of the high-affinity component of the IL-2 receptor (IL-2Rα, or CD25) by TCR signaling is transient, such that ongoing antigen recognition is required for efficient IL-2 signaling. One consequence of IL-2 signaling is the expression of the anti-apoptotic survival factor Bcl-2, which prevents activation of the **intrinsic (or mitochondrial) pathway of apoptosis** that leads to assembly of the apoptosome (see Section 9-21 and Fig. 9.45). Thus, loss of IL-2 production and/or loss of CD25 result in down-regulation of Bcl-2 and heightened susceptibility to intrinsic apoptotic death. Moreover, most naive T cells lose expression of the specific component of the IL-7 receptor, **IL-7Rα (CD127)**, soon after activation. Like IL-2 signaling, IL-7 signaling activates STAT5, which promotes expression of Bcl-2. Thus, as IL-2 signaling is lost with the decline in antigen, effector T cells cannot be 'rescued' by IL-7 signaling and may undergo activation of the intrinsic pathway of apoptosis (see Fig. 9.45). However, other pathways must be important, as mice deficient for IL-2Rβ also undergo clonal expansion and contraction, and mice with enforced expression of IL-7Rα are not rescued from clonal contraction.

A second mechanism that can contribute to effector T-cell death is activated by signaling via members of the TNF receptor superfamily, such as Fas (CD95), which can activate the **extrinsic (or death receptor) pathway of apoptosis** (see Fig. 9.45). Coupling of Fas signaling to the apoptosis pathway is inhibited by the cellular caspase 8–like inhibitory protein (c-FLIP), which is induced by TCR signaling. As TCR signaling is lost, c-FLIP expression declines, and Fas signaling can now be coupled to the **death-inducing signaling complex (DISC)**, resulting in Fas ligand (FasL)-induced apoptosis. Loss-of-function mutations in *Fas* or *FasL* lead to the increased survival of lymphocytes and is one cause of the disease **autoimmune lymphoproliferative syndrome, or ALPS** (see Section 9-21).

The relative contribution of the intrinsic and extrinsic apoptotic pathways to effector T-cell loss appears to depend on the infectious agent, but they appear to be complementary mechanisms, as mice with specific deficiencies targeting one of these two pathways have milder defects in T-cell clearance than mice with deficiencies of both. Irrespective of the apoptotic pathway induced, dying T cells are rapidly cleared by phagocytes that recognize the membrane lipid phosphatidylserine on their surface. This lipid is normally found only on the inner surface of the plasma membrane, but in apoptotic cells it rapidly redistributes to the outer surface, where it can be recognized by specific receptors on many cells. Thus, not only is the pathogen removed at the end of infection, but also most of the pathogen-specific effector T cells are also removed. Some of the pathogen-specific effector T cells survive, however, and provide the basis for memory T-cell responses, as will be discussed in the next part of the chapter.

Summary.

Effector CD4 T cells develop in response to, and subsequently amplify and sustain, innate immune responses that are induced by pathogens. Pathogen-derived antigens are transported to local lymphoid organs by migratory dendritic cells or freely in lymph to be taken up by lymphoid-resident DCs and are presented to antigen-specific naive T cells that continually recirculate through the lymphoid organs. T-cell priming and the differentiation of effector T cells occurs here, and the effector T cells either leave the lymphoid organ to provide cell-mediated immunity at sites of infection in the tissues or remain in the lymphoid organ to participate in humoral immunity by activating antigen-binding B cells. Distinct types of CD4 T cells develop in response to infection by different types of pathogens, and their development is influenced largely by the cytokines produced by innate sensor cells and ILCs that are activated early in the response.

Effector CD4 T cells serve to amplify and enhance early innate responses orchestrated by ILCs, while T_{FH} cells that develop in concert with each subset of effector T cells direct the production of high-affinity antibodies that arm innate effector cells for heightened pathogen elimination. T_H1 responses promote the development and activation of classical, M1 macrophages to protect against intracellular pathogens. T_H2 responses are directed against infections by parasites such as helminths and promote the development and activation of alternative, M2 macrophages and the recruitment of eosinophils and basophils to sites of infection. T_H17 cells are integral to the clearance of extracellular bacteria and fungi by orchestrating sustained neutrophil recruitment and production of antimicrobial peptides by epithelial cells of barrier tissues such as the intestines, lungs, and skin. CD8 T cells have an important role in protective immunity, especially in protecting the host against infection by viruses and intracellular infections by *Listeria* and other microbial pathogens that have special means for entering the host cell's cytoplasm. Primary CD8 T-cell responses to pathogens usually require CD4 T-cell help but can occur in response to some pathogens without such help. The patterns of antipathogenic response are not fixed, and effector T cells retain plasticity for adapting their response as pathogens alter their survival strategy in response to pressure from the immune system. Ideally, the adaptive immune response eliminates the infectious agent, at which time the expanded clonal populations of effector T cells contract, retaining only small populations of long-lived memory cells, which provide the host with a state of protective immunity against reinfection with the same pathogen.

Immunological memory.

In this part of the chapter, we will examine how long-lasting, protective immunity is maintained after an infection has been successfully eliminated. Immunological memory is a defining consequence of an adaptive immune response; it enables the immune system to respond more rapidly and effectively to pathogens that have been encountered previously and prevents them from causing disease. Memory responses, called secondary immune responses, **tertiary immune responses**, and so on, depending on the number of exposures to antigen, differ from primary responses in rapidity of onset, location, and magnitude. As we will see, immunological memory results from the persistence of antigen-experienced memory T cells that are retained long term at increased clonal precursor frequencies, have altered patterns of recirculation, and more rapidly express their effector functions upon re-challenge by antigen. Selective survival of T-cell clones with higher affinity for pathogen-associated antigens also increases the sensitivity of recall responses to low levels of antigen, and thus to lower pathogen numbers. Similar changes also occur in the B-cell compartment, resulting in increases in the quantity and affinity of pathogen-specific antibodies in a recall, or memory, response.

11-17 Immunological memory is long lived after infection or vaccination.

It has long been appreciated that individuals exposed to a given infectious agent become immune to that agent; they are protected from subsequent challenges by that specific infectious agent but not from challenges by other infectious agents to which they have not been exposed. The phenomenon was first recorded by the ancient Greeks and has been the basis for vaccination programs for more than 200 years. Most children in developed countries are now vaccinated against a number of viral infections (for example, measle, mumps, rubella, and varicella) and bacterial infections (for example, diphtheria and pertussis). Before vaccination was widespread, many were naturally exposed to these pathogens and developed acute, potentially dangerous illnesses. Whether through vaccination or infection, children exposed to these agents acquire long-term or, in some cases, lifelong protection from reinfection; this state of protection is a consequence of immunological memory.

Although immunological memory has been recognized for centuries, its mechanistic underpinnings have only begun to be elucidated recently. Within the past few decades it has become established that immune memory reflects the generation of a small, heterogeneous population of specialized **memory cells** formed during a primary adaptive immune response that can persist for extended periods in the absence of the antigen that originally induced them. Although some infectious agents are never cleared entirely, most are, yet the immune cells that were generated to protect against reinfection are long lived. The idea that immunological memory does not depend on repeated exposure to infection has been supported by observations of populations of people living on remote islands. In that setting, a virus such as measles can cause an epidemic, infecting all people living on the island at that time, after which the virus disappears for many years. On reintroduction from outside the island, the virus does not affect the original population but causes disease in those people born since the first epidemic.

The duration of immunological memory has been estimated in people who received vaccines early in life and have been examined for responses to the immunizing agent much later. Experimental studies in mice have also been used to estimate the duration of immune memory. Perhaps the most compelling data in humans have come from studies of those who received vaccinia, the virus used to immunize against smallpox (**Fig. 11.22**). Because smallpox was eradicated by 1977, it is presumed that the responses of vaccinated individuals represent true immunological memory and are not due to restimulation from time to time by the smallpox virus. One study found strong vaccinia-specific CD4 and CD8 T-cell memory responses as long as 75 years after the original immunization, and from the strength of these responses it was estimated that the memory response had an approximate half-life—that is, the time required for a response to diminish to 50% of its original strength—of between 8 and 15 years. By contrast with T-cell memory, titers of antivirus antibody remained stable, almost without measurable decline. Similar to the geographical isolation studies, these findings indicate that immunological memory need not be maintained by repeated exposure to infectious virus, implying that memory is sustained by long-lived, antigen-specific lymphocytes that were induced by the original exposure and persist until a second encounter with the pathogen. As will be discussed later, the developmental origins of memory cells remain the subject of considerable debate, but, at least for memory T cells, it is clear that subsets with differing circulatory behaviors and differing potential for immediate effector functions upon re-challenge by antigen are a common feature.

11-18 MHC tetramers and adoptive transfers of clonal T-cell populations have enabled the study of T-cell memory.

Immunological memory can be measured experimentally in various ways. Historically, analysis of T-cell memory relied on *in vivo* or *ex vivo* assays of T-cell function rather than a direct identification of antigen-specific memory T cells. Some assays of T-cell effector function, particularly those of CD4 T cells, such as providing help to B cells or macrophages, can take several days to perform. For this reason, such assays are not optimal for distinguishing memory T cells from preexisting effector cells, because memory cells may be reactivated during the time frame of the assay.

Two general approaches have been employed in recent years to better define the development and general features of antigen-specific memory T cells: adoptive transfers of limited numbers of naive, monoclonal CD4 or CD8 T cells derived from mice carrying specific T-cell receptor (TCR) transgenes of known peptide:MHC specificity that can be tracked during an antigenic challenge (see Appendix I, Section A-31); and the use of MHC tetramers (see Appendix I, Section A-24). In adoptive transfer studies, antibodies specific to the transgenic TCR or a congenic marker expressed by the transferred T cells, but not by the host T cells, allow the transferred cells to be tracked. MHC tetramers measure the frequency of all endogenous clones with a given peptide:MHC specificity but do not distinguish between different T-cell clones of the same specificity. Therefore, they identify a polyclonal population. MHC tetramers were generated for MHC class I molecules first, in the mid-late 1990s, but are now also available for some MHC class II molecules. Although adoptive transfers of TCR-transgenic T cells permits analysis of a single clonal population, this approach is limited to studies in mice, whereas the use of MHC tetramers allows the study of antigen-specific T cells in both mice and in humans.

Studies using both adoptive transfers of TCR-transgenic T cells and MHC tetramers have allowed a direct analysis of population dynamics during the formation and persistence of antigen-specific memory T cells and of their phenotypic and functional characteristics. In the example shown in **Fig. 11.23**, T-cell responses to infection by the intracellular bacteria *Listeria monocytogenes* in mice were analyzed with MHC class II tetramers specific to the toxin **listeriolysin O (LLO)**. In the naive T-cell repertoire of the mouse, there are approximately 100 LLO-specific CD4 T cells, which undergo ~1000-fold expansion into effector T cells during the **expansion phase** of about a week

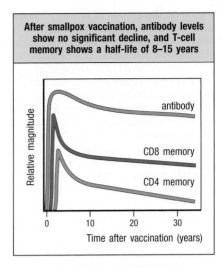

After smallpox vaccination, antibody levels show no significant decline, and T-cell memory shows a half-life of 8–15 years

antibody

CD8 memory

CD4 memory

Relative magnitude

Time after vaccination (years)

Fig. 11.22 Antiviral immunity after smallpox vaccination is long lived. Because smallpox has been eradicated, recall responses measured in people who were vaccinated for smallpox can be taken to represent true memory in the absence of reinfection. After smallpox vaccination, antibody levels show an early peak with a period of rapid decay, which is followed by long-term maintenance that shows minimal decay. CD4 and CD8 T-cell memory is long lived but gradually decays, with a longer half-life for CD8 T cells.

Fig. 11.23 Generation of memory T cells after an infection. After an infection, in this case with an attenuated strain of *Listeria monocytogenes*, the number of T cells specific for the listeriolysin (LLO) virulence factor increases dramatically and then falls back to give a sustained low level of memory T cells. T-cell responses are detected by binding of an MHC tetramer consisting of an LLO peptide bound by I-A^b. The left panel shows the primary response of CD4 T cells that are LLO-specific, and the right panel shows the contraction and memory phase. Approximately 100 T cells in the naive T-cell repertoire expand to about 100,000 effector cells by day 7 (~1000-fold expansion), and then contract to about 7000 memory cells by day 25 (~93% cell loss). These memory cells then slowly decay to ~500 cells by day 450. Data courtesy of Marc Jenkins.

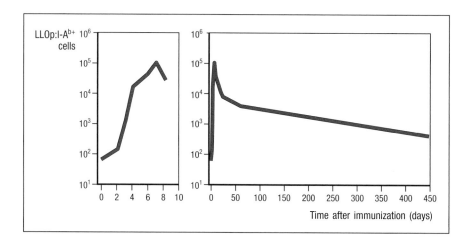

after infection. When the infection is eliminated, a rapid **contraction phase** follows in which LLO-specific T cells are reduced by about 10- to 20-fold over the course of a few weeks. This is followed by a much longer **memory phase**, which results in a population of memory T cells with a half-life of about 60 days, resulting in a frequency about 10-fold higher than that in the naive repertoire after approximately one-half the life span of the mouse (450 days). Similar studies of CD8 T cells in mice infected by lymphocytic choriomeningitis virus (LCMV) show a similar pattern of T-cell expansion, contraction, and memory phases, albeit with greater amplitude of cell number increase at the peak of expansion and in the memory phase, as well as a longer memory-cell half-life.

Studies of humans immunized with the yellow fever virus (YFV) vaccine using peptide:MHC class I tetramers have established that, at least for CD8 T cells, the half-life of individual cells that underwent clonal expansion in response to the YFV vaccine was approximately 3 months, and the average half-life of cell division of these cells was over a year during the memory phase. Thus, memory CD8 T cells in humans demonstrate remarkably slow cell turnover, surviving for extended periods without a requirement for cell division. Accordingly, at any point in time the large majority of memory cells are in an intermitotic phase. In comparison, mouse memory CD8 T cells divide, on average, about 10 times more frequently than memory CD8 T cells in humans, although still quite infrequently.

11-19 The developmental origins of memory T cells parallel those of effector T cells.

Characterization of the numbers and functions of clonal T-cell populations enabled by adoptive transfer and the use of MHC tetramers has established that while there is substantial heterogeneity in the output of the clonal T-cell response, in comparison to their naive precursors the number of memory T cells that persist long-term after antigen clearance is approximately 10- to 100-fold higher. Moreover, at the population level, memory T cells are more sensitive to antigen, they proliferate more rapidly and robustly in response to the same antigen dose, and they more rapidly display heightened effector responses (for example, production of IFN-γ) compared to their naive precursors. Thus, the clonal progeny of naive T cells that become long-lived memory T cells persist at increased numbers and with increased functional capabilities. As we will see in the next section, memory T cells also have a greater range of surveillance capabilities compared to naive T cells; that is, they are not restricted to searching for antigen in secondary lymphoid tissues (see Section 11-20). Collectively, these properties provide a basis for more rapid and effective clonal T-cell responses in secondary and subsequent challenges by the same antigen.

The precise origins of the small fraction of cells that persist as memory T cells as the effector T-cell response subsides has been difficult to determine. Despite approaches that allow the tracking of clonal populations over the course of infection and after its resolution, the heterogeneous nature of the clonal response and the relative rarity of long-lived memory cells has made delineation of memory T-cell development challenging. However, two general models for memory T-cell development have gained favor (**Fig. 11.24**). In one model, often referred to as the **linear model of memory-cell development**, memory T cells arise from effector T cells as the primary immune response subsides. In a second model, often referred to as the **branching (or asymmetric division) model of memory-cell development**, an antigen-activated naive T cell gives rise to daughter cells that preferentially commit to either the effector- or memory-cell program.

Of course, as with many models of lineage development, these two models are not mutually exclusive, and the developmental origins of individual memory T cells may combine features of both. However, key experimental observations using adoptive transfer studies of CD4 or CD8 T cells in mice indicate that at least some memory T cells arise from effector T-cell precursors, supporting the linear model. In one study that tracked the fate of T_H1 cells and CTLs that expressed an IFN-γ reporter transgene in response to LCMV infection, memory T cells arose from both CD4 and CD8 effector T cells that expressed the IFN-γ

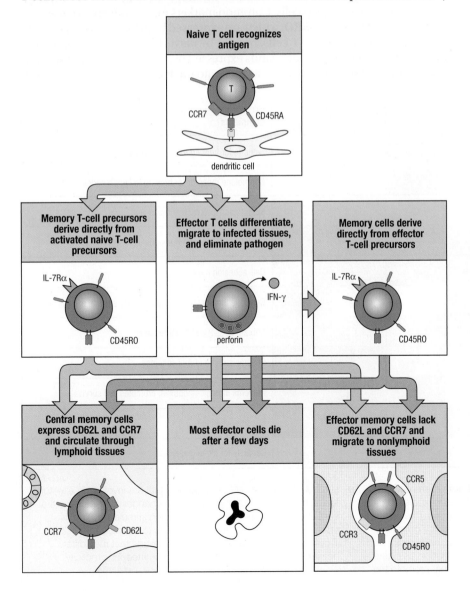

Fig. 11.24 Alternative models for the development of central memory T (T_{CM}) cell and effector memory T (T_{EM}) cell subsets. Memory T cells can arise from activated effector cells (linear model of memory-cell development; red arrows) or directly from activated naive T cells (asymmetric, or branching, model of memory-cell development; green arrows). In both models, most effector T cells generated in a primary response die after the primary response. Two types of memory T cells can arise from a primary T-cell response, irrespective of their origins: central memory T (T_{CM}) cells and effector memory T (T_{EM}) cells. Central memory cells (T_{CM}) express CD62L and CCR7 and recirculate in peripheral lymphoid tissues similarly to naive T cells. When they recognize antigen in lymphoid tissues, a recall response is initiated, and the cells rapidly undergo effector T-cell differentiation over the course of days. Effector memory cells (T_{EM}) lack CD62L and CCR7 and recirculate primarily in blood. They are rapidly recruited into inflamed tissues where they initiate effector T-cell responses after restimulation by cognate antigen. Note that these two models are not mutually exclusive. That is, in a given immune response, both pathways may contribute to the memory T-cell pool.

reporter, demonstrating that long-lived memory CD4 and CD8 T cells could arise from effector T cells. In a second study, it was found that epigenetic repression of genes universally expressed by naive but not effector CD8 T cells, including those encoding L-selectin (CD62L), CCR7, and the IL-7 receptor (CD127), was reversed in memory cells that also bore epigenetic imprinting of genes indicative of mature CTL differentiation—IFN-γ, perforin, and granzymes. This study concluded that memory T cells could arise by 'dedifferentiation' of effector T cells, thereby re-acquiring at least some characteristics of naive T cells. Although these studies did not refute the branching model of memory-cell development, they indicate that at least some memory T cells arise from effector T cells.

11-20 Memory T cells are heterogeneous and include central memory, effector memory, and tissue-resident subsets.

Changes in cell-surface proteins that occur on memory T cells are significant and have been used to characterize major subsets with different tissue recirculation and recall characteristics (**Fig. 11.25**). While some surface molecules are common to all memory T cells, others are subset-specific and identify memory T cells that share properties with naive or effector T cells. Three subsets of memory T cells have been identified. They include both CD4 and CD8 T cells: **central memory T (T_{CM})** cells; **effector memory T (T_{EM})** cells; and **tissue-resident memory T (T_{RM})** cells. Common markers for all antigen-experienced T cells are **CD44** and **CD45RO**, which are expressed both by effector T cells and by each subset of memory T cells, but not by naive T cells. CD44 is a receptor for hyaluronic acid and other ligands expressed by endothelial cells and extracellular matrix glycoproteins; it may facilitate the localization of these cells to

Protein/Function	Naive	Effector	T_{CM}	T_{EM}	T_{RM}	Comments
CD62L	+++	–	+++	–	–	Selectin for homing to lymph nodes
CCR7	+++	–	+++	–	–	Chemokine receptor for homing to lymph nodes
CD45RA	+++	+	+	+	+	Modulates T-cell receptor signaling
CD45R0	+	+++	+++	+++	+++	Modulates T-cell receptor signaling
CD44	+	+++	+++	+++	+++	Cell-adhesion molecule
CD69	–	+++	–	–	+++	C-type lectin; down-modulates S1PR1 surface expression
CD122	+	++	++	++	++	Subunit of IL-2 and IL-15 receptors
CD127	++	–	++	+++	+++	Specific subunit of IL-7 receptor
Bcl-2	++	+/–	+++	+++	+++	Prevents intrinsic apoptosis; promotes cell survival
IFN-γ, IL-4, or IL-17	–	+++	+	++	+++	Effector cytokines
Proliferation	+++	+	+++	++	+	Capacity for clonal expansion

Fig. 11.25 Expression of many proteins alters when naive T cells become memory T cells. Proteins that are expressed differently in naive T cells, effector T cells, and memory T cell subsets (T_{CM}, T_{EM}, and T_{RM}) include adhesion molecules, which govern interactions with antigen-presenting cells and endothelial cells; chemokine receptors, which affect migration to lymphoid tissues and sites of inflammation; proteins and receptors that promote the survival of memory cells; and proteins that are involved in effector functions, such as granzyme B. Some changes also increase the sensitivity of the memory T cell to antigen stimulation. This list represents a general picture that applies to both CD4 and CD8 T cells in mice and humans, but some details that may differ between these sets of cells have been omitted for simplicity.

peripheral tissues, although its exact function is not known. Different isoforms of **CD45**, a cell-surface tyrosine phosphatase expressed on all hematopoietic cells, are also useful in distinguishing naive from effector and memory T cells. In humans, the CD45RO isoform identifies effector and memory cells and is produced by alternative splicing that removes three exons encoded in the CD45 extracellular domain, whereas the **CD45RA** isoform includes at least one of these exons and identifies naive T cells. The functional consequences of the alternatively spliced isoforms are unclear.

Surface markers that distinguish memory T-cell subsets are related to recirculation and tissue localization and reflect the different surveillance patterns of each of the three major subsets (**Fig. 11.26**). Each subset has distinct activation characteristics. T_{CM} cells are characterized by expression of L-selectin (CD62L) and CCR7, which are also expressed by naive T cells, and direct their recirculation through the T-cell zones of secondary lymphoid tissues (see Section 9-3). T_{CM} cells primarily migrate from the blood into the secondary lymphoid organs, then into the lymphatic system and back into the blood, a migratory pattern like that of naive T cells. However, T_{CM} cells differ from naive T cells in their heightened sensitivity to antigen recognition and rapid expression of CD40 ligand (CD40L) in recall responses, although they are slower to acquire other effector functions (for example, production of cytokines) compared with other memory subsets. T_{EM} cells lack expression of L-selectin (CD62L) and CCR7 but express high levels of β_1 and β_2 integrins, and so are specialized for rapidly entering inflamed tissues. They also express receptors for inflammatory chemokines and can rapidly mature into effector T cells that secrete large amounts of effector cytokines (for example, IFN-γ, IL-4, or IL-17) early after restimulation with antigen. At steady state, many T_{EM} cells appear to

Fig. 11.26 Naive and memory T cells have distinct migratory patterns, enabling their surveillance of different tissue compartments for infection. Like naive T cells, T_{CM} cells recirculate between blood, the T-cell zones of secondary lymphoid organs, and lymph. T_{EM} cells recirculate between nonlymphoid tissues, lymph, lymph nodes (where they might pass through via the sinuses without entering the T-cell zone), and blood; some T_{EM} cells remain in blood circulation and migrate only through the spleen. T_{RM} cells do not recirculate but rather are confined to a single tissue.

recirculate primarily in blood, bypassing secondary lymphoid organs, except the spleen, altogether. However, a recently identified subset of T_{EM} cells that is distinguished by expression of intermediate levels of the chemokine receptor CX3CR1 (CX3CR1^{int}) can migrate at steady state from the blood into peripheral nonlymphoid tissues, and then via lymphatics and secondary lymphoid tissues back to blood (see Fig. 11.26). This subset of T_{EM} cells, referred to as peripheral memory T (T_{PM}) cells, has been described only for CD8 T cells and would appear suited for surveillance of nonlymphoid tissues.

In contrast to central and effector memory cells, T_{RM} cells compose a substantial fraction of memory T cells that do not migrate, but rather take up long-term residency in various barrier sites (see Fig. 11.26 and **Fig. 11.27**). Like T_{EM} cells, T_{RM} cells lack CCR7 but express other chemokine receptors (for example, CXCR3, CCR9) that allow migration into peripheral tissues, such as the dermis or lamina propria of the intestine. In these sites, T_{RM} cells express CD69, which reduces S1PR1 expression, thereby promoting retention in tissues. Some T_{RM} cells, particularly CD8 T_{RM} cells, can enter and reside within the epithelium of barrier tissues (for example, skin and GI tract). TGF-β production by epithelial cells induces T_{RM} to express integrin $\alpha_E\beta_7$ (CD103), which binds E-cadherin expressed by the epithelium and is required for T_{RM} retention. Because T_{RM} cells resemble effector T cells in being rapidly responsive to either TCR signaling or cytokines (see Section 11-13), they function in many ways like ILCs. That is, they are tissue-resident, sensor-responder cells that provide local tissue surveillance and can initiate a particular immune module response locally and rapidly upon pathogen challenge—whether by the same pathogen to which they initially responded or by other pathogens of the same class. However, unlike ILCs, T_{RM} cells are not seeded into nonlymphoid tissues developmentally, rather they seed nonlymphoid tissues only after a T-cell effector response in that tissue. Although T_{RM} cells are confined to nonlymphoid tissues, they are not static within these tissues; they continually migrate slowly within their nonlymphoid tissue of residence, actively surveying for signals that indicate a pathogen threat.

Fig. 11.27 Tissue-resident memory T cells are a major immune compartment that surveys peripheral tissues for reinfection by pathogens. After activation and priming in lymphoid tissues, activated CD8 and CD4 T cells enter the blood and enter tissues in response to various chemokines, as shown here for entry into the dermis, guided by expression of CXCR3. The reexpression of CD69 by T cells caused by antigen or other unknown signals leads to decreased S1PR1 surface expression, promoting retention of these cells in the dermis. In response to TGF-β, some cells induce integrin $\alpha_E\beta_7$ (CD103), which binds E-cadherin expressed by epithelial cells, promoting entry and retention of T cells in the epidermis, where many CD8 T_{RM} cells reside. Estimates indicate that T_{RM} cells may outnumber the recirculating T cells that migrate through the body.

The distinction between T_{CM}, T_{EM}, and T_{RM} memory populations has been made both in humans and in the mouse. However, within each subset there may be further heterogeneity. For example, among the CCR7-expressing T_{CM} population are cells with differing expression of other markers, particularly chemokine receptors. A subset of the CCR7-positive T_{CM} cells also expresses CXCR5, similarly to T_{FH} cells, although it is not yet clear whether these memory cells can provide help to B cells in the germinal center. Moreover, there is interconversion between memory T-cell subsets. Thus, on restimulation by cognate antigen, T_{CM} cells can rapidly lose expression of CCR7 and differentiate into T_{EM} cells. T_{EM} cells are also heterogeneous in the chemokine receptors they express and have been classified according to chemokine receptors typical of T_H1 cells (CCR5), T_H17 cells (CCR6), and T_H2 cells (CCR4). T_{CM} cells do not appear committed to particular effector lineages, and even T_{EM} cells are not fully committed to the T_H1, T_H17, or T_H2 lineage, although there is some correlation between their eventual output of T_H1, T_H17, or T_H2 cells and the chemokine receptors expressed. Further stimulation with antigen seems to drive the differentiation of T_{EM} cells gradually into the distinct effector T-cell lineages.

11-21 Circulating memory T cells acquire heightened sensitivity to IL-7 and/or IL-15 and undergo metabolic reprogramming to survive long-term.

A principal feature of circulating memory T cells (T_{CM} and T_{EM} cells) is their longevity without a requirement for antigenic stimulation. They share with naive T cells two attributes that promote their long-term survival: expression of receptors for pro-survival cytokines and altered metabolic programming. Like naive T cells, circulating memory T cells express the α subunit of the IL-7 receptor (IL-7Rα, or CD127), which pairs with constitutively expressed common γ chain (γ_c; CD132) to allow them to respond to the pro-survival cytokine IL-7. Expression of IL-7Rα is down-regulated during effector T-cell differentiation but is retained or reacquired by those cells destined to become memory T cells. The importance of IL-7Rα in the maintenance of T cells that become long-term survivors after their response to antigen has been demonstrated in multiple studies. For example, the experiment shown in **Fig. 11.28** examines mice infected with lymphocytic choriomeningitis virus (LCMV). Around day 7

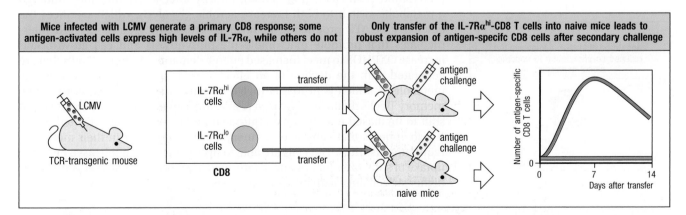

Fig. 11.28 Expression of the IL-7 receptor (IL-7Rα) indicates which CD8 effector T cells can generate robust memory responses. Mice expressing a T-cell receptor (TCR) transgene specific for a viral antigen from lymphocytic choriomeningitis virus (LCMV) were infected with the virus, and effector cells were collected on day 11. Effector CD8 T cells expressing high levels of IL-7Rα (IL-7Rα^{hi}; blue) were separated and transferred into one group of naive mice, and effector CD8 T cells expressing low IL-7Rα (IL-7Rα^{lo}; green) were transferred into another group. Three weeks after transfer, the mice were challenged with a bacterium engineered to express the original viral antigen, and the numbers of responding transferred T cells (detected by their expression of the transgenic TCR) were measured at various times after challenge. Only the transferred IL-7Rα^{hi} effector cells could generate a robust expansion of CD8 T cells after the secondary challenge.

Fig. 11.29 Memory and naive T cells have different requirements for survival. For their survival in the periphery, naive T cells require periodic stimulation with the cytokine IL-7 and with self antigens presented by self MHC molecules. On priming with its specific antigen, a naive T cell divides and differentiates. Most of the progeny differentiate into relatively short-lived effector cells that have lost expression of the IL-7 receptor (green), but some effector cells retain or reexpress the receptor and become long-lived memory T cells. These cells can be maintained by IL-7 (and in some cases, IL-15; not shown) and are less dependent on contact with self peptide:self MHC complexes for survival compared with naive T cells. APC, antigen-presenting cell.

after infection, a small population of approximately 5% of CD8 antigen-activated T cells express high levels of IL-7Rα. Adoptive transfer of these IL-7Rα^{hi} cells, but not IL-7Rα^{lo} effector T cells, provided functional CD8 T-cell memory to uninfected mice. This experiment suggests that memory T cells arise from effector T cells that maintain or reexpress IL-7Rα, perhaps because they compete more effectively for the survival signals delivered by IL-7. Indeed, memory T cells are more sensitive to IL-7 signaling than are naive T cells, due at least in part to their higher expression of IL-7Rα (see Fig. 11.25). As discussed in Section 11-16, this leads to increased expression of the anti-apoptotic factor Bcl-2, which is also increased in memory T cells compared to naive T cells.

In addition to IL-7, a subset of memory CD8 T cells also requires IL-15 for survival. Consequently, whereas both CD4 and CD8 circulating memory T cells require IL-7 for survival, some CD8 T cells also require IL-15 for survival. Further, as illustrated in **11.29**, while naive T cells require contact with self peptide:self MHC complexes in addition to cytokine stimulation for their long-term survival, it appears that memory T cells are less dependent on contact with self peptide:self MHC than are naive T cells. Nevertheless, memory T cells still respond to contact with peptide:MHC complexes to become reactivated during a secondary encounter with pathogen, but they are more sensitive to restimulation by antigen than are naive T cells, at least in part due to their higher expression of the co-stimulatory receptor CD28. As noted previously, memory T cells, particularly T$_{RM}$ cells, may be activated in a 'bystander' manner by certain inflammatory cytokines; that is, without a requirement for antigen stimulation—akin to ILCs.

As discussed in Chapter 9, a shift in T-cell metabolism accompanies the developmental transition from naive to effector T cells (see Section 9-9). Naive T cells are quiescent and depend primarily on glycolysis for oxidative phosphorylation (OXPHOS) (**Fig. 11.30**). Shortly after activation, they undergo a metabolic switch to both increase aerobic glycolysis, which sacrifices the efficiency of ATP production in favor of producing glucose-derived intermediates that promote macromolecule biosynthesis and cell growth, and increase OXPHOS to meet increased energy demands. Memory T cells that are generated with the decline of an effector response revert to a low-energy metabolism, which is primarily fueled by fatty acids, not glucose. However, memory T cells retain an increased respiratory capacity to enable a more rapid shift to increased energy consumption should they become activated again. It also appears that subsets of memory T cells may differ in their metabolic requirements. Thus, T$_{RM}$ cells are able to up-regulate mechanisms to enhance uptake of substrates for enhanced fatty acid oxidation, perhaps reflecting their higher surveillance activity at homeostasis.

11-22 CD4 T-cell help is required for CD8 T-cell memory and involves CD40 and IL-2 signaling.

There is experimental evidence that CD4 T cells play an important role in programming optimal CD8 T-cell memory. In the experiment shown in **Fig. 11.31**, the primary and memory CD8 T-cell responses were compared between wild-type mice and mice that lack expression of MHC class II, and which therefore

Naive T cell	Effector T cell	Memory T cell
T-cell activation Hours	Effector T cells Days	Memory T cells Weeks to years
Metabolic reprograming Cell-cycle entry	Rapid cell division Effector differentiation	Homeostatic proliferation Long-lived memory

■ **Glycolysis**   ■ **Oxidative phosphorylation**   □ **Fatty acid oxidation**

Fig. 11.30 The differentiation of naive T cells into effector and memory T cells is accompanied by shifts in their metabolism. Naive T cells have very low energetic demands that are met by a low-level oxidative phosphorylation (OXPHOS; represented by blue shading) within mitochondria of pyruvate that is derived from the breakdown (glycolysis; red shading) of glucose—their principal energy source—but also from a limited oxidation of acetyl-CoA that is derived from fatty acids (fatty acid oxidation, or FAO; yellow). Upon activation, T cells undergo a shift from a catabolic to anabolic metabolism to accommodate their impending transition to rapid cell division necessary for clonal expansion and effector differentiation. The increased need for macromolecule biosynthesis (for example, DNA, ribosomal RNA, proteins) is met by an increase in glycolysis, which, together with an increase in OXPHOS, provides the increased biosynthetic and energetic needs of developing effector T cells. (The height of the colored panels denotes the relative capacity of the indicated pathways.) As the T-cell response wanes, the surviving memory T cells shift their metabolism back to a catabolic state dominated by low energy consumption fueled principally by FAO, not glycolysis. However, memory T cells retain an increased number and functional reserve of mitochondria, and thus greater respiratory capacity to enable long-term survival and a rapid transition to a proliferative, anabolic metabolism upon antigen reencounter.

have a defect in CD4 T cells. In this experiment, the CD8 T-cell response was measured against a protein, ovalbumin, carried by an experimental strain of *Listeria monocytogenes*. After 7 days of infection, both types of mice showed equivalent expansion and activity of antigen-specific effector CD8 T cells. But mice with a defect in CD4 T cells generated much weaker secondary responses, characterized by the presence of far fewer expanding memory CD8 T cells after a secondary challenge. These results imply a role for CD4 T cells either in the initial programming of CD8 T cells or during the secondary memory response.

Further experiments suggest that this CD4 T-cell help for generation of memory CD8 T cells is necessary during the initial priming of naive CD8 T cells. Memory CD8 T cells that developed in the absence of CD4 help were transferred into wild-type mice. After transfer, the recipient mice were challenged again, whereupon the CD8 T cells showed a reduced ability to proliferate even though the recipient mice expressed MHC class II. This result indicates that CD4 T-cell help is required during the priming of CD8 T cells and not simply at the time of secondary responses. This requirement for CD4 help in CD8 memory generation has also been demonstrated by experiments in which CD4 T cells were depleted by treatment with antibody or in which mice were deficient in the CD4 gene.

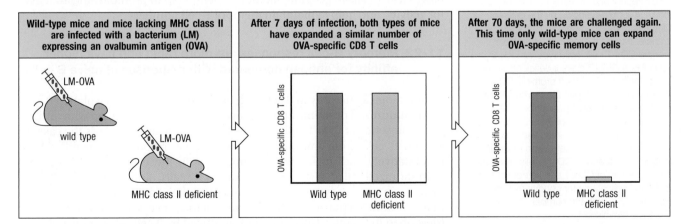

Fig. 11.31 CD4 T cells are required for the development of functional CD8 memory T cells. Mice that do not express MHC class II molecules (MHC class II deficient) fail to develop CD4 T cells. Wild-type and MHC class II–deficient mice were infected with *Listeria monocytogenes* expressing the model antigen ovalbumin (LM-OVA). After 7 days, the number of OVA-specific CD8 T cells can be measured by using specific MHC tetramers that contain an OVA peptide, and therefore bind to T-cell receptors that react with

this antigen. After 7 days of infection, mice lacking CD4 T cells were found to have the same number of OVA-specific CD8 T cells as wild-type mice. However, when mice were allowed to recover for 60 days—a time during which memory T cells could develop—and were then re-challenged with LM-OVA, the mice lacking CD4 T cells failed to expand CD8 memory cells specific to OVA, whereas there was a strong CD8 memory response in the wild-type mice.

Memory CD8 T cells are allowed to develop in mice infected with LCMV

LCMV

LCMV-specific CD8 memory T cells are transferred into wild-type mice and mice that lack CD4 T cells due to absence of MHC class II

CD8 T cells

CD8 T cells

wild-type mouse

MHC class II–deficient mouse

Memory CD8 T cells are maintained in mice with CD4 T cells, but not in mice that lack CD4 T cells

Number of CD8 memory T cells

20   40   60

Time (days)

Fig. 11.32 CD4 T cells promote the maintenance of CD8 memory cells. The dependence of memory CD8 T cells on CD4 T cells is shown by the different lifetimes of the memory cells after their transfer into host mice that either have normal CD4 T cells (wild type) or lack CD4 T cells (MHC class II deficient). In the absence of MHC class II proteins, CD4 T cells fail to develop in the thymus. When CD8 memory T cells specific for LCMV were isolated from donor mice 35 days after infection with the virus and transferred into these hosts, memory cells were maintained only in mice that had CD4 T cells. The basis for this action of CD4 T cells is not yet clear but has implications for conditions such as HIV/AIDS in which the number of CD4 T cells is diminished.

The mechanism underlying this requirement for CD4 T cells is not completely understood, although recent studies indicate that the CD8 and CD4 T cells must be activated by the same dendritic cell. Specifically, CD4 T-cell 'help' for CD8 T-cell memory generation appears to occur in the context of antigen presentation by lymph-node resident cDC1 cells that receive antigen from migratory cDCs and recruit primed CD4 cells for help. It may involve two types of signals received by the CD8 T cell from the CD4 T cell that is activated on the same cDC1 cell—those received through CD40 and those received through the IL-2 receptor. CD8 T cells that do not express CD40 are unable to generate memory T cells. Although many cells could potentially express the CD40 ligand needed to stimulate CD40, CD4 T cells are most likely the source of this signal.

A requirement for IL-2 signaling in the programming of CD8 memory was discovered by using CD8 T cells that were unable to respond to IL-2 because of a genetic deficiency in the IL-2Rα subunit. Because IL-2Rα signaling is required for the development of T_{reg} cells, mice lacking IL-2Rα develop a lymphoproliferative disorder. However, this disorder does not develop in mice that are mixed bone-marrow chimeras harboring both wild-type and IL-2Rα–deficient cells, and these chimeras can be used to study the behavior of IL-2Rα–deficient cells. When these chimeric mice were infected with LCMV and their responses were tested, memory CD8 responses were found to be defective specifically in the T cells lacking IL-2Rα.

The experiment shown in **Fig. 11.32** indicates that distinct from their effect in programming naive CD8 T cells, CD4 T cells also provide help in maintaining the number of CD8 memory T cells. In this case, CD8 memory T cells that had been programmed in normal mice were transferred into immunologically naive mice that either expressed or lacked MHC class II. Transfer of CD8 memory cells into mice lacking MHC class II resulted in a more rapid decrease in the number of memory CD8 T cells in comparison with a similar transfer into wild-type mice. In addition, CD8 effector cells transferred into mice lacking MHC class II had a relative impairment of CD8 effector functions. These experiments imply that CD4 T cells activated by MHC class II–expressing antigen-presenting cells during an immune response have a significant impact on the quantity and quality of the CD8 T-cell response, even when they are not needed for the initial CD8 T-cell activation. Thus, CD4 T cells help to program naive CD8 T cells to generate memory T cells, help to promote efficient effector activity, and help to maintain memory T-cell numbers.

11-23 Memory B-cell responses are more rapid and have higher affinity for antigen compared with responses of naive B cells.

Immunological memory in B cells can be examined *in vitro* by isolating B cells from immunized or unimmunized mice and restimulating them with antigen in the presence of CD4 T cells specific for the same antigen. As is the case for T cells, B cells from immunized mice produce responses that differ both quantitatively and qualitatively compared with those of naive B cells from unimmunized mice (**Fig. 11.33**). Akin to T cells, antigen-specific B cells increase in frequency by up to 100-fold after their initial priming in the primary immune response. Further, because of the process of affinity maturation (described in Chapter 10), antibodies produced by B cells of immunized mice typically have a higher affinity for antigen than that of antibodies produced by unprimed B lymphocytes. The response from immunized mice is due to **memory B cells** that arise in the primary response.

Memory B cells can arise from the germinal center reaction during a primary response and may have undergone isotype switching and somatic mutations there. But memory B cells can also arise independently of the germinal center reaction from short-lived, antibody-producing cells produced in the primary

	Source of B cells	
	Unimmunized donor **Primary response**	**Immunized donor** **Secondary response**
Frequency of antigen-specific B cells	$1:10^4$ to $1:10^5$	$1:10^2$ to $1:10^3$
Isotype of antibody produced	IgM > IgG	IgG, IgA
Affinity of antibody	Low	High
Somatic hypermutation	Low	High

Fig. 11.33 The generation of secondary antibody responses from memory B cells is distinct from the generation of the primary antibody response. These responses can be studied and compared by isolating B cells from immunized and unimmunized donor mice and stimulating them in culture in the presence of antigen-specific effector T cells. The primary response usually consists of antibody molecules made by plasma cells derived from a quite diverse population of precursor B cells specific for different epitopes of the antigen and with receptors that have a range of affinities for the antigen. The antibodies are of relatively low affinity overall, with few somatic mutations. The secondary response derives from a far more limited population of high-affinity B cells that have undergone significant clonal expansion. Their receptors and antibodies have high affinity for the antigen and show extensive somatic mutation. The overall effect is that although there is usually only a 10- to 100-fold increase in the frequency of activatable B cells after priming, the quality of the antibody response is radically altered, in that these precursors induce a far more intense and effective response.

response. In either case, they circulate through the blood and take up residence in the spleen and lymph nodes, where they are poised to generate more rapid and robust antibody production in recall responses. Memory B cells express some markers that distinguish them from naive B cells and plasma cells. One marker of memory B cells is simply the expression of a class-switched surface immunoglobulin isotype (that is, IgG, IgA, or IgE); naive B cells express only surface IgM and IgD. In contrast, plasma cells have very low surface immunoglobulin altogether. In humans, a useful marker of memory B cells is **CD27**, a member of the TNF receptor family that is also expressed by naive T cells and binds the TNF family ligand **CD70**, which is expressed by dendritic cells (see Section 9-13).

A primary antibody response is characterized by the initial, rapid production of IgM and a slightly delayed IgG response due to time required for class switching (**Fig. 11.34**). The secondary antibody response is characterized in its first few days by the production of relatively small amounts of IgM antibody and much larger amounts of IgG antibody, with some IgA and IgE. At the beginning of the secondary response, antibodies are made by memory B cells that were generated in the primary response and have already switched from IgM

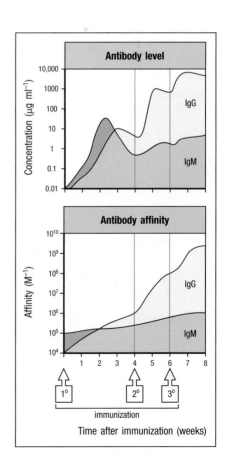

Fig. 11.34 Both the affinity and the amount of antibody increase with repeated immunization. The upper panel shows the increase in antibody concentration with time after primary (1°), secondary (2°), and tertiary (3°) immunizations. The lower panel shows the increase in the affinity of the antibodies (affinity maturation). Affinity maturation is seen largely in IgG antibody (as well as in IgA and IgE, which are not shown) coming from mature B cells that have undergone isotype switching and somatic hypermutation to yield higher-affinity antibodies. The blue shading represents IgM on its own, the yellow shading IgG, and the green shading the presence of both IgG and IgM. Although some affinity maturation occurs in the primary antibody response, most arises in later responses to repeated antigen injections. Note that these graphs are on a logarithmic scale; it would otherwise be impossible to represent the overall increase of around 1 millionfold in the concentration of specific IgG antibody from its initial level.

to another isotype (IgG, IgA, or IgE) that is expressed on their surface. This is reminiscent of the accelerated effector T-cell responses made by CD4 T_{EM} cells that are generated in a primary response and activated to generate a rapid T_H1, T_H2, or T_H17 cytokine response upon recall. Memory B cells express somewhat higher levels of MHC class II molecules and the co-stimulatory ligand B7.1 than do naive B cells. This helps memory B cells acquire and present antigen more efficiently to T_{FH} cells than do naive B cells, thereby recruiting more rapid and robust T-cell help to accelerate and increase antibody production compared with primary responses. The secondary response is characterized by a more vigorous and earlier generation of plasma cells than in the primary response, thus accounting for the almost immediate abundant production of IgG (see Fig. 11.34).

11-24 Memory B cells can reenter germinal centers and undergo additional somatic hypermutation and affinity maturation during secondary immune responses.

During a secondary exposure to infection, antibodies persisting from a primary immune response are available immediately to bind the pathogen and mark it for degradation by complement or by phagocytes. If the antibody can completely neutralize the pathogen, a secondary immune response may not occur. Otherwise, excess antigens will bind to receptors on B cells and initiate a secondary response in the secondary lymphoid organs. Memory B cells recirculate through the same secondary lymphoid compartments as naive B cells, principally the follicles of the spleen, lymph nodes, and the Peyer's patches of the gut mucosa. B cells with the highest avidity for antigen are activated first. Thus, memory B cells, which were selected previously for their avidity to antigen, make up a substantial component of the secondary response.

Besides responding more rapidly, memory B cells can reenter germinal centers during secondary immune responses and undergo additional somatic hypermutation and affinity maturation, as described in Sections 10-6 through 10-8. As in primary responses, secondary B-cell responses begin at the interface between the T-cell and B-cell zones, where memory B cells that have acquired antigen can present peptide:MHC class II complexes to helper T cells. This interaction initiates proliferation of both the B cells and T cells. Reactivated memory B cells that have not yet undergone differentiation into plasma cells migrate into the follicle and become germinal center B cells, undergoing additional rounds of proliferation and somatic hypermutation before differentiating into antibody-secreting plasma cells. Because B cells with the higher-affinity antigen receptors will more efficiently acquire and present antigen to antigen-specific T_{FH} cells in the germinal center, the affinity of the antibodies produced during secondary and tertiary responses rises progressively (see Fig. 10.14).

11-25 In immune individuals, secondary and subsequent responses are mainly attributable to memory lymphocytes.

In the normal course of an infection, a pathogen proliferates to a level sufficient to elicit an adaptive immune response and then stimulates the production of effector T cells and antibodies that eliminate the pathogen from the body. Most of the effector T cells then die, and antibody levels gradually decline, because the antigens that elicited the response are no longer present at the level needed to sustain it. We can think of this as feedback inhibition of the response. Memory T and B cells remain, however, and maintain a heightened ability to mount a response to a recurrence of infection with the same pathogen.

Antibody and memory lymphocytes remaining in an immunized individual can have the effect of reducing the activation of naive T and B cells on a subsequent encounter with the same antigen. In fact, passively transferring antibody to a naive recipient can be used to inhibit naive B-cell responses to that same antigen. This phenomenon has been put to practical use to prevent Rh⁻ mothers from making an immune response to an Rh⁺ fetus, which can result in **hemolytic disease of the newborn** (see Appendix I, Section A-7). If anti-Rh antibody is given to the mother before she is first exposed to her child's Rh⁺ red blood cells, her response will be inhibited. The mechanism of this suppression is likely to involve the antibody-mediated clearance and destruction of fetal red blood cells that have entered the mother, thus preventing naive T cells and B cells from mounting an immune response. Presumably, the anti-Rh antibody is in excess over antigen, so that not only is antigen eliminated, but immune complexes are not formed to stimulate naive B cells through Fc receptors. Memory B-cell responses are, however, not inhibited by antibody, so the Rh⁻ mothers at risk must be identified and treated before a primary response has occurred. Because of their high affinity for antigen and alterations in their B-cell receptor signaling requirements, memory B cells are much more sensitive to the small amounts of antigen that cannot be efficiently cleared by the passive anti-Rh antibody. The ability of memory B cells to be activated to produce antibody, even when exposed to preexisting antibody, also allows secondary antibody responses to occur in individuals who are already immune.

These suppressive mechanisms might also explain a phenomenon called **original antigenic sin**. This term was coined to describe the tendency of people to make antibodies only against the epitopes expressed on the first influenza virus variant to which they are exposed, even in subsequent infections with viral variants that have additional, highly immunogenic, epitopes (**Fig. 11.35**). Antibodies against the original virus will tend to suppress responses of naive B cells specific for the new epitopes. This might benefit the host by using only those B cells that can respond most rapidly and effectively to the virus. This pattern is broken only if the person is exposed to an influenza virus that lacks all epitopes seen in the original infection, because now no preexisting antibodies bind the virus, and naive B cells are able to respond.

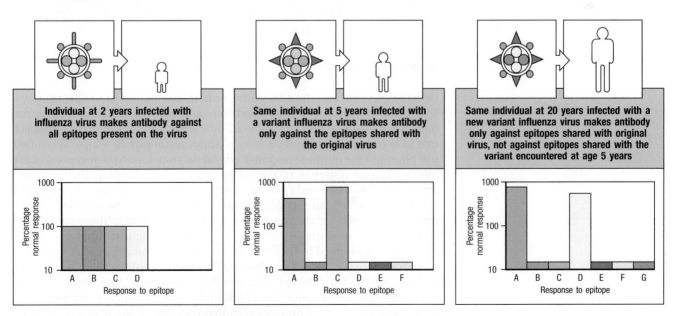

Fig. 11.35 When individuals who have been infected with one variant of influenza virus are infected with a second or third variant, they make antibodies only against epitopes that were present on the initial virus. A child infected for the first time with an influenza virus at 2 years of age makes a response to all epitopes (left panel). At age 5 years, the same child exposed to a different influenza virus responds preferentially to those epitopes shared with the original virus and makes a smaller than normal response to new epitopes on the virus (center panel). Even at age 20 years, this commitment to respond to epitopes shared with the original virus, and the subnormal response to new epitopes, is retained (right panel). This phenomenon is called original antigenic sin.

A similar suppression of naive T-cell responses by antigen-specific memory T cells can occur in the setting of infection by LCMV in the mouse or dengue virus in humans. Mice that were primed with one strain of LCMV responded to a subsequent infection with a second strain of LCMV by expanding CD8 T cells that reacted to antigens specific for the first strain. However, this type of effect was not observed when responses to variable ovalbumin antigenic epitopes were examined in the setting of recurrent infections using the bacterial pathogen *Listeria monocytogenes*, suggesting that the suppression caused by 'original antigenic sin' does not occur in all immune responses.

Summary.

Protective immunity against reinfection is one of the most important consequences of adaptive immunity and results from the establishment of populations of long-lived memory B cells and memory T cells. These antigen-specific memory cells arise from the populations of lymphocytes that expand dramatically during the primary infection and survive at higher frequencies than naive lymphocytes. Both their increased frequency and their capacity to respond more rapidly to restimulation by the same antigen contribute to protective immunity, which can be transferred to naive recipients by memory B and T cells. Memory lymphocytes are maintained by their expression of receptors for cytokines, such as IL-7 and IL-15, that provide survival signals. Memory B cells can be distinguished by changes in their immunoglobulin genes that are due to isotype switching and somatic hypermutation; secondary and subsequent immune responses are characterized by antibodies with increasing affinity for the antigen. The advent of receptor-specific reagents, such as MHC tetramers and TCR transgenic mice, has allowed for the direct analysis of the expansion and differentiation of effector and memory T cells. We now recognize that T-cell memory is complex, and memory T cells are quite heterogeneous, having central memory, effector memory, and tissue-resident memory subtypes. While CD8 T cells can generate effective primary responses in the absence of help from CD4 T cells, CD4 T cells have an integral role in regulating CD8 T-cell memory. These issues will be critical in understanding, for example, how to design more effective vaccines for diseases such as HIV/AIDS that depend on CTL responses for pathogen clearance.

Summary to Chapter 11.

Vertebrates resist infection by pathogenic microorganisms in several ways. The innate defenses can act immediately and may succeed in repelling the infection, but if not, they are followed by a series of induced early responses that help to contain the infection as adaptive immunity develops. These first two phases of the immune response rely on the nonclonotypic receptors of the innate immune system to recognize the presence of infection. They are summarized in **Fig. 11.36** and covered in detail in Chapters 2 and 3, respectively. Several specialized subsets of immune cells, which can be viewed as intermediates between innate and adaptive immunity, act next. These specialized subsets include the innate lymphoid cells, or ILCs, which are rapid responders to cytokines produced by innate sensor cells. ILCs produce, in turn, cytokines that they share with specific subsets of T cells to coordinate the recruitment and/or activation of different types of resident and circulating innate immune cells to initiate distinct modules of immunity. The third phase of an immune response is the adaptive immune response (see Fig. 11.36), which is mounted in the secondary lymphoid tissue that serves the particular site of infection and takes several days to develop—reflecting the time required for antigen-activated T lymphocytes to proliferate and differentiate into effector cells of

Phases of the immune response		
Innate phase (Immediate: 0–4 hours)	**Induced innate phase** (Early: 4–96 hours)	**Adaptive immune phase** (Late: >96 hours)
Nonspecific Innate No memory No specific T cells	Nonspecific + specific Inducible No memory No specific T cells	Specific Inducible Memory Specific T cells

	Innate phase (Immediate: 0–4 hours)	**Induced innate phase** (Early: 4–96 hours)	**Adaptive immune phase** (Late: >96 hours)
Barrier functions	Skin, epithelia, mucins, acid	Local inflammation (C5a) Local TNF-α	IgA antibody in luminal spaces IgE antibody on mast cells Local inflammation
Response to extracellular pathogens	Phagocytes Alternative and MBL complement pathway Lysozyme Lactoferrin Peroxidase Defensins	Mannose-binding lectin C-reactive protein T-independent B-cell antibody Complement	IgG antibody and Fc receptor–bearing cells IgG, IgM antibody + classical complement pathway
Response to intracellular bacteria	Macrophages	Activated NK-dependent macrophage activation IL-1, IL-6, TNF-α, IL-12	T-cell activation of macrophages by IFN-γ
Response to virus-infected cells	Natural killer (NK) cells	IFN-α and IFN-β IL-12–activated NK cells	Cytotoxic T cells IFN-γ

Fig. 11.36 The components of the three phases of the immune response against different classes of microorganisms. The mechanisms of innate immunity that operate in the first two phases of the immune response are described in Chapters 2 and 3, and thymus-independent (T-independent) B-cell responses are covered in Chapter 10. The immediate and early phases contribute to the initiation of adaptive immunity, and they influence the functional character of the antigen-specific effector T cells and antibodies that appear on the scene in the late phase of the response. There are striking similarities in the effector mechanisms at each phase of the response; the main change is in the recognition structure used.

different subsets and for T_{FH} cells to migrate to B-cell zones to provide help for B cells. Once an adaptive immune response has developed, the effector T cells and antibodies are dispersed via the circulation and recruited into the infected tissues; the infection is usually controlled, and the pathogen is contained or eliminated. The final effector mechanisms used to clear an infection depend on the type of infectious agent and the corresponding immune module elicited, such that the type of T cells or antibodies produced in the adaptive immune phase are tailored for the elimination of the type of inciting pathogen (see Fig. 11.36).

An effective adaptive immune response leads to a state of protective immunity. This state consists of the presence of effector cells and molecules produced in the initial (or primary) response and of immunological memory. Immunological memory is manifested as a heightened ability to respond to pathogens that have previously been encountered and successfully eliminated. Memory T and B lymphocytes have the property of being able to transfer immune memory to naive recipients. The mechanisms that maintain immunological memory include certain cytokines, such as IL-7 and IL-15, as well as homeostatic interactions between the T-cell receptors on memory cells and self peptide:self MHC complexes. The artificial induction of immunological memory and long-lived protective immunity by vaccination is one of the most outstanding accomplishments of immunology in the field of medicine, as will be discussed further in Chapter 16. However, as we will see in Chapter 13, many pathogens do not induce protective immunity that completely eliminates the pathogen, so we will need to learn what prevents this before we can prepare effective vaccines against these pathogens.

Discussion Questions

11.1 Subsets of innate lymphoid cells (ILCs) and T cells share a number of developmental and functional features. What are the cytokines produced by innate sensor cells that target different subsets of ILCs and effector T cells, and what are the principal cellular sources of theses cytokines? What cytokines are elicited from ILCs and effector T cells activated by these inductive cytokines? What innate effector cells are preferentially targeted by the cytokines that are produced by different ILCs and activated effector T cells? What key transcription factors are shared between ILCs and T-cell subsets?

11.2 Chemokine networks are key to the coordination of innate and adaptive immune-cell recruitment to sites of infection. Describe the sets of chemokines and their receptors that distinguish different immune modules, and identify the innate and adaptive immune cells that express them.

11.3 Although there are similarities in functionalities of subsets of ILCs and the CD4 and CD8 effector T cells, there are also important differences. Describe how these types of cells differ, and speculate how these differences may confer unique functional features on each cell population.

11.4 What are the changes in expression of trafficking molecules that accompany the transitions from naive to effector and effector to memory phenotypes of CD4 and CD8 T cells? What trafficking molecules direct T cells to different tissues?

11.5 Why have some subsets of CD4 T cells evolved to retain greater developmental plasticity? How might this contribute to host defense? Immune regulation? Immune-mediated disease?

11.6 Describe the two prevailing models for the development of memory T cells. How might these different models affect strategies for vaccine development?

11.7 Describe the role of antibody isotypes in conferring antigen recognition on different innate immune effector cells. How does this integration of innate and adaptive immune functions converge to eradicate pathogens?

Section references.

11-1   The course of an infection can be divided into several distinct phases.

Mandell, G., Bennett, J., and Dolin, R. (eds): *Principles and Practice of Infectious Diseases*, 5th ed. New York: Churchill Livingstone, 2000.

Zhang, S.Y., Jouanguy, E., Sancho-Shimizu, V., von Bernuth, H., Yang, K., Abel, L., Picard, C., Puel, A., and Casanova, J.L.: Human Toll-like receptor-dependent induction of interferons in protective immunity to viruses. *Immunol. Rev.* 2007, **220**:225–236.

11-2   The effector mechanisms that are recruited to clear an infection can be organized into immune modules.

Fearon, D.T., and Locksley, R.M.: The instructive role of innate immunity in the acquired immune response. *Science* 1996, **272**:50–53.

Gasteiger, G., and Rudensky, A.Y.: Interactions between innate and adaptive lymphocytes. *Nat. Rev. Immunol.* 2014, **14**:631–639.

Janeway, C.A., Jr.: The immune system evolved to discriminate infectious nonself from noninfectious self. *Immunol. Today* 1992, **13**:11–16.

11-3   Subsets of ILCs are early responders of the immune response.

Cortez, V.S., Robinette, M.L., and Colonna, M.: Innate lymphoid cells: new insights into function and development. *Curr. Opin. Immunol.* 2015, **32**:71–77.

McKenzie, A.N.J., Spits, H., and Eberl, G.: Innate lymphoid cells in inflammation and immunity. *Immunity* 2014, **41**:366–374.

Neill, D.R., Wong, S.H., Bellosi, A., Flynn, R.J., Daly, M., Langford, T.K., Bucks, C., Kane, C.M., Fallon, P.G., Pannell, R., *et al.*: Nuocytes represent a new innate effector leukocyte that mediates type-2 immunity. *Nature* 2010, **464**:1367–1370.

Sonnenberg, G.F., and Hepworth, M.R.: Functional interactions between innate and adaptive immunity. *Nat. Rev. Immunol.* 2019, **19**:599–613.

Sonnenberg, G.F., Monticelli, L.A., Elloso, M.M., Fouser, L.A, and Artis, D.: CD4+ lymphoid tissue-inducer cells promote innate immunity in the gut. *Immunity* 2011, **34**:7122–134.

Vivier, E., Artis, D., Colonna, M., Diefenbach, A., Di Santo, J.P., Eberl, G., Koyasu, S., Locksley, R.M., McKenzie, A.N., Mebius, R.E., *et al.*: Innate lymphoid cells: 10 years on. *Cell* 2013, **174**:1054–1066.

11-4   Effector T cells are guided to specific tissues and sites of infection by changes in their expression of adhesion molecules and chemokine receptors.

Griffith, J.W., Sokol, C.L., and Luster, A.D.: Chemokines and chemokine receptors: positioning cells for host defense and immunity. *Annu. Rev. Immunol.* 2014, **32**:659–702.

Hidalgo, A., Peired, A.J., Wild, M.K., Vestweber, D., and Frenette, P.S.: Complete identification of E-selectin ligands on neutrophils reveals distinct functions of PSGL-1, ESL-1, and CD44. *Immunity* 2007, **26**:477–489.

MacKay, C.R., Marston, W., and Dudler, L.: Altered patterns of T-cell migration through lymph nodes and skin following antigen challenge. *Eur. J. Immunol.* 1992, **22**:2205–2210.

Mantovani, A., Bonecchi, R., and Locati, M.: Tuning inflammation and immunity by chemokine sequestration: decoys and more. *Nat. Rev. Immunol.* 2006, **6**:907–918.

Mueller, S.N., Gebhardt, T., Carbone, F.R., and Heath, W.R.: Memory T cell subsets, migration patterns, and tissue residence. *Annu. Rev. Immunol.* 2013, **31**:137–161.

Sallusto, F., Kremmer, E., Palermo, B., Hoy, A., Ponath, P., Qin, S., Forster, R., Lipp, M., and Lanzavecchia, A.: Switch in chemokine receptor expression upon TCR stimulation reveals novel homing potential for recently activated T cells. *Eur. J. Immunol.* 1999, **29**:2037–2045.

11-5   Pathogen-specific effector T cells are progressively enriched at sites of infection where they may undergo further maturation to acquire full effector function.

Jenkins, M.K., Khoruts, A., Ingulli, E., Mueller, D.L., McSorley, S.J., Reinhardt, R.L., Itano, A., and Pape, K.A.: In vivo activation of antigen-specific CD4 T cells. *Annu. Rev. Immunol.* 2001, **19**:23–45.

11-6 T$_H$1 cells coordinate and amplify the host response to intracellular pathogens through classical activation of macrophages.

Bekker, L.G., Freeman, S., Murray, P.J., Ryffel, B., and Kaplan, G.: TNF-alpha controls intracellular mycobacterial growth by both inducible nitric oxide synthase-dependent and inducible nitric oxide synthase-independent pathways. *J. Immunol.* 2001, 166:6728–6734.

Ehlers, S., Kutsch, S., Ehlers, E.M., Benini, J., and Pfeffer, K.: Lethal granuloma disintegration in mycobacteria-infected TNFRp55$^{-/-}$ mice is dependent on T cells and IL-12. *J. Immunol.* 2000, 165:483–492.

Hsieh, C.S., Macatonia, S.E., Tripp, C.S., Wolf, S.F., O'Garra, A., and Murphy, K.M.: Development of T$_H$1 CD4$^+$ T cells through IL-12 produced by *Listeria*-induced macrophages. *Science* 1993, 260:547–549.

Muñoz-Fernández, M.A., Fernández, M.A., and Fresno, M.: Synergism between tumor necrosis factor-α and interferon-γ on macrophage activation for the killing of intracellular *Trypanosoma cruzi* through a nitric oxide-dependent mechanism. *Eur. J. Immunol.* 1992, 22:301–307.

Murray, P.J., and Wynn, T.A.: Protective and pathogenic functions of macrophage subsets. *Nat. Rev. Immunol.* 2011, 11:723–737.

Stout, R.D., Suttles, J., Xu, J., Grewal, I.S., and Flavell, R.A.: Impaired T cell-mediated macrophage activation in CD40 ligand-deficient mice. *J. Immunol.* 1996, 156:8–11.

11-7 Activation of macrophages by T$_H$1 cells must be tightly regulated to avoid tissue damage.

Duffield, J.S.: The inflammatory macrophage: a story of Jekyll and Hyde. *Clin. Sci.* 2003, 104:27–38.

Labow, R.S., Meek, E., and Santerre, J.P.: Model systems to assess the destructive potential of human neutrophils and monocyte-derived macrophages during the acute and chronic phases of inflammation. *J. Biomed. Mater. Res.* 2001, 54:189–197.

Wigginton, J.E., and Kirschner, D.: A model to predict cell-mediated immune regulatory mechanisms during human infection with *Mycobacterium tuberculosis*. *J. Immunol.* 2001, 166:1951–1967.

11-8 Chronic activation of macrophages by T$_H$1 cells mediates the formation of granulomas to contain intracellular pathogens that cannot be cleared.

James, D.G.: A clinicopathological classification of granulomatous disorders. *Postgrad. Med. J.* 2000, 76:457–465.

11-9 Defects in type 1 immunity reveal its important role in the elimination of intracellular pathogens.

Berberich, C., Ramirez-Pineda, J.R., Hambrecht, C., Alber, G., Skeiky, Y.A., and Moll, H.: Dendritic cell (DC)-based protection against an intracellular pathogen is dependent upon DC-derived IL-12 and can be induced by molecularly defined antigens. *J. Immunol.* 2003, 170:3171–3179.

Biedermann, T., Zimmermann, S., Himmelrich, H., Gumy, A., Egeter, O., Sakrauski, A.K., Seegmuller, I., Voigt, H., Launois, P., Levine, A.D., *et al.*: IL-4 instructs T$_H$1 responses and resistance to *Leishmania major* in susceptible BALB/c mice. *Nat. Immunol.* 2001, 2:1054–1060.

Neighbors, M., Xu, X., Barrat, F.J., Ruuls, S.R., Churakova, T., Debets, R., Bazan, J.F., Kastelein, R.A., Abrams, J.S., and O'Garra, A.: A critical role for interleukin 18 in primary and memory effector responses to *Listeria monocytogenes* that extends beyond its effects on interferon gamma production. *J. Exp. Med.* 2001, 194:343–354.

11-10 T$_H$2 cells coordinate type 2 responses to expel intestinal helminths and repair tissue injury.

Artis, D., and Grencis, R.K.: The intestinal epithelium: sensors to effectors in nematode infection. *Mucosal Immunol.* 2008, 1:252–264.

Fallon, P.G., Ballantyne, S.J., Mangan, N.E., Barlow, J.L., Dasvarma, A., Hewett, D.R., McIlgorm, A., Jolin, H.E., and McKenzie, A.N.J.: Identification of an interleukin (IL)-25-dependent cell population that provides IL-4, IL-5, and IL-13 at the onset of helminth expulsion. *J. Exp. Med.* 2006, 203:1105–1116.

Finkelman, F.D., Shea-Donohue, T., Goldhill, J., Sullivan, C.A., Morris, S.C., Madden, K.B., Gauser, W.C., and Urban, J.F., Jr.: Cytokine regulation of host defense against parasitic intestinal nematodes. *Annu. Rev. Immunol.* 1997, 15:505–533.

Humphreys, N.E., Xu, D., Hepworth, M.R., Liew, F.Y., and Grencis, R.K.: IL-33, a potent inducer of adaptive immunity to intestinal nematodes. *J. Immunol.* 2008, 180:2443–2449.

Liang, H.-E., Reinhardt, R.L., Bando, J.K., Sullivan, B.M., Ho, I.-C., and Locksley, R.M.: Divergent expression patterns of IL-4 and IL-13 define unique functions in allergic immunity. *Nat. Immunol.* 2012, 13:58–66.

Maizels, R.M., Pearce, E.J., Artis, D., Yazdanbakhsh, M., and Wynn, T.A.: Regulation of pathogenesis and immunity in helminth infections. *J. Exp. Med.* 2009, 206:2059–2066.

Ohnmacht, C., Schwartz, C., Panzer, M., Schiedewitz, I., Naumann, R., and Voehringer, D.: Basophils orchestrate chronic allergic dermatitis and protective immunity against helminths. *Immunity* 2010, 33:364–374.

Saenz, S.A., Noti, M., and Artis, D.: Innate immune cell populations function as initiators and effectors in Th2 cytokine responses. *Trends Immunol.* 2010, 31:407–413.

Sullivan, B.M., and Locksley, R.M.: Basophils: a nonredundant contributor to host immunity. *Immunity.* 2009, 30:12–20.

Van Dyken, S.J., and Locksley, R.M.: Interleukin-4- and interleukin-13-mediated alternatively activated macrophages: roles in homeostasis and disease. *Annu. Rev. Immunol.* 2013, 31:317–343.

11-11 T$_H$17 cells coordinate type 3 responses to enhance the clearance of extracellular bacteria and fungi.

Aujla, S.J., Chan, Y.R., Zheng, M., Fei, M., Askew, D.J., Pociask, D.A., Reinhart, T.A., Mcallister, F., Edeal, J., Gaus, K., *et al.*: IL-22 mediates mucosal host defense against Gram-negative bacterial pneumonia. *Nat. Med.* 2008, 14:275–281.

Basu, R., O'Quinn, D.B., Silberger, D.J., Schoeb, T.R., Fouser, L., Ouyang, W., Hatton, R.D., and Weaver, C.T.: Th22 cells are an important source of IL-22 for host protection against enteropathogenic bacteria. *Immunity* 2012, 37:1061–1075.

Fossiez, F., Djossou, O., Chomarat, P., Flores-Romo, L., Ait-Yahia, S., Maat, C., Pin, J.J., Garrone, P., Garcia, E., Saeland, S., *et al.*: T cell interleukin-17 induces stromal cells to produce proinflammatory and hematopoietic cytokines. *J. Exp. Med.* 1996, 183:2593–2603.

Happel, K.I., Zheng, M., Young, E., Quinton, L.J., Lockhart, E., Ramsay, A.J., Shellito, J.E., Schurr, J.R., Bagby, G.J., Nelson, S., *et al.*: Cutting edge: roles of Toll-like receptor 4 and IL-23 in IL-17 expression in response to *Klebsiella pneumoniae* infection. *J. Immunol.* 2003, 170:4432–4436.

LeibundGut-Landmann, S., Gross, O., Robinson, M.J., Osorio, F., Slack, E.C., Tsoni, S.V., Schweighoffer, E., Tybulewicz, V., Brown, G.D., Ruland, J., *et al.*: Syk- and CARD9-dependent coupling of innate immunity to the induction of T helper cells that produce interleukin 17. *Nat. Immunol.* 2007, 8:630–638.

Ouyang, W., Kolls, J.K., and Zheng, Y.: The biological functions of T helper 17 cell effector cytokines in inflammation. *Immunity* 2008, 28:454-467.

Romani, L.: Immunity to fungal infections. *Nat. Rev. Immunol.* 2011, 11:275–288.

Sonnenberg, G.F., Monticelli, L.A., Elloso, M.M., Fouser, L.A., and Artis, D.: CD4$^+$ lymphoid tissue-inducer cells promote innate immunity in the gut. *Immunity* 2011, 34:122–134.

Zheng, Y., Valdez, P.A., Danilenko, D.M., Hu, Y., Sa, S.M., Gong, Q., Abbas, A.R., Modrusan, Z., Ghilardi, N., De Sauvage, F.J., *et al.*: Interleukin-22 mediates early host defense against attaching and effacing bacterial pathogens. *Nat. Med.* 2008, 14:282–289.

11-12 Effector T cells continue to respond to maturational and maintenance signals as they carry out their effector functions in target tissues.

Cua, D.J., Sherlock, J., Chen, Y., Murphy, C.A., Joyce, B., Seymour, B., Lucian, L., To, W., Kwan, S., Churakova, T., *et al.*: Interleukin-23 rather than interleukin-12 is the critical cytokine for autoimmune inflammation of the brain. *Nature* 2003, 421:744–748.

Ghilardi, N., Kljavin, N., Chen, Q., Lucas, S., Gurney, A.L., and De Sauvage, F.J.: Compromised humoral and delayed-type hypersensitivity responses in IL-23-deficient mice. *J. Immunol.* 2004, 172:2827–2833.

Harbour, S.N., DiToro, D.F., Witte, S.J., Zindl, C.L., Gao, M., Schoeb, T.R., Jones, G.W., Jones, S.A., Hatton, R.D., and Weaver, C.T.: T$_H$17 cells require ongoing classic IL-6 receptor signaling to retain transcriptional and functional identity. *Sci. Immunol.* 2020, 5, eaaw2262.

Park, A.Y., Hondowicz, B.D., and Scott, P.: IL-12 is required to maintain a Th1 response during *Leishmania major* infection. *J. Immunol.* 2000, 165:896–902.

Yap, G., Pesin, M., and Sher, A.: Cutting edge: IL-12 is required for the maintenance of IFN-γ production in T cells mediating chronic resistance to the intracellular pathogen *Toxoplasma gondii*. *J. Immunol.* 2000, 165:628–631.

11-13 Effector T cells can be activated to release cytokines independently of antigen recognition.

Guo, L., Junttila, I.S., and Paul, W.E.: Cytokine-induced cytokine production by conventional and innate lymphoid cells. *Trends Immunol.* 2012, 33:598–606.

Kohno, K., Kataoka, J., Ohtsuki, T., Suemoto, Y., Okamoto, I., Usui, M., Ikeda, M., and Kurimoto, M.: IFN-gamma-inducing factor (IGIF) is a costimulatory factor on the activation of Th1 but not Th2 cells and exerts its effect independently of IL-12. *J. Immunol.* 1997, 158:1541–1550.

11-14 Effector CD4 T cells demonstrate plasticity and cooperativity that enable adaptation during antipathogen responses.

Basu, R., Hatton, R.D., and Weaver, C.T.: The Th17 family: flexibility follows function. *Immunol. Rev.* 2013, 252:89–103.

Lee, S.-J., McLachlan, J.B., Kurtz, J.R., Fan, D., Winter, S.E., Bäumler, A.J., Jenkins, M.K., and McSorley, S.J.: Temporal expression of bacterial proteins instructs host CD4 T cell expansion and Th17 development. *PLoS Pathog.* 2012, 8:e1002499.

Lee, Y.K., Turner, H., Maynard, C.L., Oliver, J.R., Chen, D., Elson, C.O., and Weaver, C.T.: Late developmental plasticity in the T helper 17 lineage. *Immunity* 2009, 30:92–107.

Murphy, K.M., and Stockinger, B.: Effector T cell plasticity: flexibility in the face of changing circumstances. *Nat. Immunol.* 2010, 11:674–680.

O'Shea, J.J., and Paul, W.E.: Mechanisms underlying lineage commitment and plasticity of helper CD4+ T cells. *Science* 2010, 327:1098–1102.

11-15 Integration of cell- and antibody-mediated immunity is critical for protection against many types of pathogens.

Baize, S., Leroy, E.M., Georges-Courbot, M.C., Capron, M., Lansoud-Soukate, J., Debre, P., Fisher-Hoch, S.P., McCormick, J.B., and Georges, A.J.: Defective humoral responses and extensive intravascular apoptosis are associated with fatal outcome in Ebola virus-infected patients. *Nat. Med.* 1999, 5:423–426.

11-16 Resolution of an infection is accompanied by the death of most effector T cells and persistence of a small number of long-lived memory T cells.

Bouillet, P., and O'Reilly, L.A.: CD95, BIM and T cell homeostasis. *Nat. Rev. Immunol.* 2009, 9:514–519.

Chowdhury, D., and Lieberman, J.: Death by a thousand cuts: granzyme pathways of programmed cell death. *Annu. Rev. Immunol.* 2008, 26:389–420.

Siegel, R.M.: Caspases at the crossroads of immune-cell life and death. *Nat. Rev. Immunol.* 2006, 6:308–317.

Strasser, A.: The role of BH3-only proteins in the immune system. *Nat. Rev. Immunol.* 2005, 5:189–200.

11-17 Immunological memory is long lived after infection or vaccination.

Akondy, R.S., Fitch, M., Edupuganti, S., Yang, S., Kissick, H.T., Li, K.W., Youngblood, B., Abdelsamad, H.A., McGuire, D.J., Cohen, K.W., *et al.*, Origin and

differentiation of human memory CD8 T cells after vaccination. *Nature* 2017, 552:362–367.

Black, F.L., and Rosen, L.: Patterns of measles antibodies in residents of Tahiti and their stability in the absence of re-exposure. *J. Immunol.* 1962, 88:725–731.

Hammarlund, E., Lewis, M.W., Hanifin, J.M., Mori, M., Koudelka, C.W., and Slifka, M.K.: Antiviral immunity following smallpox virus infection: a case-control study. *J. Virol.* 2010, 84:12754–12760.

Hammarlund, E., Lewis, M.W., Hansen, S.G., Strelow, L.I., Nelson, J.A., Sexton, G.J., Hanifin, J.M., and Slifka, M.K.: Duration of antiviral immunity after smallpox vaccination. *Nat. Med.* 2003, 9:1131–1137.

MacDonald, H.R., Cerottini, J.C., Ryser, J.E., Maryanski, J.L., Taswell, C., Widmer, M.B., and Brunner, K.T.: Quantitation and cloning of cytolytic T lymphocytes and their precursors. *Immunol. Rev.* 1980, 51:93–123.

Murali-Krishna, K., Lau, L.L., Sambhara, S., Lemonnier, F., Altman, J., and Ahmed, R.: Persistence of memory CD8 T cells in MHC class I-deficient mice. *Science* 1999, 286:1377–1381.

Seddon, B., Tomlinson, P., and Zamoyska, R.: Interleukin 7 and T cell receptor signals regulate homeostasis of CD4 memory cells. *Nat. Immunol.* 2003, 4:680–686.

11-18 MHC tetramers and adoptive transfers of clonal T-cell populations have enabled the study of T-cell memory.

Pepper, M., Pagán, A.J., Igyártó, B.Z., Taylor, J.J., and Jenkins, M.K.: Opposing signals from the Bcl6 transcription factor and the interleukin-2 receptor generate T helper 1 central and effector memory cells. *Immunity* 2011, 35:583–595.

Pagán, A.J., Pepper, M., Chu, H.H., Green, J.M., and Jenkins, M.K.: CD28 promotes CD4+ T cell clonal expansion during infection independently of its YMNM and PYAP motifs. *J. Immunol.* 2012, 189:2909–2917.

Hataye, J., Moon, J.J., Khoruts, A., Reilly, C., and Jenkins, M.K.: Naive and memory CD4+ T cell survival controlled by clonal abundance. *Science* 2006, 312:114–116.

11-19 The developmental origins of memory T cells parallel those of effector T cells.

Harrington, L.E., Janowski, K.M., Oliver, J.R., Zajac, A.J., and Weaver, C.T.: Memory CD4 T cells emerge from effector T-cell progenitors. *Nature* 2008, 452:356–360.

Restifo, N.P., and Gattinoni, L.: Lineage relationship of effector and memory T cells. *Curr. Opin. Immunol.* 2013, 25:1–8.

Wherry, E.J., Teichgraber, V., Becker, T.C., Masopust, D., Kaech, S.M., Antia, R., von Andrian, U.H., and Ahmed, R.: Lineage relationship and protective immunity of memory CD8 T cell subsets. *Nat. Immunol.* 2003, 4:225–234.

Youngblood, B., Hale, S., Kissick, H.T., Ahn, E., Xu, X., Wieland, A., Araki, K., West, E.E., Ghonheim, H.E., Fan, Y., *et al.*: Effector CD8 T cells dedifferentiate into long-lived memory cells. *Nature* 2017, 552:404–409.

11-20 Memory T cells are heterogeneous and include central memory, effector memory, and tissue-resident subsets.

Cerottini, J.C., Budd, R.C., and MacDonald, H.R.: Phenotypic identification of memory cytolytic T lymphocytes in a subset of Lyt-2+ cells. *Ann. N.Y. Acad. Sci.* 1988, 532:68–75.

Farber, D.L., Yudanin, N.A., and Restifo, N.P.: Human memory T cells: generation, compartmentalization and homeostasis. *Nat. Rev. Immunol.* 2014, 14:24–35.

Kaech, S.M., Tan, J.T., Wherry, E.J., Konieczny, B.T., Surh, C.D., and Ahmed, R.: Selective expression of the interleukin 7 receptor identifies effector CD8 T cells that give rise to long-lived memory cells. *Nat. Immunol.* 2003, 4:1191–1198.

Mueller, S.N., Gebhardt, T., Carbone, F.R., and Heath, W.R.: Memory T cell subsets, migration patterns, and tissue residence. *Annu. Rev. Immunol.* 2012, 31:137–161.

Sallusto, F., Geginat, J., and Lanzavecchia, A.: Central memory and effector memory T cell subsets: function, generation, and maintenance. *Annu. Rev. Immunol.* 2004, 22:745–763.

Sallusto, F., Lenig, D., Forster, R., Lipp, M., and Lanzavecchia, A.: **Two subsets of memory T lymphocytes with distinct homing potentials and effector functions.** *Nature* 1999, **401**:708–712.

Schenkel, J.M., and Masopust, D.: **Tissue-resident memory T cells.** *Immunity* 2014, **41**:886–897.

Skon, C.N., Lee, J.Y., Anderson, K.G., Masopust, D., Hogquist, K.A., and Jameson, S.C.: **Transcriptional downregulation of S1pr1 is required for the establishment of resident memory CD8+ T cells.** *Nat. Immunol.* 2013, **14**:1285–1293.

11-21 Circulating memory T cells acquire heightened sensitivity to IL-7 and/or IL-15 and undergo metabolic reprogramming to survive long-term.

Akondy, R.S., Monson, N.D., Miller, J.D., Edupuganti, S., Teuwen, D., Wu, H., Quyyumi, F., Garg, S., Altman, J.D., Del Rio, C., *et al.*: **The yellow fever virus vaccine induces a broad and polyfunctional human memory CD8+ T cell response.** *J. Immunol.* 2009, **183**:7919–7930.

Bradley, L.M., Atkins, G.G., and Swain, S.L.: **Long-term CD4+ memory T cells from the spleen lack MEL-14, the lymph node homing receptor.** *J. Immunol.* 1992, **148**:324–331.

Kaech, S.M., Hemby, S., Kersh, E., and Ahmed, R.: **Molecular and functional profiling of memory CD8 T cell differentiation.** *Cell* 2002, **111**:837–851.

Kassiotis, G., Garcia, S., Simpson, E., and Stockinger, B.: **Impairment of immunological memory in the absence of MHC despite survival of memory T cells.** *Nat. Immunol.* 2002, **3**:244–250.

Ku, C.C., Murakami, M., Sakamoto, A., Kappler, J., and Marrack, P.: **Control of homeostasis of CD8+ memory T cells by opposing cytokines.** *Science* 2000, **288**:675–678.

Rogers, P.R., Dubey, C., and Swain, S.L.: **Qualitative changes accompany memory T cell generation: faster, more effective responses at lower doses of antigen.** *J. Immunol.* 2000, **164**:2338–2346.

Wherry, E.J., Teichgraber, V., Becker, T.C., Masopust, D., Kaech, S.M., Antia, R., von Andrian, U.H., and Ahmed, R.: **Lineage relationship and protective immunity of memory CD8 T cell subsets.** *Nat. Immunol.* 2003, **4**:225–234.

11-22 CD4 T-cell help is required for CD8 T-cell memory and involves CD40 and IL-2 signaling.

Bourgeois, C., and Tanchot, C.: **CD4 T cells are required for CD8 T cell memory generation.** *Eur. J. Immunol.* 2003, **33**:3225–3231.

Bourgeois, C., Rocha, B., and Tanchot, C.: **A role for CD40 expression on CD8 T cells in the generation of CD8 T cell memory.** *Science* 2002, **297**:2060–2063.

Janssen, E.M., Lemmens, E.E., Wolfe, T., Christen, U., von Herrath, M.G., and Schoenberger, S.P.: **CD4 T cells are required for secondary expansion and memory in CD8 T lymphocytes.** *Nature* 2003, **421**:852–856.

Shedlock, D.J., and Shen, H.: **Requirement for CD4 T cell help in generating functional CD8 T cell memory.** *Science* 2003, **300**:337–339.

Sun, J.C., Williams, M.A., and Bevan, M.J.: **CD4 T cells are required for the maintenance, not programming, of memory CD8 T cells after acute infection.** *Nat. Immunol.* 2004, **5**:927–933.

Tanchot, C., and Rocha, B.: **CD8 and B cell memory: same strategy, same signals.** *Nat. Immunol.* 2003, **4**:431–432.

Williams, M.A., Tyznik, A.J., and Bevan, M.J.: **Interleukin-2 signals during priming are required for secondary expansion of CD8 memory T cells.** *Nature* 2006, **441**:890–893.

11-23 Memory B-cell responses are more rapid and have higher affinity for antigen compared with responses of naive B cells.

Andersson, B.: **Studies on the regulation of avidity at the level of the single antibody-forming cell. The effect of antigen dose and time after immunization.** *J. Exp. Med.* 1970, **132**:77–88.

Berek, C., and Milstein, C.: **Mutation drift and repertoire shift in the maturation of the immune response.** *Immunol. Rev.* 1987, **96**:23–41.

Bergmann, B., Grimsholm, O., Thorarinsdottir, K., Ren, W., Jirholt, P., Gjertsson, I., and Mårtensson, I.L.: **Memory B cells in mouse models.** *Scand. J. Immunol.* 2013, **78**:149–156.

Davie, J.M., and Paul, W.E.: **Receptors on immunocompetent cells. V. Cellular correlates of the "maturation" of the immune response.** *J. Exp. Med.* 1972, **135**:660–674.

Eisen, H.N., and Siskind, G.W.: **Variations in affinities of antibodies during the immune response.** *Biochemistry* 1964, **3**:996–1008.

Good-Jacobson, K.L., and Tarlinton, D.M.: **Multiple routes to B-cell memory.** *Int. Immunol.* 2012, **24**:403–408.

Klein, U., Rajewsky, K., and Küppers, R.: **Human immunoglobulin (Ig)M+IgD+ peripheral blood B cells expressing the CD27 cell surface antigen carry somatically mutated variable region genes: CD27 as a general marker for somatically mutated (memory) B cells.** *J. Exp. Med.* 1998, **188**:1679–1689.

Takemori, T., Kaji, T., Takahashi, Y., Shimoda, M., and Rajewsky, K.: **Generation of memory B cells inside and outside germinal centers.** *Eur. J. Immunol.* 2014, **44**:1258–1264.

11-24 Memory B cells can reenter germinal centers and undergo additional somatic hypermutation and affinity maturation during secondary immune responses.

Bende, R.J., van Maldegem, F., Triesscheijn, M., Wormhoudt, T.A., Guijt, R., and van Noesel, C.J.: **Germinal centers in human lymph nodes contain reactivated memory B cells.** *J. Exp. Med.* 2007, **204**:2655–2665.

Dal Porto, J.M., Haberman, A.M., Kelsoe, G., and Shlomchik, M.J.: **Very low affinity B cells form germinal centers, become memory B cells, and participate in secondary immune responses when higher affinity competition is reduced.** *J. Exp. Med.* 2002, **195**:1215–1221.

Goins, C.L., Chappell, C.P., Shashidharamurthy, R., Selvaraj, P., and Jacob, J.: **Immune complex-mediated enhancement of secondary antibody responses.** *J. Immunol.* 2010, **184**:6293–6298.

Kaji, T., Furukawa, K., Ishige, A., Toyokura, I., Nomura, M., Okada, M., Takahashi, Y., Shimoda, M., and Takemori, T.: **Both mutated and unmutated memory B cells accumulate mutations in the course of the secondary response and develop a new antibody repertoire optimally adapted to the secondary stimulus.** *Int. Immunol.* 2013, **25**:683–695.

11-25 In immune individuals, secondary and subsequent responses are mainly attributable to memory lymphocytes.

Fazekas de St Groth, B., and Webster, R.G.: **Disquisitions on original antigenic sin. I. Evidence in man.** *J. Exp. Med.* 1966, **140**:2893–2898.

Fridman, W.H.: **Regulation of B cell activation and antigen presentation by Fc receptors.** *Curr. Opin. Immunol.* 1993, **5**:355–360.

Klenerman, P., and Zinkernagel, R.M.: **Original antigenic sin impairs cytotoxic T lymphocyte responses to viruses bearing variant epitopes.** *Nature* 1998, **394**:482–485.

Mongkolsapaya, J., Dejnirattisai, W., Xu, X.N., Vasanawathana, S., Tangthawornchaikul, N., Chairunsri, A., Sawasdivorn, S., Duangchinda, T., Dong, T., Rowland-Jones, S., *et al.*: **Original antigenic sin and apoptosis in the pathogenesis of dengue hemorrhagic fever.** *Nat. Med.* 2003, **9**:921–927.

Pollack, W., Gorman, J.G., Freda, V.J., Ascari, W.Q., Allen, A.E., and Baker, W.J.: **Results of clinical trials of RhoGAm in women.** *Transfusion* 1968, **8**:151–153.

Zehn, D., Turner, M.J., Lefrançois, L., and Bevan, M.J.: **Lack of original antigenic sin in recall CD8+ T cell responses.** *J. Immunol.* 2010, **184**:6320–6326.

The Barrier Immune System

12

Previous chapters have focused on the immune response against pathogens, primarily examining responses in peripheral lymph nodes that drain infected tissues. Although most internal tissues are normally free of microbes, the barrier tissues of the body—the skin and various mucosal tissues, such as the gastrointestinal, respiratory, and urogenital tracts—are in continual contact with the external world and have ongoing encounters with microbes beginning immediately after birth and persisting throughout life. In addition to providing the greatest surface area across which pathogens can invade, these tissues are normally populated by a diverse community of resident microorganisms—the **commensal microbiota**. The requirement to contend with the commensal microbiota while performing physiological functions that expose these tissues to a wide range of environmental antigens (for example, ingestion of dietary antigens in the gastrointestinal tract; inspiration of airborne antigens in the respiratory tract) presents unique challenges to the maintenance of immune homeostasis at these sites; immune cells in barrier tissues must tolerate the commensal microbiota while maintaining the ability to mount robust responses against pathogenic microbes. In this chapter we consider specialized features of the immune system at these barrier tissues, with primary emphasis on those features invested by the mucosae—the **mucosal immune system**.

The mucosal immune system—in particular, that of the gut—may well have been the first part of the adaptive immune system to arise in evolution, possibly developing to contend with the vast populations of commensal microorganisms that coevolved with vertebrates to provide nutrient and nonnutrient benefits: primarily bacteria, but also fungi, viruses, and parasites, particularly worms (helminths). Organized lymphoid tissues and antibodies are first found in vertebrates in the gut of primitive cartilaginous fishes, and two important central lymphoid organs—the **thymus** and the avian **bursa of Fabricius**—have developmental origins related to the gut. It has therefore been suggested that the mucosal immune system of the gut represents the original vertebrate immune system, and that the spleen and lymph nodes are later specializations. Here we consider the unique features of the barrier immune system, focusing primarily on the gastrointestinal tract but also considering other barrier tissues such as the pulmonary tract and the nonmucosal barrier tissue, skin.

Organization of the mucosal immune system.

The main line of defense against invasion by microbes at mucosal tissues is the epithelium that covers their surfaces. In some sites the mucosal epithelium is composed of multiple layers (for example, oral cavity, nasal cavity, nasopharynx), but in sites such as the intestines and the lower airways of the respiratory tract, the epithelium is a single cell layer thick to facilitate nutrient uptake and gas exchange, respectively. Especially in these sites, where the physiological role of the tissue depends on free exchange of molecules between the 'outside' and 'inside,' the epithelium can be breached relatively easily. Epithelial barrier function is therefore supplemented by molecules provided by the epithelium itself, such as mucus and antimicrobial peptides, as well as the cells and molecules of the mucosal immune system. Each of these components is integrated into a layered defense that restrains the entry of microbes while allowing physiological activities to proceed.

The epithelium is not just a passive barrier between the external and internal environments; it is central to sensing the environment and communicating with immune cells to induce mucosal immune responses. Throughout this chapter, we focus on the unique relationship of the mucosal epithelia with the innate and adaptive mucosal immune systems and on how these two arms of immunity are integrated with epithelial function at homeostasis and in host defense. Many of the anatomic and immunological principles underlying the mucosal immune system apply to all mucosal tissues. Here we will focus primarily on the intestines as our main example, as it is the largest and best-studied mucosal immune system. Unique aspects of respiratory mucosa and skin barrier immunity will be considered later.

12-1 The mucosal immune system protects the internal surfaces of the body.

The mucosal immune system comprises the internal body surfaces that are lined by a mucus-covered epithelium—the gastrointestinal (GI) tract, the upper and lower respiratory tract, and the urogenital tract. It also includes the biliary tract, middle ear, and exocrine glands, such as the conjunctivae and lacrimal glands of the eye, the salivary glands, and the lactating breast (**Fig. 12.1**). The surfaces of mucosal tissues are covered by epithelia that range from a single cell layer thick—such as the simple columnar epithelium composed of **enterocytes**, or intestinal epithelial cells, that line the intestines—to multiple layers, such as the nonkeratinized stratified squamous epithelium of the esophagus and vagina (**Fig. 12.2**). The mucosal surfaces represent an enormous area to be protected. Collectively, the mucosal tissues of humans have a surface area of almost 400 m^2, roughly 200 times that of the skin. Although

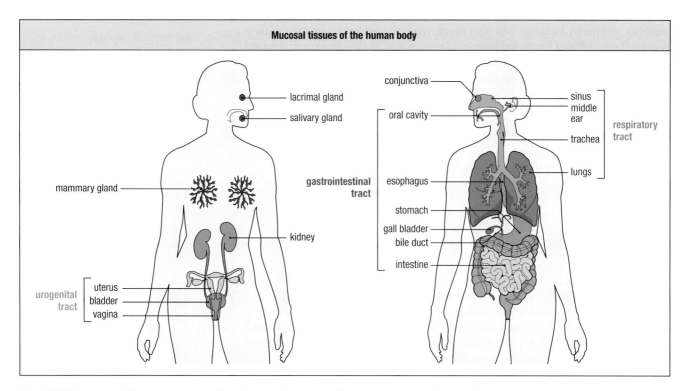

Fig. 12.1 The mucosal immune system. The tissues of the mucosal immune system are the lymphoid organs and cells associated with the gastrointestinal, respiratory, and urogenital tracts, as well as the oral cavity, pharynx, middle ear, and the glands associated with these tissues, such as the salivary glands and lacrimal glands. The lactating breast is also considered part of the mucosal immune system.

	Mucosae			Skin
Simple columnar epithelium	**Pseudostratified columnar epithelium**	**Nonkeratinized stratified squamous epithelium**		**Keratinized stratified squamous epithelium**

Fig. 12.2 A variety of different types of epithelium line the barrier tissues. Shown are the major types of epithelium that cover different barrier tissues of the body. Each type of epithelium has a relatively high cell-turnover rate (several days to a few weeks), reflecting exposure to environmental injury. All basal epithelial cells rest on a basement membrane that separates the epithelium from the underlying tissue, such as the lamina propria of the intestinal tract or the dermis of the skin. In several tissues, more than one type of epithelium is found. In the gastrointestinal (GI) tract, the major segments are covered by a simple columnar epithelium that is a single cell layer thick (for example, stomach, intestines, biliary tract), whereas the oral cavity, esophagus, and rectum are covered by nonkeratinized stratified squamous epithelium composed of multiple layers of epithelial cells. Similarly, the upper respiratory tract (nasal sinuses, tonsils, pharynx, and larynx) is covered by nonkeratinized stratified squamous epithelium, whereas the branching conducting airways (trachea, bronchi, bronchioles) are covered by pseudostratified columnar epithelium that is generally one to two cells thick. Note that the epithelium covering alveoli, the small terminal pockets in the lung where gas exchange occurs, is primarily a very thin simple squamous epithelium (one cell layer thick; not shown) to facilitate movement of O_2 and CO_2 across the epithelium. In the female genital tract (not shown), the uterus and cervical canal are covered by columnar epithelium, whereas the vagina is covered by nonkeratinized stratified squamous epithelium. A characteristic of the simple columnar and pseudostratified mucosal epithelia is the presence of mucus-producing goblet cells. The skin is composed of two major compartments—the epidermis and the dermis—which are separated by the basement membrane. The epidermis is further subdivided into four layers of keratinocytes, so named because of the high content of the filamentous structural protein, keratin, that is increasingly abundant in these cells as they mature toward the surface of the skin. Keratin is highly abundant in the outer layer of dead cells and contributes to the skin's water impermeability and barrier. SM, submucosa.

the skin is a barrier tissue, it is not moist and mucus-covered, and hence not a mucosal tissue. It is covered instead by layers of dying and dead interdigitating 'squames' (literally, scales), or **keratinocytes**—flattened cells that compose its multilayered keratinized squamous epithelium (see Fig. 12.2), as will be discussed later.

In accord with the large surface area of mucosal tissues, the mucosal immune system forms the largest part of the body's immune tissues. Approximately three-quarters of all lymphocytes in the body are found in the mucosae and they produce the majority of immunoglobulin in healthy individuals. The mucosae are continually exposed to antigens and other materials that enter from the environment or are produced by resident microbes. When compared with lymph nodes and spleen (which we will refer to as the **systemic immune system** in this

Fig. 12.3 Distinctive features of the mucosal immune system. The mucosal immune system is larger, encounters a wider range of antigens, and encounters them much more frequently than the rest of the immune system—what we call in this chapter the systemic immune system. This is reflected in distinctive anatomic features, specialized mechanisms for the uptake of antigen, and unusual effector and regulatory responses that are designed to prevent unwanted immune responses to food and other innocuous antigens.

Distinctive features of the mucosal immune system	
Anatomic features	Intimate interactions between mucosal polarized epithelia and lymphoid tissues
	Discrete compartments of diffuse lymphoid tissue and more organized structures such as Peyer's patches, isolated lymphoid follicles, and tonsils
	Specialized antigen-uptake mechanisms, e.g., M cells in Peyer's patches, adenoids, and tonsils
	Broad surface area in contact with environmental agents/microbes
Effector mechanisms	Activated/memory T cells predominate even in the absence of infection
	Multiple activated 'natural' effector/regulatory T cells present
	Production of mucins and mucus
	Secretory IgA antibodies
	Production of antimicrobial peptides (AMPs)
	Presence of distinctive microbiota
Immunoregulatory environment	Active down-regulation of immune responses (e.g., to food and other innocuous antigens) predominates at homeostasis
	Inhibitory macrophages and tolerance-inducing dendritic cells
	High number of FoxP3$^+$ T$_{reg}$ cells and FoxP3$^-$ T$_R$1 cells

chapter), the mucosal immune system has many unique and unusual features (**Fig. 12.3**).

Because of their physiological functions in food absorption (the intestines), gas exchange (the lungs), sensory activities (eyes, nose, mouth, and throat), and reproduction (prostate, uterus, and vagina), many mucosal surfaces are thin and permeable barriers to the interior of the body. The importance of these tissues to life means that effective defense mechanisms are essential to protect them from invasion. Equally significant is that their fragility and permeability create obvious vulnerability to infection, and it is not surprising that the vast majority of infectious agents invade via these routes. Diarrheal diseases, acute respiratory infections, pulmonary tuberculosis, measles, whooping cough, and worm infestations continue to be the major causes of death throughout the world, especially in infants in developing countries. To these must be added the human immunodeficiency virus (HIV), a pathogen whose natural route of entry via a mucosal surface is often overlooked, as well as other sexually transmitted infections, such as syphilis (**Fig. 12.4**).

The mucosal surfaces are also portals of entry for a vast array of foreign antigens that must be tolerated to prevent untoward immune activation and immune-mediated disease. This is perhaps best illustrated by the gut, which is exposed to enormous quantities of food proteins—an estimated 30–35 kg per year per person. Moreover, the healthy large and small intestines are colonized by hundreds of species of microbes that live in symbiosis with their host, known as commensal microorganisms, or commensal microbiota. The microbiota consists of complex communities that have coevolved with their mammalian hosts over hundreds of millions of years. Bacteria dominate the commensal microbiota, and at least 10^{13} bacteria are present in the colon contents, making them the most numerous cells in the body—outnumbering the total number of cells of the host. Substantial populations of archaea, fungi, and bacterial viruses (bacteriophages) are also found in the healthy intestine, as are parasites such as worms (helminths) in countries with less advanced

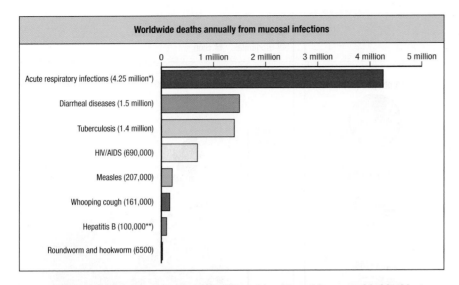

Fig. 12.4 Mucosal infections are one of the biggest health problems worldwide. Most of the pathogens that cause death throughout the world either infect mucosal surfaces or enter the body through the mucosae. Respiratory infections are caused by numerous bacteria (such as *Streptococcus pneumoniae* and *Haemophilus influenzae*, which cause pneumonia; and *Bordetella pertussis*, the cause of whooping cough) and viruses (such as influenza, SARS-CoV-2, and respiratory syncytial virus). The bacterium *Mycobacterium tuberculosis*, which causes tuberculosis, also enters through the respiratory tract. Measles manifests itself as a systemic disease, but it originally enters via the oral or respiratory route. A variety of diarrheal diseases (for example, rotavirus, *Vibrio cholerae*, and *Shigella*) are transmitted via the fecal–oral route, often by contaminated food or drinking water. The human immunodeficiency virus (HIV) that causes AIDS is sexually transmitted through the mucosa of the urogenital or lower intestinal tracts or is secreted into breast milk and passed from mother to child in this way. Hepatitis B is also a sexually transmitted virus. Both HIV and hepatitis B can also be transmitted via IV drug use, although this is not a mucosal route of infection. Finally, parasitic worms inhabiting the intestine cause chronic debilitating disease and premature death. Most of these deaths, especially those from acute respiratory and diarrheal diseases, occur in children under 5 years old in the developing world, and there are still no effective vaccines against many of these pathogens. Numbers shown are best estimates for 2019 based on data from multiple sources (e.g., The Global Burden of Disease; World Health Organization; U.S. Centers for Disease Control and Prevention).
*Note that this estimate predates the SARS-CoV-2 pandemic.
**Does not include deaths from liver cancer or cirrhosis resulting from chronic hepatitis infections.

sanitation. The host provides the microbiota with a warm, nutrient-rich environment, and in return, the microbiota provides key functions that benefit the host. In normal circumstances these organisms do no harm, and many are beneficial to their hosts, having important metabolic functions, as well as being essential for normal immune function and providing a buffer against potential pathogens. Other mucosal tissues are also colonized by substantial populations of resident commensal organisms, as is the skin (**Fig. 12.5**).

Because food and the commensal microbiota contain many foreign antigens, they can be recognized by the adaptive immune system and normally induce antigen-specific immune tolerance. Inappropriate responses to these antigens are potentially damaging to the host and are the cause of a number of common diseases, including **celiac disease** (caused by an aberrant immune response to the wheat protein **gluten**; discussed in Chapter 14) and inflammatory bowel diseases such as **Crohn's disease** (due to a dysregulated response to commensal bacteria; discussed further later and in Chapter 15). As we shall see, the innate and adaptive mucosal immune systems of the intestinal immune system have developed multiple strategies to accommodate these 'friendly' antigens while retaining robust host defense against pathogens, including opportunistic pathogens that are normal constituents of the commensal microbiota. Similar issues are faced at other mucosal surfaces, such as the respiratory tract

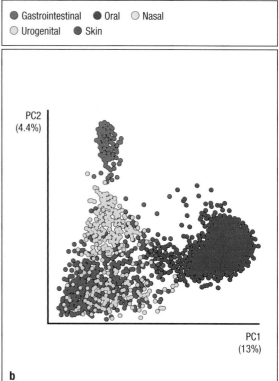

Fig. 12.5 Composition of the commensal microbiota at different barrier surfaces in healthy humans. Panel a: The different sizes of the pie charts for different sites reflect the number of distinct bacterial phyla typically present at those sites. The color key indicates the five bacterial phyla that make up the majority of commensal species. Ubiquitous commensal bacteria include *Lactobacillus* and *Clostridium* spp. (Firmicutes), *Bacteroides fragilis* (Bacteroidetes), *Bifidobacterium* spp. (Actinobacteria), *Escherichia coli* (Proteobacteria), and *Akkermansia* spp. (Verrucomicrobia). The numbers in parentheses denote the number of independent strains. Panel b: Principal component analysis of the microbiota isolated from the indicated human tissues in different individuals, plotting the first and second principal components (PC1 and PC2, respectively).

The primary component of microbiota variation between individuals is body area (that is, site location) and accounts for 13% of the variation in microbial identity among site-specific samples taken from different individuals. The colon contains the greatest number of different species (more than 1000 as estimated from individual surveys). Although not shown because it is more difficult to sample, the commensal microbiota of the human small intestine are distinct from and less diverse than those of the large intestine, dominated by members of Firmicutes and Proteobacteria phyla, particularly Lactobacillaceae and Enterobacteriaceae family members, respectively. Note that the values shown are derived from surveys of the Western countries/Western diets; the microbiota composition shifts contingent on diet and other factors.

and genital tract. Here, protective immunity against pathogens is essential, but many of the antigens entering these tissues are harmless, being derived from commensal organisms, pollen, other innocuous environmental material, and, in the lower urogenital tract, seminal fluid.

12-2 Immune cells of the mucosal immune system are located both within and outside of specialized lymphoid tissues in proximity to the epithelium.

The deployment of immune cells in mucosal tissues can be divided into inductive and effector sites—that is, sites where immune cells are initially activated and sites where they act directly in support of the barrier function of the epithelium. Like all other tissues in the body, lymphatics that drain the mucosal tissues deliver antigens to regional lymph nodes, such as the **mesenteric lymph nodes**, which serve as inductive sites for the small intestine and proximal colon, or the cervical lymph nodes, which serve as inductive sites for the oral and nasal cavities, for example. In addition, the mucosae contain inductive sites with organizational features similar to those of other peripheral lymphoid tissues, but they lack afferent lymphatics and receive antigens directly across the overlying epithelium with which they are in direct contact, as will

Components of the mucosa-associated lymphoid tissue (MALT)		
Region	**Components**	**Regional lymph nodes**
GALT (gut-associated lymphoid tissue)	Peyer's patches, cecal patch (mice), appendix (human), and isolated lymphoid follicles (ILFs) or solitary intestinal lymphoid tissue (SILT)	Mesenteric lymph nodes (small intestine, cecum, proximal and middle colon), caudal and iliac lymph nodes (distal colon)
NALT (nasal-associated lymphoid tissue)	Tonsils of Waldeyer's ring (encircling the nasopharynx and oropharynx in humans and composed of nasopharyngeal, tubal, palatine, and lingual tonsils) and ILFs in nasal mucosa. Mice lack tonsils but do have paired NALT structures in floor of nasal cavity	Cervical lymph nodes
BALT (bronchus-associated lymphoid tissue)	Not typically present in uninfected adults, as the lower airways are sterile, but develops in respiratory infections	Peribronchial and mediastinal lymph nodes

Fig. 12.6 Components of the mucosa-associated lymphoid tissue (MALT).

be discussed below; these are collectively referred to as **mucosa-associated lymphoid tissue (MALT)** (**Fig. 12.6**). Although organized lymphoid tissue is not typically present in the nose or lower respiratory tract in adult humans (unless infection is present), it is present in children and in some species such as mice; in the nose it is called the **nasal- (or nasopharynx-) associated lymphoid tissue (NALT)**, while in the lower respiratory tract it is known as the **bronchus-associated lymphoid tissue (BALT)**. The best-studied mucosal lymphoid tissue—and the largest in mass—is that associated with the gastrointestinal tract, or gut, known as the **gut-associated lymphoid tissue (GALT)**, the bulk of which resides in the intestines. Because the intestines comprise several anatomically defined segments with distinct functions—extending in the small intestine from the duodenum to jejunum and ileum, and in the large intestine from cecum to colon (**Fig. 12.7**)—there are regional differences in the environmental exposure and response of the associated immune tissues. There are also microanatomic differences that reflect regional specialization and affect the local immune response.

The GALT includes the **Peyer's patches**, which are most prevalent in the distal small intestine; **isolated lymphoid follicles (ILFs)**, also known as solitary isolated lymphoid tissue (SILT), which are smaller structures found throughout the small and large intestine; and, in humans, the **appendix** (**Fig. 12.8**; and see Fig. 12.7). (Similar to the human appendix is the cecal patch in mice, found near the tip of the blind pouch, or cecum, that is the beginning part of the large intestine; *cecum* is derived from the Latin for 'blind.') Each of these components of the GALT is located within the wall of the intestine; the patches and larger ILFs extend from the intestinal epithelium through the full thickness of the mucosa to the submucosa, whereas smaller ILFs are fully contained within the mucosa; that is, bound below by the muscularis mucosa. In mice, but not typically in humans, Peyer's patches (and the cecal patch) are visible to the naked eye and have a distinctive appearance, forming dome-like aggregates of lymphoid cells that project into the intestinal lumen (see Fig. 1.24). There are approximately 100–300 Peyer's patches in the human small intestine, concentrated in the distal small intestine, or ileum. Peyer's patches are much richer in B cells than the systemic peripheral lymphoid organs, with each consisting of multiple B-cell follicles that contain active germinal centers (that is, secondary B-cell follicles). T-cell zones are situated between and immediately below the follicles. This is in contrast to ILFs, which typically contain a single follicle or a less organized aggregate of B cells, without a distinct T-cell zone. In humans, Peyer's patches may consist of more than a hundred B-cell follicles, although they vary in size with age, peaking in adolescence and declining thereafter.

Fig. 12.7 Anatomy of the gastrointestinal tract. Left panel: Shown are the different tissues of the gastrointestinal tract, extending from the end of the esophagus to the rectum. The different segments of the small intestine (duodenum, jejunum, and ileum) generally lack discrete transition zones, as do the segments of the large intestine (cecum, ascending colon, transverse colon, descending colon, and rectum), although the duodenum refers to the C-shaped segment that receives bile and pancreatic enzymes as it courses around the head of the pancreas (not shown) before connecting to the jejunum at the duodenojejunal flexure. The cecum is delimited from the colon at the level of the ileocecal valve, which delivers contents of the ileum to the large intestine. The major lymphatic drainage of the intestines, from mid-duodenum through mid-colon, flows to the mesenteric lymph nodes then to the intestinal lymphatic duct and thoracic duct before reentering the bloodstream. The vascular drainage of the intestines is unusual in that it is first delivered to the liver via the hepatic portal vein prior to returning to the right side of the heart. The liver therefore processes the entire venous drainage of the intestines and plays a contributory role in restraining immune responses to the commensal microbiota. Right panel: Schematic of the layers of the small and large intestine, highlighting relationships between the mucosa (encompassing the epithelium, lamina propria, and the thin, inner layer of muscle—the muscularis mucosa), the submucosa (between the muscularis mucosa and the thicker, outer circular and longitudinal muscle layers—the muscularis externa), the thin serosa that forms the outer surface of the intestines, and the mesentery, which supports the intestines along one edge and through which the major blood vessels, lymphatics, and nerves that serve the intestines pass. The larger arteries, veins, lymphatic vessels, and nerves that supply the intestine from the mesentery penetrate the outer muscle layers and travel through the submucosa, sending smaller branches through the muscularis mucosa to supply the lamina propria. As the name implies, the mesenteric lymph nodes are embedded within adipose tissue that fills the mesentery (not shown).

A feature common to all MALT, including GALT, that distinguishes it from conventional lymph nodes is the absence of afferent lymphatics or a capsule. This organization is essential to the function of the GALT as an important site for the initiation of immune responses in the gut, enabling direct sampling of luminal antigens that are transported across the specialized epithelium overlying the Peyer's patches and ILFs—the **follicle-associated epithelium (FAE)**. Contained within the FAE are specialized epithelial cells called **microfold cells**

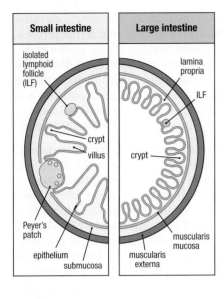

Fig. 12.8 Architecture of the small and large intestinal mucosae. Illustrated here is a cross section of the small and large intestines, highlighting the organization of tissue compartments and the relationship of the gut-associated lymphoid tissue—Peyer's patches in the small intestine and isolated lymphoid follicles in the small and large intestine—to the epithelium, the mucosa, and the submucosa. The mucosae of the small (left panel) and large (right panel) intestines are distinguished by the organization of the former into numerous villi (fingerlike projections into the intestinal lumen that increase the surface area for digestion of food and nutrient absorption), which alternate with crypts. This is in contrast to the large intestine, which generally lacks villi and is composed of crypts that are separated by very limited lamina propria. The epithelium comprises a single cell layer that is replaced continually by new cells derived from stem cells in the base of the crypts. The tissue layer bounded by the epithelium above and a slender layer of smooth muscle below (the muscularis mucosa) is called the lamina propria. Lymphocytes are found in several discrete compartments in the intestine, with the organized lymphoid tissues such as Peyer's patches and isolated lymphoid follicles forming what is known as the gut-associated lymphoid tissue (GALT). These tissues lie within the wall of the intestine itself, separated from the contents of the intestinal lumen by the single layer of epithelium. The draining lymph nodes for most of the small and large intestines are the mesenteric lymph nodes, which are connected to Peyer's patches and the intestinal mucosa by afferent lymphatic vessels; they are the largest collection of lymph nodes in the body. The outer wall of the small and large intestines is composed of thicker external muscle layers—a circular and a longitudinal layer that are known collectively as the muscularis externa—that provide the propulsive force, or peristalsis, that moves the luminal contents along the intestinal tract.

(M cells) (**Fig. 12.9**; and see **Fig. 1.24** and **Section 12-4**), which transport intact bacteria, abiotic particulates, and soluble antigens within vacuoles across their cell bodies. The area immediately beneath the FAE, the subepithelial dome, is rich in dendritic cells and lymphocytes, which are in intimate contact with the FAE. Unlike the enterocytes that make up the rest of the intestinal epithelium,

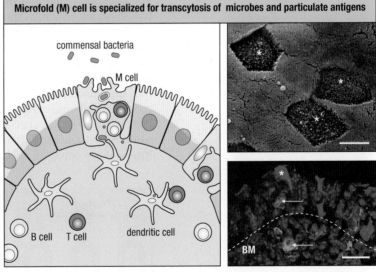

Fig. 12.9 The epithelium overlying lymphoid tissues within the intestinal mucosa is specialized for uptake of particulate antigens. The left panel depicts the continuous epithelium of the small intestine, here seen overlying a villus, crypts, and an isolated lymphoid follicle, or ILF. The epithelium over the ILF, similar to that overlying Peyer's patches (not shown), is referred to as follicle-associated epithelium, or FAE, and contains isolated microfold (M) cells. M cells, highlighted in the middle panel, are specialized for the transport of intact microbes and large particles in vacuoles across their cell bodies to be released to convoluted basolateral membranes that form 'pockets' within the epithelial layer, allowing close contact with lymphocytes and other cells. This favors the local transport of antigens that have been taken up from the intestine by the M cells and their delivery to dendritic cells for antigen presentation. The top right micrograph shows a scanning electron microscopy (SEM) image that highlights microvilli differences in M cells (identified by asterisks; pseudocolored purple) relative to neighboring enterocytes (pseudocolored tan) on the luminal surface of a Peyer's patch. At bottom right, an immunofluorescence micrograph of Peyer's patch follicle epithelium shows M cells identified by expression of peptidoglycan recognition protein-S (PGRP-S; red, example highlighted by asterisk) interacting with processes extended across the basement membrane (BM; indicated by dotted line) by CX3CR1-expressing myeloid cells (green; arrows). M-cell pockets in the epithelium are inferred from the presence of basolateral B and T cells (DAPI; blue). The white scale bars indicate 12.5 μm (top right micrograph) and 25 μm (bottom right micrograph), respectively. Photomicrographs courtesy of Dr. David Lo.

cells that compose the follicle-associated epithelium do not secrete digestive enzymes or mucins, and so lack the thick layer of surface mucus (the glycocalyx) found covering conventional epithelial cells, and the M cells have a folded luminal surface instead of microvilli (see Fig. 1.24 and Section 12.4). These cells are therefore directly exposed to microorganisms and particles within the gut lumen and, because of their ability to transport large antigenic particles and intact microbes across their cell bodies within vesicles, are a preferred route by which microbes and their antigens enter the Peyer's patches from the lumen.

Unlike Peyer's patches, which are found mainly in the distal ileum, several thousand ILFs can be identified microscopically throughout the small and large intestines, but they are more abundant in the large intestine, correlating with the greater load of commensal microorganisms there. Like Peyer's patches, these follicles are also covered by a follicle-associated epithelium containing M cells (see Fig. 12.9). However, ILFs contain mainly B cells and develop only after birth in response to antigen stimulation due to colonization of the gut by commensal microorganisms (**Fig. 12.10**). Peyer's patches, in contrast, are already present in the fetal gut, although their full development is completed only after colonization by the intestinal microbiota after birth. In the mouse gut, and perhaps in humans, isolated lymphoid follicles arise from small aggregates in the intestinal wall called **cryptopatches**, which are composed of dendritic cells and **lymphoid tissue inducer (LTi) cells**, a type of ILC3 (see Section 9-2 and Section 11-3). Cryptopatches undergo maturation into ILFs only after signals from the developing microbiota stimulate the recruitment of B cells. Peyer's patches and ILFs are connected by efferent lymphatics to regional lymph nodes, such as the mesenteric lymph nodes. This allows antigens taken up across the FAE to stimulate local responses in the Peyer's patch or ILF, as well as distally in the draining lymph node.

The small intestine and the proximal large intestine drain to the mesenteric lymph nodes, which, as the name implies, are located in the mesentery, a connective tissue that tethers the intestine to the rear wall of the abdomen and contains the vasculature, nerves, and lymphatics that supply the intestines (see Fig. 12.7). Although not technically part of the GALT, these lymph nodes are in communication with the GALT via efferent lymphatics, as indicated earlier. They also drain the effector sites within the intestine, described later. The mesenteric lymph nodes represent the largest collection of lymph nodes in the body and play a crucial role in initiating and shaping immune responses to intestinal antigens. The ILFs and lamina propria of the distal large intestine drain to separate nodes known as the caudal and inguinal lymph nodes

Fig. 12.10 Inductive sites of the GALT. The inductive sites of the GALT include cryptopatches (first panel), which are collections of dendritic cells and lymphoid tissue inducer (LTi) cells clustered near the bases of intestinal crypts at the time of birth that mature in response to signals from the developing microbiota after birth; isolated lymphoid follicles (ILFs), or solitary isolated lymphoid tissue (SILT) (second panel), which are single aggregates of lymphoid tissue that arise from cryptopatches and are found within the mucosa throughout the small and large intestine; and Peyer's patches (third panel), which are present in the distal ileum and are composed of larger aggregates of lymphoid tissue that contain multiple germinal centers.

found close to the bifurcation of the descending aorta on the posterior wall of the lower abdominal cavity. The mesenteric lymph nodes and Peyer's patches differentiate independently of the systemic immune system during fetal development, and their development involves distinct chemokines and receptors of the tumor necrosis factor (TNF) family (see Section 9-2). The differences between the GALT and the systemic lymphoid organs are thus imprinted early in life.

In addition to the inductive sites discussed above, the barrier function of the intestines is supported by effector sites that contain innate and adaptive immune cells that migrate through or reside within the intestinal epithelium itself or in the underlying layer of connective tissue called the intestinal lamina propria (**Fig. 12.11**; see also Fig. 12.8). The intestinal epithelium and lamina propria are referred to as effector sites because the preponderance of

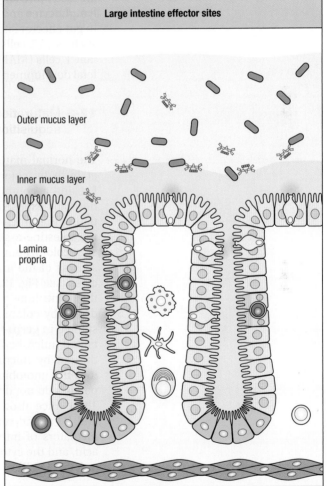

Fig. 12.11 Effector sites of the GALT. The effector sites of the small (left panel) and large (right panel) intestine include the single-cell layer of the intestinal epithelium, in which resides a variety of conventional and unconventional T cells, the so-called intraepithelial lymphocytes (IELs); and the lamina propria, which is populated by innate immune cells (for example, macrophages, dendritic cells) and effector T cells, as well as antibody-secreting cells (plasma cells). (Note that because B cells are not present in the epithelium, the alternate term, intraepithelial T cells, or IETs, is increasingly gaining favor, although we will use the conventional term, IELs, here.) There are also smaller numbers of ILCs, mast cells, and eosinophils in the lamina propria. Lymphatics drain from the lamina propria to the regional lymph nodes (for example, mesenteric lymph nodes). Although not strictly an effector site, the mucus layers overlying the intestinal epithelium (a single layer in the small intestine and two layers in the large intestine) contain antimicrobial peptides (AMPs; primarily small intestine), secreted lectins (for example, peptidoglycan protein ZG16; primarily large intestine), and secreted immunoglobulins (for example, SIgA) that provide an important barrier against interactions between luminal microbes and the mucosa. Note that different types of epithelial cells highlighted here (for example, goblet cells, Paneth cells, enteroendocrine cells, and so forth) will be discussed later in Section 12-4). SIgA, secretory immunoglobulin A; ISC, intestinal stem cell.

adaptive immune cells within them are effector cells that either have migrated there after recognition of antigen in inductive lymphoid tissues of the GALT or regional lymph nodes or, in the case of the epithelium, have populated the site directly from the thymus as functionally competent effector cells around the time of birth. The intestinal epithelium harbors a substantial number of conventional and unconventional T cells, so-called **intraepithelial lymphocytes (IELs)**, as well as some innate lymphoid cells (ILCs), which will be discussed further in Section 12-5. The intestinal lamina propria is diffusely populated by macrophages and dendritic cells that are strategically located beneath the epithelium, and it also contains antigen-experienced effector and regulatory T cells, as well as antibody-producing plasma cells, which are most numerous in the small intestine. Indeed, at homeostasis the largest number of effector T cells and antibody-producing B cells is found in the intestinal mucosa. The intestinal lamina propria also contains smaller numbers of ILCs and type 2 innate effector cells, including eosinophils, basophils, and mast cells, which are also more abundant in the small intestine. In addition, a variety of innate lymphocytes and lymphoid cells on the innate-adaptive spectrum are found in gut effector sites. These are cells that express invariant antigenic receptors, such as γδ T cells, invariant NKT (iNKT) cells, and mucosal-associated invariant T cells (MAIT cells), many of which populate the lamina propria during fetal development in preparation for colonization of the gut by the microbiota.

12-3 Maturation of the gut-associated lymphoid tissue is driven by acquisition of the commensal microbiota.

The normal maturation of the intestinal mucosa and the GALT is initiated at birth by colonization of the intestines by the commensal microbiota. Lacking a commensal microbiota, the preterm infant is germ-free, but is normally exposed to the vaginal microbiota of the mother during birth, initiating the process of intestinal colonization. Although Peyer's patches and the intestine-associated lymph nodes develop *in utero*, ILFs develop only after colonization by the commensal microbiota, and all of the GALT requires sensing of the intestinal microbiota to become fully populated by lymphocytes (see Fig. 12.10). Similarly, other components of the intestinal mucosa that contribute to the establishment of host–microbiota commensalism are driven by colonization of the neonate at birth. This process has been best studied in **germ-free mice** (or **gnotobiotic mice**), which are raised in a contained, microbe-free environment so that there is either no colonization of the gut by microorganisms or colonization only by microbes introduced into the gnotobiotic chamber. In the intestines of germ-free mice, Peyer's patches do not develop normally, and isolated lymphoid follicles are absent. These mice also have severely reduced numbers of intestinal T lymphocytes and ILCs, and very few IgA-secreting plasma cells. They also have reduced mediators of intestinal immunity, such as antimicrobial peptides, retinoic acid, and the cytokines IL-7, IL-22, IL-25, IL-33, and thymic stromal lymphopoietin (TSLP).

As we learned in Chapter 9 (see Section 9-2), preparation for the adaptation to microbial colonization requires the actions of lymphoid tissue inducer (LTi) cells. This subset of ILC3 cells is instrumental in organizing development of the GALT, as well as other lymphoid tissues in the body (see Fig. 9.2). During fetal development, LTi cells disseminate to sites of future lymphoid tissue development in the gut, recruited by the chemokine CXCL13, a product of specialized stromal cells. Activation of these stromal cells by lymphotoxin (LT-$\alpha_1\beta_2$) expressed on LTi cells initiates the development of structural components of the Peyer's patches, as well as the recruitment and partitioning of B and T cells into B-cell follicles and T-cell zones. ILF development is similarly dependent on LTi cells but is initiated after birth when cells in cryptopatches are stimulated to recruit lymphocytes in response to microbial stimuli from the developing microbiota (see Fig. 12.10). Thus, ILFs develop from crypto-patches only after colonization by the intestinal microbiota. As discussed later, LTi cells continue to contribute to the intestinal response to the microbiota beyond their role in the perinatal development of the GALT, as do other subsets of ILCs that seed the intestines—and other barrier tissues—during the perinatal period.

Like the GALT, the intestinal epithelium of the newborn undergoes changes to accommodate to the microbiota. For example, expression of TLR-4, the receptor for lipopolysaccharide (LPS)—a major pathogen-associated molecular pattern (PAMP) expressed by Gram-negative bacteria—is significantly up-regulated prior to birth. Soon after exposure to the developing microbiota, however, intestinal epithelial cells (IECs) rapidly down-regulate TLR-4 and other components of its signaling apparatus to attenuate signaling at the IEC apical membrane. Nevertheless, TLR-4 remains expressed within endocytic vesicles where it can sense bacterial invasion and induce a pro-inflammatory response. An additional immune mechanism that prepares the neonate for microbial colonization is the seeding of the intestinal epithelium by intraepithelial lymphocytes (IELs) before birth. As we will see in Section 12-5, localization of IELs within the epithelium enables them to respond rapidly to help limit bacterial translocation, maintain epithelial barrier integrity, and promote repair of the epithelium after injury.

At maturity, the intestines maintain the largest number and diversity of commensal microbes in or on the body, harboring several hundred species of commensal bacteria alone. The greatest density of microbiota along the intestinal tract is in the distal ileum and large intestine, particularly in the cecum. Over the first year or so of life, however, there are marked and often erratic shifts in the intestinal microbiota as it transitions from a more limited consortium dominated by so-called **pioneer bacterial species**—primarily facultative anaerobes dominated by Proteobacteria, such as *E. coli*, which can thrive in a more aerobic microbiota-naive intestine—to a more diverse consortium dominated by strict anaerobes, such as Firmicutes (for example, *Clostridium* spp.) and Bacteroidetes (for example, *Bacteroides fragilis*), that occurs in concert with a reduction of oxygen levels in the superficial intestinal mucosa and the lumen (**Fig. 12.12**).

Another major driver of maturation of the intestinal microbiota is the transition from a liquid to solid diet that occurs with weaning from breast milk. Prior to the introduction of solid food, breast milk provides a specialized mix of nutrients and antimicrobial proteins that influence the ecology of the neonatal microbiota, as well as maternal secretory IgA (SIgA), the specificities of which have been shaped by the mother's microbiota. In essence, the mother's mucosal immune memory is transmitted to her child. Thus, in infants delivered transvaginally, the intestinal microbiota not only is seeded by maternal

Fig. 12.12 Stages of microbial colonization of the neonatal intestines after birth. The newborn human begins to be colonized with commensal microbes during the process of birth and immediately after. The large-intestinal microbiota is initially colonized by members of the Proteobacteria phylum, particularly Enterobacteriaceae, which are facultative anaerobes that can thrive in the relatively oxygen-rich intestinal environment of the newborn. Initially, the bacterial composition is dominated by relatively few species. In the days to weeks that follow, strict anaerobic bacteria come to dominate the microbial community, and the number of different species grows. During the first month, Actinobacteria, particularly Bifidobacteriaceae, begin to predominate, but the introduction of solid foods at around 4–6 months is accompanied by an expansion of members of the Firmicutes phylum, dominated by clostridial species of the Lachnospiraceae, Clostridiaceae, and Ruminococcaceae families. Members of the Ruminococcaceae family continue to increase in abundance over the ensuing months. By 2–3 years of age, the composition of the large intestinal microbiota consists mainly of members of the Bacteroidetes (for example, Bacteroidaceae) and Firmicutes (for example, Lachnospiraceae and Ruminococcaceae) phyla, strict anaerobes that continue to stably dominate the microbiota into adulthood. Relative proportions of major bacterial phyla are depicted in circles at each stage of development. Note that although there is relatively less diversity in the species that compose the intestinal microbiota early after birth compared to later (bacterial diversity), there is greater variability in composition between individuals early after birth compared to later (interindividual diversity).

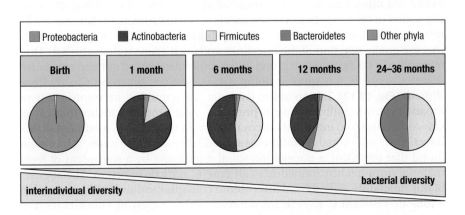

bacteria, but also its composition may be shaped by maternal SIgA, which is influenced, in turn, by the mother's microbiota. The transition to solid foods introduces new substrates, such as complex carbohydrates, that serve as fuel for a transition of the microbiota to its mature composition. As different constituents of the microbiota have different nutrient and metabolic features, the foods ingested can result in marked alterations in the composition of the microbiota.

In humans, two major phyla of anaerobic bacteria—Firmicutes and Bacteroidetes—come to dominate the mature intestinal microbiota, although significant Proteobacteria, Actinobacteria, Verrucomicrobia, and Archaea are also found (see Fig. 12.5). Trillions of these microorganisms normally exist in a beneficial symbiotic relationship with the host known as **mutualism**, reflecting the benefits that both microbes and host derive from their sharing of resources. Microbiota–host mutualism dates back almost 500 million years to the rise of jawed vertebrates, with the result that the microbiota has coevolved with their hosts over many millennia. Indeed, it is speculated that the development of an adaptive immune system in vertebrates may have allowed them to accommodate to a complex intestinal microbiota and generate the bacterial bioreactor as a mechanism to extend the range of foods from which they derive energy, providing a competitive survival advantage. This has produced, in essence, a superorganism that includes humans and their microbiota.

The microbiota has an essential role in maintaining health. Its collective genome, or **microbiome**, contains more than 10 times the number of genes encoded in the human genome, including many genes that encode enzymes that metabolize dietary constituents such as cellulose and produce essential cofactors such as vitamin K_1. **Short-chain fatty acids (SCFAs)**, such as acetate, propionate, and especially **butyrate**, produced by anaerobic commensal bacteria during the metabolism (fermentation) of complex dietary carbohydrates, are an essential source of energy for colonic enterocytes as substrates for the tricarboxylic acid (TCA) cycle. Host benefits derived from the commensal microbiota extend beyond those related to nutrition, however. The microbiota also plays an important role in protection against pathogens by competing for colonization niches and nutrient resources, collectively referred to as **colonization resistance**. Indeed, the normal microbiota contains bacterial species that can cause pathology if not continually restrained by other members of the collective. These **opportunistic pathogens** include a number of Gram-negative and Gram-positive bacteria of the Enterobacteriaceae family, such as *E. coli*, *Klebsiella pneumoniae*, and *Proteus mirabilis*, which can cause serious disease if they extend beyond the confines of the intestinal lumen.

This protective role of the intestinal microbiota is dramatically illustrated by the adverse effects of broad-spectrum antibiotics, which can kill large numbers of commensal gut bacteria, thereby creating an ecological niche for bacteria that would not otherwise be able to successfully compete. The disproportionate expansion of relatively minor constituents of the microbiota that are normally restrained by the collective is called **dysbiosis**, which can disrupt the normal metabolic function of the intestines and even cause serious disease. One example of a bacterium that grows in the antibiotic-treated gut and can cause severe disease is the spore-forming, Gram-positive anaerobe ***Clostridium difficile*** (Fig. 12.13). This organism is an increasing problem in countries where broad-spectrum antibiotic use is prevalent, as it produces toxins that cause severe diarrhea and intestinal mucosal injury. In many cases, treatment of this infection by additional antibiotics is not effective. In these cases, it has been found that providing a normal intestinal microbiota by a transplant of fecal material from healthy individuals can cure *C. difficile* infection. The success of this procedure, called **fecal microbiota transplantation (FMT)**, in treating antibiotic-resistant *C. difficile* infection has led to a growing consideration of

| The colon is colonized by large numbers of commensal bacteria | Antibiotics kill many of these commensal bacteria | *Clostridium difficile* gains a foothold and produces toxins that cause mucosal injury | Neutrophils and red blood cells leak into gut between injured epithelial cells | Connective tissue degradation leads to colitis and pseudomembrane formation |

Fig. 12.13 Infection by *Clostridium difficile*. Treatment with antibiotics can cause massive disruption of the intestinal microbiota by killing many commensal bacteria that normally colonize the colon and contribute to colonization resistance. This allows pathogenic bacteria to proliferate and to occupy an ecological niche that is normally occupied by harmless commensal bacteria. *Clostridium difficile* is an example of a toxic pathogen that can cause severe bloody diarrhea in patients treated with antibiotics. Damage to the epithelium leads to an exudate of necrotic material and fibrin that forms a thin yellow-white layer on the luminal surface of the colon, referred to as a pseudomembrane. This infection is often treated with antibiotics that target *C. difficile*, but newer therapies aimed at restoring the normal composition of the microbiota by transplantation of feces from normal donors (fecal microbiota transplantation, or FMT) have shown considerable promise.

its use for the treatment of other gastrointestinal and extraintestinal diseases thought to be linked to a dysbiotic microbiota, including inflammatory bowel disease (IBD), obesity, metabolic syndrome, and diabetes, and even CNS disorders such as Parkinson's disease and multiple sclerosis.

Summary.

The barrier tissues of the body are continually exposed to an enormous diversity of antigens derived from the environment and the commensal microbiota. While *in utero*, the developing fetus is largely insulated from these antigens, but immediately after birth, the newborn must contend with them, beginning an interaction that affects the development and function of the mucosal immune system and persists throughout life. Specializations of the immune system at mucosal tissues facilitate free interactions with these antigens while maintaining the epithelial integrity to prevent microbes from breaching the epithelium.

The anatomy of the epithelium differs regionally, but most of the surface of mucosal tissues is covered by a single layer of epithelial cells. A unique adaptation of mucosal tissues is their deployment of inductive lymphoid tissues, such as Peyer's patches and isolated lymphoid follicles, which lack afferent lymphatics and instead receive antigens directly across specialized epithelial cells that separate them from the lumens of the mucosae. These components of the mucosa-associated lymphoid tissue, or MALT, complete their development in response to microbes that populate the mucosae after birth and are central to the lifelong maintenance of immune tolerance to the commensal microbiota. Maintenance of the commensal microbiota confers benefits to the host, including certain nutrients and vitamins and colonization resistance against potential pathogens, but dysregulation of the microbiota, or dysbiosis, can lead to disease. The mucosal tissues are also major sites of entry of pathogens, and, as in other tissues, draining lymph nodes also serve the mucosal tissues as sites for the induction of adaptive immunity against pathogens and commensals alike. As a reflection of their important role on the front lines, barrier tissues contain the largest number of effector B and T cells in the body and produce the largest quantity of antibody.

Innate immune defenses of the intestinal immune system.

The GI tract is one of the body's most extensive portals for the entry of microbes, whether commensals or pathogens. As such, it has evolved specialized barrier defenses with which to restrain the microbiota and minimize pathogen threats while maintaining its functions of nutrient and water uptake. The innate defenses in the gut are also tuned toward anti-inflammatory responses through regulatory networks that promote efficient removal of microbes that traverse the epithelium without untoward production of pro-inflammatory factors (for example, cytokines and chemokines). The strategy is one of a layered defense that integrates the mucus layer; an epithelium that contains resident immune cells, produces antimicrobial factors, and transports antibodies into the lumen; and a lamina propria populated by innate and adaptive immune cells positioned for rapid responses to microbial threats and poised for tissue repair should barrier breaches occur. Here we consider the innate components of this layered defense and examine their role in maintaining a defensive posture while promoting coexistence with the microbiota.

12-4 The intestines are lined by a diversity of epithelial cell types that develop from a common progenitor and play distinct roles in mucosal immunity.

Central to intestinal host defense is the epithelium, which is an active sensor of, and conduit for, interactions between the host and the 'external' environment; that is, the contents of the intestinal lumen—both ingested (food) and resident (commensal microbiota). The intestinal epithelium is a simple columnar epithelium that is one cell thick and is polarized such that it distinguishes the external and internal environments. It performs a complex role in balancing the uptake of nutrients and water with its barrier function of excluding commensal and pathogenic microbes. It is composed of a diversity of cell types that, although derived from a common stem-cell precursor, play distinct roles in these varied functions. The mix of intestinal epithelial cell (IEC) types varies along the length of the intestines, as does the microanatomy of their deployment, corresponding to regional variation in the dominant functions of segments of the small and large intestines. In the small intestine, the epithelium covers fingerlike projections, or villi, which markedly increase the surface area for absorption of food (**Fig. 12.14**). The height of villi is greatest in the proximal small intestine and decreases progressively along the axis from the duodenum to the ileum, reflecting the greater role of the proximal and middle small intestine in nutrient uptake. Each villus is supported by a dense network of small blood vessels, nerves, and a single **lacteal**—a closed-ended lymphatic vessel that conducts lymph and immune cells, as well as absorbed nutrients (for example, lipids), from the lamina propria to regional lymph nodes (see Fig. 12.14). Individual villi are surrounded by multiple invaginations, called crypts, which are shared by surrounding villi and are sites for the production of new epithelial cells, as we will consider momentarily. In the large intestine, villi are scarce; most of the large intestinal mucosa is composed of tightly apposed crypts between which there is scant lamina propria at homeostasis. The absorptive surface of the large intestine is therefore reduced, reflecting its more limited role in nutrient uptake in favor of its role in water regulation and waste elimination, as well as support of the commensal microbiota.

In both the small and large intestine, the crypts are the 'nursery' for production of new epithelial cells (**Fig. 12.15**; and see Fig. 12.11). Because of the substantial mechanical, chemical, and microbial stresses to which the intestinal

Fig. 12.14 Relationship of the vasculature, lymphatics, and nerve fibers in the intestinal mucosa. The intestines are specialized for nutrient uptake and fluid regulation while performing immunoregulatory functions and defense against potential enteric pathogens. Supporting these various functions is a network of vascular, lymphatic, and nervous system components that supply the different layers of the intestines. Small branches from the network of small arteries and veins that course along the submucosa penetrate the muscularis mucosa to generate an intricate network of arterioles, capillaries, and venules that supply the lamina propria and through which innate immune cells and effector lymphocytes are delivered. Small lymphatic vessels originate in the lamina propria and course through the submucosa and the mesentery to deliver lymph and immune cells to regional lymph nodes (for example, mesenteric lymph nodes). Shown in these panels is the relationship of these structures in small intestinal villi. Generally, a single blind lymphatic vessel called a lacteal is found centrally in the villus and invested by a capillary network and nerve fibers. Dietary fat absorption is also carried out by lacteals and is uniquely promoted by lacteal contractions that are controlled by the autonomic nervous system. Left panel: Schematic of the relationship of the intestinal epithelium to the vascular and lymphatic vessels and nerve fibers. Middle panel: Intestinal whole-mount immunofluorescence image showing lacteals (red) and blood capillaries and venules (green). Right panel: Upper, immunostaining of villus blood capillaries (red) and nerve fibers (green) highlighting the close association of nerve fibers and capillaries; lower, immunostaining of an intestinal villus lacteal (red), smooth muscle cells (blue), and macrophages (green). The white scale bars indicate 100 μm (middle panel) and 50 μm (upper and lower right panels), respectively.

epithelium is subjected, its turnover is among the most rapid in the body, with the lifetime of most IECs averaging 3–5 days from their generation in the depths of crypts to their shedding into the lumen from the mucosal surface. Regeneration is from a small population of continually cycling, self-renewing stem cells, called **intestinal stem cells (ISCs)**, or crypt base columnar (CBC) cells, which reside at the bottom, or base, of the crypts and are identified by their expression of leucine-rich repeat–containing G protein–coupled receptor 5 (LGR5), which recognizes the R-spondin family of ligands. The strategic location of these cells as distant as anatomically possible from the intestinal lumen and the small opening through which the crypt connects with the intestinal lumen are thought to protect ISCs from insults and reflects their critical role in resupplying the epithelium at both homeostasis and during infection. Progeny of ISCs destined for differentiation into mature IECs are rapidly dividing cells that populate the lower and middle crypts, so-called transit-amplifying (TA) cells, which, in turn, give rise to the two major groups of IECs: absorptive IECs and secretory IECs. Within these two major subsets of differentiated IECs, at least six cell types are recognized: absorptive enterocytes and

Fig. 12.15 Development of intestinal epithelial cells (IECs). In the intestines, stem cells marked by expression of LGR5 (leucine-rich repeat–containing G protein–coupled receptor 5; a component of the WNT receptor) reside in the base of each crypt and give rise to progeny that develop as they ascend along the crypt walls (curved arrows). The stem cells divide continually to generate rapidly proliferating transit-amplifying (TA) cells, which occupy much of the remainder of the base of the crypts (lower third to half of crypt). Developing TA cells are fated to one of two major subsets of mature IECs: absorptive or secretory cells. Notch signals determine whether stem cells differentiate toward the absorptive fate (Notch on) or toward the secretory fate (Notch off). The absorptive subset includes mature enterocytes and microfold (M) cells (not shown). The secretory subset includes goblet cells, tuft cells, enteroendocrine cells, and, in the small intestines, Paneth cells. Epithelial turnover occurs every 3–5 days in the small intestine and 5–7 days in the large intestine, with senescent cells being lost at the tips of villi in the small intestine (upper panel) or from the surface between adjacent crypts in the large intestine (lower panel) by a process referred to as anoikis. Anoikis is a form of apoptotic or programmed cell death that is induced when anchorage-dependent epithelial cells detach from the basement membrane. The hierarchy of cell differentiation is shown in the tree on the right of each panel and indicates the predominance of absorptive enterocytes in the small intestine and goblet cells in the colon. In the small intestine, new Paneth cells are supplied from TA cells every 3–6 weeks and migrate to position themselves between the LGR5+ stem cells, where they provide a niche that supports the survival and differentiation of the stem cells.

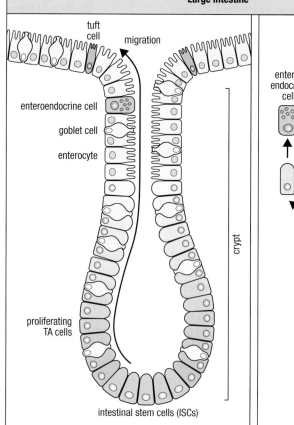

Features of intestinal epithelial cell types				
Cell	**Lineage**	**Cell markers**	**Tissue site(s)**	**Major functions**
Crypt base columnar (CBC)	Intestinal stem cell	LGR5	Small intestine Large intestine	Self-renewal Production of all intestinal epithelial cell types
Absorptive enterocyte	Absorptive	Sucrose isomaltase Lactase	Small intestine Large intestine	Uptake of nutrients and fluids Microbial and metabolic sensing Transport of secretory immunoglobulins
Microfold (M) cell	Absorptive	RANK	Small intestine Large intestine	Antigen uptake Bacterial translocation
Goblet cell	Secretory	MUC2, Trefoil factor	Small intestine Large intestine	Production of mucins Antigen uptake
Paneth cell	Secretory	Lysozyme	Small intestine	Support for intestinal stem cells Secretion of antimicrobial peptides (AMPs)
Tuft cell	Secretory	IL-25	Small intestine Large intestine	Sensing of helminthic odorants and succinate Mobilization of type 2 ILCs via IL-25 and eicosanoid release
Enteroendocrine cell	Secretory	Chromogranin A	Small intestine Large intestine	Respond to multiple nutrient and microbial-secreted products to release hormones and neurotransmitters

Fig. 12.16 Features of intestinal epithelial cell subsets.

M cells (absorptive subset); and goblet cells, Paneth cells, enteroendocrine cells, and tuft cells (secretory subset) (Fig. 12.15 and **Fig. 12.16**).

In accord with its specialization for nutrient and fluid uptake, the absorptive enterocyte, or simply enterocyte (from the Greek *enterikos*, meaning 'intestine'), is the most abundant cell type in both small and large intestines (see Figs. 12.15 and 12.16). To enhance its absorptive function, the enterocyte projects microvilli toward the intestinal lumen to increase surface area, and it expresses a range of enzymes and transporters tasked with breaking down and taking up nutrients from food. Enterocytes also are critical sensor cells of the innate immune system, reflecting their dominance on the front line separating the external from internal environments. As for all IECs, an important aspect of the barrier function is the network of intercellular junctions that bind individual cells to each other (**Fig. 12.17**). Organized near the luminal surface of IECs, these tight junctions are formed by complexes of a number of members of the claudin and occludin families of junctional transmembrane proteins that are linked to the epithelial-cell cytoskeleton to form a continuous seal between adjacent cells. This results in a selective, semipermeable structure that generally restricts the passage of molecules between IECs to ions, small solutes, and water. In addition to regulating the flow of these molecules across the epithelium, tight junctions organize the polarity of IECs and create an 'outside,' or apical, surface of enterocytes that faces the intestinal lumen and an 'inside,' or basolateral, surface, which rests on a basement membrane and enables communication with the underlying lamina propria.

This partitioning of the cell surface of IECs is important for its responses to microbial threats, as different pattern-recognition receptors (PRRs), such as TLRs, are differentially arrayed between the apical and basolateral cell membranes. As an example, **TLR-5**, which senses bacterial flagellins—a component of the flagella that provide motility for bacteria and are often expressed by pathogenic strains—is preferentially arrayed on the basolateral surface of enterocytes where it can detect microbes that have breached the barrier and alert the IECs to secrete antimicrobial factors, such as antimicrobial peptides (AMPs), as well as cytokines and alarmins that activate innate and adaptive

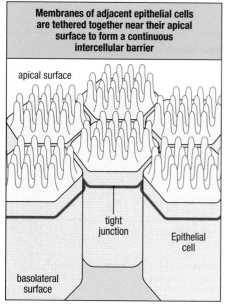

Membranes of adjacent epithelial cells are tethered together near their apical surface to form a continuous intercellular barrier

apical surface

tight junction

Epithelial cell

basolateral surface

Adhesion complexes create a seal preventing most molecules from passing through the intercellular space

The transmembrane proteins claudin and occludin associate with zonulin (ZO) proteins that interact with the actin cytoskeleton to regulate the permeability of tight junctions

claudin

ZO proteins

actin

occludin

Fig. 12.17 Polarization of IECs is organized by a set of cell–cell adhesion molecules that compose tight junctions. Adjacent IECs form tight junctions that are essential to the function of the intestinal barrier and the regulation of movement of ions, solutes, and water across the intestinal epithelium. Tight junctions also partition the plasma membrane and embedded proteins into apical and basolateral domains that have distinct functions in epithelial sensing of microbes, transepithelial signaling, and immune functions (left panel). Tight junctions are primarily composed of claudins and occludins, transmembrane proteins that undergo homotypic adhesions between adjacent IECs near their apical surfaces to form a continuous 'ribbon' that seals the intercellular junction (middle panel). The intracellular domains of these complexes are linked to the IEC actin filament network via zonulin (ZO) proteins, allowing reorganization of the actin skeleton to regulate the permeability of the tight junctions.

immune cells. Thus, in addition to their role in nutrient uptake, enterocytes are active participants in immune responses in the intestines, acting as critical innate sensor and effector cells.

Although the IECs that compose the follicle-associated epithelium (FAE) are a subset of enterocytes, the developmental relationship of microfold (M) cells to enterocytes is less clear. M cells represent a small fraction of all IECs (<1%). Their development is controlled by local B cells and RANK ligand (RANKL), a member of the tumor necrosis factor (TNF) superfamily (see Section 7-23). As indicated earlier (see Section 12-2), M cells are highly specialized for sampling particulate antigens from the intestinal lumen. In contrast to absorptive enterocytes, the apical surface of M cells is devoid of microvilli and lacks a glycocalyx, and because M cells reside in the mucus-depleted follicle-associated epithelium, they are in direct contact with the luminal contents so as to facilitate sampling of the molecules and microbes found there (see Fig. 12.9). M cells also express receptors that bind SIgA, facilitating the uptake of bacteria coated with SIgA (see Section 12.9). M cells have a remarkable ability to shuttle intact microbes across the epithelium in vesicles that deliver their contents to the subepithelial dome where they can be sampled by dendritic cells, a process referred to as **transcytosis** (meaning literally 'across the cell'). The basolateral surfaces of M cells are highly invaginated to form large pockets typically occupied by B and T cells, as well as dendritic cells. This enables the immune system to actively interrogate the microbiota as part of the general mechanism to promote tolerance to nonharmful components of the consortium by inducing regulatory T cells (T_{reg} cells) or SIgA to antigens of commensal microbes, as we will discuss further later (see Section 12-10). As we will also see, some pathogens utilize the M cell as a ferry to cross the epithelial barrier and gain access to the host, even though this feeds them into the heart of the intestinal adaptive immune system.

The second most abundant IEC is the **goblet cell**, so named because of the large secretory vacuole that occupies much of the cytoplasmic space in mature cells (see Figs. 12.15 and 12.16). The goblet cell's primary function is the production of mucins, which are heavily charged, glycosylated, secreted or cell-associated glycoproteins that are organized into the gel-like mucus layer that coats the intestinal epithelium (**Fig. 12.18**); because mucus is the defining feature of mucosal tissues, the goblet cell is the defining secretory cell of the mucosae. The physicochemical properties of mucus—both slippery and sticky—make

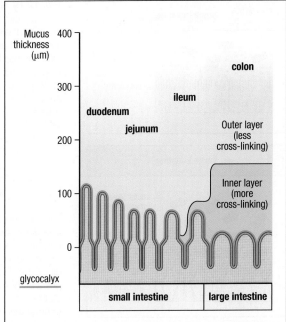

Fig. 12.18 Structure and organization of mucins and mucus.
The defining feature of most mucosal tissues is their production of mucus, which is composed of different mucins, glycoproteins with greater than 50% of their mass contributed by O-glycans. There are two major types of mucins: transmembrane mucins, which are anchored to the surface of mucosal epithelial cells, and gel-forming mucins, which are released from the cell surface. Mucus is produced by goblet cells, which are specialized for the production of mucins and for assembly and secretion of mucin polymers that form mucus. Left panel: The major mucin in the intestines is MUC2, a gel-forming mucin. Monomers of MUC2 have C- and N-terminal domains that enable homodimerization and homotrimerization, respectively, and an elongated central portion that is rich in prolines, as well as serines and threonines that undergo heavy O-glycosylation during synthesis to form a rigid rod with a bottlebrush-like structure that binds water and gives mucus its lubricating gel-like properties. Shown in the

series of left panels is the assembly of the MUC2 mucin into dimeric forms via disulfide bonding of C-termini cysteine knot domains in the endoplasmic reticulum (ER), O-glycosylation (green; protein core black) in the Golgi apparatus, formation of a netlike sheet by trimerization of N-terminal domains via disulfide bonds in the trans Golgi network (TGN), and a schematic picture of the secreted MUC2 polymer. The polymerized mucin is compacted in the goblet-cell granules and undergoes expansion upon secretion to form extended sheets that can be further cross-linked to produce a netlike, three-dimensional lattice. The MUC2 mucin is anchored in the goblet cells such that the mucus remains attached until cleaved by a host protease (meprin-β in the small intestine) to release the gel lattice from the cell. Right panel: The thickness and structure of mucus is different along the length of the intestines, correlating somewhat with the density of the commensal microbiota from which the epithelium is protected.

it a lubricant that reduces mechanical stress on the epithelium by the flow of material in the lumen while also trapping microbes to block their interaction with the epithelium and facilitate their removal by the normal, rhythmic muscular contractions of the intestines, termed peristalsis. Mucus also provides a scaffolding for retention of SIgA and AMPs that reinforce this physical barrier. Intestinal mucus also serves as a substrate for colonization of harmless commensal bacteria that provide a microbial buffer against pathogens.

Mucus thickness varies along the duodenal–colonic axis of the intestines (Fig. 12.18 and **Fig. 12.19**). The mucus layer is thinner and focally discontinuous in the proximal small intestine, becoming thicker and continuous in the ileum. In the large intestine, the mucus layer becomes thicker still, several times thicker than in the proximal small intestine. This correlates with the density of goblet cells in the different regions of the intestine, which generally has an inverse relationship with the length of villi (and therefore absorptive function) and a direct relationship with the abundance of commensal bacteria; the density of both goblet cells and bacteria is greatest in the large intestine, and the density of each declines proximally. Also, in the large intestine there are two functionally distinct mucus layers: a thinner, more compact, firmly adherent inner layer that is generally devoid of microbes, and a thicker, more loosely structured, nonadherent outer layer that can be colonized by microbes. The inner, compact layer is generally lacking in the small intestine.

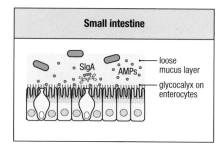

Small intestine

loose mucus layer

glycocalyx on enterocytes

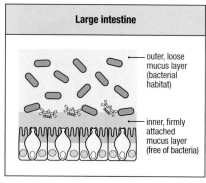

Large intestine

outer, loose mucus layer (bacterial habitat)

inner, firmly attached mucus layer (free of bacteria)

OML

IML

Fig. 12.19 The organization of mucus differs in the small and large intestine. Enterocytes, the major cell type in the intestinal epithelium, have transmembrane mucins covering their apical cell membrane. These mucins reach further out into the intestinal lumen than any other membrane protein and generate a local, attached glycan-rich diffusion barrier, called the glycocalyx, which protects the enterocyte cell membrane. Upper panel: In the upper small intestine, where most digestion and absorption of food takes place, the MUC2 mucin is typically cleaved and detached from the cell surface, allowing the mucus to be transported distally. The mucus lattice is also less densely cross-linked, such that the mucus layer is relatively porous, enabling efficient nutritional uptake. Middle panel: In the large intestine, mucus is composed of two distinct layers: a more densely cross-linked inner layer that is attached to the cells, and an outer, more porous layer in which commensal bacteria can reside. The inner mucus layer is most prominent in the distal colon where it has a stratified structure of layered sheets composed of MUC2 multimers. This dense, well-organized structure is anchored to the epithelium and limits bacterial penetration by having pore sizes smaller than bacteria, creating a zone that is almost completely free from bacteria. Remarkably, the inner mucus layer of the colon can be replaced every hour. The inner colonic mucus layer is converted to a detached, less dense outer mucus layer by the actions of secreted proteases. This allows the mucus to move with the fecal stream, providing lubrication to protect the epithelium from mechanical damage. The mucin glycans of the outer mucus layer also create a specialized niche that fosters colonization by harmless commensal bacteria that harvest the mucin glycans for food. Lower panel: Immunostaining of the colon highlights the mucus layers. Goblet cells in the colon are identified with an anti-MUC2 antibody (green). The section is counterstained with 4′,6-diamidino-2-phenylindole (DAPI) to visualize epithelial-cell nuclei (pale blue). Note that the inner stratified mucus layer is linked via MUC2-stained threads to the goblet cells of the surface epithelia. OML, outer mucus layer; IML, inner mucus layer. Asterisks indicate representative goblet-cell vacuoles. The white scale bar in the lower panel indicates 25 μm.

Although bacteria can penetrate the loose, outer layer of mucus, they are normally kept away from the surface of the epithelial cells, and the cross-linking of the inner layer in the large intestine is such that the pores generated are too small for bacteria to penetrate. Defects in this structure compromise antimicrobial defense, and some enteric pathogens produce mucolytic enzymes that allow them to disrupt the mucus structure to invade.

Although there are many different mucins, the dominant mucin in the intestines is the secreted mucin **MUC2**, which undergoes cross-linking with itself and membrane-bound mucins to form the compact inner layer (see Figs. 12.18 and 12.19). Proteolytic cleavage of the MUC2 polypeptide backbone in the outer layer results in a less compact structure that is amenable to colonization by components of the microbiota. Indeed, mucin glycans serve as nutrients for several keystone anaerobic bacterial species of the large intestinal commensal microbiota (for example, *Bifidobacterium* and *Bacteroides* spp.). The breakdown of these glycans by bacterial fermentation generates short-chain fatty acids (SCFAs), such as propionate and butyrate, which are principal fuel sources for IECs, representing a positive IEC–microbiota feedback loop that promotes retention of these protective bacterial species in the healthy gut. Other fermentation products of mucin degradation (for example, acetate and lactate) that are generated by commensal bacteria are toxic to some pathogenic bacteria, providing an indirect mechanism by which mucus participates in host defense. In contrast to most of the intestinal epithelium, the follicle-associated epithelium that is associated with Peyer's patches and isolated lymphoid follicles is devoid of goblet cells and is not covered by mucus, thereby facilitating sampling of the luminal contents. Notably, there is functional heterogeneity among goblet cells. In the large intestine, the entrance to the colonic crypts is bordered by so-called **sentinel goblet cells**, which, upon sensing pathogens, stimulate a simultaneous release of mucins from other goblet cells in the crypt that is under assault, resulting in an expulsive jet of mucus that flushes the crypt to eject invading microbes. This phenomenon appears to be coordinated by cell-to-cell communication via gap junctions, which are distinct from tight junctions and are specialized structures that provide regulable

Antimicrobial proteins produced in the intestinal mucosa			
Family (examples)	**Mechanism of action**	**Cellular source**	**Microbial targets**
α-Defensins (humans) Cryptidins (mice)	Cell membrane disruption	Paneth cells Neutrophils Macrophages	Gram+ and Gram− bacteria, fungi, protozoa, viruses
β-Defensins (e.g., BD1, BD2, BD3)	Cell membrane disruption	Enterocytes	Gram+ and Gram− bacteria, fungi, protozoa, viruses
Calprotectin (S100A8–S100A9)	Metal chelation	Enterocytes Neutrophils	Gram+ and Gram− bacteria, fungi, viruses
C-type lectins (e.g., REG3β, REG3γ)	Cell membrane disruption	Paneth cells Enterocytes	Gram+ and Gram− bacteria
Lysozyme	Cleavage of bacterial cell wall peptidoglycan	Paneth cells	Gram+ > Gram− bacteria
Phospholipase A$_2$	Cleavage of bacterial cell membrane phospholipids	Paneth cells Macrophages	Gram+ bacteria

Fig. 12.20 Antimicrobial proteins that contribute to innate defense of the intestinal mucosa. A variety of antimicrobial proteins are produced in the intestinal mucosa. These include small, typically cationic antimicrobial peptides (AMPs) that insert into bacterial cell walls (e.g., defensins), as well as enzymes (e.g., lysozyme) that cleave components of bacterial cell walls or cell membranes. These proteins are produced by both intestinal epithelial cells (IECs), including Paneth cells of the small intestine and non-Paneth epithelial cells in the small and large intestines, and myeloid cells, such as macrophages and neutrophils that infiltrate the intestines during inflammation.

pores between adjacent IECs to enable rapid cell-to-cell communication. Also, as we will detail later (see Section 12-9), goblet cells play an important role in the delivery of soluble antigens across the epithelium to underlying dendritic cells.

Paneth cells are a population of secretory IECs that reside in the base of crypts in the small intestine, where they are intercalated between ISCs (see Figs. 12.11, 12.15, and 12.16). They develop from early secretory cell progenitors and have two major functions: the production of antimicrobial peptides, both at homeostasis and in response to pathogen-induced activation; and the provision of maintenance signals for ISCs. Paneth cells are characterized by an abundance of intracytoplasmic secretory granules containing a diversity of antimicrobial factors (**Fig. 12.20**), some of which are secreted at homeostasis and appear to help in maintaining a sterile crypt and reinforcing the mucus layer to restrain bacterial incursion and protect the ISCs (**Fig. 12.21**). Paneth cells can also respond directly to PAMPs, as they express TLRs and NODs and they are highly autophagic. Defects in Paneth-cell function lead to reduced bacterial defense and are believed to be important in susceptibility to inflammatory bowel disease in humans due to the penetration of microbes across the mucus barrier (see Section 15-17). Notably, Paneth cells are not found in the large intestine. However, a similar cell has been identified in contact with ISCs in colonic crypts, and it appears to serve Paneth-like cell functions, although it lacks the large cytoplasmic granules characteristic of Paneth cells.

Intestinal **tuft cells**, so named for the characteristic 'tuft' of microvilli they project into the lumen, are a chemosensory type of IEC related to odorant and taste receptors in the upper airways and tongue (see Figs. 12.15 and 12.16; see also Fig. 11.3). Tuft cells are specialized for recognition of molecules produced by helminths and are therefore key sensor IECs that promote type 2 immune responses (see Section 11-3). They are relatively rare, representing less than 1% of all IECs, although their numbers increase during helminthic infections.

Enteroendocrine cells (EECs) are a second type of chemosensory IEC that, like tuft cells, are primarily dispersed throughout the superficial, or lumen-facing, intestinal epithelium (see Figs. 12.11, 12.15, and 12.16). EECs are specialized for sensing a range of nutrients in the intestinal lumen that stimulate their release of hormones and/or neurotransmitters to regulate digestion, absorption, and satiety in the gut, as well as local and systemic metabolism. Like tuft cells, EECs compose less than 1% of all IECs, but because of the large number

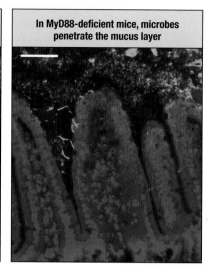

Fig. 12.21 Microbial signals activate the production of antimicrobial peptides that restrain bacterial encroachment of the intestinal epithelium. The antimicrobial defense of the intestinal mucosa provided by mucus is enhanced by factors produced by both epithelial and immune cells. Particularly in the small intestine, with its thinner, more porous mucus layer and absence of a microbe-excluding inner mucus layer, bacteria are kept away from the epithelial cells by the continual renewal of mucus and presence of antibacterial agents, such as defensins and secretory IgA (SIgA), which form a gradient owing to their slow diffusion through the mucus. This produces a 'killing field' that bacteria must traverse if they are to reach the epithelium. The highest concentration of antimicrobial peptides (AMPs) is in the crypts and at the crypt openings, as these components are largely produced by the Paneth cells at the bottom of the crypts in the small intestine. The production of AMPs is contingent on recognition of microbial products—as shown in mice deficient in the TLR signaling component MyD88 in IECs, which results in the loss of physical separation of bacteria from the small intestinal epithelium (left through right panels). Similarly, deficiency of the antimicrobial C-type lectin REG3γ, which targets Gram-positive bacteria, allows these bacteria to penetrate the mucus layer (not shown). The two right panels show bacteria (green) detected by fluorescence *in situ* hybridization (FISH) and epithelial-cell nuclei (blue) labeled with DAPI. The white scale bars indicate 50 μm.

of cells in the intestinal epithelium, EECs represent the largest collection of endocrine cells in the body. There is considerable heterogeneity in EECs, with at least eight subtypes that are distinguished by the nutrient receptors they express and the hormones and neurotransmitters they release when stimulated. Although the roles of EECs in intestinal immunity are still being defined, the innervation of some EECs by nerve fibers that communicate with the central nervous system suggests that, in addition to their roles in regulating intestinal physiology at homeostasis, EECs may also contribute to **neuroimmune interactions** that regulate certain immune responses.

12-5 The intestinal epithelium contains conventional and unconventional T cells that are focused on barrier maintenance and defense.

The epithelial cells of the intestines are not alone on the front line. Compared to most other epithelia in the body, the epithelium of barrier tissues, including the intestines, is unusual in harboring a substantial number of conventional and unconventional (innate-like) T cells, or intraepithelial lymphocytes (IELs), as well as small numbers of ILC1 cells (**Fig. 12.22** and **Fig. 12.23**). At birth, unconventional T cells are the dominant IELs, as they populate the epithelium perinatally and expand in response to colonization by the intestinal microbiota immediately after birth. As an increasing number of antigen-experienced conventional T cells take up residency in the epithelium throughout life, the balance between unconventional and conventional IELs shifts, such that conventional T cells become a greater fraction of the total with age. Because population of the epithelium by conventional T cells is controlled more by the history of antigenic exposure, the ratios of

Lymphocytes called intraepithelial lymphocytes (IELs) are positioned within the intestinal epithelium

Intestinal lumen

enterocyte

IEL

basement membrane

Lamina propria

Immunofluorescent staining demonstrates that most IELs are CD8⁺, whereas most T cells in the lamina propria are CD4⁺

At higher magnification, the IELs can be seen to lie within the epithelial layer between epithelial cells

Fig. 12.22 Intraepithelial lymphocytes.
The epithelium of the intestines contains a large population of lymphocytes known as intraepithelial lymphocytes (IELs; shown for small-intestinal villus in left panel). The immunofluorescent micrograph in the center panel is of a section of small-intestinal villi highlighting that most of the lymphocytes in the epithelium are CD8 T cells (green), whereas most in the underlying lamina propria are CD4 T cells (red). The intestinal epithelial cells (IECs) are stained blue. Those IECs with dark vacuoles are goblet cells; the dark vacuoles are the mucin-containing vacuoles. Magnification ×400. The electron micrograph in the right panel shows that the IELs lie between epithelial cells (EC) on the basement membrane (BM) separating the lamina propria (LP) from the epithelium. One IEL can be seen having crossed the basement membrane into the epithelium, leaving a trail of cytoplasm in its wake. Magnification ×8000.

conventional to unconventional IELs can vary considerably between individuals, and in the same individual, throughout life. Normally, very few IELs are actively dividing, and there is a limited contribution of circulating cells to the IEL compartment.

IELs are intercalated between and therefore are in immediate contact with IECs, situated beneath the tight junctions that bind IECs and above the basement membrane on which the IECs rest (see Fig. 12.22). The number and composition of IELs differs regionally along the intestinal tract; the highest density of IELs is found in the proximal small intestine and gradually decreases toward the ileum and the colon. In the healthy proximal small intestine, there is about one IEL for every 10 epithelial cells at homeostasis, the highest density of IELs among the barrier tissues. This number drops to about one IEL per 50 IECs in the colon. The difference in density largely reflects the greater proportion of non-crypt epithelium in the proximal small intestine, where the luminal or surface epithelium contains a greater density of IELs. Because of the tremendous surface area of the intestinal epithelium, IELs are one of the single largest populations of T cells in the body.

Notably, IELs are not static, rather they are highly motile within the intestinal epithelium, reflecting their surveillance function. Because of their disposition within the barrier epithelium itself and their fully mature effector status, IELs are both early sensors of changes in the epithelium resulting from environmental exposures and rapid responders that target epithelial cells for altered function or destruction so as to maintain barrier integrity. IELs participate in host defense against pathogens, in epithelial repair, and in homeostatic interactions with the epithelium, microbiota, and nutrients. They may play an important role in the removal of IECs that have sustained genotoxic stress or DNA damage that is not adequately repaired by the DNA damage response, thereby removing IECs at risk for malignant transformation. Here, we will focus on the populations of T cells that make up the large majority of IELs.

Innate-like, unconventional T cells (for example, invariant TCRγδ and oligoclonal TCRαβ T cells) take up residence within the intestinal epithelium

Fig. 12.23 Interactions between IECs and IELs. A variety of T cells are resident in the intestinal epithelium, including unconventional TCRγδ and TCRαβ cells that recognize butyrophilins (BTNs) and nonclassical MHC molecules (upper panels, left and right), as well as conventional TCRαβ cells that recognize peptide antigens presented by classical MHC molecules (lower left panel). Small numbers of ILC1 cells can also be found within the intestinal epithelium (lower right panel). Nearly all of these cells have cytocidal functions, irrespective of their recognition characteristics, and are mobile within the epithelial layer, allowing them to survey IECs for alterations that signal a need for IEC removal. TL, thymus leukemia antigen; β, IL-2Rβ; γ$_c$, common gamma chain; AHR, aryl hydrocarbon receptor.

immediately before and after birth. They are also referred to as thymic-derived, or natural, IELs (nIELs) (Fig. 12.23, upper panels, and **Fig. 12.24**), reflecting their development in, and immigration directly from, the thymus, without having to pass through organized lymphoid tissues to acquire their full effector functions (see Section 8-XX). In contrast, conventional T cells migrate into the intestinal epithelium only after their activation by specific antigen in the GALT or gut-associated lymph nodes; these T cells are therefore referred to as induced, or peripheral, IELs (pIELs) (Fig. 12.23, lower left panel, and Fig. 12.24). (Note that this terminology resembles that of the two major subsets of T$_{reg}$ cells—natural, or thymic, and induced, or peripheral, T$_{reg}$ cells.) pIELs derive from conventional CD4 and CD8 T cells, thus their T-cell receptors (TCRs) recognize foreign peptides bound to conventional MHC I or MHC II molecules, respectively. In contrast, TCRαβ nIELs are responsive to a diversity of MHC molecules, including MHC I and MHC II molecules as well as non-classical MHC I molecules (for example, MHC Ib), albeit through recognition mechanisms that do not appear to require specific peptides (see Chapter 6). Similarly, TCRγδ nIELs, which constitute the largest fraction of IELs in the intestines, are not activated by classical peptide:MHC recognition.

Although the variety of structures recognized by each type of nIEL is still an area of discovery, it is clear that this recognition diversity considerably expands the range of external and internal signals that can be sensed within the intestinal epithelial compartment. Nevertheless, most IEL types, both conventional and unconventional, share similar functionality in bolstering barrier defense and maintaining barrier function; most IELs are characterized by the expression of effector capabilities typical of innate and adaptive cells of the cytotoxicity

Characteristics of intraepithelial lymphocytes				
IEL subset	**Co-receptor expression**	**TCR repertoire**	**NK receptors**	**Antigenic ligands**
Unconventional TCRγδ nIEL	CD4⁻CD8⁻ CD8αα	TCRVγ7 > TCRVγ4 (mouse) TCRVγ1 (human)	NKG2 family CD94 LY49 family (mouse) KIR family (human)	BTNLs (mouse, ? human) MULT1, H60a, Qa-1 (mouse) CD1, MICA, MICB, ULBP (human)
Unconventional TCRαβ nIEL	CD4⁻CD8⁻ CD8αα	Oligoclonal	NKG2 family CD94 LY49 family (mouse) KIR family (human)	MHC I, MHC II (mouse, human) Non-classical MHC I (mouse) MICA, MICB, ULBP (human)
Conventional TCRαβ pIEL	CD8⁺CD8αα CD4⁺CD8αα	Diverse	None	Peptide:MHC I Peptide:MHC II
ILC1	CD4⁻CD8⁻	None	NKG2 family CD94 LY49 family (mouse) KIR family (human)	MULT1, H60a, Qa-1 (mouse) MICA, MICB, ULBP (human)

Fig. 12.24 Characteristics of intraepithelial lymphocytes.

immune module (see Section 11-2) (**Fig. 12.25**). Thus, common properties of IELs are their cytolytic capability (reflected in their expression of perforin and granzyme B) and expression of type 1 cytokines (for example, IFN-γ, TNF-α and FasL), which are activated in response to antigen recognition or to the local production of the cytokines IL-12, IL-18, and IL-15. Accordingly, a major function of nIELs and pIELs is their recognition and destruction of IECs that display properties of infection, damage, or stress. IELs can also express anti-microbial peptides, and at least a subset of nIELs is programmed for IL-17 production when activated. Additionally, IELs can express epithelial growth factors, such as epidermal growth factor (EGF), which promotes epithelial proliferation and repair in response to IEC damage.

The developmental origins of conventional and unconventional IELs are distinct. Although both subsets undergo selection in the thymus, neither TCRγδ nor TCRαβ nIELs undergo typical positive and negative selection like conventional TCRαβ T cells. Like most TCRγδ cells in the body, TCRγδ cells destined for residence in the intestinal epithelium exit the thymus as double-negative T cells; that is, prior to the double-positive stage of thymic selection (see Section 8-18). This includes TCRγδ cells with invariant use of $V_\gamma 7$, which represent the majority of intestinal nIELs in mice, as well as a smaller fraction of TCRγδ cells that express invariant $V_\gamma 4$. Each of these populations arise as part of the second programmed wave of TCRγδ cell development around the time of birth (see Section 8-18).

In contrast to TCRγδ nIELs, positive selection of TCRαβ nIELs requires recognition of MHC molecules. However, unlike conventional TCRαβ cells, TCRαβ nIELs appear to recognize many MHCs, including nonclassical MHC I and MHC I–like molecules (for example, CD1), rather than just a single one. Their intrathymic selection by unrestricted MHC molecules has been termed **agonist selection**, indicating the absence of classical TCR recognition of a specific peptide:MHC ligand. Instead, the TCRs of TCRαβ nIELs appear to be promiscuous for a range of different MHC molecules and are therefore broadly cross-reactive with MHC, including nonself MHC molecules.

Concurrent with their selection in the thymus, unconventional TCRγδ and TCRαβ cells fated for the intestinal epithelium up-regulate the integrin $\alpha_4\beta_7$, which directs them to the intestines rather than to peripheral lymphoid organs. They also up-regulate **CCR9** or **CCR10**, which directs them to the epithelium of the small or large intestine in response to **CCL25** or **CCL28**, respectively. They remain double-negative in the intestine but are induced by the high local concentrations of TGF-β produced by IECs to express the **CD8αα** homodimer and

Fig. 12.25 Effector functions of intraepithelial lymphocytes. Peripheral IELs (pIELs; top panels) are generally conventional CD8 cytotoxic T cells that recognize peptides derived from viruses or other intracellular pathogens bound to classical MHC class I molecules on infected epithelial cells. pIELs express an αβ TCR and the CD8αβ heterodimer co-receptor. Natural IELs (nIELs) carrying the CD8αα homodimer (bottom panels) recognize MIC-A and MIC-B using the receptor NKG2D and are activated by IL-15. Human epithelial cells that have been stressed by infection or altered cell growth or by a toxic peptide from the protein α-gliadin (a component of gluten) up-regulate expression of the nonclassical MHC class I molecules MIC-A and MIC-B and produce IL-15. Both types of IELs can kill by releasing perforin and granzyme. Apoptosis of epithelial cells can also be induced by the binding of Fas ligand on the T cell to Fas on the epithelial cell.

α$_E$ integrin (CD103), which pairs with β$_7$ integrin to form α$_E$β$_7$, which, in turn, binds E-cadherin expressed by IECs (see Figs. 12.23 and 12.24). CD8αα binds the nonclassical MHC class Ib molecule **thymus leukemia antigen (TL)**, which is expressed by IECs. Indeed, nearly all intraepithelial T cells, both nIELs and pIELs, express CD8αα, which appears both to down-modulate TCR signaling to prevent overreactivity of IELs to IEC antigens and to promote NK-like killing of damaged or stressed IECs. CD8αα may also serve as a survival signal to IELs.

Unlike nIELs, pIELs arise extrathymically from conventional CD4 and CD8 T cells after cognate antigen recognition in lymphoid tissues associated with the intestines. The precise signals that determine whether antigen-induced CD4 or CD8 T cells will become intraepithelial residents is not completely understood, but critical to their homing to the epithelial compartment is their expression of $\alpha_E\beta_7$ integrin (CD103) and CD8$\alpha\alpha$ induced by TGF-β signaling in the intestinal mucosa (see Figs. 12.23 and 12.24). In the case of CD4 pIELs, many appear to be derived from FoxP3$^+$ T$_{reg}$ cells that down-regulate FoxP3, whereas CD8 T cells retain much of their transcriptional program. Because both CD4 and CD8 pIELs retain expression of their native co-receptor, they acquire CD4$^+$CD8$\alpha\alpha^+$ and CD8$^+$CD8$\alpha\alpha^+$ phenotypes and retain responsiveness to cognate peptide:MHC II and peptide:MHC I complexes, respectively. This implies IECs must have the capacity to process and present foreign antigens on MHC I and MHC II molecules. Indeed, in response to IFN-γ signaling, IECs can up-regulate CIITA, the master transcriptional regulator of classical antigen-presenting pathways, and thus appear able to gain antigen-presenting cell (APC) functions, thereby enabling recognition by CD8 or CD4 pIELs.

As discussed in Chapter 6, the ligands recognized by unconventional T cells are heterogeneous and include both unique recognition receptors and those shared with other immune cells (see Sections 6-16 through 6-20). Both subsets of nIELs express molecules typical of the NKG2 family of NK-cell receptors, including NKG2D, an activating receptor that recognizes a subset of nonclassical MHC Ib molecules that are induced on intestinal epithelial cells in response to cellular injury, stress, or ligation of TLRs (see Section 6-16). In addition, as indicated earlier, TCR$\alpha\beta$ nIELs express cross-reactive TCRs capable of responding to broad changes in expression of classical and nonclassical MHC molecules in a cognate peptide–independent manner. This suggests TCR$\alpha\beta$ nIELs may be activated by alterations in MHC expression in a manner akin to NK cells.

As for TCR$\gamma\delta$ nIELs, it was recently shown that an important ligand for the dominant TCRVγ7 nIELs in mice is a heterodimer of BTNL1 and BTNL6, members of the **butyrophilin (BTN)** gene family. These ligands are structurally related to the B7 family of co-stimulatory molecules and are expressed on IECs but do not appear to engage receptors of the CD28 family. Rather, butyrophilins bind domains on invariant TCRs of some unconventional T cells, as has been shown for a subset of human TCR$\gamma\delta$ cells, thereby providing an activating signal via the $\gamma\delta$ TCR (**Fig. 12.26**). The TCR-liganding function of

Fig. 12.26 Butyrophilins activated by phosphoantigens mediate interactions between IECs and some $\gamma\delta$ T cells. Most butyrophilins (BTNs) expressed by IECs contain a cytosolic B30.2 (PRYSPRY) domain, which, when bound by phosphoantigens derived from microbes taken up by IECs or from endogenous sources in transformed cells, induces heterodimerization of two different butyrophilin molecules (left panel). This causes a reorientation of the BTN extracellular domains, enabling recognition by $\gamma\delta$ TCRs expressed by a subset of nIELs (middle panel), activating their cytolytic function and resulting in the killing of the IEC and its clearance by macrophages (right panel).

| Microbial (or self) phosphoantigens taken up by epithelial cell bind heterodimeric B30.2 domains of butyrophilin (BTN), resulting in "inside-out" signaling | Recognition of reoriented butyrophilin V-like domains by $\gamma\delta$ TCR activates cytocidal function of T cell, targeting IEC | IEC undergoes apoptotic death, releasing alarmins and chemokines that attract CX3CR1-bearing macrophage, resulting in removal of IEC |

B30.2
BTN
IEC
$\gamma\delta$ IEL
nonpeptide diphosphoantigens
$\gamma\delta$ TCR
apoptotic IEC
macrophage

some butyrophilin family molecules is dependent on an intracellular domain, termed B30.2. This domain binds a variety of nonpeptide diphosphate (pyrophosphate)-containing molecules, or phosphoantigens, which are products of microbes or transformed epithelial cells. Butyrophilins thus appear to be a form of pattern-recognition receptor that can detect foreign or self phosphoantigens and generate an 'inside-out' signal; that is, the TCR recognizes metabolites inside IECs via allosteric modulation of the BTN extracellular domains. Exactly how these ligands are regulated on IECs and whether this family of ligands is generic for different TCRγδ subsets is currently unknown. However, deletion of BTNL1 leads to selective loss of TCR Vγ7 nIELs in mice, indicating that this signal is required for their maintenance.

Important for both the development and maintenance of all subsets of nIELs and pIELs is expression by the epithelium of IL-15, which is produced in response to the microbiota and is 'trans-presented' to IELs in a complex with the IL-15Rα chain (see Fig. 12.23). That is, IL-15 produced by IECs is bound to the IEC surface by IL-15Rα, and this complex induces signaling via the IL-2Rβ and γc subunits expressed on IELs. The necessity for IL-15 in IEL maintenance is evident from the loss of IELs in either IL-15– or IL-15R–deficient mice. IL-15 signaling induces IEL expression of the **aryl hydrocarbon receptor (AHR)**, a transcription factor activated by various environmental ligands derived from cruciferous vegetables, microbiota metabolites, and xenobiotics that is expressed with subsets of ILC3 cells and T_H17 cells. IL-15 also induces IELs to express **Tbet**, which is also expressed by T_H1 cells and ILC1 cells. Both of these transcription factors are required for the maintenance and function of IELs. Mice that lack the AHR or Tbet have reduced numbers of IELs and show loss of nIELs, along with abnormalities in epithelial barrier repair, reinforcing the view that these unusual lymphocytes play important roles in the innate immune response to local materials in the intestine.

12-6 Innate lymphoid cells and unconventional lymphocytes are present in GALT and in the lamina propria and are rapid responders to microbes that breach the epithelium.

Just as the intestinal epithelium is populated by IELs in the perinatal period, so too are the GALT and intestinal lamina propria populated by tissue-resident innate lymphoid cells (ILCs) and innate-like lymphocytes. As discussed in Chapter 11 (see Section 11-3), in addition to cytotoxic ILCs (NK cells), three main groups of 'helper' ILCs are recognized (see Fig. 11.5)—ILC1, ILC2, and ILC3—each of which preferentially distributes to barrier tissues around birth. The composition of ILCs within the intestinal mucosa is dependent on the microbial exposure of the host, but in more industrialized countries where gastrointestinal worm infestation is less common, ILC3 cells are the most prominent. Most ILC3 cells are found in the GALT, but there are also ILC3 cells within the lamina propria.

Beyond the function of the LTi subset of ILC3 cells in the development of the GALT, ILCs play a central role in the early response to pathogen encroachment in the mature intestinal tissues and may also contribute to the homeostatic function of intestinal epithelial stem cells, although this is an area of ongoing study. There is an increasing appreciation of heterogeneity within ILC subsets, and at least two major mature ILC3 subsets are recognized: LTi-like ILC3 cells that lack NK receptors (NK-cell receptor negative, or NCR⁻) and non-LTi ILC3 cells that express NK receptors (NK-cell receptor positive, or NRC⁺). In humans, NCR⁻, LTi-like ILC3 cells are thought to preferentially express IL-17, whereas NCR⁺ ILC3 cells produce IL-22. In mice, there is greater overlap in cytokine expression profiles by these subsets. The development and function of both subsets is controlled by the transcription factors RORγt and AHR. Like all ILC3 cells, those in the intestines produce IL-17 and IL-22 in response to IL-23 and

IL-1β, which are produced primarily by local dendritic cells and inflammatory macrophages. As we will see in Section 12-20, IL-22 produced by ILC3 cells is indispensable for host protection in certain types of bacterial infections, where it acts on the epithelium to alter IEC development and stimulate production of antimicrobial peptides that restrain bacterial growth and prevent breach of the epithelium in advance of the adaptive response. Notably, similarly to T$_H$17 cells, with which they share many properties, ILC3 cells can be induced to transition to ILC1-type cells that lose expression of RORγt in favor of Tbet expression, resulting in a type 1 functional program. Indeed, most of the ILC1 cells that come to populate the intestinal mucosa appear to derive from ILC3 cells.

As we learned in Section 11-3, IL-5 and IL-13 produced by ILC2 cells in response to IL-33, TSLP, and IL-25 produced by enterocytes and/or tuft cells form an important layer of T cell–independent responses to helminth parasites in the intestine and may contribute to food allergies (see Chapter 14). CD1-restricted **invariant NKT (iNKT) cells** and **mucosal-associated invariant T (MAIT) cells** (see Sections 6-18 and 6-19) are also present in the lamina propria and account for 2–3% of lamina propria T cells in the human small intestine. As their names imply, both iNKT cells and MAIT cells express an invariant TCRα chain paired with a limited range of TCRβ chains. iNKT cells recognize lipids and glycolipids complexed with CD1d, whereas MAIT cells recognize metabolites of vitamin B derived mainly from the microbial riboflavin metabolism pathway complexed with MR1.

Summary.

The intestinal epithelium is composed of a diversity of cell types, each with specific functions in intestinal physiology and mucosal immunity. All intestinal epithelial cells (IECs) develop from common progenitors (intestinal stem cells, or ISCs) that reside in the base of the intestinal crypts and differentiate as they move from the base of the crypts toward the surface. There are two major developmental branches: absorptive and secretory. Absorptive enterocytes are most numerous and include absorptive enterocytes and M cells. Secretory enterocytes include goblet cells, Paneth cells (in the small intestine; not in the large intestine), tuft cells, and enteroendocrine cells. Each of these cell types contributes to innate immunity, albeit through mechanisms that reflect their specific functions. Most IECs have a high rate of turnover and must be continually replenished from the ISC pool.

A central feature of the intestinal mucosa—and other mucosal tissues—is the production of mucus, which is produced by goblet cells. Mucus plays an important role in protecting the epithelium from mechanical injury and from interactions with microbes. It provides a physical barrier but also retains molecules produced by or transported across the epithelium, including a diversity of antimicrobial peptides (AMPs) and secretory IgA (SIgA).

The integrity of the intestinal epithelium is supported by both innate and adaptive immune cells. The epithelium itself is populated by a range of natural and peripheral intraepithelial lymphocytes (nIELs and pIELs), including both conventional and unconventional TCRαβ and TCRγδ subsets. IELs actively survey the epithelium and respond by eliminating infected or damaged cells by cytolytic targeting. Beneath the epithelium there are substantial numbers of resident macrophages and dendritic cells that can take up microbes that traverse the epithelium and can eliminate them or ferry them to immune inductive sites to initiate adaptive immune responses. Intestinal phagocytes that sense pathogens can also release cytokines that activate innate lymphoid cells (ILCs) present within mucosal lymphoid tissues, such as in isolated lymphoid follicles (ILFs), as well as in the lamina propria.

The role of adaptive immunity in regulating the intestinal mucosal immune system at homeostasis.

As is evident from the foregoing discussion, three principal tasks of the intestinal mucosa are nutrient and water absorption, maintenance of the commensal microbiota, and defense against pathogens. The balance between nutrient uptake and accommodation to the microbiota, which are constant needs, and defense of the host, a less frequent need, represents a daunting challenge. The adaptive immune system plays a central role in navigating this balance, informed by signals from the epithelium and the array of innate immune cells that are integrated into the intestinal mucosa. Perhaps in no other tissue in the body is the necessity for the maintenance of immune tolerance more imperative: the diversity of foreign antigens present in food and the commensal bacteria is immense but must be tolerated.

A simple solution would be complete partitioning of these antigens from adaptive immune cells. Indeed, the innate defenses are sufficiently robust that much of the host response to the microbiota progresses without involvement of CD4 T cell–dependent responses. Further, a portion of the secretory IgA (SIgA) that contributes to the partitioning of commensal organisms away from the epithelium is generated in isolated lymphoid follicles (ILFs) without help from T cells. However, complete exclusion of foreign antigens within food and the microbiota is not possible, and in fact, the system has evolved to actively sample the luminal antigens through the specialized mucosal lymphoid tissues, such as Peyer's patches and ILFs. Accordingly, the mucosal immune system has acquired strategies to recognize and respond to innocuous antigens in a way that minimizes inflammation, unless absolutely necessary.

As the foreign antigens derived from food and the commensal microbiota are extracellular and therefore primarily presented by MHC II, it is the CD4 T-cell response that is central to the induction of homeostatic adaptive immunity in the intestines. As we will see, in the intestines, induction of T-cell immunity strongly favors the development of T_{reg} cells at homeostasis, reflecting unique properties of the antigen-presenting cells (APCs) in the gut and the route by which antigen is introduced—including the delivery of innocuous antigens to intestinal APCs via SIgA. Here, we will discuss mechanisms active in the intestinal mucosa that promote noninflammatory recognition of antigens by macrophages and dendritic cells, followed by a consideration of the induction of T_{reg} cells and SIgA-producing B cells.

12-7 The mucosal immune system must establish and maintain tolerance to harmless foreign antigens.

Antigens within food and commensal bacteria normally do not induce an inflammatory immune response, despite the lack of central (thymic) tolerance to them (**Fig. 12.27**). The mucosal immune system's environment is inherently

Fig. 12.27 Immune priming and tolerance are different outcomes of intestinal exposure to antigen. The intestinal immune system generates protective immunity against antigens that are presented during infections by pathogenic organisms. IgA antibodies are produced within the GALT, serum IgG and IgA are made in draining lymph nodes, and the appropriate effector T cells are activated in the intestine and elsewhere. When the antigen is encountered again, there is effective memory, ensuring rapid protection. Antigens from food proteins induce tolerance locally and systemically, with little or no IgA antibody production. T cells are not activated, and subsequent responses to challenge are suppressed. In the case of commensal bacteria, there is local secretory IgA (SIgA) production, but typically no systemic antibody responses, and peripheral regulatory T cells) (pT_{reg} cells) rather than effector T cells are activated.

	Protective immunity	Mucosal tolerance
Antigen	Invasive bacteria, viruses, toxins	Food proteins; commensal bacteria
Primary Ig production	Intestinal IgA and IgG Specific Ab present in serum	Some local IgA Low or no Ab in serum
Primary T-cell response	Local and systemic effector and memory T cells	pT_{reg} cell induction; no local effector T-cell response
Response to antigen reexposure	Enhanced (memory) response	Low or no response or systemic response

tolerogenic—a barrier to the development of nonliving vaccines, which need to overcome local regulatory mechanisms. Food proteins are not digested completely in the intestine; significant amounts are absorbed into the body in an immunologically relevant form. The default response to oral administration of a protein antigen is the development of a phenomenon known as **oral tolerance**. This is a form of **peripheral tolerance** that renders the systemic and mucosal immune systems relatively unresponsive to subsequent exposures to the same antigen. It can be demonstrated experimentally in mice by feeding them a foreign protein such as ovalbumin (**Fig. 12.28**). When the animals are then challenged with the antigen in adjuvant via a nonmucosal route, such as injection into the skin, the normal immune response one would expect is blunted. This suppression of systemic immune responses is long lasting and is antigen specific; responses to other antigens are not affected. A similar suppression of subsequent immune responses is observed after the administration of proteins into the respiratory tract, giving rise to the general concept of **mucosal tolerance**, because the usual response to such antigens is delivered via a mucosal surface. Systemic T-cell responses can also be inhibited by feeding humans protein antigens that they have not encountered previously, although it has proven an ineffective strategy for reversing reactivity to antigens to which individuals are already sensitized, such as food allergens. Thus, although mucosal tolerance can be used to avoid inflammatory disease in experimental animal models of type 1 diabetes mellitus, arthritis, and encephalomyelitis, clinical trials in humans have been less successful and have given way to other therapies, as we will discuss in greater detail in Chapters 14 and 16.

Various mechanisms are likely to account for oral tolerance to protein antigens, although the preferential generation of peripheral regulatory T (pT$_{reg}$) cells appears to be dominant. Antigens delivered to the GALT or draining lymph nodes generally induce antigen-specific FoxP3$^+$ T$_{reg}$ cells at homeostasis. As we will learn, migratory dendritic cells of the intestinal mucosa are conditioned by the local cytokine environment to produce two factors that induce T$_{reg}$ cell differentiation from naive CD4 T-cell precursors—retinoic acid and TGF-β—without producing pro-inflammatory signals, such as IL-1, IL-6, IL-23, or IL-12, which would otherwise stimulate the differentiation of effector CD4 T cells, such as T$_H$17 or T$_H$1 cells. These same pT$_{reg}$ cell–inducing factors also induce the expression of homing molecules that direct the migration of pT$_{reg}$ cells back to the intestinal mucosa, where they act to repress subsequent exposure to their cognate antigens. Although it is known that these same factors are also essential for the suppression of systemic immune responses to the same antigens, the mechanisms responsible for this link between the mucosal and peripheral immune systems are not yet understood. One plausible mechanism is that pT$_{reg}$ cells that have been primed in the intestines encounter antigen peripherally as they circulate from the intestines via draining lymph into the bloodstream. Alternatively, there is evidence that orally administered antigens can be found in lymph and the bloodstream, enabling access to resident dendritic cells in peripheral lymph nodes, although this remains to be proven. Notably, unlike soluble antigens, microbial antigens generally induce tolerance that is confined to the intestine; the systemic immune system normally remains ignorant of them, which may reflect their containment by the GALT and draining lymph nodes. Importantly, at times oral tolerance induction can fail, as is believed to occur in celiac disease (discussed in detail in Section 14-17) and peanut allergies (discussed in Sections 14-10 and 14-12).

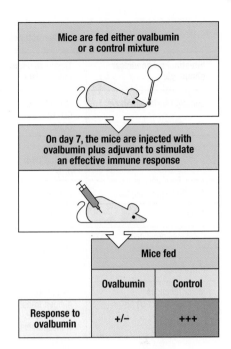

Fig. 12.28 Tolerance to antigens can be generated experimentally by oral administration. Mice are fed for 2 weeks with 25 mg of either ovalbumin or a control protein. Seven days later, the mice are immunized subcutaneously with ovalbumin plus an adjuvant, and after 2 weeks, the serum antibodies and T-cell function are measured. Mice that were fed ovalbumin have a lower ovalbumin-specific systemic immune response than that of mice fed the control protein.

The figure shows: "Mice are fed either ovalbumin or a control mixture" → "On day 7, the mice are injected with ovalbumin plus adjuvant to stimulate an effective immune response" →

Mice fed		
	Ovalbumin	Control
Response to ovalbumin	+/−	+++

Celiac Disease Case Study

12-8 Macrophages and dendritic cells have complementary roles in the maintenance of immune tolerance in the intestines.

Both inductive and effector sites within the intestinal mucosa contain abundant macrophages and dendritic cells (DCs). Indeed, the lamina propria of the healthy intestines contains the largest population of macrophages and

Characteristics of major mononuclear phagocytes in the intestines			
Intestinal mononuclear phagocyte	**Tissue-resident macrophage**	**Conventional dendritic cell 1 (cDC1)**	**Conventional dendritic cell 2 (cDC2)**
Common surface markers	MHC class II CD11c CCR2	MHC class II CD11c CCR2	MHC class II CD11c CCR2
Unique surface markers	CX3CR1 FcγRI (CD64) $\alpha_v\beta_8$	XCR1	SIRPα
Key inducing cytokines	CSF1 (M-CSF)	FLT3L	FLT3L
TLRs	TLR-4^{lo}, various	TLR-3$^+$, various	TLR-3$^-$, various
Cytokines produced	TGF-β (activation) (IL-10)	IL-12	IL-6, IL-23, TGF-β
Prevalence	Abundant	Frequent	Abundant
Major functions	"Silent" bacterial uptake and destruction Antigen transfer to migratory DCs Efferocytosis Transepithelial antigen sampling	Antigen presentation to naive CD8 T cells	Antigen presentation to naive CD4 T cells

Fig. 12.29 Characteristics of major mononuclear phagocytes in the intestines.

conventional dendritic cells (cDCs) in the body, with the highest number residing in the small intestine. A major historical confounder in understanding the origins and function of macrophages and DCs in the intestines has been the crossover in expression of several markers between the two lineages in this tissue. Thus, the classical macrophage marker, F4/80, is expressed by some cDCs in the intestines, and many intestinal macrophages express the DC marker CD11c (**Fig. 12.29**). However, recent studies indicate that while both intestinal macrophages and DCs express CD11c and class II MHC, unlike most DCs in this site, intestinal macrophages generally lack expression of α_E integrin (CD103). Instead, intestinal macrophages have been found to express **FcγRI** (CD64; see Fig. 10.38) and, in the mouse, **CX3CR1**, the receptor for the chemokine CX3CL1 (fractalkine); most intestinal DCs do not. On the basis of these markers, it is clear that intestinal macrophages are dependent on colony stimulating factor 1 (CSF1; also known as M-CSF) for their development and survival; in contrast, intestinal DCs are dependent on FLT3 ligand (FLT3L). Accordingly, CD64$^+$CD11c$^+$MHC II$^+$ cells are tissue-resident and display characteristic macrophage morphology, with abundant cytoplasm and intracytoplasmic vacuoles, while CD64$^-$CD11c$^+$MHC II$^+$ cells are migratory and localize to the GALT and mesenteric lymph nodes in a CCR7-dependent manner to participate in T-cell priming.

In contrast to many other tissues, where macrophages seed early in life and are maintained by local turnover, intestinal macrophages continually differentiate within the intestinal lamina propria from circulating Ly6C^{hi} monocytes that are recruited there by homeostatic chemokines recognized by CCR2 (for example, CCL2, CCL8). The transition from incoming monocytes to mature macrophages takes several days, and although the mature cells typically have a tissue life span of days to weeks, some studies have shown that a minority of macrophages can persist for several months. In the intestines, macrophages are much more prevalent than cDCs and represent ∼75% of all mononuclear phagocytes. They are positioned immediately under the epithelium and are highly phagocytic and microbicidal, and thus ideally suited to ingest and degrade any microbes or other particulates that penetrate the epithelial barrier. They also clear dying epithelial cells, which are found in large numbers in the intestine—an inevitable consequence of the high turnover of most IECs.

As mentioned earlier, intestinal macrophages, unlike macrophages in other parts of the body, are conditioned by the intestinal microenvironment to be non-inflammatory; they do not produce significant quantities of inflammatory cytokines (for example, TNF-α, IL-1β, IL-6) or reactive oxygen or nitrogen species in response to phagocytosis or exposure to stimuli such as bacteria or TLR ligands. They also lack receptors for IgA, complement, and the signaling components of the IgG receptor, and they have limited antigen-presentation capacity. Because of their anti-inflammatory properties, these cells are sometimes referred to as **inflammation-anergic macrophages**. Unlike other tissue macrophages, these cells appear to be terminally differentiated and do not give rise to M1 or M2 macrophages (see Section 11-6). Like other immune cells in the gut, intestinal macrophages are conditioned by exposure to the commensal microbiota, as evidenced by decreased numbers and lower turnover of these cells in germ-free mice and mice treated with broad-spectrum antibiotics.

The terminal differentiation of intestinal macrophages from incoming monocytes is regulated by TGF-β signaling. TGF-β is abundant in the intestinal lamina propria, where it is produced in its latent form by IECs, stromal cells, T_{reg} cells, mast cells, and macrophages themselves, and binds to the extracellular matrix. Once in the mucosa, signaling via TGF-β receptor 1 (TGF-βRI) and TGF-β receptor 2 (TGF-βRII) on incoming monocytes is essential for their differentiation into intestinal macrophages. The up-regulation of genes that are characteristic of the homeostatic profile of intestinal macrophages, such as CX3CR1 and CD11c, and the down-regulation of others, such as Ly6C, is mediated by the TGF-β–TGF-βR axis. Also up-regulated by TGF-β signaling is $\alpha_v\beta_5$ integrin, which is used by intestinal macrophages to ingest apoptotic cells in a process referred to as **efferocytosis** (Latin for 'to bury'). This integrin also activates latent TGF-β, and the process of efferocytosis induces TGF-β expression by intestinal macrophages, providing a feed-forward mechanism by which macrophage uptake of apoptotic cells contributes to tissue homeostasis. In this regard, apoptotic up-regulation of the ligand for CX3CR1 (that is, CX3CL1) by apoptotic epithelial cells serves to attract tissue macrophages to ensure their prompt removal, contributing also to their positioning immediately beneath the epithelium. CX3CR1 and $\alpha_v\beta_5$ integrin also contribute to the extension of **transepithelial dendrites (TEDs)**, cellular processes that extend across the epithelium to sample the luminal contents without perturbing tight junctions and epithelial integrity, as will be discussed further in Section 12-9.

While TGF-β signaling is required for induction of the inflammation-anergic phenotype of intestinal macrophages, IL-10 signaling also contributes by down-regulating components of TLR signaling, including MyD88, TRIF, and TRAF6, as well as CD14, a component of the LPS recognition complex. Thus, despite expressing TLR-3 and TLRs 5–9, intestinal macrophages have impaired abilities to activate MyD88-dependent and -independent NFκB signaling downstream of TLR ligation. IL-10 signaling also up-regulates inhibitors of NFκB signaling. Although intestinal macrophages can express IL-10, they appear to be a minor source, as macrophage-specific deletion of IL-10 does not disrupt intestinal homeostasis. Instead, CD4 T cells, particularly FoxP3[+] T_{reg} cells and FoxP3[−] T regulatory 1 (T_R1) cells, appear to be the major source of IL-10 that restrains intestinal macrophages from assuming a pro-inflammatory function (see Section 12-10). Thus, T cell–specific deletion of IL-10 and macrophage-specific deletion of the IL-10 receptor both lead to severe intestinal inflammation. Dietary and microbiota-derived metabolites, such as the short-chain fatty acid butyrate, can also repress the expression of pro-inflammatory cytokines.

In the inflamed intestines, whether the inflammation is caused by infection or immune-mediated disease (for example, inflammatory bowel disease), the accelerated influx of monocytes from the circulation results in a large number of phagocytic cells that express high levels of CD14, CD11c, and MHC II (CD14^hiCD11^hiMHC II^hi cells) and couple TLR signaling to an inflammatory response. These cells can produce abundant pro-inflammatory cytokines, such as TNF-α, IL-1β, IL-6, and IL-23, as well as chemokines that recruit both innate and adaptive immune cells. Monocytes recruited by inflammatory signals also demonstrate enhanced antigen processing and presentation capabilities, and they deploy the typical array of functional Fc and complement receptors. Notably, the CX3CR1^{hi} resident macrophages that persist in an inflammatory setting retain their anti-inflammatory signature, consistent with their fixed, terminal differentiation.

Dendritic cells that populate the intestinal mucosa at homeostasis share many features with those in other tissues. At homeostasis, these cells actively sample antigens transported across the epithelium, and they spend a relatively short time in the intestine before migrating into T-cell zones of the GALT or draining lymph nodes. As elsewhere, migration of dendritic cells to lymph nodes depends on the chemokine receptor CCR7 (see Fig. 9.7). It is estimated that 5–10% of the mucosal DC population emigrates to mesenteric lymph nodes every day, allowing constant delivery of antigens from the mucosa to lymph nodes. However, intestinal DCs differ from peripheral DCs in two fundamental ways: first, in the GALT, the lines between migratory and lymphoid tissue–resident DCs are somewhat blurred because of the close proximity of the antigen-sampling regions beneath the follicle-associated epithelium (FAE) to T-cell zones and the lack of afferent lymphatics; and second, at homeostasis, intestinal DCs are conditioned by the TGF-β–rich microenvironment to induce primarily noninflammatory adaptive immune responses dominated by the production of peripheral T_{reg} cells and T follicular helper (T_{FH}) cells that favor B-cell class switching to secretory IgA. These functions are critical to the induction of antigen-specific immune tolerance of food and the commensal microbiota, and they reinforce the anti-inflammatory tone of the intestines in a complementary, reinforcing feedback loop with intestinal macrophages. We will discuss further the role of DCs in maintaining homeostasis in Section 12-10.

12-9 The intestines have multiple routes for uptake and delivery of antigen to antigen-presenting cells.

A key challenge to the intestinal immune system is the task of surveying the immense intestinal surface area for the diversity of soluble, particulate, and microbial luminal antigens to which it must respond—all while maintaining an intact barrier. The intestinal mucosa must monitor what is 'out there' so that it can regulate its external and internal environments while remaining vigilant for potential threats. Accordingly, multiple mechanisms for the uptake of luminal antigens have evolved. These follow two general routes: across the specialized follicle-associated epithelium (FAE) that overlies Peyer's patches and ILFs; and across the non-FAE intestinal epithelium that overlies the lamina propria (**Fig. 12.30**). In both locations, antigens can be transported directly across the epithelial cells themselves (transepithelial transport, or transcytosis), between epithelial cells through regulated passages within the tight junctions (paracellular transport), or via transepithelial processes of macrophages and DCs that extend across the epithelium between IECs (phagocyte-mediated transport). Finally, antigens can be delivered across the epithelium in association with dying epithelial cells that are taken up by phagocytes. Although many luminal antigens are sampled as 'free' molecules, microbial antigens in particular are often taken up bound to secretory IgA (SIgA). Whereas antigens taken up across the non-FAE epithelium are transported to regional lymph nodes via afferent lymphatics, as is the case for other tissues, those taken up across the FAE epithelium are typically transported directly to the underlying GALT, which lacks afferent lymphatics but shares with other lymphoid tissues a similar network of reticular cells and conduits through which antigens are delivered for recognition by naive T cells (see Section 9-4).

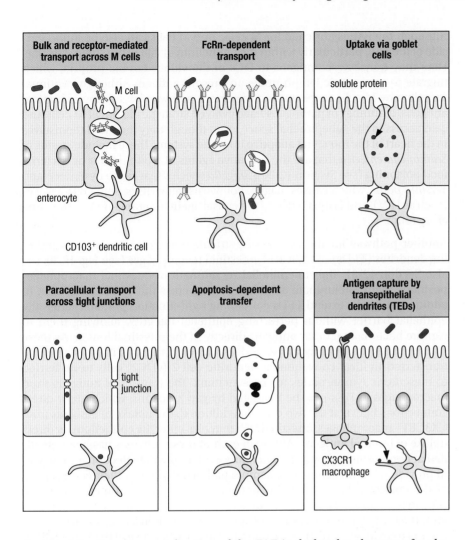

Fig. 12.30 Routes of antigen uptake in the intestines. Top row, first panel: Particulate antigens, such as bacteria, can be transported directly across M cells, either free or bound by SIgA via receptor-mediated transport. Second panel: Enterocytes can capture and internalize antigen:antibody complexes by means of the neonatal Fc receptor (FcRn) on their surface and transport them across the epithelium by transcytosis. Lamina propria dendritic cells express FcRn and other Fc receptors and capture and internalize the complexes. Third panel: During the process of exocytosis of mucin granules by goblet cells, soluble antigens can be endocytosed and transported across the goblet cell to CD103$^+$ dendritic cells in the lamina propria that dock with the secreting goblet cell. Bottom row, first panel: Small, soluble antigens can be transported across the tight junctions that seal the apical borders of adjacent enterocytes, enabling antigen uptake by a dendritic cell beneath the epithelium, a process called paracellular transport, or 'leak.' Second panel: Enterocytes infected with a pathogen can undergo apoptosis and be phagocytosed by a dendritic cell. Third panel: Mononuclear phagocytes can extend cellular processes called transepithelial dendrites (TEDs) between the cells of the epithelium without disturbing its integrity. These cells, thought to be primarily CX3CR$^+$ macrophages, may internalize antigen and pass it to neighboring conventional dendritic cells for presentation to T cells.

As noted previously, specialization of the FAE includes the absence of a glycocalyx and the presence of M (microfold) cells. M cells continually sample luminal antigens that range from macromolecules and small particulates to viruses and whole bacteria particles. This material is transported through the interior of the cell in membrane-bound vesicles to the basolateral cell membrane, where it is released. The basal cell membrane of an M cell makes close contacts with processes of dendritic cells to facilitate local antigen presentation within Peyer's patches and ILFs (see Fig. 12.30; see also Fig. 12.9). These dendritic cells are recruited to the subepithelial dome, or even into the FAE, in response to chemokines that are released constitutively by FAE epithelial cells; CCL20 and CCL9 produced by FAE cells bind to their receptors (CCR6 and CCR1, respectively) on dendritic cells. Although many antigens are taken up by macropinocytosis and micropinocytosis, intact microbes in particular can be taken up by receptor-mediated endocytosis. For a number of bacteria this may involve specific recognition of the bacterial FimH protein found in type 1 pili by a glycoprotein (GP2) on the M cell or receptors that recognize SIgA bound to the bacteria. Because antigens delivered via M cells promote SIgA responses in the GALT, the receptor-mediated uptake of SIgA-coated microbes provides a positive feedback loop for SIgA production. In addition to receptor-mediated uptake of SIgA-bound antigens by the M cell, non-M cells of both FAE and non-FAE express the **neonatal Fc receptor (FcRn)**, which binds and transcytoses IgG bidirectionally across the epithelium. Although primarily a pathway to import maternal IgG from breast milk to the newborn for passive transfer of antibodies (see Section 10-17), this mechanism can also mediate the uptake of IgG-bound antigens, as well as transport IgG from the lamina propria into the lumen, typically in the context of infections (see Section 12-20).

**Figure panel labels:**

Bulk and receptor-mediated transport across M cells
M cell
enterocyte
CD103$^+$ dendritic cell

FcRn-dependent transport

Uptake via goblet cells
soluble protein

Paracellular transport across tight junctions
tight junction

Apoptosis-dependent transfer

Antigen capture by transepithelial dendrites (TEDs)
CX3CR1 macrophage

Although the FAE is enriched for M cells, rare M cells can also be found outside of the FAE, particularly within the epithelium of villi of the small intestine. Here they transcytose antigens to DCs in the villous lamina propria, which migrate to mesenteric lymph nodes to present antigen. Although continual sampling by M cells represents an important pathway for sensing of luminal antigens, a number of pathogens have evolved strategies to target M cells and gain access to the subepithelial space, even though they then find themselves in the heart of the intestinal adaptive immune system. These include strains of *Salmonella enterica* that are the causative agents of typhoid fever or bacterial food poisoning (see Section 12-20); *Shigella* species that cause dysentery; and *Yersinia pestis*, which causes plague. Poliovirus, reoviruses, some retroviruses (such as HIV), and prions (such as the causal agent of scrapie) follow the same entry route.

Another pathway for the uptake of particulate antigens is via transepithelial dendrites (TEDs) of CX3CR1$^+$ intestinal macrophages (see Fig. 12.30; see also Section 12-8). The subepithelial recruitment of intestinal macrophages positions them to eliminate any bacteria that cross the epithelial barrier. In addition, they can extend TEDs containing tight-junction proteins across the epithelial barrier without perturbing epithelial integrity, allowing them to capture bacteria and other antigens directly in the intestinal lumen. As these macrophages are nonmigratory, antigens taken up in this manner must be transferred to local conventional dendritic cell 2 (cDC2) cells to be ferried to mesenteric lymph nodes for presentation. The transfer of antigens from macrophages to DCs may be mediated by gap junctions, which allow direct connections between the two cells. In addition to the uptake of antigens from CX3CR1$^+$ macrophages, intestinal DCs may also enter the epithelium for direct uptake of luminal antigens. Although each of these activities has been identified at homeostasis, they are particularly evident during infection and appear to provide a key mechanism to sample pathogens prior to their compromise of the epithelial barrier. Finally, antigen derived from apoptotic epithelial cells may be processed by cross-presenting dendritic cells (see Section 6-5) for induction of immune responses against enteric (that is, intestinal) viruses, such as rotaviruses, which cause diarrheal disease because of their specialized ability to infect enterocytes.

While the pathways described above play important roles in the acquisition of particulate antigens, including microbes, other pathways appear to dominate in the uptake of soluble antigens at homeostasis; the relatively limited surface area of follicle-associated epithelium and the small number of M cells restricts the flux of antigens that can be sampled via this route, and direct TED-mediated uptake at homeostasis is limiting. Recently, it was found that in addition to their role in secreting mucins, goblet cells have an important role in the transport of soluble antigens across the epithelial barrier. This occurs via **goblet cell–associated passages (GAPs)** that conduct low-molecular-mass soluble antigens (<70 kDa) to underlying CD103$^+$ cDC2 cells in the lamina propria (see Fig. 12.29). Precisely how antigen is transferred to DCs is unclear, but it appears to be linked to the process of goblet-cell secretion; when goblet-cell mucin secretion is stimulated, there is increased antigen uptake by goblet cells. DCs that have taken up antigen by this mechanism are found to contain goblet-cell proteins, indicating that goblet-cell components are transferred to DCs along with the luminal antigens. Importantly, in mice in which goblet cells were deleted, luminal antigen delivery to lamina-propria dendritic cells was undetectable, indicating that GAPs are a major pathway for soluble-antigen delivery at homeostasis and likely play a central role in oral-tolerance induction.

Another route for the uptake of soluble antigens is via **paracellular transport**, also referred to as paracellular 'leak.' As discussed in Section 12-4, because of the network of tight junctions between adjacent IECs, the intestinal epithelium is a selectively permeable barrier, allowing water, solutes, small molecules, and ions through, but preventing the transit of larger proteins (see Fig. 12.17). However, the permeability of tight junctions can be regulated by the differential expression of certain claudin proteins (for example, claudin-2), allowing macromolecules up to 10 kDa to traverse the epithelium. In the small intestine, paracellular transport appears to vary between villi at homeostasis, suggesting that it is actively regulated locally. Small antigens delivered via paracellular transport are not taken up efficiently by intestinal DCs. Instead, they are transported via lacteals and lymphatics to mesenteric lymph nodes, where they are delivered to resident DCs via reticular conduits (see Section 9-4). In inflammatory intestinal disease, such Crohn's disease or ulcerative colitis, increased permeability and disruption of tight junctions results in increased paracellular leak, possibly contributing to a breakdown in tolerance to antigens of the commensal microbiota.

12-10 Intestinal dendritic cells favor the induction of antigen-specific T_{reg} cells that are critical for the maintenance of mucosal immune homeostasis.

Peripheral FoxP3$^+$ T_{reg} cells are central players in intestinal immune tolerance to food and the commensal microbiota and are preferentially induced in the gut at homeostasis. Although thymic-derived regulatory T cells (tT$_{reg}$ cells) circulate to GALT and mesenteric lymph nodes, just as they do to peripheral lymphoid tissues, the dominant T_{reg} cells in the intestinal tissues are pT$_{reg}$ cells, which express a distinct TCR repertoire that reflects their development in response to nonself antigens taken up from the intestines, not to self antigens expressed in the thymus. These two populations can be distinguished by expression of the transcription factor helios and the surface receptor neuropilin-1 (NRP1), both of which are preferentially expressed by FoxP3$^+$ tT$_{reg}$ cells, but not by pT$_{reg}$ cells; hence the majority of T_{reg} cells in the intestines are typically FoxP3$^+$helios$^-$NRP1$^-$ pT$_{reg}$ cells. Global deficits in FoxP3$^+$ T_{reg} cells, such as those seen in people or mice with mutations in the FOXP3 gene, are associated with systemic autoimmunity that includes **inflammatory bowel disease (IBD)** and food allergies (see Section 15-4). In mice deficient for a conserved intronic enhancer element in the Foxp3 gene called CNS1 (conserved nucleotide sequence 1), which controls the development of pT$_{reg}$ cells, but not tT$_{reg}$ cells, there is intestine-specific breakdown in tolerance that results in inflammation and an imbalance in the microbiota in the colon. Thus, intestinal immune homeostasis is primarily controlled by pT$_{reg}$ cells responsive to antigens introduced via the gut.

As elsewhere, conventional dendritic cells (cDCs) are important in initiating and shaping immune responses in mucosal tissues. They are deployed both in intestinal lymphoid tissues (that is, GALT) and throughout the lamina propria. Both of the major subtypes of conventional dendritic cells (cDC1 and cDC2) are present in the intestine (see Fig. 12.29; see also Section 6-5 and Section 9-6). Given their dominant role in presentation of extracellular antigens, including those derived from food and commensal microbes, cDC2 cells are critical to the induction of T_{reg} cells in the gut. As mentioned earlier (see Section 12-8), the anti-inflammatory, pro-regulatory behavior of mucosal dendritic cells in the healthy gut is promoted by factors that are constitutively produced in the mucosal microenvironment. These include thymic stromal lymphopoietin (TSLP) produced by IECs; short-chain fatty acids (SCFAs), such as butyrate, which are produced by anaerobic commensal bacteria; prostaglandin E2 (PGE2) produced by stromal cells; neuropeptides, such as vasointestinal peptide (VIP), produced by local neurons; IL-10 produced by intestinal macrophages and FoxP3$^+$ T_{reg} cells; and TGF-β and retinoic acid (RA) produced

Fig. 12.31 Factors controlling the function of conventional dendritic cells in the intestinal lamina propria. The differentiation and function of dendritic cells in the intestinal lamina propria are affected by products of bacteria, epithelial cells, stromal cells, and neuronal cells, as well as dietary and microbial metabolites. Major factors that induce a pro-tolerogenic DC functional state include TGF-β, IL-10, retinoic acid, and TSLP. Circulating pre-DCs can acquire a tolerogenic phenotype in response to epithelial-cell production of retinoic acid (RA; derived from vitamin A), transforming growth factor-β (TGF-β), and thymic stromal lymphopoietin (TSLP), to active bacterial metabolites such as short-chain fatty acids (SCFAs) and niacin, as well as to specific microbial products, such as zymosan (β-glucan). Immune and nonimmune cells produce IL-10, TGF-β, prostaglandin E2 (PGE2), RA, and vasoactive intestinal peptide (VIP), which can influence cDC function.

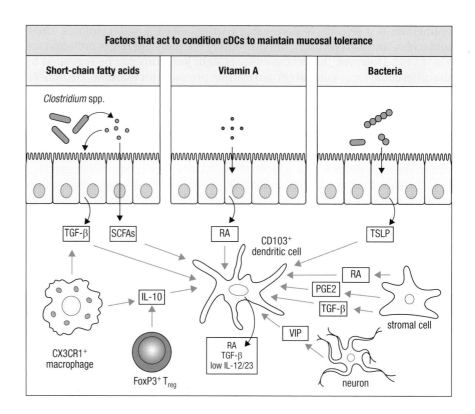

by IECs and stromal cells (**Fig. 12.31**). The collective action of these factors induces the expression by intestinal DCs of RA and TGF-β, both of which are critical to the induction of FoxP3$^+$ pT$_{reg}$ cells (see Section 9-15 and Fig. 9.37).

Because vitamin A (retinol), the substrate from which RA is generated, cannot be synthesized and must be absorbed by the intestine from the diet, pT$_{reg}$ cell induction is dependent on a dietary factor. Retinol stored in the liver and delivered to the small intestine via bile provides an additional source for the local generation of retinoic acid in the intestines. Production of RA from vitamin A requires the sequential actions of enzymes expressed by intestinal DCs: alcohol dehydrogenases (ADHs) and retinal dehydrogenases (RALDHs). RA is a ligand for a nuclear receptor, retinoic acid receptor (RAR), activation of which promotes the development of pT$_{reg}$ cells while strongly repressing the differentiation of T$_H$17 cells (see Fig. 9.37). RA also induces the expression of gut-specific homing receptors, including α$_4$β$_7$ and CCR9 (see Section 12-11). The induction of regulatory T cells in intestinal tissues is also dependent on TGF-β, which is produced by migratory and lymphoid tissue–resident cDC2 cells that take up antigens in the lamina propria and GALT, respectively. TGF-β also induces expression of the integrin α$_E$β$_7$ (CD103) on developing T$_{reg}$ cells. The combined effects of RA and TGF-β therefore, are to induce the differentiation of FoxP3$^+$ pT$_{reg}$ cells and to direct their trafficking to the intestines.

After trafficking to the intestines, pT$_{reg}$ cells can acquire additional functional features that are important in maintaining immune homeostasis. It is thought that this transition involves further differentiative signals received when T$_{reg}$ cells enter effector sites in the intestines, such as the lamina propria. Referred to as **effector regulatory T (eT$_{reg}$) cells**, these cells are characterized by their expression of the anti-inflammatory cytokines IL-10 and TGF-β, both of which contribute to the tolerogenic nature of homeostatic intestinal cDCs in a positive feedback loop and are indispensable for restraining inflammatory responses to the commensal microbiota in the large intestine. Studies that examined the expression of FoxP3 and IL-10 in tissues throughout the body using transgenic reporter mice found that the highest frequency of IL-10–expressing cells in

T_{reg} cells are highly enriched in the intestinal mucosa				
	CD4+FoxP3−		CD4+FoxP3+	
	IL-10−	IL-10+	IL-10−	IL-10+
Mesenteric LNs	80–90%	~1%	5–10%	~1%
Small intestine	70–80%	5–10%	5–10%	5–10%
Large intestine	60–70%	3–5%	10–15%	15–20%
Large intestine, GF	80–90%	~1%	5–10%	~1%

Fig. 12.32 T_{reg} cell subsets are major populations in the large and small intestines. Flow cytometry was used to analyze T_{reg} cell subsets in murine intestines and mesenteric lymph nodes, defined by concordant or differential expression of IL-10 and FoxP3 within the total fraction of CD4 T cells. The analysis of large intestinal cells compared those isolated from conventionally housed and germ-free (GF) mice. LNs, lymph nodes.

the body was in the intestines (**Fig. 12.32**), particularly in the large intestine, where it is primarily expressed by FoxP3+helios−NRP1− pT$_{reg}$ cells at homeostasis. The functional importance of IL-10 expression by eT$_{reg}$ cells has been demonstrated in studies in which selective deletion of the gene *Il10* in FoxP3+ T cells resulted in spontaneous inflammation of the large intestine, or colitis. Thus, IL-10 produced by eT$_{reg}$ cells is important for immune homeostasis in the large intestine.

Elegant experiments in the 1990s led to the now generally accepted idea that T cells with the potential to respond to commensal microbiota are present in normal animals but are usually kept in check through active repression by T$_{reg}$ cells (**Fig. 12.33**). In these studies, the transfer of naive CD4 T cells into immunodeficient mice led to spontaneous IBD, or colitis, unless a separate population that included T$_{reg}$ cells was co-transferred. The cell types that drove this disease were later shown to be microbiota-reactive T$_H$17 and T$_H$1 cells

Cells transferred	Microbiota	Disease
Unfractionated CD4+ T cells	+	No
CD4+CD45RB^{hi} T cells (naive)	+	Colitis
CD4+CD45RB^{hi} T cells + CD4+CD45RB^{lo} T cells (includes T$_{reg}$ cells)	+	No
CD4+CD45RB^{hi} T cells + IL-10–deficient CD4+CD45RB^{lo} T cells (includes T$_{reg}$ cells)	+	Colitis
CD4+CD45RB^{hi} T cells	−	No

Normal	Colitis
	M SM ME

Fig. 12.33 T cells with the potential to produce inflammation in response to commensal bacteria are present in normal animals, but are controlled by regulatory T cells. Transfer of total (unfractionated) CD4+ T cells from a normal mouse into an immunodeficient mouse, such as one lacking the gene *Rag1* (*Rag1−/−*), will lead to reconstitution of the CD4 T-cell compartment. However, if naive CD4 T cells (CD4+CD45RB^{hi}) are isolated from the total CD4 T-cell population and transferred, the recipient mice develop severe inflammation of the colon. This is prevented by co-transferring CD4+CD45RB^{lo} T cells that were removed during the isolation of the naive (CD45RB^{hi}) fraction of the total CD4+ T-cell population. The CD4+CD45RB^{lo} fraction comprises nearly all of the T$_{reg}$ cells within the CD4 T-cell population. If the CD4+CD45RB^{lo} fraction is isolated from IL-10–deficient mice, the protective effect of these cells is lost. The intestinal inflammation caused by naive CD4+ T cells requires the presence of the microbiota; it does not occur in germ-free mice or in mice treated with antibiotics. These experiments demonstrate that some CD4+ T cells in normal animals are capable of provoking inflammatory responses against the intestinal microbiota, but they are normally held in check by regulatory T cells. Shown in the two right panels are examples of the histopathology of the normal mouse colon (left) and the colitic colon (right), the latter demonstrating a much thickened mucosa (M) due to elongation of the crypts and dense infiltrates of inflammatory cells, as well as the expansion of the submucosa (SM) and thickening of the muscularis externa (ME).

that developed from the transferred naive CD4 T cells. That the inflammatory response was directed against the intestinal microbiota was demonstrated by the absence of disease in germ-free mice. An essential requirement for IL-10 expression by T_{reg} cells in preventing disease was found, as the transfer of T_{reg} cells deficient in IL-10 failed to control the development of colitis. Similar studies have shown that T_{reg} cells deficient for TGF-β are impaired in their prevention of colitis. Accordingly, mutations in the genes *IL10RA*, *IL10RB*, *TGFBR1*, or *TGFBR2* in humans are associated with severe early-onset inflammatory bowel disease, such as Crohn's disease, presumably due, at least in part, to defects in the function of eT_{reg} cells reactive to commensal microbial antigens.

12-11 Lymphocytes primed within the mucosal immune system are directed to return to the mucosal tissue by tissue-specific adhesion molecules and chemokine receptors.

The destination of naive T cells and B cells circulating in the bloodstream is not predetermined, and like those in other peripheral lymphoid tissues, the cells destined to be primed in the GALT or mesenteric lymph nodes enter through **high endothelial venules (HEVs)** (see Fig. 9.4). As in the systemic immune system, this process is controlled largely by the chemokines **CCL21** and **CCL19**, which are released from stromal cells in these sites and bind the receptor **CCR7** on naive lymphocytes. In the Peyer's patches and ILFs, this process is assisted by the binding of the mucosal vascular addressin **MAdCAM-1** on HEVs to the **L-selectin** expressed on naive T cells. **CXCR5** responding to **CXCL13** produced in B-cell areas is also important for recruitment of naive B cells to Peyer's patches and ILFs. As in other peripheral lymphoid tissues, if the naive lymphocytes do not see their antigen, they do not down-regulate **sphingosine 1-phosphate receptor 1 (S1PR1)**, and they return to the bloodstream via the lymphatics. If they encounter antigen in the GALT or regional lymph nodes, they are imprinted by intestinal DCs to return to the intestinal lamina propria.

Although some T and B lymphocytes initially activated in Peyer's patches or ILFs may migrate directly to adjacent parts of the lamina propria, most leave via the lymphatics, pass through mesenteric lymph nodes, and eventually end up in the thoracic duct. From there they circulate in the bloodstream (**Fig. 12.34**) and selectively reenter the intestinal lamina propria via small blood vessels. Gut-specific homing by antigen-stimulated T and B cells is determined in large part by the expression of the integrin $\alpha_4\beta_7$, which binds

Fig. 12.34 Priming of naive T cells and the redistribution of effector T cells in the intestinal immune system. Naive T cells express the chemokine receptor CCR7 and L-selectin, which direct their entry into Peyer's patches and isolated lymphoid follicles (ILFs) via high endothelial venules (HEVs). In T-cell areas, they encounter antigen that has been transported into the lymphoid tissue by M cells and is presented by local dendritic cells. During activation, and under the selective control of signals from dendritic cells activated locally by TGF-β, the T cells lose L-selectin and acquire the chemokine receptor CCR9 and the integrin $\alpha_4\beta_7$. After activation, but before full differentiation, the primed T cells exit from the Peyer's patch via the draining lymphatics, passing through the mesenteric lymph node to enter the thoracic duct. The thoracic duct empties into the bloodstream, delivering the activated T cells back to the wall of the small intestine. Here T cells bearing CCR9 and $\alpha_4\beta_7$ are attracted specifically to leave the bloodstream and enter the lamina propria of the villus.

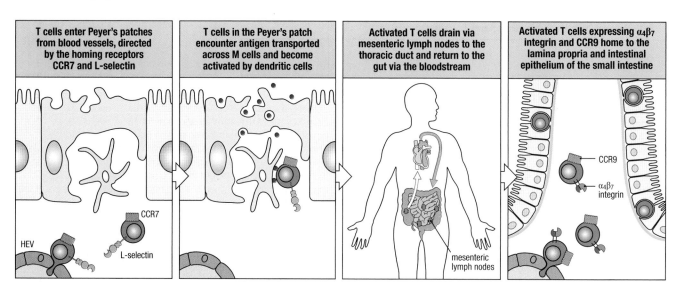

T cells enter Peyer's patches from blood vessels, directed by the homing receptors CCR7 and L-selectin

T cells in the Peyer's patch encounter antigen transported across M cells and become activated by dendritic cells

Activated T cells drain via mesenteric lymph nodes to the thoracic duct and return to the gut via the bloodstream

Activated T cells expressing $\alpha_4\beta_7$ integrin and CCR9 home to the lamina propria and intestinal epithelium of the small intestine

CCR7

L-selectin

HEV

mesenteric lymph nodes

CCR9

$\alpha_4\beta_7$ integrin

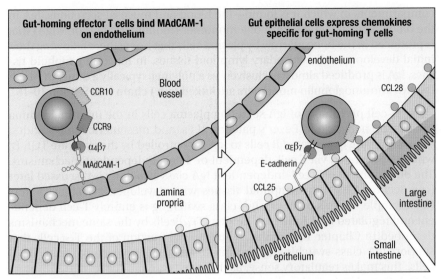

Fig. 12.35 Molecular control of intestine-specific homing of lymphocytes. Left panel: T and B lymphocytes primed by antigen in the Peyer's patches or mesenteric lymph nodes arrive as effector lymphocytes in the bloodstream supplying the intestinal wall (see Fig. 12.34). The lymphocytes express the integrin $\alpha_4\beta_7$, which binds specifically to MAdCAM-1 expressed selectively on the endothelium of blood vessels in mucosal tissues. This provides the adhesion signal needed for the emigration of cells into the intestinal lamina propria. Right panel: If primed in the GALT or lymph nodes draining the small intestine, the effector lymphocytes also express the chemokine receptor CCR9, which allows them to respond to CCL25 (yellow circles) produced by epithelial cells of the small intestine; this enhances their selective recruitment to the small intestine. Effector lymphocytes that have been primed in the GALT or lymph nodes draining the large intestine do not express CCR9 but instead express CCR10. CCR10 may respond to CCL28 (green circles) produced by colon epithelial cells to fulfill a similar function. Lymphocytes destined to enter the epithelial layer no longer express the $\alpha_4\beta_7$ integrin and instead express the $\alpha_E\beta_7$ integrin. The receptor for this is E-cadherin on intestinal epithelial cells (IECs). These interactions may help to retain lymphocytes in the epithelium once they have entered the lamina propria or the epithelium.

to MAdCAM-1 expressed on microvessels of intestinal tissues (**Fig. 12.35**). Homing of these lymphocytes to the small intestinal or large intestinal mucosa is further regulated by differential expression of the chemokine receptors, including CCR9 or CCR10, which respectively bind the homeostatic chemokine CCL25 (small intestine) or CCL28 (large intestine) produced by the local epithelium. The chemokine receptor–like orphan G-coupled protein receptor 15 (GCPR15) also appears to be important for trafficking of effector T cells to the large intestine, although its ligand(s) is not yet known. Notably, the epithelium of the lactating breast also expresses CCL28. In this way, SIgA-producing B lymphoblasts primed to commensal microbial antigens in the large intestine are recruited to the breast where they produce maternal SIgA, which is passively transferred to the nursing neonate.

12-12 Secretory IgA is the dominant class of antibody associated with the mucosal immune system at homeostasis.

The dominant class of antibody in the mucosal immune system is immunoglobulin A (IgA), which is produced locally by plasma cells in the lamina propria, including that of the intestines. Hundreds of thousands of IgA-producing plasma cells are present in the normal human intestine, and they produce 3–4 g of IgA each day, by far the most of any immunoglobulin class produced in the gut. This continual production of large quantities of IgA occurs in the absence of pathogenic invasion and is driven almost entirely by recognition of the commensal microbiota. The nature of IgA differs between the two main compartments in which it is found—the blood and mucosal secretions. IgA in the blood is mainly in the form of a monomer (monomeric IgA, or MIgA) that is produced in the bone marrow by plasma cells that home there following their initial development in secondary lymphoid tissues. In mucosal lymphoid tissues, IgA is produced almost exclusively as a polymer, typically a dimer in which the two immunoglobulin monomers are linked by a **J chain** (see Section 10-16).

Naive B-cell precursors of IgA-secreting plasma cells in the intestinal lamina propria are activated in Peyer's patches, ILFs, and mesenteric lymph nodes. Class switching of activated B cells to IgA is controlled by the cytokine TGF-β, whether generated via T cell–dependent or T cell–independent mechanisms. The development of T cell–independent IgA class switching is discussed later (see Section 12-13). In lymphoid tissues with developed germinal centers (for example, Peyer's patches), IgA class switching is entirely T-cell dependent and regulated by **T follicular helper (T_{FH})** cells by the same mechanisms described in Chapter 10. Notably, a substantial fraction of the T_{FH} cells that support IgA class switching in the intestines appears to derive from pT_{reg} cells. This makes regulatory sense, as these cells are producers and activators of TGF-β, and by inducing the production of SIgA to antigens they recognize, they provide a self-reinforcing positive feedback loop, due to the fact that delivery of antigens in complex with SIgA favors the generation of pT_{reg} cells. In this regard, it has been shown in mice that depletion of T_{reg} cells leads to a decline in IgA$^+$ plasma cells and intestinal IgA over a few days, indicating that intestinal plasma cells are relatively short-lived and that T_{reg} cells are critical for their maintenance and/or their replacement.

Unlike mice, which produce a single isotype of monomeric and dimeric IgA, humans produce two IgA isotypes, IgA1 and IgA2. The ratio of IgA1 to IgA2 varies markedly depending on the tissue, being about 10:1 in the blood and upper respiratory tract, about 3:2 in the small intestine, and 2:3 in the colon. Some common pathogens of the respiratory mucosa (such as *Haemophilus influenzae*) and the genital mucosa (such as *Neisseria gonorrhoeae*) produce proteolytic enzymes that can cleave IgA1, whereas IgA2 is cleavage-resistant. The higher proportion of plasma cells secreting IgA2 in the large intestine might result because the high density of commensal microorganisms at this site drives the production of cytokines that cause its selective class switching. The IgA isotype produced in mice is most like human IgA2.

IgA-expressing B plasmablasts produced in the GALT or regional lymph nodes express the mucosal homing integrin $\alpha_4\beta_7$ and the chemokine receptors CCR9 or CCR10, which cause them to localize to the small or large intestinal lamina propria. Once there, these cells undergo final differentiation into plasma cells that synthesize IgA dimers and secrete them into the subepithelial space (**Fig. 12.36**). To reach antigens in the gut lumen, the dimeric IgA must be transported across the epithelium by the **polymeric immunoglobulin receptor (pIgR)** (see Section 10-16). pIgR is expressed constitutively on the basolateral surfaces of immature epithelial cells located at the base of intestinal crypts where it binds dimeric IgA. pIgR transports the dimeric IgA to the luminal surface of the epithelium, where it is released by proteolytic cleavage of the extracellular domain of the receptor. Part of the cleaved pIgR remains associated with IgA and is known as **secretory component (SC)**. The resulting antibody is protected from proteolytic cleavage and is referred to as secretory IgA (SIgA) (see Section 10-16). The same pathway is used to transport pentameric IgM across the intestinal epithelium—so-called secretory IgM (SIgM)—which appears to play an important role in the colonization of the intestines by the commensal microbiota early in life.

In some animals there is a second route of IgA secretion into the intestine—the **hepatobiliary route**. Dimeric IgA that has not bound pIgR is taken up into venules in the lamina propria, which drain intestinal blood to the liver via the portal vein (see Fig. 12.7). In the liver, the portal vein delivers the dimeric IgA

Binding of IgA to receptor on basolateral face of epithelial cell	Endocytosis	Transcytosis to apical face of epithelial cell	Release of IgA dimer at apical face of epithelial cell

Fig. 12.36 Transcytosis of IgA antibody across epithelia is mediated by the polymeric Ig receptor (pIgR), a specialized transport protein. Most IgA antibody is synthesized in plasma cells lying just beneath epithelial basement membranes of the gut, the respiratory epithelia, the tear and salivary glands, and the lactating mammary gland. The IgA dimer, linked by a J chain, diffuses across the basement membrane and is bound by the pIgR on the basolateral surface of the epithelial cell. The bound complex undergoes transcytosis, by which it is transported in a vesicle across the cell to the apical surface. There the pIgR is cleaved, leaving the extracellular IgA-binding component bound to the IgA molecule as the so-called secretory component. Although not shown, carbohydrate on the secretory component binds to mucins in mucus and holds the IgA at the epithelial surface. The residual part of pIgR that remains cell-associated is nonfunctional and is internalized and degraded. IgA is transported across epithelia in this way into the lumina of several organs that are in contact with the external environment. Pentameric IgM, which is also linked by a J chain, is similarly transported across mucosal epithelia by pIgR and released in association with the secretory component.

to sinusoids that are lined by a fenestrated endothelium containing 'holes' that allow the antibodies direct access to underlying hepatocytes, which express pIgR on their surface. IgA is taken up into the hepatocytes and transported by transcytosis into an adjacent bile duct. In this way, secretory IgA can be delivered back to the duodenum via the common bile duct. This hepatobiliary route allows dimeric IgA to eliminate antigens that have invaded the lamina propria and have been bound there by IgA. Although highly efficient in rats and other rodents, this route does not seem to be of great significance in humans and other primates, in whom hepatocytes do not express pIgR.

IgA secreted into the gut lumen binds to the layer of mucus coating the epithelial surface via carbohydrate determinants in secretory component. There it prevents invasion by pathogenic organisms and also has a crucial role in maintaining the homeostatic balance between the host and the commensal microbiota. IgA does this in a number of ways (**Fig. 12.37**). First, it inhibits microbial adherence to the epithelium, its ability to bind bacteria being assisted by the unusually wide and flexible angle between the Fab pieces of the IgA molecule, particularly the IgA1 isotype, allowing very efficient bivalent binding to large antigens such as bacteria. Secretory IgA also aggregates bacteria such that they are less able to penetrate the network of mucins in the mucus. Secretory IgA can also neutralize microbial toxins or enzymes.

In addition to its activities in the lumen, IgA can neutralize bacterial lipopolysaccharide and viruses it encounters within endosomes inside epithelial cells, as well as across the epithelial barrier in the lamina propria after bacteria and viruses have penetrated there. The resulting IgA:antigen complexes are then reexported into the gut lumen. From there they are excreted from the body. Complexes containing dimeric IgA formed in the lamina propria can also be excreted via the hepatobiliary route described earlier. In addition to enabling the elimination of antigens, the formation of IgA:antigen complexes can enhance the uptake of luminal antigen by M cells and local dendritic cells, via binding of carbohydrate residues on IgA to lectin receptors such as Dectin-1

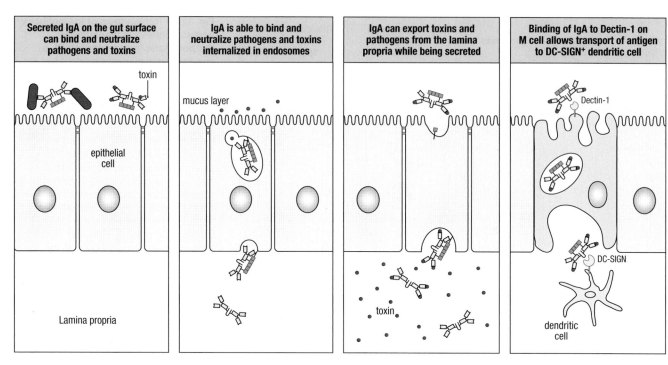

Secreted IgA on the gut surface can bind and neutralize pathogens and toxins	IgA is able to bind and neutralize pathogens and toxins internalized in endosomes	IgA can export toxins and pathogens from the lamina propria while being secreted	Binding of IgA to Dectin-1 on M cell allows transport of antigen to DC-SIGN⁺ dendritic cell

Fig. 12.37 Mucosal IgA has several functions in epithelial surfaces. First panel: IgA adsorbs on the layer of mucus covering the epithelium, where, in addition to aggregating commensal bacteria (not shown), it can neutralize pathogens and their toxins, preventing their access to tissues and inhibiting their functions. Second panel: Pathogens and toxins internalized by the epithelial cell can meet and be neutralized by IgA in endosomes. Third panel: Toxins or pathogens that have reached the lamina propria encounter pathogen-specific IgA there, and the resulting complexes are reexported into the lumen across the epithelial cell as the dimeric IgA is secreted. Fourth panel: Antigen bound to secretory IgA in the lumen can bind via carbohydrate residues on the Fc portion of IgA to Dectin-1 on M cells in Peyer's patches and be transported to underlying dendritic cells.

and DC-SIGN, respectively. In addition to these antigen-specific effects, secretory IgA can restrict the entry of bacteria in a nonspecific manner, because the high carbohydrate content of the Fc part of the IgA heavy chain allows it to act as a decoy for receptors that bacteria use to bind carbohydrates on the epithelial surface. Importantly, SIgA has little capacity to activate the classical pathway of complement or to act as an opsonin, and so does not induce inflammation. Uptake of IgA:antigen complexes by dendritic cells also induces these cells to produce anti-inflammatory IL-10. Together these properties mean that IgA can limit the penetration of microbes into the mucosa without risking inflammatory damage to these fragile tissues, something that would be potentially harmful in the intestine. For the same reasons, secretory IgA fosters the beneficial symbiosis between the host and its commensal microbiota.

12-13 T cell–independent processes can contribute to IgA production in some species.

A significant proportion of intestinal SIgA is derived from T cell–independent B-cell activation and class switching. This is clearly true in mice, and probably similar in humans, although experimental support for the latter is more limited. T cell–independent B-cell activation depends on activation of the innate immune system by the products of commensal microbes and results from the direct interaction of B cells with intestinal cDCs and follicular dendritic cells in isolated lymphoid follicles. Most of this SIgA production seems to involve lymphocytes of the B-1 subset (see Section 8-10), which arise from precursor B cells in the peritoneal cavity and migrate to the intestinal wall in response to microbial constituents such as lipopolysaccharide (LPS). Once in the mucosa, TGF-β–dependent class switching to IgA occurs under the influence of local factors, including IL-6, retinoic acid, and BAFF and APRIL (see Fig. 10.6), which bind to TACI on B cells, substituting for signals otherwise supplied by CD4 helper T cells (see Section 10-1). Intestinal epithelial cells produce BAFF and APRIL, while local macrophages, DCs, and eosinophils may contribute by producing APRIL, IL-6, and TGF-β.

The IgA antibodies produced in these T cell–independent responses are generally of more limited diversity and lower affinity, with little evidence of somatic hypermutation. They are nevertheless an important source of 'natural' antibodies directed at commensal bacteria and may play a particularly important role in modulating the developing intestinal microbiota in neonates prior to establishment of more mature T- and B-cell responses. With progressive maturation of the immune system during the first years of life, there is a shift to a greater fraction of SIgA contributed by T-dependent B-cell activation and class switching; hence, a greater proportion of SIgA has undergone somatic hypermutation with increasing age. T-independent SIgA production in the intestines may offer a glimpse into the evolutionary history of specific antibody responses in the mucosa, and it appears to serve as a 'backup' for the generation of SIgA when T cell–dependent IgA production is compromised, as it is in AIDS or in individuals with an inherited deficiency of CD40.

12-14 IgA deficiency is relatively common in humans but may be compensated for by secretory IgM.

Selective deficiency of IgA production is one of the most common inherited, or primary, immune deficiencies in humans, occurring in about 1 in 500 to 700 Caucasians. (It is somewhat rarer in other ethnic groups.) The most frequent genetic mutation that has been identified in this condition is in the TACI receptor for BAFF. A slightly higher incidence of respiratory infections, atopy (a tendency for allergic reactions to harmless environmental antigens), and autoimmune disease has been reported in older people with IgA deficiency. However, most individuals with IgA deficiency are not overly susceptible to infections. The dispensability of IgA probably reflects the ability of IgM to replace IgA as the predominant antibody in secretions, and increased numbers of IgM-producing plasma cells are indeed found in the intestinal mucosa of IgA-deficient people. Because IgM is a J chain–linked polymer, IgM produced in the gut mucosa is bound efficiently by the pIgR and is transported across epithelial cells into the gut lumen as secretory IgM. The importance of this backup mechanism has been shown in knockout mice. Animals lacking IgA alone have a normal phenotype, but those lacking the pIgR are susceptible to mucosal infections. They also show increased penetration of commensal bacteria into tissues and a consequent systemic immune response to these bacteria. Genetic absence of the pIgR has never been reported in humans, suggesting that such a defect is lethal.

12-15 Large numbers of antigen-experienced T cells are present in the intestinal lamina propria even in the absence of disease.

Most of the T cells in the healthy lamina propria have been activated by dendritic cells and express markers of effector or memory T cells. Just as for T_{reg} cells and B cells, the largest deployment of effector T cells at homeostasis is in the intestines. The T-cell population of the lamina propria has a ratio of CD4 to CD8 T cells of 3:1 or more, similar to that in systemic lymphoid tissues. In industrialized countries, where intestinal helminth infections are less common, the major effector T-cell subsets resident in the gut express cytokines characteristic of T_H17 and T_H1 cells. And like T_{reg} cells and B cells, the development of these effector subsets is largely dependent on the dominant component of the microbiota—bacteria. T_H17 cells in particular, in their role as responders to extracellular antigens, are particularly abundant, due in part to their developmental ties to pT_{reg} cells with which they share a requirement for the abundant intestinal cytokine, TGF-β (see Section 9-14). Their large number likely reflects the constant state of immune recognition of the microbiota and other environmental antigens that takes place in the intestine. At least some T_H17 cells in the lamina propria appear to be resident memory (T_{RM}) cells, although the proportion varies depending on the antigenic exposure history. Cytokines produced by intestinal T_H17 cells are important components of intestinal homeostasis and defense. IL-17 is needed for full expression of the polymeric immunoglobulin receptor involved in secretion of IgA into the lumen, while IL-22 stimulates intestinal epithelial cells to produce antimicrobial peptides that help maintain epithelial barrier integrity. Effector CD8 T cells are also present in the normal lamina propria and are capable of both cytokine production and cytotoxic activity when a protective immune response to a pathogen is required.

Whether at steady state, in response to infection, or in the context of chronic inflammation induced by inflammatory bowel disease (IBD), the intestine contains, in addition to effectors that express IL-17, cells that express IFN-γ, or both IL-17 and IFN-γ. Although a fraction of these T cells is generated in response to the microbiota and are therefore presumed to be specific for antigens of the commensal flora, their developmental origins and functions remain incompletely defined. Notably, however, in contrast to T_H1 and T_H2 cells, T_H17 cells retain the capacity for divergent cytokine expression profiles and function after their commitment to the T_H17 pathway and can give rise to IL-17$^+$IFN-γ$^+$ effectors, as well as IL-17$^-$IFN-γ$^+$ effectors that resemble classical T_H1 cells, so-called T_H17/T_H1 cells (see Section 11-14 and Fig. 11.21). This has been demonstrated for both human and mouse T_H17 cells and has raised the possibility that many of the IFN-γ–producing 'T_H1' cells in the intestine arise from the T_H17 pathway. While the relative contributions of T_H17 and T_H17/T_H1 cells to host defense or inflammatory disease remain to be elucidated, IFN-γ–producing cells are required for disease pathogenesis in at least some mouse models of IBD. Although these T_H17/T_H1 cells share many features of classical T_H1 cells, gene-expression analyses indicate important differences that are likely to have implications for immune disease mediated by these cells. This suggests generic categorization of IFN-γ–producing CD4 T cells as 'T_H1' cells is an oversimplification, and so further studies aimed at dissecting the contributions of branches of the T_H17 pathway to immune protection or pathogenesis will be important.

In any other situation, the presence of such large numbers of differentiated effector T cells would suggest the presence of a pathogen and likely would lead to inflammation. The fact that it does not so do in the healthy lamina propria is because the generation of T_H1, T_H17, and cytotoxic T cells is balanced by the presence of substantial numbers of IL-10–producing T cells. In the large intestine, these are almost entirely FoxP3$^+$ T_{reg} cells, whereas in the small intestine, FoxP3$^+$ T_{reg} cells and FoxP3$^-$ CD4 T cells (T_R1) produce IL-10 and are likely involved in preventing unrestrained effector T cell–driven inflammation, as occurs in IBD.

12-16 Priming of lymphocytes in one mucosal tissue may induce protective immunity at other mucosal surfaces.

Not all parts of the mucosal immune system use the same tissue-specific chemokines, allowing localized compartmentalization of lymphocyte recirculation within the system. Thus, effector T and B cells primed in lymphoid organs draining the small intestine (mesenteric lymph nodes and Peyer's patches) are most likely to return to the small intestine; similarly, those primed in the respiratory tract migrate most efficiently back to the respiratory mucosa. This programming of tissue homing is useful in returning antigen-specific effector cells to the mucosal organ in which they will be most effective in fighting an infection or controlling immune responses against foreign proteins and commensals. Nevertheless, some lymphocytes that have been primed in the GALT, for example, can also circulate as effector cells to other mucosal tissues such as the respiratory tract, urogenital tract, and lactating breast. This overlap between mucosal recirculation routes gave rise to the idea of a **common mucosal immune system**, which is distinct from other parts of the immune system. Although this is now understood to be an oversimplification, it does have important implications for vaccine development, because it may enable immunization by one mucosal route to be used to protect against infection at another mucosal surface. An important example of this is the induction of SIgA antibody production in the lactating breast by natural infection or vaccination of mucosal surfaces such as the intestine. As we have seen, this is because the vasculature of the lactating breast expresses MAdCAM-1 and chemokines recognized by CCR10 (see Section 12-11). This "cross-talk" is a crucial means of generating protective immunity that can be transmitted to nursing infants by passive transfer of the antibodies in maternal milk. A further example has been shown in experimental animals, in which nasal immunization has a special ability to prime immune responses in the urogenital tract against HIV. The mechanisms behind this are currently unknown.

Summary.

A fundamental challenge of the intestinal immune system is the maintenance of tolerance in the face of considerable nonpathogenic antigenic challenges, both microbial and nonmicrobial. Multiple mechanisms contribute to this, but central to immune homeostasis in the intestines is the delivery of antigens under conditions that favor the differentiation of pT_{reg} cells and SIgA-producing plasma cells—adaptive immune cells that both reinforce non-inflammatory responses to their inductive antigens. This is achieved by the creation of a microenvironment rich in anti-inflammatory cytokines, principal among which are TGF-β, which is produced by IECs and stromal cells, and IL-10, which is produced primarily by pT_{reg} cells themselves. Among other local factors important to intestinal immune homeostasis is retinoic acid (RA), which is produced from vitamin A by IECs and stromal cells, as well as cDCs that are conditioned in the intestines. TGF-β has potent actions on macrophages and cDCs, but also has direct effects on developing T cells and B cells to favor pT_{reg} cell differentiation and IgA class-switching, respectively, as does RA. IL-10 potently suppresses the production of pro-inflammatory cytokines by intestinal macrophages, playing a nonredundant role in maintaining the anti-inflammatory tone of the intestinal mucosa. The critical role of pT_{reg} cells and IL-10 has been demonstrated in murine studies wherein deletion of either results in spontaneous intestinal inflammation. SIgA promotes intestinal homeostasis as a non-complement-fixing antibody isotype that promotes pro-tolerogenic delivery of antigens to which it binds.

Many of the same factors that contribute to tolerogenic adaptive immunity in the intestines also promote homing of lymphocytes to effector sites in the intestinal mucosa. Thus, TGF-β and RA both contribute to the expression of integrins (for example, $\alpha_4\beta_7$) and chemokine receptors (for example, CCR9 and CCR10) that direct lymphocytes to the intestines, ensuring that pT_{reg} cells and IgA plasmablasts are directed to the site where they can reinforce tolerance to the antigens that induced their differentiation. Importantly, expression of the mucosal addressin (MadCAM-1) and chemokines that can attract gut-primed B cells by the lactating breast provides an important mechanism for delivery of maternal SIgA reactive to the mother's microbiota to her newborn, providing a mechanism to transmit immune tolerance to her offspring.

The intestinal immune response in host defense and immune-mediated disease.

Although major functions of the intestinal immune response are the control of interactions with the commensal microbiota and barrier surveillance and repair at homeostasis, host defense against a variety of infectious agents is also a critical function. Despite the array of innate immune mechanisms in the gut and stiff competition from the indigenous microbiota, the gut is nevertheless a frequent site of infection by a wide variety of pathogenic organisms. These include many viruses; enteric bacteria such as enteropathogenic *E. coli*, *Vibrio*, *Salmonella*, and *Shigella* species, and *Listeria monocytogenes*; protozoans such as *Entamoeba histolytica*; multicellular helminth parasites such as tapeworms and pinworms; and fungi. These pathogens cause disease in different ways, and, as elsewhere in the body, the key to generating protective immunity is the activation of appropriate aspects of the innate and adaptive immune systems.

As in other tissues, the intestines must be able to generate a spectrum of immune responses tailored to individual pathogens, as discussed in the last chapter. Not surprisingly, many microbes have evolved means of adapting to and subverting these host responses. To ensure an adequate response to pathogens, the mucosal immune system needs to be able to recognize and respond to any foreign antigen, but it must not produce the same effector response to harmless antigens (from food or commensals). A major role of the intestinal immune system is to balance these competing demands. As we have highlighted previously, both innate and adaptive responses to intestinal infection are initiated through, and integrated with, the intestinal epithelium. In the last chapter, we highlighted features of type 2 immunity in the intestines (see Section 11-10). In this part of the chapter, we will consider several types of enteric bacterial infections to highlight some of the different strategies taken by pathogens to penetrate the intestinal defenses, along with mechanisms available to resist these pathogens. In the final part of the chapter, we will consider viral infections of the respiratory tract and fungal infection of the skin to highlight features of barrier defense against these types of pathogens.

12-17 Enteric pathogens elicit 'danger signals' by activating pattern-recognition receptors that are sequestered in the intestinal epithelium.

Central to the response of innate and adaptive immune cells in the intestinal tissues is the assessment of relative threat of those microbes that interact with and traverse the epithelial barrier. As we have seen, at homeostasis there is continual, albeit low-level transcytosis of commensal microbes. However, because these microbes enter in an orderly fashion, transported in large part across M cells, their recognition generally favors the induction of tolerance. Moreover, the large majority of commensal bacteria pose little risk to the host because they are strict anaerobes that cannot persist outside of the low-oxygen environment of the intestinal lumen, especially in the large intestine, where most reside. Although the surface epithelium of the intestines is relatively hypoxic—due to high oxygen consumption induced by the metabolism of short-chain fatty acids produced by commensal anaerobes—the more aerobic environment of host tissues, including the deeper lamina propria, prevents the growth of these anaerobes. However, a small but persistent fraction of the intestinal microbiota includes facultative anaerobes, particularly Enterobacteriaceae family members from the phylum Proteobacteria, which can thrive outside the intestinal lumen and retain the potential for serious disease should they traverse the epithelium in substantial numbers and disseminate as opportunistic pathogens. Similarly, most bacterial pathogens are facultative anaerobes that can thrive outside the gut lumen. The sensing of these organisms by the intestinal mucosa is therefore of paramount importance to host defense.

A central mechanism for discriminating friend from foe at the intestinal barrier is, as in most tissues, the activation of pattern-recognition receptors (PRRs), such as Toll-like receptors (TLRs). However, because TLRs that sense bacteria are down-modulated in the intestines to accommodate to the commensal microbiota, there are special adaptations of the intestinal epithelium that allow bugs to reach the border, but not cross it, except via M cells that direct them directly to the GALT. Central to this balancing act is the partitioning of PRRs within the polarized epithelium. Thus, while some receptors that sense microbes at the apical surface of IECs are down-modulated, these same receptors are retained within intracellular vacuoles, as well as in the IEC cytosol and at basolateral surfaces, such that penetration of microbes into or across the epithelial barrier elicits pro-inflammatory responses, ignited by signals from the epithelium itself (**Fig. 12.38**). TLRs in intracellular vacuoles or at the basolateral surface of IECs detect intracellular pathogens or extracellular pathogens and their products that have been internalized by endocytosis or have penetrated the epithelium. Moreover, IECs express a variety of cytosolic sensors, as described in Chapter 3, which are activated when microorganisms or their products enter the cytoplasm. These include the **nucleotide-binding and oligomerization domain (NOD)** proteins NOD1 and NOD2, as well as cGAS and STING, among others (see Sections 3-9 and 3-10; Figs. 3.18 and 3.19). NOD1 recognizes a diaminopimelic acid–containing peptide that is found only in the cell walls of Gram-negative bacteria. NOD2 recognizes a muramyl

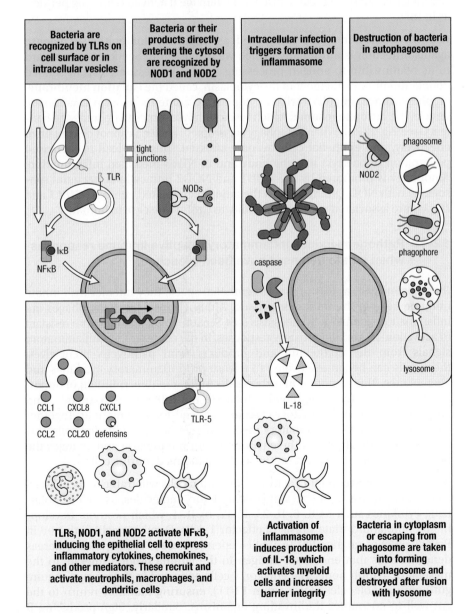

Fig. 12.38 Epithelial cells have a primary role in innate defense against pathogens. TLRs are present in intracellular vesicles or on the basolateral or apical surfaces of epithelial cells, where they recognize different components of invading bacteria. Cytoplasmic NOD1 and NOD2 detect cell-wall peptides from bacteria. TLRs and NODs activate NFκB (see Fig. 3.19), inducing epithelial cells to produce CXCL8, CXCL1 (GROα), CCL1, and CCL2, which attract neutrophils and macrophages, and CCL20, which attracts dendritic cells. Many types of cell damage can activate an inflammasome (see Section 3-11), which in turn activates pro-caspase 1 and produces IL-18. Bacteria that invade the epithelial-cell cytoplasm or escape into the cytosol from phagosomes can induce autophagy. The organisms become ubiquitinated, leading to the recruitment of adaptor proteins that attract the phagophore, forming an autophagosome. Fusion with lysosomes then leads to destruction of the cargo within the autophagosome. NOD2 can also trigger autophagosome formation by binding directly to adaptor proteins, including the Crohn's disease–associated molecule ATG16L1.

Figure panel headers and labels:

Bacteria are recognized by TLRs on cell surface or in intracellular vesicles

Bacteria or their products directly entering the cytosol are recognized by NOD1 and NOD2

Intracellular infection triggers formation of inflammasome

Destruction of bacteria in autophagosome

tight junctions

TLR

NODs

IκB

NFκB

CCL1 CXCL8 CXCL1
CCL2 CCL20 defensins

TLR-5

caspase

IL-18

phagosome

NOD2

phagophore

lysosome

TLRs, NOD1, and NOD2 activate NFκB, inducing the epithelial cell to express inflammatory cytokines, chemokines, and other mediators. These recruit and activate neutrophils, macrophages, and dendritic cells

Activation of inflammasome induces production of IL-18, which activates myeloid cells and increases barrier integrity

Bacteria in cytoplasm or escaping from phagosome are taken into forming autophagosome and destroyed after fusion with lysosome

dipeptide found in the peptidoglycans of most bacteria, as well as structures in certain viruses and mycobacteria. Epithelial cells defective in NOD2 are less resistant to infection by intracellular bacteria. Mice lacking NOD2 also show increased translocation of bacteria across the epithelium. A defect in recognition of the commensal microbiota by NOD2 also seems to be important in some cases of Crohn's disease, as up to 15% of Caucasian individuals carry a mutation in the NOD2 gene that renders the NOD2 protein nonfunctional.

Crohn's Disease

Ligation of TLRs or NOD proteins in IECs stimulates the production of cytokines, such as IL-18, and the production of chemokines. It can also modulate the production of antimicrobial peptides, mucins, and tight junctions, whether through direct actions or by indirect actions of cytokines induced by local immune cells that act, in turn, on the epithelium. Epithelial cells also express members of the intracellular **NOD-like receptor (NLR)** family, including NLRC4 and NLRP6, which can form **inflammasomes** (see Fig. 12.38). As described in Section 3-11, the formation of an inflammasome leads to activation of caspase 1, which cleaves pro-IL-18 to produce the active cytokine (see Fig. 3.20). While the cell targets activated by IL-18 (for example, macrophages) contribute to epithelial defense against bacterial invasion by promoting barrier integrity, these cells can cause tissue damage if activated for long periods, as in IBD.

One mechanism recently recognized as important for epithelial defense against infection is **autophagy**, which we discussed in Section 6-6 in regard to its relationship to antigen processing. In this process, a crescent-shaped double-membrane fragment in the cytoplasm, called the **isolation membrane**, or **phagophore**, engulfs various cytoplasmic contents to form a complete vesicle, the **autophagosome**, which fuses with lysosomes to degrade the contents (see Fig. 12.38). When autophagy is disrupted, bacteria cannot be contained effectively, and epithelial cells become stressed. This can lead to increased penetration of bacteria into the body and to NFκB-mediated inflammation. Autophagy is promoted by the NOD1 and NOD2 intracellular bacterial sensors. As with NOD2, mutations in the autophagy-related genes *ATG16L1* and *IRGM1* are associated with susceptibility to Crohn's disease in humans.

12-18 Pathogens induce inflammatory adaptive immune responses when innate defenses have been breached.

If pathogens gain access to the subepithelial space, they interact with innate immune cells in the underlying tissue. Although resident macrophages are inflammation-anergic at homeostasis (see Section 12-8), and therefore resistant to activation of pro-inflammatory responses, in the context of pro-inflammatory signals from the epithelium and products from pathogens themselves, these cells can become activated to release pro-inflammatory cytokines and chemokines. This response, in turn, results in the rapid recruitment of monocytes from the circulating blood, which are not inflammation-anergic, and amplifies the pro-inflammatory cascade in a feed-forward manner. Together with the cascade of inflammatory mediators released by epithelial cells, this process dramatically alters the environment of the mucosa and changes the behavior of local antigen-presenting cells, including dendritic cells.

As described in Section 9-8, activated dendritic cells will traffic to local T-cell zones and express high levels of co-stimulatory molecules, as well as polarizing cytokines such as IL-6, IL-23, IL-12, or IL-4, which promote development of the appropriate subset of effector T cells. Dendritic cells activated in Peyer's patches migrate to the T cell–dependent areas of the patch, whereas dendritic cells that encounter antigen in the lamina propria migrate to the mesenteric lymph node. The effector T cells activated in these ways acquire gut-homing molecules (see Section 12-11), ensuring that they return to the gut wall to encounter the invading organisms. Similarly, SIgA-producing B lymphocytes are generated in Peyer's patches and mesenteric lymph nodes, giving rise to plasma cells that accumulate in the lamina propria. IgA secretion into the lumen is enhanced in response to infection because pIgR expression is enhanced by TLR ligands and pro-inflammatory cytokines. In a number of infections, B cells undergo class switching to IgG, generating intestinal plasma cells that produce complement-fixing IgG isotypes that enhance the eradication of the invading microbes, as we discuss later in Section 12-20.

The activated myeloid cells found in the inflamed mucosa may also contribute to amplifying and sustaining the functions of effector T and B cells that arrive in the mucosa. For example, IL-1 and IL-23 produced by recently arrived monocytes appear to be important for the survival and function of local T_H17 cells. Pro-inflammatory myeloid cells also produce mediators such as IL-6, TNF-α, and nitric oxide, which help drive IgA switching and secondary expansion of mucosal B cells.

12-19 Effector T-cell responses in the intestine protect the function of the epithelium.

Once activated, the effector T cells that accumulate in the intestine behave much like their counterparts elsewhere in the body, producing cytokines and generating cytolytic activity as appropriate to the pathogen. What is different is that a major aim of the protective immune response in the intestine is tailored to preserving the integrity and function of the epithelial barrier. This is achieved in a number of ways, depending on the nature of the pathogen.

In viral infections, CD8 cytotoxic T cells among intraepithelial lymphocytes kill infected epithelial cells (see Fig. 12.25), triggering their replacement by uninfected cells derived from the rapidly dividing stem cells in the crypts. A similar process can occur during other forms of protective immune responses, with cytokines from CD4 effector T cells directly stimulating stem cells in the colonic crypts to accelerate epithelial-cell generation and modulate the developmental trajectory of IECs toward either the secretory pathway (for example, in response to helminths) or the absorptive pathway (for example, in response to extracellular bacteria). This forces the replacement of infected cells and generates a moving target for organisms that are attempting to attach to the surface of the epithelium. It also expands the types of cells best suited to combat particular types of pathogens.

As an example, the production of IL-13 by ILC2 cells and T_H2 cells during parasitic infections increases the number of goblet cells and enhances their production of mucus, and also expands the number of tuft cells that contribute to a positive feedback loop by producing IL-25, which enhances production of IL-13 from ILC2 cells and T_H2 cells. Conversely, IL-22 produced by T_H17 cells contributes to defense against extracellular bacteria and fungi by promoting a shift in the type of mucin produced by goblet cells, promoting the cell death and sloughing of infected IECs and stimulating the production of antimicrobial peptides by Paneth cells and other IECs, as we discuss in the next section. Finally, these mediators and others can enhance the peristaltic action of the intestine and its outward secretion of fluid, washing out pathogens within the lumen of the intestine. Together these processes aim to generate a hostile and unstable environment for the pathogen, reducing its ability to invade and damage the epithelial barrier.

12-20 Noninvasive and invasive enteric bacterial pathogens use different strategies to colonize the intestines.

Bacterial pathogens elicit different host defenses contingent on their pattern of intestinal infection. Some bacterial pathogens are invasive; that is, they

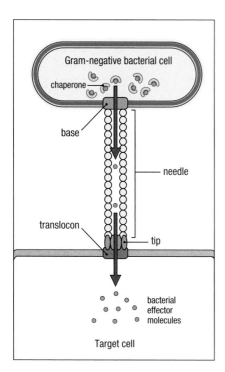

Fig. 12.39 Pathogenic bacteria use specialized secretion systems to inject effector molecules into host cells. A number of pathogenic Gram-negative bacteria use a complex, needle-like protein assembly—a type III or IV secretion system, or injectisome—to inject virulence proteins into target cells to compromise host defenses and establish infection. These 'nanoinjectors' are assembled from more than 20 proteins and are composed of a base that spans the two bacterial membranes, a needle that is anchored in the base and is formed by the polymerization of repeating α-helical subunits, and a tip complex that serves as a docking structure for the translocon, which penetrates the host-cell membrane to allow bacterial effector proteins to pass into the host cell.

typically penetrate the intestinal epithelial barrier and are able to disseminate beyond the mucosa. Other bacterial pathogens are noninvasive and neither traverse the intestinal epithelium nor disseminate. Enteric bacterial pathogens can also differ in the region of the intestinal tract they colonize. In any case, in order for enteropathogens to gain access to the host, they must first adhere to the epithelium, whether or not they subsequently traverse it. In the small intestine, which lacks the thick, two-layer mucus defense present in the large intestine, the opportunity for directly engaging the epithelium is greater, and, in the case of the proximal small intestine or follicle-associated epithelium overlying Peyer's patches and ILFs, there is scant mucus to prevent it. Indeed, as we shall see, like bacterial constituents of the commensal microbiota, several enteric pathogens specifically target M cells as an entry point to cross the epithelium. Thus, the epithelium can serve as both barrier and gateway for enteropathogens.

Enteropathogenic bacteria have evolved a variety of strategies for colonization and/or invasion of the intestinal epithelium, most of which are organism-specific. The bacterial molecules that mediate these properties are typically encoded by a cluster of genes called a pathogenicity island, which is either present on an extrachromosomal plasmid or integrated into the bacterial genome flanked by genetic mobility elements, enabling transfer between bacteria. The factors encoded within these elements that confer pathogenicity are referred to as virulence factors. Although each pathogen has developed distinctive ways to colonize the intestine, the expression of molecules that promote their attachment to, and/or internalization by, intestinal epithelial cells is a common feature. These include fimbriae (that is, specialized pili) and/or adhesins that bind host-membrane molecules. Many Gram-negative bacteria also assemble a needle-like protein structure, or **injectisome**, such as a type III secretion system (T3SS) or a type IV secretion system (T4SS) (**Fig. 12.39**), through which a wide spectrum of bacterial proteins, or effectors, is injected into host cells, including receptors for enhanced binding of the bacterium. In addition to their role in bacterial adhesion, these bacterial effectors can also target cellular pathways in IECs to modulate host-cell signaling pathways to facilitate pathogen replication and spread. However, as discussed earlier (see Section 12-17), these bacterial effectors can also activate intracellular pattern-recognition receptors that initiate host immunity. Some bacteria also use injectisomes, particularly type VI secretion systems (T6SSs), to deliver effectors to other bacteria and kill them in a type of interbacterial warfare that allows the pathogen to outcompete commensals.

Here we consider two noninvasive bacterial pathogens that attach to the intestinal epithelium, but do not invade. *Vibrio cholerae*, a Gram-negative, flagellum-expressing (motile) bacterium, is the causative agent of cholera, a prominent diarrheal disease that affects more than 2 million people and causes more than 75,000 deaths annually worldwide, particularly in underdeveloped regions with poor sanitation. Although most strains of *V. cholerae* are nonpathogenic free-living aquatic bacteria, pathogenic strains express at least two virulence factors that result in human disease: cholera toxin (CT) and the adhesin toxin-coregulating pilus (TCP). Both are required for virulence; TCP mediates initial attachment of *V. cholerae* to IECs of the small intestine, and CT mediates the pathogenic effect of cholera. Cholera toxin is a multi-subunit exotoxin composed of a pentameric binding subunit (CTB) and a monomeric active subunit (CTA). CTB binds to the cell-surface ganglioside GM1, which is widely expressed. The binding of CTB to the surface of an IEC stimulates endocytosis of the toxin and cleavage of CTB from the CTA subunit. The CTA subunit is delivered into the host cell where it activates adenylate cyclase, resulting in accumulation of intracellular cyclic AMP (cAMP). This stimulates the robust secretion of chloride ions and blocks the uptake of sodium chloride, causing a massive efflux of water. The resulting efflux of water and electrolytes results in severe diarrhea and dehydration that can be lethal, particularly for infants and small children. Infection by *V. cholerae* stimulates long-lasting immunity that is thought to be mediated primarily by neutralizing SIgA antibodies that block the bacteria's attachment to the small-intestinal epithelium. Because of its potency in delivering antigens to the intestinal mucosa, the CTB subunit of cholera toxin has been explored as a mucosal adjuvant for antigens linked to it for delivery to the intestines.

Another noninvasive bacterial pathogen that causes diarrheal disease is enteropathogenic *E. coli* (EPEC). Although *E. coli* strains are normal constituents of the commensal microbiota, enteropathogenic *E. coli* strains contain a pathogenicity island called the locus of enterocyte effacement (LEE), so-named because it comprises the genes responsible for attaching and effacing lesions, a feature of EPEC characterized by tight adherence of the bacterium to enterocytes that results in characteristic destruction of microvilli (**Fig. 12.40**). The LEE pathogenicity island encodes multiple virulence factors, including components of a T3SS, which is used to deliver bacterial effectors into enterocytes. LEE also encodes two genes required for the attachment of EPEC to enterocytes: intimin and a translocated intimin receptor (Tir) to which intimin binds to establish firm adhesion to the cell surface of IECs. Unlike *V. cholerae*, which stimulates remarkably little inflammation in the involved small-intestinal mucosa, EPEC, which colonizes the large intestine, induces colonic inflammation (colitis) that resolves only when the infection is cleared.

The immune response to EPEC has been modeled in mice using the highly related rodent pathogen, *Citrobacter rodentium*. Host defense against *C. rodentium* infection is dominated by a type 3 response that is initiated when the bacterium penetrates the mucus layer in the distal colon and interacts with colonic enterocytes (see Fig. 12.40). *C. rodentium* does not express a flagellum and is thus nonmotile, so how it is able to traverse the thick, two-layer colonic mucus barrier is unknown. However, during the process of traversing the mucus layers, the bacterium assembles its T3SS from proteins encoded in the LEE, allowing it to dock to an epithelial cell. Adhesion is stabilized by injection of the Tir protein, which inserts into the apical plasma membrane of the IEC where it can bind intimin on the bacterial surface. This adhesion is strengthened by creation of a pedestal formed from disruption and effacement of host-cell microvilli by other bacterial effectors injected into the IEC, enabling a broad area of contact between pedestal and bacterium—hence the term 'attaching and effacing' bacterial pathogen. Detection of bacterial effectors injected into the cytosol of the IECs is thought to initiate the IEC's programmed death, resulting in the phagocytosis of dying bacteria-laden cells by subepithelial CX3CR1+ macrophages and cDC2 cells. TEDs projected across the infected epithelium by these phagocytes may also contribute by direct uptake of the pathogen. The local production of IL-1β and IL-23 by activated mononuclear phagocytes activates ILC3s within the mucosa, which, in turn, release type 3 cytokines, including IL-17 and IL-22, as described in Chapter 11 (see Section 11-3). The induction of IL-22 by ILC3 cells is particularly important to the innate immune response to *C. rodentium*, as mice deficient for either IL-22 or IL-23 rapidly succumb to infection prior to induction of an adaptive immune response. However, the adaptive response is also indispensable for host protection, as mice deficient for CD4 T cells or B cells succumb to infection, albeit later, after the earlier innate phase of the response.

The adaptive immune response against *C. rodentium* is dependent on the development of pathogen-specific TH17 cells that produce IL-22, which are recruited to the lamina propria of the infected segment of the large intestine and are required to fully amplify the protection of the epithelium initiated by ILC3 cells. Indeed, as the host response progresses, CD4 T cells become the major source of IL-22. The adaptive response also contributes *Citrobacter*-specific IgG antibodies, which are transported across the epithelium to bind the bacterium in the intestinal lumen. This IgG, which is dependent on FcRn

Fig. 12.40 Innate and adaptive phases of the host response to attaching and effacing enteropathogenic bacteria. Certain Gram-negative human enteric pathogens, such as pathogenic strains of *E. coli*, are typically noninvasive, but they cause intestinal inflammation by their colonization of the intestinal epithelium. This infection is modeled in mice by *Citrobacter rodentium,* which is very similar to enteropathogenic *E. coli*. These bacteria can penetrate the inner mucus layer and attach to the superficial surface of epithelial cells in the colon, thereby inducing a type 3 immune response (first upper panel). During attachment to an IEC, the bacterium uses a type III secretion system (T3SS; see Fig. 13.39) to inject bacterial effector molecules into the epithelial cell, including the translocated intimin receptor (Tir), to which the bacterial surface protein intimin binds to establish firm attachment (insets, first two lower panels). In the process, the attached bacterium causes loss (effacement) of microvilli on the IEC, hence the term 'attaching and effacing' bacteria. Recognition of the attached bacteria by epithelial cells and epithelial-cell pyroptosis results in the release of chemokines and cytokines that recruit mononuclear phagocytes, which take up

infected IECs and bacteria. The ensuing release of IL-23 and IL-1β causes the activation of ILC3 cells to release IL-22, which acts on the intestinal epithelium to induce protective responses, including the release of antimicrobial peptides (AMPs) and the recruitment of neutrophils, which restrain bacterial growth (second upper panel). Trafficking of bacterial antigen–laden dendritic cells to draining lymph nodes induces the development of TH17 cells and bacteria-specific IgG-producing plasmablasts, which migrate to the inflamed colon via the bloodstream (second two lower panels). In the colon, they further amplify the protective response via the release of greater amounts of IL-22 (TH17 cells) and IgG antibodies, which are transported across the epithelium by the neonatal Fc receptor (FcRn; not shown) (third upper panel). Inflammatory cytokines stimulate increased cell turnover in the crypts, resulting in increased depth of crypts (crypt hyperplasia), as well as the emptying of goblet cells and their decreased differentiation (so-called goblet cell 'hypoplasia'). Secreted IgG binds to bacteria, fixing complement and recruiting neutrophils into the intestinal lumen where they destroy the bacteria, resolving the infection (fourth panel).

for transepithelial transport from the lamina propria into the lumen, opsonizes bacteria and leads to their clearance by neutrophils recruited to the infection site by CCR2-activating chemokines and complement fragments (see Fig. 12.40). In normal mice, the infection is completely cleared within 3–4 weeks, and IgG-dependent protective immunity is generated.

In contrast to noninvasive bacterial pathogens, invasive bacteria can penetrate the intestinal epithelium to cause local injury or disseminate from the intestinal mucosa to cause systemic disease. Examples include *Listeria*, *Shigella*, and *Salmonella* spp., among others. Although we have previously considered *Listeria monocytogenes* in the context of systemic immunity (see Chapter 11), it is normally transmitted via the intestinal tract. *L. monocytogenes* is a food-borne, aerobic, Gram-positive rod, an intracellular pathogen that has evolved mechanisms to escape killing within phagocytes (see Section 11-6). It uses the virulence factor internalin A to initially establish a foothold within IECs of the small intestine. Internalin A binds to E-cadherin, which is normally expressed beneath tight junctions and therefore inaccessible to the bacterium. However, E-cadherin becomes luminally accessible around goblet cells during their exocytosis of mucins, and *L. monocytogenes* is then able to bind and be internalized into endocytic vesicles. *L. monocytogenes* may take advantage of the goblet cell–associated passage (GAP) pathway to be transcytosed to the basolateral surface of the epithelium, from which it can spread to other epithelial cells and to macrophages. Another *L. monocytogenes* virulence factor, **listeriolysin O (LLO)**, is a pore-forming toxin that allows *L. monocytogenes* to escape phagolysosomes within macrophages to enter the cytosol, where it avoids intracellular killing and replicates. Once in macrophages, *L. monocytogenes* can be transported out of the gut to systemic tissues, where it can spread cell-to-cell without exposure to the extracellular environment (see Section 13-22), rendering antibody responses ineffectual. Cell-to-cell transmission is achieved by *L. monocytogenes*–induced polymerization of actin filaments within the host-cell cytoplasm that propel the bacterium to the cell membrane, where it forms protrusions into neighboring cells that can be internalized, and from which the bacterium can again escape, initiating another cycle of cell-to-cell dissemination. The host response to *L. monocytogenes*, an obligate intracellular pathogen, bridges type 1 and cytotoxic immunity (see Section 11-6).

Shigella dysenteriae is a nonmotile, Gram-negative rod that causes shigellosis, or bacillary dysentery, which is transmitted via the fecal–oral route. Shigellosis is a major enteric infection in developing countries, where it causes as many as 150 million cases and 100,000 deaths each year. Like *Listeria*, *Shigella* spp. are intracellular pathogens that have evolved mechanisms for escape from phagolysosomes and use a similar actin-mediated propulsion to spread cell-to-cell and evade host immunity. However, *Shigella* uses the M cell for transport across the intestinal epithelium of the ileum and colon (**Fig. 12.41**), where it is delivered to subepithelial dome macrophages, which it is able to infect and

ANIMATION 11.2

Fig. 12.41 *Shigella flexneri* infects intestinal epithelial cells to cause bacillary dysentery. *Shigella flexneri* binds to M cells and is translocated beneath the gut epithelium (first panel). The bacteria infect intestinal epithelial cells from their basal surface and are released into the cytoplasm (second panel). Muramyl tripeptides containing diaminopimelic acid in the cell walls of shigellae bind to and oligomerize the protein NOD1. Oligomerized NOD1 binds the serine/threonine kinase RIPK2 and activates the NFκB pathway (see Fig. 3.19), leading to the transcription of genes for chemokines and cytokines (third panel). Activated epithelial cells release the chemokine CXCL8, which acts as a neutrophil chemoattractant (fourth panel). IκB, inhibitor of κB; IKK, IκB kinase.

kill. The release of the bacterium from macrophages allows it to spread locally to intestinal epithelial cells via their basolateral surfaces. By activating intracellular sensors of IECs such as NOD1 as it migrates from cell to cell, *Shigella* stimulates a robust innate immune response that, along with direct bacterial damage, causes extensive damage to the epithelium. *Shigella* also releases Shiga toxin, an exotoxin that injures local endothelial cells, resulting in bloody diarrhea; it can also affect the microvasculature in other organs, such as the kidney, to produce hemolytic uremic syndrome (HUS), so named for its intravascular destruction of red blood cells (hemolysis) and damage to kidney function (uremia). Although the more virulent *Shigella* spp. such as *Shigella dysenteriae* can cause considerable local injury of the intestinal mucosa, they do not typically disseminate beyond the intestines. As for *L. monocytogenes*, eradication of *Shigella* is dependent on type 1 and cytotoxic immunity; antibody responses are poorly induced and nonprotective.

Like *Shigella*, *Salmonella enterica* serovar Typhi, the causative agent of typhoid fever in humans, targets the M cells of Peyer's patches to traverse the intestinal epithelium, although it is also able to directly invade other enterocytes and can be taken up by TEDs of subepithelial mononuclear phagocytes (**Fig. 12.42**). *Salmonella enterica* serovar Typhi is a food-borne, Gram-negative, rod-shaped facultative anaerobe that infects only humans. It is equipped with multiple flagella and is highly motile. *Salmonella* uses both type III and type VI secretion systems to cause disease. Expression of the T6SS is induced first to destroy

Fig. 12.42 *Salmonella enterica* serovar Typhimurium is an important cause of food poisoning and penetrates the epithelial layer in three ways. *Salmonella enterica* serovar Typhimurium adheres to and enters M cells, which it then kills by causing apoptosis (top left panel). It then can infect macrophages and gut epithelial cells. TLR-5 expressed by the epithelial basal membrane can bind *Salmonella* flagellin, activating the NFκB pathway. After uptake by macrophages in the lamina propria, invasive *Salmonella* induces caspase 1 activation, promoting production of IL-1β and IL-18. CXCL8 is also produced by the infected macrophages, and together these mediators recruit and activate neutrophils (lower left panel). Salmonellae can also invade gut epithelial cells directly by adhering to the luminal epithelial surface via fine threadlike protrusions called fimbriae (top middle panel). The cell processes extended between epithelial cells by mononuclear phagocytes may be infected by salmonellae in the lumen and thus effectively breach the epithelial layer (top right panel). Dendritic cells in the lamina propria may take up antigen from infected macrophages and carry those antigens to the draining mesenteric lymph node to prime the adaptive immune response (lower right panel). If containment processes in the lymph node fail, salmonellae can invade beyond the intestine and its lymphoid tissues and enter the bloodstream to cause systemic infection.

commensal bacteria to clear a niche for infection. This is down-regulated as the T3SS is expressed. As for EPEC, the T3SS is important in the attachment of the bacterium to host cells, although *Salmonella* can also enter IECs after attachment. As we learned in Chapter 11 (see Section 11-14), *Salmonella* are facultative intracellular pathogens that can shift from an extracellular lifestyle to an intracellular lifestyle as they try to evade first a type 3 and then a type 1 host immune response, respectively. By adapting to survival within migratory dendritic cells, *Salmonella* can be transported with their phagocyte host to regional lymph nodes and, if not contained there, can disseminate widely.

12-21 Dysregulated immune responses to commensal bacteria provoke intestinal disease.

Because of their antigenic memory and longevity, effector CD4 T cells are a liability when inappropriately directed against self antigens or, in the case of the microbiota, the 'extended' self that includes antigens of the commensal microbiota. Indeed, in view of the enormous number of antigens encoded in the collective genome (microbiome) of the intestinal microbiota, it is remarkable that dysregulated effector responses against the microbiota are the exception. When they do occur, the result is inflammatory bowel disease (IBD), including Crohn's disease (CD) and **ulcerative colitis (UC)**. Although these two types of IBD have distinct clinical and histopathologic features, both are characterized by aberrant immune responses to antigens of the intestinal microbiota. In all experimental models of IBD, the intestinal damage depends on the presence of commensal bacteria; it can be prevented by administration of broad-spectrum antibiotics and does not occur in germ-free animals. As in autoimmunity directed against host self antigens (see Chapter 15), dysregulated CD4 T-cell responses to antigens of the microbiota lead to chronic, typically relapsing and remitting disease that reflects the immune system's inability to eliminate the antigens that drive the abnormal response.

Many genes that are associated with susceptibility to Crohn's disease in humans encode proteins that regulate innate immunity. When these regulatory processes fail, systemic immune responses are generated against antigens from commensal bacterial, such as **flagellin**, the monomer that polymerizes to form bacterial flagella. Studies of both mouse models and humans with CD reveal a remarkably similar reactivity to specific flagellin epitopes expressed by *Clostridium* spp. that appear to be immunodominant despite their minor representation within the commensal flora. Why these commensals are common targets in a large subset of individuals with CD—but not UC—is unknown, but it likely reflects unique properties that place them in specific geographic niches in the microbiota and/or in intimate contact with the immune system, where their expression of flagella, which is atypical for commensal bacteria, makes them unusually proficient at inducing effector responses rather than regulatory responses.

In view of their prominent role in adaptive immune responses to the intestinal microbiota and propensity for generating inflammation promoted by both IL-17 and IFN-γ, it is not surprising that T_H17 cells have emerged as leading contributors to IBD pathogenesis. Prior to the discovery of T_H17, CD and UC were viewed in the context of T_H1- and T_H2-centric mechanisms, respectively, but increasingly, data from genome-wide association studies (GWASs) implicate the contributions of the T_H17 pathway in both disorders. Indeed, it is fitting that IL-23, discovery of which revolutionized views on the immunopathogenesis of autoimmunity and led to discovery of T_H17 cells, was the first cytokine linked to IBD by GWASs, as variants of its receptor (IL-23R) have been found to confer both protection and susceptibility to CD and UC. As the number of GWASs and next-generation sequencing studies has proliferated, so too has the number of genes linked to the T_H17 pathway in IBD (see Section

15-14). This has been supplemented by genes of innate and adaptive immune pathways that are integrated with, and control, T_H17 responses, spanning the gamut from epithelial barrier integrity maintenance and restitution to microbial sensing to immunomodulatory cytokines.

Summary.

Despite robust mechanisms that favor immune tolerance at homeostasis, as a major portal for the entry of pathogens the intestinal mucosa must be able to respond rapidly to all classes of pathogens. Thus, cytotoxic, type 1, type 2, or type 3 responses are each efficiently induced in response to enteric pathogens. How this is achieved in the face of a dominant tolerogenic tone is not completely understood, but a major contributor is the generation of pro-inflammatory signals generated by the intestinal epithelium upon sensing pathogen invasion. Polarization of the epithelium into apical (lumen-facing) and basolateral (internal tissue–facing) surfaces by the tight-junctional apparatus allows distribution of pattern-recognition receptors into endosomal/cytosolic and basolateral compartments where they sense microbes that have violated epithelial integrity but remain relatively insensate with respect to microbes in the mucus layer or lumen.

For invasive pathogens that directly violate the integrity of the intestinal epithelium, they must first transit or avoid the mucus barrier. A number of pathogens have evolved mechanisms that direct them to target mucosal sites that are relatively mucus-free, such as the small-intestinal villi or the follicle-associated epithelium and M cells of Peyer's patches and ILFs. Others have evolved mechanisms, which are not fully understood, by which they can penetrate the mucus layers to gain access to epithelial cells. Whatever the mechanism, the result is the production by the activated epithelium of pro-inflammatory signals that override the tolerogenic tone of the homeostatic mucosa to activate local ILCs and recruit circulating monocytes and granulocytes that further amplify inflammatory signals and promote adaptive immune effector responses.

Immunity at other barrier tissues.

Like the intestines, other barrier tissues present a considerable surface area for interaction with the external environment. Indeed, infections of the respiratory tract and skin are among the most common, and respiratory infections cause more deaths than do any other type of infection (see Fig. 12.4). While the innate and adaptive immune cells that participate in barrier immunity in these tissues are similar, there are anatomic differences in the organs and the epithelia that invest them that deserve special consideration. Moreover, the unique physiological functions of these tissues present special challenges for the immune system. Here, we briefly examine features of the respiratory tract and skin that bear on these challenges.

12-22 Anatomy and mucosal immunity of the airways.

Although there are many similarities in mucosal immunity of the gastrointestinal and respiratory tracts, there are also important differences that reflect their unique anatomy and physiological functions. The primary function of the respiratory tract is gas exchange—the intake of oxygen and release of CO_2. Because life is not supported by even a brief interruption in this function, the lungs, where gas exchange occurs, are continually exposed to 5–10 liters of air per minute at rest. The respiratory tract is divided into upper and

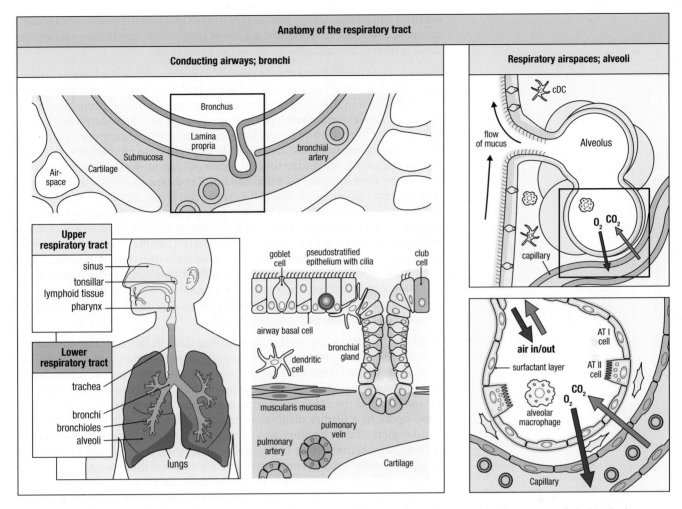

Fig. 12.43 Anatomy of the respiratory tract. The respiratory tract includes the nasal passages and sinuses, the pharynx, and the trachea, which branches into bronchi that divide further into smaller and smaller bronchioles (inset, left panel). These end in small clusters of air sacs, called alveoli, where gas exchange occurs. The large and small conducting airways in the chest cavity (trachea, bronchi, and bronchioles) are lined by a pseudostratified epithelium, which rests on a basement membrane underlaid by the lamina propria (left panel). The respiratory epithelium in the conducting airways includes goblet cells, club cells, and the more numerous respiratory epithelial cells, which have cilia on their apical surface that beat rhythmically to propel the mucus layer toward the pharynx where it can be expectorated or swallowed. The mucus is produced by goblet cells in the epithelium and in bronchial glands within the mucosa, which also produce antimicrobial peptides, similarly to crypts of the intestinal tract. Immune cells are present within the epithelium and lamina propria of the conducting airways.

Under normal conditions, the airways are sterile below the larynx, and no organized lymphoid tissues are present within the mucosa. However, there are extensive lymphatics that drain to regional lymph nodes (bronchial and mediastinal lymph nodes), and the upper airways contain nasal-associated lymphoid tissue (NALT) and tonsillar tissues. The respiratory epithelium progressively thins to a single layer of columnar cells with fewer goblet cells in the smallest airways. The terminal bronchioles and alveoli lack goblet cells and are not covered by mucus. Alveoli are lined by two types of epithelium (right panel): type I alveolar cells (AT I), a very thin, squamous epithelium that covers most of the alveolar surface and is adapted for gas exchange; and type II alveolar cells (AT II), cuboidal cells that produce surfactant, which reduces the surface tension of the alveolar lining to prevent the airspaces from collapsing. A specialized macrophage, the alveolar macrophage, resides in the alveolus and is responsible for clearing any inhaled particles or pathogens.

lower segments, separated by the vocal cords of the larynx (**Fig. 12.43**). Like the intestines, the upper respiratory tract—including the nose and nasal sinuses, pharynx, and larynx above the vocal cords—is populated by a commensal microbiota that develops after birth. Unlike the intestines, which harbor a preponderance of anaerobes, particularly in the large intestine, a greater contribution by facultative anaerobes is found in the upper respiratory tract. The lower respiratory tract includes the conducting airways—the larynx below the vocal cords, trachea, and branching bronchi and bronchioles—through which air is conducted in inspiration and expiration, as well as the respiratory airspaces, including alveoli, in which gas exchange between the inspired air and blood occurs. Collectively, all the pulmonary tissues distal to the two major bronchi compose the lungs. Importantly, the lower respiratory tract is normally sterile; there is no resident microbiota below the vocal cords.

The larger conducting airways are lined by a pseudostratified columnar epithelium, which becomes progressively thinner and transitions to a simple columnar epithelium in the smaller conducting airways (terminal bronchioles; see Fig. 12.2). The dominant cell types in these airways are ciliated columnar cells, goblet cells, club cells, and airway basal cells. In addition, there are small numbers of respiratory tuft cells (also called brush cells) and neuroendocrine cells. Goblet cells, tuft cells, and neuroendocrine cells serve similar functions in the respiratory tract as in the GI tract. The basal cells are stem cells that differentiate to replenish all epithelial cell types in the larger airways (that is, above the bronchioles). Goblet cells become less numerous as the airways become smaller and are lost in the terminal bronchioles (the smallest airways). **Club cells** (formerly called Clara cells) are secretory cells that appear in the bronchioles, increasing in number as the goblet cells decrease in number. They produce a serous product that lubricates the bronchiole as the mucus layer terminates approaching the respiratory airspaces. They also produce antimicrobial factors (for example, lysozyme) and serve as stem cells for repopulation of the epithelium of the distal airways.

As in the intestines, the wall of conducting airways beneath the epithelium includes the lamina propria, muscularis mucosa, and submucosa (see Fig. 12.43). In contrast to the GI tract, where the outer wall is composed of muscle layers that produce the peristaltic waves that propel the luminal contents downstream, the outer wall of the conducting airways is supported by cartilage, which keeps them open. In a further distinction from the GI tract, the respiratory tract is blind-ended; that is, inspired air and any particulates or microbes that it contains must be eliminated by transport back up through the airways or locally by phagocytic cells. A central mechanism for clearance of the airways is the **mucociliary escalator**, a term that refers to the constant propulsion of mucus produced by goblet cells (and, in the larger conducting airways, bronchial glands) up and out of the respiratory tract by the constant unidirectional beating of cilia of the ciliated columnar cells. This constant clearance mechanism is enhanced by coughing and sneezing, which can propel air, particulates, and inhaled microbes from the airways at speeds up to 100 miles per hour.

The alveoli are lined by two epithelial cell types: type I and type II alveolar cells (AT I and AT II cells) (see Fig. 12.43). Most of the surface area of the alveoli is lined by the AT I cells, which are simple squamous cells that facilitate gas exchange with surrounding alveolar capillaries. AT II cells are more cuboidal and produce a surfactant composed of a variety of phospholipids and glycoproteins that reduces the surface tension of the alveolus to facilitate reinflation after exhalation. Although more numerous than AT I cells, AT II cells cover far less surface area due to their smaller footprint on the alveolar basement membrane. Within alveoli are **alveolar macrophages**, which reside in the alveolar lumen, where they act to scavenge small particulates that are deposited there, including microbes. Like macrophages at other mucosal sites, alveolar macrophages are anti-inflammatory at homeostasis, as gas exchange is highly sensitive to thickening of the space between the alveolar lumen and surrounding capillaries (the alveolo-capillary membrane). This is due to the production of TGF-β by alveolar epithelial cells, which is activated and 'presented' to alveolar macrophages by $\alpha_v\beta_6$ integrin expressed on the surface of AT I cells. The turnover of alveolar macrophage populations is very slow at steady state, and renewal is largely dependent on local cell division. However, as for tissue-resident macrophages in the airways and the gut, renewal of alveolar macrophages during inflammatory processes occurs via incoming monocytes.

As in the GI tract, the respiratory airways are populated by a complement of innate and adaptive immune cells that are found within the lamina propria and the epithelium itself. These cells include conventional dendritic cells (cDCs), plasmacytoid DCs (pDCs), resident CX3CR1$^+$ macrophages, ILCs, T cells, and antibody-secreting plasma cells. Notably, the antibody isotypes that predominate in the upper and lower respiratory tract differ: in the upper respiratory tract, SIgA dominates, whereas in the lower respiratory tract, IgG is dominant, transported across the epithelium by pIgR and FcRn, respectively. This difference likely reflects the presence of a commensal microbiota in the upper respiratory tract, but not in the lower tract. As in the intestines, most intraepithelial T cells, including both conventional and nonconventional T cells, express CD8, whereas CD4 T cells dominate in the lamina propria. Also, the mucus layer contains SIgA and antimicrobial peptides that restrain invasion by microbes. Moreover, airway macrophages and dendritic cells (DCs) are located immediately beneath and within the airway epithelium and can extend cellular projections (transepithelial dendrites, or TEDs) into the airway lumen as they do within the gut.

However, unlike the intestinal mucosa, the respiratory mucosa of adults does not typically contain lymphoid tissues. While isolated lymphoid follicles can be found within the walls of the larger airways in childhood (bronchus-associated lymphoid tissue, or BALT), these are lacking in adults. Thus, the induction of adaptive immune responses in the adult respiratory tract, as in nonmucosal tissues, is initially mediated by draining lymph nodes (hilar, parabronchial, and mediastinal lymph nodes). Effector T and B cells primed in these sites return to the lung effector sites, such as lamina propria and the respiratory epithelium. As in the intestines, at homeostasis the immunologic 'tone' of these inductive sites in the upper airways favors the generation of FoxP3$^+$ T$_{reg}$ cells and SIgA-expressing plasma cells, due to similar mechanisms (retinoic acid and TGF-β) that trigger the generation of cDC2 cells that promote these tolerogenic mechanisms. However, in response to infections, BALT can be induced rapidly in the lower airways. After BALT is established, it generates B-cell areas containing germinal centers and T-cell areas around high endothelial venules that are organized similarly to other MALT—including an overlying FAE and M cells—and supports the induction of adaptive immune responses as in other mucosal tissues.

12-23 Respiratory immunity to inhaled pathogens; respiratory viruses.

The extensive surface area ($\sim$70 m^2 in adult humans), high rate of continual air exchange with the environment ($\sim$10,000 liters per day), and absence of a competing microbiota in the lower airways make the respiratory tract a major portal for the entry of infectious agents. At all barrier sites, the types of microbial exposure shape the types of disease, and, in the respiratory tract, pathogens generally enter suspended in air as particulates. This favors infections by organisms that can be transmitted in small droplets or as free particles—particularly bacteria and viruses.

The efficiency of the airways in removing particulates is size-dependent. The larger the particle, the less likely it is to be deposited in the smaller airways and alveoli. Larger particles are blocked by hairs in the nostrils, and particles with an aerodynamic diameter greater than 10 μm (roughly the size of an activated T cell) are cleared by the upper airways, especially when inhaled through the nose. This is due to the extensive mucus-coated 'baffles' formed by the turbinate bones, which project into the nasal passages and nasal sinuses and provide a large surface mucosal surface that helps to trap particulates that flow over them. In the lower respiratory tract, particulates and microbes entrapped by mucus in the conducting airways are directed by cilia toward the back of the throat, where they can be expectorated or swallowed. Most particles that do pass to the conducting airways are efficiently removed from the air by the highly branching nature of the tracheobronchial tree; with more than 20 generations of branches, the likelihood is great that even smaller particulates (1–5 μm) will

Major respiratory viral pathogens					
Viruses	**Genome**	**Receptors**	**Cellular tropism**		**Disease**
			Primary	**Secondary**	
Influenza virus	(−) ssRNA	Sialylated glycan	Epithelial cells	DCs, macrophages, fibroblasts	Influenza epidemics and pandemics
Respiratory syncytial virus (RSV)	(−) ssRNA	GAG	Epithelial cells	Macrophages, T cells	Infant 'colds'
Adenovirus	dsDNA	CAR	Epithelial cells	Fibroblasts	Bronchitis, croup, viral pneumonia
Rhinovirus	(+) ssRNA	ICAM-1	Epithelial cells	Macrophages	Upper respiratory infections, sinusitis
Coronavirus	(+) ssRNA	APN, ACE2, DPP4	Epithelial cells	Type I alveolar epithelial cells	Common cold Severe acute respiratory syndrome (SARS-CoV, SARS-CoV-2, MERS)
Coxsackie virus	(+) ssRNA	CARs	Epithelial, vascular endothelial cells	–	Sore throat, upper respiratory infections
Paramyxovirus (Parainfluenza)	(−) ssRNA	Gangliosides, sialylated glycoproteins	Epithelial cells	–	Parainfluenza

Fig. 12.44 Major respiratory viral pathogens. See text for details. Abbreviations: APN, aminopeptidase N; ACE2, angiotensin-converting enzyme 2; CAR, Coxsackie–adenovirus receptor; DPP4, dipeptidyl peptidase 4; GAG, glycosaminoglycan; ICAM-1, intracellular adhesion molecule-1.

be trapped in the mucus blanket and removed. However, those microbes that express receptors that allow their attachment to the respiratory epithelial cells (RECs) can establish a foothold if they penetrate the mucus layer—especially those that are delivered deeper into the airways and thus have a longer distance to travel to be cleared by the mucociliary escalator. Finally, particles less than ~1 μm in size (roughly the size of a bacterium) can be delivered to the terminal respiratory airways and alveoli, which are devoid of a mucus coating. In this instance, the last line of defense is alveolar macrophages, which are efficient at disposing of inhaled bacteria, but less able to eliminate viruses.

Common respiratory pathogens include a variety of viruses (**Fig. 12.44**). While some of these cause relatively mild, self-limiting upper respiratory infections (for example, rhinovirus), others frequently cause more serious lower respiratory infections (for example, respiratory syncytial virus, parainfluenza). Here we consider influenza and coronavirus, two classes of viral pathogens that cause disease that can be mild or life-threatening, depending on the particular strain. Both are RNA viruses, meaning that the viral genome is encoded by RNA, not DNA, and therefore must be replicated by RNA polymerases, which have a greater error rate than DNA polymerase (see Section 13-25). As a consequence, the mutation rate for these viruses is greater than for DNA viruses. The alteration of viral proteins—and thus of viral antigens that are the targets of immune recognition—resulting from these proofreading mutations is referred to as **antigenic drift** (**Fig. 12.45**). Moreover, because the influenza RNA genome is segmented, and the virus's two major surface proteins—**hemagglutinin** and **neuraminidase**—are encoded on different segments, new viral strains can be generated by reassortment of the linear genetic elements encoding these two proteins when more than one strain of influenza infects the same cell. Consequently, prior B- and T-cell immunity generated from exposure to one strain of the virus may not be protective against the newly generated strain. The rapid changes in viral antigens caused by these reassortments of viral gene segments is referred to as **antigenic shift**. Similar assortment of viral nucleoproteins may also affect shifts in host recognition by T cells. Accordingly, influenza is prone to develop pandemics because prior herd immunity may not be protective against these new strains.

ANIMATION 12.1

ANIMATION 12.2

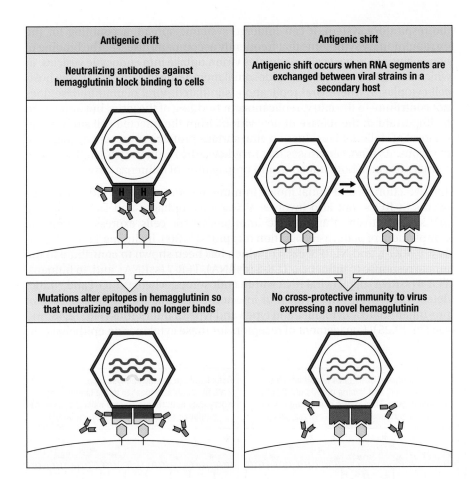

Antigenic drift	Antigenic shift
Neutralizing antibodies against hemagglutinin block binding to cells	Antigenic shift occurs when RNA segments are exchanged between viral strains in a secondary host
Mutations alter epitopes in hemagglutinin so that neutralizing antibody no longer binds	No cross-protective immunity to virus expressing a novel hemagglutinin

Fig. 12.45 Two types of variation allow repeated infection with type A influenza virus. Neutralizing antibody that mediates protective immunity is directed at the viral surface protein hemagglutinin (H), which is responsible for viral binding to and entry into cells. Antigenic drift (left panels) involves the emergence of point mutants with altered binding sites for protective antibodies on the hemagglutinin. The new virus can grow in a host that is immune to the previous strain of virus, but as T cells and some antibodies can still recognize epitopes that have not been altered, the new variants cause only mild disease in previously infected individuals. Antigenic shift (right panels) is a rare event involving the reassortment of the segmented RNA viral genomes of two different influenza viruses, probably in a bird or a pig. These antigen-shifted viruses have large changes in their hemagglutinin, and therefore T cells and antibodies produced in earlier infections are not protective. These shifted strains cause severe infection that spreads widely, causing the influenza pandemics that occur every 10–50 years. There are eight RNA molecules in each viral genome, but for simplicity only three are shown.

Individual strains of influenza are identified by type and the combination of hemagglutinin (H) and neuraminidase (N) variants. There are three major types of influenza that infect humans (A, B, C), two of which, types A and B, are responsible for most seasonal human disease. In general, type B strains cause less virulent infections; type A strains are the only viruses known to cause flu pandemics. At least 18 type A hemagglutinin and 11 neuraminidase subtypes have been identified to date, resulting in more than a hundred influenza A subtypes, which are identified by their combination of H and N usage [for example, influenza A (H3N2)]. Seasonal influenza viruses cause 3–5 million serious infections and up to a half million or more deaths worldwide each year. The outbreaks typically occur in the winter, when people are clustered indoors, facilitating spread from person to person. Influenza viruses also infect other species (for example, birds, pigs), which can be a source of further antigenic shifts due to **zoonotic** infections; that is, the transmission of a related infectious agent from other animals to humans. When this occurs, the existing immunity within humans can be ineffective, resulting in particularly lethal pandemics. A prime example is the swine flu pandemic of 1918, which was caused by an influenza A (H1NI) strain and caused an estimated 40 million deaths worldwide.

The attachment of influenza virus to the respiratory epithelium is mediated by the viral hemagglutinin surface molecule, which recognizes sialic acid residues on host-cell surface glycoproteins. Because of the broad expression of sialic acid on the cells of many tissues, the **cellular tropism**, or ability of the virus to infect specific host-cell types, is broad. Therefore, the route of delivery of influenza, typically in microdroplets inhaled via the airways, determines its localization to the respiratory tract more than its targeting to a particular cell type in the respiratory tract. And because the virus can infect cells outside the respiratory system, it can undergo systemic spread, accounting for the extrapulmonary symptoms that frequently accompany disease. The binding of hemagglutinin to host cells stimulates virion uptake into endocytic vesicles, in which the virus fuses with the endosomal membrane to gain entry to the host-cell cytoplasm, where viral replication is initiated. Viral neuraminidase does not contribute to the entry, replication, or budding of the virus, but appears to be important in the release of new virions from the infected cell surface and removal of sialic acid residues on viral surface proteins to prevent aggregation of virions. As for other viruses that invade via the respiratory tract, RECs are a primary target of both infection and propagation of influenza virus.

The detection of, and initial innate immune response against, influenza virus occurs in RECs, but also involves airway macrophages and DCs, including pDCs. Collectively, these innate immune sensor cells express a complete complement of pattern-recognition receptors (PRRs), including TLR-3, TLR-7, TLR-8, RIG-I, and NLRP3, each of which has been shown to contribute to the innate response to influenza. TLR-3 (dsRNA), TLR-7 (ssRNA), and, in humans, TLR-8 (ssRNA) detect viral RNA within endosomes, whereas RIG-I and NLRP3 detect virus within the cytosol of infected cells. This triggers the release of pro-inflammatory cytokines and type I and type III interferons (**Fig. 12.46**; and see Fig. 13.25). Engagement of receptors for these cytokines on epithelial cells

Fig. 12.46 The immune response to respiratory viruses. Virus infection of respiratory epithelial cells (RECs) is first detected by cytosolic and/or endosomal pattern-recognition receptors (PRRs) in the infected epithelial cells (not shown). Recognition of the invading virus by the PRRs leads sensor cells to produce type I interferons (IFN-αβ) and type III interferon (IFN-λ), as well as pro-inflammatory cytokines, such as IL-18, and chemokines, such as CC-chemokine ligand 2 (CCL2; not shown) (left panel). Viral recognition by plasmacytoid dendritic cells in the mucosa also stimulates the release of type I interferons, which acts on epithelial cells and local mononuclear phagocytes to amplify their production of inflammatory mediators, including TNF-α. These soluble mediators promote the recruitment of monocytes and activate type 1 and type 2 conventional dendritic cells, which ingest viral particles and deliver antigen to draining lymph nodes where they release IL-12 and induce T_H1 and CTL responses, as well as B-cell responses to induce the development of IgG-producing antibodies (middle panel). Migration of CTLs, T_H1 cells, and plasmablasts from draining lymph nodes to the infected respiratory mucosa results in lysis of virally infected cells and the prevention of cell-to-cell spread of virus through antibody-mediated blockade of viral attachment (right panel).

and other cell types present in the lungs (for example, pDCs, γδ T cells, and NK cells) induces intracellular resistance mechanisms to viral replication and also amplifies the initial innate response and contributes to the release of chemokines that promote the recruitment of circulating inflammatory cells, such as pro-inflammatory monocytes and neutrophils. These signals also activate resident cells in the airways that can kill infected epithelial cells, such as NK cells and intraepithelial lymphocytes, as well as initiate the adaptive immune response. The uptake of dying RECs by cDC1 cells is important for the induction of an influenza-specific cytotoxic T lymphocyte (CTL) response, which is coordinated with a T helper type 1 response induced either by the same cDC1 cells or by cDC2 cells on which type I interferons have acted. This results in the recruitment of CTLs and T_H1 cells to the respiratory mucosa where they act to eliminate infected cells and amplify the IFN response by releasing type II interferon (IFN-γ), which also enhances local antigen presentation of viral antigens. There is also production of IgG-producing plasmablasts that traffic to the respiratory mucosa where they mature and produce antibodies that target the elimination of free virus by phagocytes.

Antibody responses to the influenza virus surface glycoproteins, particularly those directed against hemagglutinin, also block viral attachment and are therefore neutralizing, conferring protection against cell-to-cell transmission of the influenza virus during active infection, as well as preventing viral reinfection after recovery from initial infection. Antigenic sites on the head domain of hemagglutinin that contribute to binding of the virus to the sialic acid residues on host cells are the dominant target of the neutralizing antibody response and are immunodominant compared to other viral B-cell epitopes; they block the interactions of hemagglutinin with host-cell sialic acid residues, thereby preventing viral attachment and entry into RECs. The importance of antibodies in protection against influenza infection was discovered in the 1930s, when it was found that the transfer of serum from infected individuals was protective. The relatively rapid mutation of the gene encoding hemagglutinin results in antigenic drift, which is a principal reason that influenza virus vaccines have to be updated yearly. This is also true for new pandemic viruses that result from antigenic shift, for which antigenically matched vaccines have to be produced. This is despite the fact that antibody responses against influenza virus are typically robust and long lasting.

In view of the importance of the antibody response to protection against influenza, it is evident that B-cell help mediated by T_{FH} cells is central to a protective host response. Cytotoxic T cells (CTLs) are also required for optimal clearance of influenza virus. The CTL response targets antigenic components of the influenza viral core, or nucleocapsid, that include nucleoprotein (NP), membrane protein M1, and the viral polymerases, which, because of their conserved function to viral replication are less tolerant of antigenic drift. Thus, in contrast to the antibody response, the CTL response is more conserved across different influenza virus strains and subtypes. This may mitigate against the severity of disease caused by new viral strains in individuals who have been infected by influenza previously. Because current vaccines use killed virus, which provokes good antibody responses but not CTL responses, there is interest in developing better vaccines that also provide cross-protective immunity by eliciting robust CTL memory responses.

Another RNA virus family that can elicit mild or severe respiratory disease is the Coronaviridae, or coronaviruses, literally, 'crown' viruses, so named because of the appearance of their surface glycoproteins when viewed by electron microscopy (**Fig. 12.47**). Coronaviruses have the largest genomes of known RNA viruses (~25 to 32 kb; roughly twice the size of the influenza virus genome) and cause disease ranging from the common cold to life-threatening **severe acute respiratory syndrome,** or **SARS**. There are two major subfamilies of coronavirus, Torovirinae and Coronavirinae, the latter of which includes the *Alphacoronavirus* and *Betacoronavirus* genera that typically infect only

SARS-CoV-2	Spike protein structure	RBDs of spike protein subunits exist in closed and open conformations on virion surface
		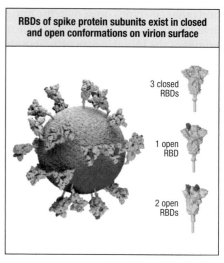

Fig. 12.47 Structure of the SARS-CoV-2 virion, the cause of the COVID-19 SARS pandemic. SARS-CoV-2, the causative agent of the COVID-19 SARS pandemic, is an enveloped plus-stranded RNA virus with a large nucleoprotein (NP)-encapsidated genome (left panel). The virion is roughly spherical and measures about 100 nm in diameter. The viral lipid membrane includes three transmembrane proteins: the spike protein (S), which is a trimer of identical subunits, and two smaller proteins, a membrane protein (M) and an envelope protein (E). The structure of the spike protein solved by cryo-electron microscopy (cryo-EM) is shown in the middle panel. In its closed conformation (shown), the receptor-binding domains (RBDs) of each subunit are folded down on the apical surface of the S-protein trimer, preventing binding to the cellular receptor targeted by the virus—angiotensin-converting enzyme 2 (ACE2). ACE2 is an ectoenzyme that is expressed by cells lining the airways of the lungs, as well as by other cells in the body, such as certain endothelial cells that line blood vessels. Although not highlighted here, each S-protein subunit is composed of two fragments—an S1 fragment that contains the RBD and an S2 fragment that contains the fusion domain—that are generated by proteolytic cleavage during virion assembly. The RBDs and the stalk region, at the S-protein base, are identified. The RBDs of each subunit of the S protein can open spontaneously to permit binding to ACE2, as modeled in the right panel. At any point in time, most S proteins expose none of the RBDs in open conformation (3 closed RBDs), with fewer numbers of S proteins exposing one (1 open RBD) or two (2 open RBDs) binding domains (highlighted in purple). Note that the stalk region at the base of the S protein is highly flexible, allowing the head of the protein to tilt freely on the virion surface. Binding of the S protein to ACE2 on a target cell results in cleavage of the S2 fragment by a host-cell surface serine protease (for example, transmembrane serine protease 2, or TMPRSS2), which is thought to trigger to dissociation of the S1 fragment and refolding of the S2 fragment into a conformation that mediates fusion of the viral membrane with the host-cell membrane, resulting in virion uptake by the host cell.

mammals and are causes of human disease. Strains of both alphacoronaviruses and betacoronaviruses can cause the common cold. Less common strains of betacoronaviruses cause SARS, of which there have been three major outbreaks to date: SARS coronavirus (SARS-CoV; 2002–2004); Middle East respiratory syndrome coronavirus (MERS-CoV; 2012–2015); and most recently, SARS-CoV-2 (late 2019–present). The viral syndrome caused by SARS-CoV-2 has been referred to as **coronavirus disease-2019,** or **COVID-19,** reflecting its date of emergence.

Just as for influenza, the factors that determine the virulence of different strains of coronavirus are not well understood, although the emergence of zoonotic infections against which there is little preexisting immunity appears contributory. Although not proven, bats appear to be the likely source of each of the coronavirus strains that have caused the outbreaks responsible for SARS-CoV, MERS-CoV, and SARS-CoV-2. Whereas MERS-CoV originated in the Middle East and has remained largely endemic to the Arabian Peninsula where endemic infection of camels serves as a reservoir for transmission to humans, both SARS-CoV and SARS-CoV-2 originated in China and may have been amplified in, and been transmitted to, humans by intermediate hosts yet to be identified.

Although the scope of the initial SARS-CoV outbreak (~8000 cases and ~800 deaths worldwide) has now been dramatically eclipsed by SARS-CoV-2 (at least 175 million cases and over 3 million deaths worldwide to date), both of these pathogens, and all other strains of coronavirus, are primarily transmitted via respiratory spread. While MERS-CoV has diverged and uses the host ecto-enzyme dipeptidyl peptidase 4 (DPP4) for virion attachment, SARS-CoV and SARS-CoV-2 use **angiotensin-converting enzyme 2 (ACE2)**, an ectoenzyme that is preferentially expressed on the apical surface of airway epithelial cells. Attachment of these viruses to DPP4 or ACE2 is mediated by the **coronavirus spike protein (S)**, a homotrimeric envelope protein that is the dominant pro-tein expressed on the virus surface—the one responsible for the 'crown' motif for which the virus is named (see Fig. 12.47). The S protein has two fragments that are separated by a protease cleavage site: the S1 region contains the receptor-binding domain (RBD), and the S2 region mediates membrane fusion.

Binding of the S protein to the host cell stimulates its uptake into endosomes, wherein its cleavage by host proteases exposes the S2 fragment that causes viral membrane fusion with the endosomal membrane, triggering release of the viral genome into the host-cell cytosol. At least for SARS-CoV-2, the spike protein can bind ACE2 of multiple mammalian species, including bats, cats, civet cats, swine, ferrets, nonhuman primates, and possibly dogs, in addition to humans. Pangolins, which are scale-covered, ant-eating mammals that are a protected species that is traded illegally in Asia and elsewhere, have been implicated as an intermediate host in some studies. The distribution of the ACE2 viral receptor to epithelial cells of alveoli (in addition to those of the air-ways), like that of sialic acid residues targeted by influenza virus, may contrib-ute to the severe respiratory syndromes that strains of each of these types of virus can cause by direct injury to the alveoli. In a further parallel with influ-enza virus, ACE2 is expressed by other epithelial cells of the body, including the epithelium of the intestines, which can be the primary site of infection if the virus is ingested rather than inhaled in respiratory droplets or a second-ary site of involvement after spread from the lungs. ACE2 is also expressed by endothelial cells and may mediate infection of blood vessels.

In contrast to influenza, the coronavirus genome is not segmented, but rather is a single continuous positive-sense RNA strand (see Fig. 12.44), such that the virus may undergo antigenic drift but not antigenic shift. There is insufficient information at present as to the rate of antigenic drift in SARS-CoV-2. However, early evidence indicates that the virus has mutated several times during the current pandemic, producing several substrains that are more infectious than the parent strain. Indeed, it has been found that much of the antigenic drift observed in coronaviruses is focused on the RBD of the S1 fragment of the spike protein, which mediates attachment to the ACE2 host-cell receptor. Because the RBD of each monomer of the spike protein is an extended loop that projects from its surface and is not critical for its structural integrity, muta-tions in RBDs can occur rapidly without threat to virion integrity and function. In the case of SARS-CoV-2, the affinity of the RBD for ACE2 is substantially higher than that of SARS-CoV, suggesting a mechanism for its more efficient spread and rapid emergence as a pandemic. Thus, somewhat similar to influ-enza, the virus may be able to alter the antigenic targets of the host antibody response to evade blockade of virion uptake. In the case of SARS-CoV-2 this may be particularly selected for in bats, which represent ~20% of all mamma-lian species and live in dense populations that facilitate rapid selection of new strain variants that can sustain propagation within the host community.

Although there is limited information at present on details of the host immune response to SARS-CoV-2, there is reason to believe that the host response shares many features with the response to influenza, in which both neutral-izing antibodies and CTLs play central roles (see Fig. 12.46). Neutralizing antibodies against SARS-CoV and MERS-CoV have been characterized from survivors of these infections, and some cross-protective antibodies against SARS-CoV-2 have been identified in individuals previously infected by SARS-CoV. Indeed, there is some indication that prior exposure to less pathogenic strains of betacoronaviruses that cause the common cold and also use ACE2 as a host receptor can afford at least partial protection against SARS-CoV-2. Although some reports have suggested that protective antibody responses to SARS-CoV-2 may, for unknown reasons, be short-lived, experience from SARS-CoV and MERS-CoV indicates that at least some neutralizing antibodies persist for many years, raising the possibility that the vaccines that have recently been implemented for SARS-CoV-2 may provide long-lived protection. Especially in view of the global health crisis caused by SARS-CoV-2, the potential for vaccines that induce neutralizing antibody responses against multiple variants of the RBD are an area of active investigation, although greater conservation of non-RBD components of the virus that are targeted by CTLs may also hold promise (see Chapter 16).

12-24 Cutaneous immunity.

Our focus so far has been on the immune responses at mucosal surfaces of the intestines and respiratory tract. Although not a mucosal tissue, the skin is nevertheless a highly important barrier. Unlike the intestinal and respiratory tracts, the skin develops from ectoderm rather than endoderm, and though smaller in total surface area than these mucosal tissues, it is the largest organ of the body by weight. Although the skin contributes to the generation of essential metabolites, including active vitamin D, and plays a major role in regulating body temperature and sensing the external environment, its main function is protective. Thus, in contrast to the GI and respiratory tracts, where physiological functions necessitate a thin epithelium that facilitates exchange with the external environment, the skin forms a tight but not impermeable seal that is ideal for providing protection against physical damage (for example, lacerations and radiative and chemical threats), microbial incursion, and water loss. However, despite structural differences between skin and other barrier tissues, many of the immune-cell populations present in skin are similar to those in other barrier tissues as are the host-protective strategies, although there are some unique features of skin immunity that we will highlight here.

The skin consists of the outer epidermis and the inner dermis (**Fig. 12.48**; and see Fig. 12.2), which are in many ways analogous in function to the epithelium and lamina propria, respectively, of mucosal tissues. However, unlike the single-cell epithelium of the intestines or the pseudostratified epithelium of the respiratory tract, the epithelium of the skin lacks goblet cells and, therefore, mucus. Similarly, the skin lacks standing inductive lymphoid tissues, such as the Peyer's patches and ILFs of the intestinal tract, and given that SIgA is a specialized adaptation of mucosal tissues, it is absent in skin. Rather, the first line of defense of the skin is the continually proliferating keratinocytes—so named because of their high content of keratin, a highly cross-linked fibrous protein that is a major structural component of epidermal cells as well as hair and nails. Keratinocytes differentiate as they mature toward the skin surface to create an outer, densely keratinized and cross-linked matrix of anucleated, dead squamous cells, which are continually sloughed and replaced. This outermost layer, or stratum, of the epidermis is the stratum corneum, which is composed of dead keratinocytes sealed by extracellular lipids, which prevents fluid loss and acts as a relatively impenetrable barrier. The stratum corneum is replaced about every 10 days. The other layers of the skin include (from outside, in) the stratum granulosum and stratum spinosum, which are populated by immune cells, and the stratum basale, which is attached to the basement membrane and acts as a reservoir for renewal of the superficial layers of keratinocytes. Another epithelial cell type is the melanocyte, which produces pigment granules that are transferred to developing keratinocytes; melanocyte pigment absorbs UV irradiation to protect skin cells from solar damage. The underlying dermal tissue consists of fibroblasts within a connective matrix that supports hair follicles, some glands, and nerve endings and has a rich supply of

Fig. 12.48 Immune components of barrier function in skin.
The skin is composed of two major compartments—the epidermis and the dermis—which are separated by a basement membrane. The outermost layer is the epidermis, which is composed of layers of increasingly differentiated keratinocytes that can be subdivided into four layers, or strata—the stratum corneum, stratum granulosum, stratum spinosum, and stratum basale. The cellular composition of the epidermis is dominated by keratinocytes, which account for ~90% of all cells in the epidermal compartment. Other epithelial cell types include the hair follicle epithelium and melanocytes, which produce pigment that is transferred to developing keratinocytes to protect from UV irradiation from the sun. Other cells that reside in the human epidermis are Langerhans cells and CD8+ TCRαβ tissue-resident memory T (T$_{RM}$) cells. The murine epidermis also contains dendritic epidermal T cells (DETCs), which are natural intraepithelial lymphocytes (nIELs) that express TCRγδ and populate the epidermis near the time of birth and are absent in human epidermis. Owing to the presence of blood and lymphatic vessels, through which circulating lymphocytes are trafficked to and from the skin, the cellular composition of the dermal compartment is more diverse than that of the epidermis. Dermis-residing immune cells include dermal dendritic cells, γδ T cells, αβ T cells, innate lymphoid cells (ILCs), mast cells, macrophages, B cells, and natural killer (NK) cells. The dermis also provides structural support for the skin and, as such, consists of fibroblasts and connective tissue.

lymphatic and blood vessels. This vascularization enables the extravasation of circulating immune cells mostly to the dermis but also to the epidermis.

Keratinocytes account for ~90% of the cells in the epidermis, although this percentage varies from site to site, depending on skin thickness. Included among the remaining cells are epidermal immune cells, primarily Langerhans cells and T cells. In mice, intraepidermal T cells are dominated by a γδ T-cell subset termed dendritic epidermal T cells (DETCs), which are unconventional T cells with a restricted antigenic specificity (Vγ3+Vδ1+). They populate the skin from the thymus before birth (see Section 8-XX), and they remain there as long-lived resident T cells. DETC precursors up-regulate expression of CCR10 before exiting the thymus to home to the epidermis in response to CCL27 expressed by keratinocytes. Functionally, DETCs are thought to regulate epidermal repair during wound healing, and they may act as innate immune sensor cells. There is no direct equivalent of DETCs in human skin, although the epidermis of humans does contain $\gamma\delta$ T cells that appear to be functionally comparable to DETCs in the mouse. Both species contain $\alpha\beta$ T cells in the epidermis, which, akin to the shift from unconventional to conventional T_{RM} cells in the intestinal epithelium with age (see Section 12-5), tend to replace the $\gamma\delta$ T cells throughout life, depending on the history of antigenic exposure. This has led to speculation that skin $\gamma\delta$ cells present at birth represent a primitive adaptive immune system that is replaced by $\alpha\beta$ T_{RM} cells contingent on an individual's exposure to skin pathogens.

The dermis is enriched in collagen and elastic fibers, which provide the structural framework for vascular and lymphatic vessels that deliver circulating immune cells to and from the skin. Immune cells that reside in the dermis under steady-state conditions are similar to those in the lamina propria of mucosal tissues: cDCs, tissue-resident macrophages, ILCs, $\gamma\delta$ T cells, $\alpha\beta$ T cells, B cells, macrophages, and natural killer (NK) cells. There are also small numbers of innate effector cells, such as mast cells. Dermal $\gamma\delta$ T cells are considerably more diverse than their epidermal counterparts, and although their activating ligands are incompletely characterized, they appear to be mainly restricted by host stress proteins, such as MICA and NKG2B. Dermal $\alpha\beta$ T cells are largely memory cells that have homed to the skin after activation and differentiation in draining lymph nodes. Although details of the signals that imprint skin-trafficking features are not completely understood, some evidence suggests that vitamin D, the active form of which is generated locally in the skin in response to UVB radiation, may imprint T cells to traffic to skin, as in the programming of gut T cells by retinoic acid derived from vitamin A. In any case, up-regulation of E-selectin ligands, such as cutaneous lymphocyte antigen (CLA; see Section 11-14), and CXCR3, CCR4, CCR8, and CCR10 are contributory.

A unique feature of immunity induced in the skin is the contribution of **Langerhans cells (LCs)**. While cDCs from dermis elicit the activation of CD4 and CD8 T cells in draining lymph nodes, cDCs are not typically positioned in the epidermis, where LCs constitute the largest single population of antigen-presenting cells in the entire skin. Like tissue-resident macrophages in mucosal tissues, LCs are derived from monocytic, not dendritic, cell precursors and are a long-lived, self-renewing population that populates the epidermis before birth. Langerhans cells are particularly enriched in the stratum spinosum of the epidermis. Like resident macrophages at mucosal sites, LCs constantly extend and retract dendrites between keratinocytes while maintaining barrier integrity by establishing tight junctions with adjacent keratinocytes. However, unlike mucosa-resident macrophages, LCs are migratory upon activation by inflammatory signals received from keratinocytes (for example, IL-1β and TNF-α) and traffic to draining lymph nodes where they can activate naive T cells. LCs may directly present antigen, but they can also transfer antigens transported from the epidermis to resident lymphoid DCs.

Although there is evidence supporting a role for LCs in the initiation of a variety of adaptive immune responses (for example, type 1 and type 3), LCs have limited ability to phagocytose bacteria and are particularly important in antiviral immunity in the skin. Nevertheless, cutaneous infection models with the type 3 pathogens *Candida albicans* or *Staphylococcus aureus* have demonstrated clear roles for LCs in priming protective CD4 T-cell responses. Moreover, activation of LCs in response to ionizing radiation has been shown to prime skin-tropic T_{reg} cells. In humans, but not mice, LCs also express high levels of the invariant MHC-like molecule CD1a and appear particularly adapted to present lipid antigens to T cells. Thus, LCs appear especially adapted to activate immunity to topical sensitizers that do not reach the dermis, such as the poison ivy lipid urushiol.

Like other barrier tissues, the skin harbors a resident microbiota that is established soon after birth and plays an important role in shaping local immunity in the skin. Across the $\sim 2\,m^2$ of the skin surface of humans resides a diversity of bacteria, fungi, and viruses (see Fig. 12.5 and Fig. 12.48). Like the commensal microbiota in other sites, the skin microbiota provides colonization resistance to limit pathogen invasion and promote homeostasis. The latter includes the induction of populations of FoxP3$^+$ T_{reg} cells that maintain local tolerance. As in the GI and respiratory tracts, this reflects the local production and activation of TGF-β by keratinocytes. Thus, T_{reg} cells specific for components of the skin microbiota arise early in neonatal life in response to skin colonization. Cutaneous T_{reg} cells reside principally in the dermis, where they constitute one of the highest frequencies of T_{reg} cells within the body. In addition to their role in accommodating to the skin microbiota, cutaneous T_{reg} cells also appear to play an important role in non-immunological functions in skin. They have been shown to regulate cutaneous wound healing and the function of stem cells in hair follicles. Accordingly, soon after a skin wound occurs, skin T_{reg} cells accumulate in large numbers at the affected site, where they limit the effector T-cell response and promote epidermal regeneration via production of ligands of the epidermal growth factor receptor pathway. A large fraction of T_{reg} cells in skin is found near hair follicles, which serve as a major habitat for skin-resident microbes. T_{reg} cell responses in that niche may contribute to the development of hair follicles soon after birth and may promote the resident commensal microbes to thwart occupation of the niche by pathogens.

Shifts in composition of the skin microbiota, or dysbiosis, have been documented in many skin inflammatory disorders and are likely cofactors in the etiology of many immune skin disorders. For example, atopic dermatitis, a chronic inflammatory disorder of the skin, has long been associated with colonization of the skin by *Staphylococcus aureus*. Similarly, enrichment in *Streptococcus* spp. was observed in skin lesions of psoriasis. Defined microorganisms or microbial communities could potentially contribute to the initiation or amplification of skin pathologies through several mechanisms. Local expansion of defined members of the skin microbiota with enhanced inflammatory potential could alter tissue homeostasis. For example, *S. aureus* isolates that release δ-toxin trigger local allergic responses as the δ-toxin induces degranulation of dermal mast cells, which in turn promotes both innate and adaptive type 2 immune responses. *S. aureus* α-toxin can also promote IL-17 production from human CD4 T cells, a property that could be explained by the ability of this toxin to induce IL-1β production by monocytes. The skin milieu and defined factors such as vitamin B$_{12}$ can have a profound effect on the metabolism of the skin microbiota and thus the prevention or promotion of colonization by pathogens. Additional studies will be needed to better understand the role of shifts in the skin microbiota in promoting immune-mediated disease in skin.

12-25 The sensory nervous system communicates with the immune system to enhance defense against infections in the skin.

In this section, we will describe a recently recognized mechanism that enhances the immune barrier of the skin. This involves neuroimmune interactions between the peripheral nervous system and dendritic cells in the epidermis that act to activate immune defenses not only at the direct site of infection but also at neighboring skin regions that are innervated by these neurons (**Fig. 12.49**). This mechanism involves c-fiber sensory neurons, which are unmyelinated small-diameter neurons that carry sensory information, often in the form of pain, to indicate damage. Such neurons are called nociceptive neurons (from the Latin *nocere*, 'to do harm'). Among these neurons is a

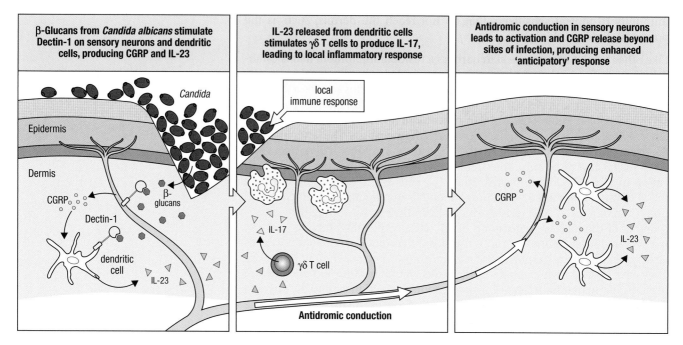

| β-Glucans from *Candida albicans* stimulate Dectin-1 on sensory neurons and dendritic cells, producing CGRP and IL-23 | IL-23 released from dendritic cells stimulates γδ T cells to produce IL-17, leading to local inflammatory response | Antidromic conduction in sensory neurons leads to activation and CGRP release beyond sites of infection, producing enhanced 'anticipatory' response |

Fig. 12.49 Communication between nociceptive sensory neurons and dermal dendritic cells enhances the strength of immune responses. Left panel: When the skin barrier is breached through damage, environmental organisms, such as *Candida albicans,* can establish a local infection. This organism can be recognized directly by cells in the skin through the detection of β-glucans by the lectin receptor Dectin-1, which is expressed by dendritic cells and by TRPV1$^+$ sensory neurons. Activation of these neurons leads to their release of calcitonin gene–related peptide (CGRP), which acts on dermal dendritic cells to enhance their IL-23 production. Middle panel: Dermal dendritic cells are frequently located close to the axons of sensory neurons. CGRP released by these neurons enhances the IL-23 produced by dermal DCs, which in turn acts on various T-cell populations, including local dermal γδ T cells, to produce IL-17 family cytokines that promote local antifungal defense. Right panel: Activation of a sensory neuron by local infection also can stimulate action potentials that conduct information toward the neuronal cell body and, at branches, can conduct information by antidromic activation back toward the terminals of the sensory neuron in noninfected regions of skin. This provides for enhanced type 3 responses in anticipation of further infectious spread.

subtype expressing the transient receptor potential cation channel subfamily V member 1 (TRPV1), which is a receptor for capsaicin, the molecule in chili peppers that induces its burning sensation. Further, some TRPV1$^+$ neurons also express the sodium ion channel Na$_V$1.8, and it is this subset that seems to be important in this neuroimmune pathway.

The role of the nervous system in cutaneous defense against pathogens was recognized in an experimental system of skin inflammation induced by cutaneous administration of imiquimod (IMQ), a small compound that activates TLR-7. Normally, IMQ administration to skin produces an inflammatory response that is dependent on the production of IL-23 by dermal dendritic cells. This IL-23 can activate the production of IL-17 from local T cells, predominantly dermal γδ T cells, and leads to measurable skin thickening in regions such as the ear. As we introduced in Section 9-14, extracellular bacteria and fungi, common microbes encountered by the skin, typically induce type 3 responses, in which IL-17 family cytokines help recruit neutrophils and other cells that are effective in eliminating these types of organisms. When sensory neurons expressing TRPV1 were eliminated prior to treatment with IMQ by the administration of resiniferatoxin (RTX), a toxin and extremely strong agonist of TRPV1, it was discovered that IMQ no longer induced inflammation in treated skin. However, the administration of IL-23 to skin treated with IMQ restored its ability to induce inflammation. Further, the majority of dermal dendritic cells were located close to TRPV1$^+$ sensory fibers. These findings suggested that TRPV1 sensory neurons somehow regulated the ability of dermal dendritic cells to produce IL-23.

These findings were later extended to the setting of skin infection by the environmental fungus *Candida albicans*, which typically induces a type 3 response involving IL-23 and IL-17 production. Recognition of *C. albicans* is mediated, at least in part, by **Dectin-1**, a C-type lectin family member (CLEC7A) that recognizes polysaccharides known as β-glucans, which are derived from the cell walls of bacteria and fungi, and even plants. In addition to its expression by dendritic cells, Dectin-1 also appears to be expressed by dermal keratinocytes and TRPV1$^+$ sensory neurons (see Fig. 12.49), suggesting that each of these cells might recognize β-glucans released by the cell walls of *C. albicans*. Indeed, it was found that infection by *C. albicans* activated neurons to release calcitonin gene–related peptide (CGRP), which acts to facilitate IL-23 production by dermal dendritic cells by an unknown mechanism. A second component of neuronal sensing of *C. albicans* seems to involve the purinoreceptor P2X3, which recognizes extracellular ATP. ATP can be released from keratinocytes activated by Dectin-1 signaling in response to β-glucans made by *C. albicans*. Additionally, some evidence suggests that some strains of *Candida* may directly release significant amounts of ATP. In either case, the combination of signaling by Dectin-1 and P2X3 leads to release of CGRP, promoting enhanced IL-23 from dermal dendritic cells, thus enhancing type 3 immunity in the vicinity of these cells.

Besides promoting IL-23 production by dendritic cells locally at the site of infection, the activation of TRPV1$^+$ neurons by *C. albicans* also has an important secondary benefit. Because sensory neurons extend branches into an entire region of skin, the activation of one branch of a sensory neuron can lead to active nerve conduction through its entire sensory field, which can enhance immune activation to areas of skin outside the initial site of infection. This effect was discovered in clever experiments that used optogenetics in which a channelrhodopsin, a light receptor activated by blue light, was selectively expressed in TRPV1$^+$ neurons of mice. Activation of neurons in a small region by shining a small focus of light onto a small patch of skin was observed to result in enhanced responses to *C. albicans* not only in the region activated by light, but also in adjacent regions of uninfected skin. This expansion of the area in which immunity is heightened occurs by conduction of nerve potential throughout the area served by the sensory neurons. This form of conduction is called antidromic nerve conduction, meaning that a nerve signal passes from the peripheral site of stimulation, first toward a neuronal cell body, but then into other local regions at the sites of axonal branching (see Fig. 12.49). In this way, the communication between sensory neurons and immune cells can provide an anticipatory response at sites not yet infected. Although this is still an active area of research, the anticipatory response is likely due to the release of CGRP by neurons induced by this antidromic conduction at distant sites independently of Dectin-1 signaling.

Summary.

Among barrier tissues, the respiratory tract is unique in that its major surface geography—the lower respiratory tract—is normally sterile; it is devoid of a commensal microbiota, reflecting the requirement for close contact between the airspaces and the blood to accomplish its major physiological function of gas exchange. Much of the protection from pathogens—and from commensals inhaled from the upper respiratory tract—lies in the unusual anatomy of the respiratory tract, which is highly efficient at trapping inhaled particulates of varying sizes and transporting them out of the airspaces via the mucociliary escalator. As in the gut, a tolerogenic tone is strongly favored in the respiratory tract to prevent the dire consequences attendant to overexuberant inflammation in the airways and airspaces, compromise of which can be rapidly fatal. These consequences, coupled with the relative ease of airborne spread of respiratory pathogens, accounts for the fact that respiratory infections are the greatest cause of death among all mucosal infections. This is painfully evident in the COVID-19 pandemic that has recently gripped the world and has emphatically exposed the need for better vaccine strategies that prevent, rather than treat, airborne infections.

The skin differs from other barrier sites in the keratinized epithelium of its epidermis, reflecting its exposure to the greatest physical injury among barrier tissues and its role in minimizing water loss. The epidermis also represents a formidable barrier to pathogen entry, unless it is physically damaged (for example, by cuts or burns) or penetrated by other organisms (for example, insects that transmit microbial pathogens). Unlike many mucosal tissues, such as the intestines, which harbor lymphoid tissues that are in direct contact with the epithelium and its local microbiota, the skin does not normally contain local lymphoid tissues; adaptive immunity in the skin is initiated in draining lymph nodes. Unique to the skin is its population by a specialized resident macrophage, the Langerhans cell, which appears to be important in delivering antigens acquired in the epidermis to lymph nodes. Intraepidermal lymphoid cells, including conventional T_{RM} cells and unconventional $\gamma\delta$ T cells, likely play important roles in immune defense, but the unconventional $\gamma\delta$ T cells, including DETCs in mice, also have an important role in injury repair—representing an important immune function in supporting barrier function in a tissue so exposed to physical injury. The skin is also among the most important sensory organs of the body, literally the main interface with the outside world. Recent discoveries highlight the remarkable interplay of the neural and immune networks in skin that appear to enhance local immunity.

Summary to Chapter 12.

The barrier immune system is an extensive and diverse apparatus that has a crucial role in health, not just by protecting physiologically vital organs but also by helping to regulate the immunological tone to preserve immunological tolerance to nonthreatening antigens. Because of their extensive exposure to the external environment, the skin and mucosal surfaces of the body are at greatest risk of infection and possess unique, site-specific characteristics that distinguish their immune mechanisms from nonbarrier tissues. These include, but are not limited to: the immediate juxtaposition of mucosal epithelium and lymphoid tissue; immune regulation of mucus production that characterizes mucosal tissues; specialized antigen uptake mechanisms; a standing population of activated/memory lymphocytes and innate lymphoid cells (ILCs) even in the absence of infection; a diverse population of conventional and unconventional T cells resident within epithelia; the production of dimeric secretory IgA as the predominant antibody in mucosal tissues; and the down-regulation of immune responses to innocuous antigens such as food antigens and commensal microorganisms. Many of the most remarkable advances in immunobiology are being made in studies of barrier immunity, where there is a growing understanding both of the complexity of the role of innate and adaptive immune cells in supporting the mutualism between the host and the commensal microbiota and of the import of neuroimmune interactions that likely reflect the central role of barrier tissues in sensing, responding to, and protecting the host from the outside world.

Discussion Questions

12.1 Describe the different pathways by which antigens are taken up in the intestines.

12.2 Describe the processes that normally promote non-inflammatory immunity against antigens of the commensal microbiota in the intestines.

12.3 What factors contribute to the trafficking of T cells primed in the GALT to the intestinal mucosa?

12.4 Discuss how dendritic cells in intestinal tissues differ from their counterparts in other tissues, and describe how their

functions are adapted to the local challenges faced by the immune system in the gut.

12.5 Describe the unique anatomic features of the respiratory tract that contribute to the lack of a commensal microbiota in the lungs.

12.6 An unusual aspect of the intestine is the close interaction between epithelial cells and cells of the immune system. Outline how these interactions help shape immune responses to the different kinds of antigens encountered by the gut.

General references.

Hooper, L.V., Littman, D.R., and Macpherson, A.J.: **Interactions between the microbiota and the immune system.** *Science* 2012, **336**:1268–1273.

Maynard, C.L., Elson, C.O., Hatton, R.D. and Weaver, C.T.: **Reciprocal interactions of the intestinal microbiota and immune system.** *Nature* 2012, **489**:231–241.

Mestecky, J., Strober, W., Russell, M.W., Kelsall, B.L., Cheroutre, H., and Lambrecht, B.N. (eds): *Mucosal Immunology,* 4th ed. Amsterdam: Academic Press/Elsevier, 2015.

Mowat, A.M.: **Anatomical basis of tolerance and immunity to intestinal antigens.** *Nat. Rev. Immunol.* 2003, **3**:331–341.

Smith, P.D., Blumberg, R.S., and MacDonald, T.T.: *Principles of Mucosal Immunology,* 2nd ed. Boca Raton: CRC Press, 2020.

Section references.

12-1   The mucosal immune system protects the internal surfaces of the body.

Brandtzaeg, P.: **Function of mucosa-associated lymphoid tissue in antibody formation.** *Immunol. Invest.* 2010, **39**:303–355.

Cerutti, A., Chen, K., and Chorny, A.: **Immunoglobulin responses at the mucosal interface.** *Annu. Rev. Immunol.* 2011, **29**:273–293.

Corthesy, B.: **Role of secretory IgA in infection and maintenance of homeostasis.** *Autoimmun. Rev.* 2013, **12**:661–665.

Fagarasan, S., Kawamoto, S., Kanagawa, O., and Suzuki, K.: **Adaptive immune regulation in the gut: T cell-dependent and T cell-independent IgA synthesis.** *Annu. Rev. Immunol.* 2010, **28**:243–273.

Matsunaga, T., and Rahman, A.: **In search of the origin of the thymus: the thymus and GALT may be evolutionarily related.** *Scand. J. Immunol.* 2001, **53**:1–6.

Naz, R.K.: **Female genital tract immunity: distinct immunological challenges for vaccine development.** *J. Reprod. Immunol.* 2012, **93**:1–8.

Randall, T.D.: **Bronchus-associated lymphoid tissue (BALT) structure and function.** *Adv. Immunol.* 2010, **107**:187–241.

12-2   Immune cells of the mucosal immune system are located both within and outside of specialized lymphoid tissues in proximity to the epithelium.

Baptista, A.P., Olivier, B.J., Goverse, G., Greuter, M., Knippenberg, M., Kusser, K., Domingues, R.G., Veiga-Fernandes, H., Luster, A.D., Lugering, A., *et al.*: **Colonic patch and colonic SILT development are independent and differentially regulated events.** *Mucosal Immunol.* 2013, **6**:511–521.

Brandtzaeg, P., Kiyono, H., Pabst, R., and Russell, M.W.: **Terminology: nomenclature of mucosa-associated lymphoid tissue.** *Mucosal Immunol.* 2008, **1**:31–37.

Eberl, G., and Sawa, S.: **Opening the crypt: current facts and hypotheses on the function of cryptopatches.** *Trends Immunol.* 2010, **31**:50–55.

Lee, J.S., Cella, M., McDonald, K.G., Garlanda, C., Kennedy, G.D., Nukaya, M., Mantovani, A., Kopan, R., Bradfield, C.A., Newberry, R.D., *et al.*: **AHR drives the development of gut ILC22 cells and postnatal lymphoid tissues via pathways dependent on and independent of Notch.** *Nat. Immunol.* 2012, **13**:144–151.

Macpherson, A.J., McCoy, K.D., Johansen, F.E., and Brandtzaeg, P.: **The immune geography of IgA induction and function.** *Mucosal Immunol.* 2008, **1**:11–22.

Pabst, O., Herbrand, H., Worbs, T., Friedrichsen, M., Yan, S., Hoffmann, M.W., Korner, H., Bernhardt, G., Pabst, R., and Forster, R.: **Cryptopatches and isolated lymphoid follicles: dynamic lymphoid tissues dispensable for the generation of intraepithelial lymphocytes.** *Eur. J. Immunol.* 2005, **35**:98–107.

Randall, T.D.: **Bronchus-associated lymphoid tissue (BALT) structure and function.** *Adv. Immunol.* 2010, **107**:187–241.

Randall, T.D., and Mebius, R.E.: **The development and function of mucosal lymphoid tissues: a balancing act with micro-organisms.** *Mucosal Immunol.* 2014, **7**:455–466.

Suzuki, K., Kawamoto, S., Maruya, M., and Fagarasan, S.: **GALT: organization and dynamics leading to IgA synthesis.** *Adv. Immunol.* 2010, **107**:153–185.

12-3   Maturation of the gut-associated lymphoid tissue is driven by acquisition of the commensal microbiota.

Alexander, K.L., Targan, S.R., and Elson, C.O.: **Microbiota activation and regulation of innate and adaptive immunity.** *Immunol. Rev.* 2014, **260**:206–220.

Arpaia, N., Campbell, C., Fan, X., Dikiy, S., van der Veeken, J., deRoos, P., Liu, H., Cross, J.R., Pfeffer, K., Coffer, P.J., *et al.*: **Metabolites produced by commensal bacteria promote peripheral regulatory T-cell generation.** *Nature* 2013, **504**:451–455.

Belkaid, Y., and Hand, T.W.: **Role of the microbiota in immunity and inflammation.** *Cell* 2014, **157**:121–141.

Chung, H., Pamp, S.J., Hill, J.A., Surana, N.K., Edelman, S.M., Troy, E.B., Reading, N.C., Villablanca, E.J., Wang, S., Mora, J.R., *et al.*: **Gut immune maturation depends on colonization with a host-specific microbiota.** *Cell* 2012, **149**:1578–1593.

Maynard, C.L., Elson, C.O., Hatton, R.D., and Weaver, C.T.: **Reciprocal interactions of the intestinal microbiota and immune system.** *Nature* 2012, **489**:231–241.

Peterson, D.A., McNulty, N.P., Guruge, J.L., and Gordon, J.I.: **IgA response to symbiotic bacteria as a mediator of gut homeostasis.** *Cell Host Microbe* 2007, **2**:328–339.

12-4   The intestines are lined by a diversity of epithelial cell types that develop from a common progenitor and play distinct roles in mucosal immunity.

Barker, N.: **Adult intestinal stem cells: critical drivers of epithelial homeostasis and regeneration.** *Nat. Rev. Mol. Cell Biol.* 2014, **15**:19–33.

Gehart, H., and Clevers, H.: Tales from the crypt: new insights into intestinal stem cells. *Nat. Rev. Gastroenterol. Hepatol.* 2018, **16**:19–34.

Johansson, M.E.V., and Hansson, G.C.: Immunological aspects of intestinal mucus and mucins. *Nat. Rev. Immunol.* 2016, **16**, 639–649.

Johansson, M.E.V., Sjövall, H., and Hansson, G.C.: The gastrointestinal mucus system in health and disease. *Nat. Rev. Gastroenterol. Hepatol.* 2013, **10**:352–361.

Peterson, L.W., and Artis, D.: Intestinal epithelial cells: regulators of barrier function and immune homeostasis. *Nat. Rev. Immunol.* 2014, **14**:141–153.

Veiga-Fernandes, H., and Mucida, D.: Neuro-immune interactions at barrier surfaces. *Cell* 2016, **165**:801–811.

12-5 The intestinal epithelium contains conventional and unconventional T cells that are focused on barrier maintenance and defense.

Agace, W.W., Roberts, A.I., Wu, L., Greineder, C., Ebert, E.C., and Parker, C.M.: Human intestinal lamina propria and intraepithelial lymphocytes express receptors specific for chemokines induced by inflammation. *Eur. J. Immunol.* 2000, **30**:819–826.

Cheroutre, H., Lambolez, F., and Mucida, D.: The light and dark sides of intestinal intraepithelial lymphocytes. *Nat. Rev. Immunol.* 2011, **11**:445–456.

Eberl, G., and Sawa, S.: Opening the crypt: current facts and hypotheses on the function of cryptopatches. *Trends Immunol.* 2010, **31**:50–55.

Hayday, A., Theodoridis, E., Ramsburg, E., and Shires, J.: Intraepithelial lymphocytes: exploring the Third Way in immunology. *Nat. Immunol.* 2001, **2**:997–1003.

Jiang, W., Wang, X., Zeng, B., Liu, L., Tardivel, A., Wei, H., Han, J., MacDonald, H.R., Tschopp, J., Tian, Z., et al.: Recognition of gut microbiota by NOD2 is essential for the homeostasis of intestinal intraepithelial lymphocytes. *J. Exp. Med.* 2013, **210**:2465–2476.

Li, Y., Innocentin, S., Withers, D.R., Roberts, N.A., Gallagher, A.R., Grigorieva, E.F., Wilhelm, C., and Veldhoen, M.: Exogenous stimuli maintain intraepithelial lymphocytes via aryl hydrocarbon receptor activation. *Cell* 2011, **147**:629–640.

Pobezinsky, L.A., Angelov, G.S., Tai, X., Jeurling, S., Van Laethem, F., Feigenbaum, L., Park, J.H., and Singer, A.: Clonal deletion and the fate of autoreactive thymocytes that survive negative selection. *Nat. Immunol.* 2012, **13**:569–578.

12-6 Innate lymphoid cells and unconventional lymphocytes are present in GALT and in the lamina propria and are rapid responders to microbes that breach the epithelium.

Buonocore, S., Ahern, P.P., Uhlig, H.H., Ivanov, I.I., Littman, D.R., Maloy, K.J., and Powrie, F.: Innate lymphoid cells drive interleukin-23-dependent innate intestinal pathology. *Nature* 2010, **464**:1371–1375.

Klose, C.S., Kiss, E.A., Schwierzeck, V., Ebert, K., Hoyler, T., d'Hargues, Y., Goppert, N., Croxford, A.L., Waisman, A., Tanriver, Y., et al.: A T-bet gradient controls the fate and function of CCR6–RORγt+ innate lymphoid cells. *Nature* 2013, **494**:261–265.

Kruglov, A.A., Grivennikov, S.I., Kuprash, D.V., Winsauer, C., Prepens, S., Seleznik, G.M., Eberl, G., Littman, D.R., Heikenwalder, M., Tumanov, A.V., et al.: Nonredundant function of soluble LTα3 produced by innate lymphoid cells in intestinal homeostasis. *Science* 2013, **342**:1243–1246.

Le Bourhis, L., Dusseaux, M., Bohineust, A., Bessoles, S., Martin, E., Premel, V., Core, M., Sleurs, D., Serriari, N.E., and Treiner, E.: MAIT cells detect and efficiently lyse bacterially-infected epithelial cells. *PLoS Pathog.* 2013, **9**:e1003681.

Mortha, A., Chudnovskiy, A., Hashimoto, D., Bogunovic, M., Spencer, S.P., Belkaid, Y., and Merad, M.: Microbiota-dependent crosstalk between macrophages and ILC3 promotes intestinal homeostasis. *Science* 2014, **343**:1249288.

Spits, H., and Cupedo, T.: Innate lymphoid cells: emerging insights in development, lineage relationships, and function. *Annu. Rev. Immunol.* 2012, **30**:647–675.

12-7 The mucosal immune system must establish and maintain tolerance to harmless foreign antigens.

Cassani, B., Villablanca, E.J., Quintana, F.J., Love, P.E., Lacy-Hulbert, A., Blaner, W.S., Sparwasser, T., Snapper, S.B., Weiner, H.L., and Mora, J.R.: Gut-tropic T cells that express integrin α4β7 and CCR9 are required for induction of oral immune tolerance in mice. *Gastroenterology* 2011, **141**:2109–2118.

Coombes, J.L., Siddiqui, K.R., Arancibia-Carcamo, C.V., Hall, J., Sun, C.M., Belkaid, Y., and Powrie, F.: A functionally specialized population of mucosal CD103+ DCs induces Foxp3+ regulatory T cells via a TGF-β and retinoic acid-dependent mechanism. *J. Exp. Med.* 2007, **204**:1757–1764.

Du Toit, G., Roberts, G., Sayre, P.H., Bahnson, H.T., Radulovic, S., Santos, A.F., Brough, H.A., Phippard, D., Basting, M., Feeney, M., et al.: Randomized trial of peanut consumption in infants at risk for peanut allergy. *N. Engl. J. Med.* 2015, **372**:803–813.

Huang, G., Wang, Y., and Chi, H.: Control of T cell fates and immune tolerance by p38α signaling in mucosal CD103+ dendritic cells. *J. Immunol.* 2013, **191**:650–659.

Mowat, A.M., Strobel, S., Drummond, H.E., and Ferguson, A.: Immunological responses to fed protein antigens in mice. I. Reversal of oral tolerance to ovalbumin by cyclophosphamide. *Immunology* 1982, **45**:105–113.

12-8 Macrophages and dendritic cells have complementary roles in the maintenance of immune tolerance in the intestines.

Bain, C.C., and Mowat, A.M.: Macrophages in intestinal homeostasis and inflammation. *Immunol. Rev.* 2014, **260**:102–117.

Bain, C.C., Bravo-Blas, A., Scott, C.L., Geissmann, F., Henri, S., Malissen, B., Osborne, L.C., Artis, D., and Mowat, A.M.: Constant replenishment from circulating monocytes maintains the macrophage pool in adult intestine. *Nat. Immunol.* 2014, **15**:929–937.

Cerovic, V., Bain, C.C., Mowat, A.M., and Milling, S.W.F.: Intestinal macrophages and dendritic cells: what's the difference? *Trends Immunol.* 2014, **35**:270–277.

Farache, J., Koren, I., Milo, I., Gurevich, I., Kim, K.W., Zigmond, E., Furtado, G.C., Lira, S.A., and Shakhar, G.: Luminal bacteria recruit CD103+ dendritic cells into the intestinal epithelium to sample bacterial antigens for presentation. *Immunity* 2013, **38**:581–595.

Jaensson-Gyllenback, E., Kotarsky, K., Zapata, F., Persson, E.K., Gundersen, T.E., Blomhoff, R., and Agace, W.W.: Bile retinoids imprint intestinal CD103+ dendritic cells with the ability to generate gut-tropic T cells. *Mucosal Immunol.* 2011, **4**:438–447.

Matteoli, G.: Gut CD103+ dendritic cells express indoleamine 2,3-dioxygenase which influences T regulatory/T effector cell balance and oral tolerance induction. *Gut* 2010, **59**:595–604.

Persson, E.K., Scott, C.L., Mowat, A.M., and Agace, W.W.: Dendritic cell subsets in the intestinal lamina propria: ontogeny and function. *Eur. J. Immunol.* 2013, **43**:3098–3107.

Salazar-Gonzalez, R.M., Niess, J.H., Zammit, D.J., Ravindran, R., Srinivasan, A., Maxwell, J.R., Stoklasek, T., Yadav, R., Williams, I.R., Gu, X., et al.: CCR6-mediated dendritic cell activation of pathogen-specific T cells in Peyer's patches. *Immunity* 2006, **24**:623–632.

Schlitzer, A., McGovern, N., Teo, P., Zelante, T., Atarashi, K., Low, D., Ho, A.W., See, P., Shin, A., Wasan, P.S., et al.: IRF4 transcription factor-dependent CD11b+ dendritic cells in human and mouse control mucosal IL-17 cytokine responses. *Immunity* 2013, **38**:970–983.

Scott, C.L., Bain, C.C., Wright, P.B., Schien, D., Kotarsky, K., Persson, E.K., Luda, K., Guilliams, M., Lambrecht, B.N., Agace, W.W., et al.: CCR2+CD103− intestinal dendritic cells develop from DC-committed precursors and induce interleukin-17 production by T cells. *Mucosal Immunol.* 2015, **8**:327–339.

Smith, P.D., Smythies, L.E., Shen, R., Greenwell-Wild, T., Gliozzi, M., and Wahl, S.M.: Intestinal macrophages and response to microbial encroachment. *Mucosal Immunol.* 2011, **4**:31–42.

Travis, M.A., Reizis, B., Melton, A.C., Masteller, E., Tang, Q., Proctor, J.M., Wang, Y., Bernstein, X., Huang, X., Reichardt, L.F., et al.: Loss of integrin αvβ8 on dendritic cells causes autoimmunity and colitis in mice. *Nature* 2007, **449**:361–365.

Uematsu, S., Jang, M.H., Chevrier, N., Guo, Z., Kumagai, Y., Yamamoto, M., Kato, H., Sougawa, N., Matsui, H., Kuwata, H., et al.: Detection of pathogenic intestinal bacteria by Toll-like receptor 5 on intestinal CD11c+ lamina propria cells. *Nat. Immunol.* 2006, **7**:868–874.

Vicente-Suarez, I., Larange, A., Reardon, C., Matho, M., Feau, S., Chodaczek, G., Park, Y., Obata, Y., Gold, R., Wang-Zhu, Y., *et al.*: **Unique lamina propria stromal cells imprint the functional phenotype of mucosal dendritic cells.** *Mucosal Immunol.* 2015, **8**:141–151.

Watchmaker, P.B., Lahl, K., Lee, M., Baumjohann, D., Morton, J., Kim, S.J., Zeng, R., Dent, A., Ansel, K.M., Diamond, B., *et al.*: **Comparative transcriptional and functional profiling defines conserved programs of intestinal DC differentiation in humans and mice.** *Nat. Immunol.* 2014, **15**:98–108.

12-9 The intestines have multiple routes for uptake and delivery of antigen to antigen-presenting cells.

Anosova, N.G., Chabot, S., Shreedhar, V., Borawski, J.A., Dickinson, B.L., and Neutra, M.R.: **Cholera toxin, *E. coli* heat-labile toxin, and non-toxic derivatives induce dendritic cell migration into the follicle-associated epithelium of Peyer's patches.** *Mucosal Immunol.* 2008, **1**:59–67.

Hase, K., Kawano, K., Nochi, T., Pontes, G.S., Fukuda, S., Ebisawa, M., Kadokura, K., Tobe, T., Fujimura, Y., Kawano, S., *et al.*: **Uptake through glycoprotein 2 of FimH+ bacteria by M cells initiates mucosal immune response.** *Nature* 2009, **462**:226–230.

Jang, M.H., Kweon, M.N., Iwatani, K., Yamamoto, M., Terahara, K., Sasakawa, C., Suzuki, T., Nochi, T., Yokota, Y., Rennert, P.D., *et al.*: **Intestinal villous M cells: an antigen entry site in the mucosal epithelium.** *Proc. Natl. Acad. Sci. USA* 2004, **101**:6110–6115.

Kulkarni, D.H., Gustafsson, J.K., Knoop, K.A., McDonald, K.G., Bidani, S.S., Davis, J.E., Floyd, A.N., Hogan, S.P., Hsieh, C-S., and Newberry, R.D.: **Goblet cell associated antigen passages support the induction and maintenance of oral tolerance.** *Mucosal Immunol.* 2020, **13**:271–282.

Lelouard, H., Fallet, M., de Bovis, B., Meresse, S., and Gorvel, J.P.: **Peyer's patch dendritic cells sample antigens by extending dendrites through M cell-specific transcellular pores.** *Gastroenterology* 2012, **142**:592–601.

Mabbott, N.A., Donaldson, D.S., Ohno, H., Williams, I.R., and Mahajan, A.: **Microfold (M) cells: important immunosurveillance posts in the intestinal epithelium.** *Mucosal Immunol.* 2013, **6**:666–677.

Salazar-Gonzalez, R.M., Niess, J.H., Zammit, D.J., Ravindran, R., Srinivasan, A., Maxwell, J.R., Stoklasek, T., Yadav, R., Williams, I.R., Gu, X., *et al.*: **CCR6-mediated dendritic cell activation of pathogen-specific T cells in Peyer's patches.** *Immunity* 2006, **24**:623–632.

Sato, S., Kaneto, S., Shibata, N., Takahashi, Y., Okura, H., Yuki, Y., Kunisawa, J., and Kiyono, H.: **Transcription factor Spi-B-dependent and -independent pathways for the development of Peyer's patch M cells.** *Mucosal Immunol.* 2013, **6**:838–846.

Zhao, X., Sato, A., Dela Cruz, C.S., Linehan, M., Luegering, A., Kucharzik, T., Shirakawa, A.K., Marquez, G., Farber, J.M., Williams, I., *et al.*: **CCL9 is secreted by the follicle-associated epithelium and recruits dome region Peyer's patch CD11b+ dendritic cells.** *J. Immunol.* 2003, **171**:2797–2803.

12-10 Intestinal dendritic cells favor the induction of antigen-specific T_{reg} cells that are critical for the maintenance of mucosal immune homeostasis.

Arpaia, N., Campbell, C., Fan, X., Dikiy, S., van der Veeken, J., deRoos, P., Liu, H., Cross, J.R., Pfeffer, K., Coffer, P.J., *et al.*: **Metabolites produced by commensal bacteria promote peripheral regulatory T-cell generation.** *Nature* 2013, **504**:451–455.

Atarashi, K., Tanoue, T., Oshima, K., Suda, W., Nagano, Y., Nishikawa, H., Fukuda, S., Saito, T., Narushima, S., Hase, K., *et al.*: **T_{reg} induction by a rationally selected mixture of Clostridia strains from the human microbiota.** *Nature* 2013, **500**:232–236.

Belkaid, Y., and Hand, T.W.: **Role of the microbiota in immunity and inflammation.** *Cell* 2014, **157**:121–141.

Hadis, U., Wahl, B., Schulz, O., Hardtke-Wolenski, M., Schippers, A., Wagner, N., Muller, W., Sparwasser, T., Forster, R., and Pabst, O.: **Intestinal tolerance requires gut homing and expansion of FoxP3+ regulatory T cells in the lamina propria.** *Immunity* 2011, **34**:237–246.

Kato, L.M., Kawamoto, S., Maruya, M., and Fagarasan, S.: **The role of the adaptive immune system in regulation of gut microbiota.** *Immunol. Rev.* 2014, **260**:67–75.

Macia, L., Thorburn, A.N., Binge, L.C., Marino, E., Rogers, K.E., Maslowski, K.M., Vieira, A.T., Kranich, J., and Mackay, C.R.: **Microbial influences on epithelial integrity and immune function as a basis for inflammatory diseases.** *Immunol. Rev.* 2012, **245**:164–176.

Maynard, C.L., Elson, C.O., Hatton, R.D., and Weaver, C.T.: **Reciprocal interactions of the intestinal microbiota and immune system.** *Nature* 2012, **489**:231–241.

Peterson, D.A., McNulty, N.P., Guruge, J.L., and Gordon, J.I.: **IgA response to symbiotic bacteria as a mediator of gut homeostasis.** *Cell Host Microbe* 2007, **2**:328–339.

Round, J.L., and Mazmanian, S.K.: **Inducible Foxp3+ regulatory T-cell development by a commensal bacterium of the intestinal microbiota.** *Proc. Natl. Acad. Sci. USA* 2010, **107**:12204–12209.

Shale, M., Schiering, C., and Powrie, F.: **CD4+ T-cell subsets in intestinal inflammation.** *Immunol. Rev.* 2013, **252**:164–182.

Zigmond, E., Bernshtein, B., Friedlander, G., Walker, C.R., Yona, S., Kim, K.W., Brenner, O., Krauthgamer, R., Varol, C., Müller, W., *et al.*: **Macrophage-restricted interleukin-10 receptor deficiency, but not IL-10 deficiency, causes severe spontaneous colitis.** *Immunity* 2014, **40**:720–733.

12-11 Lymphocytes primed within the mucosal immune system are directed to return to the mucosal tissue by tissue-specific adhesion molecules and chemokine receptors.

Agace, W.: **Generation of gut-homing T cells and their localization to the small intestinal mucosa.** *Immunol. Lett.* 2010, **128**:21–23.

Hu, S., Yang, K., Yang, J., Li, M., and Xiong, N.: **Critical roles of chemokine receptor CCR10 in regulating memory IgA responses in intestines.** *Proc. Natl. Acad. Sci. USA* 2011, **108**:E1035–E1044.

Kim, S.V., Xiang, W.V., Kwak, C., Yang, Y., Lin, X.W., Ota, M., Sarpel, U., Rifkin, D.B., Xu, R., and Littman, D.R.: **GPR15-mediated homing controls immune homeostasis in the large intestine mucosa.** *Science* 2013, **340**:1456–1459.

Macpherson, A.J., Geuking, M.B., Slack, E., Hapfelmeier, S., and McCoy, K.D.: **The habitat, double life, citizenship, and forgetfulness of IgA.** *Immunol. Rev.* 2012, **245**:132–146.

Mikhak, Z., Strassner, J.P., and Luster, A.D.: **Lung dendritic cells imprint T cell lung homing and promote lung immunity through the chemokine receptor CCR4.** *J. Exp. Med.* 2013, **210**:1855–1869.

Mora, J.R., and von Andrian, U.H.: **Differentiation and homing of IgA-secreting cells.** *Mucosal Immunol.* 2008, **1**:96–109.

Pabst, O., and Bernhardt, G.: **On the road to tolerance—generation and migration of gut regulatory T cells.** *Eur. J. Immunol.* 2013, **43**:1422–1425.

12-12 Secretory IgA is the dominant class of antibody associated with the mucosal immune system at homeostasis.

Fritz, J.H., Rojas, O.L., Simard, N., McCarthy, D.D., Hapfelmeier, S., Rubino, S., Robertson, S.J., Larijani, M., Gosselin, J., Ivanov, II, *et al.*: **Acquisition of a multifunctional IgA+ plasma cell phenotype in the gut.** *Nature* 2012, **481**:199–203.

Hirota, K., Turner, J.E., Villa, M., Duarte, J.H., Demengeot, J., Steinmetz, O.M., and Stockinger, B.: **Plasticity of Th17 cells in Peyer's patches is responsible for the induction of T cell-dependent IgA responses.** *Nat. Immunol.* 2013, **14**:372–379.

Karlsson, M.R., Johansen, F.E., Kahu, H., Macpherson, A., and Brandtzaeg, P.: **Hypersensitivity and oral tolerance in the absence of a secretory immune system.** *Allergy* 2010, **65**:561–570.

Kawamoto, S., Maruya, M., Kato, L.M., Suda, W., Atarashi, K., Doi, Y., Tsutsui, Y., Qin, H., Honda, K., Okada, T., *et al.*: **Foxp3 T cells regulate immunoglobulin A selection and facilitate diversification of bacterial species responsible for immune homeostasis.** *Immunity* 2014, **41**:152–165.

Lin, M., Du, L., Brandtzaeg, P., and Pan-Hammarstrom, Q.: **IgA subclass switch recombination in human mucosal and systemic immune compartments.** *Mucosal Immunol.* 2014, **7**:511–520.

Moor, K., Diard, M., Sellin, M.E., Felmy, B., Wotzka, S.Y., Toska, A., Bakkeren, E., Arnoldini, M., Bansept, F., and Dal Co, A.: High-avidity IgA protects the intestine by enchaining growing bacteria. *Nature* 2017, **544**:498–502.

Woof, J.M., and Russell, M.W.: Structure and function relationships in IgA. *Mucosal Immunol.* 2011, **4**:590–597.

Yel, L.: Selective IgA deficiency. *J. Clin. Immunol.* 2010, **30**:10–16.

12-13 T cell–independent processes can contribute to IgA production in some species.

Barone, F., Vossenkamper, A., Boursier, L., Su, W., Watson, A., John, S., Dunn-Walters, D.K., Fields, P., Wijetilleka, S., Edgeworth, J.D., *et al.*: IgA-producing plasma cells originate from germinal centers that are induced by B-cell receptor engagement in humans. *Gastroenterology* 2011, **140**:947–956.

Fagarasan, S., Kawamoto, S., Kanagawa, O., and Suzuki, K.: Adaptive immune regulation in the gut: T cell-dependent and T cell-independent IgA synthesis. *Annu. Rev. Immunol.* 2010, **28**:243–273.

Lin, M., Du, L., Brandtzaeg, P., and Pan-Hammarstrom, Q.: IgA subclass switch recombination in human mucosal and systemic immune compartments. *Mucosal Immunol.* 2014, **7**:511–520.

Tezuka, H., Abe, Y., Asano, J., Sato, T., Liu, J., Iwata, M., and Ohteki, T.: Prominent role for plasmacytoid dendritic cells in mucosal T cell-independent IgA induction. *Immunity* 2011, **34**:247–257.

12-14 IgA deficiency is relatively common in humans but may be compensated for by secretory IgM.

Karlsson, M.R., Johansen, F.E., Kahu, H., Macpherson, A., and Brandtzaeg, P.: Hypersensitivity and oral tolerance in the absence of a secretory immune system. *Allergy* 2010, **65**:561–570.

Yel, L.: Selective IgA deficiency. *J. Clin. Immunol.* 2010, **30**:10–16.

12-15 Large numbers of antigen-experienced T cells are present in the intestinal lamina propria even in the absence of disease.

Belkaid, Y., Bouladoux, N., and Hand, T.W.: Effector and memory T cell responses to commensal bacteria. *Trends Immunol.* 2013, **34**:299–306.

Brandtzaeg, P.: Mucosal immunity: induction, dissemination, and effector functions. *Scand. J. Immunol.* 2009, **70**:505–515.

Cao, A.T., Yao, S., Gong, B., Elson, C.O., and Cong, Y.: Th17 cells upregulate polymeric Ig receptor and intestinal IgA and contribute to intestinal homeostasis. *J. Immunol.* 2012, **189**:4666–4673.

Cauley, L.S., and Lefrancois, L.: Guarding the perimeter: protection of the mucosa by tissue-resident memory T cells. *Mucosal Immunol.* 2013, **6**:14–23.

Cheroutre, H., and Lambolez, F.: Doubting the TCR coreceptor function of CD8αα. *Immunity* 2008, **28**:149–159.

Maynard, C.L., and Weaver, C.T.: Intestinal effector cells in health and disease. *Immunity* 2009, **31**:389–400.

Sathaliyawala, T., Kubota, M., Yudanin, N., Turner, D., Camp, P., Thome, J.J., Bickham, K.L., Lerner, H., Goldstein, M., Sykes, M., *et al.*: Distribution and compartmentalization of human circulating and tissue-resident memory T cell subsets. *Immunity* 2013, **38**:187–197.

12-16 Priming of lymphocytes in one mucosal tissue may induce protective immunity at other mucosal surfaces.

Agnello, D., Denimal, D., Lavaux, A., Blondeau-Germe, L., Lu, B., Gerard, N.P., Gerard, C., and Pothier, P.: Intrarectal immunization and IgA antibody-secreting cell homing to the small intestine. *J. Immunol.* 2013, **190**:4836–4847.

Brandtzaeg, P.: Induction of secretory immunity and memory at mucosal surfaces. *Vaccine* 2007, **25**:5467–5484.

Czerkinsky, C., and Holmgren, J.: Mucosal delivery routes for optimal immunization: targeting immunity to the right tissues. *Curr. Top. Microbiol. Immunol.* 2012, **354**:1–18.

Ruane, D., Brane, L., Reis, B.S., Cheong, C., Poles, J., Do, Y., Zhu, H., Velinzon, K., Choi, J.H., Studt, N., *et al.*: Lung dendritic cells induce migration of protective T cells to the gastrointestinal tract. *J. Exp. Med.* 2013, **210**:1871–1888.

12-17 Enteric pathogens elicit 'danger signals' by activating pattern-recognition receptors that are sequestered in the intestinal epithelium.

Cliffe, L.J., Humphreys, N.E., Lane, T.E., Potten, C.S., Booth, C., and Grencis, R.K.: Accelerated intestinal epithelial cell turnover: a new mechanism of parasite expulsion. *Science* 2005, **308**:1463–1465.

Kinnebrew, M.A., Buffie, C.G., Diehl, G.E., Zenewicz, L.A., Leiner, I., Hohl, T.M., Flavell, R.A., Littman, D.R., and Pamer, E.G.: Interleukin 23 production by intestinal CD103+CD11b+ dendritic cells in response to bacterial flagellin enhances mucosal innate immune defense. *Immunity* 2012, **36**:276–287.

Prescott, D., Lee, J., and Philpott, D.J.: An epithelial armamentarium to sense the microbiota. *Semin. Immunol.* 2013, **25**:323–333.

Sokol, H., Conway, K.L., Zhang, M., Choi, M., Morin, B., Cao, Z., Villablanca, E.J., Li, C., Wijmenga, C., Yun, S.H., *et al.*: Card9 mediates intestinal epithelial cell restitution, T-helper 17 responses, and control of bacterial infection in mice. *Gastroenterology* 2013, **145**:591–601.

Sonnenberg, G.F., Fouser, L.A., and Artis, D.: Functional biology of the IL-22-IL-22R pathway in regulating immunity and inflammation at barrier surfaces. *Adv. Immunol.* 2010, **107**:1–29.

Turner, J.E., Stockinger, B., and Helmby, H.: IL-22 mediates goblet cell hyperplasia and worm expulsion in intestinal helminth infection. *PLoS Pathog.* 2013, **9**:e1003698.

12-18 Pathogens induce inflammatory adaptive immune responses when innate defenses have been breached.

Bain, C.C., and Mowat, A.M.: Macrophages in intestinal homeostasis and inflammation. *Immunol. Rev.* 2014, **260**:102–117.

Farache, J., Koren, I., Milo, I., Gurevich, I., Kim, K.W., Zigmond, E., Furtado, G.C., Lira, S.A., and Shakhar, G.: Luminal bacteria recruit CD103+ dendritic cells into the intestinal epithelium to sample bacterial antigens for presentation. *Immunity* 2013, **38**:581–595.

Persson, E.K., Scott, C.L., Mowat, A.M., and Agace, W.W.: Dendritic cell subsets in the intestinal lamina propria: ontogeny and function. *Eur. J. Immunol.* 2013, **43**:3098–3107.

Salazar-Gonzalez, R.M., Niess, J.H., Zammit, D.J., Ravindran, R., Srinivasan, A., Maxwell, J.R., Stoklasek, T., Yadav, R., Williams, I.R., Gu, X., *et al.*: CCR6-mediated dendritic cell activation of pathogen-specific T cells in Peyer's patches. *Immunity* 2006, **24**:623–632.

Uematsu, S., Jang, M.H., Chevrier, N., Guo, Z., Kumagai, Y., Yamamoto, M., Kato, H., Sougawa, N., Matsui, H., Kuwata, H., *et al.*: Detection of pathogenic intestinal bacteria by Toll-like receptor 5 on intestinal CD11c+ lamina propria cells. *Nat. Immunol.* 2006, **7**:868–874.

12-19 Effector T-cell responses in the intestine protect the function of the epithelium.

Cliffe, L.J., Humphreys, N.E., Lane, T.E., Potten, C.S., Booth, C., and Grencis, R.K.: Accelerated intestinal epithelial cell turnover: a new mechanism of parasite expulsion. *Science* 2005, **308**:1463–1465.

Kinnebrew, M.A., Buffie, C.G., Diehl, G.E., Zenewicz, L.A., Leiner, I., Hohl, T.M., Flavell, R.A., Littman, D.R., and Pamer, E.G.: Interleukin 23 production by intestinal CD103+CD11b+ dendritic cells in response to bacterial flagellin enhances mucosal innate immune defense. *Immunity* 2012, **36**:276–287.

Sokol, H., Conway, K.L., Zhang, M., Choi, M., Morin, B., Cao, Z., Villablanca, E.J., Li, C., Wijmenga, C., Yun, S.H., *et al.*: Card9 mediates intestinal epithelial cell restitution, T-helper 17 responses, and control of bacterial infection in mice. *Gastroenterology* 2013, **145**:591–601.

Sonnenberg, G.F., Fouser, L.A., and Artis, D.: Functional biology of the IL-22-IL-22R pathway in regulating immunity and inflammation at barrier surfaces. *Adv. Immunol.* 2010, **107**:1–29.

Turner, J.E., Stockinger, B., and Helmby, H.: IL-22 mediates goblet cell hyperplasia and worm expulsion in intestinal helminth infection. *PLoS Pathog.* 2013, 9:e1003698.

12-20   Noninvasive and invasive enteric bacterial pathogens use different strategies to colonize the intestines.

Geddes, K., Rubino, S.J., Magalhaes, J.G., Streutker, C., Le Bourhis, L., Cho, J.H., Robertson, S.J., Kim, C.J., Kaul, R., Philpott, D.J., *et al.*: Identification of an innate T helper type 17 response to intestinal bacterial pathogens. *Nat. Med.* 2011, 17:837–844.

Prescott, D., Lee, J., and Philpott, D.J.: An epithelial armamentarium to sense the microbiota. *Semin. Immunol.* 2013, 25:323–333.

Satpathy, A.T., Briseño, C.G., Lee, J.S., Ng, D., Manieri, N.A., Kc, W., Wu, X., Thomas, S.R., Lee, W.L., Turkoz, M., *et al.*: Notch2-dependent classical dendritic cells orchestrate intestinal immunity to attaching-and-effacing bacterial pathogens. *Nat. Immunol.* 2013, 14:937–948.

Silberger, D.J., Zindl, C.L., and Weaver, C.T. *Citrobacter rodentium:* a model enteropathogen for understanding the interplay of innate and adaptive components of type 3 immunity. *Mucosal Immunol.* 2017, 10:1108–1117.

Song-Zhao, G.X., Srinivasan, N., Pott, J., Baban, D., Frankel, G., and Maloy, K.J.: Nlrp3 activation in the intestinal epithelium protects against a mucosal pathogen. *Mucosal Immunol.* 2014, 7:763–774.

12-21   Dysregulated immune responses to commensal bacteria provoke intestinal disease.

Zigmond, E., Bernshtein, B., Friedlander, G., Walker, C.R., Yona, S., Kim, K.W., Brenner, O., Krauthgamer, R., Varol, C., Müller, W., *et al.*: Macrophage-restricted interleukin-10 receptor deficiency, but not IL-10 deficiency, causes severe spontaneous colitis. *Immunity* 2014, 40:720–733.

12-22   Anatomy and mucosal immunity of the airways.

Guilliams, M., Lambrecht, B.N., and Hammad, H.: Division of labor between lung dendritic cells and macrophages in the defense against pulmonary infections. *Mucosal Immunol.* 2013, 6:464–473.

Sato, S., and Kiyono, H.: The mucosal immune system of the respiratory tract. *Curr. Opin. Virol.* 2012, 2:225–232.

12-23   Respiratory immunity to inhaled pathogens; respiratory viruses.

Braciale, T.J., Sun, J., and Kim, T.S.: Regulating the adaptive immune response to respiratory virus infection. *Nat. Rev. Immunol.* 2012, 12:295–305.

Holt, P.G., Strickland, D.H., Wikström, M.E., and Jahnsen, F.L.: Regulation of immunological homeostasis in the respiratory tract. *Nat. Rev. Immunol.* 2008, 8:142–152.

Iwasaki, A., Foxman, E.F., and Molony, R.D.: Early local immune defences in the respiratory tract. *Nat. Rev. Immunol.* 2017, 17:7–20.

Krammer, F., Smith, G.J.D., Fouchier, R.A.M., Peiris, M., Kedzierska, K., Doherty, P.C., Palese, P., Shaw, M.L., Treanor, J., Webster, R.G., and García-Sastre, A.: Influenza. *Nat. Rev. Dis. Primers* 2018, 4:3.

Subbarao, K., and Mahanty, S.: Respiratory virus infections: understanding COVID-19. *Immunity* 2020, 52:905–909.

12-24   Cutaneous immunity.

Belkaid, Y., and Tamoutounour, S.: The influence of skin microorganisms on cutaneous immunity. *Nat. Rev. Immunol.* 2016, 16:353–366.

Ho, A.W., and Kupper, T.S.: T cells and the skin: from protective immunity to inflammatory skin disorders. *Nat. Rev. Immunol.* 2019, 19:490–502.

Kabashima, K., Honda, T., Ginhoux, F., and Egawa, G.: The immunological anatomy of the skin. *Nat. Rev. Immunol.* 2019, 19:19–30.

12-25   The sensory nervous system communicates with the immune system to enhance defense against infections in the skin.

Cohen, J.A., Edwards, T.N., Liu, A.W., Hirai, T., Jones, M.R., Wu, J., Li, Y., Zhang, S., Ho, J., Davis, B.M., *et al.*: Cutaneous TRPV1+ neurons trigger protective innate type 17 anticipatory immunity. *Cell* 2019, 178:919–932.

Kashem, S.W., Riedl, M.S., Yao, C., Honda, C.N., Vulchanova, L., and Kaplan, D.H.: Nociceptive sensory fibers drive interleukin-23 production from CD301b⁺ dermal dendritic cells and drive protective cutaneous immunity. *Immunity* 2015, 43:515–526.

Maruyama, K., Takayama, Y., Kondo, T., Ishibashi, K.I., Sahoo, B.R., Kanemaru, H., Kumagai, Y., Martino, M.M., Tanaka, H., Ohno, N., *et al.*: Nociceptors boost the resolution of fungal osteoinflammation via the TRP channel-CGRP-Jdp2 axis. *Cell Rep.* 2017, 19:2730–2742.

Maruyama, K., Takayama, Y., Sugisawa, E., Yamanoi, Y., Yokawa, T., Kondo, T., Ishibashi, K.I., Sahoo, B.R., Takemura, N., Mori, Y., *et al.*: The ATP transporter VNUT mediates induction of Dectin-1-triggered *Candida* nociception. *iScience* 2018, 6:306–318.

Riol-Blanco, L., Ordovas-Montanes, J., Perro, M., Naval, E., Thiriot, A., Alvarez, D., Paust, S., Wood, J.N., and von Andrian, U.H.: Nociceptive sensory neurons drive interleukin-23-mediated psoriasiform skin inflammation. *Nature* 2014, 510:157–161.

Failures of Host Defense Mechanisms

13

In the normal course of an infection, the infectious agent first triggers an innate immune response. The foreign antigens of the infectious agent, enhanced by signals from innate immune cells, then induce an adaptive immune response that ultimately clears the infection and establishes a state of protective immunity. This does not always happen, however. In this chapter we examine circumstances in which there are failures of host defense, whether due to immune defects in an abnormal host, as occurs in immunodeficiency, or to the evasion or subversion of immune defenses in normal hosts by pathogens. Finally, we will consider the special case in which the immune defenses of a normal host are impaired by one infectious agent that leads to more generalized susceptibility to infection, as occurs in the acquired immune deficiency syndrome (AIDS) caused by the human immunodeficiency virus (HIV).

In the first part of the chapter, we examine **primary (or inherited) immunodeficiency**, in which host defense fails because of an inherited defect in a gene (or genes) that results in the elimination or impaired function of one or more components of the immune system, leading to heightened susceptibility to infection with particular classes of pathogens. Immunodeficiency diseases caused by defects in T- or B-lymphocyte development, phagocyte function, and complement components have all been discovered. In the second part of the chapter, we briefly consider mechanisms by which pathogens evade or subvert specific components of the immune response to avoid elimination, so-called **immune evasion**. In the last part of the chapter, we consider how infection by HIV subverts the immune system and can lead to AIDS, an example of **secondary (or acquired) immunodeficiency**. The study of circumstances and mechanisms by which the immune system can fail has already contributed greatly to our understanding of host defense mechanisms and is providing insight into new methods of controlling or preventing infectious diseases, including AIDS.

IN THIS CHAPTER

Immunodeficiency diseases.

Evasion and subversion of immune defenses.

Acquired immune deficiency syndrome.

Immunodeficiency diseases.

Immunodeficiencies occur when one or more components of the immune system are impaired; immunodeficiencies are classified as primary (inherited, or congenital) or secondary (acquired). Primary immunodeficiencies (PIDs), or inborn errors of immunity, are caused by the inheritance of damaging variants in any of a large number of genes that are involved in or control immune responses. They affect the development of immune cells, their function, or both. Clinical features of these disorders are highly variable, although a common feature is recurrent and often overwhelming infections in very young children. As will be discussed, many of the infectious agents that come to clinical attention in these individuals do not typically cause disease in those with a normal immune system and are referred to as **opportunistic pathogens**, while other infectious agents also cause disease in normal individuals but occur more frequently and with greater severity in those with impaired immunity.

Secondary immunodeficiencies are not inherited, rather they are acquired as a consequence of other diseases—including infectious diseases themselves, medical interventions that impair the immune response, or environmental factors such as nutritional deficiency. They are far more common than primary immunodeficiencies. Some forms of immunodeficiency principally affect immune regulatory pathways. Defects of this type can lead to allergy, abnormal proliferation of lymphocytes, autoimmunity, and certain types of cancer, and will be discussed in other chapters. Here, we will mainly focus on those immunodeficiencies that predispose to infection.

Primary immunodeficiencies can be classified on the basis of the components of the immune system involved. However, because of the integration of many aspects of immune defense, defects in one component of the immune system can affect the function of others. Therefore, primary defects in innate immunity can lead to defects in adaptive immunity, and vice versa. Nevertheless, it is instructive to consider immune defects in the context of the major types of immunity affected, as these can lead to distinct patterns of infection and clinical disease. By examining which infectious diseases accompany a particular immunodeficiency, we gain insights into components of the immune system that are important in the response to particular agents. The inherited immunodeficiencies also reveal how interactions between different immune cell types contribute to the immune response and to the development of T and B lymphocytes. Finally, these inherited diseases can lead us to the defective gene, often revealing new information about the molecular basis of immune processes and providing the necessary information for diagnosis, genetic counseling, and also the possibility of gene therapy for cure.

13-1 Primary immunodeficiency diseases are caused by inherited gene variants that typically cause recurrent infections early in life.

Before the advent of antibiotics, most individuals with inherited immune defects died in infancy or early childhood because of their susceptibility to particular classes of pathogens. Such cases were not easily identified because many normal infants also died of infection. In the modern era, individuals with immune deficiency first come to clinical attention through a history of recurrent infection, often by the same or similar pathogens. The type of infection hints at which part of the immune system is deficient—and often highlights the interlinked functions of different components of the innate and adaptive immune systems. Recurrent infection by **pyogenic, or pus-forming, bacteria** suggests a defect in antibody, complement, or phagocyte function. This reflects the fact that the normal pathway of host defense against such bacteria is the binding of antibody followed by the fixation of complement, which allows the opsonized bacteria to be taken up by phagocytic cells and killed. Breaking any of the links in this chain of events can cause a similar immunodeficient state. Alternatively, a history of persistent fungal skin infection, such as cutaneous candidiasis, or recurrent viral infections suggests a defect in host defense mediated by specific functions of T lymphocytes, whereas global T-cell dysfunction impairs both B-cell responses and aspects of innate immunity, giving rise to broad defects in host defense.

Since the beginning of the 21st century, the identification of new primary immunodeficiencies (PIDs) has accelerated, reflecting the relative ease in identifying dysfunctional gene variants since completion of the first draft of the human genome in 2001 and the increasing affordability of human genome sequencing, as well as new information on the function of immune genes that has been developed from mouse studies. More than 350 primary immunodeficiencies have now been described, involving almost 2% of the ~20,000 genes encoded in the human genome. These disorders are typically **monogenic disorders**—the result of a single damaging gene variant—and can be autosomal recessive, autosomal dominant, or X-linked. Disease caused by decreased expression or function of a gene product, whether resulting in complete (**amorphic**) or partial (**hypomorphic**) loss-of-function (LOF) variants, are far more common than diseases caused by gain-of-function (GOF, or **hypermorphic**) variants. And most PIDs are the result of recessive gene variants, whether caused by mutations in genes on autosomes or the X chromosome. As males have only one X chromosome, all males who inherit an X chromosome carrying an affected gene will have disease. In contrast, female carriers with only one affected X chromosome are typically healthy.

Gene targeting in mice (see Appendix I, Section A-36) has created many immunodeficient states that continue to add to our knowledge of the contribution of individual gene products to normal immune function. Nevertheless, human immunodeficiency diseases remain the best source of insight into the normal pathways of defense against infectious diseases and immune regulation. Immunodeficiencies also teach us about the redundancy of defense mechanisms against infectious disease. By chance, the first person to be reported with a hereditary deficiency of complement (C2 deficiency) was an immunologist who showed no evidence of immune compromise. This teaches us that there are multiple protective immune mechanisms against infection, such that a defect in one component of immunity might be compensated for by other components. Thus, although there is abundant evidence that complement deficiency increases susceptibility to pyogenic infection, not every human with complement deficiency suffers from recurrent infections.

Nine general categories of PIDs are now recognized (**Fig. 13.1**) and are grouped on the basis of the major immune cell type or pathway affected. None is very common (IgA deficiency, the most common, affects ~1 in 500 Caucasians), and some are extremely rare (single cases or family identified). Examples of these diseases are described in subsequent sections on the basis of the causal defects and their impact on innate and adaptive immunity.

13-2 Defects in T-cell development can result in severe combined immune deficiencies.

The pathways leading to the development of circulating naive T cells and B cells are summarized in **Fig. 13.2**. Individuals with defects in T-cell development are highly susceptible to a broad range of infectious agents, demonstrating the central role of T-cell differentiation and maturation in adaptive immune

Major category	Example	Gene defect	Inheritance	Cells affected	Immune defect	Antibody levels	Common infections/ other features
Combined immunodeficiencies (CIDs) limited to the immune system	γc deficiency	IL2RG	XL	T cells, NK cells	Deficient T-cell and NK-cell development	Low	General susceptibility to opportunistic and standard pathogens
	RAG-1 or RAG-2 deficiency	RAG1; RAG2	AR	T cells, B cells	Deficient T- and B-cell development	Low	General susceptibility to opportunistic and standard pathogens
CIDs with defects in tissues outside the immune system	FOXN1 deficiency; Nude phenotype	FOXN1	AR	Thymic epithelium, T cells	Deficient T-cell development	Decreased	General susceptibility to opportunistic and standard pathogens
	Job syndrome	STAT3	AD	T$_H$17 and T$_{FH}$ cells	Defective T$_H$17 and T$_{FH}$ cell development	High IgE	Extracellular bacteria, mucocutaneous candidiasis, bone development abnormalities
Antibody deficiencies	Bruton's X-linked agammaglobulinemia (XLA)	BTK	XL	B cells	Absent mature B cells	Low	Pyogenic bacteria and enteroviruses
	AID deficiency	AICDA	AR	B cells	Defective Ig class-switching and somatic hypermutation	IgG and IgA low; IgM increased	Bacterial infections, enlarged germinal centers
	Selective IgA deficiency	Unknown	?	B cells	Deficient clas-switched IgA B cells	Low–absent IgA; other isotypes	Typically asymptomatic
Immune dysregulation	Perforin deficiency	PRF1	AR	CTLs and NK cells	Impaired CTL and NK-cell cytotoxicity	Normal	Fever, hepatosplenomegaly
	IL-10 deficiency	IL10	AR	Multiple	No IL-10	Normal	Inflammatory bowel disease (IBD)
Phagocyte defects	Elastase deficiency	SCN1	AD	Neutrophils	Neutrophil deficiency	Normal	Severe bacterial infections; myelodysplasia/leukemia
	GATA2 deficiency	GATA2	AD	Monocytes and DCs	Monocyte and DC deficiency	Normal	Susceptibility to mycobacteria, HPV, histoplasmosis; myelodysplasia/leukemia
Innate immunity defects	IL-12p40 deficiency	IL12B	AR	DCs, monocytes, and macrophages	IFN-γ secretion	Normal	Mycobacterial and *Salmonella* infections
	IFN-γ receptor 1 deficiency	IFNGR1	AR/AD	Multiple	IFN-γ signaling	Normal	Mycobacterial and *Salmonella* infections
Autoinflammatory disorders	Muckle–Wells syndrome	NLRP3	AD (GOF)	Neutrophils and monocytes	Inflammasome hyperactivity	Normal	Recurrent fever, urticaria
Complement deficiencies	C1q deficiency	C1QA	AR	Apoptotic cells	Deficient activation of classical complement pathway	Normal	Infections by encapsulated bacteria (e.g., *Streptococcus pneumoniae, Klebsiella pneumoniae*), immune- complex disease (e.g., SLE)
	MASP deficiency	MASP2	AR	None	Deficient activation of lectin complement pathway	Normal	Pyogenic bacteria, autoimmunity
Phenocopies of inborn errors of immunity	APECED syndrome	AIRE	AR	T cells	Impaired negative selection of T cells	Normal, with autoantibodies	Chronic mucocutaneous candidiasis, multiple endocrinopathies

Fig. 13.1 Human immunodeficiency syndromes. Examples of categories, specific gene defects, inheritance patterns, consequences for the immune system, and resulting disease susceptibilities are listed for some common and some rare human immunodeficiency syndromes. Severe combined immune deficiency (SCID) can be due to many different defects, as summarized in Fig. 13.2 and described in the text. AD, autosomal dominant; APECED, autoimmune polyendocrinopathy–candidiasis–ectodermal dystrophy; AR, autosomal recessive; GOF, gain-of-function; XL, X-linked.

responses to virtually all microbes. Because such individuals make neither T cell–dependent antibody responses nor cell-mediated immune responses, and thus cannot develop immunological memory, they are said to suffer from **severe combined immune deficiency (SCID).**

X-linked SCID (XSCID) is the most frequent form of SCID and is caused by mutations in the gene *IL2RG* on the X chromosome, which encodes the

X-linked Severe Combined Immunodeficiency

Fig. 13.2 Defects in T-cell and B-cell development that cause immunodeficiency. The pathways leading to development of circulating naive T cells and B cells are shown. Mutations in genes that cause human immunodeficiency diseases are indicated in red boxes. These include mutations in genes that encode T cell–intrinsic or B cell–intrinsic proteins (for example, γ_c, CD3λ, BTK), as well as mutations in genes that encode proteins expressed on the thymic epithelium (for example, TAP-1 or CIITA), defects that impair thymic development and thus T-cell development. BCR, B-cell receptor; CLP, common lymphoid progenitor; HSC, hematopoietic stem cell; MZ B cell, marginal zone B cell; pre-BCR, pre-B-cell receptor; pre-TCR, pre-T-cell receptor; RS-SCID, radiation-sensitive SCID; SCID, severe combined immune deficiency; TCR, T-cell receptor; XSCID, X-linked SCID.

interleukin-2 receptor (IL-2R) common gamma chain (γ_c). γ_c is required in all receptors of the IL-2 cytokine family (IL-2, IL-4, IL-7, IL-9, IL-15, and IL-21). Individuals with XSCID thus have defects in signaling of all IL-2-family cytokines and, owing to the defects in IL-7 and IL-15, T cells and NK cells fail to develop normally (see Fig. 13.2). B-cell numbers, on the other hand, are normal, but due to the absence of T-cell help, their function is not. Individuals with XSCID are overwhelmingly male; in females who are carriers of the mutation, T-cell and NK-cell progenitors in which X-inactivation has preserved the wild-type *IL2RG* allele progress through development to establish a normal mature immune repertoire. XSCID is known as the 'bubble boy disease' after David

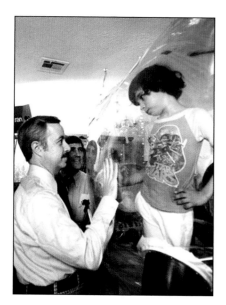

Fig. 13.3 The boy in the bubble. David Vetter was a well-known patient with X-linked SCID who raised public awareness of immunodeficiency diseases. He spent nearly the entirety of his life in specially fabricated plastic barriers to protect him from the threat of pathogens, giving rise to the moniker 'the boy in the bubble.' This photo, taken at his family's home, shows David, age 7, at his first introduction to Dr. William Shearer, a pediatric immunologist who would be a principal in David's care for the remainder of his life. In the background is Dr. Buford Nichols, another member of David's medical team. David succumbed at age 12 to complications of a bone marrow transplant. Photo courtesy of David's mother, Carol Ann Demaret.

Vetter (**Fig. 13.3**), a boy who lived for more than a decade in a protective, **gnotobiotic** ('known organisms') environment that excluded outside microbes. He died from complications of lymphoproliferative disease caused by the causative agent of infectious mononucleosis—Epstein–Barr virus—soon after a bone marrow transplant was performed to reconstitute his immune system. A clinically and immunologically indistinguishable type of SCID is associated with an inactivating mutation in the kinase Jak3 (see Sections 8-1 and 8-14), which physically associates with γ_c and transduces signaling through γ_c-chain cytokine receptors. This autosomal recessive mutation also impairs the development of T and NK cells, but the development of B cells is unaffected.

Other immunodeficiencies in mice have pinpointed more precisely the roles of individual cytokines and their receptors in T-cell and NK-cell development. For example, mice with targeted mutations in the β_c gene (*IL2RB*) defined a key role for IL-15 as a growth factor for the development of NK cells, as well as a role for this cytokine in T-cell maturation and trafficking. Mice with targeted mutations in IL-15 itself or the α chain of its receptor also have no NK cells and relatively normal T-cell development, but they show a more specific T-cell defect, primarily limited to impaired maintenance of memory CD8 T cells. This is in contrast to deficiencies of MCM4 or GINS1 in humans, which result in a selective deficiency of NK cells.

Although gene variants in *IL2RA* that result in deficiency of the third component of the IL-2 receptor [IL-2Rα (CD25)] impair the development and function of effector T cells (see Section 9-10) and result in immune deficiency and increased infections, these aspects are overshadowed by multi-organ autoimmune disease. The latter is due to defective development and function of regulatory T (T_{reg}) cells, which constitutively express IL-2Rα and require ongoing IL-2 signaling (see Section 15-15).

Humans with a deficiency of the IL-7 receptor α chain (IL-7Rα) have no T cells but normal levels of NK cells, illustrating that IL-7 signaling, while essential for T-cell development, is not essential for the development of NK cells (see Fig. 13.2). Notably, mice with a gene-targeted deficiency of the IL-7 receptor share with humans a deficiency of T cells, but also lack B cells, which is not the case in humans. This illustrates the species-specific role of certain cytokines and provides a cautionary note against extrapolating findings from mice to humans. In humans and mice whose T cells show defective production of IL-2 after receptor stimulation, most T-cell development itself is normal, although there is impaired development of FoxP3$^+$ T_{reg} cells, which predisposes to immune regulatory abnormalities and autoimmunity (see Chapter 15). The more limited effects of individual cytokine signaling defects are in contrast to the global defects in T- and NK-cell development in individuals with XSCID.

As in all serious T-cell deficiencies, individuals with XSCID do not make effective antibody responses to most antigens, although their B cells seem normal. Most, but not all, naive IgM-positive B cells from female carriers of XSCID have inactivated the defective X chromosome rather than the normal one, showing that B-cell development is affected by, but is not wholly dependent on, the γ_c chain. Mature memory B cells that have undergone class switching have inactivated the defective X chromosome almost without exception. This might reflect the fact that the γ_c chain is also part of the receptor for IL-21, signaling through which is important for the maturation of class-switched B cells (see Section 10-1).

13-3 SCID can also be due to defects in the purine salvage pathway.

Variants of autosomal recessive SCID that arise from defects in enzymes of the salvage pathway of purine synthesis include **adenosine deaminase (ADA) deficiency** and **purine nucleotide phosphorylase (PNP) deficiency**

Adenosine Deaminase Deficiency

(**Fig. 13.4**; and see Fig. 13.2). ADA catalyzes the conversion of adenosine and deoxyadenosine to inosine and deoxyinosine, respectively, and its deficiency results in the accumulation of deoxyadenosine and its precursor, S-adenosylhomocysteine, which are toxic to developing T and B cells. PNP catalyzes the conversion of inosine and guanosine to hypoxanthine and guanine, respectively. PNP deficiency, which is a rarer form of SCID, also causes the accumulation of toxic precursors but affects developing T cells more severely than B cells. In both diseases, the development of **lymphopenia**, or decreased numbers of lymphocytes, is progressive after birth, resulting in profound lymphopenia within the first few years of life. Because both enzymes are housekeeping proteins expressed by many cell types, the immune deficiency associated with each of these inherited defects is part of a broader clinical syndrome.

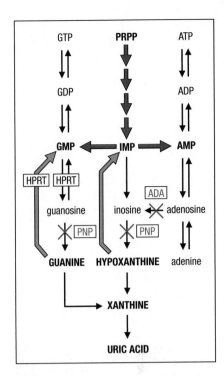

Fig. 13.4 Inherited defects in the purine salvage pathway cause SCID. Outline of purine *de novo* synthesis, salvage, and degradation. The principal precursors, intermediates, and products are boldface. Red arrows indicate synthesis, and blue arrows indicate salvage. Black arrows indicate the conversion of nucleotides to nucleosides and bases, and the conversion of nucleosides to nucleotides. More than 90% of purines are recovered from the salvage pathway rather than being generated from *de novo* synthesis. Inherited deficiencies of adenosine deaminase (ADA) or purine nucleotide phosphorylase (PNP) lead to severe combined immune deficiency (SCID) because of accumulation of purine salvage intermediates that are toxic to developing B and T cells. ADP, adenosine diphosphate; AMP, adenosine monophosphate, or adenylate; ATP, adenosine triphosphate; GDP, guanosine diphosphate; GMP, guanosine monophosphate, or guanylate; GTP, guanosine triphosphate; HPRT, hypoxanthine-guanine phosphoribosyl transferase; IMP, inosine monophosphate, or inosylate; PRPP, phosphoribosyl pyrophosphate.

13-4 Defects in antigen receptor gene rearrangement can result in SCID.

Another group of autosomally inherited defects leading to SCID is caused by failures of DNA rearrangement that prevent successful generation of T- and B-cell antigen receptors during lymphocyte development. Mutations in either the *RAG1* or *RAG2* gene that result in nonfunctional proteins cause arrest of lymphocyte development because of absence of positive selection at the pro- to pre-T cell and pro- to pre-B-cell transitions due to a failure of V(D)J recombination. This results in a complete lack of both T cells and B cells in affected individuals. Because the effects of RAG deficiencies are limited to lymphocytes that undergo antigen receptor gene rearrangement, NK-cell development is not impaired.

Some children with hypomorphic mutations in either *RAG1* or *RAG2* can make a small amount of functional RAG protein, allowing limited V(D)J recombination. This group includes individuals with a distinctive and severe disease called **Omenn syndrome**, which, in addition to increasing susceptibility to multiple opportunistic infections, has clinical features very similar to graft-versus-host disease (GVHD) wherein the individual's T cells mount a response against his or her own tissues. This is characterized clinically by rashes, eosinophilia, diarrhea, and enlargement of the lymph nodes (see Section 15-25). An explanation for this phenotype is that low levels of *RAG* activity result in limited T-cell receptor gene recombination. Interestingly, no B cells are found, suggesting that B cells have more stringent requirements for *RAG* activity. Because of the limited number of successfully rearranged T-cell receptors, the repertoire of T cells is highly restricted in individuals with Omenn syndrome, and there is activation and clonal expansion of the limited number of specificities present. The clinical features strongly suggest that these peripheral T cells are autoreactive and are responsible for the graft-versus-host phenotype.

A subset of individuals with autosomal recessive SCID are characterized by an abnormal sensitivity to ionizing radiation. They produce very few mature B and T cells because of the failure of DNA rearrangement in their developing lymphocytes; only rare VJ or VDJ joints are seen, and most of these are abnormal. This type of SCID is due to defects in ubiquitous DNA repair proteins involved in repairing DNA double-strand breaks, which are generated not only during antigen receptor gene rearrangement (see Section 5-4) but also by ionizing radiation. Owing to the increased radiosensitivity in these individuals, this class of SCID is called **radiation-sensitive SCID (RS-SCID)** to distinguish it from SCID due to lymphocyte-specific defects. Defects in the genes for Artemis, DNA protein kinase catalytic subunit (DNA-PKcs), or DNA ligase 4 cause RS-SCID (see Fig. 13.2). Because defects in repair of DNA breaks increase the risk of translocations during cell division that can lead to

Omenn Syndrome

malignant transformation, individuals with RS-SCID variants are also more likely to develop cancer.

13-5 Defects in signaling from T-cell antigen receptors can cause severe immunodeficiency.

Several gene defects have been described that interfere with signaling through the T-cell receptor (TCR) and thus block the activation of T cells early in thymic development (see Fig. 13.2). Individuals with mutations in the CD3δ, CD3ε, or CD3ζ chains of the CD3 complex have defective pre-TCR signaling and fail to progress to the double-positive stage of thymic development, resulting in SCID. Another lymphocyte signaling defect that leads to severe immunodeficiency is caused by mutations in the tyrosine phosphatase CD45. Humans and mice with CD45 deficiency show a marked reduction in peripheral T-cell numbers and also abnormal B-cell maturation. Severe immunodeficiency also occurs in individuals who make a defective form of the cytosolic protein tyrosine kinase ZAP-70, which transmits signals from the T-cell receptor (see Section 7-10). CD4 T cells emerge from the thymus in normal numbers, whereas CD8 T cells are absent. However, the CD4 T cells that mature fail to respond to antigenic stimuli.

Wiskott–Aldrich Syndrome

Wiskott–Aldrich syndrome (WAS), which is caused by a defect in the gene *WAS* on the X chromosome that encodes WAS protein (WASp), has shed new light on the molecular basis of signaling and immune synapse formation between various cells in the immune system. Although the disease affects platelets and was first described as a blood-clotting disorder, it also causes immunodeficiency that is characterized by reduced T-cell numbers, defective NK-cell cytotoxicity, and a failure of antibody responses (see Section 7-19). WASp is expressed in all hematopoietic cell lineages and is a key regulator of lymphocyte and platelet development and function through its transduction of receptor-mediated signals that induce reorganization of the cytoskeleton (see Section 9-18). Several signaling pathways downstream of the T-cell receptor are known to activate WASp (see Sections 7-19 and 9-18). Activation of WASp in turn activates the Arp2/3 complex, which is essential for initiating actin polymerization that is critical for immune synapse formation and the polarized release of effector molecules by T cells (see Sections 7-19 and 9-18). In individuals with WAS, and in mice whose *Was* gene has been knocked out, T cells fail to respond normally to T-cell receptor signaling. It has also recently been suggested that WASp is required for the suppressive function of natural T_{reg} (nT_{reg}) cells, and this may help explain why individuals with WASp are susceptible to autoimmune diseases.

13-6 Genetic defects in thymic development or function that block T-cell development result in combined immunodeficiencies.

A disorder of thymic development associated with SCID and a lack of body hair has been known for many years in mice; the mutant strain is descriptively named *nude* (see Section 8-11). A small number of children have been described with the same phenotype. In both mice and humans this syndrome is caused by mutations in the gene *FOXN1*, which encodes a transcription factor selectively expressed in skin and thymus. FOXN1 is necessary for the differentiation of thymic epithelium and the formation of a functional thymus. In individuals with a mutation in *FOXN1*, the lack of thymic function prevents normal T-cell development. B-cell development is normal in individuals with the mutation, yet B-cell responses are deficient because of the lack of T cells, and the response to nearly all pathogens is profoundly impaired.

DiGeorge Syndrome

DiGeorge syndrome is another disorder in which the thymic epithelium fails to develop normally, resulting in SCID. The genetic abnormality underlying this complex developmental disorder is a deletion within one copy of chromosome 22. The deletion varies between 1.5 and 5 megabases in size, with the smallest deletion that causes the syndrome containing approximately 24 genes. The relevant gene within this interval is *TBX1*, which encodes the transcription factor T-box 1. DiGeorge syndrome is caused by the deletion of a single copy of this gene, such that individuals with this disorder are **haploinsufficient** for *TBX1*. Without the proper inductive thymic environment, T cells cannot mature and, in individuals with this syndrome, both cell-mediated immunity and T cell–dependent antibody production are impaired.

Defects in the expression of MHC molecules can lead to severe immunodeficiency as a result of effects on the positive selection of T cells in the thymus (see Fig. 13.2). Individuals with **bare lymphocyte syndrome (BLS)** lack expression of either MHC class II or MHC class I molecules, so-called BLS II or BLS I, respectively. These are also referred to simply as **MHC class II deficiency** or **MHC class I deficiency**. In the case of MHC class II deficiency, the thymus lacks MHC class II molecules. Hence, CD4 T cells cannot be positively selected, and few develop. The antigen-presenting cells in these individuals also lack MHC class II molecules, and so the few CD4 T cells that do develop cannot be stimulated by antigen. MHC class I expression is normal, and CD8 T cells develop normally. However, such individuals suffer from severe immunodeficiency, illustrating the central importance of CD4 T cells in adaptive immunity to most pathogens.

MHC Class II Deficiency
MHC Class I Deficiency

MHC class II deficiency is caused not by mutations in the MHC genes themselves but by mutations in one of several genes encoding gene-regulatory proteins that are required for the transcriptional activation of MHC class II genes. Four complementing gene defects (known as groups A, B, C, and D) have been defined in individuals who fail to express MHC class II molecules, indicating that the products of at least four different genes are required for the normal expression of these proteins. Genes corresponding to each complementation group have been identified: the *MHC class II transactivator*, or *CIITA*, is mutated in group A, and the genes *RFXANK*, *RFX5*, and *RFXAP* are mutated in groups B, C, and D, respectively (see Fig. 13.2). These last three encode proteins that are components of a multimeric complex, RFX, which is involved in the control of gene transcription. RFX binds a DNA sequence called an X-box, which is present in the promoter region of all MHC class II genes.

A more limited immunodeficiency has been observed in a small number of individuals who have almost no cell-surface MHC class I molecules (i.e., MHC class I deficiency, or BLSI). In contrast to those with MHC class II deficiency, affected individuals have normal levels of mRNA encoding MHC class I molecules and normal production of MHC class I proteins, but very few of the proteins reach the cell surface. This condition is due either to mutations in *TAP1* or *TAP2*, which encode the subunits of the peptide transporter responsible for transporting peptides generated in the cytosol into the endoplasmic reticulum where they are loaded into nascent MHC class I molecules, or to mutations in *TAPBP*, which encodes tapasin, another component of the peptide transporter complex (see Section 6-4). Although the reduction in MHC class I molecules on the surface of thymic epithelial cells results in reduced numbers of CD8 T cells (see Fig. 13.2), people with MHC class I deficiency are not abnormally susceptible to viral infections. This is surprising given the key role of MHC class I presentation and of cytotoxic CD8 T cells in combating viral infections. There is, however, evidence for TAP-independent pathways for the presentation of certain peptides by MHC class I molecules, and the clinical phenotype of *TAP1*- and *TAP2*-deficient individuals indicates that these pathways may be sufficient to allow sufficient development and function of CD8 T cells to control viruses.

Autoimmune Polyendocrinopathy–Candidiasis–Ectodermal Dystrophy (APECED)

Some defects in thymic cells lead to a phenotype with other effects besides those of immunodeficiency. The gene *AIRE* encodes a transcription factor that enables thymic epithelial cells to express many self proteins that mediate efficient negative selection (see Section 8-25). Defects in *AIRE* lead to a T-cell repertoire that includes cells autoreactive to self antigens, causing a complex syndrome called **APECED (autoimmune polyendocrinopathy–candidiasis–ectodermal dystrophy)**, which is characterized by autoimmunity, developmental defects, and immunodeficiency (see Chapter 15). As will be discussed in Section 13-12, an important aspect of the immunodeficiency component of this syndrome results from the break in self-tolerance, which leads to blocking autoantibodies against key cytokines involved in host defense, including IFN-γ, IL-17, and IL-22.

13-7 Defects in B-cell development result in deficiencies in antibody production that cause an inability to clear extracellular bacteria.

In addition to inherited defects in proteins that are crucial to both T-cell and B-cell development, such as RAG-1 and RAG-2, defects that are specific to B-cell development have also been identified (see Fig. 13.2). Individuals with these defects are characterized by an inability to cope with extracellular bacteria and some viruses whose efficient clearance requires specific antibodies. Pyogenic bacteria, such as staphylococci and streptococci, have polysaccharide capsules that impair recognition by the receptors on macrophages and neutrophils that stimulate phagocytosis. These bacteria escape elimination by the innate immune response and are successful extracellular pathogens, but they can be cleared by an adaptive immune response. Opsonization by antibody and complement enables phagocytes to ingest and destroy the bacteria. The principal effect of deficiencies in antibody production is therefore a failure to control infections by pyogenic bacteria. Susceptibility to some viral infections, notably those caused by enteroviruses, is also increased because of the importance of antibodies in neutralizing viruses that enter the body through the gut.

X-linked Agammaglobulinemia

The first description of an immunodeficiency disease was Ogden C. Bruton's account, in 1952, of the failure of a male child to produce antibodies. Because inheritance of this condition is X-linked and is characterized by the complete absence of immunoglobulin in the serum (**agammaglobulinemia**), it was called **Bruton's X-linked agammaglobulinemia (XLA)** (see Fig. 13.2). Since then, autosomal recessive variants of agammaglobulinemia have been described. Infants with these diseases are usually identified as a result of recurrent infections with pyogenic bacteria, such as *Streptococcus pneumoniae*, and enteroviruses that typically occur after weaning in breast-fed infants, or much earlier in infants that are not breast-fed. In this regard, it should be noted that normal infants have a transient deficiency in immunoglobulin production in the first 3–12 months of life (**Fig. 13.5**). Nevertheless, antibody levels in the normal newborn infant are comparable to those of the mother at birth because of the transplacental transport of maternal IgG (see Section 10-17). Breast-fed infants also receive maternal antibodies from breast milk that are protective until their endogenous antibody production begins to be established. After the infant is weaned, maternal IgG is catabolized and gradually decreases until there is no longer a maternal contribution to the infant's circulating IgG. In infants who are not breast-fed, the delay in production of endogenous IgG results in low levels in circulation between the ages of 3 months and 1 year. This can lead to a period of heightened susceptibility to infection, especially in premature babies, who are often formula-fed and begin with lower levels of maternal IgG, and also reach immune competence later after birth. Because of the transient protection afforded newborn infants by maternal antibodies,

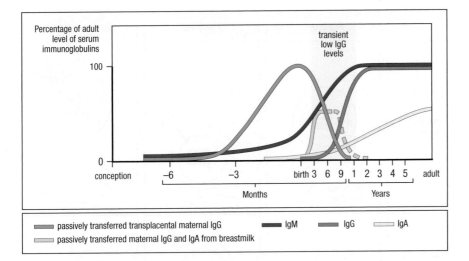

Percentage of adult
level of serum
immunoglobulins

transient
low IgG
levels

100

0

conception   −6   −3   birth 3 6 9   1 2 3 4 5   adult

Months   Years

▬▬ passively transferred transplacental maternal IgG   ▬▬ IgM   ▬▬ IgG   ▭ IgA
▬▬ passively transferred maternal IgG and IgA from breastmilk

Fig. 13.5 Immunoglobulin levels in newborn infants are primarily contributed by passive transfer from the mother. Babies are born with high levels of maternal IgG, which is transported across the placenta from the mother during gestation. After birth, the production of IgM by the newborn increases almost immediately; the production of IgG by the infant, however, does not begin for about 6 months, during which time the maternal IgG that had been transferred transplacentally falls and is supplemented by maternal IgG in breast milk that is taken up in the neonatal gut. Maternal IgA is also supplied in breast milk and contributes to immune protection and establishment of the intestinal microbiome in the newborn. In infants that are not breast-fed, IgG levels are low from about the age of 3 months to 1 year, which can lead to heightened susceptibility to disease.

XLA is typically detected several months after birth, contingent on whether they are breast-fed or not, and thus when maternal antibody levels in the infant have declined.

The defective gene in XLA encodes a protein tyrosine kinase called BTK (Bruton's tyrosine kinase), which is a member of the Tec family of kinases that transduce signals through the pre-B-cell receptor (pre-BCR; see Section 7-20). As discussed in Section 8-4, the pre-BCR is composed of successfully rearranged μ heavy chains complexed with the surrogate light chain (composed of λ5 and VpreB) and with the signal-transducing subunits Igα and Igβ. Stimulation of the pre-BCR recruits cytoplasmic proteins, including BTK, which convey signals required for the proliferation and differentiation of pre-B cells. In the absence of BTK function, B-cell maturation is largely arrested at the pre-B-cell stage (see Fig. 13.2; see also Section 8-4), resulting in profound B-cell deficiency and agammaglobulinemia. Some B cells do mature, however, perhaps as a result of compensation by other Tec kinases.

During embryonic development, females randomly inactivate one of their two X chromosomes. Because BTK is required for B-lymphocyte development, only cells in which the normal allele of *BTK* is active develop into mature B cells. Thus, in all B cells in female carriers of a mutant *BTK*, the active X chromosome is the normal one and the abnormal X chromosome is inactivated. This fact allowed female carriers of XLA to be identified even before the nature of the BTK protein was known. In contrast, the active X chromosomes in the T cells and macrophages of carriers are an equal mixture of normal and *BTK* mutant X chromosomes. Nonrandom X-inactivation only in B cells shows conclusively that the gene *BTK* is required for the development of B cells but not the other cell types, and that BTK must act in the B cells themselves rather than in stromal or other cells required for B-cell development (**Fig. 13.6**).

Autosomal recessive deficiencies in other components of the pre-BCR also block early B-cell development and cause severe B-cell deficiency and congenital agammaglobulinemia similar to that of XLA. These disorders are much rarer than XLA and result from mutations in the gene that encodes the heavy chain (*IGHM*), which is the second most common cause of agammaglobulinemia, or in the genes that encode λ5 (*IGLL1*), Igα (*CD79A*), or Igβ (*CD79B*). Mutations that cripple the B-cell receptor signaling adaptor, B-cell linker protein (encoded by *BLNK*), also cause the arrest of early B-cell development that results in B-cell deficiency.

Individuals with pure B-cell defects resist many pathogens other than pyogenic bacteria. Fortunately, the latter can be suppressed with antibiotics and with monthly infusions of human immunoglobulin collected from a large pool

Fig. 13.6 The product of the gene *BTK* is important for B-cell development. In X-linked agammaglobulinemia (XLA), a protein tyrosine kinase of the Tec family called BTK, which is encoded on the X chromosome, is defective. In normal individuals, B-cell development proceeds through a stage in which the pre-B-cell receptor, consisting of μλ5:VpreB (see Section 8-3), transduces a signal via BTK, triggering further B-cell development. In males with XLA, no signal can be transduced and, although the pre-B-cell receptor is expressed, the B cells develop no further. In female mammals, including humans, one of the two X chromosomes in each cell is permanently inactivated early in development. Because the choice of which chromosome to inactivate is random, half of the pre-B cells in a carrier female will have inactivated the chromosome with the wild-type *BTK,* meaning that they can express only the defective *BTK* and cannot develop further. Therefore, in the carrier, mature B cells always have the nondefective X chromosome active. This is in sharp contrast to all other cell types, which have the nondefective X chromosome active in only half of their cells. Nonrandom X-inactivation in a particular cell lineage is a clear indication that the product of the X-linked gene is required for the development of cells of that lineage. It is also sometimes possible to identify the stage at which the gene product is required, by detecting the point in development at which X-inactivation develops bias. Using this kind of analysis, one can identify carriers of X-linked traits such as XLA without needing to know the nature of the mutant gene.

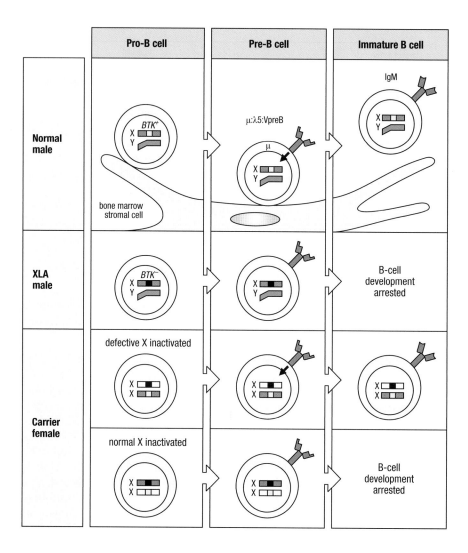

of donors. Because there are antibodies against many common pathogens in this pooled immunoglobulin, it serves as a fairly successful shield against infection.

13-8 Combined immunodeficiencies (CIDs) can be caused by defects in T-cell differentiation and function that impair activation of B cells, dendritic cells and macrophages, and innate effector cells.

After their development in the thymus or bone marrow, T and B cells require antigen-driven activation and differentiation to mount effective immune responses. Similar to defects in early T-cell development, defects in T-cell activation and differentiation that occur after thymic selection can have an impact on cell-mediated immunity, antibody responses, or both, the latter resulting in CID. In the case of B cells, cell-intrinsic defects in their activation and differentiation result in defects in antibody responses but have limited effects on cell-mediated immunity. A shared feature of PIDs that result from impaired T-dependent antibody responses, whether caused by defects in T-cell helper function or B cell–intrinsic defects, is a deficiency of class-switched antibody isotypes (that is, IgG, IgA, and IgE) that is typically accompanied by a compensatory increase in production of IgM antibodies, referred to as **hyper IgM syndrome**.

The most common cause of hyper IgM syndrome is **CD40 ligand deficiency**, or X-linked hyper IgM syndrome, which is a form of CID caused by mutations

 CD40 Ligand Deficiency

Fig. 13.7 Defects in T-cell and B-cell activation and differentiation cause immunodeficiencies. The pathways leading to activation and differentiation of naive T cells and B cells are shown. The protein products of genes known to be mutated in the relevant human immunodeficiency diseases are indicated in red boxes. BCR, B-cell receptor; CD40L, CD40 ligand; CID, combined immunodeficiency; CVIDs, common variable immunodeficiencies; TCR, T-cell receptor. Note that the defect in cytoskeletal function in Wiskott–Aldrich syndrome (WAS) affects immune-cell function at many steps in this schema and is not included in the figure for the sake of clarity.

in the gene encoding CD40 ligand, or CD154 (*CD40LG*) (**Fig. 13.7**). CD40 ligand is normally expressed on activated CD4 T cells, enabling them to deliver a key activating signal to classical antigen-presenting cells—B cells, dendritic cells, and macrophages—via engagement of CD40 (see Section 10-4). In individuals with damaging variants of *CD40LG*, T$_{FH}$ cells fail to activate naive B cells to undergo differentiation into germinal center B cells, resulting in failed heavy-chain class switching, somatic hypermutation, and germinal center formation (**Fig. 13.8**). This results in severe reductions in circulating levels of all antibody isotypes except IgM, causing heightened susceptibility to infections that require high-affinity, class-switched antibodies for their clearance.

Because CD40 signaling is also required for the complete activation of dendritic cells and macrophages, including the heightened production of IL-12, which is important for the production of IFN-γ by T$_H$1 cells and NK cells (see Sections 11-3 and 11-6), individuals with CD40 ligand deficiency also have defects in type 1 immunity and thus manifest a form of CID, as well as hyper IgM syndrome. Inadequate cross-talk between T cells and dendritic cells via CD40L–CD40 interaction can lead to lower levels of co-stimulatory molecules on dendritic cells, thus impairing their ability to stimulate naive T cells (see Sections 9-11 and 9-13). Thus, in addition to their susceptibility to infection by extracellular pathogens that require class-switched antibodies, such as pyogenic bacteria, the individuals also have defects in the clearance of intracellular pathogens, such as mycobacteria, and are particularly prone to opportunistic infections by *Pneumocystis jirovecii*, which is normally killed by activated macrophages. Not unexpectedly, a similar syndrome has been identified in individuals with damaging variants in the gene encoding CD40 (*CD40*), which has been found in rare cases with an autosomal recessive variant of CID and hyper IgM syndrome (see Fig. 13.7). Here, the defective expression of CD40 by B cells, dendritic cells, and macrophages causes their inability to be activated by CD40 ligand, resulting in disease that closely phenocopies CD40 ligand deficiency.

Another CID is characterized by elevations in IgE, referred to as **hyper IgE syndrome (HIES)**, or **Job syndrome**. The most common example is **STAT3 deficiency**, which is characterized by recurrent skin and pulmonary infections caused by pyogenic bacteria, chronic mucocutaneous candidiasis

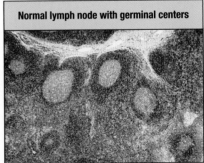

Fig. 13.8 Individuals with CD40 ligand deficiency are unable to activate B cells to form germinal centers. Lymphoid tissues in individuals with CD40 ligand deficiency, which manifests as a deficiency of high-affinity, class-switched antibody isotypes and hyper IgM syndrome, are devoid of germinal centers (top panel), unlike a normal lymph node (bottom panel). B-cell activation by T cells is required both for isotype switching and for the formation of germinal centers, where extensive B-cell proliferation takes place.

(noninvasive fungal infection of the skin and mucosal surfaces), very high serum concentrations of IgE, chronic eczematous dermatitis or skin rash, and skeletal and dental abnormalities. The inherited defect is an autosomal dominant loss-of-function variant of STAT3, which is activated downstream of several cytokine receptors, including those for IL-6, IL-21, IL-22, and IL-23, and is central to the differentiation and/or function of T_{FH} cells, T_H17 cells, and ILC3 cells, as well as B cells. Because T_{FH} cells are deficient in these individuals, T-cell help for B cells is compromised, resulting in poor production of most class-switched antibodies. The exception is IgE, which is abnormally elevated, hence the designation of this disease as an HIES variant of CID. The cause of the elevated IgE is not understood, and it is unclear why these individuals fail to have heightened allergic responses despite the elevated IgE. Because of the defect in development of T_H17 cells and ILC3 function, recruitment of neutrophils normally orchestrated by IL-17 is defective, as is production of IL-22, the receptor for which normally activates STAT3 signaling in epithelial cells of the skin and mucosal barriers to enhance antimicrobial resistance (see Sections 11-3 and 12-20). This is thought to underlie the impaired defense against extracellular bacteria and fungi at barrier epithelia.

13-9 B cell–specific activation defects cause hyper IgM syndromes that are limited to defects in the antibody response.

Some variants of hyper IgM syndrome are due to intrinsic defects in the process of B-cell activation that impair normal development of the germinal center response, resulting in defective class switch recombination and/or somatic hypermutation. Individuals with these variants are susceptible to severe extracellular bacterial infections, but because T-cell differentiation and function are spared, they have no increased susceptibility to intracellular pathogens or opportunistic agents, such as *P. jirovecii,* and thus do not have CID. One such variant is due to loss-of-function mutations in activation-induced cytidine deaminase (AID), which is required for both isotype class switching and somatic hypermutation in B cells (see Fig. 13.7 and Section 10-7). In individuals with autosomally inherited defects in the gene that encodes AID (*AICDA*), hyper IgM syndrome is accompanied by the accumulation of defective germinal center B cells in abnormal germinal centers, causing enlargement of the lymph nodes and spleen. Other variants of B cell–intrinsic hyper IgM syndrome have been identified in individuals with autosomal recessive defects in genes that encode factors involved in class switch recombination in B cells, including the DNA repair enzyme uracil-DNA glycosylase (UNG; see Section 10-10) and the chromatin remodeling complex INO80; these individuals have normal AID function and normal somatic hypermutation, but defective class switching.

13-10 Common variable immunodeficiency results from a variety of inherited defects that cause more limited defects in the antibody response.

Other examples of predominantly antibody deficiency include the most common forms of PID, referred to as **common variable immunodeficiencies (CVIDs)**. CVIDs are a clinically and genetically heterogeneous group of disorders that often go undiagnosed until late childhood or adulthood because the immune deficiency is relatively mild. Thus, CVIDs are sometimes referred to as late-onset hypogammaglobulinemias. Unlike other types of immunoglobulin deficiency, CVID is characterized by variable deficiencies in two or more antibody isotypes. Although the genetic basis for CVID is unknown in the large majority of cases, in the minority in which the affected gene has been identified, most result from B cell–intrinsic defects.

Defects in genes encoding receptors for the B-cell maturation and survival factors BAFF and APRIL, BAFF-R (*TNFRSF13C*) and TACI (*TNFRSF13B*), are among the identified gene variants known to cause B cell–intrinsic abnormalities that result in CVID (see Fig. 13.7 and Section 10-3). Individuals with these variants typically have decreased circulating IgG and IgA, with or without decreased IgM, but they have quite variable clinical presentations. Although some of these individuals have recurrent bacterial infections, many are asymptomatic. Other individuals with inherited B cell–intrinsic defects that result in CVID have damaging variants of the genes encoding CD19, CD21, and CD81, which are components of the B-cell co-receptor (see Section 7-20 and Fig. 13.7).

13-11 Unidentified genetic defects cause isotype-specific antibody deficiencies.

Selective **IgA deficiency**, the most common PID, exists in both sporadic and familial forms, and both autosomal recessive and autosomal dominant inheritance have been described. The etiology of IgA deficiency in most individuals is not understood, and many of these individuals are asymptomatic. In IgA-deficient individuals who do develop recurrent infections, an associated defect in one of the IgG subclasses (typically IgG2 and/or IgG4) is often found. Because secretory IgA is thought to play a role in homeostatic regulation of the microbiota in mucosal tissues (for example, the intestinal tract), there is an increased incidence of microbiota-associated immune-mediated disease in these individuals (for example, inflammatory bowel disease).

Similarly to individuals with selective IgA deficiency, individuals with selective **IgM deficiency** have normal levels of the other immunoglobulin isotypes and lack a defined genetic basis for their PID. In contrast to IgA deficiency, however, selective IgM deficiency is rare, and these individuals tend to have recurrent bacterial infections in infancy that are often severe, particularly those caused by encapsulated organisms, such as *Pneumococcus* species.

13-12 Normal pathways for host defense against different infectious agents are pinpointed by genetic deficiencies of cytokine pathways central to type 1/T$_H$1 and type 3/T$_H$17 responses.

Inherited defects in cytokines that are involved in the development and function of different effector T-cell subsets have been defined, as have defects in the receptors or the signaling pathways through which they act. In contrast to the T-cell immunodeficiencies considered earlier, here we consider deficiencies that do not have major defects in antibody production. A small number of families have been discovered that have individuals who suffer from persistent and sometimes fatal attacks by intracellular pathogens normally restrained by type 1 immunity, especially *Mycobacterium*, *Salmonella*, and *Listeria* species. These microbes are specialized for survival within macrophages, and their eradication requires enhanced microbicidal activities induced by IFN-γ produced by type 1 cells: NK cells, ILC1 cells, and T$_H$1 cells (see Section 11-2). Accordingly, susceptibility to these infections is conferred by a variety of inherited mutations that impair or abolish the function of IL-12 or IFN-γ, key cytokines in the development and functions of type 1 cells (**Fig. 13.9**). Individuals with mutations in the genes encoding the p40 subunit of IL-12 (*IL12B*), the IL-12 receptor β$_1$ chain (*IL12RB1*), and the two subunits (R1 and R2) of the IFN-γ receptor (*IFNGR1* and *IFNGR2*) have been identified. Although affected individuals have heightened susceptibility to the more virulent *Mycobacterium tuberculosis*, they suffer more frequently from the

Interferon-γ
Receptor Deficiency

Fig. 13.9 Inherited defects in effector cytokine pathways that impair type 1/T$_H$1 and type 3/T$_H$17 immunity. Shown are pathways in IL-12, IL-23, and IFN-γ signaling for which inherited defects have been described. Note that defects in IL-12p40 (p40) and IL-12Rβ1 result in impaired function of both ILC1 cells/NK cells/T$_H$1 cells and ILC3 cells/T$_H$17 cells because these subunits are shared, respectively, by IL-12 and IL-23, and their receptors. Also, because STAT1 is activated by the receptors of type II interferon (IFN-γ) and type I interferons (IFN-α and IFN-β, not shown), defects in STAT1 result in impaired antibacterial and antiviral immune defense, whereas deficiency in either of the IFN-γ receptor subunits (IFN-γR1 or IFN-γR2) primarily results in impaired defense against intracellular bacteria.

Fig. 13.10 Immune deficiencies with defects in T$_H$17/ILC3 function. Nearly all T$_H$17/ILC3 immune deficiencies result in chronic mucocutaneous candidiasis (CMC). *Deficiencies of IL-12p40 and IL-12Rβ1 also result in T$_H$1/ILC1/NK cell deficits. †It is currently unclear whether STAT1 gain-of-function mutations cause ILC3 deficits in addition to reduced numbers of T$_H$17 cells.

non-tuberculous, or atypical, opportunistic strains of mycobacteria, such as *Mycobacterium avium*, likely due to the greater prevalence of atypical strains in the environment. They may also develop disseminated infection after vaccination with *Mycobacterium bovis* bacillus Calmette–Guérin (BCG), the strain of *M. bovis* that is used as a live vaccine against *M. tuberculosis*. Because the IL-12p40 subunit is shared by IL-12 and IL-23, IL-12p40 deficiency results in a broader infectious disease risk due to defective type 1 and type 3 (T$_H$17/ILC3) functions (**Fig. 13.10;** see also Fig. 13.9). Similarly, deficiency of IL-12Rβ1 chain, which is shared by the IL-12 and IL-23 receptors, results in broader susceptibilities than the deficiencies of IFN-γ or its receptor.

Disease	Mutated gene	Inheritance	Immune phenotype	Associated infections
STAT3 deficiency; hyper IgE syndrome (Job syndrome)	*STAT3*	Autosomal dominant	Deficit of IL-17–producing T$_H$17 and ILC3 cells; hyper IgE	CMC, *Staphylococcus aureus*, *Aspergillus*
IL-12p40 deficiency	*IL12B*	Autosomal recessive	Deficit of IL-17–producing T$_H$17 and ILC3 cells*	Intracellular and extracellular bacteria, CMC
IL-12Rβ deficiency	*IL12RB1*	Autosomal recessive	Deficit of IL-17–producing T$_H$17 and ILC3 cells*	Intracellular and extracellular bacteria, CMC
IL-17RA deficiency	*IL17RA*	Autosomal recessive	No IL-17 response	CMC, pyogenic bacteria
IL-17F deficiency (partial)	*IL17F*	Autosomal recessive	Impaired IL-17F function	CMC, pyogenic bacteria
CARD9 deficiency	*CARD9*	Autosomal recessive	Deficit of IL-17–producing T$_H$17 and ILC3 cells	CMC and severe *Candida/* dermatophyte infections
STAT1 gain-of-function (GOF) mutation	*STAT1*	Autosomal dominant	Deficit of IL-17–producing T$_H$17 and ILC3 cells†	CMC, pyogenic bacteria
APECED syndrome	*AIRE*	Autosomal recessive	Neutralizing antibodies: IL-17A, IL-17F +/– IL-22	CMC

Autosomal recessive loss-of-function mutations in *STAT1* impair IFN-γ receptor signaling and are also associated with increased susceptibility to infections by mycobacterial and other intracellular bacteria (see Fig. 13.9). However, because of the shared function of STAT1 in IFN-α receptor signaling in response to IFN-α and IFN-β (type I interferons), individuals with STAT1 defects are also susceptible to viral infections. Notably, individuals with partial loss of function of STAT1 have been identified who are susceptible to mycobacterial infections, but not viral infections, suggesting a more stringent requirement of STAT1 in protection against the former.

In addition to the T_H17-related defects described earlier for STAT3-deficient HIES (see Section 13-8), other defects in cytokine-mediated functions of this pathway have been identified that lack the hyper IgE component. Whereas heightened susceptibility to intracellular bacteria is a feature common to immunodeficiencies that impair type 1 immunity, heightened susceptibility to infections by fungi (e.g., *Candida albicans*) and pyogenic bacteria (e.g., *Staphylococcus aureus*) are characteristics of these type 3 deficiencies. This reflects the specialized function of T_H17 cells and ILC3 cells in barrier defense against fungi and extracellular bacteria. Inherited deficiencies in IL-17RA, the shared receptor component for homodimeric and heterodimeric IL-17F–IL-17A ligands, as well as deficiency of IL-17F itself, confer susceptibility to these infectious agents and thus identify a key role for IL-17 cytokines in host defense against them. A similar susceptibility to chronic mucocutaneous candidiasis and pyogenic bacteria has been found in individuals with autosomal dominant, gain-of-function mutations in *STAT1*. Because T_H17 cell development is impaired by STAT1 signaling downstream of several cytokine receptors (for example, type I and type II IFN receptors), individuals with these mutations have impaired type 3 defenses because of heightened STAT1 activity. Note that this is in contrast to individuals with loss-of-function *STAT1* mutations, who are predisposed to intracellular bacterial infections because of defective type 1 immunity.

In addition to inherited defects in effector cytokine genes, some forms of immunodeficiency result in the production of neutralizing autoantibodies against these cytokines. This results in infectious risks similar to those caused by primary cytokine deficiencies. Most individuals with APECED syndrome (caused by defects in *AIRE*; see Section 13-6) develop chronic mucocutaneous candidiasis that is due to the development of autoantibodies against IL-17A, IL-17F, and/or IL-22. Individuals with neutralizing autoantibodies against IFN-γ who have impaired protection against atypical mycobacteria have also been reported, consistent with impaired type 1 responses in these individuals.

13-13 Inherited defects in the cytolytic pathway of lymphocytes can cause uncontrolled lymphoproliferation and inflammatory responses to viral infections.

Cytotoxic granules are formed from components of late endosomes and lysosomes. Once formed, there are multiple steps in the exocytosis of cytotoxic granules from cytotoxic cells and their delivery to target cells. The importance of the cytolytic pathway in immune regulation is highlighted by inherited defects that impair key steps in either the formation or exocytosis of cytotoxic granules (**Fig. 13.11**). These result in a severe and often fatal condition, known as **hemophagocytic lymphohistiocytic (HLH) syndrome**, which manifests as uncontrolled activation and expansion of CD8 T lymphocytes and macrophages that infiltrate multiple organs, causing tissue necrosis and organ failure. The hyperactive immune response is thought to reflect the inability of cytotoxic cells to destroy infected targets, and possibly themselves, after an initiating viral infection, particularly by a herpes family virus such as Epstein–Barr virus (EBV). In this regard it is notable that despite the impaired release

Hemophagocytic Lymphohistiocytic Syndrome

Fig. 13.11 Defects in components involved in the exocytosis of cytotoxic granules cause familial hemophagocytic lymphohistiocytosis (FHL) syndromes. After antigen recognition, there is polarization of perforin-containing cytotoxic granules of the cytotoxic T lymphocyte (CTL) toward the target cell at the site of immunological synapse formation. Cytotoxic granules are transported along microtubules to the plasma membrane, where they dock through a Rab27a-dependent interaction. Docked vesicles are primed by Munc13-4–mediated triggering of a conformational change in syntaxin 11, which is part of a large SNARE (soluble *N*-ethylmaleimide–sensitive factor accessory protein receptor) complex connecting the docked vesicle with the plasma membrane. Through the actions of Munc18-2, a fusion reaction is initiated via the syntaxin 11–containing SNARE complex that releases the contents of the cytotoxic granules into the synapse-bounded intercellular space, allowing perforin-mediated pore formation in the target-cell plasma membrane. The sites in the exocytic pathway that are affected by inherited defects in each of the proteins highlighted in red are indicated, as are the associated familial hemophagocytic lymphohistiocytosis syndromes.

Chediak–Higashi
Syndrome

of cytotoxic granules, the release of IFN-γ by cytotoxic T lymphocytes (CTLs) and NK cells of individuals with this disorder is not typically impaired, which contributes to the heightened activity of macrophages and the associated inflammatory disorder caused by an increased release of pro-inflammatory cytokines such TNF, IL-6, and macrophage colony-stimulating factor (M-CSF). The activated macrophages phagocytose blood cells, including erythrocytes and leukocytes, which gives the syndrome its name.

There are multiple autosomal recessive variants of HLH, also referred to as **familial hemophagocytic lymphohistiocytosis (FHL)**, that are distinguished by the protein in the cytolytic pathway that is affected (see Fig. 13.11). Examples include inherited deficiencies of the following: the cytotoxic granule protein perforin, which is required for pore formation in the target cell (and when defective is associated with the syndrome FHL2); the priming protein, Munc13-4 (FHL3); syntaxin 11 (FHL4), a member of the SNARE family of proteins that mediate membrane fusion; and Munc18-2 (FHL5), a protein involved in the reorganization of SNARE proteins to activate the fusion process. Because components of the biogenesis and exocytosis of cytotoxic granules are shared with other secretory vesicles, such as lysosomes, additional immune defects can occur in affected individuals, as can nonimmune defects. In particular, a subset of the immunodeficiencies that affect cytotoxic granule function are also characterized by partial loss of skin pigmentation. This is due to defects in vesicular transport proteins that are also required for the formation or exocytosis of melanosomes, organelles that store the skin pigment melanin in melanocytes. Examples of these immunodeficiencies include **Chediak–Higashi syndrome**, caused by autosomal recessive mutations in the protein LYST (or CHS1), which regulates lysosomal trafficking, and **Griscelli syndrome**, caused by mutations in a small GTPase, Rab27a, which is integral to the tethering of certain vesicles, including cytotoxic granules, to cytoskeletal structures to enable their intracellular trafficking.

In Chediak–Higashi syndrome, abnormal giant lysosomes and granules accumulate in T lymphocytes, myeloid cells, platelets, and melanocytes. The hair is typically a metallic silver color, vision is poor because of abnormalities in retinal pigment cells, and platelet dysfunction causes increased bleeding. Because the phagocytes of these individuals have defective phagolysosomal fusion, the individuals experience defective killing of intracellular and extracellular pathogens. In addition, they have defective cytolytic activity of CTLs and NK cells, thought to be due to the abnormal enlargement of cytotoxic granules that fail to dock properly. Affected children therefore suffer early in life from severe, recurrent infections by a range of bacteria and fungi. This is typically followed by development of hemophagocytic lymphohistiocytosis, often triggered by viral infection such as EBV, leading to an accelerated phase of the disease. Three variants of Griscelli syndrome have been identified, each caused by a distinct gene defect: in the type 2 variant (*RAB27A* mutation), the defect results in both immunodeficiency and pigment abnormalities; in types 1 and 3, only the pigment abnormalities are found. Although the immune defects in children with type 2 Griscelli syndrome have much in common with those of Chediak–Higashi syndrome, their myeloid cells lack the giant intracellular granules that are characteristic of the latter.

13-14 X-linked lymphoproliferative syndrome is associated with fatal infection by Epstein–Barr virus and the development of lymphomas.

In some primary immunodeficiencies, there is unique susceptibility to a single pathogen. Such is the case for two rare X-linked immunodeficiencies with a similar lymphoproliferative defect that results from vulnerability to a herpes family virus, the Epstein–Barr virus (EBV), albeit via independent mechanisms. EBV specifically infects B cells and typically causes a self-limiting infection in normal individuals, which is the result of active control of the virus by the actions of NK cells, NKT cells, and cytotoxic T cells that have specificity for B cells expressing EBV antigens. After the development of immunity to EBV, the virus is not completely cleared, but is maintained in a latent state in infected B cells (see Section 13-27). In the presence of certain types of immunodeficiency, however, this control can break down, resulting in overwhelming EBV infection (severe infectious mononucleosis) that is accompanied by unrestrained proliferation of EBV-infected B cells and cytotoxic T cells, hypogammaglobulinemia (low levels of circulating immunoglobulins), and the potential for the development of lethal, non-Hodgkin's B-cell lymphomas. These occur in the rare immunodeficiency **X-linked lymphoproliferative (XLP) syndrome**. XLP syndrome results from mutations in one of two X-linked genes: the SH2 domain–containing gene 1A (*SH2D1A*), which encodes SAP [signaling lymphocyte activation molecule (SLAM)-associated protein], or the X-linked inhibitor of apoptosis gene (*XIAP*).

In XLP1, which accounts for approximately 80% of individuals with this syndrome, the defect in SAP results in defective coupling of immune-cell receptors of the SLAM family to the Src family tyrosine kinase Fyn in T cells, NKT cells, and NK cells (**Fig. 13.12**). SLAM family members interact through

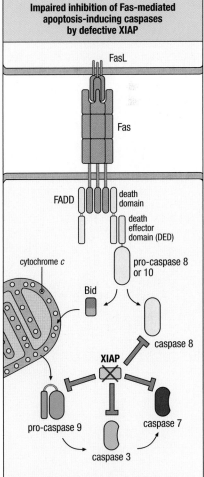

Fig. 13.12 X-linked lymphoproliferative (XLP) syndrome is caused by inherited defects in SAP and XIAP, resulting in abnormal SLAM and TNF family receptor signaling, respectively. SLAM is an immune receptor family, members of which are expressed by T cells, B cells, NK cells, dendritic cells, and macrophages. Signaling is initiated via homotypic or heterotypic interactions between family members. SLAM signaling recruits the Src homology 2 (SH2) domain–containing factor SAP, which recognizes tyrosine-based motifs in the cytoplasmic domain of SLAM to activate the Src-related tyrosine kinase Fyn (left upper panel). Fyn then phosphorylates additional tyrosine residues of SLAM to recruit additional signaling components. Mutation in SAP in individuals with XLP1 (right upper panel) disrupts activation of Fyn and SLAM signaling, thereby impairing T- and NK-cell cytotoxicity, which results in severe Epstein–Barr virus (EBV) infections (fulminant infectious mononucleosis, or FIM) and lymphoma. Defective SLAM signaling also impairs up-regulation of expression of the T-cell co-stimulator ICOS (inducible co-stimulatory protein) in T_{FH} cells, which results in impaired antibody responses. Activation of apoptosis-inducing caspases by TNF family receptors, such as Fas, is normally inhibited by XIAP (lower panel). XIAP interacts with both initiator caspases (8 and 9) and executioner caspases (3 and 7) to inhibit their actions, such as cleavage and activation of the Bcl-2 family sentinel protein, Bid. In individuals with XLP2, XIAP is defective, resulting in abnormal regulation of caspase activation that leads to the complex clinical phenotype, which includes lymphoproliferation and defective control of EBV virus.

X-linked
Lymphoproliferative
Syndrome

homotypic or heterotypic binding to modulate the outcome of interactions between T cells and antigen-presenting cells and between NK cells and their target cells. In the absence of SAP, ineffective EBV-specific cytotoxic T-cell and NK-cell responses are made, and there is severe deficiency of NKT cells, indicating that SAP has a nonredundant role in the control of EBV infection and the development of NKT cells. There is unchecked proliferation of EBV-reactive cytotoxic T cells and NK cells that results in systemic macrophage activation, inflammation, and hemophagocytic features similar to those that occur in immunodeficiencies caused by defects in the cytolytic pathway (see Section 13-13). Moreover, defective SLAM signaling between T_{FH} cells and B cells of individuals with XLP1 causes impaired T-dependent antibody responses and hypogammaglobulinemia.

Defects in the XIAP protein, which normally binds the TNF receptor–associated factors TRAF1 and TRAF2 and inhibits the activation of apoptosis-inducing caspases (see Section 7-23), leads to a similar X-linked syndrome called **XLP2** (see Fig. 13.12). XIAP deficiency results in the enhanced apoptosis and turnover of activated T cells and NK cells. Paradoxically, this leads to a lymphoproliferative phenotype similar to that of XLP1, the basis of which is not well understood. As in XLP1, there is severe depletion of NKT cells in XLP2, indicating that, like SAP, XIAP is required for the normal maintenance of these cells. Also as in XLP1, there is defective control of EBV infection in XLP2, although this is less prominent. The exact reason for the impaired suppression of EBV in these immunodeficiencies remains to be defined.

13-15 Immunodeficiency is caused by inherited defects in the development of dendritic cells.

Dendritic cells (DCs) are specialized antigen-presenting cells that link innate and adaptive immunity through their central role in activating naive T cells. We have already considered PIDs that include impaired functions of DCs (for example, IL-12p40 deficiency, CD40 deficiency; see Sections 13-12 and 13-8). Here we consider PIDs associated with impaired development of DCs. Our understanding of the diversity and function of DCs has advanced rapidly from studies of mice having lineage-specific, gene-targeted deletions of transcription factors that result in the loss of subsets of these cells, and from the defects in protection against specific pathogens that result as a consequence of the loss of specific DC subsets (see Section 9-7). In humans, where study of the development and function of DCs is more challenging, and in whom clinical workup for dendritic-cell deficiencies has not been a standard component of PID patient studies, the identification of PIDs that result from damaging variants in genes that impact DC development has lagged. Moreover, while defects in transcription factors that affect DC development have begun to be identified, these often affect other immune-cell lineages, complicating the immunodeficiency phenotype.

An autosomal dominant mutation in GATA2 has been identified in the largest group of individuals that have an inherited deficiency of dendritic cells. Affected individuals develop a progressive loss of all subsets of dendritic cells (conventional and plasmacytoid) and monocytes, as well as reduced numbers of B cells and NK cells, a condition that has been termed DCML (dendritic cell, monocyte, B and NK lymphoid) deficiency. Although T-cell numbers are normal in these individuals, their function becomes impaired as dendritic cells are lost. The loss of products of several hematopoietic lineages, but not all, suggests redundancy of the function of GATA2 in unaffected lineages. The basis for the progressive decline in products of the affected lineages is unknown but is thought to reflect a role for GATA2 in maintaining stem-cell progenitors that seed these populations. Given the deficiency of all dendritic and monocyte cells, the immune defects in these individuals are diverse, as are pathogen susceptibilities. These individuals also have a substantial risk of hematologic malignancies.

Rare inherited defects in interferon regulatory factor 8 (IRF8) are associated with developmental abnormalities of monocytes and dendritic cells. In an autosomal recessive form, there is loss of monocytes and all types of circulating dendritic cells (conventional and plasmacytoid dendritic cells), as well as NK-cell deficiency. This suggests a difference in the role of IRF8 in the development of human and mouse DCs, as deficiency of the latter targeted to myeloid cells results in a relatively specific deficiency of type 1 conventional dendritic cells (cDC1 cells). Because dendritic cells are the primary antigen-presenting cells for naive T cells, this deficiency in humans results in impaired development of effector T cells, and these individuals are susceptible to a range of severe opportunistic infections early in life, including those caused by intracellular bacteria, viruses, and fungi.

13-16 Defects in complement components and complement-regulatory proteins cause defective humoral immune function and tissue damage.

The diseases discussed so far are mainly due to defects that have substantial impact on the adaptive immune system. In the next few sections we look at selected PIDs that are limited to cells and molecules of the innate immune system. We start with the complement system, which can be activated by any of three pathways that converge on the cleavage and activation of complement component 3 (C3), allowing it to bind covalently to pathogen surfaces where it acts as an opsonin (discussed in Chapter 2). Not surprisingly, the spectrum of infections associated with complement deficiencies overlaps substantially with that seen in individuals with deficiencies in antibody production. In particular, there is increased susceptibility to extracellular bacteria that require opsonization by antibody and/or complement for efficient clearance by phagocytes (**Fig. 13.13**). Defects in the activation of C3 by any of the three pathways, as well as defects in C3 itself, are associated with increased susceptibility to infection by a range of pyogenic bacteria, including *Streptococcus*

Fig. 13.13 Defects in complement components are associated with susceptibility to certain infections and the accumulation of immune complexes. Defects in the early components of the alternative pathway and in C3 lead to susceptibility to extracellular pathogens, particularly pyogenic bacteria. Defects in the early components of the classical pathway predominantly affect the processing of immune complexes and the clearance of apoptotic cells, leading to immune-complex disease. Deficiency of mannose-binding lectin (MBL), the recognition molecule of the mannose-binding lectin pathway, is associated with bacterial infections, mainly in early childhood. Defects in the membrane-attack components are associated only with susceptibility to strains of *Neisseria* species, the causative agents of meningitis and gonorrhea, implying that the effector pathway is important chiefly in defense against these organisms.

pneumoniae, emphasizing the role of C3 as a central effector that promotes the phagocytosis and clearance of encapsulated bacteria.

In contrast, defects in the membrane-attack components of complement (C5–C9) downstream of C3 activation have more limited effects and result almost exclusively in susceptibility to *Neisseria* species. A similar susceptibility to *Neisseria* species is found in individuals with defects in the alternative complement pathway components, factor D and factor P, indicating that defense against these bacteria, which can survive intracellularly, is largely mediated via antibody-independent extracellular lysis by the membrane-attack complex. Data from large population studies in Japan, where endemic *Neisseria meningitidis* infection is rare, show that the risk each year of infection with this organism is approximately 1 in 2,000,000 to a normal person. This compares with a risk of 1 in 200 to a person in the same population who has an inherited deficiency of one of the membrane-attack complex proteins—a 10,000-fold increase in risk.

The early components of the classical complement pathway are particularly important for the elimination of immune complexes and apoptotic cells, which can cause significant pathology in autoimmune diseases such as systemic lupus erythematosus. This aspect of inherited complement deficiency is discussed in Chapter 15. Deficiency of mannose-binding lectin (MBL), which initiates complement activation independently of antibody (see Section 2-6), is relatively common (found in more than 5% of the population). In the majority of individuals who have reduced but not absent levels, MBL deficiency is often clinically silent. However, in those with complete MBL deficiency, there is increased susceptibility to bacterial infections, such as pneumonia or meningitis in early childhood. A similar phenotype is found in individuals with defects in the gene that encodes the MBL-associated serine protease-2 (*MASP2*).

Another set of complement-related diseases is caused by defects in complement-control proteins (**Fig. 13.14**). Deficiencies in decay-accelerating factor (DAF) or protectin (CD59), membrane-associated control proteins that protect the surfaces of the body's cells from complement activation, lead to destruction of red blood cells, resulting in the disease **paroxysmal nocturnal hemoglobinuria**, as discussed in Section 2-17. Deficiencies in soluble complement-regulatory proteins such as factor I and factor H have various outcomes. Homozygous **factor I deficiency** is a rare defect that results in uncontrolled activity of the alternative pathway C3 convertase, leading to a *de facto* C3 deficiency (see Section 2-16). Deficiencies in membrane cofactor of proteolysis (MCP), factor I, or factor H can also cause a condition known as **atypical hemolytic uremic syndrome**, so called because it leads to lysis of red blood cells (hemolysis) and impaired kidney function (uremia).

A striking consequence of the loss of a complement-regulatory protein is seen in individuals with C1-inhibitor defects, which cause the syndrome known as **hereditary angioedema (HAE)** (see Section 2-16). Deficiency of C1 inhibitor results in a failure to regulate both the blood clotting and complement activation pathways, leading to excessive production of vasoactive mediators that cause fluid accumulation in the tissues (edema) and local laryngeal swelling that can result in suffocation.

13-17 Defects in phagocytic cells result in widespread bacterial infections.

Deficiencies in phagocyte numbers or function can be associated with severe immunodeficiency; indeed, a total absence of neutrophils is incompatible with survival in a normal environment. Phagocyte immunodeficiencies can be grouped into four general types: deficiencies in phagocyte production, phagocyte adhesion/motility, phagocyte activation by pattern-recognition receptors

Systemic Lupus Erythematosus

Hereditary Angioedema

Complement protein	Effects of deficiency
C1, C2, C4	Immune-complex disease
C3	Susceptibility to encapsulated bacteria
C5–C9	Susceptibility to *Neisseria*
Factor D, Factor P (properdin)	Susceptibility to encapsulated bacteria and *Neisseria* but no immune-complex disease
Factor I	Similar effects to deficiency of C3
MCP, factor I, or factor H	Atypical hemolytic uremic syndrome
Polymorphisms in factor H	Age-related macular degeneration
DAF, CD59	Autoimmune-like conditions, including paroxysmal nocturnal hemoglobinuria
C1INH	Hereditary angioedema (HAE)

Fig. 13.14 Defects in complement-control proteins are associated with a range of diseases.

Disease	Examples	Gene defect	Inheritance	Immune defect	Common infections
Severe congenital neutropenia	Elastase-2 deficiency (SCN1)	*ELANE*	AD	Neutrophil deficiency	Severe pyogenic bacterial infections
	GFI-1 deficiency (SCN2)	*GFI1*	AD		Severe pyogenic bacterial infections
	HAX1 deficiency (SCN3, or Kostmann's disease)	*HAX1*	AR		Severe pyogenic bacterial infections
	G6PC3 deficiency (SCN4)	*G6PC3*	AR		Severe pyogenic bacterial infections
Leukocyte adhesion deficiency	β2 integrin deficiency (LAD-1)	*ITGB2*	AR	Defective leukocyte extravasation	Ulcerating skin infections without pus
	GDP-fucose transporter deficiency (LAD-2)	*SLC35C1*	AR		Recurrent bacterial infections
	Kindlin-3 deficiency (LAD-3)	*FERMT3*	AR		Severe bacterial infections
TLR/IL-1R signaling defects	MyD88 deficiency	*MYD88*	AR	Impaired TLR and IL-1 receptor signaling	Noninvasive bacterial infections, skin and respiratory tract
	IRAK4 deficiency	*IRAK4*	AR		Noninvasive bacterial infections, skin and respiratory tract
	TLR-3 deficiency	*TLR3*	AD or AR	Impaired types I and III interferon responses	Herpes simplex and varicella-zoster encephalitis
	TRAF3 deficiency	*TRAF3*	AD		Herpes simplex and varicella-zoster encephalitis
Non-TLR PRR signaling defect	CARD9 deficiency	*CARD9*	AR	Defective phagocyte recognition of fungi; impaired T$_H$17 response	Invasive fungal infections
Chronic granulomatous disease	X-linked CGD	*CYBB*	XL	Impaired intracellular killing in neutrophils and monocyte/macrophages	Severe, recurrent bacterial infections of barrier tissues

Fig. 13.15 Defects in phagocytic cells are associated with persistence of bacterial infection, as well as some fungal and viral infections. Defects in neutrophil development caused by congenital neutropenias (for example, elastase-2 deficiency; HAX1 deficiency) result in profound defects in antibacterial defense. Impairment of the leukocyte integrins with a common β$_2$ subunit (CD18) or defects in the selectin ligand sialyl-Lewis^X prevent phagocytic cell adhesion and migration to sites of infection (leukocyte adhesion deficiency). Inability to transmit signals through Toll-like receptors (TLRs), due to defects in MyD88 or IRAK4, for example, or through non-TLR sensor molecules (for example, CARD9 deficiency) impairs the proximal sensing of many infectious agents by innate immune cells. The respiratory burst is defective in chronic granulomatous disease [for example, deficiency of NADP oxidase 2 (NOX2), which is encoded by *CYBB*], as well as in glucose-6-phosphate dehydrogenase (G6PD) deficiency and myeloperoxidase (MPO) deficiency (the latter two not shown). In chronic granulomatous disease (CGD), infections persist because neutrophil and macrophage activation is defective, leading to chronic stimulation of CD4 T cells and hence to granulomas. These diseases illustrate the critical role of phagocytes in removing and killing pathogenic bacteria. AD, autosomal dominant; AR, autosomal recessive; XL, X-linked.

(PRRs), and phagocyte killing of microorganisms (**Fig. 13.15**). We consider each in turn.

Inherited deficiencies of neutrophil production (**neutropenias**) are classified as either **severe congenital neutropenia (SCN)** or **cyclic neutropenia**. In severe congenital neutropenia, which can be inherited as a dominant or recessive trait, the neutrophil count is persistently less than 0.5×10^9 per liter of blood (normal numbers are 3×10^9 to 5.5×10^9 per liter). Cyclic neutropenia is characterized by fluctuation in neutrophil numbers from near normal to very low or undetectable with an approximate cycle time of 21 days, resulting in periodicity of infectious risk. The most common variant, SCN1, is caused by sporadic or autosomal dominant mutations of the gene that encodes neutrophil elastase (*ELANE*), a component of the azurophilic, or primary, granules involved in the degradation of phagocytosed microbes. Altered targeting of defective elastase-2 to granules causes apoptosis of developing myelocytes and a developmental block at the promyelocyte–myelocyte stage. Some mutations of *ELA2* cause cyclic neutropenia; how the mutant elastase causes a 21-day cycle in neutropenia is still a mystery. A rare autosomal dominant variant, SCN2, is caused by mutations in the oncogene *GFI1*, which encodes a transcriptional repressor that acts on *ELA2*. This finding arose from the

Severe Congenital Neutropenia

unexpected observation that mice lacking the protein Gfi-1 are neutropenic because of overexpression of *Ela2*.

Autosomal recessive forms of SCN have also been identified. Deficiency of the mitochondrial protein HAX1 leads to increased apoptosis in developing myeloid cells, resulting in a severe neutropenia referred to as SCN3, or **Kostmann's disease** (see Fig. 13.15). The heightened sensitivity of developing neutrophils to apoptosis is highlighted by SCN4, which is associated with genetic defects in glucose metabolism. Individuals with recessive mutations in the genes encoding the glucose-6-phosphatase catalytic subunit 3 (*G6PC3*) also demonstrate increased apoptosis during granulocyte development that results in neutropenia. Acquired neutropenia associated with chemotherapy, malignancy, or aplastic anemia is also associated with a similar spectrum of severe pyogenic bacterial infections. Finally, neutropenia can also be a feature of other PIDs, including CD40 ligand deficiency, CVID, XLA, Wiskott–Aldrich syndrome, and GATA2 deficiency. In some individuals with these PIDs, there is formation of autoantibodies that lead to accelerated destruction of neutrophils.

Leukocyte Adhesion Deficiency

Defects in the migration of phagocytic cells to extravascular sites of infection can cause serious immunodeficiency. Leukocytes reach such sites by emigrating from blood vessels in a tightly regulated process (see Fig. 3.30). Deficiencies in the molecules involved in each stage of this process can prevent neutrophils and macrophages from penetrating infected tissues and are referred to as **leukocyte adhesion deficiencies (LADs)** (see Fig. 13.15). Deficiency in the leukocyte integrin common β_2 subunit CD18, which is a component of LFA-1, MAC-1, and p150:p95, prevents the migration of leukocytes into an infected site by abolishing the cells' ability to adhere tightly to the endothelium. Because it was the first LAD to be characterized, it is now referred to as type 1 LAD, or LAD-1, and is the most common variant of LAD. Reduced rolling of leukocytes on the endothelium has been described in rare individuals who lack the sialyl-Lewis^X antigen because of a deficiency in the GDP-fucose–specific transporter that is involved in the biosynthesis of sialyl-Lewis^X and other fucosylated ligands for the selectins. This is referred to as type 2 LAD, or LAD-2. Type 3 LAD, or LAD-3, results from deficiency of kindlin-3, a protein involved in the induction of the high-affinity binding state of β integrins required for firm adhesion. Each variant of LAD has an autosomal recessive pattern of inheritance and causes severe, life-threatening bacterial or fungal infections early in life that are characterized by impaired wound healing and, in pyogenic bacterial infections, the absence of pus formation. The infections that occur in these individuals are resistant to antibiotic treatment. LAD-3 is also associated with defects in platelet aggregation that cause increased bleeding.

Interleukin-1 Receptor– Associated Kinase 4 Deficiency

A key step in the activation of innate immune cells, including phagocytes, is their recognition of microbial-associated molecular patterns through pattern-recognition receptors (PRRs), such as Toll-like receptors, or TLRs (see Section 3-5). Several primary immunodeficiencies have been identified that are caused by defects in intracellular signaling components of TLRs. Signaling through all TLRs except TLR-3 requires the adaptor protein MyD88, which recruits and activates the kinases IRAK4 and IRAK1 required for downstream activation of the NFκB and MAP kinase pathways (see Fig. 13.15; see also Section 3-7). Autosomal recessive mutations in the genes encoding MyD88 or IRAK4 have a similar phenotype: recurrent, severe peripheral and invasive infections by pyogenic bacteria that elicit little inflammation, known as a **'cold' pyogenic infection**. Because TLRs and IL-1 family receptors are structurally related and are part of the same superfamily (IL-1 receptor/TLR superfamily), many of the signaling functions of MyD88 and IRAK4 molecules are shared with IL-1 family receptors. Thus, at least part of the immune defect in individuals with inherited abnormalities in these molecules may be attributed to aberrant signaling by IL-1 family members. Notably, increased viral infections are not typical in individuals with MyD88 mutations, despite this protein's role in signaling by each of the nucleic acid–sensing TLRs except TLR-3 (for example, TLR-7, TLR-8, and TLR-9). This indicates that activation of interferon regulatory factors (IRFs) that induce interferon responses downstream of these TLRs remains intact despite the defects in MyD88.

Remarkably, of the 10 TLRs found in humans, defects in only one—TLR-3—have been definitively linked to a PID (see Fig. 13.15). While defects in other TLRs have been identified (for example, TLR-4), they have not been associated with an overt immunodeficiency phenotype, likely reflecting a substantial level of redundancy. On the other hand, individuals with hemizygous (dominant) and homozygous (recessive) mutations in the gene encoding TLR-3, which senses double-stranded RNA, have recurrent herpes simplex virus 1 (HSV-1) or varicella-zoster virus (VZV) infections of the central nervous system (HSV or VZV encephalitis) because of impaired production of type I and type III interferons that act to limit viral infection of the CNS by enhancing blood–brain barrier function. Also, cells of the nervous system preferentially express the type III IFN receptor component, IFNLR1, rather than the type I IFN receptor, and rely on type III IFNs produced downstream of TLR-3 signaling to enhance antiviral resistance in the CNS.

Recurrent Herpes Simplex Encephalitis

Individuals with inherited deficiencies in molecules involved in TLR-3 signaling (for example, TRIF, TRAF3, TBK1, and IRF3), are similarly susceptible to herpes viral encephalitis, as are individuals with mutations in the TLR-transport protein UNC93B1, which is required for the transport of TLR-3 from the endoplasmic reticulum to the endolysosome. Notably, leukocytes from these individuals have no defect in their response to TLR-3 ligands or HSV-1, indicating redundancy of TLR-3 function in these cells, but not in those of the central nervous system. Similarly, these individuals show only a limited predisposition to other viral infections, implying the existence of TLR-3–independent protection against most other types of viral infection.

Genetic defects that affect signaling by PRRs other than TLRs have been described. CARD9 is an adaptor molecule involved in signaling downstream of C-type lectin receptors expressed on myeloid cells (see Fig. 13.15). Dectin-1, Dectin-2, and macrophage-inducible C-type lectin (MINCLE) each recognize fungal-associated molecular patterns that signal through CARD9 to induce secretion of pro-inflammatory cytokines, including IL-6 and IL-23. Autosomal recessive CARD9 deficiency results in impaired T_H17 cell responses to fungi, with the result that these individuals, similar to those with inborn errors of IL-17 immunity (for example, IL-17RA deficiency and IL-17F deficiency; see Section 13-12), suffer chronic mucocutaneous candidiasis. However, in addition, these individuals suffer more invasive infections by *Candida* spp. and dermatophytes, which are ubiquitous filamentous fungi that normally cause common superficial skin and nail infections, such as tinea pedis ('athlete's foot').

Most of the other known defects in phagocytic cells affect either their ability to ingest microbes or their ability to destroy microbes once ingested (see Fig. 13.15). Individuals with **chronic granulomatous disease (CGD)** are highly susceptible to bacterial and fungal infections and form granulomas as a result of an inability to kill bacteria ingested by phagocytes (see Fig. 13.15; see also Section 3.2). The defect in this case is in the production of reactive oxygen species (ROS) such as the superoxide anion. Discovery of the molecular defect in this disease gave weight to the idea that these agents killed bacteria directly; this notion has since been challenged by the finding that the generation of ROS is not itself sufficient to kill target microorganisms. It is now thought that ROS cause an influx of K^+ ions into the phagocytic vacuole, increasing the pH to the optimal level for the action of microbicidal peptides and proteins, which are the key agents in killing the invading microorganism.

Chronic Granulomatous Disease

Genetic defects affecting any of the constituent proteins of the NADPH oxidase expressed in neutrophils and monocytes (see Section 3-2) can cause

Disease (common abbreviation)	Clinical features	Inheritance	Mutated gene	Protein (alternative name)
Familial Mediterranean fever (FMF)	Periodic fever, serositis (inflammation of the pleural and/or peritoneal cavity), arthritis, acute-phase response	Autosomal recessive	*MEFV*	Pyrin
TNF receptor–associated periodic syndrome (TRAPS) (also known as familial Hibernian fever)	Periodic fever, myalgia, rash, acute-phase response	Autosomal dominant	*TNFRSF1A*	TNF-α 55 kDa receptor (TNFR-I)
Pyogenic arthritis, pyoderma gangrenosum, and acne (PAPA)		Autosomal dominant	*PSTPIP1*	CD2-binding protein 1
Muckle–Wells syndrome	Periodic fever, urticarial rash, joint pains, conjunctivitis, progressive deafness	Autosomal dominant	*NLRP3*	Cryopyrin
Familial cold autoinflammatory syndrome 1 (FCAS1) (familial cold urticaria)	Cold-induced periodic fever, urticarial rash, joint pains, conjunctivitis			
Chronic infantile neurologic cutaneous and articular syndrome (CINCA)	Neonatal-onset recurrent fever, urticarial rash, chronic arthropathy, facial dysmorphia, neurologic involvement			
Hyper IgD syndrome (HIDS)	Periodic fever, elevated IgD levels, lymphadenopathy	Autosomal recessive	*MVK*	Mevalonate synthase
Blau syndrome	Granulomatous inflammation of skin, eye, and joints	Autosomal dominant	*NOD2*	NOD2

Fig. 13.16 The autoinflammatory diseases. CD2-binding protein 1 is also known as PSTPIP1.

Hereditary Periodic Fever Syndromes

chronic granulomatous disease. Individuals with these diseases have an inability to clear certain bacteria, which in some cases leads to the formation of granulomas. Deficiencies in glucose-6-phosphate dehydrogenase (G6PD) and myeloperoxidase (MPO) also impair intracellular bacterial killing and lead to a similar, although less severe, phenotype.

13-18 Mutations in the molecular regulators of inflammation can cause uncontrolled inflammatory responses that result in 'autoinflammatory disease.'

There are a small number of diseases in which mutations in genes that control the life, death, and pro-inflammatory cytokine release of monocytes and neutrophils are associated with severe inflammatory disease. Although they do not lead to immunodeficiency, we have included them here because they are single-gene defects affecting a crucial aspect of innate immunity—the inflammatory response. These conditions represent a failure of the mechanisms that normally limit inflammation and are known as **autoinflammatory diseases**, which can lead to inflammation even in the absence of infection (**Fig. 13.16**).

One group of autoinflammatory diseases is characterized by dysregulation of the inflammasome. These disorders result either from impaired dampening of inflammasome activity or intrinsic hyperactivity of the inflammasome, which normally regulates apoptosis and release of pro-inflammatory cytokines such as IL-1β by myeloid cells in response to inflammation and the stress response (see Section 3-11 and Figs. 3.20 and 3.21). Patients with **familial Mediterranean fever (FMF)** suffer episodic attacks of severe inflammation, which can occur at various sites throughout the body and are associated with fever, an acute-phase response (see Section 3-9), and severe malaise. The pathogenesis of FMF was a mystery until its cause was discovered to result from impaired expression of the gene *MEFV* (so named for its association with Mediterranean fever), which encodes a protein called **Pyrin**. Pyrin, and the pyrin domains of NLRPs, exemplified by NLRP3 (or cryopyrin), interact to restrain inflammasome activity. The absence of functional

Pyrin, as occurs in FMF, leads to unregulated inflammatory cytokine release and defective apoptosis, resulting in uncontrolled local and systemic inflammation (see Fig. 13.16). Mutations in the gene encoding PSTPIP1 (proline-serine-threonine phosphatase-interacting protein 1), which interacts with Pyrin, are associated with another dominantly inherited autoinflammatory syndrome—**pyogenic arthritis, pyoderma gangrenosum, and acne (PAPA)**. The defective variants of *PSTPIP1* result in increased binding of Pyrin to PSTPIP1, which is thought to sequester Pyrin and limits its normal regulatory function.

Muckle–Wells syndrome and **familial cold autoinflammatory syndrome 1 (FCAS1)** are caused by gain-of-function mutations of *NLRP3*, whereas **familial cold autoinflammatory syndrome 2 (FCAS2)** results from gain-of-function mutations in *NLRP12* (see Fig. 13.16). Hyperactivity of NLRP3 or NLRP12 resulting from these mutations leads to unregulated overproduction of pro-inflammatory cytokines. Individuals with these dominantly inherited syndromes present with episodes of fever—which is induced by exposure to cold in the case of FCAS—as well as urticarial rash, joint pains, and conjunctivitis. Damaging variants of *NLRP3* are also associated with the autoinflammatory disorder **chronic infantile neurologic cutaneous and articular syndrome (CINCA)**, in which short recurrent fever episodes in infancy are common, although severe arthropathic, neurologic, and dermatologic symptoms predominate. Because a common feature of each of these disorders is inflammasome-mediated elevation of IL-1β production, treatment with anti-inflammatory agents such as NSAIDs and corticosteroids can be effective, and patients often respond dramatically to the drugs that block IL-1 signaling, including anakinra, an injectable, recombinant preparation of the IL-1 receptor antagonist (IL-1RA), and the fully human anti-IL-1β monoclonal antibody canakinumab (see Section 16-27).

A disease with similar clinical manifestations, but caused by non-inflammasome-related defects, is **TNF receptor–associated periodic syndrome (TRAPS)** (see Fig. 13.16). As the name implies, TRAPS is caused by mutations in the gene encoding TNF-α receptor I (*TNFRSF1A*). Patients with TRAPS have reduced levels of TNFR-I, which leads to increased levels of pro-inflammatory TNF-α in the circulation because it is not regulated by binding to this receptor. This increase, in turn, leads to elevation of other pro-inflammatory cytokines, including IL-1β. The disease responds to therapeutic blockade with anti-TNF agents, such as etanercept, a recombinant form of the TNF receptor; adalimumab and infliximab, human TNF-blocking monoclonal antibodies; and IL-1β blockade by anakinra and canakinumab.

13-19 Factor-replacement therapies, hematopoietic stem-cell transplantation, and gene therapy can be used successfully to correct genetic defects.

In some PIDs, immune deficiency is amenable to factor-replacement therapy, which is the periodic administration of a recombinant or natural protein that is deficient in an individual to restore functional levels. For example, periodic administration of recombinant adenosine deaminase (ADA) or IFN-γ has been used successfully to treat patients who have ADA-deficient SCID and some patients who have chronic granulomatous disease, respectively. Similarly, immunoglobulins pooled from healthy donors, called intravenous Ig (IVIG) therapy, can be administered via injection to patients who have agammaglobulinemia variants or CVID. Advances in the design and engineering of recombinant monoclonal antibodies is also enabling more targeted Ig-replacement therapies for individuals whose PID makes them particularly susceptible to certain types of infections that can be prevented by neutralizing antibodies.

Hematopoietic stem-cell transplant. One MHC allele shared

MHC$^{a \times b}$ T cells   MHC^b

Donor cells undergo selection on MHC^b in the recipient thymus

MHC^b-restricted T cells can be activated by MHC$^{a \times b}$ APC and recognize infected MHC^b cells

Graft-Versus-Host Disease

Fig. 13.17 The donor and the recipient of a hematopoietic stem cell (HSC) graft must share at least some MHC molecules to restore immune function. An HSC transplant from a genetically different donor is illustrated in which the donor marrow cells share some MHC molecules with the recipient. The shared MHC type is designated 'b' and illustrated in blue; the MHC type of the donor HSCs that is not shared is designated 'a' and illustrated in yellow. In the recipient, developing donor lymphocytes are positively selected on MHC^b-expressing thymic epithelial cells and are negatively selected by the recipient's stromal epithelial cells and at the cortico-medullary junction by encounter with dendritic cells derived from both the donor HSCs and residual recipient dendritic cells. The negatively selected cells are shown as apoptotic cells. The donor-derived antigen-presenting cells (APCs) in the periphery can activate T cells that recognize MHC^b molecules; the activated T cells can then recognize the recipient's infected MHC^b-bearing cells.

It is also possible to correct the defects in lymphocyte development that lead to SCID and some other immunodeficiency phenotypes by replacing the defective cellular component, generally by hematopoietic stem cell (HSC) transplantation (**Fig. 13.17**; see also Section 15-25). The main difficulties in these therapies result from human leukocyte antigen (HLA) polymorphism. To be useful, the graft must share some HLA alleles with the host. As we learned in Section 8-21, the HLA alleles expressed by the thymic epithelium determine which T cells can be positively selected. When HSCs are used to restore immune function to individuals with a normal thymic stroma, both the T cells and the antigen-presenting cells are derived from the graft. Therefore, unless the graft shares at least some HLA alleles with the recipient, the T cells that are selected on host thymic epithelium cannot be activated by graft-derived antigen-presenting cells. There is also a danger that mature, post-thymic T cells that contaminate donor HSCs prepared from the peripheral blood or bone marrow might recognize the host as foreign and attack it, causing **graft-versus-host disease (GVHD)** (**Fig. 13.18**). This can be overcome by depleting the donor graft of mature T cells. For immunodeficiency diseases other than SCID where there are residual T cells and NK cells in the recipient, some form of myeloablative treatment (destruction of the bone marrow, typically using cytotoxic drugs or irradiation) is often carried out before transplantation, both to generate space for engraftment of the transplanted HSCs and to minimize the threat of **host-versus-graft disease (HVGD)** (see Fig. 13.18). The intensity of the myeloablative regimen is dependent on the nature of the immunodeficiency. For diseases where persistence of the patient's cells can be tolerated, engraftment of only a fraction of donor HSCs is sufficient for cure, and non-myeloablative chemotherapy may suffice prior to HSC transplantation. In conditions that require complete elimination of the patient's blood cells and full engraftment of donor cells (for example, XLP), more intensive (myeloablative) chemotherapy may be required.

Because many of the gene defects that cause inherited immunodeficiencies have been identified, an alternative therapeutic approach is **somatic gene therapy**. This strategy involves the isolation of HSCs from the patient's bone marrow or peripheral blood, introduction of a normal copy of the defective gene by the use of a viral vector, and reinfusion of the corrected stem cells into the patient. Initially, retroviral vectors were used for gene-therapy trials, but use of these ceased because of severe complications in some patients. Although the genetic defect was corrected in patients with X-linked SCID, CGD, and WAS who received this treatment, some patients developed leukemia because of insertion of the retrovirus within a proto-oncogene. The inability to control the site in the genome in which retrovirally encoded genes insert and the use of viral vectors with strong promoters that can transactivate neighboring genes make this treatment problematic. More recently, the use of self-inactivating retroviral and lentiviral vectors for gene correction has shown promise as a means of avoiding this complication. As an example, retrovirally mediated gene therapy for SCID caused by ADA deficiency is now approved in

Europe and has not shown the complications of some previous gene-therapy treatments. New efforts to implement CRISPR-mediated gene editing without off-target gene effects is a rapidly evolving technology. This approach offers the promise of 'repairing' specific gene defects in patient-derived stem cells *ex vivo* before reinfusion, but it is not yet established. Until better methods for introduction of corrected genes into self-renewing stem cells are identified, allogeneic HSC transplantation will remain the standard treatment for many primary immunodeficiencies.

13-20 Noninherited, secondary immunodeficiencies are major predisposing causes of infection and death.

The primary immunodeficiencies have taught us much about the biology of specific immune-system proteins. Fortunately, these conditions are rare. In contrast, secondary immunodeficiency is relatively common. Malnutrition devastates many populations around the world, and a major feature of malnutrition is secondary immunodeficiency. Secondary immunodeficiency particularly affects cell-mediated immunity, and death in famines is frequently caused by infection. Measles, which itself causes immunosuppression, is an important cause of death in malnourished children. In the developed world, measles is an unpleasant illness, but major complications are uncommon. In contrast, measles in the malnourished has a high mortality. Tuberculosis is another important infection in the malnourished. In mice, protein starvation causes immunodeficiency by affecting antigen-presenting cell function, but in humans it is not clear how malnourishment specifically affects immune responses. Links between the endocrine and immune systems may provide part of the answer. Adipocytes (fat cells) produce the hormone leptin, levels of which are related directly to the amount of fat present in the body; leptin levels therefore fall during starvation when fat is consumed. Both mice and humans with genetic leptin deficiency have reduced T-cell responses, and in mice the thymus atrophies. In both starved mice and those with inherited leptin deficiency, these abnormalities can be reversed by the administration of leptin.

Secondary immunodeficiency states are also associated with hematopoietic tumors, such as leukemia and lymphomas. Myeloproliferative diseases, such as leukemia, can be associated with deficiencies of neutrophils (neutropenia) or an excess of immature myeloid progenitors that lack functional properties of mature neutrophils, either of which increases susceptibility to bacterial and fungal infections. Destruction or invasion of peripheral lymphoid tissue by lymphomas or metastases from other cancers can promote opportunistic infections.

Congenital asplenia (a rare inherited absence of the spleen), surgical removal of the spleen, or destruction of spleen function by certain diseases is associated with a lifelong predisposition to overwhelming infection by *S. pneumoniae*, graphically illustrating the role of mononuclear phagocytic cells within the spleen in the clearance of this organism from blood. Individuals who have lost spleen function should be vaccinated against pneumococcal infection and are often counseled to take prophylactic antibiotics throughout their lives.

Secondary immunodeficiency is also a complication of certain medical therapies. A major complication of cytotoxic drugs used to treat cancer is immunosuppression and increased susceptibility to infection. Many of these drugs kill all dividing cells, including normal cells of the bone marrow and lymphoid systems. Infection is thus one of the major side effects of cytotoxic drug therapy. Immune suppression to induce host tolerance of solid-organ allografts, such as kidney or heart transplants, also carries a substantial increased risk for infection and even for malignancy.

Fig. 13.18 Grafting of bone marrow can be used to correct immunodeficiencies caused by defects in lymphocyte maturation, but two problems can arise. First, if there are mature T cells in the bone marrow, they can attack cells of the host by recognizing their MHC antigens, causing graft-versus-host disease (top panel). This can be prevented by T-cell depletion of the donor bone marrow (center panel). Second, if the recipient has competent T cells, these can attack the bone marrow stem cells (bottom panel). This causes failure of the graft by the usual mechanism of transplant rejection (see Chapter 15).

Congenital Asplenia

The growing use of biologic therapies to treat some forms of allograft rejection, malignancies, autoimmune disease, and autoinflammatory disorders (see Section 16-27) has led to an increased risk of infection because of their immunosuppressive effects, while illuminating how specific pathways are involved in immunity to particular infections. For example, administration of antibodies that block TNF-α in patients with rheumatoid arthritis, inflammatory bowel disease, or TRAPS has been associated with infrequent but increased instances of infectious complications, including the risk of *de novo* infections (for example, *Listeria monocytogenes* and certain opportunistic infections, such as *Pneumocystis jirovecii*), as well as reactivation of latent *Mycobacterium tuberculosis* or varicella-zoster virus infection. Because of the risk of reactivation of latent tuberculosis in these patients, pretreatment screening for a positive TB test is now routine prior to anti-TNF therapy, as is screening for certain latent viral infections. Similarly, use of rituximab—a depleting monoclonal antibody that targets the CD20 co-receptor component on B cells and is used to treat some B-cell lymphomas and leukemias (see Section 16-19) and patients who have certain forms of allograft rejection or autoimmunity—carries a significant risk for reactivation of active hepatitis B virus infection, as well as JC virus reactivation, which causes progressive multifocal leukoencephalopathy (PML), a highly lethal CNS infection. Similar to the widening use of biologics, the advent of pharmacologic inhibitors of JAK kinases ('jakinibs') that impair STAT signaling in immune cells in the treatment of these diseases increases the risk of infectious complications and may also provide insights into the immune pathways that utilize them. As the use of biologic and jakinib-based therapies grows, so too will the risk of infectious complications due to secondary immunodeficiencies.

Summary.

Genetic defects can occur in almost any molecule involved in the immune response. These defects give rise to characteristic immunodeficiency diseases, which, although rare, provide much information about the development and functioning of the immune system in normal humans. Inherited immunodeficiencies illustrate the vital role of the adaptive immune response and T cells, in particular, without which cell-mediated immunity and humoral immunity both fail. Inherited immunodeficiencies have provided information about the separate roles of B lymphocytes in humoral immunity and of T lymphocytes in cell-mediated immunity, the importance of phagocytes and complement in humoral immunity and innate immunity, and the specific functions of a growing number of cell-surface and signaling molecules in the adaptive immune response. There are also some inherited immune disorders whose causes we still do not understand. The study of these diseases will undoubtedly teach us more about the normal immune response and its control. Acquired defects in the immune system—the secondary immunodeficiencies—are much more common than the primary inherited immunodeficiencies. In the next part of this chapter, we briefly consider general mechanisms by which successful pathogens evade or subvert immune defenses, and in the final part of the chapter, we detail how extreme subversion of the immune system by one pathogen, the human immunodeficiency virus (HIV), has created a major pandemic characterized by the acquired immune deficiency syndrome (AIDS) in affected individuals.

Evasion and subversion of immune defenses.

In the previous part of the chapter, we learned how specific defects in immune pathways lead to infection, often by microbes that would normally be defeated by a healthy immune system. These 'opportunistic' infections often dominate the clinical expression of inherited immunodeficiencies because the causative organisms are ubiquitous and abundant in the environment. A minority of microbes are true pathogens that can infect those with normal immune defenses. A defining feature of pathogens is their ability to avoid immune destruction by components of the innate and adaptive immune systems, at least long enough to replicate in the infected host and spread to new hosts. At one end of the spectrum are pathogens that establish an acute infection, replicate quickly, and find a new host before they are cleared by a successful immune response; at the other end are pathogens that establish chronic infections, persisting long-term in the host while evading elimination by immune defenses. Successful pathogens use different strategies to these ends and over millions of years of coevolution with their hosts have evolved remarkably diverse strategies for avoiding detection and destruction by the immune system, often employing several strategies that subvert immunity at multiple points. The anti-immune strategies employed by pathogens are as sophisticated as the immune system itself. They must be in order for pathogens to achieve success against the diverse strategies that vertebrates have evolved to ensure host protection.

Viruses, bacteria, and protozoan (unicellular) or metazoan (multicellular) parasites can all act as pathogens. While fungi and helminthic (metazoan) parasites are major causes of common skin infections and intestinal worm infestation, respectively, they do not typically cause life-threatening infections in normal people and will not be considered further here. In contrast, a select number of viruses, bacteria, and protozoan parasites are the major causes of morbidity and mortality due to infectious agents. The human immunodeficiency virus (HIV, cause of AIDS), *Mycobacterium tuberculosis* (cause of tuberculosis), and *Plasmodium falciparum* (cause of malaria) are the three greatest infectious disease threats to humans; each of these pathogens infects more than 100 million people worldwide and kills 1 million to 2 million people annually. Although the strategies for survival within, and propagation between, hosts differ for each type of pathogen, many of the innate and adaptive immune mechanisms employed to thwart the pathogen are the same. Here we briefly consider the lifestyle and principal immune responses elicited by different types of pathogens and the strategies the pathogens employ to evade or subvert the immune system.

13-21 Extracellular bacterial pathogens have evolved different strategies to avoid detection by pattern-recognition receptors and destruction by antibody, complement, and antimicrobial peptides.

Extracellular bacterial pathogens replicate outside of host cells, whether on the surfaces of barrier tissues they colonize (for example, gastrointestinal or respiratory tracts) or in tissue spaces or blood after invasion across barrier epithelia. There are both Gram-negative and Gram-positive pathogenic species. As discussed in Section 11-11, these bacteria typically elicit type 3 immunity, which orchestrates neutrophilic responses, the development of opsonizing and complement-fixing antibodies, and the production of antimicrobial peptides by barrier epithelial cells and immune cells that clear these microbes from barrier epithelia and prevent their invasion. Some of the microbial-associated molecular patterns (MAMPs) expressed by Gram-negative and Gram-positive bacteria are distinct, but they share similar immune-cell activating properties.

Gram-negative pathogens contain lipopolysaccharide (LPS), a potent activator of TLR-4, in their outer cell membrane, whereas the cell walls of both Gram-positive and Gram-negative pathogens contains peptidoglycans, which activate TLR-2 and NOD1 and NOD2. One strategy of immune evasion used by these pathogens, therefore, is the shielding of their surface MAMPs to avoid detection of the MAMPs by pattern-recognition receptors (PRRs) on immune cells (**Fig. 13.19**).

Bacterial strategy	Mechanism	Result	Examples
Extracellular bacteria			
Shielding or inhibition of MAMPs	Capsular polysaccharide	Block detection of lipopolysaccharide (LPS)	*K. pneumoniae*
	Hypoacylation of lipid A	Antagonism of TLR-4	*P. gingivalis*
	Coating of bacterium by host proteins (e.g., fibrin)	Block detection of peptidoglycan	*S. aureus*
Antigenic variation	Modulation of expressed pili, fimbriae	Antibodies that block bacterial attachment become ineffective	*N. gonorrhoeae, E. coli*
Inhibition of opsonization	Secretion of complement-degrading factors	Cleavage of complement components	*N. meningitidis, P. aeruginosa, S. aureus*
	Capsular polysaccharide	Block fixation of complement	*S. pneumoniae, H. influenzae, K. pneumoniae*
	Expression of Fc-binding surface molecules (e.g., Protein A)	Prevents binding of antibody to Fc receptors of phagocytes	*S. aureus*
	Production of biofilms	Shielding of bacteria from phagocytosis	*S. epidermidis, S. aureus, P. aeruginosa*
Inhibition/scavenging of reactive oxygen species (ROS)	Secretion of catalase and superoxide dismutase	Neutralize ROS produced by NADPH and myeloperoxidase (MPO)	*S. aureus, B. abortus*
Resistance to antimicrobial peptides (AMPs)	Secretion of AMP-degrading peptidases	Cleavage of AMPs	*E. coli*
	Modulation of cell membrane phospholipids	Prevents binding, functional insertion of AMPs in cell membrane	*S. aureus*
Intracellular bacteria			
Antigenic variation	Modulation of expressed pili, fimbriae	Antibodies that block bacterial attachment become ineffective	*Salmonella* spp.
Inhibition of MAMP recognition/ signaling	Production of peptidoglycan hydrolase	Block detection of peptidoglycan by NODs	*L. monocytogenes*
	Secretion of intracellular toxins	Block NFκB and MAP kinase signaling pathways	*Y. pestis*
Resistance to anti-microbial peptides	Secretion of AMP-degrading peptidases	Cleavage of AMPs	*Y. pestis*
	Modulation of cell membrane phospholipids	Prevents binding, functional insertion of AMPs in cell membrane	*Salmonella* spp.
Inhibition of fusion of phagosome with lysosome	Release of bacterial cell wall components	Inhibits phago-lysosomal fusion	*M. tuberculosis, M. leprae, L. pneumophila*
Survival within phagolysosome	Waxy, hydrophobic cell wall containing mycolic acids and other lipids	Resistance against lysosomal enzymes	*M. tuberculosis, M. leprae*
Escape from phagosome	Production of hemolysins (e.g., listeriolysin O)	Lysis of phagosome; escape into cytosol	*L. monocytogenes, Shigella* spp.

Fig. 13.19 Mechanisms used by bacteria to subvert the host immune system.

Several Gram-negative pathogens modify the lipid A core of LPS with carbo-hydrates and other moieties that interfere with TLR-4 binding. Indeed, some bacteria produce variants of lipid A that act as TLR-4 antagonists rather than agonists. Both Gram-negative and Gram-positive pathogens have evolved mechanisms to modulate recognition of the peptidoglycan fragments by the intracellular PRRs, NOD1 and NOD2 (see Section 3-8), which impairs innate immune activation. NOD1 normally detects γ-glutamyl diaminopimelic acid (iE-DAP), which is found in peptidoglycans produced by Gram-negative and rod-shaped Gram-positive pathogens such as *Salmonella* and *Listeria*, respectively. NOD2 normally detects muramyl dipeptide, which is a component of peptidoglycans of most bacteria. Bacteria can modify the glycans found in the peptidoglycans of their cell walls to avoid cleavage by lysozyme, which is normally involved in the release of peptidoglycan fragments sensed by NOD receptors. They can also modify the stem peptides of peptidoglycans, which contribute to NOD1 recognition. Finally, some bacteria produce hydrolases that degrade peptidoglycan in a manner to render it less detectable by NOD receptors.

A limited number of Gram-positive pathogens can also shield their outer cell membrane with a thick carbohydrate capsule. In addition to inhibiting recognition of peptidoglycan and activation of the alternative pathway of complement, the capsule prevents antibody and complement deposition on the bacterial cell membrane, thereby avoiding direct damage by the membrane-attack complex of the complement cascade. The capsule also impairs clearance of the pathogen by phagocytes (see Fig. 13.19). A similar strategy is employed by both Gram-negative and Gram-positive bacteria, including those that lack a capsule, through the secretion of extracellular polymeric substances (EPSs) to create **biofilms**, which protect them from immune clearance. Biofilms are composed of exopolysaccharides (for example, cellulose), proteins, and nucleic acids and in which are embedded a community of bacteria—as opposed to free-living, or planktonic, cells (**Fig. 13.20**). While the latter are more easily phagocytosed and delivered to lysosomal compartments where they can be destroyed, bacteria embedded within biofilms are more difficult to ingest and

Fig. 13.20 The formation of biofilms by bacteria restrains immune clearance. Biofilms represent one mechanism by which microbes evade host immune defenses. They can form on either living tissues (biotic surface) or foreign material introduced into the body (abiotic surface), such as intravenous catheters or medical implants, and provide a source for recurrent seeding of the host by microbes. Biofilms form when free-living, or planktonic, microbial cells—in this case the Gram-negative bacterium *Pseudomonas aeruginosa*—attach to a surface or tissue (bacterial adhesion; shown is attachment to fibronectin in a tissue) and grow on it, producing an extracellular matrix (glycocalyx, or extracellular polymeric substance; EPS) that is composed of secreted proteins, glycans, and lipids, as well as the extravasated DNA (eDNA) of dying cells. This supports the microbial community and shields it from antimicrobial defenses, including antibodies, complement, and phagocytic cells. The photos (right panels) are scanning electron micrographs of a biofilm of *Pseudomonas aeruginosa* on an abiotic surface. Note the strands of glycocalyx (EPS) that connect and envelope individual bacteria. The upper and lower scale bars indicate 1 μm and 10 μm, respectively.

Fig. 13.21 Host defense against *Streptococcus pneumoniae* is type specific. The different strains of *S. pneumoniae* have antigenically distinct capsular polysaccharides. The capsule prevents effective phagocytosis until the bacterium is opsonized by specific antibody and complement, allowing phagocytes to destroy it. Antibody against one type of *S. pneumoniae* does not cross-react with the other types, so an individual immune to one type has no protective immunity to a subsequent infection with a different type. An individual must generate a new adaptive immune response each time he or she is infected with a different type of *S. pneumoniae*.

Streptococcus pneumoniae

There are many types of *S. pneumoniae*, which differ in their capsular polysaccharides

| Individual infected with one type of *S. pneumoniae* | Antibody response clears infection | Subsequent infection with a different type of *S. pneumoniae* is unaffected by response to first type | New antibody response clears second infection |

destroy. In addition to resisting host-clearance mechanisms, biofilms also enable long-term colonization on surfaces of host tissues by facilitating the sharing of resources within the mini-consortium of cooperating bacteria.

In the case of *Streptococcus pneumoniae*, an important cause of bacterial pneumonia, the carbohydrate capsule also serves as a platform for **antigenic variation** to modulate the expression of surface antigenic epitopes recognized by antibody. More than 90 known types of *S. pneumoniae* are distinguished by differences in the structure of their polysaccharide capsules. The different types are distinguished by using specific antibodies as reagents in serological tests and so are often known as **serotypes**. Infection with one serotype can lead to type-specific immunity, which protects against reinfection by that type but not by a different serotype. Thus, from the point of view of the adaptive immune system, each serotype of *S. pneumoniae* represents a distinct organism, with the result that essentially the same pathogen can cause disease many times in the same individual (**Fig. 13.21**). Similarly, antigenic variation mediated by DNA rearrangement also occurs in bacteria and helps to account for the success of *Neisseria* species (which cause gonorrhea and meningitis) and enteropathogenic *Escherichia coli*. Fimbriae or pili are expressed on the bacterial surface and used for attachment to host-cell surfaces and are major antigenic targets for antibody-mediated blockade of bacterial attachment and colonization. The gene locus encoding the expressed *Neisseria* pilus (*pilE*) can undergo recombination with partial pilin genes stored in 'silent' (*pilS*) loci to generate a constantly shifting pilus for display on the bacterial surface. By constantly changing the expressed pilus, the bacterium evades antibody-mediated immune clearance.

Among other anti-immune strategies used by extracellular pathogens are strategies to inhibit different aspects of the complement cascade. Because complement is central to the clearance of most extracellular bacteria, these pathogens have evolved multiple strategies to interfere with different components of each pathway of complement activation. Examples include expression of Fc-binding proteins that block activation of the classical pathway of complement (for example, Protein A); mechanisms to inactivate the C3 convertase, which impacts all complement pathways; decoration of the bacterial surface with host inhibitors of complement (for example, factor H and C4b-binding protein, or C4BP); and the release of proteases that can cleave key complement components (**Fig. 13.22**; see also Section 2-18). Bacterial proteases that can cleave antibody bound to the bacterial surface also exist (for example, staphylokinase, or SAK). These bacteria have also evolved mechanisms to defeat antimicrobial peptides (AMPs), such as defensins and cathelicidins. These small cationic and amphipathic peptides exert their antimicrobial activity by inserting into negatively charged cell membranes to generate pores that lyse the bacterium (see Section 2-4). Pathogens can alter their cell membrane composition to minimize AMP binding and can also produce proteases that degrade the AMPs.

An unusual feature of Gram-negative pathogens, including both extracellular and intracellular bacteria, is their capacity to inject immune modulatory

Fig. 13.22 Pathogenic bacteria target multiple steps in the complement cascade to subvert immunity. Extracellular pathogens can subvert all three branches of the complement cascade (lectin, classical, and alternative pathways) to evade immune destruction. Highlighted are several products of the Gram-positive bacteria, *Staphylococcus aureus,* which is remarkably versatile in the products it makes to inhibit different steps in the complement cascade. Examples of bacterial proteins produced by *S. aureus* and the sites of their actions in each cascade are indicated in red boxes: SAK (staphylokinase) cleaves IgG and removes it from the bacterial surface, while SSL10 (staphylococcal superantigen-like protein 10) binds IgG and blocks initiation of the classical pathway; Sbi (second immunoglobulin binding protein) and Spa (staphylococcal protein A) block C1q binding to the Fc portion of immunoglobulin, also blocking initiation of the classical pathway, while Sbi can also interfere with activation of the alternative pathway; SCIN (staphylococcal complement inhibitor) stabilizes C3 convertase in an inactive state; Ecb (extracellular complement-binding protein) and Efb (extracellular fibrinogen-binding protein) bind C3d and inactivate both C3 and C5, preventing C5 convertase activity; and CHIPS (chemotaxis inhibitory protein of staphylococcus) blocks the C5a receptor on phagocytes.

bacterial proteins directly into host cells via specialized structures: the type III and type IV secretion systems (T3SS and T4SS, respectively), as discussed in Chapter 12 (see Section 12-20 and Fig. 12.39). These needle-like structures, or **injectisomes**, assemble on the bacterial surface and dock with the plasma membrane of target cells to provide a conduit through which bacterial proteins are secreted directly into the cytosol of host cells. A range of bacterial virulence factors that aid in subverting the host immune response are delivered via this mechanism, including bacterial factors that block signaling cascades central to the inflammatory response: NFκB and MAP kinases. Among the most remarkable of these are the Yersinia outer proteins (Yops) produced by *Yersinia pestis*, the causative agent of bubonic plague. Secretion of several of these factors (for example, YopH, YopE, YopO, and YopT) into phagocytes disrupts the actin cytoskeleton, which is essential for phagocytosis. The essential roles played by T3SS or T4SS in immune subversion by a number of Gram-negative pathogens are demonstrated by the loss of pathogenicity of mutant bacteria lacking components of these structures.

13-22 Intracellular bacterial pathogens can evade the immune system by seeking shelter within phagocytes.

To avoid the major effectors directed against extracellular bacteria—complement and antibodies—some bacterial pathogens have evolved specialized mechanisms for surviving within macrophages, using these phagocytes as their primary host cell and as a vehicle for dissemination within the host. This 'Trojan horse' strategy is achieved by three general tactics: blockade of phagosome–lysosome fusion; escape from the phagosome into the cytosol; and resistance to killing mechanisms within the phagolysosome. *Mycobacterium tuberculosis*, for example, is taken up by macrophages but prevents the fusion of the phagosome with the lysosome, protecting itself from the bactericidal actions of the lysosomal contents. Other bacteria, such as *Listeria monocytogenes*, escape from the phagosome into the cytoplasm of the macrophage, where they multiply. They then spread to adjacent cells in the tissue without emerging into the extracellular environment. They do this by hijacking the cytoskeletal protein actin, which assembles into filaments at the rear of the bacterium. The actin filaments drive the bacteria forward into vacuolar projections to adjacent cells; the vacuoles are then lysed by the *Listeria*, releasing the bacteria into the cytoplasm of the adjacent cell. Moreover, *Listeria* has been shown to induce the expression of phosphatidylserine on the outer membrane leaflet of bacteria-containing blebs that protrude from infected cells; the expression of phosphatidylserine is normally recognized by phagocytes as a signal for the uptake of apoptotic cell debris. In this way, *Listeria* is delivered directly to phagocytic cells, thereby avoiding attack by antibodies.

After uptake, *Salmonella* species use a type III secretion system to secrete effectors such as SifA into the host cytosol and membranes in order to alter the composition of the *Salmonella*-containing vacuole so as to avoid destruction. Remarkably, *Salmonella* can also inject factors that delay the apoptotic death of host macrophages, prolonging the phagocytes' life spans until their bacterial cargo can be delivered to new cellular hosts. Other actions of intracellular bacteria counter reactive oxygen species or microbicidal peptides delivered into the phagolysosome by the ingesting phagocyte.

As a trade-off for their intracellular lifestyle, intracellular bacteria risk activation of immune effectors that target these pathogens: NK cells and T cells. As discussed in Section 11-6, a major function of the type 1 immune response is activation of NK cells and T_H1 cells that activate phagocytes for enhanced intracellular killing by secretion of IFN-γ or expression of CD40L. Additionally,

Infection with *Mycobacterium leprae* can result in different clinical forms of leprosy
There are two polar forms, tuberculoid and lepromatous leprosy, but several intermediate forms also exist

Tuberculoid leprosy	Lepromatous leprosy
Organisms present at low to undetectable levels	Organisms show florid growth in macrophages
Low infectivity	High infectivity
Granulomas and local inflammation. Peripheral nerve damage	Disseminated infection. Bone, cartilage, and diffuse nerve damage
Normal serum immunoglobulin levels	Hypergammaglobulinemia
Normal T-cell responsiveness. Specific response to *M. leprae* antigens	Low or absent T-cell responsiveness. No response to *M. leprae* antigens

Fig. 13.23 T-cell and macrophage responses to *Mycobacterium leprae* are sharply different in the two polar forms of leprosy. Infection with *M. leprae*, whose cells stain as small, dark red dots in the photographs, can lead to two very different forms of disease. In tuberculoid leprosy (left), growth of the organism is well controlled by T$_H$1-like cells that activate infected macrophages. The tuberculoid lesion contains granulomas and is inflamed, but the inflammation is local and causes only local effects, such as peripheral nerve damage. In lepromatous leprosy (right), infection is widely disseminated, and the bacilli grow uncontrolled in macrophages; in the late stages of disease there is major damage to connective tissues and to the peripheral nervous system. Cytokines typically produced by T$_H$2 cells (IL-4, IL-5, and IL-10) dominate in the lepromatous form, whereas cytokines produced by T$_H$1 cells (IL-2, IFN-γ, and TNF-β dominate in the tuberculoid form. It therefore seems that T$_H$1-like cells predominate in tuberculoid leprosy, and T$_H$2-like cells predominate in lepromatous leprosy. IFN-γ would be expected to activate macrophages, enhancing the killing of *M. leprae*, whereas IL-4 can actually inhibit the induction of bactericidal activity in macrophages.

those intracellular pathogens that have evolved mechanisms to escape the phagosome, such as *Listeria*, generate cytosolic peptides that feed the MHC class I antigen presentation pathway and thus induce cytotoxic T-cell responses that target their host cell for destruction. In leprosy, a disease caused by skin and peripheral nerve infection with *Mycobacterium leprae*, effective host defense requires macrophage activation by NK and T$_H$1 cells (**Fig. 13.23**). Like *M. tuberculosis*, *M. leprae* is able to persist and grow in macrophage vesicles and is normally restrained, but not cleared, by a type 1 host response. In individuals who mount normal type 1 immune responses, few live bacteria are found, little antibody is produced, and, although skin and peripheral nerves are damaged by the inflammatory responses associated with macrophage activation, the disease progresses slowly and the individuals typically survive. Because of its similarities to tuberculosis, this variant is called tuberculoid leprosy. This is in contrast to lepromatous leprosy, in which type 1 responses to *M. leprae* are deficient, and an ineffective type 2 response is mounted instead. This results in abundant growth of the bacterium in macrophages and gross tissue destruction that is eventually fatal if untreated. Although high levels of antibacterial antibodies are produced in individuals with lepromatous leprosy, probably due to the high bacterial load, the antibodies are ineffective at controlling infection because they do not reach the intracellular bacteria.

13-23 Immune evasion is also practiced by protozoan parasites.

Most common protozoan parasites, such as *Plasmodium* and *Trypanosoma* species, have complex life cycles: part of the life cycle occurs in humans, and part occurs in an intermediate host, such as an arthropod vector (for example, mosquitoes, flies, or ticks). Transmission of these organisms by their intermediate host is unusual, in that the normal barriers to infection are bypassed when the infectious agent is directly delivered to blood. Thus, many of the normal innate immune defenses associated with barrier function are completely bypassed during infection. Further, the most successful of these organisms have developed complex and varied immune-evasion strategies that often result in 'hide-and-seek' type chronic infections characterized by episodic disease manifestations, despite their eliciting antibody- and cell-mediated adaptive immune responses.

As described earlier for some bacterial pathogens (see Section 13-21), *Trypanosoma brucei*, a causative agent of trypanosomiasis, or sleeping sickness, has evolved a remarkable capacity for antigenic variation to evade the antibody response elicited in infected humans. The trypanosome is coated with a single type of glycoprotein, the variant-specific glycoprotein (VSG), which elicits a potent protective antibody response that rapidly clears most of the parasites. The trypanosome genome, however, contains about 1000 VSG genes, each encoding a protein with distinct antigenic properties. A VSG gene is expressed by being placed into the active expression site in the parasite genome. Only one VSG gene is expressed at a time, and it can be changed by a gene rearrangement that places a new VSG gene into the expression site (**Fig. 13.24**). So, under the selective pressure of an effective host antibody response, the few trypanosomes within the population that express a different VSG escape elimination and multiply to cause a recurrence of disease. Antibodies are then made against the new VSG, and the whole cycle is repeated, resulting in periods of active and quiescent disease. The chronic cycles of antigen clearance lead to immune-complex damage and inflammation, and eventually to neurological damage, resulting finally in the coma that gives sleeping sickness its name. The cycles of evasive action make trypanosome infections very difficult for the immune system to defeat, and they are a major health problem in Africa.

Caused by *Plasmodium* species, malaria is another serious and widespread disease. Like *Trypanosoma brucei*, *Plasmodium* species vary their antigens to avoid elimination by the immune system. In addition, plasmodia undergo different parts of their life cycle in different cellular hosts within humans. Initial infection occurs by the sporozoite form of the organism, which is transmitted by the bite of an infected mosquito and targets hepatocytes in the liver. Here, the organism replicates rapidly to produce merozoites that burst from infected hepatocytes to infect circulating red blood cells. Thus, as the immune system focuses its efforts on the eradication of the parasite in the liver, the parasite morphs and escapes to its second cellular host, red blood cells. And because red blood cells are the only cells in the body that lack MHC class I molecules, antigens produced by the merozoites within infected red blood cells escape detection by CD8 T cells, preventing cytotoxic destruction of the infected cells. This represents one of the most elegant adaptations to evade cell-mediated immunity.

Immune subversion is also practiced by protozoan parasites. *Leishmania major*, which is transmitted to dermal tissues of humans by the bite of sandflies, is an obligate intracellular parasite that replicates within tissue macrophages.

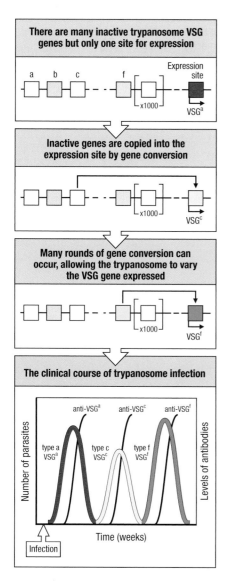

Fig. 13.24 Antigenic variation in trypanosomes allows them to escape immune surveillance. The surface of a trypanosome is covered with a variant-specific glycoprotein (VSG). Each trypanosome has about 1000 genes encoding different VSGs, but only the gene in a specific expression site within the telomere at one end of the chromosome is active. Although several genetic mechanisms have been observed for changing the VSG gene expressed, the usual mechanism is gene conversion. An inactive gene, which is not at the telomere, is copied and transposed into the telomeric expression site, where it becomes active. When an individual is first infected, antibodies are raised against the VSG initially expressed by the trypanosome population. A small number of trypanosomes spontaneously switch their VSG gene to a new type, and although the host antibody eliminates the initial variant, the new variant is unaffected. As the new variant grows, the whole sequence of events is repeated.

Like other intracellular pathogens that reside within phagocytic vesicles, *L. major* requires a type 1 immune response for its eradication. Through mechanisms that are incompletely understood, *L. major* specifically inhibits the production of IL-12 by its macrophage host, thereby inhibiting the production of IFN-γ by NK cells and inhibiting the differentiation and function of T_H1 cells. In addition, *L. major* has been shown to actively induce IL-10–producing T_{reg} cells to suppress clearance of the infection.

13-24 Many viruses target type I and type III interferon pathways to impair host antiviral defense.

Viruses are both the simplest and most diverse of pathogens. They can replicate only within nucleated cells, relying on host cellular machinery to replicate and propagate themselves. As obligate intracellular pathogens, viruses activate receptors that recognize nonmammalian DNA and RNA structures in endosomal vesicles during virus entry into the cell (for example, TLRs 3, 7, 8, and 9) or cytosolic PRRs that detect viral genomic DNA or RNA and their intermediates during viral replication (for example, RIG-I, MDA-5, cGAS, IFI16, and NOD2) (**Fig. 13.25**). While the endosomal TLRs are especially prevalent on innate sensor cells—including dendritic cells, monocyte/macrophages, granulocytes, and barrier epithelial cells—the cytosolic sensors are ubiquitously expressed. Viral recognition directly induces production of type I and type III interferons, which up-regulate cell-intrinsic antiviral **restriction factors** that impair different aspects of viral replication in both infected and uninfected cells. Although the signaling outputs of the type I and type III interferon receptors are nearly identical (see Section 3-22), their cellular distribution differs such that the type I receptor (IFNAR; IFN-α/β) is nearly ubiquitous, whereas the type III receptor (IFNLR; IFN-λ 1, 2, 3, or 4) is restricted to epithelial cells of mucosal barrier tissues, such as the gastrointestinal, respiratory, and urogenital tracts, and to hepatocytes in the liver and neuronal cells.

Although many cell types produce type I interferons, plasmacytoid dendritic cells are specialized for high levels of type I interferon production early in viral infections and, along with NK cells, play a central role in early antiviral host defense before the adaptive response matures. The type I interferons engage multiple arms of adaptive immunity by promoting: differentiation of T_{FH} cells that provide help for production of opsonizing and complement-fixing virus-specific antibodies that block viral entry into uninfected cells and activate complement to destroy enveloped viruses; differentiation of T_H1 cells, which produce type II interferon (IFN-γ) to enhance intracellular interference pathways, MHC class I and class II antigen processing and presentation, and inflammatory responses; and differentiation of cytolytic CD8 T cells, which destroy virally infected cells and also produce IFN-γ.

Viruses have evolved a remarkable diversity of strategies to impair interferon responses. The fact that most viruses devote at least a part of their limited genomes to gene products that target interferon production and/or signaling indicates the importance of this cytokine family in host antiviral defense. Examples of virally encoded proteins that interfere with nearly every step of these pathways have been described (see Fig. 13.25), whether targeting the receptors that recognize them, the signaling pathways that induce interferons, the receptors for interferons, or the signals shared downstream of their receptors that activate target cells to up-regulate cell-intrinsic antiviral actions.

13-25 RNA viruses use different mechanisms of antigenic variation to keep a step ahead of the adaptive immune system.

In addition to the diverse strategies employed by viruses to overcome interferon-induced host defense, some of the strategies used by viruses are specific

Fig. 13.25 The induction of and response to type I interferons are major targets for immune subversion by viruses. Several pattern-recognition receptors that recognize microbial forms of DNA and RNA produced in the course of viral infection and replication activate the production of type I and type III interferons by the infected cell. Heterodimeric receptors for these cytokines (IFNAR1/IFNAR2 or IFNLR1/IL10RB, respectively) are expressed on nearly all cells of the body and activate STAT1 and STAT2 to amplify production of type I and type III interferons and induce expression of restriction factors that block replication of viruses. Shown in the red boxes and the accompanying key are sites in the interferon signaling cascades at which the indicated viruses interfere.

A – Adenovirus	K – HSV-2
B – Dengue virus	L – Influenza A virus
C – Ebola virus	M – KSHV
D – HAV	N – Measles virus
E – HBV	O – Poliovirus
F – HCV	P – Rotavirus
G – HCoV	Q – RSV
H – HIV-1	R – SARS-CoV
I – HPV	S – Sendai virus
J – HSV-1	T – Vaccinia virus

to the type of viral genome. RNA viruses must replicate their genomes using RNA polymerases, which lack the proofreading ability of DNA polymerase. A consequence is that RNA viruses have a greater rate of mutation than DNA viruses, with the practical consequence that RNA viruses cannot support large genomes. However, this also affords them opportunities for rapidly altering antigenic epitopes targeted by the adaptive immune system as a mechanism for immune evasion. Further, some RNA viruses have segmented genomes, which lend themselves to reassortment during viral replication. Both of these mechanisms are used by influenza virus, a common seasonal respiratory pathogen that causes acute infections and has been responsible for several major pandemics. At any one time, a single virus type is responsible for most cases of influenza throughout the world. The human population gradually develops protective immunity to this virus type, chiefly through the production of neutralizing antibody directed against the viral hemagglutinin, the main surface protein of the influenza virus, which is responsible for viral binding to and entry into cells. Because the virus is rapidly cleared from immune individuals, it might be in danger of running out of potential hosts were it not able to use both mutation mechanisms to alter its antigenic type (see Section 12-23 and Fig. 12.45).

The first mutation mechanism, caused by point mutations in the genes encoding the two major viral surface glycoproteins—hemagglutinin and neuraminidase—is called **antigenic drift** (see Section 12-23 and Fig. 12.45). Every 2–3 years a variant flu virus arises with mutations that allow it to evade neutralization by the antibodies present in the population. Other mutations may affect epitopes in viral proteins that are recognized by T cells, particularly cytotoxic CD8 T cells, with the consequence that cells infected with the mutant virus also escape destruction. People immune to the old flu virus are thus susceptible to the new variant, but because the changes in the viral proteins are relatively minor, there is still some cross-reaction with antibodies and memory T cells produced against the previous variant, and most of the population still has some level of immunity. Thus, epidemics resulting from antigenic drift are typically mild.

Antigenic changes in influenza virus that result from reassortment of the eight segments of its RNA genome are known as **antigenic shifts** and result in major changes in the hemagglutinin expressed by the virus (see Section 12-23 and Fig. 12.45). Antigenic shifts result from co-infection of a host cell by two (or more) variants of influenza, often in a nonhuman viral host, such as a bird or a pig—hence the terms avian or swine flu, respectively. Antigenic shift can lead to reassortment of the segmented RNA genome of the human influenza virus and animal influenza viruses in an animal host, in which, for example, the hemagglutinin gene from the animal virus replaces the hemagglutinin gene in the human virus. These new, antigen-shifted viruses have large changes in their surface proteins (for example, hemagglutinin), and therefore T cells and antibodies produced in earlier infections are not protective. Accordingly, new strains that result from antigen shifts can cause severe infection that spreads rapidly and widely, causing the global influenza pandemics that occur every 10–50 years. These pandemics are typically associated with more severe disease, often with substantial mortality, because the new viral proteins are recognized poorly, if at all, by antibodies and T cells directed against the previous variant.

Hepatitis C virus (HCV) is an RNA virus that can cause both acute and chronic infections of the liver. Although complete resolution of HCV may occur in ~20–40% of individuals with acute hepatitis, as is the case for hepatitis B virus, or HBV (a DNA virus), hepatitis C can cause chronic hepatitis, liver cirrhosis, and in some cases hepatocellular carcinoma. HCV is the most common cause of blood-borne chronic infection in the United States and the leading viral cause of liver cirrhosis and liver transplantation. As with influenza virus, HCV has a high capacity for mutation of immune epitopes that allow it to evade elimination. The RNA polymerase that the HCV uses to replicate its genome lacks proofreading capacity. This contributes to a high viral mutation rate that can change viral antigenicity; rapid alteration of T-cell epitopes selects for escape variants of HCV that evade cytolytic T-cell responses. However, unlike influenza, the viral surface glycoprotein responsible for binding of HCV to hepatocytes (E2, which binds CD81) presents a difficult target against which to produce effective neutralizing antibodies, due both to its heavy glycosylation in the region of CD81 binding and its high rate of mutation. Antibody responses against HCV are therefore of limited effectiveness, which has impaired the development of an effective vaccine. Fortunately, new antiviral therapies (direct-acting antivirals, or DAAs) that target multiple steps in the virus life cycle have replaced older interferon-based therapies and now have a cure rate of ~95%.

13-26 DNA viruses use multiple mechanisms to subvert CTL and NK-cell responses.

Of all the pathogens, DNA viruses that can establish chronic infections have evolved the greatest diversity of mechanisms for subverting or escaping immune defenses (**Fig. 13.26**). Unlike RNA viruses, DNA viruses have relatively low mutation rates and are thus less able to employ antigenic variation

Fig. 13.26 Mechanisms used by viruses of the herpes and pox families to subvert the host immune system.

Viral strategy	Specific mechanism	Result	Virus examples
Inhibition of inflammatory response	Viral interference in interferon induction and signaling	Impedes interferon response	HCV, HBV, herpesviruses, adenovirus
	Virally encoded chemokine receptor homolog, e.g., β-chemokine receptor	Sensitizes infected cells to effects of β-chemokine; advantage to virus unknown	Cytomegalovirus
	Virally encoded soluble cytokine receptor, e.g., IL-1 receptor homolog, TNF receptor homolog, interferon-γ receptor homolog	Blocks effects of cytokines by inhibiting their interaction with host receptors	Vaccinia Rabbit myxoma virus
	Viral inhibition of adhesion molecule expression, e.g., LFA-3, ICAM-1	Blocks adhesion of lymphocytes to infected cells	Epstein–Barr virus
	Protection from NFκB activation by short sequences that mimic TLRs	Blocks inflammatory responses elicited by IL-1 or bacterial pathogens	Vaccinia
Blocking of antigen processing and presentation	Inhibition of MHC class I expression	Impairs recognition of infected cells by cytotoxic T cells	Herpes simplex Cytomegalovirus
	Inhibition of peptide transport by TAP	Blocks peptide association with MHC class I	Herpes simplex
Inhibition of humoral immunity	Virally encoded Fc receptor	Blocks effector functions of antibodies bound to infected cells	Herpes simplex Cytomegalovirus
	Virally encoded complement receptor	Blocks complement-mediated effector pathways	Herpes simplex
	Virally encoded complement control protein	Inhibits complement activation by infected cell	Vaccinia
Immunosuppression of host	Virally encoded cytokine homolog of IL-10	Inhibits T_H1 lymphocytes Reduces interferon-γ production	Epstein–Barr virus

to evade immune defenses. However, because their lower rate of mutation allows them to support much larger genomes, these viruses have been able to accommodate a remarkable number of viral genes that encode proteins that can subvert nearly every aspect of antiviral defense. In the case of pox viruses, adenovirus, and especially herpesviruses, large DNA viruses that will be our focus here, more than 50% of the genome can be dedicated to immune evasion-related genes. Further, some of these viruses, particularly the herpesviruses, have evolved mechanisms that allow them to enter a state known as **latency**, in which the virus is not actively replicated. In the latent state, the virus does not cause disease; however, because no viral peptides are produced to load MHC class I molecules that signal the virus's presence to cytolytic T cells, it cannot be eliminated and can establish life-long infections. As we will discuss in Section 13-27, latent infections can be reactivated, resulting in recurrent illness. Of the eight types of herpesviruses that infect humans, at least one of the five most common types—herpes simplex virus (HSV)-1 and HSV-2 (both of which can cause labial and genital herpes), Epstein–Barr virus (EBV; which causes infectious mononucleosis), varicella-zoster virus (which causes chickenpox and shingles), and cytomegalovirus (CMV)—infects nine out of 10 people and typically establishes lifelong latency. Here we highlight major mechanisms by which these viruses succeed.

Central to the long-term survival of the DNA viruses is evasion of CTLs and NK cells. The presentation of viral peptides by MHC class I molecules at a cell surface signals CD8 T cells to kill the infected cell. Many of the large DNA viruses evade immune recognition by producing proteins called **immunoevasins**, which prevent the appearance of viral peptide:MHC class I complexes on the infected cell (**Fig. 13.27**). Indeed, at least one viral inhibitor of every key step in the processing and presentation of peptide:MHC class I complexes has been described. Some immunoevasins block peptide entry into the endoplasmic reticulum (ER) by targeting the TAP transporter (**Fig. 13.28**, top panel). Viral proteins can also prevent peptide:MHC complexes from reaching the cell surface by retaining MHC class I molecules in the ER (Fig. 13.28, middle panel). Several viral proteins catalyze the degradation of newly synthesized MHC class I molecules by a process known as **dislocation**, which initiates the pathway normally used to degrade misfolded ER proteins by directing them back

ANIMATION 13.1

Fig. 13.27 Immunoevasins produced by viruses interfere with the processing of antigens that bind to MHC class I molecules.

Virus	Protein	Category	Mechanism
Herpes simplex virus 1	ICP47	Blocks peptide entry to endoplasmic reticulum	Blocks peptide binding to TAP
Human cytomegalovirus (HCMV)	US6		Inhibits TAP ATPase activity and blocks peptide release into endoplasmic reticulum
Bovine herpesvirus	UL49.5		Inhibits TAP peptide transport
Adenovirus	E19	Retention of MHC class I in endoplasmic reticulum	Competitive inhibitor of tapasin
HCMV	US3		Blocks tapasin function
Murine cytomegalovirus (CMV)	m152		Down-regulation of host MHC class I
HCMV	US2	Degradation of MHC class I (dislocation)	Transports some newly synthesized MHC class I molecules into cytosol
Murine gamma-herpesvirus 68	mK3		E3 ubiquitin ligase activity
Murine CMV	m4	Binds MHC class I at cell surface	Interferes with recognition by cytotoxic lymphocytes by an unknown mechanism

Viral evasins US6 and ICP47 block antigen presentation by preventing peptide movement through the TAP peptide transporter

Adenovirus protein E19 competes with tapasin and inhibits peptide loading onto nascent MHC class I proteins

The mK3 protein of murine γ-herpesvirus is an E3 ubiquitin ligase that targets MHC class I for degradation by the proteasome

Fig. 13.28 The peptide-loading complex in the endoplasmic reticulum is targeted by viral immunoevasins. The top panel shows blockade of peptide entry to the endoplasmic reticulum (ER). The cytosolic ICP47 protein from herpes simplex virus (HSV)-1 prevents peptides from binding to TAP in the cytosol, whereas the US6 protein from human CMV interferes with the ATP-dependent transfer of peptides through TAP. The middle panel shows the retention of MHC class I molecules in the ER by the adenovirus E19 protein. This binds certain MHC molecules and retains them in the ER through an ER-retention motif, at the same time competing with tapasin to prevent association with TAP and peptide loading. The bottom panel shows how the murine gamma-herpesvirus mK3 protein, an E3 ubiquitin ligase, targets newly synthesized MHC class I molecules. mK3 associates with tapasin:TAP complexes and directs the addition of ubiquitin subunits with K48 linkages (see Section 7-5) to the cytoplasmic tail of the MHC class I molecule. The polyubiquitination of the cytoplasmic tail of the MHC class I molecule initiates the process of degradation of the MHC molecule by the proteasomal pathway.

into the cytosol (Fig. 13.28, bottom panel). By preventing the formation of stably assembled and folded peptide:MHC class I complexes, these viral proteins divert the peptide:MHC class I complexes into the ER-associated degradation (ERAD) pathway for disposal. Through these multiple mechanisms, viral factors impair or completely block the presentation of viral peptides to CTLs. The actions of viral inhibitors are not limited to the MHC class I pathway, as viral inhibitors of the MHC class II processing pathway have also been described; these inhibitors ultimately target CD4 T cells. Finally, as many viruses target cells other than dendritic cells, their antigens come to the attention of CD8 T cells via cross-presentation by cDC1 cells. Viral mechanisms that interfere with this pathway are not well understood, although it is known that because the viruses are not required to persist in dendritic cells, the viruses can block recognition and destruction of their cellular hosts even after primed CTL effectors have been generated.

In addition to their role in the acute innate response to viral infection, a major function of NK cells is the recognition and cytolysis of cells that have down-regulated MHC class I molecules to evade detection by CTLs. Accordingly, viruses that target the MHC class I pathway have also evolved mechanisms to repress the cytolytic activity of NK cells. Strategies here include, but are not limited to, expression of viral homologs of MHC class I that engage killer inhibitory receptors (KIRs) and leukocyte inhibitory receptors (LIRs). For example, human CMV produces a homolog of HLA class I called UL18, which binds LIR-1 on NK cells and provides an inhibitory signal that blocks NK-cell cytolysis. Viral products have been defined that also antagonize activating receptors on NK cells, as well as inhibit NK-cell effector pathways.

DNA viruses have evolved mechanisms to subvert additional functions of the immune system. The mechanisms used include the expression of viral homologs of cytokines or chemokines and their receptors, and viral proteins that bind cytokines or their receptors to inhibit their actions (**Fig. 13.29**). Poxviruses (for example, smallpox, vaccinia) in particular have evolved a remarkable array of decoy viral receptors for cytokines and chemokines. As noted previously, because all three types of interferons (types I, II, and III) are major effector cytokines in antiviral defense, diverse viral strategies are centered on the inhibition of this family of cytokines, whether by production of decoy receptors or inhibitory binding proteins, inhibition of JAK–STAT signaling by IFN receptors, inhibition of cytokine transcription, or interference with transcription factors induced by IFNs (see Fig. 13.29). Viral homologs of immunosuppressive cytokines are also produced. CMV and EBV impair antiviral responses by producing homologs of the cytokine IL-10, which down-regulate the production of several pro-inflammatory cytokines by immune cells, including IFN-γ, IL-12 and IL-23, IL-1, IL-6, and TNF-α. This can promote tolerogenic rather than immunogenic adaptive responses to viral antigens. Several viruses also interfere with chemokine responses by producing either decoy chemokine receptors or chemokine homologs that interfere

Fig. 13.29 Poxviruses and herpesviruses target cytokines, chemokines, and their receptors as mechanisms of immune evasion. Shown are examples of virally produced cytokines (upper panel) and chemokines (lower panel) that interfere with a variety of immune activating or repressive pathways to interfere with host defense. In addition to blocking binding of chemokines to their target receptor, each of the viral products shown in the lower panels also blocks the glycosaminoglycan (GAG)-binding domain of the targeted chemokines, thereby preventing chemokine binding to cell surfaces or the extracellular matrix.

with natural ligand-induced signaling through chemokine receptors (see Fig. 13.29). Collectively, herpesviruses and poxviruses produce more than 40 viral homologs of receptors belonging to the seven transmembrane-spanning G protein–coupled chemokine receptor (viral GPCR; vGPCR) superfamily.

13-27 Viruses that establish latency persist in vivo by ceasing to replicate until immunity wanes.

As mentioned in the previous section, a major class of viral agents that cause latent infections in humans are the herpesviruses—large, enveloped DNA viruses characterized by the ability to establish lifelong infections. While we have considered a number of strategies by which these viruses subvert immunity, they have also evolved mechanisms to maintain their genome within the nucleus of infected cells indefinitely without replicating. In contrast to an actively **lytic, or productive, phase** of the viral life cycle, wherein the virus

Primary infection

trigeminal
ganglion

Recurrence of infection

Latent phase

Fig. 13.30 Persistence and reactivation of herpes simplex virus infection. The initial infection in the skin is cleared by an effective immune response, but residual infection persists in sensory neurons such as those of the trigeminal ganglion, whose axons innervate the lips. When the virus is reactivated, usually by some environmental stress and/or alteration in immune status, the skin in the area served by the nerve is reinfected from virus in the ganglion, and a new cold sore results. This process can be repeated many times.

Acute Infectious
Mononucleosis

replicates and lyses its cellular host, a herpesvirus can establish latency, or a **lysogenic phase**, by expression of a small region of its genome called the latency-associated transcript (LAT). LAT encodes factors that repress expression of other viral genes, thereby preventing immune recognition of the viral proteins those genes encode. LAT also interferes with apoptotic death of the host cell, thereby prolonging the cell's life span—and that of the viral genome it harbors. An example is herpes simplex virus (HSV), the cause of cold sores, which infects epithelial cells and then spreads to sensory neurons serving the infected area. An effective immune response controls the epithelial infection, but the virus persists in a latent state in the sensory neurons. Factors such as sunlight, bacterial infection, or hormonal changes reactivate the virus, which then travels down the axons of the sensory neuron and reinfects the epithelial tissues (**Fig. 13.30**). At this point, the immune response again becomes active and controls the local infection by killing the epithelial cells, producing a new sore. This cycle can be repeated many times.

There are two reasons why the sensory neuron remains infected: first, the virus is quiescent and generates few virus-derived peptides to present on MHC class I molecules; second, neurons carry very low levels of MHC class I molecules, which makes it harder for cytotoxic CD8 T cells to recognize infected neurons and attack them. The low level of MHC class I expression is beneficial because it reduces the risk that neurons, which have a limited capacity for regeneration, will be targeted inappropriately by cytotoxic T cells. It does, however, make neurons attractive as cellular reservoirs for persistent infections. Herpesviruses often enter latency: varicella-zoster virus, which causes chickenpox, remains latent in one or a few dorsal root ganglia after the acute illness is over and can be reactivated by stress or immunosuppression. It then spreads down the nerve and reinfects the skin to cause the disease **herpes zoster**, or **shingles**, which is marked by the reappearance of the classic varicella rash in the area of skin served by the infected dorsal root. Unlike herpes simplex virus, which reactivates frequently, varicella-zoster virus usually reactivates only once in a lifetime in an immunocompetent host.

Yet another herpesvirus, the Epstein–Barr virus (EBV), establishes a persistent infection in most individuals. EBV enters latency in B cells after a primary infection that often passes without being diagnosed. In a minority of infected individuals, the initial acute infection of B cells is more severe, causing the disease known as **infectious mononucleosis**, or glandular fever. EBV infects B cells by binding to CR2 (CD21), a component of the B-cell co-receptor complex, and to MHC class II molecules. In the primary infection, most of the infected cells proliferate and produce virus, leading in turn to the proliferation of antigen-specific T cells and the excess of mononuclear white cells in the blood that gives the disease its name. Virus is released from the B cells, destroying them in the process, and virus can be recovered from saliva. The infection is eventually controlled by virus-specific cytotoxic CD8 T cells, which kill the infected proliferating B cells. A fraction of memory B lymphocytes become latently infected, however, and EBV remains quiescent in these cells.

These two forms of infection (subclinical infections and infectious mononucleosis) are accompanied by quite different patterns of expression of viral genes. EBV has a large DNA genome encoding more than 70 proteins. Many of these are required for viral replication and are expressed by the replicating virus, providing a source of viral peptides by which infected cells can be recognized. In a latent infection, the virus survives within the host B cells without replicating, and a very limited set of viral proteins is expressed. One of these is the Epstein–Barr virus nuclear antigen 1 (EBNA-1), which is needed to maintain the viral genome. EBNA-1 interacts with the proteasome (see Section 6-6) to prevent its own degradation into peptides that would otherwise elicit a T-cell response.

Latently infected B cells can be isolated by culturing B cells from individuals who have apparently cleared their EBV infection: in the absence of T cells, latently infected cells retaining the EBV genome become transformed into so-called immortal cell lines, the equivalent of tumorigenesis *in vitro*. Infected B cells occasionally undergo malignant transformation *in vivo*, giving rise to a B-cell lymphoma called Burkitt's lymphoma. In this lymphoma, expression of the peptide transporters TAP-1 and TAP-2 is down-regulated (see Section 6-3), and so cells are unable to process endogenous antigens for presentation on HLA class I molecules (the human MHC class I). This deficiency provides one explanation for how these tumors escape attack by cytotoxic CD8 T cells. Individuals with acquired and inherited immunodeficiencies of T-cell function have an increased risk of developing EBV-associated lymphomas, presumably as a result of a failure of immune surveillance.

13-28 DNA and RNA viruses can induce exhaustion of CTL and NK cell responses, thereby impairing the antiviral response.

In addition to immune-evasion mechanisms, both HCV and HBV, and members of the herpesvirus family (for example, CMV), among others, have been shown to promote chronic infection by inducing 'exhaustion' of antiviral CD8 T cells and NK cells (**Fig. 13.31**). In the case of an inability to completely clear antigen, such as occurs with viruses that can evade immune clearance and/or establish latency, or in the setting of chronic type I IFN signaling, CTLs and NK cells undergo an altered programming that impairs their proliferation and function. Such cells are characterized by their expression of a set of immune checkpoint inhibitory receptors, including CTLA-4, LAG-3, TIM-3, or the programmed death-1 (PD-1) receptor (see Section 7-25), which deliver signals that suppress CTL and NK-cell effector functions when activated by their ligands. It is thought that this mechanism has evolved to restrain immune-mediated damage to host cells. Evidence that immune checkpoint inhibition represents an active mechanism to restrain NK and CD8 T-cell function comes from studies showing that blockade of the PD-L1–PD-1 interaction or CTLA-4 can restore antiviral effector function and decrease viral load. A similar mechanism of immune-cell exhaustion is shared with failed antitumor responses, where effective immune-evasion strategies by malignant cells activate this program in NK and CD8 T cells. New immunotherapies that block these inhibitory pathways (**checkpoint blockade**) are showing considerable promise in the treatment of malignancies (see Section 16-13) and are also being studied for efficacy in treating some chronic viral infections.

Summary.

Infectious agents can cause recurrent or persistent disease by avoiding normal host-defense mechanisms or by subverting these mechanisms to promote their own replication. There are many different ways of evading or subverting

Fig. 13.31 Chronic viral infection can induce exhaustion of CTLs and NK cells. When the immune system is unable to successfully clear a viral infection, chronic stimulation of cytolytic T cells (left panel) and NK cells (right panel) results in the up-regulation of a set of inhibitory receptors that repress activation of the cytolytic machinery of these cells, resulting in impaired antiviral immunity.

the immune response. Antigenic variation, latency, resistance to immune effector mechanisms, and suppression of the immune response all contribute to persistent and medically important infections. In some cases, the immune response is part of the problem: some pathogens use immune activation to spread infection, and others would not cause disease if it were not for the immune response. Each of these mechanisms teaches us something about the nature of the immune response and its weaknesses, and each requires a different medical approach to prevent or to treat infection.

Acquired immune deficiency syndrome.

The most extreme example of immune subversion by a pathogen is the **acquired immune deficiency syndrome (AIDS)** caused by the **human immunodeficiency virus (HIV)**. The disease is characterized by a progressive loss of CD4 T cells, which, when sufficiently depleted, results in high susceptibility to opportunistic infections and certain malignancies. To date, the earliest documented case of HIV infection in humans was identified in a sample of serum from Kinshasa (Democratic Republic of the Congo) that was stored in 1959. It was not until 1981, however, that the first cases of AIDS were officially reported. Because the disease seemed to be spread by contact with body fluids, the cause was suspected to be a new virus, and by 1983 the causative agent, HIV, was isolated and identified.

There are at least two types of HIV—HIV-1 and HIV-2—that are closely related. While both viruses are transmitted by sexual contact and blood-borne exposure (for example, blood transfusion, shared needles), HIV-1 replicates to higher viral loads in blood and is therefore more easily transmitted; HIV-1 has a high rate of transmission from mother to child, which is uncommon in HIV-2. Although in individuals who progress to AIDS, disease is indistinguishable, HIV-1 progresses to AIDS more rapidly and with greater incidence than HIV-2. HIV-1 is therefore by far the most prevalent cause of AIDS worldwide. And while both HIV-1 and HIV-2 are endemic to West Africa, HIV-2 is rarely found elsewhere.

Both HIV-1 and HIV-2 seem to have originally spread to humans from other primate species in Africa. Viral genome sequencing of isolates suggests that the primate precursor of HIV-1, simian immunodeficiency virus (SIV), has passed to humans on at least four independent occasions from chimpanzees or western gorillas, whereas HIV-2 originated in the sooty mangabey (**Fig. 13.32**). The best estimate is that the most prevalent of the four major variants of HIV-1, group M (responsible for ~99% of HIV-1 infections worldwide), was transmitted to humans from chimpanzees in the first half of the 20th

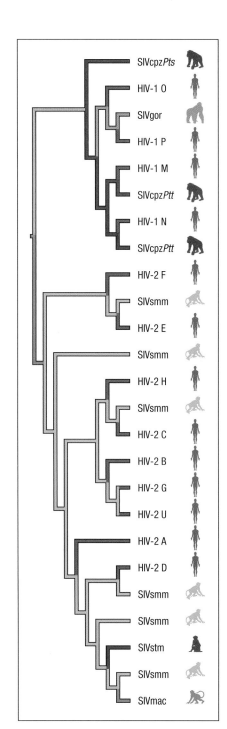

Fig. 13.32 Phylogenetic origins of HIV-1 and HIV-2. HIV-1 shows marked genetic variability and is classified on the basis of genomic sequence into four major groups: M (main), O (outlier), N (non-M, non-O), and P (non-M, non-N, non-O), which are further diversified into subtypes, or clades, that are designated by the letters A to K. In different parts of the world, different subtypes predominate. Phylogenetic analyses of chimpanzee simian immunodeficiency virus (SIVcpz), gorilla SIV (SIVgor), and HIV-1 sequences demonstrate that the four groups of HIV-1 (M, N, O, and P) originated from four independent cross-species transmission events: two transfers of SIVcpz*Ptt* from central chimpanzees (subspecies *Pan troglodytes troglodytes,* or *Ptt*) gave rise to HIV-1 groups M and N, while two transfers of SIVgor from western lowland gorillas (subspecies *Gorilla gorilla gorilla*) gave rise to HIV-1 groups O and P. Similarly, separate zoonotic transmissions of SIVsmm from sooty mangabey monkeys to humans are responsible for at least nine different lineages of HIV-2 (groups A–H and a newly described lineage, U). SIVstm and SIVmac resulted from experimental infections of stump-tailed macaques and rhesus macaques with SIVsmm, respectively. Abbreviations: cpz*Pts*, chimpanzee *Pan troglodytes schweinfurteii;* cpz*Ptt,* chimpanzee *Pan troglodytes troglodytes*; mac, macaque; SIV, simian immunodeficiency virus; smm, sooty mangabey monkey; stm, stump-tailed macaque.

century; transmission of group O also dates to the early 20th century, whereas the two other HIV-1 variants (groups N and P) appear to have been transmitted more recently. As for other zoonotic infections where there has been insufficient time for pathogen and host to coevolve to an equilibrium that attenuates virulence, SIV is generally less pathogenic in its nonhuman primate host than is HIV in its human host. Thus, whereas development of AIDS is nearly universal in HIV-1–infected humans that do not receive treatment, development of AIDS in SIV-infected nonhuman primates is considerably more variable, with some primates failing to develop disease at all, whereas others, such as chimpanzees, do develop AIDS—indicating that they, like humans, were infected by SIV relatively recently.

HIV infection does not immediately cause AIDS. Without treatment, the average time to development of AIDS after infection of adults is several years. The long delay between infection and development of symptomatic immune deficiency reflects the unusual cellular host for viral replication—CD4 T cells, as well as the nature of the immune response to the virus. HIV is now pandemic, and despite great strides made in treatment and prevention that have followed from a greater understanding of the pathogenesis and epidemiology of the disease, almost 690,000 people died of AIDS-related causes in 2020, and an estimated 38 million are infected by HIV worldwide, presaging the death of many from AIDS for years to come (**Fig. 13.33**). In sub-Saharan Africa, which accounts for more than two-thirds of the global incidence, 1 in every 20 adults is infected. Indeed, prior to the development of effective therapies for preventing both the progression of HIV to AIDS and its transmission, HIV/AIDS had become the most deadly single infectious agent in the short time following its identification as a new human pathogen. However, as we will see, despite the elusiveness of a cure for HIV/AIDS or development of an effective vaccine, the success of current therapies in preventing transmission of the virus has resulted in an accelerating decline in the incidence of new cases of HIV infections worldwide since its peak in 1997, and the number of annual deaths from HIV/AIDS has also steadily declined since its peak in the early 2000s. Among the regions with the most rapid declines in incidence of new infections

Fig. 13.33 The incidence of new HIV infection is increasing more slowly in many regions of the world, but AIDS is still a major disease burden. The number of individuals living with HIV/AIDS is large and continues to grow, although the number of new infections in 2020 decreased by more than one-third since the peak of the epidemic. Worldwide, in 2020, it is estimated that there were around 38 million individuals infected with HIV, including some 1.5 million new cases, 160,000 of which were in children. There were approximately 690,000 deaths from AIDS in 2020, a decrease of almost 40% since the peak in 2005. New infections in children have declined almost 70% since 2000, with 160,000 new cases in 2020. (AIDS Epidemic Update, UNAIDS/World Health Organization, 2021.)

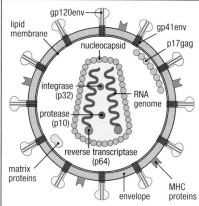

Fig. 13.34 The virion of human immunodeficiency virus (HIV). The virus illustrated is HIV-1, the leading cause of AIDS. The virion is roughly spherical and measures 120 nm in diameter, or about 60 times smaller than the T cells it infects. The HIV envelope protein (Env), which binds the host cell, is composed of a trimer of gp120:gp41 heterodimers. The three viral enzymes that are packaged in the virion—reverse transcriptase, integrase, and protease—are shown schematically in the viral capsid. The p17gag protein is a structural component of the nucleocapsid core of the virus. In reality, many molecules of these enzymes are contained in each virion.

ANIMATION 13.2

is sub-Saharan Africa. Still, there are focal areas of increasing incidence (for example, Eastern Europe and Central Asia).

13-29 HIV is a retrovirus that establishes a chronic infection that slowly progresses to AIDS.

HIV is an enveloped RNA virus whose structure is shown in **Fig. 13.34**. Each virus particle, or virion, is decorated with a trimeric viral envelope protein that is used by the virus to infect target cells and contains two copies of an RNA genome and numerous copies of viral enzymes that are required to establish infection in the cellular host. HIV is an example of a **retrovirus**, so named because the viral genome must be transcribed from RNA into DNA in the infected cell—the reverse (*retro*) of the usual pattern of transcription—by the viral **reverse transcriptase** enzyme. This generates a DNA intermediate that is integrated into the host-cell chromosomes to enable viral replication. RNA transcripts produced from the integrated viral DNA serve both as mRNAs to direct the synthesis of viral proteins and later as the RNA genomes of new viral particles. These escape from the cell by budding from the plasma membrane, each enclosed in a membrane envelope.

HIV belongs to a group of retroviruses called the **lentiviruses**, from the Latin *lentus*, meaning 'slow,' because of the gradual course of the diseases that they cause. These viruses persist and continue to replicate for many years before causing overt signs of disease. In the case of HIV, the virus targets cells of the immune system itself, producing an initial acute infection that is often associated with symptoms initially but is then controlled to the point that infection is not apparent—but rarely leading to an immune response that can prevent ongoing replication of the virus. Thus, although the initial acute infection does seem to be controlled by the immune system, HIV establishes latency within cells of the immune system and replicates periodically to infect new cells for many years. As will be discussed later, this ultimately depletes key cells of the immune system—particularly CD4 T cells, resulting in immune deficiency, or AIDS, which leads to opportunistic infections and/or malignancy that cause death.

13-30 HIV infects and replicates within cells of the immune system.

A defining characteristic of HIV is its ability to infect and replicate within cells of the immune system. Three immune cell types are the primary targets of HIV uptake: CD4 T cells, macrophages, and dendritic cells. And while it is clear that macrophages and dendritic cells can pass the virus on to other cells, it remains controversial whether these cells support viral replication. In any case, CD4 T cells support the great majority of viral replication.

HIV's ability to enter particular cell types, known as its cellular **tropism**, is determined by the expression of specific receptors for the virus on the surface of those cells. HIV enters cells by means of its envelope (Env) protein, a complex of two noncovalently associated viral glycoproteins, gp120 and gp41, which form trimers that are embedded in the viral membrane (see Fig. 13.34 and also Fig. 13.36 later). The gp120 subunits of trimeric gp120:gp41 complexes bind with high affinity to the cell-surface molecule CD4, which is expressed on CD4 T cells, and to a lesser extent on subsets of dendritic cells and macrophages. Before fusion and entry of the virus, gp120 must also bind a co-receptor on the host cell. The major co-receptors are the chemokine receptors CCR5 and CXCR4 (**Fig. 13.35**). While CCR5 is predominantly expressed on subsets of effector memory (T_{EM} and T_{RM}) CD4 T cells, dendritic cells, and macrophages, CXCR4 is expressed primarily by naive and central memory (T_{CM}) CD4 T cells. After initial binding to CD4, gp120 undergoes a conformational change that

Fig. 13.35 HIV virions target different co-receptors expressed by distinct cell targets. In addition to the CD4 molecule, HIV virions must bind a chemokine co-receptor to initiate viral entry and infection. HIV virions that bind the CCR5 chemokine receptor (so-called R5 variants) target effector memory (T$_{EM}$) and resident memory (T$_{RM}$) CD4 T cells, as well as dendritic cells and macrophages (hence, 'M-tropic')—all of which express the CCR5 co-receptor. R5 variants of HIV are thought to represent the major population of virus that establishes initial infection. HIV virions that bind the CXCR4 chemokine receptor (so-called X4 variants) target naive and central memory (T$_{CM}$) CD4 T cells. X4 variants of HIV emerge after initial infection to expand the pool of T-cell targets within the T-cell repertoire. The photographic image (bottom panel) shows a pseudocolored scanning electron micrograph of HIV virions (yellow) infecting a CD4 T cell (blue).

R5 virus (M-tropic)

X4 virus (T-tropic)

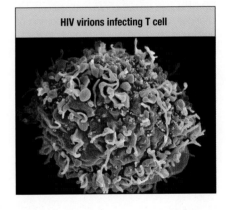

HIV virions infecting T cell

exposes a high-affinity site that is bound by the co-receptor (**Fig. 13.36**). This, in turn, causes gp41 to refold and insert a portion of its structure (fusion peptide) into the plasma membrane of the target cell, inducing fusion of the viral envelope with the cell's plasma membrane. This allows the viral nucleocapsid, composed of the viral genome and associated viral proteins, to enter the host-cell cytoplasm (**Fig. 13.37**). As will be discussed later, the particular chemokine co-receptor bound by a given viral particle is of importance in the transmission of HIV between individuals and its propagation within an infected person.

Once the virus has entered cells, it replicates similarly to other retroviruses. Reverse transcriptase transcribes the viral RNA into a complementary DNA (cDNA) copy. The viral cDNA, which encodes nine genes (**Fig. 13.38**), is then integrated into the host-cell genome by viral integrase, which recognizes and partially cleaves repetitive DNA sequences, called long terminal repeats (LTRs), that reside at each end of the viral genome. LTRs are required for the integration of the provirus into the host-cell DNA and contain binding sites for gene-regulatory proteins that control expression of the viral genes. The integrated cDNA copy is known as the **provirus**.

Like the genomes of other retroviruses, the HIV genome is small, with three major genes—*gag*, *pol*, and *env*. The gene *gag* encodes the structural proteins of the viral nucleocapsid core, *pol* encodes the enzymes involved in viral replication, and *env* encodes the viral envelope glycoproteins (see Fig. 13.38). The *gag* and *pol* mRNAs are translated to give polyproteins—long polypeptide chains that are then cleaved by the **viral protease** (encoded by *pol*) into individual functional proteins. Thus, *pol* alone encodes the three major enzymes that are required for viral replication: reverse transcriptase, integrase, and viral protease. The product of the *env* gene, gp160, has to be cleaved by a host-cell protease into gp120 and gp41, which are then assembled as trimers in the viral envelope. HIV has six other, smaller, regulatory genes encoding proteins that affect viral replication and infectivity in various ways. Two of these, Tat and Rev, perform regulatory functions that are essential early in the viral replication cycle. The remaining four—Nef, Vif, Vpr, and Vpu—are essential for efficient virus production *in vivo*.

HIV can complete its replication cycle in the host cell to produce progeny virus, or, like other retroviruses and herpesviruses, establish a latent infection in which the provirus remains quiescent. What determines whether infection of a cell results in latency or a productive infection is unclear, but it is thought to be related to the activation state of the cell infected. As we will discuss in the next section, transcription of the provirus after integration is initiated by host transcription factors, which are induced by immune-cell activation. Thus, infection of a cell that becomes dormant soon after infection might favor viral latency, whereas infection of activated cells favors productive viral replication. This has important consequences in the case of CD4 T cells, which, unlike macrophages and dendritic cells, are very long-lived and can provide a reservoir of latent HIV provirus that can be activated when the T cells are reactivated, even years after initial infection. Because macrophages and dendritic cells in tissues are short-lived cells that do not divide, latency in these host cells would be short-lived. Thus, long-lived latency of HIV is primarily a consequence of the tropism of the virus for CD4 T cells. The combined features of tropism for CD4

Fig. 13.36 Structural basis for binding of the HIV envelope gp120:gp41 trimer to CD4 and co-receptors. The ability of HIV to infect host cells requires sequential interactions between the viral envelope (Env) protein and CD4 and the CCR5 or CXCR4 co-receptors of the host. Shown are cryo-electron microscopy (cryo-EM) solved structures of the HIV Env trimer, composed of three heterodimers of gp120 (gray structures) and gp41 (red structures). Prior to binding CD4 on the host-cell surface (left panel), the HIV Env trimer is in a 'closed' conformation, with variable sequence loops (V1 and V2, purple; and V3, blue) arranged on the apical surface in a manner that occludes the co-receptor binding site for CCR5 or CXCR4. Upon binding of CD4 to its binding site on gp120 (orange patches), gp120 undergoes conformational changes that lead to an 'open' conformation (right panel) that results from peripheralization of the variable loops to expose co-receptor binding sites (highlighted by light gray ovals), allowing binding to CCR5 or CXCR4. Repositioning of gp120 domains induced by CD4 binding also relieves constraints on gp41 that results in the refolding of the gp41 subunit and exposure of its fusogenic domain. Current structural studies support a model in which co-receptor binding stabilizes CD4-induced gp120 conformational changes to expose the fusogenic domain of gp41 and bring it in close proximity to the target membrane to induce fusion.

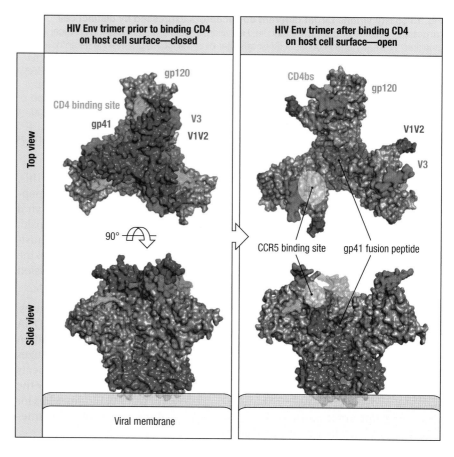

T cells and activation-dependent transcription of the provirus are central to the pathogenesis of HIV and its characteristic progressive depletion of CD4 T cells that leads to AIDS.

13-31 Activated CD4 T cells are the major source of HIV replication.

HIV provirus requires activation of the host cell to complete its replication cycle and produce infectious virions that can infect other cells. This is due to a requirement for transactivation of proviral gene expression by transcription factors of the host cell. Two host transcription factors can initiate transcription of the viral genome: NFκB and nuclear factor of activated T cells (NFAT). Both of these factors require cellular activation for their translocation to the nucleus, where they bind DNA and induce gene transcription (see Sections 7-14 and 7-16). While NFκB is expressed in all of the immune cells infected by HIV, NFAT is primarily activated in CD4 T cells, enabling transactivation of the provirus by an additional factor in this cell host. This, coupled with the fact that CD4 T cells are long-lived and more abundant in immune tissues, contributes to CD4 T cells being the major cellular source for HIV replication. Here we consider the mechanism by which transcription of the HIV provirus is regulated in CD4 T cells.

As discussed in Sections 7-14 and 7-16, activation of T cells by antigen induces activation and nuclear translocation of NFAT and NFκB; activation of effector memory T cells by cytokines can also activate NFκB in the absence of antigen (see Fig. 13.37). Thus, in addition to antigen-dependent activation of HIV provirus transcription by NFAT and NFκB , provirus might be activated independently of TCR stimulation in memory CD4 T cells via NFκB alone, as it is in infected macrophages and dendritic cells. Binding of NFAT and NFκB initiates transcription of viral RNA by binding to promoters in the proviral LTR. The viral transcript is spliced in various ways to produce mRNAs for translation of viral proteins (see Fig. 13.38).

Fig. 13.37 The life cycle of HIV. Top row: The virus binds to CD4 using gp120, which is altered by CD4 binding so that it now also binds a chemokine receptor that acts as a co-receptor for viral entry. This binding releases gp41, which causes fusion of the viral envelope with the cell membrane and release of the viral core into the cytoplasm. Once in the cytoplasm, the viral core releases the RNA genome, which is reverse-transcribed into double-stranded complementary DNA (cDNA) using the viral reverse transcriptase. The double-stranded cDNA migrates to the nucleus in association with the viral integrase and the Vpr protein and is integrated into the cell genome, becoming a provirus. Bottom row: Activation of CD4 T cells induces the expression of the transcription factors NFκB and NFAT, which bind to the proviral long terminal repeat (LTR) and initiate transcription of the HIV genome. The first viral transcripts are extensively processed, producing spliced mRNAs encoding several regulatory proteins, including Tat and Rev. Tat both enhances transcription from the provirus and binds to the RNA transcripts, stabilizing them in a form that can be translated. Rev binds the RNA transcripts and transports them to the cytosol. As levels of Rev increase, less extensively spliced and unspliced viral transcripts are transported out of the nucleus. The singly spliced and unspliced transcripts encode the structural proteins of the virus, and unspliced transcripts, which are also the new viral genomes, are packaged with these proteins to form many new virus particles.

At least two of the viral proteins—Tat and Rev—serve to enhance production of the viral genome (see Fig. 13.37). Tat binds to a transcriptional activation region (TAR) in the 5′ LTR. This recruits cellular cyclin T1 and its partner, cyclin-dependent kinase 9 (CDK9), to form a complex that phosphorylates RNA polymerase and enhances its ability to generate full-length transcripts

Fig. 13.38 The genomic organization of HIV. Like all retroviruses, HIV-1 has an RNA genome flanked by long terminal repeats (LTRs) involved in viral integration and in regulation of transcription of the viral genome. The genome can be read in three frames, and several of the viral genes overlap in different reading frames. This allows the virus to encode many proteins in a small genome. The three main protein products—Gag, Pol, and Env—are synthesized by all infectious retroviruses. The known functions of the different genes and their products are listed. The products of *gag, pol,* and *env* are known to be present in the mature viral particle, together with the viral RNA. The mRNAs for Tat, Rev, and Nef proteins are produced by splicing of viral transcripts, so their genes are split in the viral genome. In the case of Nef, only one exon, shown in yellow, is translated.

Gene		Gene product/function
gag	Group-specific antigen	Core proteins and matrix proteins
pol	Polymerase	Reverse transcriptase, protease, and integrase enzymes
env	Envelope	Transmembrane glycoproteins. gp120 binds CD4 and CCR5; gp41 is required for virus fusion and internalization
tat	Transactivator	Positive regulator of transcription
rev	Regulator of viral expression	Allows export of unspliced and partially spliced transcripts from nucleus
vif	Viral infectivity	Affects particle infectivity
vpr	Viral protein R	Transport of DNA to nucleus. Augments virion production. Cell-cycle arrest
vpu	Viral protein U	Promotes intracellular degradation of CD4 and enhances release of virus from cell membrane
nef	Negative-regulation factor	Augments viral replication *in vivo* and *in vitro*. Decreases CD4, MHC class I and II expression

of the viral genome. In this way, Tat provides a positive feedback circuit for rapid amplification of productive viral replication. Rev is important for shuttling unspliced viral RNA transcripts out of the nucleus by binding to a specific viral RNA sequence, the Rev response element (RRE). Eukaryotic cells have mechanisms to prevent the export of incompletely spliced mRNA transcripts from the nucleus. This could pose a problem for the retrovirus, which is dependent on export of unspliced mRNA species that encode the full complement of viral proteins, as well as the viral RNA genome. While export of a fully spliced mRNA transcript that encodes Tat and Rev occurs early after viral infection by means of the normal host cellular mechanisms of mRNA export, the export of later, unspliced viral transcripts requires Rev to prevent their destruction by the host cell.

The success of viral replication also depends on the proteins Nef, Vif, Vpu, and Vpr. These viral products appear to have evolved to defeat host immune mechanisms of viral clearance, as well as antiviral restriction factors—host cellular proteins that function in a cell-autonomous manner to inhibit replication of retroviruses. Nef (negative-regulation factor) performs multiple critical functions in the viral life cycle. It acts early in the viral life cycle to sustain T-cell activation and the establishment of a persistent state of HIV infection, in part by lowering the threshold for T-cell receptor signaling and down-regulating expression of the inhibitory co-stimulatory receptor CTLA-4. Combined, these actions result in a greater and more sustained T-cell activation that promotes viral replication. Nef also contributes to immune evasion of infected cells by down-regulating expression of MHC class I and class II molecules, making actively infected cells less likely to induce an antiviral immune response or be killed by cytotoxic T cells. In addition, Nef promotes the clearance of surface CD4 molecules, which otherwise would bind to the virion during budding and interfere with virion release. Vif (viral infectivity factor) acts to overcome a cytidine deaminase called APOBEC, which catalyzes the conversion of deoxycytidine to deoxyuridine in reverse-transcribed viral cDNA, thereby destroying its ability to encode viral proteins. Vpu (viral protein U) is unique to HIV-1 and variants of SIV and is required to overcome a cellular factor called tetherin, which inserts into both the plasma membrane of the host cell and the envelope of the mature virion to block its release. The function of Vpr (viral protein R) is not fully understood, but it may target the restriction factor SAMHD1, a cellular protein that inhibits HIV-1 infection by limiting the intracellular pool of deoxynucleoside triphosphate (dNTP) molecules available for viral cDNA synthesis by reverse transcriptase.

13-32 There are several routes by which HIV is transmitted and establishes infection.

Infection with HIV occurs after the transfer of body fluids from an infected person to an uninfected one. HIV infection is most commonly spread by sexual intercourse. Transmission by the exchange of contaminated needles used for intravenous drug delivery or by the therapeutic use of infected blood or blood products also occurs, although the latter route of transmission has largely been eliminated in countries where blood products are routinely screened for HIV. An important route of virus transmission is from an infected mother to child, which can occur *in utero*, during birth, or through breast milk. Rates of transmission from an untreated infected mother to her child vary (from about 15 to 45%), depending on the viral load in the mother and whether the mother breast-feeds the child, as breast-feeding increases the risk of transmission. The use of antiretroviral drugs to decrease maternal viral load during pregnancy dramatically reduces the transmission rate to the child (see Section 13-41).

The virus can be transmitted as free infectious particles or via infected cells for which the virus has tropism (for example, CD4 T cells and dendritic cells). Infected cells are found in blood, but can also be present in semen or vaginal secretions, as well as breast milk; free virus is present in blood, semen, vaginal fluid, or mother's milk. As we discuss in the next section, HIV virions can differentially express gp120 variants that bind either CCR5 or CXCR4, thereby influencing the cell types infected. In the genital and gastrointestinal mucosae, which are the dominant sites of primary infection by sexual transmission, HIV virions establish infection initially in a small number of mucosal immune cells that express CCR5—effector memory CD4 T cells, dendritic cells, and macrophages (see Fig. 13.35). The virus replicates locally in these cells before spreading via T cells or dendritic cells (mucosal macrophages are nonmigratory) to lymph nodes draining the mucosa. The lymphoid compartment of mucosal tissues is enriched for T_H1 and T_H17 cells, which express CCR5 (naive T cells and T_H2 cells do not), so initial viral replication is favored in these subsets of CD4 T cells. After accelerated replication in regional lymph nodes, where there is a high concentration of CD4 T cells, the virus disseminates widely via the bloodstream and gains broader access to the gut-associated lymphoid tissue (GALT), where the highest number of CD4 T cells in the body reside.

13-33 HIV variants with tropism for different co-receptors play different roles in transmission and progression of disease.

To establish infection in a new host, the HIV virion must contact a CD4-expressing immune cell. The cell type targeted is determined by the affinity of the virion's gp120 variant for the different chemokine co-receptors: CCR5 or CXCR4. Accordingly, the two major tropism variants of HIV are referred to as R5 and X4, respectively (see Fig. 13.35). Because CCR5 dominates on CD4-expressing immune cells resident at the major sites of viral transmission—sites that are constantly exposed to commensal microbes and thus harbor large numbers of activated immune cells (mucosal tissues of the female and male genital tracts or rectum for sexual transmission; upper gastrointestinal tract for

Fig. 13.39 Dendritic cells can initiate infection by transporting HIV from mucosal surfaces to lymphoid tissue. HIV adheres to the surface of intraepithelial dendritic cells by the binding of viral gp120 to DC-SIGN (left panel). It gains access to dendritic cells at sites of mucosal injury or possibly to dendritic cells that have protruded between epithelial cells to sample the external world; HIV can also bind directly to some epithelial cells and is transported across them to subepithelial dendritic cells (not shown). Dendritic cells internalize HIV virions into mildly acidic early endosomes and migrate to lymphoid tissue (center panel). HIV virions are translocated back to the cell surface, and when the dendritic cell encounters CD4 T cells in a secondary lymphoid tissue, the HIV is transferred to the T cell (right panel).

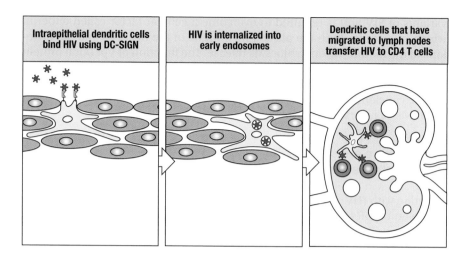

mother-to-child transmission)—CCR5-tropic, R5 strains of virus are typically required for transmission and dominate early in infection.

Before HIV can contact CD4-expressing immune cells in the genital and intestinal mucosae, it must traverse the epithelium of these tissues. Here, the CCR5-tropic variants of the virus also have an advantage. Infection occurs across two types of epithelium: the stratified, or multilayered, squamous epithelium that lines the mucosae of the vagina, foreskin of the penis, ectocervix, oropharynx, and esophagus; or the single-layered columnar epithelium lining the endocervix, rectum, and upper GI tract. Epithelial cells of the rectum and endocervix can express CCR5 and have been shown to selectively translocate R5, but not X4, HIV variants through the epithelial monolayer. Other molecules expressed by epithelial cells also participate; gp120-binding glycosphingolipids expressed by epithelial cells of the vaginal or ectocervical mucosae also foster transcytosis of virus across the epithelium. The rate at which virus can cross epithelial barriers to establish infection is fast. SIV virus has been shown to penetrate the cervicovaginal epithelium within 30–60 minutes of exposure.

In addition to direct transcytosis across epithelial cells, the interdigitating processes of dendritic cells that ramify between epithelial cells provide an avenue for HIV to traverse the epithelium. A complex ferrying mechanism seems to transfer HIV picked up by dendritic cells to CD4 T cells in lymphoid tissue. HIV can attach to dendritic cells by the binding of viral gp120 to C-type lectin receptors such as langerin (CD207), the mannose receptor (CD206), and DC-SIGN. A portion of the bound virus is rapidly taken up into vacuoles, where it can remain for days in an infectious state. In this way the virus is protected and remains stable until it encounters a susceptible CD4 T cell, whether in the local mucosal environment or after being carried to draining lymphoid tissue (**Fig. 13.39**). Finally, at some mucosal sites, CCR5-expressing CD4 T cells reside within the epithelium (intraepithelial T cells) and have been shown to be sites of early viral replication. Thus, HIV can infect CD4 T cells either directly or via dendritic cells that interact with CD4 T cells.

During the **acute phase** of infection, which typically lasts for several weeks and is characterized by an influenza-like illness in about half of those infected (the rest remaining asymptomatic), there is rapid replication of the virus, primarily in CCR5-expressing CD4 T cells (**Fig. 13.40**). This period is marked by an abundance of virus circulating in the blood (viremia) and the rapid decline of CCR5-expressing CD4 T cells, the latter due primarily to the extensive death of CD4 T cells in the GALT that are killed by viral cytopathic effects (macrophages and dendritic cells appear more resistant to lysis by replicating virus). The depletion of immune cells in the gut might compound the rapid production of virus in the GALT by fostering increased immune-cell activation because of barrier breakdown and translocation of constituents of the microbiota. Because of

Fig. 13.40 The typical course of untreated infection with HIV.
The first few weeks are typified by an acute influenza-like viral illness, sometimes called seroconversion disease, with high titers of virus in the blood. An adaptive immune response follows, which controls the acute illness and largely restores levels of CD4 T cells but does not eradicate the virus. This is the asymptomatic phase, which typically lasts 5–10 years without treatment. Opportunistic infections and other symptoms become more frequent as the CD4 T-cell count in peripheral blood falls, beginning at about 500 cells μl^{-1}. The disease then enters the symptomatic phase. When CD4 T-cell counts fall below 200 cells μl^{-1}, the individual is said to have AIDS. Note that CD4 T-cell counts are measured for clinical purposes in cells per microliter (cells μl^{-1}), rather than cells per milliliter (cells ml^{-1}), the unit used elsewhere in this book.

the high viral titers and preponderance of R5 strains during the acute phase of infection, the risk of viral transmission to uninfected contacts during this time is especially high.

The acute phase and its high viremia reside in virtually all individuals once an adaptive immune response is established (see Fig. 13.40). Cytolytic CD8 T cells specific for viral antigens develop and kill HIV-infected cells, and virus-specific antibodies become detectable in the serum of those infected (**seroconversion**). The development of a CTL response results in early control of the virus, resulting in a sharp drop in viral titers and a rebound of CD4 T-cell counts. The level of virus that persists in blood plasma at this stage of infection, referred to as the **viral set point**, is usually a good indicator of future disease progression. At this point, the disease transitions to a clinically latent phase, or **asymptomatic phase**, marked by low viremia and slowly declining CD4 T-cell numbers, typically over several years. During this time the virus continues to actively replicate, but it is held in check, principally by HIV-specific CD8 T cells and antibodies.

Under strong selective pressure brought by the antiviral antibody response, there is selection for HIV **escape mutants** that express altered envelope variants no longer neutralized by existing anti-envelope antibodies. This gives rise to many different viral variants in a single infection and to even broader variation within the population as a whole. Late in infection, in approximately 50% of cases, the dominant viral type switches from R5 to X4 variants that infect T cells via CXCR4 co-receptors. This is followed by a rapid decline in CD4 T-cell count and progression to AIDS. The exact mechanism by which this shift in viral tropism leads to accelerated loss of CD4 T cells is not completely understood, although the expression of the CXCR4 co-receptor by both naive and memory CD4 T cells may play a role by expanding the pool of HIV-susceptible T cells. On balance, then, R5 variants appear critical for transmission of the virus from infected to uninfected individuals, whereas X4 variants that emerge under selective pressure exerted by the antiviral immune response contribute to the progression of disease within an infected individual.

13-34 A genetic deficiency of the co-receptor CCR5 confers resistance to HIV infection.

Evidence for the importance of CCR5 in transmission of HIV infection has come from studies of individuals with a high risk of exposure to HIV-1 who remain seronegative. Lymphocytes and macrophages from these individuals are highly resistant to HIV infection in cultures inoculated with HIV. The resistance of these individuals to HIV infection is explained by the discovery that they are homozygous for a nonfunctional variant of CCR5, called Δ32, caused by a 32-base-pair deletion from the coding region that leads to a frameshift mutation and a truncated protein. The frequency of this mutant allele in Caucasians is high at 0.09 (that is, about 10% of members of this population are heterozygous carriers of the allele and about 1% are homozygous). The mutant allele has not been found in Japanese or in black Africans from Western or Central Africa. Whether heterozygous deficiency of CCR5 provides some protection against infection by HIV is controversial, but it appears to contribute to a modest, if any, reduction in progression rates. In addition to the structural polymorphism of the gene, variations in the promoter region of the CCR5 gene have been associated with different rates of disease progression. The high incidence of the *CCR5Δ32* allele in Caucasians predating the HIV pandemic suggests selection for this variant in a past epidemic. Both smallpox and bubonic plagues have been put forward as possible selective agents, but this is as yet unproven.

13-35 An immune response controls but does not eliminate HIV.

Infection with HIV generates an immune response that contains the virus but only very rarely, if ever, eliminates it. A time course of the response of various adaptive immune elements to HIV in adults is shown in **Fig. 13.41**, together with the levels of infectious virus in plasma. As was noted earlier, in the acute phase, virus-mediated cytopathicity results in a substantial depletion of CD4 T cells, particularly in mucosal tissues. There is a good initial recovery of T-cell numbers outside mucosal tissues and transition to the asymptomatic phase of disease as the immune response develops and curbs viral replication (see Fig. 13.40). However, replication of the virus persists and, after a variable period lasting from a few months to more than 20 years, the CD4 T-cell numbers fall too low to maintain effective immunity, and AIDS develops (defined as less than 200 CD4 T cells per microliter in peripheral blood) (see Fig. 13.40). Several factors conspire to progressively deplete CD4 T cells until they can no longer maintain immunity: destruction by cytotoxic lymphocytes directed against HIV-infected cells, immune activation (direct and indirect) that induces activation of latent virus, ongoing viral cytopathic effects, and insufficient T-cell regeneration in the thymus. In this section we consider the roles of cytotoxic

Fig. 13.41 The immune response to HIV. Infectious virus is present at relatively low levels in the peripheral blood of infected individuals during a prolonged asymptomatic phase, during which the virus is replicated persistently in lymphoid tissues. During this period, CD4 T-cell counts gradually decline (see Fig. 13.40), although antibodies and cytotoxic CD8 T cells directed against the virus remain at high levels. Two different antibody responses are shown in the figure, one to the envelope protein (Env) of HIV, and one to the core protein p24. Eventually, the levels of antibody and HIV-specific cytotoxic T lymphocytes (CTLs) also decline, and there is a progressive increase in infectious HIV in the peripheral blood.

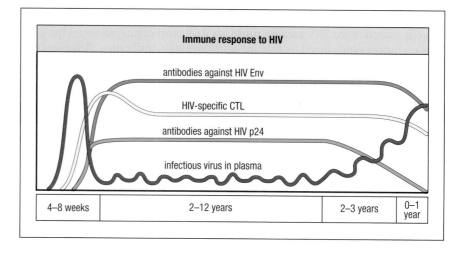

Immune response to HIV

antibodies against HIV Env

HIV-specific CTL

antibodies against HIV p24

infectious virus in plasma

| 4–8 weeks | 2–12 years | 2–3 years | 0–1 year |

CD8 T cells, CD4 T cells, antibodies, and other immune factors in mounting the immune response to HIV infection that initially contains the infection, but ultimately fails.

Studies of peripheral blood cells from infected individuals reveal cytotoxic T cells specific for viral peptides that can kill infected cells *in vitro*. *In vivo*, cytotoxic T cells are recruited to sites of HIV replication, where they are thought to kill many productively infected cells before any infectious virus is released, thereby containing viral load at the quasi-stable levels that are characteristic of the asymptomatic period. Evidence for the clinical importance of the control of HIV-infected cells by cytotoxic CD8 T cells comes from studies relating the numbers and activity of CD8 T cells to viral load. There is also direct evidence from experiments in macaques infected with SIV that cytotoxic CD8 T cells control retrovirus-infected cells; treatment of infected animals with monoclonal antibodies that remove CD8 T cells is rapidly followed by a large increase in viral load.

In addition to direct cytotoxicity mediated by recognition of cells infected with virus, a variety of factors produced by CD4, CD8, and NK cells are important in antiviral immunity. Chemokines that bind CCR5, such as CCL5, CCL3, and CCL4, are released at the site of infection by CD8 T cells and inhibit virus spread by competing with R5 strains of HIV-1 for the engagement of co-receptor CCR5, whereas CXCL12 can compete with R4 strains for binding to CXCR4. Cytokines such as IFN-α and IFN-γ may also be involved in controlling virus spread.

Evidence shows that in addition to being a major target for HIV infection, CD4 T cells also have an important role in the host response to HIV-infected cells. An inverse correlation is found between the strength of CD4 T-cell proliferative responses to HIV antigen and viral load. In addition, the type of effector CD4 T-cell response mounted against the virus appears to be important. There is an inverse correlation with viral load and control of acute infection in individuals whose CD4 T cells express greater T_H1 type activity, including production of IFN-γ and granzyme B. Like CD8 T cells, HIV-specific T_H1 cells can have lytic activity that contributes to clearance of HIV-infected targets. Moreover, CD4 T cells from individuals who do not progress to AIDS long after infection by HIV show strong antiviral proliferative responses. Finally, early treatment of acutely infected individuals with antiretroviral drugs is associated with a recovery in CD4 proliferative responses to HIV antigens. If antiretroviral therapy is stopped, the CD4 responses persist in some of these individuals and are associated with reduced levels of viremia. However, infection continues to persist in these individuals, and immunological control of the infection will ultimately fail. If CD4 T-cell responses are essential for the control of HIV infection, then the fact that HIV is tropic for these cells and kills them may explain the inability of the host immune response to control the infection in the long term.

Antibodies against HIV proteins are generated early in the course of infection, but, like T cells, are ultimately unable to clear the virus. As for viral T-cell epitopes, the virus shows a high capacity for generating escape mutants under the selective pressure of the antibody response. Two aspects of the antibody response appear to be important: (1) generating neutralizing antibodies against gp120 and gp41 envelope viral antigens in order to block viral attachment or entry into CD4-positive target cells, and (2) generating non-neutralizing antibodies that, like some neutralizing antibodies, target infected cells for antibody-dependent cell-mediated cytotoxicity (ADCC). Although neutralizing antibodies are eventually produced in nearly all who are HIV-infected, the relative inaccessibility of viral epitopes on the gp120 protein that bind CD4 and chemokine co-receptors (see Fig. 13.36) hampers the development of such antibodies for a prolonged period (typically months); this buys the virus time to generate escape mutants before the neutralizing antibodies can be produced. Indeed, the generation of so-called **broadly neutralizing antibodies**, which can block infection by multiple viral strains, is typically found in those with high viral titers, emphasizing the fact that these antibodies cannot significantly modify established disease. Analyses of effective neutralizing antibodies to HIV indicate that they have undergone extensive somatic hypermutation that is rarely induced before the first year after infection. Nevertheless, analysis of these antibodies has identified a number of 'vulnerable' sites on the HIV gp120:gp41 envelope trimer that interfere with viral attachment and entry into target cells. The passive administration of some broadly neutralizing antibodies against HIV can protect experimental animals from mucosal infection by HIV, offering hope that a vaccine that can induce broadly neutralizing antibodies might be developed that could prevent new infections.

In contrast to neutralizing antibodies, which develop late in infection and appear to play a modest role in restraining viral replication, there is growing evidence that non-neutralizing antibodies that recruit ADCC by NK cells, macrophages, and neutrophils develop early in infections and are important in restraining viral replication in concert with the actions of cytolytic CD8 T cells. Again, however, the high rate of mutability of the virus allows it to stay a step ahead and persist. The mutations that occur as HIV replicates can allow resulting virus variants to escape recognition by CTLs or antibodies and are important in contributing to the long-term failure of the immune system to contain the infection. An immune response is often dominated by T or B cells specific for particular epitopes—**immunodominant** epitopes—and mutations in immunodominant HIV peptides presented by MHC class I molecules have been found, as have mutations in the epitopes targeted by neutralizing and non-neutralizing antibodies. Mutant peptides have been found to inhibit T cells responsive to the wild-type epitope, thus allowing both the mutant and wild-type viruses to survive.

While the immune response to HIV is ultimately unsuccessful, its importance in restraining disease progression is clear. This is perhaps best exemplified in the tragic case of children infected with HIV perinatally, in whom the course of disease is much more fulminant than in adults. This reflects a poor immune response to the virus in the acute phase of infection due to immaturity of the neonatal immune system, as well as infection by a viral strain that has already evaded an immune system that is genetically close to that of the child. In essence, the poor immune response results in the lack of a latent phase, leading rapidly to AIDS.

13-36 Lymphoid tissue is the major reservoir of HIV infection.

In view of the active, ongoing immune response to HIV infections and the advent of antiretroviral therapies that efficiently blunt viral replication (see Section 13-39), it is important to identify the reservoirs that allow the virus to persist. Although HIV load and turnover are usually measured in terms of the RNA present in virions in the blood, the major reservoir of HIV infection appears to be lymphoid tissue. Here, in addition to infected CD4 T cells, macrophages, and dendritic cells, HIV is also trapped in the form of immune complexes on the surface of follicular dendritic cells in germinal centers. These cells are not themselves infected but may act as a reservoir of infective virions that can persist for months, if not longer. Although tissue macrophages and dendritic cells seem able to harbor replicating HIV without being killed by it, these cells are short-lived and are not thought to be major reservoirs of latent infection. However, they appear to be important in spreading virus to other tissues, such as the brain, where infected cells in the central nervous system may contribute to the virus's long-term persistence.

From studies of patients receiving antiretroviral treatment, it is estimated that more than 95% of the virus that can be detected in the plasma is derived from productively infected CD4 T cells that have a very short half-life—about 2 days.

Virus-producing CD4 T cells are found in the T-cell areas of lymphoid tissues, and these T cells are thought to succumb to infection while being activated in an immune response. Latently infected memory CD4 T cells that become reactivated by antigen also produce virus that can spread to other activated CD4 T cells. In addition to cells that are productively or latently infected, a further large population of cells is infected by defective proviruses, which do not produce infectious virus. Unfortunately, latently infected memory CD4 T cells have an extremely long mean half-life of around 44 months. This means drug therapy that effectively eliminates viral replication would have to be administered for more than 70 years to completely clear the virus. Practically, then, infected patients will never be able to eliminate an HIV infection and require treatment for life.

13-37 Genetic variation in the host can alter the rate of HIV disease progression.

It became clear early in the HIV/AIDS pandemic that the course of the disease could vary widely. Indeed, while nearly all untreated HIV-infected individuals progress to AIDS and ultimately die from opportunistic infections or cancer, not all do. A small percentage of people exposed to the virus seroconvert, but do not seem to have progressive disease. Their CD4 T-cell counts and other measures of immune competence are maintained for decades without antiretroviral therapy. Among these are **long-term nonprogressors**, who, despite detectable viral loads, fail to progress to AIDS over many years, and **elite controllers**, who have unusually low levels of circulating virus (undetectable by some clinical assays despite ongoing low-level viral replication) and represent less than 1% of infected individuals. These individuals have been the subjects of a number of studies to determine how they are able to control their infection without therapy. Another group consists of individuals who engage in high-risk behaviors that repeatedly expose them to infection yet remain virus- and disease-free. Although evidence of prior HIV infection has been reported in such individuals, it is unclear whether these individuals were ever truly infected with infectious virus or were exposed to highly attenuated or defective strains unable to successfully establish infection. In any case, study of these individuals is of considerable interest as it could provide a better understanding of how the host immune response might better control the virus and define what genetic factors might predispose to a protective host response. It might also provide mechanistic insights that could guide development of better vaccines.

Although genetic variation in the virus itself can affect the outcome of infection, a growing number of host gene variants are being defined that impact the rate of progression of HIV infection toward AIDS. The implementation of genome-wide association studies (GWASs) and, more recently, better high-throughput tools to define individual genetic variation (for example, exome and whole-genome sequencing) are accelerating discovery of genetic variations that distinguish highly susceptible and resistant individuals (**Fig. 13.42**). As discussed in Section 13-34, one of the clearest cases of host genetic variation affecting HIV infection is a mutant allele of *CCR5*, *CCR5Δ32*, that when homozygous effectively blocks HIV-1 infection and when heterozygous may slow AIDS progression. Genetic polymorphisms in the HLA class I locus, particularly in the genes *HLA-B* and *HLA-C*, are another major factor in determining disease progression and are currently the strongest predictors of HIV control. Evidence from GWASs has mapped polymorphisms to the peptide-binding groove of HLA class I molecules as key determinants defining disease progression. Polymorphisms outside of the peptide-binding groove as well as those in noncoding regions that control the expression levels of HLA molecules are also implicated. The HLA class I alleles HLA-B57, HLA-B27, and HLA-B13, among others, are

Genes that influence progression to AIDS				
Gene	**Allele**	**Mode**	**Effect**	**Mechanism of action**
HIV entry				
CCR5	Δ32	Recessive	Prevents infection	Knockout of CCR5 expression
		Dominant	Prevents lymphoma (L)	Decreases available CCR5
			Delays AIDS	
	P1	Recessive	Accelerates AIDS (E)	Increases CCR5 expression
CCR2	I64	Dominant	Delays AIDS	Interacts with and reduces CXCR4
CCL5	In1.1c	Dominant	Accelerates AIDS	Decreases CCL5 expression
CXCL12	3′A	Recessive	Delays AIDS (L)	Impedes CCR5–CXCR4 transition (?)
CXCR6	E3K	Dominant	Accelerates P. jirovecii pneumonia (L)	Alters T-cell activations (?)
CCL2-CCL7-CCL11	H7	Dominant	Enhances infection	Stimulates immune response (?)
Cytokine anti-HIV				
IL10	5′A	Dominant	Limits infection	Decreases IL-10 expression
			Accelerates AIDS	
IFNG	−179T	Dominant	Accelerates AIDS (E)	
Acquired immunity, cell mediated				
HLA	A, B, C	Homozygous	Accelerates AIDS	Decreases breadth of HLA class I epitope recognition
	B*27	Codominant	Delays AIDS	Delays HIV-1 escape
	B*57			
	B*35-Px		Accelerates AIDS	Deflects CD8-mediated T-cell clearance of HIV-1
Acquired immunity, innate				
KIR3DS1	3DS1	Epistatic with HLA-Bw4	Delays AIDS	Clears HIV+, HLA− cells (?)

Fig. 13.42 Genes that influence progression to AIDS in humans.
Abbreviations: E, an effect that acts early in progression to AIDS; L, acts late in AIDS progression; ?, plausible mechanism of action with no direct proof.

associated with a better prognosis, whereas HLA-B35 and HLA-B07 are associated with more rapid disease progression. Homozygosity of HLA class I genes (*HLA-A, HLA-B,* and *HLA-C*) is also associated with more rapid progression, presumably because the T-cell response to infection is less diverse. Remarkably, one of the strongest associations with viral control is a single-nucleotide polymorphism (SNP) 35 kb upstream of the *HLA-C* locus; this polymorphism confers greater immune control that correlates with increased expression levels of HLA-C—with the greater control presumably being due to enhanced presentation of viral peptides to CD8 T cells. Certain polymorphisms of the killer cell immunoglobulin-like receptors (KIRs) present on NK cells (see Section 3-26), in particular the receptor KIR-3DS1 in combination with certain alleles of *HLA-B*, also delay the progression to AIDS. Mutations that affect the production of cytokines such as IFN-γ and IL-10 have also been implicated in the restriction of HIV progression.

Fig. 13.43 A variety of opportunistic pathogens and cancers can kill individuals with AIDS. Infections are the major cause of death in AIDS, with respiratory infection with *P. jirovecii* and mycobacteria being the most prominent. Host defense against most of these pathogens requires effective macrophage activation by CD4 T cells or effective cytotoxic T cells. Opportunistic pathogens are present in the normal environment but cause severe disease primarily in immunocompromised hosts, such as individuals with AIDS or individuals with cancer. Individuals with AIDS are also susceptible to several rare cancers, such as Kaposi's sarcoma [associated with human herpesvirus 8 (HHV8)] and various lymphomas, suggesting that immune surveillance of the causative herpesviruses by T cells can normally prevent such tumors (see Chapter 16).

Infections	
Parasites	*Toxoplasma* spp. *Cryptosporidium* spp. *Leishmania* spp. *Microsporidium* spp.
Intracellular bacteria	*Mycobacterium tuberculosis* *Mycobacterium avium* *intracellulare* *Salmonella* spp.
Fungi	*Pneumocystis jirovecii* *Cryptococcus neoformans* *Candida* spp. *Histoplasma capsulatum* *Coccidioides immitis*
Viruses	Herpes simplex Cytomegalovirus varicella-zoster

Malignancies
Kaposi's sarcoma – (HHV8)   Non-Hodgkin's lymphoma, including   EBV-positive Burkitt's lymphoma   Primary lymphoma of the brain

13-38 The destruction of immune function as a result of HIV infection leads to increased susceptibility to opportunistic infection and eventually to death.

When CD4 T-cell numbers decline below a critical level, cell-mediated immunity is lost, and infections with a variety of opportunistic microbes appear (**Fig. 13.43**). Typically, resistance is lost early to oral *Candida* species and to *Mycobacterium tuberculosis*, which cause thrush (oral candidiasis) and tuberculosis, respectively. Later, individuals suffer from shingles (caused by the activation of latent varicella-zoster virus), from aggressive EBV-induced B-cell lymphomas, and from Kaposi's sarcoma, a tumor of endothelial cells that probably results both from a response to cytokines produced in the infection and a herpesvirus called Kaposi's sarcoma herpesvirus (KSHV, or HHV8). Since the earliest recognition of AIDS, pneumonia caused by *Pneumocystis jirovecii* (previously called *P. carinii*) has been the most common opportunistic infection; it was typically fatal before effective antifungal therapy was introduced. Co-infection by hepatitis C virus is common and associated with more rapid progression of hepatitis. In the final stages of AIDS, infection with cytomegalovirus or a member of the *Mycobacterium avium* group of bacteria is more prominent. It is important to note that not all individuals with AIDS get all of these infections or tumors, and there are other tumors and infections that are less prominent but still significant. Figure 13.43 lists the most common opportunistic infections and tumors, which are typically controlled until the CD4 T-cell counts drop toward zero.

13-39 Drugs that block HIV replication lead to a rapid decrease in titer of infectious virus and an increase in CD4 T cells.

Studies with drugs that block HIV replication indicate that the virus is replicating rapidly at all phases of infection, including the asymptomatic phase. Three viral proteins in particular have been the target of drugs aimed at arresting viral replication. These are viral reverse transcriptase, which is required for synthesis of the provirus; viral integrase, which is required for insertion of the viral provirus into the host genome; and viral protease, which cleaves viral polyproteins to produce virion proteins and viral enzymes. Reverse transcriptase is inhibited by nucleoside analogs such as zidovudine (ZDV; also known as azidothymidine, or AZT), which was the first anti-HIV drug to be licensed in the United States. Inhibitors of reverse transcriptase, integrase, and protease prevent infection of uninfected cells; cells that are already infected can continue to produce virions because, once the provirus is established, reverse transcriptase and integrase are not needed to make new virus particles, and while the viral protease acts at a very late maturation step of the virus, inhibition of the protease does not prevent virus from being released. However, in all cases, further cycles of infection by released virions are blocked, and replication is therefore prevented.

The introduction of combination therapy with a cocktail of viral protease inhibitors and nucleoside analogs, also known as combination antiretroviral therapy, or cART (previously referred to as highly active antiretroviral therapy, or HAART), has dramatically reduced mortality and morbidity in patients with HIV infection (**Fig. 13.44**). Patients treated with cART show a rapid and

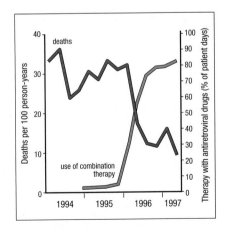

Fig. 13.44 The mortality in advanced HIV infection fell in the United States in parallel with the introduction of combination antiretroviral therapy. The graph shows the number of deaths, expressed each calendar quarter as the deaths per 100 person-years. Figure based on data from F. Palella.

Fig. 13.45 The time course of reduction of HIV circulating in the blood during drug treatment. The production of new HIV particles can be arrested for prolonged periods by treatment using combinations of protease inhibitors and viral reverse-transcriptase inhibitors. After the initiation of such treatment, virus production is curtailed as the infected cells die and no new cells are infected. The half-life of virus decay occurs in three phases. The first phase has a half-life ($t_{1/2}$) of about 2 days, reflecting the half-life of productively infected CD4 T cells, and lasts for about 2 weeks, during which time viral production declines as the lymphocytes that were productively infected at the onset of treatment die. Released virus is rapidly cleared from the circulation, where it has a half-life of 6 hours, and there is a decrease in virus levels in plasma of more than 95% during this first phase. The second phase typically lasts for about 4 months, and the virus has a half-life of about 2 weeks. During this phase, virus is released from infected macrophages and from resting, latently infected CD4 T cells stimulated to divide and develop productive infection. It is thought that there is then a third phase of unknown length that results from the reactivation of integrated provirus in memory T cells and other long-lived reservoirs of infection. This reservoir of latently infected cells might remain present for many years. Measurement of this phase of viral decay is impossible at present because viral levels in plasma are below detectable levels (dotted line).

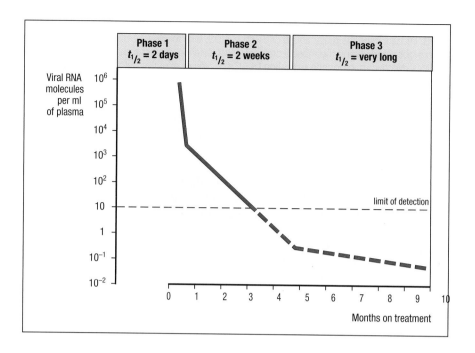

dramatic reduction in viremia, eventually maintaining levels of HIV RNA close to the limit of detection (50 copies per milliliter of plasma) for extended periods with continual therapy—in most cases, indefinitely (**Fig. 13.45**). It is unclear how the virus particles are removed so rapidly from the circulation after the initiation of cART. It seems most likely that they are opsonized by specific antibody and complement and removed by cells of the mononuclear phagocyte system. Opsonized HIV particles may also be trapped in lymphoid follicles on the surface of follicular dendritic cells.

cART is also accompanied by a slow but steady increase in CD4 T cells, despite the fact that many other compartments of the immune system remain compromised. Three complementary mechanisms have been established for the recovery in CD4 T-cell numbers. One is a redistribution of memory CD4 T cells from lymphoid tissues into the circulation as viral replication is controlled; this occurs within weeks of starting treatment. A second one is a reduction in the abnormal levels of immune activation as HIV infection is controlled; this mechanism is associated with reduced killing of infected CD4 T cells by cytotoxic T lymphocytes. The third mechanism is much slower and is caused by the emergence of new naive T cells from the thymus, which is indicated by the presence of T-cell receptor excision circles (TRECs) in these later-arriving cells (see Section 5-10).

Although cART is effective at inhibiting HIV replication, thereby preventing the progression to AIDS and greatly decreasing transmission by those infected, it is ineffective at eradicating all viral stores. Cessation of cART therefore leads to a rapid rebound of virus multiplication, so that patients require treatment indefinitely. This, coupled with the side effects and high cost of cART, has stimulated investigation into other targets to block viral replication (**Fig. 13.46**), as well as ways of eliminating viral reservoirs to eradicate infection permanently. New classes of anti-HIV replication drugs include **viral entry inhibitors**, which block the binding of gp120 to CCR5 or block viral fusion by inhibiting gp41, and **viral integrase inhibitors**, which block the insertion of the reverse-transcribed viral genome into the host DNA. Other approaches under development include efforts to enhance the activity of HIV restriction factors, such as APOBEC (see Section 13-31), which causes extensive mutation of newly formed HIV cDNA to destroy its ability to replicate.

Fig. 13.46 Possible targets for interference with the HIV life cycle. In principle, HIV could be attacked by therapeutic drugs at multiple points in its life cycle: virus entry, reverse transcription of viral RNA, insertion of viral cDNA into cellular DNA by the viral integrase, cleavage of viral polyproteins by the viral protease, and assembly and budding of infectious virions. As yet, only drugs that inhibit reverse transcriptase and protease action have been developed. Combination therapy using different kinds of drugs is more effective than using a single drug.

Given the success of cART in blocking active viral replication, the inability of existing therapies to purge reservoirs of latently infected cells has become the greatest barrier to a cure. To overcome this, strategies are being considered that would induce viral replication in latently infected cells in combination with measures to enhance immune clearance of virus and infected cells. Examples of ways to activate latent virus include the administration of cytokines that activate viral transcription and replication (for example, IL-2, IL-6, and TNF-α) and the use of agents that target epigenetic modifiers, such as histone deacetylase (HDAC) inhibitors, to activate latent provirus. To date, however, no clinical trial using agents that target latent viral reservoirs has shown a significant reduction in viral load over that gained from cART treatment alone. Indeed, it was recently discovered that the activation of viral replication in latently infected cells is intrinsically stochastic, so that many immune cells harboring latent provirus will fail to activate viral replication in any given cycle of cellular activation. This adaptation of HIV to avoid elimination of latently infected cells could represent a formidable barrier to strategies aimed at 'flushing out' latent virus so that it can be eliminated.

An alternative strategy for cure has been highlighted by an American HIV patient, Timothy Ray Brown, who underwent hematopoietic stem-cell transplantation (HSCT) for treatment of leukemia while studying in Berlin (hence, referred to as the **Berlin patient**). By identifying a stem-cell donor who was homozygous for the *CCR5Δ32* co-receptor mutation, Brown's doctor was able to reconstitute him with immune cells resistant to viral propagation. Brown's CD4 T-cell counts rebounded, and he was found to be free of any evidence of HIV infection after cessation of antiretroviral therapy post-transplant. He remained virus-free for more than 10 years, suggesting that he was the first person to be cured of infection via HSCT. He ultimately died from recurrence of the leukemia for which he originally received HSCT. In view of the large number of infected individuals worldwide, the risk of complications with HSCT, and the rarity of HLA-matched CCR5-deletant donors, it is unlikely that this will be a practical approach for cure at the population level. And although the advent of gene-therapy approaches to effectively delete the CCR5 co-receptor in patients' own hematopoietic stem cells has raised the possibility of HSCT using autologous CCR5-deficient stem cells, the relative risk of HSCT compared to cART remains unfavorable. Moreover, there is a risk of progression or reinfection post-transplant by CXCR4-tropic viral variants. This outcome

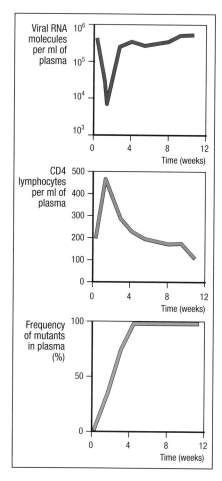

Fig. 13.47 Resistance of HIV to protease inhibitors develops rapidly. After the administration of a single protease inhibitor drug to a patient with HIV, there is in plasma a precipitous fall in levels of viral RNA, with a half-life of about 2 days (top panel). This is accompanied by an initial rise in the number of CD4 T cells in peripheral blood (center panel). Within days of starting the drug, mutant drug-resistant variants can be detected in plasma (bottom panel) and in peripheral blood lymphocytes. After only 4 weeks of treatment, viral RNA levels and CD4 lymphocyte levels have returned to their original pre-drug levels, and 100% of plasma HIV is present as the drug-resistant mutant.

does, however, dramatically establish that eradication of a latency reservoir combined with blockade of viral replication—whether by genetic or therapy-mediated interventions—might achieve a permanent cure.

13-40 In the course of infection, HIV accumulates many mutations, which can result in the outgrowth of drug-resistant variants.

The rapid replication of HIV, with the generation of 10^9 to 10^{10} virions every day, is coupled with a mutation rate of approximately 3×10^{-5} per nucleotide base per cycle of replication, and thus leads to the generation of many variants of HIV in a single infected individual in the course of a day. This high mutation rate arises from the error-prone nature of retroviral replication and poses a formidable challenge to the immune system. Reverse transcriptase lacks the proofreading mechanisms of cellular DNA polymerases, and the RNA genomes of retroviruses are copied into DNA with relatively low fidelity. Thus, although primary infection is typically established by a single founder virus, numerous variants of HIV, called **quasi-species**, rapidly develop within an infected individual. This phenomenon was first recognized in HIV and has since proved to be common to all lentiviruses.

As a consequence of its high variability, HIV rapidly develops resistance to antiviral drugs, much as it develops escape mutants that evade T-cell recognition (see Sections 13-33 and 13-35). When a drug is administered, viral variants with mutations that confer resistance emerge and multiply until the previous levels of virus are regained. Resistance to some viral protease inhibitors requires only a single mutation and appears after only a few days (**Fig. 13.47**); resistance to some inhibitors of reverse transcriptase develops in a similarly short time. In contrast, resistance to the nucleoside analog zidovudine takes months to develop, as it requires three or four mutations in the viral reverse transcriptase. Because of the relatively rapid appearance of resistance to anti-HIV drugs, successful drug treatment has typically depended on combination therapy, where the chance of simultaneous resistance mutations in multiple HIV proteins is virtually nil. Nevertheless, monotherapy with newer-generation antiretroviral agents has proven effective in patients with low viral loads at the onset of treatment.

13-41 HIV treatment and prophylaxis are leading to a decline in the spread of HIV and AIDS.

It is now well established that the spread of HIV can be prevented if antiretroviral drugs are taken regularly by those already infected and those who are uninfected but at risk for exposure. The advent of cART represented a major advance in blocking the transmission of HIV from infected people because of its ability to greatly reduce viral titers in body fluids—so-called treatment as prevention. Moreover, the prophylactic use of antiretroviral drugs (referred to as pre-exposure prophylaxis, or **PrEP**) by individuals at high risk for contracting HIV has demonstrated considerable effectiveness in preventing infection by the virus. When taken daily, the combination of two orally administered reverse transcriptase inhibitors has demonstrated more than 90% reduction in the risk of sexually transmitted HIV infection in at-risk populations. Moreover, use of antiretroviral therapy immediately post-exposure—for example, in hospital workers exposed to contaminated blood by accidental needlestick—substantially reduces the risk of acquiring HIV. Although an early concern with PrEP was the risk of developing drug resistance in those who do contract HIV while on PrEP, particularly in individuals with poor adherence to the dosing regimen, the experience to date has shown that this risk is quite modest. Current trials of new PrEP strategies that are based on long-acting formulations administered monthly instead of daily may further reduce the risk of poor compliance and increase efficacy.

However, not everyone infected with or at risk of contracting HIV has access to cART, as it is expensive and requires ongoing treatment. Further, many of those infected are unaware that they carry the virus. Even where cART is unavailable, access to regular screening for those at risk is critical to inform those infected so they can take measures to avoid passing the virus to others. This, in turn, requires strict confidentiality and mutual trust. A barrier to the control of HIV is the reluctance of individuals to find out whether they are infected, especially as one of the consequences of a positive HIV test is stigmatization by society. Here, education becomes an important component of the prevention strategy, both to remove the stigma and provide guidance on how transmission of the virus can be prevented.

In addition to cART, precautions that can be taken by uninfected individuals are relatively inexpensive and involve measures to protect against contact with body fluids, such as semen, blood, blood products, or breast milk, from people who are infected. It has been repeatedly demonstrated that this is sufficient to prevent infection, as exemplified by health-care workers who care for AIDS patients for long periods without seroconversion or signs of infection. The routine use of condoms greatly reduces the risk of HIV transmission, as does restraint from breast-feeding by infected mothers of newborns. Male circumcision also reduces transmission rates, as the foreskin is a major site of viral entry in uncircumcised males. Additional measures that have been considered include the use of microbicidal gels or suppositories, improvements in which have led to products that show promise in recent trials. Some of these agents can also reduce the transmission of other sexually transmitted diseases (for example, genital herpes) that increase the risk of HIV transmission.

13-42 Vaccination against HIV remains an attractive solution but poses many difficulties.

The effectiveness of cART both in preventing transmission from those infected with HIV and as prophylaxis for those uninfected but at risk has profoundly altered the natural history and transmission rates of HIV infection (**Fig. 13.48**). Nevertheless, a safe and effective vaccine for the prevention of HIV infection and AIDS remains a major goal. Ideally, an effective vaccine would elicit both broadly neutralizing antibodies that block viral entry into target cells (that is, anti-gp120) and effective cytolytic T-cell responses to prevent and control HIV infection. However, no such vaccine has yet been developed, and its attainment is fraught with difficulties that have not been faced in the development of vaccines against other diseases.

The main problem is the nature of the infection itself, featuring a virus that directly undermines the central component of adaptive immunity—the CD4 T cell—and that proliferates and mutates extremely rapidly to cause sustained infection in the face of strong cytotoxic T-cell and antibody responses. The development of vaccines that could be administered to individuals already infected, to boost immune responses and prevent progression to AIDS, has been considered, as have prophylactic vaccines that would prevent initial infection. The development of therapeutic vaccination in those already infected would be extremely difficult. As discussed earlier (see Section 13-40), HIV evolves in individuals by the selective proliferation of mutant viruses that escape recognition by antibodies and cytotoxic T cells. The ability of the virus to persist in latent form as a transcriptionally silent provirus invisible to the immune system might also prevent even an immunized person from clearing an infection once it has been established.

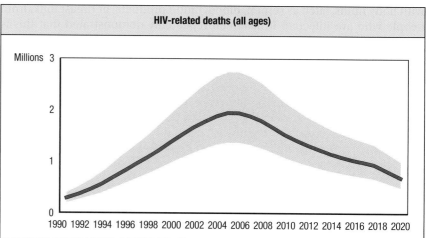

Fig. 13.48 The incidence of new HIV infections and HIV-related deaths worldwide is declining due to effective nonvaccine prevention and antiretroviral therapy. The introduction of effective antiretroviral drugs and their more widespread use, both for treatment of infected individuals and prevention of infection in those at high risk, has begun to stem the tide of the HIV pandemic.

There has been more hope for prophylactic vaccination to prevent new infection. But even here, the lack of protection of the normal immune response and the sheer scale of sequence diversity among HIV strains in the infected population—there are currently thousands of different HIV strains circulating in the human population—remain significant challenges. Individuals infected with one strain of virus do not seem to be resistant to closely related strains, and cases of superinfection, where two strains simultaneously infect the same cell, have also been described. This is compounded by the intrinsic difficulty in generating broadly neutralizing antibodies against HIV envelope glycoproteins (see Section 13-35). Further, there remains uncertainty over what form protective immunity to HIV might take. It is now believed that induction of both effective antibody and T-cell responses will be required to achieve protective immunity, although which epitopes might provide the best targets and how best to induce them remain undefined. Finally, the time from conception to design to performance of complete clinical trials of vaccines against HIV takes years, slowing the rate of progress; to date, few major clinical vaccine trials have been completed, and those have failed.

However, against this discouraging background, progress has been made, and there remains hope that successful vaccines might yet be developed. Various strategies are being tried in an attempt to develop vaccines against HIV, varying from delivery of recombinant HIV proteins, plasmid DNA vaccination with HIV genes (see Section 16-9), delivery of HIV genes in viral vectors, to combinations thereof. Many successful vaccines against other viral diseases contain a live attenuated strain of the virus, which raises an immune response but does not cause disease (see Section 16-4). There are substantial difficulties in the development of live attenuated vaccines against HIV, not least the worry of recombination between vaccine strains and wild-type viruses that would lead to a reversion to virulence. An alternative approach is the use of other viruses, such as vaccinia or adenovirus, to deliver and express HIV genes that elicit B- and T-cell responses against HIV antigens. Because these viral vectors have already demonstrated safety in other human vaccination studies, they have been obvious choices for initial trials. Recently, there has been encouraging, albeit limited, success with this type of approach in combination with boosts using recombinant gp120. Delivery of HIV *gag, pol,* and *env* genes via a canarypox viral vector followed by boosts with HIV gp120 were shown to reduce the risk of infection in a modest but significant number of high-risk vaccine recipients. This represents the first demonstration of any degree of efficacy in a large HIV vaccine trial to date, and a confirmatory study is ongoing. Perhaps as important, data from this study have provided insights into the type of immune response that correlates with protection, indicating that the induction of non-neutralizing antibodies that elicit ADCC (for example, IgG3 isotype) might provide protection. Because neutralizing antibodies against HIV have proven so difficult to elicit, this provides encouragement that they might not be required. Further, a study that used a cytomegalovirus (CMV) vector to deliver SIV genes to rhesus monkeys showed that potent CTL responses were induced. Although these CTL responses did not prevent infection by a pathogenic SIV strain, they did result in clearance of virus in about half of the monkeys vaccinated after its systemic spread. This unprecedented result suggests that the viral vector used for delivery of HIV genes—in this case a vector that produces HIV antigens for prolonged periods after vaccination—might play an important role in the type and amplitude of the antiviral CD8 T-cell response elicited, and protection might be achieved by an effective T-cell response alone. Additional studies will be needed to determine whether combination vaccines that elicit the appropriate non-neutralizing antibodies and robust CD8 T-cell responses might achieve protection even in the absence of neutralizing antibodies.

In addition to the biological obstacles to developing effective HIV vaccines, there are difficult ethical issues. It would be unethical to conduct a vaccine trial without concurrent efforts to minimize the exposure of a population to HIV. In view of rapid adaptation worldwide of pre-exposure prophylaxis (PrEP) as the standard of care for preventing viral spread, future vaccine trials will have difficulty determining efficacy in the face of active cART use. The effectiveness of a vaccine can be assessed only in a population in which the exposure rate to the virus is high enough to assess whether vaccination protects against infection. Given the dramatic successes of cART as a transmission blocker and a prophylactic, it is conceivable that HIV/AIDS could be eradicated without the successful development of a vaccine, assuming there was universal screening for HIV and universal availability and use of cART.

Summary.

Infection with the human immunodeficiency virus (HIV) is the cause of acquired immune deficiency syndrome (AIDS). Although substantial gains in curbing the rate of spread of HIV have been made, this worldwide epidemic continues to spread, especially through heterosexual contact in less-developed countries. HIV is an enveloped retrovirus that replicates in cells of the immune system. Viral entry requires the presence of CD4 and a particular chemokine receptor, and the viral cycle is dependent on transcription factors found in activated T cells. Infection with HIV causes a loss of CD4 T cells and an acute viremia that rapidly subsides as cytotoxic T-cell responses develop, but HIV infection is not eliminated by this immune response. HIV establishes a state of persistent infection in which the virus is continually replicating in newly infected cells. Current treatment consists of combinations of antiviral drugs that block viral replication and cause a rapid decrease in virus levels and a slow increase in CD4 T-cell counts. The main effect of HIV infection is the destruction of CD4 T cells, which occurs through the direct cytopathic effects of HIV infection and through killing by cytotoxic CD8 T cells. As the CD4 T-cell counts wane, the body becomes progressively more susceptible to opportunistic infection. Eventually, most untreated HIV-infected individuals develop AIDS and die; however, a small minority, so-called long-term nonprogressors, remain healthy for many years with no apparent ill effects of infection. From these individuals we hope to be able to learn how infection with HIV can be controlled. The existence of these individuals, and of others who seem to have been naturally immunized against infection, gives hope that it will be possible to develop effective vaccines against HIV.

Summary to Chapter 13.

Whereas most infections elicit protective immunity, successful pathogens have developed some means of at least partly resisting the immune response and can cause serious, sometimes persistent, disease. Some individuals have inherited deficiencies in different components of the immune system, making them highly susceptible to certain classes of infectious agents. Persistent infections and inherited immunodeficiency diseases illustrate the importance of innate and adaptive immunity in effective host defense and present ongoing challenges for immunological research. The human immunodeficiency virus (HIV), which leads to acquired immune deficiency syndrome (AIDS), combines the characteristics of a persistent infectious agent with the ability to create immunodeficiency in its human host, a combination that is usually slowly lethal to the individual. The key to fighting new pathogens such as HIV is to increase our understanding of the basic properties of the immune system and its role in combating infection.

Discussion Questions

13.1 Why do some primary immunodeficiency diseases preferentially affect males? List the most common examples.

13.2 How are primary immunodeficiencies that affect either the complement system or B-cell development similar and different?

13.3 What do people with inherited and acquired immunodeficiencies teach us about the normal mechanism of host protection against opportunistic infections?

13.4 List examples of immunodeficiencies that primarily affect T lymphocytes. Why do these generally affect immune responses more severely than do deficiencies involving B cells only?

13.5 Compare and contrast the host response to intracellular versus extracellular bacterial pathogens.

13.6 List the different ways in which viruses can evade the immune system. Which of these strategies leads to chronic infection, and why?

13.7 Compare antigenic drift and antigenic shift in the context of influenza infections and pandemics. How do these different types of antigenic variation occur?

13.8 How do HIV accessory proteins (Nef, Vif, Vpu, and Vpr) protect the virus from immune clearance?

13.9 How does infection by HIV cause AIDS?

13.10 Why can HIV infection not be cured by current drug therapies? Why is it difficult to make an HIV vaccine?

General references.

Alcami, A., and Koszinowski, U.H.: **Viral mechanisms of immune evasion.** *Immunol. Today* 2000, **21**:447–455.

Bousfiha, A., Jeddane, L., Picard, C., Al-Herz, W., Ailal, F., Chatila, T., Cunningham-Rundles, C., Etzioni, A., Franco, J.L., Holland, S.N., *et al.*: **Human inborn errors of immunity: 2019 update of the IUIS phenotypical classification.** *J. Clin. Immunol.* 2020, **40**:66–81.

De Cock, K.M., Mbori-Ngacha, D., and Marum, E.: **Shadow on the continent: public health and HIV/AIDS in Africa in the 21st century.** *Lancet* 2002, **360**:67–72.

Finlay, B.B., and McFadden, G.: **Anti-immunology: evasion of the host immune system by bacterial and viral pathogens.** *Cell* 2006, **124**:767–782.

Lederberg, J.: **Infectious history.** *Science* 2000, **288**:287–293.

Notarangelo, L.D.: **Primary immunodeficiencies.** *J. Allergy Clin. Immunol.* 2010, **125**:S182–S194.

Notarangelo, L.D., Bacchetta, R., Casanova, J.-L., and Su, H.C. **Human inborn errors of immunity: an expanding universe.** *Sci. Immunol.* 2020, **5**:eabb1662.

Xu, X.N., Screaton, G.R., and McMichael, A.J.: **Virus infections: escape, resistance, and counterattack.** *Immunity* 2001, **15**:867–870.

Section references.

13-1 Primary immunodeficiency diseases are caused by inherited gene variants that typically cause recurrent infections early in life.

Carneiro-Sampaio, M., and Coutinho, A.: **Immunity to microbes: lessons from primary immunodeficiencies.** *Infect. Immun.* 2007, **75**:1545–1555.

Cunningham-Rundles, C., and Ponda, P.P.: **Molecular defects in T- and B-cell primary immunodeficiency diseases.** *Nat. Rev. Immunol.* 2005, **5**:880–892.

Koss, M., Bolze, A., Brendolan, A., Saggese, M., Capellini, T.D., Bojilova, E., Boisson, B., Prall, O.W.J., Elliott, D.A., Solloway, M., *et al.*: **Congenital asplenia in mice and humans with mutations in a Pbx/Nkx2-5/p15 module.** *Dev. Cell* 2012, **22**:913–926.

Marodi, L., and Notarangelo, L.D.: **Immunological and genetic bases of new primary immunodeficiencies.** *Nat. Rev. Immunol.* 2007, **7**:851–861.

13-2 Defects in T-cell development can result in severe combined immune deficiencies.

Buckley, R.H., Schiff, R.I., Schiff, S.E., Markert, M.L., Williams, L.W., Harville, T.O., Roberts, J.L., and Puck, J.M.: **Human severe combined immunodeficiency: genetic, phenotypic, and functional diversity in one hundred eight infants.** *J. Pediatr.* 1997, **130**:378–387.

Leonard, W.J.: **The molecular basis of X linked severe combined immunodeficiency.** *Annu. Rev. Med.* 1996, **47**:229–239.

Leonard, W.J.: **Cytokines and immunodeficiency diseases.** *Nat. Rev. Immunol.* 2001, **1**:200–208.

Stephan, J.L., Vlekova, V., Le Deist, F., Blanche, S., Donadieu, J., De Saint-Basile, G., Durandy, A., Griscelli, C., and Fischer, A.: **Severe combined immunodeficiency: a retrospective single-center study of clinical presentation and outcome in 117 patients.** *J. Pediatr.* 1993, **123**:564–572.

13-3 SCID can also be due to defects in the purine salvage pathway.

Hirschhorn, R.: **Adenosine deaminase deficiency: molecular basis and recent developments.** *Clin. Immunol. Immunopathol.* 1995, **76**:S219–S227.

13-4 Defects in antigen receptor gene rearrangement can result in SCID.

Bosma, M.J., and Carroll, A.M.: **The SCID mouse mutant: definition, characterization, and potential uses.** *Annu. Rev. Immunol.* 1991, **9**:323–350.

Fugmann, S.D.: **DNA repair: breaking the seal.** *Nature* 2002, **416**:691–694.

Gennery, A.R., Cant, A.J., and Jeggo, P.A.: **Immunodeficiency associated with DNA repair defects.** *Clin. Exp. Immunol.* 2000, **121**:1–7.

Moshous, D., Callebaut, I., de Chasseval, R., Corneo, B., Cavazzana-Calvo, M., Le Deist, F., Tezcan, I., Sanal, O., Bertrand, Y., Philippe, N., *et al.*: **Artemis, a novel DNA double-strand break repair/V(D)J recombination protein, is mutated in human severe combined immune deficiency.** *Cell* 2001, **105**:177–186.

13-5 Defects in signaling from T-cell antigen receptors can cause severe immunodeficiency.

Castigli, E., Pahwa, R., Good, R.A., Geha, R.S., and Chatila, T.A.: **Molecular basis of a multiple lymphokine deficiency in a patient with severe combined immunodeficiency.** *Proc. Natl. Acad. Sci. USA* 1993, **90**:4728–4732.

Kung, C., Pingel, J.T., Heikinheimo, M., Klemola, T., Varkila, K., Yoo, L.I., Vuopala, K., Poyhonen, M., Uhari, M., Rogers, M., *et al.*: **Mutations in the tyrosine phosphatase CD45 gene in a child with severe combined immunodeficiency disease.** *Nat. Med.* 2000, **6**:343–345.

Roifman, C.M., Zhang, J., Chitayat, D., and Sharfe, N.: **A partial deficiency of interleukin-7Rα is sufficient to abrogate T-cell development and cause severe combined immunodeficiency.** *Blood* 2000, **96**:2803–2807.

13-6 Genetic defects in thymic development or function that block T-cell development result in combined immunodeficiencies.

Coffer, P.J., and Burgering, B.M.: **Forkhead-box transcription factors and their role in the immune system.** *Nat. Rev. Immunol.* 2004, **4**:889–899.

DiSanto, J.P., Keever, C.A., Small, T.N., Nicols, G.L., O'Reilly, R.J., and Flomenberg, N.: **Absence of interleukin 2 production in a severe combined immunodeficiency disease syndrome with T cells.** *J. Exp. Med.* 1990, **171**:1697–1704.

DiSanto, J.P., Rieux Laucat, F., Dautry Varsat, A., Fischer, A., and de Saint Basile, G.: **Defective human interleukin 2 receptor γ chain in an atypical X chromosome-linked severe combined immunodeficiency with peripheral T cells.** *Proc. Natl. Acad. Sci. USA* 1994, **91**:9466–9470.

Gadola, S.D., Moins-Teisserenc, H.T., Trowsdale, J., Gross, W.L., and Cerundolo, V.: **TAP deficiency syndrome.** *Clin. Exp. Immunol.* 2000, **121**:173–178.

Gilmour, K.C., Fujii, H., Cranston, T., Davies, E.G., Kinnon, C., and Gaspar, H.B.: **Defective expression of the interleukin-2/interleukin-15 receptor β subunit leads to a natural killer cell-deficient form of severe combined immunodeficiency.** *Blood* 2001, **98**:877–879.

Grusby, M.J., and Glimcher, L.H.: **Immune responses in MHC class II-deficient mice.** *Annu. Rev. Immunol.* 1995, **13**:417–435.

Pignata, C., Gaetaniello, L., Masci, A.M., Frank, J., Christiano, A., Matrecano, E., and Racioppi, L.: **Human equivalent of the mouse Nude/SCID phenotype: long-term evaluation of immunologic reconstition after bone marrow transplantation.** *Blood* 2001, **97**:880–885.

Steimle, V., Reith, W., and Mach, B.: **Major histocompatibility complex class II deficiency: a disease of gene regulation.** *Adv. Immunol.* 1996, **61**:327–340.

13-7 Defects in B-cell development result in deficiencies in antibody production that cause an inability to clear extracellular bacteria and some viruses.

Bruton, O.C.: **Agammaglobulinemia.** *Pediatrics* 1952, **9**:722–728.

Conley, M.E.: **Genetics of hypogammaglobulinemia: what do we really know?** *Curr. Opin. Immunol.* 2009, **21**:466–471.

Lee, M.L., Gale, R.P., and Yap, P.L.: **Use of intravenous immunoglobulin to prevent or treat infections in persons with immune deficiency.** *Annu. Rev. Med.* 1997, **48**:93–102.

Notarangelo, L.D.: **Immunodeficiencies caused by genetic defects in protein kinases.** *Curr. Opin. Immunol.* 1996, **8**:448–453.

Preud'homme, J.L., and Hanson, L.A.: **IgG subclass deficiency.** *Immunodefic. Rev.* 1990, **2**:129–149.

13-8 Combined immunodeficiencies (CIDs) can be caused by defects in T-cell differentiation and function that impair activation of B cells, dendritic cells and macrophages, and innate effector cells.

Doffinger, R., Smahi, A., Bessia, C., Geissmann, F., Feinberg, J., Durandy, A., Bodemer, C., Kenwrick, S., Dupuis-Girod, S., Blanche, S., *et al.*: **X-linked anhidrotic ectodermal dysplasia with immunodeficiency is caused by impaired NFκB signaling.** *Nat. Genet.* 2001, **27**:277–285.

Durandy, A., and Honjo, T.: **Human genetic defects in class-switch recombination (hyper-IgM syndromes).** *Curr. Opin. Immunol.* 2001, **13**:543–548.

Ferrari, S., Giliani, S., Insalaco, A., Al Ghonaium, A., Soresina, A.R., Loubser, M., Avanzini, M.A., Marconi, M., Badolato, R., Ugazio, A.G., *et al.*: **Mutations of CD40 gene cause an autosomal recessive form of immunodeficiency with hyper IgM.** *Proc. Natl. Acad. Sci. USA* 2001, **98**:12614–12619.

Harris, R.S., Sheehy, A.M., Craig, H.M., Malim, M.H., and Neuberger, M.S.: **DNA deamination: not just a trigger for antibody diversification but also a mechanism for defense against retroviruses.** *Nat. Immunol.* 2003, **4**:641–643.

Minegishi, Y.: **Hyper-IgE syndrome.** *Curr. Opin. Immunol.* 2009, **21**:487–492.

Park, M.A., Li, J.T., Hagan, J.B., Maddox, D.E., and Abraham, R.S.: **Common variable immunodeficiency: a new look at an old disease.** *Lancet* 2008, **372**:489–503.

Thrasher, A.J., and Burns, S.O.: **WASP: a key immunological multitasker.** *Nat. Rev. Immunol.* 2010, **10**:182–192.

Yong, P.F., Salzer, U., and Grimbacher, B.: **The role of costimulation in antibody deficiencies: ICOS and common variable immunodeficiency.** *Immunol. Rev.* 2009, **229**:101–113.

13-9 B cell–specific activation defects cause hyper IgM syndromes that are limited to defects in the antibody response.

Durandy, A., and Honjo, T.: **Human genetic defects in class-switch recombination (hyper-IgM syndromes).** *Curr. Opin. Immunol.* 2001, **13**:543–548.

13-10 Common variable immunodeficiency results from a variety of inherited defects that cause more limited defects in the antibody response.

Park, J.H., Resnick, E.S., and Cunningham-Rundles, C.: **Perspectives on common variable immune deficiency.** *Ann. N.Y. Acad. Sci.* 2011, **1246**:41–49.

13-11 Unidentified genetic defects cause isotype-specific antibody deficiencies.

Burrows, P.D., and Cooper, M.D.: **IgA deficiency.** *Adv. Immunol.* 1997, **65**:245–276.

Gupta, S., and Gupta, A. **Selective IgM deficiency—an underestimated primary immunodeficiency.** *Front. Immunol.* 2017, **8**:1056.

Yel, L.: **Selective IgA deficiency.** *J. Clin. Immunol.* 2010, **30**:10–16.

13-12 Normal pathways for host defense against different infectious agents are pinpointed by genetic deficiencies of cytokine pathways central to type 1/T$_H$1 and type 3/T$_H$17 responses.

Browne, S.K.: **Anticytokine autoantibody-associated immunodeficiency.** *Annu. Rev. Immunol.* 2014, **32**:635–657.

Casanova, J.L., and Abel, L.: **Genetic dissection of immunity to mycobacteria: the human model.** *Annu. Rev. Immunol.* 2002, **20**:581–620.

Dupuis, S., Dargemont, C., Fieschi, C., Thomassin, N., Rosenzweig, S., Harris, J., Holland, S.M., Schreiber, R.D., and Casanova, J.L.: **Impairment of mycobacterial but not viral immunity by a germline human STAT1 mutation.** *Science* 2001, **293**:300–303.

Lammas, D.A., Casanova, J.L., and Kumararatne, D.S.: **Clinical consequences of defects in the IL-12-dependent interferon-γ (IFN-γ) pathway.** *Clin. Exp. Immunol.* 2000, **121**:417–425.

Lanternier, F., Cypowyj, S., Picard, C., Bustamante, J., Lortholary, O., Casanova, J.-L., and Puel, A.: **Primary immunodeficiencies underlying fungal infections.** *Curr. Opin. Pediatr.* 2013, **25**:736–747.

Lanternier, F., Pathan, S., Vincent, Q.B., Liu, L., Cypowyj, S., Prando, C., Migaud, M., Taibi, L., Ammar-Khodja, A., Boudghene Stambouli, O., *et al.*: **Deep

dermatophytosis and inherited CARD9 deficiency.** *N. Engl. J. Med.* 2013, **369**:1704–1714.

Newport, M.J., Huxley, C.M., Huston, S., Hawrylowicz, C.M., Oostra, B.A., Williamson, R., and Levin, M.: **A mutation in the interferon-γ-receptor gene and susceptibility to mycobacterial infection.** *N. Engl. J. Med.* 1996, **335**:1941–1949.

Puel, A., Döffinger, R., Natividad, A., Chrabieh, M., Barcenas-Morales, G., Picard, C., Cobat, A., Ouachée-Chardin, M., Toulon, A., Bustamante, J., *et al.*: **Autoantibodies against IL-17A, IL-17F, and IL-22 in patients with chronic mucocutaneous candidiasis and autoimmune polyendocrine syndrome type I.** *J. Exp. Med.* 2010, **207**:291–297.

Van de Vosse, E., Hoeve, M.A., and Ottenhoff, T.H.: **Human genetics of intracellular infectious diseases: molecular and cellular immunity against mycobacteria and salmonellae.** *Lancet Infect. Dis.* 2004, **4**:739–749.

13-13 Inherited defects in the cytolytic pathway of lymphocytes can cause uncontrolled lymphoproliferation and inflammatory responses to viral infections.

de Saint Basille, G., and Fischer, A.: **The role of cytotoxicity in lymphocyte homeostasis.** *Curr. Opin. Immunol.* 2001, **13**:549–554.

de Saint Basile, G., Ménasché, G., and Fischer, A.: **Molecular mechanisms of biogenesis and exocytosis of cytotoxic granules.** *Nat. Rev. Immunol.* 2010, **10**:568–579.

13-14 X-linked lymphoproliferative syndrome is associated with fatal infection by Epstein–Barr virus and the development of lymphomas.

Latour, S., Gish, G., Helgason, C.D., Humphries, R.K., Pawson, T., and Veillette, A.: **Regulation of SLAM-mediated signal transduction by SAP, the X-linked lymphoproliferative gene product.** *Nat. Immunol.* 2001, **2**:681–690.

Morra, M., Howie, D., Grande, M.S., Sayos, J., Wang, N., Wu, C., Engel, P., and Terhorst, C.: **X-linked lymphoproliferative disease: a progressive immunodeficiency.** *Annu. Rev. Immunol.* 2001, **19**:657–682.

Rigaud, S., Fondaneche, M.C., Lambert, N., Pasquier, B., Mateo, V., Soulas, P., Galicier, L., Le Deist, F., Rieux-Laucat, F., Revy, P., *et al.*: **XIAP deficiency in humans causes an X-linked lymphoproliferative syndrome.** *Nature* 2006, **444**:110–114.

13-15 Immunodeficiency is caused by inherited defects in the development of dendritic cells.

Bigley, V., Cytlak, U., and Collin, M.: **Human dendritic cell immunodeficiencies.** *Semin. Cell Dev. Biol.* 2019, **86**:50–61.

Collin, M., Bigley, V., Haniffa, M., and Hambleton, S.: **Human dendritic cell deficiency: the missing ID?** *Nat. Rev. Immunol.* 2011, **11**:575–583.

Hambleton, S., Salem, S., Bustamante, J., Bigley, V., Boisson-Dupuis, S., Azevedo, J., Fortin, A., Haniffa, M., Ceron-Gutierrez, L., Bacon, C.M., *et al.*: **IRF8 mutations and human dendritic-cell immunodeficiency.** *N. Engl. J. Med.* 2011, **365**:127–138.

13-16 Defects in complement components and complement-regulatory proteins cause defective humoral immune function and tissue damage.

Colten, H.R., and Rosen, F.S.: **Complement deficiencies.** *Annu. Rev. Immunol.* 1992, **10**:809–834.

Dahl, M., Tybjaerg-Hansen, A., Schnohr, P., and Nordestgaard, B.G.: **A population-based study of morbidity and mortality in mannose-binding lectin deficiency.** *J. Exp. Med.* 2004, **199**:1391–1399.

Walport, M.J.: **Complement. First of two parts.** *N. Engl. J. Med.* 2001, **344**:1058–1066.

Walport, M.J.: **Complement. Second of two parts.** *N. Engl. J. Med.* 2001, **344**:1140–1144.

13-17 Defects in phagocytic cells result in widespread bacterial infections.

Andrews, T., and Sullivan, K.E.: **Infections in patients with inherited defects in phagocytic function.** *Clin. Microbiol. Rev.* 2003, **16**:597–621.

Etzioni, A.: **Genetic etiologies of leukocyte adhesion defects.** *Curr. Opin. Immunol.* 2009, **21**:481–486.

Fischer, A., Lisowska Grospierre, B., Anderson, D.C., and Springer, T.A.: **Leukocyte adhesion deficiency: molecular basis and functional consequences.** *Immunodefic. Rev.* 1988, **1**:39–54.

Goldblatt, D., and Thrasher, A.J.: **Chronic granulomatous disease.** *Clin. Exp. Immunol.* 2000, **122**:1–9.

Klein, C., and Welte, K.: **Genetic insights into congenital neutropenia.** *Clin. Rev. Allergy Immunol.* 2010, **38**:68–74.

Netea, M.G., Wijmenga, C., and O'Neill, L.A.J.: **Genetic variation in Toll-like receptors and disease susceptibility.** *Nat. Immunol.* 2012, **13**:535–542.

Spritz, R.A.: **Genetic defects in Chediak–Higashi syndrome and the beige mouse.** *J. Clin. Immunol.* 1998, **18**:97–105.

Suhir, H., and Etzioni, A.: **The role of Toll-like receptor signaling in human immunodeficiencies.** *Clin. Rev. Allergy Immunol.* 2010, **38**:11–19.

13-18 Mutations in the molecular regulators of inflammation can cause uncontrolled inflammatory responses that result in 'autoinflammatory disease.'

Delpech, M., and Grateau, G.: **Genetically determined recurrent fevers.** *Curr. Opin. Immunol.* 2001, **13**:539–542.

Dinarello, C.A.: **Immunological and inflammatory functions of the interleukin-1 family.** *Annu. Rev. Immunol.* 2009, **27**:519–550.

Drenth, J.P., and van der Meer, J.W.: **Hereditary periodic fever.** *N. Engl. J. Med.* 2001, **345**:1748–1757.

Kastner, D.L., and O'Shea, J.J.: **A fever gene comes in from the cold.** *Nat. Genet.* 2001, **29**:241–242.

Stehlik, C., and Reed, J.C.: **The PYRIN connection: novel players in innate immunity and inflammation.** *J. Exp. Med.* 2004, **200**:551–558.

13-19 Factor-replacement therapies, hematopoietic stem-cell transplantation, and gene therapy can be used successfully to correct genetic defects.

Fischer, A., Hacein-Bey, S., and Cavazzana-Calvo, M.: **Gene therapy of severe combined immunodeficiencies.** *Nat. Rev. Immunol.* 2002, **2**:615–621.

Fischer, A., Le Deist, F., Hacein-Bey-Abina, S., Andre-Schmutz, I., de Saint, B.G., de Villartay, J.P., and Cavazzana-Calvo, M.: **Severe combined immunodeficiency. A model disease for molecular immunology and therapy.** *Immunol. Rev.* 2005, **203**:98–109.

Hacein-Bey-Abina, S., Le Deist, F., Carlier, F., Bouneaud, C., Hue, C., De Villartay, J.P., Thrasher, A.J., Wulffraat, N., Sorensen, R., Dupuis-Girod, S., *et al.*: **Sustained correction of X-linked severe combined immunodeficiency by *ex vivo* gene therapy.** *N. Engl. J. Med.* 2002, **346**:1185–1193.

Rosen, F.S.: **Successful gene therapy for severe combined immunodeficiency.** *N. Engl. J. Med.* 2002, **346**:1241–1243.

Thrasher, A.J., and Williams, D.A.: **Evolving gene therapy in primary immunodeficiency.** *Mol. Ther.* 2017, **25**:1132–1141.

13-20 Noninherited, secondary immunodeficiencies are major predisposing causes of infection and death.

Chandra, R.K.: **Nutrition, immunity and infection: from basic knowledge of dietary manipulation of immune responses to practical application of ameliorating suffering and improving survival.** *Proc. Natl. Acad. Sci. USA* 1996, **93**:14304–14307.

Lord, G.M., Matarese, G., Howard, J.K., Baker, R.J., Bloom, S.R., and Lechler, R.I.: **Leptin modulates the T-cell immune response and reverses starvation-induced immunosuppression.** *Nature* 1998, **394**:897–901.

13-21 Extracellular bacterial pathogens have evolved different strategies to avoid detection by pattern-recognition receptors and destruction by antibody, complement, and antimicrobial peptides.

Arciola, C.R., Campoccia, D., and Montanaro, L.: **Implant infections: adhesion, biofilm formation and immune evasion.** *Nat. Rev. Microbiol.* 2018, **16**:397–409.

Bhavsar, A.P., Guttman, J.A., and Finlay, B.B.: **Manipulation of host-cell pathways by bacterial pathogens.** *Nature* 2007, **449**:827–834.

Blander, J.M., and Sander, L.E.: **Beyond pattern recognition: five immune checkpoints for scaling the microbial threat.** *Nat. Rev. Immunol.* 2012, **12**:215–225.

Hajishengallis, G., and Lambris, J.D.: **Microbial manipulation of receptor crosstalk in innate immunity.** *Nat. Rev. Immunol.* 2011, **11**:187–200.

Hornef, M.W., Wick, M.J., Rhen, M., and Normark, S.: **Bacterial strategies for overcoming host innate and adaptive immune responses.** *Nat. Immunol.* 2002, **3**:1033–1040.

Lambris, J.D., Ricklin, D., and Geisbrecht, B.V.: **Complement evasion by human pathogens.** *Nat. Rev. Microbiol.* 2008, **6**:132–142.

Phillips, R.E.: **Immunology taught by Darwin.** *Nat. Immunol.* 2002, **3**:987–989.

Raymond, B., Young, J.C., Pallett, M., Endres, R.G., Clements, A., and Frankel, G.: **Subversion of trafficking, apoptosis, and innate immunity by type III secretion system effectors.** *Trends Microbiol.* 2013, **21**:430–441.

Serruto, D., Rappuoli, R., Scarselli, M., Gros, P., and van Strijp, J.A.G.: **Molecular mechanisms of complement evasion: learning from staphylococci and meningococci.** *Nat. Rev. Microbiol.* 2010, **8**:393–399.

Thammavongsa, V., Kim, H.K., Missiakas, D., and Schneewind, O.: **Staphylococcal manipulation of host immune responses.** *Nat. Rev. Microbiol.* 2015, **13**:529–543.

Vance, R.E., Isberg, R.R., and Portnoy, D.A.: **Patterns of pathogenesis: discrimination of pathogenic and nonpathogenic microbes by the innate immune system.** *Cell Host Microbe* 2009, **6**:10–21.

Yeaman, M.R., and Yount, N.Y.: **Mechanisms of antimicrobial peptide action and resistance.** *Pharmacol. Rev.* 2003, **55**:27–55.

13-22 Intracellular bacterial pathogens can evade the immune system by seeking shelter within phagocytes.

Cambier, C.J., Takaki, K.K., Larson, R.P., Hernandez, R.E., Tobin, D.M., Urdahl, K.B., Cosma, C.L., and Ramakrishnan, L.: **Mycobacteria manipulate macrophage recruitment through coordinated use of membrane lipids.** *Nature* 2014, **505**:218–222.

Clegg, S., Hancox, L.S., and Yeh, K.S.: ***Salmonella typhimurium* fimbrial phase variation and FimA expression.** *J. Bacteriol.* 1996, **178**:542–545.

Cossart, P.: **Host/pathogen interactions. Subversion of the mammalian cell cytoskeleton by invasive bacteria.** *J. Clin. Invest.* 1997, **99**:2307–2311.

Young, D., Hussell, T., and Dougan, G.: **Chronic bacterial infections: living with unwanted guests.** *Nat. Immunol.* 2002, **3**:1026–1032.

13-23 Immune evasion is also practiced by protozoan parasites.

Donelson, J.E., Hill, K.L., and El-Sayed, N.M.: **Multiple mechanisms of immune evasion by African trypanosomes.** *Mol. Biochem. Parasitol.* 1998, **91**:51–66.

Sacks, D., and Sher, A.: **Evasion of innate immunity by parasitic protozoa.** *Nat. Immunol.* 2002, **3**:1041–1047.

13-24 Many viruses target type I and type III interferon pathways to impair host antiviral defense.

Chan, Y.K., and Gack, M.U.: **Viral evasion of intracellular DNA and RNA sensing.** *Nat. Rev. Microbiol.* 2016, **14**:360–373.

McNab, F., Mayer-Barber, K., Sher, A., Wack, A., and O'Garra, A.: **Type I interferons in infectious disease.** *Nat. Rev. Immunol.* 2015, **15**:87–103.

13-25 RNA viruses use different mechanisms of antigenic variation to keep a step ahead of the adaptive immune system.

Bowie, A.G., and Unterholzner, L.: **Viral evasion and subversion of pattern-recognition receptor signalling.** *Nat. Rev. Immunol.* 2008, **8**:911–922.

Brander, C., and Walker, B.D.: **Modulation of host immune responses by clinically relevant human DNA and RNA viruses.** *Curr. Opin. Microbiol.* 2000, **3**:379–386.

Gibbs, M.J., Armstrong, J.S., and Gibbs, A.J.: **Recombination in the hemagglutinin gene of the 1918 'Spanish flu.'** *Science* 2001, **293**:1842–1845.

Hatta, M., Gao, P., Halfmann, P., and Kawaoka, Y.: **Molecular basis for high virulence of Hong Kong H5N1 influenza A viruses.** *Science* 2001, **293**:1840–1842.

Hilleman, M.R.: **Strategies and mechanisms for host and pathogen survival in acute and persistent viral infections.** *Proc. Natl. Acad. Sci. USA* 2004, **101**:14560–14566.

Laver, G., and Garman, E.: **Virology. The origin and control of pandemic influenza.** *Science* 2001, **293**:1776–1777.

13-26   DNA viruses use multiple mechanisms to subvert CTL and NK-cell responses.

Alcami, A.: **Viral mimicry of cytokines, chemokines and their receptors.** *Nat. Rev. Immunol.* 2003, **3**:36–50.

Hansen, T.H., and Bouvier, M.: **MHC class I antigen presentation: learning from viral evasion strategies.** *Nat. Rev. Immunol.* **9**:503–513.

Felix, J., and Savvides, S.N.: **Mechanisms of immunomodulation by mammalian and viral decoy receptors: insights from structures.** *Nat. Rev. Immunol.* 2017, **17**:112–129.

McFadden, G., and Murphy, P.M.: **Host-related immunomodulators encoded by poxviruses and herpesviruses.** *Curr. Opin. Microbiol.* 2000, **3**:371–378.

Paludan, S.R., Bowie, A.G., Horan, K.A., and Fitzgerald, K.A.: **Recognition of herpesviruses by the innate immune system.** *Nat. Rev. Immunol.* 2011, **11**:143–154.

Yewdell, J.W., and Hill, A.B.: **Viral interference with antigen presentation.** *Nat. Immunol.* 2002, **2**:1019–1025.

13-27   Viruses that establish latency persist *in vivo* by ceasing to replicate until immunity wanes.

Cohen, J.I.: **Epstein–Barr virus infection.** *N. Engl. J. Med.* 2000, **343**:481–492.

Hahn, G., Jores, R., and Mocarski, E.S.: **Cytomegalovirus remains latent in a common precursor of dendritic and myeloid cells.** *Proc. Natl. Acad. Sci. USA* 1998, **95**:3937–3942.

Ho, D.Y.: **Herpes simplex virus latency: molecular aspects.** *Prog. Med. Virol.* 1992, **39**:76–115.

Kuppers, R.: **B cells under the influence: transformation of B cells by Epstein–Barr virus.** *Nat. Rev. Immunol.* 2003, **3**:801–812.

Lauer, G.M., and Walker, B.D.: **Hepatitis C virus infection.** *N. Engl. J. Med.* 2001, **345**:41–52.

Macsween, K.F., and Crawford, D.H.: **Epstein–Barr virus—recent advances.** *Lancet Infect. Dis.* 2003, **3**:131–140.

Nash, A.A.: **T cells and the regulation of herpes simplex virus latency and reactivation.** *J. Exp. Med.* 2000, **191**:1455–1458.

13-28   DNA and RNA viruses can induce exhaustion of CTL and NK cell responses, thereby impairing the antiviral response.

McLane, L.M., Abdel-Hakeem, M.S., and Wherry, E. J.: **CD8 T cell exhaustion during chronic viral infection and cancer.** *Ann. Rev. Immunol.* 2019, **37**:457–495.

Wherry, E.J., and Kurachi, M.: **Molecular and cellular insights into T cell exhaustion.** *Nat. Rev. Immunol.* 2015, **15**:486–499.

Zajac, A.J., Blattman, J.N., Murali-Krishna, K., Sourdive, D.J., Suresh, M., Altman, J.D., and Ahmed, R.: **Viral immune evasion due to persistence of activated T cells without effector function.** *J. Exp. Med.* 1998, **188**:2205–2213.

13-29   HIV is a retrovirus that establishes a chronic infection that slowly progresses to AIDS.

Baltimore, D.: **The enigma of HIV infection.** *Cell* 1995, **82**:175–176.

Barre-Sinoussi, F.: **HIV as the cause of AIDS.** *Lancet* 1996, **348**:31–35.

Campbell-Yesufu, O.T., and Gandhi, R.T.: **Update on human immunodeficiency virus (HIV)-2 infection.** 2011, **52**:780–787.

Heeney, J.L., Dalgleish, A.G., and Weiss, R.A.: **Origins of HIV and the evolution of resistance to AIDS.** *Science* 2006, **313**:462–466.

Sharp, P.M., and Hahn, B.H.: **Origins of HIV and the AIDS pandemic.** *Cold Spring Harb. Perspect. Med.* 2011, **1**:a006841.

13-30   HIV infects and replicates within cells of the immune system.

Grouard, G., and Clark, E.A.: **Role of dendritic and follicular dendritic cells in HIV infection and pathogenesis.** *Curr. Opin. Immunol.* 1997, **9**:563–567.

Moore, J.P., Trkola, A., and Dragic, T.: **Co-receptors for HIV-1 entry.** *Curr. Opin. Immunol.* 1997, **9**:551–562.

Pohlmann, S., Baribaud, F., and Doms, R.W.: **DC-SIGN and DC-SIGNR: helping hands for HIV.** *Trends Immunol.* 2001, **22**:643–646.

Root, M.J., Kay, M.S., and Kim, P.S.: **Protein design of an HIV-1 entry inhibitor.** *Science* 2001, **291**:884–888.

Sol-Foulon, N., Moris, A., Nobile, C., Boccaccio, C., Engering, A., Abastado, J.P., Heard, J.M., van Kooyk, Y., and Schwartz, O.: **HIV-1 Nef-induced upregulation of DC-SIGN in dendritic cells promotes lymphocyte clustering and viral spread.** *Immunity* 2002, **16**:145–155.

Unutmaz, D., and Littman, D.R.: **Expression pattern of HIV-1 coreceptors on T cells: implications for viral transmission and lymphocyte homing.** *Proc. Natl. Acad. Sci. USA* 1997, **94**:1615–1618.

Wang, H., Barnes, C.O., Yang, Z., Nussenzweig, M.C., and Bjorkman, P.J.: **Partially open HIV-1 envelope structures exhibit conformational changes relevant for coreceptor binding and fusion.** *Cell Host Microbe* 2018, **24**:579–592.e4.

Wilen, C.B., Tilton, J.C., and Doms, R.W.: **HIV: cell binding and entry.** *Cold Spring Harb. Perspect. Med.* 2012, **2**:a006866.

Wyatt, R., and Sodroski, J.: **The HIV-1 envelope glycoproteins: fusogens, antigens, and immunogens.** *Science* 1998, **280**:1884–1888.

13-31   Activated CD4 T cells are the major source of HIV replication.

Chiu, Y.L., Soros, V.B., Kreisberg, J.F., Stopak, K., Yonemoto, W., and Greene, W.C.: **Cellular APOBEC3G restricts HIV-1 infection in resting CD4+ T cells.** *Nature* 2005, **435**:108–114.

Cullen, B.R.: **HIV-1 auxiliary proteins: making connections in a dying cell.** *Cell* 1998, **93**:685–692.

Cullen, B.R.: **Connections between the processing and nuclear export of mRNA: evidence for an export license?** *Proc. Natl. Acad. Sci. USA* 2000, **97**:4–6.

Emerman, M., and Malim, M.H.: **HIV-1 regulatory/accessory genes: keys to unraveling viral and host cell biology.** *Science* 1998, **280**:1880–1884.

Ho, Y.-C., Shan, L., Hosmane, N.N., Wang, J., Laskey, S.B., Rosenbloom, D.I.S., Lai, J., Blankson, J.N., Siliciano, J.D., and Siliciano, R.F.: **Replication-competent noninduced proviruses in the latent reservoir increase barrier to HIV-1 cure.** *Cell* 2013, **155**:540–551.

Kinoshita, S., Su, L., Amano, M., Timmerman, L.A., Kaneshima, H., and Nolan, G.P.: **The T-cell activation factor NF-ATc positively regulates HIV-1 replication and gene expression in T cells.** *Immunity* 1997, **6**:235–244.

Malim, M.H., and Bieniasz, P.D.: **HIV restriction factors and mechanisms of evasion.** *Cold Spring Harb. Perspect. Med.* **2**:a006940.

Trono, D.: **HIV accessory proteins: leading roles for the supporting cast.** *Cell* 1995, **82**:189–192.

13-32   There are several routes by which HIV is transmitted and establishes infection.

Bomsel, M., and David, V.: **Mucosal gatekeepers: selecting HIV viruses for early infection.** *Nat. Med.* 2002, **8**:114–116.

Kwon, D.S., Gregorio, G., Bitton, N., Hendrickson, W.A., and Littman, D.R.: **DC-SIGN-mediated internalization of HIV is required for trans-enhancement of T cell infection.** *Immunity* 2002, **16**:135–144.

Peckham, C., and Gibb, D.: **Mother-to-child transmission of the human immunodeficiency virus.** *N. Engl. J. Med.* 1995, **333**:298–302.

Royce, R.A., Sena, A., Cates, W., Jr., and Cohen, M.S.: **Sexual transmission of HIV.** *N. Engl. J. Med.* 1997, **336**:1072–1078.

13-33   HIV variants with tropism for different co-receptors play different roles in transmission and progression of disease.

Berger, E.A., Murphy, P.M., and Farber, J.M.: **Chemokine receptors as HIV-1 coreceptors: roles in viral entry, tropism, and disease.** *Annu. Rev. Immunol.* 1999, **17**:657–700.

Connor, R.I., Sheridan, K.E., Ceradini, D., Choe, S., and Landau, N.R.: **Change in coreceptor use correlates with disease progression in HIV-1—infected individuals.** *J. Exp. Med.* 1997, **185**:621–628.

Littman, D.R.: **Chemokine receptors: keys to AIDS pathogenesis?** *Cell* 1998, **93**:677–680.

13-34   A genetic deficiency of the co-receptor CCR5 confers resistance to HIV infection.

Gonzalez, E., Kulkarni, H., Bolivar, H., Mangano, A., Sanchez, R., Catano, G., Nibbs, R.J., Freedman, B.I., Quinones, M.P., Bamshad, M.J., *et al.*: **The influence of CCL3L1 gene-containing segmental duplications on HIV-1/AIDS susceptibility.** *Science* 2005, **307**:1434–1440.

Liu, R., Paxton, W.A., Choe, S., Ceradini, D., Martin, S.R., Horuk, R., Macdonald, M.E., Stuhlmann, H., Koup, R.A., and Landau, N.R.: **Homozygous defect in HIV-1 coreceptor accounts for resistance of some multiply exposed individuals to HIV 1 infection.** *Cell* 1996, **86**:367–377.

Samson, M., Libert, F., Doranz, B.J., Rucker, J., Liesnard, C., Farber, C.M., Saragosti, S., Lapoumeroulie, C., Cognaux, J., Forceille, C., *et al.*: **Resistance to HIV-1 infection in Caucasian individuals bearing mutant alleles of the CCR 5 chemokine receptor gene.** *Nature* 1996, **382**:722–725.

13-35   An immune response controls but does not eliminate HIV.

Baltimore, D.: **Lessons from people with nonprogressive HIV infection.** *N. Engl. J. Med.* 1995, **332**:259–260.

Barouch, D.H., and Letvin, N.L.: **CD8+ cytotoxic T lymphocyte responses to lentiviruses and herpesviruses.** *Curr. Opin. Immunol.* 2001, **13**:479–482.

Haase, A.T.: **Targeting early infection to prevent HIV-1 mucosal transmission.** *Nature* 2010, **464**:217–223.

Ho, D.D., Neumann, A.U., Perelson, A.S., Chen, W., Leonard, J.M., and Markowitz, M.: **Rapid turnover of plasma virions and CD4 lymphocytes in HIV-1 infection.** *Nature* 1995, **373**:123–126.

Liao, H.-X., Lynch, R., Zhou, T., Gao, F., Alam, S.M., Boyd, S.D., Fire, A.Z., Roskin, K.M., Schramm, C.A., Zhang, Z., *et al.*: **Co-evolution of a broadly neutralizing HIV-1 antibody and founder virus.** *Nature* 2013, **496**:469-476.

Johnson, W.E., and Desrosiers, R.C.: **Viral persistence: HIV's strategies of immune system evasion.** *Annu. Rev. Med.* 2002, **53**:499–518.

McCoy, L.E., and Burton, D.R.: **Identification and specificity of broadly neutralizing antibodies against HIV.** *Immunol. Rev.* 2017, **275**:11–20.

Pantaleo, G., Menzo, S., Vaccarezza, M., Graziosi, C., Cohen, O.J., Demarest, J.F., Montefiori, D., Orenstein, J.M., Fox, C., Schrager, L.K., *et al.*: **Studies in subjects with long-term nonprogressive human immunodeficiency virus infection.** *N. Engl. J. Med.* 1995, **332**:209–216.

Schmitz, J.E., Kuroda, M.J., Santra, S., Sasseville, V.G., Simon, M.A., Lifton, M.A., Racz, P., Tenner-Racz, K., Dalesandro, M., Scallon, B.J., *et al.*: **Control of viremia in simian immunodeficiency virus infection by CD8+ lymphocytes.** *Science* 1999, **283**:857–860.

Siliciano, R.F., and Greene, W.C.: **HIV latency.** *Cold Spring Harb. Perspect. Med.* 2011, **1**:a007096.

Sok, D., and Burton, D.R. **Recent progress in broadly neutralizing antibodies to HIV.** *Nat. Immunol.* 2018, **19**:1179–1188.

13-36   Lymphoid tissue is the major reservoir of HIV infection.

Burton, G.F., Masuda, A., Heath, S.L., Smith, B.A., Tew, J.G., and Szakal, A.K.: **Follicular dendritic cells (FDC) in retroviral infection: host/pathogen perspectives.** *Immunol. Rev.* 1997, **156**:185–197.

Chun, T.W., Carruth, L., Finzi, D., Shen, X., DiGiuseppe, J.A., Taylor, H., Hermankova, M., Chadwick, K., Margolick, J., Quinn, T.C., *et al.*: **Quantification of latent tissue reservoirs and total body viral load in HIV-1 infection.** *Nature* 1997, **387**:183–188.

Haase, A.T.: **Population biology of HIV-1 infection: viral and CD4+ T cell demographics and dynamics in lymphatic tissues.** *Annu. Rev. Immunol.* 1999, **17**:625–656.

Pierson, T., McArthur, J., and Siliciano, R.F.: **Reservoirs for HIV-1: mechanisms for viral persistence in the presence of antiviral immune responses and antiretroviral therapy.** *Annu. Rev. Immunol.* 2000, **18**:665–708.

13-37   Genetic variation in the host can alter the rate of HIV disease progression.

Piacentini, L., Biasin, M., Fenizia, C., and Clerici, M.: **Genetic correlates of protection against HIV infection: the ally within.** *J. Intern. Med.* 2009, **265**:110–124.

Walker, B.D., and Yu, X.G.: Unravelling the mechanisms of durable control of HIV-1. *Nat. Rev. Immunol.* 2013, **13**:487–498.

13-38   The destruction of immune function as a result of HIV infection leads to increased susceptibility to opportunistic infection and eventually to death.

Kedes, D.H., Operskalski, E., Busch, M., Kohn, R., Flood, J., and Ganem, D.R.: **The seroepidemiology of human herpesvirus 8 (Kaposi's sarcoma associated herpesvirus): distribution of infection in KS risk groups and evidence for sexual transmission.** *Nat. Med.* 1996, **2**:918–924.

Miller, R.: **HIV-associated respiratory diseases.** *Lancet* 1996, **348**:307–312.

Zhong, W.D., Wang, H., Herndier, B., and Ganem, D.R.: **Restricted expression of Kaposi sarcoma associated herpesvirus (human herpesvirus 8) genes in Kaposi sarcoma.** *Proc. Natl. Acad. Sci. USA* 1996, **93**:6641–6646.

13-39   Drugs that block HIV replication lead to a rapid decrease in titer of infectious virus and an increase in CD4 T cells.

Allers, K., Hütter, G., Hofmann, J., Loddenkemper, C., Rieger, K., Thiel, E., and Schneider, T.: **Evidence for the cure of HIV infection by CCR5Δ32/Δ32 stem cell transplantation.** *Blood* 2011, **117**:2791–2799.

Barouch, D.H., and Deeks, S.G.: **Immunologic strategies for HIV-1 remission and eradication.** *Science* 2014, **345**:169–174.

Boyd, M., and Reiss, P.: **The long-term consequences of antiretroviral therapy: a review.** *J. HIV Ther.* 2006, **11**:26–35.

Carcelain, G., Debre, P., and Autran, B.: **Reconstitution of CD4+ T lymphocytes in HIV-infected individuals following antiretroviral therapy.** *Curr. Opin. Immunol.* 2001, **13**:483–488.

Farber, J.M., and Berger, E.A.: **HIV's response to a CCR5 inhibitor: I'd rather tighten than switch!** *Proc. Natl. Acad. Sci. USA* 2002, **99**:1749–1751.

Ho, D.D.: **Perspectives series: host/pathogen interactions. Dynamics of HIV-1 replication *in vivo*.** *J. Clin. Invest.* 1997, **99**:2565–2567.

Kordelas, L., Verheyen, J., Esser, S., and Group, E.H.A.: **Shift of HIV tropism in stem-cell transplantation with CCR5 Delta32 mutation.** *N. Engl. J. Med.* 2014, **371**:880–882.

Lundgren, J.D., and Mocroft, A.: **The impact of antiretroviral therapy on AIDS and survival.** *J. HIV Ther.* 2006, **11**:36–38.

Perelson, A.S., Essunger, P., Cao, Y.Z., Vesanen, M., Hurley, A., Saksela, K., Markowitz, M., and Ho, D.D.: **Decay characteristics of HIV-1-infected compartments during combination therapy.** *Nature* 1997, **387**:188–191.

Wei, X., Ghosh, S.K., Taylor, M.E., Johnson, V.A., Emini, E.A., Deutsch, P., Lifson, J.D., Bonhoeffer, S., Nowak, M.A., Hahn, B.H., *et al.*: **Viral dynamics in human immunodeficiency virus type 1 infection.** *Nature* 1995, **373**:117–122.

13-40   In the course of infection, HIV accumulates many mutations, which can result in the outgrowth of drug-resistant variants.

Condra, J.H., Schleif, W.A., Blahy, O.M., Gabryelski, L.J., Graham, D.J., Quintero, J.C., Rhodes, A., Robbins, H.L., Roth, E., Shivaprakash, M., *et al.*: ***In vivo*** emergence of HIV-1 variants resistant to multiple protease inhibitors. *Nature* 1995, **374**:569–571.

Finzi, D., and Siliciano, R.F.: **Viral dynamics in HIV-1 infection.** *Cell* 1998, **93**:665–671.

Katzenstein, D.: **Combination therapies for HIV infection and genomic drug resistance.** *Lancet* 1997, **350**:970–971.

Moutouh, L., Corbeil, J., and Richman, D.D.: **Recombination leads to the rapid emergence of HIV 1 dually resistant mutants under selective drug pressure.** *Proc. Natl. Acad. Sci. USA* 1996, **93**:6106–6111.

13-41 HIV treatment and prophylaxis are leading to a decline in the spread of HIV and AIDS.

Coates, T.J., Aggleton, P., Gutzwiller, F., Des-Jarlais, D., Kihara, M., Kippax, S., Schechter, M., and van-den-Hoek, J.A.: **HIV prevention in developed countries.** *Lancet* 1996, **348**:1143–1148.

Decosas, J., Kane, F., Anarfi, J.K., Sodji, K.D., and Wagner, H.U.: **Migration and AIDS.** *Lancet* 1995, **346**:826–828.

Dowsett, G.W.: **Sustaining safe sex: sexual practices, HIV and social context.** *AIDS* 1993, **7**(suppl. 1):S257–S262.

Kirby, M.: **Human rights and the HIV paradox.** *Lancet* 1996, **348**:1217–1218.

Nelson, K.E., Celentano, D.D., Eiumtrakol, S., Hoover, D.R., Beyrer, C., Suprasert, S., Kuntolbutra, S., and Khamboonruang, C.: **Changes in sexual behavior and a decline in HIV infection among young men in Thailand.** *N. Engl. J. Med.* 1996, **335**:297–303.

Weniger, B.G., and Brown, T.: **The march of AIDS through Asia.** *N. Engl. J. Med.* 1996, **335**:343–345.

13-42 Vaccination against HIV remains an attractive solution but poses many difficulties.

Barouch, D.H.: **The quest for an HIV-1 vaccine—moving forward.** *N. Engl. J. Med.* 2013, **369**:2073–2076.

Haynes, B.F., and Burton, D.R.: **Developing an HIV vaccine.** *Science* 2017, **355**:1129–1130.

Isitman, G., Stratov, I., and Kent, S.J.: **Antibody-dependent cellular cytotoxicity and NK cell-driven immune escape in HIV Infection: implications for HIV vaccine development.** *Adv. Virol.* 2012, **212**:637208.

Letvin, N.L.: **Progress and obstacles in the development of an AIDS vaccine.** *Nat. Rev. Immunol.* 2006, **6**:930–939.

McMichael, A.J., and Koff, W.C.: **Vaccines that stimulate T cell immunity to HIV-1: the next step.** *Nat. Immunol.* 2014, **15**:319–322.

Pollard, A.J., and Bijker, E.M. **A guide to vaccinology: from basic principles to new developments.** *Nat. Rev. Immunol.* 2021, **21**:83–100.

Zolla-Pazner, S., and Cardozo, T.: **Structure-function relationships of HIV-1 envelope sequence-variable regions refocus vaccine design.** *Nat. Rev. Immunol.* 2010, **10**:527–535.

Allergic Diseases and Hypersensitivity Reactions

14

Although the adaptive immune response is critical for defense against infections, antigens not associated with infectious agents can sometimes elicit adaptive immune responses and cause disease. In one circumstance in which this happens, inherently harmless 'environmental' antigens such as pollen, food, and drugs induce hypersensitivity reactions known generally as **allergic reactions**.

In the early 1960s, the British pathologists P. G. H. Gell and R. R. A. Coombs classified hypersensitivity reactions due to immunological responses into four broad types. Type I hypersensitivity reactions represented immediate-type allergic reactions mediated by plasma 'reagin,' later identified as **IgE** antibodies, accompanied by mast-cell activation as the major final effector mechanism. Type II and type III hypersensitivity reactions were driven by antigen-specific IgG antibodies with the final effector mechanism being by cytotoxicity (type II) or by formation of immune complexes (type III). Finally, type IV hypersensitivity reactions were depicted as being driven by cellular effectors, including lymphocytes and a variety of myeloid cell types. The Gell and Coombs classification system is still in widespread use, particularly in the clinic, but we now understand that immune responses usually involve both humoral and cellular components. The classification of responses described in Chapter 11 in terms of the four types of immune-response modules is also a useful system for understanding disease pathogenesis, including allergic responses (see Fig. 11.5).

Most allergic reactions occur because the individual has become **sensitized** to an innocuous antigen—the **allergen** (such as those in food, pollen, or house dust)—by producing IgE antibodies against it. Subsequent exposure to the allergen triggers the activation of IgE-binding cells, chiefly mast cells and basophils, in the exposed tissue, leading to a series of characteristic responses. In hay fever (allergic rhinoconjunctivitis), symptoms occur when allergenic proteins derived from grass or weed pollen grains come in contact with the mucous membrane of the nose and eyes. In contrast, some hypersensitivity disorders, such as allergic contact dermatitis, serum sickness, or celiac disease, are not dependent on IgE antibodies and represent unwanted immune responses driven by IgG antibodies and/or cellular immune responses.

We are all exposed regularly to potential environmental allergens, but most of us do not develop clinically significant allergic reactions to them. However, some surveys suggest that more than half of the population shows allergic response to at least one substance in the environment. Some individuals manifest allergic responses to multiple common antigens. A predisposition to become IgE-sensitized to environmental allergens is called **atopy**; such individuals are said to be **atopic**. In this chapter, we discuss the genetic and environmental factors that may contribute to this predisposition. Genetic factors appear to play a role. If both parents are atopic, a child has a 40–60% chance of developing an IgE-mediated allergy, whereas the risk is much lower, of the order 10%, if neither parent is atopic.

IgE is prominent in the defense against extracellular parasites such as helminths and protozoa (see Section 11-10), which are prevalent in developing nations. But in developed nations, most serum IgE is directed against innocuous antigens, sometimes causing allergies (**Fig. 14.1**). Although rarely

IN THIS CHAPTER

IgE and IgE-mediated allergic diseases.

Effector mechanisms in IgE-mediated allergic reactions.

Non-IgE-mediated allergic diseases.

Fig. 14.1 IgE-mediated reactions to extrinsic antigens. All IgE-mediated responses involve mast-cell degranulation, but the symptoms experienced by the individual can be very different depending, for example, on whether the allergen is injected directly into the bloodstream, is eaten, or comes into contact with the mucosa of the ocular or respiratory tract.

IgE-mediated allergic reactions			
Reaction or disease	**Common stimuli**	**Route of entry**	**Response**
Systemic anaphylaxis	Drugs Venoms Food, e.g., peanuts Serum	Intravenous (either directly or following absorption into the blood after oral intake)	Edema Increased vascular permeability Laryngeal edema Circulatory collapse Death
Acute urticaria (wheal-and-flare)	Post-viral Animal hair Bee stings Allergy testing	Through skin Systemic	Local increase in blood flow and vascular permeability Edema
Seasonal rhinoconjunctivitis (hay fever)	Pollens (ragweed, trees, grasses) Dust-mite feces	Contact with conjunctiva of eye and nasal mucosa	Edema of conjunctiva and nasal mucosa Sneezing
Asthma	Dander (cat) Pollens Dust-mite feces	Inhalation leading to contact with mucosal lining of lower airways	Bronchial constriction Increased mucus production Airway inflammation Bronchial hyperreactivity
Food allergy	Peanuts Tree nuts Shellfish Fish Milk Eggs Soy Wheat	Oral	Vomiting Diarrhea Pruritus (itching) Urticaria (hives) Anaphylaxis (rarely)

life-threatening, allergic diseases can cause much distress and lost time from school and work, and their prevalence is increasing. Consequently, most clinical and scientific attention paid to IgE has been directed toward its pathologic roles in allergic disease rather than its protective capacity.

Here we first consider the mechanisms that favor the **sensitization** of an individual to an allergen, resulting in the production of antigen-specific IgE. We then describe the IgE-mediated allergic reaction itself, originally called the type I hypersensitivity response in a clinical classification scheme that was developed before the identification of IgE. We will also describe the pathological consequences of the interaction between an allergen and the IgE bound to the high-affinity Fcε receptor on mast cells and basophils. Finally, we consider the causes and consequences of other types of immunological hypersensitivity reactions, primarily type II and type III hypersensitivity responses.

IgE and IgE-mediated allergic diseases.

Immediate hypersensitivity reactions are those allergic reactions caused by activation of mast cells and basophils. This activation occurs when antigen binds to IgE that is already bound to the high-affinity IgE receptor **FcεRI** (see Section 10-24) expressed by these cells. IgE differs from other antibody isotypes in being predominantly localized in the tissues, where it is tightly bound to the surface cells expressing FcεRI. Binding of antigen to IgE causes cross-linking of FcεRI and the release of chemical mediators from the mast cells (**Fig. 14.2**). How an initial antibody response to environmental antigens comes to be dominated by IgE production in atopic individuals is still being worked out. In this part of the chapter, we describe the current understanding of the factors that contribute to this process.

The enzyme Der p 1 cleaves occludin in tight junctions and enters mucosa	Dendritic cell primes T cell in lymph node	IgE specific for Der p 1 travels to mucosa	Der p 1–specific IgE binds to mast cell; Der p 1 triggers mast-cell degranulation
Der p 1 is taken up by dendritic cells for antigen presentation and T-cell priming	T$_{FH}$/T$_H$2 cell induces B-cell switch to IgE production	IgE binds to FcεRI receptor on mast cell	Mast-cell granule contents cause allergic symptoms

Fig. 14.2 Sensitization to an inhaled allergen. Der p 1 is a common respiratory allergen that is found in fecal pellets of the house dust mite. When an atopic individual first encounters Der p 1, subepithelial dendritic cells ingest the allergenic protein and traffic to the draining lymph node, where T cells specific for Der p 1 are activated (first and second panels). Interaction of T$_{FH}$ cells (producing T$_H$2 cytokines such as IL-4) with Der p 1–specific B cells leads to the production of class-switched plasma cells producing Der p 1–specific IgE, which travels back to the mucosa (third panel). Here, the IgE is bound to Fc receptors on resident submucosal mast cells. On a subsequent encounter with Der p 1, the allergen binds to the mast cell–bound IgE, triggering mast-cell activation and the release of mast-cell granule contents, which cause the symptoms of the allergic reaction (last panel). Der p 1 is a protease that cleaves occludin, a protein that helps to maintain epithelial tight junctions; the enzymatic activity of Der p 1 is thought to help it pass through the epithelium.

14-1 Sensitization involves class switching to IgE production on first contact with an allergen.

To produce an allergic reaction, an individual must first be exposed to the allergen under conditions that lead to the production of IgE antibodies. Allergic symptoms occur when this individual experiences a subsequent exposure to that antigen. The different symptoms can depend on what tissues are involved. In developed countries, the most common exposure is to airborne allergens, which predominantly affect the nasal passages (allergic rhinitis), eyes (allergic conjunctivitis), or lower airways and lungs (asthma). Ingested allergens can lead to food allergy, sometimes affecting only the gastrointestinal tract, but not infrequently involving locations distant from the site of antigen entry. Reactions can occur at sites distant from the allergen entry point by transport through the blood circulation and can be limited to a single distant organ. Hives (also called urticaria) occur when allergens target the skin, wheezing (or bronchospasms) occurs when they target the lungs, and life-threatening lowering of the blood pressure (shock) occurs when they target the vascular system. Serious systemic reactions are termed **anaphylaxis**. It is not known why sensitization with a particular allergen in one individual leads to local reactions at the time of allergen challenge, whereas sensitization with the same allergen can yield anaphylaxis in another individual.

Atopic individuals often develop sensitization to many different antigens and may have many types of allergic symptoms depending on the route and quantity of allergen. Frequently, a progression can occur; for example, from atopic eczema in childhood to include allergic rhinitis and eventually asthma in later life. This progression has been termed the **atopic march**. Allergic reactions in non-atopic people, in contrast, are predominantly due to sensitization to one specific allergen, such as to bee venom or a drug such as penicillin, and can develop at any time of life. However, not all encounters with a potential allergen will lead to sensitization, and not all sensitizations will lead to a symptomatic allergic response, even in atopic individuals.

Recall that we have already described many of the signals leading to immune responses that result in production of IgE. In Section 9-15, we described the development of T_H2 cells that produce cytokines such as IL-4 and IL-5. In Section 10-12, we described how cytokines such as IL-4 can promote switching to IgE, typically in the germinal center reaction under the influence of T_{FH} cells. Presumably, conditions that favor T_H2 development also favor the emergence of T_{FH} cells producing similar cytokines, although this is an area still under active investigation. And in Section 11-10, we described how type 2 immune responses can protect against infections by parasites, particularly at vulnerable sites such as the mucosal epithelium of the lungs and intestines (see Section 12-4). Further, very recent discoveries have identified new types of cells—called Tuft cells in the intestine—in various mucosal epithelia that promote type 2 immune responses. These cells function as chemosensory cells and are sensitive to various signals that are still being identified. When activated, Tuft cells produce cytokines that enhance type 2 immune responses; one mechanism is their production of IL-25 (Section 11-3), which acts on T cells and type 2 innate lymphoid cells (ILC2 cells) to produce IL-13. IL-33, which can be produced by activated mast cells and by damaged or injured epithelial cells, also contributes to amplification of type 2 immune responses. IL-33 can act directly on T_H2 cells and ILC2 cells, augmenting their cytokine production.

Normally, allergic responses against common environmental antigens may be controlled because of the lack of signals that typically accompany infections. Dendritic cells that encounter and process antigens in the absence of 'danger' signals, such as those provoked by microbial infection, generally do not drive the development of CD4 T cells into an effector cell, such as a T_H2 cell. Instead, such dendritic cells can induce the development of antigen-specific regulatory T cells (T_{reg} cells) that contribute to a state of tolerance to the antigen (see Section 12-10). Despite a great deal of molecular understanding, it is still unknown why some individuals become strongly sensitized to particular allergens, but others do not.

Features of airborne allergens that may promote the priming of T_H2 cells that drive IgE responses	
Protein, often with carbohydrate side chains	Protein antigens induce T-cell responses
Low dose	Favors activation of IL-4–producing CD4 T cells
Low molecular mass	Allergen can diffuse out of particles into the mucosa
Highly soluble	Allergen can be readily eluted from particle
Stable	Allergen can survive in desiccated particle
Contains peptides that bind host MHC class II	Required for T-cell priming

Fig. 14.3 Properties of inhaled allergens. The typical characteristics of inhaled allergens are described in this table.

14-2 Although many types of antigens can cause allergic sensitization, proteases are common sensitizing agents.

Most airborne allergens are small, highly soluble proteins carried on dry particles such as pollen grains or dust-mite feces (**Fig. 14.3**). On contact with the mucus-covered epithelia of the eyes, nose, or airways, the allergen is eluted from the particle and is picked up by dendritic cells to provoke sensitization (see Fig. 14.2). At mucosal surfaces, allergens are typically presented to the immune system at low concentrations. It has been estimated that the maximum exposure of a person to the common pollen allergens in ragweed (*Ambrosia* species) does not exceed 1 µg per year.

However, not all allergens involve such low doses. Bee venom is a frequent cause of allergic sensitization, and individual bee stings result in the injection into the skin of 20–75 µg of bee venom. This is 1–2 orders of magnitude more than the dose of ragweed antigen that is inhaled into the airways. In the case of food allergy, ingestion of many grams of an allergenic food into the gastrointestinal tract over prolonged periods of time can lead to sensitization. Sensitization can also occur in response to injected antigens in either small or large doses. For example, before the introduction of recombinant human insulin, individuals with diabetes could develop allergy to porcine insulin, usually administered in small doses of 1–2 mg per injection. In contrast, penicillin-type drugs (including cephalosporins and other β-lactam–containing antibiotics) can lead to sensitization when administered by intramuscular or intravenous injection in the range of 1–2 g per injection.

While no physical, chemical, or functional feature has been found that is common to all allergens, many clinically significant allergens are proteases. One ubiquitous protease allergen is the cysteine protease **Der p 1**, which is present in the feces of the house dust mite, *Dermatophagoides pteronyssinus*. Der p 1 provokes allergic reactions in about 20% of the North American population. This enzyme has been found to cleave occludin, a protein component of intercellular tight junctions in the airway mucosa. The destruction of the integrity of the tight junctions between epithelial cells may allow Der p 1 to gain access to the subepithelial antigen-presenting cells such as dendritic cells, thereby inducing an immune response (see Fig. 14.2). Although still an area of active research, other activities of proteases include the activation of **nociceptors**, which are neuropeptide-producing sensory neurons present in the skin. House dust mites that have cysteine protease activity can activate these sensory neurons and induce their secretion of substance P, which can activate nearby mast cells. Cytokines secreted from mast cells can promote type 2 immune responses.

The cysteine protease papain, derived from the papaya fruit, can cause allergic reactions in workers preparing the enzyme. Allergies caused by environmental allergens present in the workplace are called **occupational allergies**. Although Der p 1 and papain are potent allergens, not all allergens are enzymes. In fact, two allergens identified from filarial worms are enzyme inhibitors, and in general, most allergenic pollen-derived proteins do not seem to possess enzymatic activity.

Some associations between allergies and proteases are indirect and somewhat coincidental. For example, high levels of IgE and multiple allergies are seen in individuals with Netherton syndrome (**Fig. 14.4**), an autosomal recessive condition caused by a mutation in the gene *SPINK5* (serine protease inhibitor Kazal-type 5). *SPINK5* encodes the serine protease inhibitor LEKTI (lymphoepithelial Kazal type–related inhibitor), which is expressed in the most differentiated viable layer of the skin (the granular cell layer), just internal to the cornified cell layer of the epidermis. Absence of LEKTI results in overly active epidermal **kallikreins**, which are proteases that can cleave desmosomes in the skin, leading to keratinocyte shedding and disturbed barrier function of the skin. It is the disturbance of the skin's barrier function—not the direct action of the protease—that leads to the production of IgE and allergies by allowing entry of antigen directly into the skin and underlying dermis, where immune responses can be initiated. A major component driving the T_H2 and IgE response is the production by the damaged epidermis of thymic stromal lymphopoietin (TSLP), which acts on T cells and dendritic cells to promote a type 2 immune response through mechanisms that are not precisely understood but are still being investigated. Mice with skin-specific deletions in the gene *Notch1* (see Section 8-14) also develop a failure in the barrier function of the skin, due to the requirement for Notch signaling for terminal keratinocyte differentiation. These mice also produce high amounts of TSLP and develop allergic manifestations in the skin.

Fig. 14.4 Netherton syndrome illustrates the association between disruption of the skin barrier and development of high levels of IgE and allergy. This 26-year-old man with Netherton syndrome, caused by a deficiency in the protease inhibitor SPINK5, had persistent erythroderma (redness of the skin), recurrent infections of the skin and other tissues, and multiple food allergies associated with high serum IgE levels. In the photograph, large erythematous plaques covered with scales and erosions are visible over the upper trunk. The epidermis in these regions is thickened and contains a perivascular infiltrate of neutrophils and mononuclear cells.

14-3 Genetic factors contribute to the development of IgE-mediated allergic disease.

For more than a decade, the genetic causes of allergy and asthma have been investigated predominantly using genome-wide association studies (GWASs). These studies examine the association of common genetic variations in the genome with a variety of clinical manifestations. The genetic variations that are mapped are typically **single-nucleotide polymorphisms, or SNPs**, which are frequently present in two forms at a genomic site. SNPs can be located in a coding region of a gene, where they may change the sequence of the encoded protein, but more frequently they are located in the intragenic regions of

Asthma susceptibility loci
Genes expressed in airway epithelial cells
Chemokines: *CCL5, CCL11, CCL24, CCL26*
Antimicrobial peptides: *DEFB1*
Secretoglobin family: *SCGB1A1*
Epithelial barrier protein: *FLG*
Genes regulating CD4 T-cell and ILC2 differentiation and function
Transcription factors: *GATA3, TBX21, RORA, STAT3, PHF11, IKZF4*
Cytokines: *IL4, IL5, IL10, IL13, IL25, IL33, TGFβ1*
Cytokine receptors: *IL2RB, IL4RA, IL5RA, IL6R, IL18R, IL1RL1, FCER1B*
Pattern-recognition receptors: *CD14, TLR2, TLR4, TLR6, TLR10, NOD1, NOD2*
Antigen presentation: *HLA-DRB1, HLA-DRB3, HLA-DQA, HLA-DQB, HLA-DPA, HLA-DPB, HLA-G*
Prostaglandin receptors: *PDFER2, PTGDR*
Genes with other functions
Proteinase or proteinase inhibitor: *USP38, SPINK5*
Signaling proteins: *IRAKM, SMAD3, PYHIN1, NOTCH4, GAB1, TNIP1*
Receptors: *ADRB2, P2X7*
Other: *DPP10, GPRA, COL29A1, ORMDL3, GSDMB, WDR36, DENND1B, RAD50, PBX2, LRRC32, AGER, CDK2*

Fig. 14.5 Susceptibility loci for asthma.
Loci that have shown linkage on the basis of GWASs or targeted gene analysis are listed, separated into genes that are expressed in epithelial cells of the airways, genes that regulate the differentiation and/ or function of CD4 T cells and ILC2 cells, and genes with other miscellaneous or unknown functions.

unknown function or in gene-regulatory regions. The medical conditions examined in GWASs have included asthma, total IgE levels, allergic sensitization, atopic dermatitis, allergic rhinitis, and food allergies. These studies have identified more than 40 loci associated with these conditions and have examined large numbers of individuals, a process that allows the discovery of SNPs with weak, but statistically significant, associations (**Fig. 14.5**). The strength of such associations is defined by the **odds ratio**. For example, an odds ratio of 10 means that the chance of having asthma is 10 times higher when a person has a particular SNP compared to individuals who have a common variant. The large size of GWASs for allergic conditions has allowed the identification of risk alleles with odds ratios less than 1.2, despite having very high statistical significance (p values). For example, a recent study into risk loci for asthma included nearly 24,000 asthma cases, more than 100,000 controls, and identified 5 new risk loci, with the largest odds ratio being 1.11. In other words, having that risk allele increases a person's chance of having asthma by a factor of 1.11 compared with a person with the common allele. Thus, their risk is increased only by 11% over normal.

Many of the risk alleles identified for allergic disorders are near genes with recognizable immunological function (see Fig. 14.5), but how any particular SNP contributes to susceptibility is frequently unknown. For example, specific alleles at the IL-33 receptor and IL-13 loci show strong association with both allergic asthma and atopic eczema. This sharing of genetic risk alleles by allergic asthma and atopic eczema is consistent with the finding that these two disorders are commonly found together in atopic families, with some family members manifesting both disorders, while other family members may manifest only atopic eczema or allergic asthma, but not both. But how this risk allele alters the biological activity of IL-33 in immune responses is unclear.

Alleles of many genes, especially genes that regulate the skin's barrier function, show linkage to atopic eczema without enhancing the risk for allergic asthma or allergic rhinoconjunctivitis, suggesting that other genetic factors can contribute to allergic responsiveness. In addition, there are differences among various ethnic groups for which susceptibility genes are most associated with a given allergic disease. Several of the chromosome regions associated with allergy or asthma are also associated with the inflammatory disease psoriasis and with autoimmune diseases, suggesting that these loci contain genes that are involved in exacerbating inflammation.

One candidate susceptibility gene for both allergic asthma and atopic eczema resides at 11q12–13 and encodes the β subunit of the high-affinity IgE receptor FcεRI. Another region associated with allergic disease, 5q31–33, contains at least four types of candidate genes that might be responsible for increased susceptibility. First, there is a cluster of tightly linked genes encoding the cytokines IL-3, IL-4, IL-5, IL-9, IL-13, and granulocyte–macrophage colony-stimulating factor (GM-CSF), which enhance IgE class switching, eosinophil survival, and mast-cell proliferation. A genetic variation in the IL-4 gene promoter that is associated with increased IgE levels in atopic individuals exhibits increased transcriptional activity in experimental systems, and so conceivably produces increased IL-4 *in vivo*. Atopy has also been associated with a gain-of-function mutation of the α subunit of the IL-4 receptor, with the mutation causing increased signaling after ligation of the receptor.

The second set of candidate genes in this region of chromosome 5 belongs to the TIM family (for T cell, immunoglobulin domain, and mucin domain). These genes encode four surface proteins expressed on T cells (Tim-1, -2, -3) and antigen-presenting cells (Tim-3, -4). In mice, Tim-3 is expressed on T_H1 cells and inhibits T_H1 responses, whereas Tim-2 is preferentially expressed in and inhibits T_H2 cells. Mouse strains with different variants of the Tim genes differ both in their susceptibility to allergic inflammation of the airways and in the production of IL-4 and IL-13 by their T cells. The third and fourth candidate genes in this part of the genome encode p40 and the β-adrenergic receptor. The p40 gene encodes the shared subunit of IL-12 and IL-23 (see Fig. 11.17) and could influence their production, while the β-adrenergic receptor gene could influence smooth muscle responsiveness to endogenous or pharmacological ligands. However, for the susceptibility locus at 5q31–33, we still do not understand how the different polymorphisms influence the complex genetics of atopy.

An inherited variation in IgE responses is linked to a particular HLA class II allele (the human MHC class II region) but affects responses to specific allergens rather than causing a general susceptibility to atopy. This results from the ability of certain HLA class II alleles to form a peptide:MHC complex with some allergens, which in atopic individuals will favor a T_H2 response. For example, IgE responses to several ragweed pollen allergens are associated with haplotypes containing the HLA class II allele DRB1*1501.

Allergic responses to drugs such as penicillin were originally thought to show no association with HLA class II or with the presence or absence of atopy. However, some drugs can interact with specific HLA alleles in a way that changes the structure of the peptide:MHC complex, and so elicit an auto-immune-type reaction. For example, a metabolite of the seizure medication carbamazepine, carbamazepine-10,11-epoxide (EPX), binds with HLA-B15:02 and the peptide bound in this HLA-B allele. The immune response to this EPX:peptide:HLA-B complex can lead to development of toxic epidermal necrolysis, a severe immune-mediated skin reaction in which widespread skin loss occurs due to necrosis, leaving the skin looking scalded.

Some genes may affect only particular aspects of allergic disease. In the skin, filaggrin contributes to normal skin barrier function by binding keratin molecules into the lipid envelope of cornifying keratinocytes. Loss-of-function mutations in the gene encoding filaggrin lead to the development of eczema. Through unknown mechanisms, filaggrin mutations also can contribute to the development of asthma. Almost half of the people in the United States who suffer from severe eczema have at least one mutated filaggrin allele. Between 7% and 10% of Caucasians carry a loss-of-function mutation in filaggrin, and the frequency of this mutation is considerably higher in individuals with asthma.

Allergic Asthma

14-4 Environmental factors may interact with genetic susceptibility to cause allergic disease.

Studies suggest that environmental factors and genetic variation each account for about 50% of the risk of developing atopy. In the past 50–60 years, atopic allergic diseases, and asthma in particular, have become more prevalent in economically advanced regions of the world, likely due to environmental changes that interact with an individual's genetic background. Although the incidence of asthma is lower in economically underdeveloped regions of Africa, Americans of African ancestry show increased asthma frequency and severity compared with Americans not of African ancestry. This shows a clear impact of environment on the expressivity of genetic influences.

One hypothesis suggests that this steady increase in allergic diseases is the result of a reduction in infectious diseases in early childhood that has occurred as populations have moved increasingly from rural into urban environments. The original proposition, first suggested in 1989 by David P. Strachan, was that infections in early life reduced atopy, and that less-hygienic environments, particularly those encountered in less-developed rural settings, predispose to more numerous infections early in childhood, which help to protect against the development of atopy and allergic asthma. Subsequently, this proposition

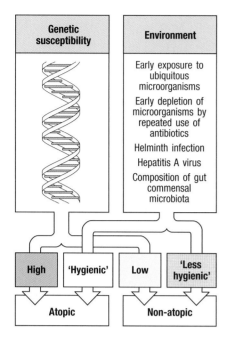

Fig. 14.6 Genes, the environment, and atopic allergic diseases. Both inherited and environmental factors are important determinants of the likelihood of developing allergic disease. Many genes are known to influence the development of asthma (see Fig. 14.5). The postulate of the 'hygiene hypothesis' is that exposure to some infections and to common environmental microorganisms in infancy and childhood drives the immune system toward a general state of non-atopy. In contrast, children who have a genetic susceptibility to atopy and who live in an environment with low exposure to infectious disease and environmental microorganisms or who received multiple courses of antibiotics in infancy and early childhood are thought not to develop efficient immunoregulatory mechanisms and to be most susceptible to the development of atopic allergic disease.

has evolved to become known as the **hygiene hypothesis** (**Fig. 14.6**) and has incorporated additional ideas. One idea was that reduced early-life exposure to microorganisms that were associated with farm animals and soil microorganisms led to changes in the intestinal microbiota, which performs an important immunomodulatory function (discussed in Chapter 12). But this idea seemed inconsistent with other evidence of a negative correlation between infection by helminths (such as hookworms and schistosomes) and the development of allergic disease. A study in Venezuela showed that children treated for a prolonged period with anti-helminthic agents had a higher prevalence of atopy than did untreated and heavily parasitized children. As helminths provoke a strong T_H2-mediated IgE response, this result was seemingly inconsistent with the original hygiene hypothesis.

This apparent inconsistency may suggest that many types of infection protect against the development of atopy. This protection could result from the production of cytokines such as IL-10 and TGF-β as part of the homeostatic responses during the infection. IL-10 and TGF-β suppress the formation of both T_H1 and T_H2 responses, and IL-10 suppresses T_H17 responses (see Sections 9-15 and 9-16). Most allergic reactions are initiated by antigens that enter through mucosal surfaces such as the respiratory or intestinal epithelium. The human mucosal immune system has evolved mechanisms of regulating responses to commensal flora and environmental antigens (such as food antigens) that involve the generation of IL-10 and TGF-β, thereby promoting the emergence of T_{reg} cells (see Chapter 12). Thus, decreased early exposure to common microbial pathogens and commensal bacteria could reduce the production of T_{reg} cells and increase the risk of an allergic response to common environmental antigens.

In support of a role for disturbed immunoregulatory pathways in susceptibility to asthma is circumstantial evidence that early exposures to certain types of childhood infections or to animals, with the important exception of the respiratory infection that we consider shortly, help to protect against the development of allergic disease. A history of infection with hepatitis A virus also may have a negative association with atopy. A possible explanation for this association is that the human counterpart of the murine Tim-1 protein (see Section 14-3) is the cellular receptor for hepatitis A virus (designated HAVCR1). The infection of T cells by hepatitis A virus could thus directly influence their differentiation and cytokine production, limiting the development of an IgE-generating response.

In contrast to these negative associations, there is a positive association between asthma in children and previous attacks of bronchiolitis associated with respiratory syncytial virus (RSV) infection. Children hospitalized with RSV infection have a skewed ratio of cytokine production away from IFN-γ toward IL-4, presumably increasing their likelihood of developing T_H2 responses and increased production of IgE. This effect of RSV appears to depend on age at first infection. But the basis for this association remains unclear. In a randomized clinical trial, prevention of RSV infection in the first year of life using an antibody to the virus (palivizumab) did not reduce the occurrence of asthma subsequently up to 6 years of age. Conceivably, some other environmental factor may represent a significant cause of asthma or the association between RSV and asthma may be due to an underlying factor associated with both susceptibility to RSV and asthma.

Other environmental factors that might contribute to the increase in atopic disease are changes in diet, allergen exposure, atmospheric pollution, and tobacco smoke. There is evidence for an interaction between allergens and pollution, particularly in genetically susceptible individuals. Diesel exhaust particles are the best-studied pollutant in this context; they increase IgE production 20- to 50-fold when combined with allergen, with an accompanying shift to T_H2 cytokine production. Reactive oxidant chemicals such as ozone are generated as a result of such pollution, and individuals less able to deal with this onslaught may be at increased risk of allergic disease. Genes that might be governing this aspect of susceptibility are *GSTP1* and *GSTM1*, members of the glutathione-*S*-transferase superfamily that are important in preventing oxidative stress. Individuals who were allergic to ragweed pollen and who carried particular variant alleles of these genes showed an increased airway hyperreactivity when challenged with the allergen-plus-diesel exhaust particles than when challenged with the allergen alone. A study in Mexico City on the effects of atmospheric ozone levels on atopic children with allergic asthma also found that the children carrying the null allele of *GSTM1* were more susceptible than noncarriers to airway hyperreactivity when exposed to given levels of ozone.

Summary.

Allergens are generally innocuous antigens that commonly provoke an IgE antibody response in susceptible individuals. Such antigens normally enter the body at very low doses by diffusion across mucosal surfaces and trigger a type 2 immune response. The differentiation of naive allergen-specific T cells into T_H2 cells and T_{FH} cells that produce cytokines such as IL-4 and IL-13 support the switching of allergen-specific B cells to the IgE isotype. The specific IgE produced in response to the allergen circulates and binds to the high-affinity receptor for IgE on mast cells and basophils, where it serves as the trigger to activate these cells upon future encounter with free allergen. The tendency for a person to overproduce IgE in response to exposure to innocuous allergens is influenced by both genetic and environmental factors. GWASs have revealed a large number of SNPs that identify alleles of many candidate genes associated with atopy and allergy. Most of these candidate genes have functions related to regulation of immune processes. However, most such alleles have a relatively weak odds ratio for their association, and in most cases the mechanism of their association is unclear. Nonetheless, once IgE has been produced in response to an allergen, subsequent exposure to the allergen triggers an allergic response, which we describe in the next part of the chapter.

Effector mechanisms in IgE-mediated allergic reactions.

Allergic reactions are triggered when allergens cross-link preformed IgE bound to the high-affinity receptor FcεRI on mast cells. Mast cells line external mucosal surfaces and serve to alert the immune system to local infection. Once activated, they induce inflammatory reactions by secreting pharmacological mediators such as **histamine** stored in preformed granules and by synthesizing prostaglandins, leukotrienes, and platelet-activating factor from the plasma membrane. Mast cells also release various cytokines and chemokines after activation and, in the case of an allergic reaction, provoke unpleasant reactions to innocuous antigens that are not associated with invading pathogens that need to be expelled.

14-5 Most IgE is cell-bound and engages effector mechanisms of the immune system by pathways different from those of other antibody isotypes.

Antibodies engage effector cells such as mast cells by binding to receptors specific for their Fc constant regions. Most antibodies engage Fc receptors only after their antigen-binding sites have bound specific antigen, forming an immune complex of antigen and antibody. IgE is an exception, because it is captured by the high-affinity Fcε receptor (FcεRI) in the absence of bound antigen. This means that, unlike other antibodies, which are found mainly in body fluids, IgE is mostly found fixed on cells that carry this receptor—mast cells in tissues, and basophils in the circulation and at sites of inflammation. The ligation of the cell-bound IgE antibody by specific multivalent antigen triggers the activation of these cells at the sites of antigen entry into the tissues. The release from these activated mast cells of inflammatory lipid mediators, cytokines, and chemokines at sites of IgE-triggered reactions recruits eosinophils and basophils to augment the allergic response. It also recruits T_H2 cells, which can then mount a local type 2 cellular response.

There are two types of Fc receptors that bind IgE. The first, FcεRI, expressed on mast cells and basophils, is a high-affinity receptor of the immunoglobulin superfamily (see Section 10-24). High levels of IgE, such as those that exist in people with allergic diseases or parasite infections, can result in a marked increase in FcεRI on the surface of mast cells, an enhanced sensitivity of such cells to activation by low concentrations of specific antigen, and a markedly increased, IgE-dependent release of chemical mediators and cytokines. When IgE bound to this receptor is cross-linked by specific antigen, it transduces an activating signal through the receptor-bound Lyn tyrosine kinase (see Section 7-20), which phosphorylates ITAMs on the intracellular domain of the receptor (**Fig. 14.7**). The phosphorylated ITAMs recruit and activate the amplifying tyrosine kinase Syk, which in turn phosphorylates and activates a broad range of downstream effector pathways. One important target is the activation of the enzyme phospholipase C-γ (PLC-γ). As in the TCR signaling pathway, this leads to the generation of IP_3 and ultimately to an increase in cytosolic calcium (see Section 7-13 and Fig. 7.18), which activates the release of the preformed secretory granules in the cell into the surrounding tissues.

Fig. 14.7 Allergens induce signaling by the FcεRI receptor to cause degranulation of mast cells. First panel: IgE specific to an allergen is bound to the high-affinity IgE receptor, FcεRI. Binding of a multivalent allergen to this IgE induces receptor cross-linking, leading to the phosphorylation by the bound kinases Fyn (not shown) and Lyn of the ITAMs in the γ chain of FcεRI, which is similar in structure to the TCR γζ chain, thus recruiting the ITAM-binding kinase Syk. Second panel: Syk phosphorylates the signaling molecule LAT, which recruits signaling components that lead to the activation of phospholipase C-γ (PLC-γ) (see Fig. 7-17). Third panel: Activated PLC-γ cleaves phosphatidylinositol 4,5-bisphosphate (PIP$_2$), generating inositol 1,4,5-trisphosphate (IP$_3$), which acts on receptors in the membrane of the endoplasmic reticulum (ER) to induce the release of calcium ions (Ca^{+2}) into the cytosol. Fourth panel: This increase in cytosolic Ca^{+2} ions induces the fusion of membranes of the preformed secretory granules in the mast-cell cytoplasm with the cell's plasma membrane (mechanisms not shown) to release the granule's contents, such as histamine, into the extracellular space.

The second IgE receptor, FcεRII, usually known as **CD23**, is a C-type lectin and is structurally unrelated to FcεRI; it binds IgE with low affinity. CD23 is present on many cell types, including B cells, activated T cells, monocytes, eosinophils, platelets, follicular dendritic cells, and some thymic epithelial cells. This receptor was thought to be crucial for the regulation of IgE levels, but mouse strains in which the gene for CD23 has been inactivated still develop relatively normal polyclonal IgE responses. Nevertheless, CD23 does seem to be involved in enhancing IgE antibody levels in some situations. Responses against a specific antigen are known to be increased in the presence of the antigen complexed with IgE, but such enhancement fails to occur in mice that lack the gene for CD23. This has been interpreted to indicate that CD23 on antigen-presenting cells has a role in the capture of antigen that is complexed with IgE.

14-6 Mast cells reside in tissues and orchestrate allergic reactions.

When Paul Ehrlich described mast cells found in the mesentery of rabbits, he called them *Mastzellen* ('fattened cells'). Like basophils, mast cells contain granules rich in acidic proteoglycans that take up basic dyes. Mast cells are derived from hematopoietic stem cells but mature locally, often residing near surfaces exposed to pathogens and allergens, such as mucosal tissues and the connective tissues surrounding blood vessels.

The major factors for mast-cell growth and development include stem-cell factor (the ligand for the receptor tyrosine kinase Kit), IL-3, and T_H2-associated cytokines such as IL-4 and IL-9. Mice with defective Kit lack differentiated mast cells, and although they produce IgE, they cannot make IgE-mediated inflammatory responses. This shows that such responses depend almost exclusively on mast cells. There are many mast-cell precursors in tissues, and they can rapidly differentiate into mature mast cells in conditions of allergic inflammation, thus aiding the continuation of the allergic response. Mast-cell growth and survival depend on the activation of phosphatidylinositol 3-kinase (PI 3-kinase) in mast cells by Kit. Pharmacological inactivation of the p110δ isoform of PI 3-kinase has been shown to protect mice against allergic responses. Inhibitors of the amplifying tyrosine kinase Syk have also shown promise as blockers of IgE-dependent mast-cell responses.

The consequences of IgE-mediated mast-cell activation depend on the dose of antigen, its route of entry, and which tissues are affected (**Fig. 14.8**). Symptoms range from the swollen eyes and rhinitis associated with contact of pollen with the conjunctiva of the eye and the nasal epithelium to the life-threatening circulatory collapse that occurs in anaphylaxis. The immediate reaction caused by mast-cell degranulation is followed, to a greater or lesser extent depending on the disease, by a more sustained inflammation, which is due to the

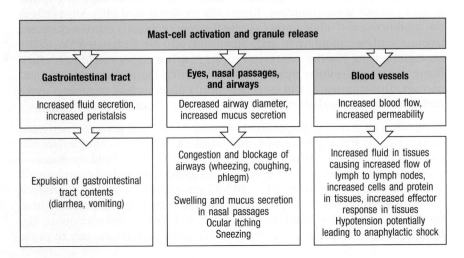

Fig. 14.8 Mast-cell activation has different effects on different tissues.

Fig. 14.9 Molecules released by activated mast cells. Mast cells release a wide variety of biologically active proteins and other chemical mediators. The enzymes and toxic mediators listed in the first two rows are released from the preformed granules. The cytokines, chemokines, and lipid mediators are mostly synthesized after activation.

Class of product	Examples	Biological effects
Enzyme	Tryptase, chymase, cathepsin G, carboxypeptidase A	Remodel connective tissue matrix
Toxic mediator	Histamine, heparin	Toxic to parasites Increase vascular permeability Cause smooth muscle contraction Anticoagulation
Cytokine	IL-4, IL-13, IL-33	Stimulate and amplify T_H2 cell response
	IL-3, IL-5, GM-CSF	Promote eosinophil production and activation
	TNF-α (some stored preformed in granules)	Promotes inflammation Stimulates cytokine production by many cell types Activates endothelium
Chemokine	CCL3	Attracts monocytes, macrophages, and neutrophils
Lipid mediator	Prostaglandins D2, E2 Leukotrienes C4, D4, E4	Smooth muscle contraction Chemotaxis of eosinophils, basophils, and T_H2 cells Increase vascular permeability Stimulate mucus secretion Bronchoconstriction
	Platelet-activating factor	Attracts leukocytes Amplifies production of lipid mediators Activates neutrophils, eosinophils, and platelets

recruitment of other effector leukocytes, notably T_H2 lymphocytes, eosinophils, and basophils.

Mast-cell degranulation begins within seconds of antigen binding, releasing an array of preformed and newly generated inflammatory mediators (**Fig. 14.9**). Granule contents include the short-lived vasoactive amine, histamine, serine esterases, and proteases such as chymase and tryptase. Histamine acts through four known receptors, H_1 through H_4, each a G protein–coupled receptor. Histamine acts via the H_1 receptor on local blood vessels to cause an immediate increase in local blood flow and vessel permeability. This leads to edema and local inflammation. Histamine is also a major stimulus for itching and sneezing, by virtue of its activation of neural receptors. By acting through H_2, H_3, and H_4 receptors on a variety of leukocytes and tissue cells, histamine participates in atopic dermatitis, chronic urticaria, and several autoimmune disorders.

Human mast cells are classified into subtypes on the basis of their protease content and tissue location. Mast cells in mucosal epithelia express tryptase as their primary serine protease. These cells are designated MC_T. Mast cells in the submucosa and other connective tissues predominantly express chymase, tryptase, carboxypeptidase A, and cathepsin G and are designated MC_{CT}. The proteases released by the mast cells activate matrix metalloproteinases, which break down extracellular matrix proteins, causing tissue disintegration and damage. These proteases can exert beneficial effects such as degrading snake and bee venoms, thus helping to suppress allergic responses to these agents.

In addition to secreting the contents of their preformed granules, activated mast cells also synthesize *de novo* and release a number of other inflammatory mediators. These include chemokines, cytokines, and lipid mediators—prostaglandins, leukotrienes, thromboxanes (collectively called eicosanoids), and platelet-activating factor. MC_T and MC_{CT} mast cells, for example, produce the cytokine IL-4, which helps perpetuate type 2 immune responses. These secreted products contribute to both acute and chronic inflammation. The lipid mediators, in particular, can act both rapidly and persistently to cause smooth muscle contraction, increased vascular permeability, and the secretion of mucus, as well as induce the influx and activation of leukocytes, which contribute to allergic inflammation.

Eicosanoids derive mainly from the membrane-associated fatty acid arachidonic acid. This is cleaved from membrane phospholipids by phospholipase A_2, which is activated at the plasma membrane as a result of cell activation. Arachidonic acid can be modified by either of two pathways to give rise to lipid mediators. Modification via the cyclooxygenase pathway produces the prostaglandins and thromboxanes, whereas leukotrienes are produced via the lipoxygenase pathway. Prostaglandin D2 is the major prostaglandin produced by mast cells; it recruits T_H2 cells, eosinophils, and basophils, all of which express its receptor (PTGDR). Prostaglandin D2 is critical to the development of allergic diseases such as asthma; polymorphisms in the gene *PTGDR* have been linked to an increased risk of developing asthma. The leukotrienes, especially C4, D4, and E4, are also important in sustaining inflammatory responses in tissues. Nonsteroidal anti-inflammatory drugs such as aspirin and ibuprofen exert their effects by preventing prostaglandin production. They inhibit the cyclooxygenases that act on arachidonic acid to form the ring structure present in prostaglandins.

Large amounts of the cytokine tumor necrosis factor (TNF)-α are also released by mast cells after activation. Some comes from stores in the granules; some is newly synthesized by the activated mast cells. TNF-α activates endothelial cells, resulting in increased expression of adhesion molecules, which in turn promotes the influx of pro-inflammatory leukocytes and lymphocytes into the affected tissue (see Chapter 3). Additionally, mast-cell TNF-α contributes importantly to the influx of leukocytes into regional lymph nodes in response to microbial infection of peripheral tissues.

14-7 Eosinophils and basophils cause inflammation and tissue damage in allergic reactions.

The inflammatory cascade produced by mast-cell activation is amplified by the recruitment of eosinophils, basophils, T_H2 lymphocytes, and B cells. Normally this reaction is a defense against parasite infection (see Section 10-25), but in an allergic reaction, it represents a pathological response to environmental antigens.

Eosinophils are granulocytic leukocytes that originate in bone marrow. They are so called because their granules, which contain arginine-rich basic proteins, are colored bright orange by the acidic stain eosin. In healthy humans, these cells represent less than 6% of the leukocytes in the circulation; most eosinophils are found in tissues, especially in the connective tissue immediately underneath respiratory, gut, and urogenital epithelium, implying a likely role for these cells in defense against invading organisms at these sites. They possess numerous cell-surface receptors, including receptors for cytokines (such as IL-5), Fcγ and Fcα receptors, and the complement receptors CR1 and CR3, through which they can be activated and stimulated to degranulate. For example, parasites coated with IgG, C3b, or IgA can cause eosinophil degranulation. In allergic tissue reactions, the large concentrations of IL-5, IL-3, and GM-CSF that are typically present are likely to contribute to degranulation.

When activated, eosinophils express two kinds of effector function. First, they can release highly toxic granule proteins and free radicals, which can kill microorganisms and parasites but also can cause significant damage to host tissues in allergic reactions (**Fig. 14.10**). Second, they can synthesize chemical mediators, including prostaglandins, leukotrienes, and cytokines. These amplify the inflammatory response by activating epithelial cells and by recruiting and activating more eosinophils and leukocytes. In chronic inflammatory

Fig. 14.10 Eosinophils secrete a range of highly toxic granule proteins and other inflammatory mediators. As for mast cells (see Fig. 14.9), enzymes and toxic mediators released by eosinophils are largely stored preformed in granules. In contrast, cytokines, chemokines, and lipid mediators are largely synthesized after eosinophil activation.

Class of product	Examples	Biological effects
Enzyme	Eosinophil peroxidase	Toxic to targets by catalyzing halogenation Triggers histamine release from mast cells
	Eosinophil collagenase	Remodels connective tissue matrix
	Matrix metalloproteinase-9	Matrix protein degradation
Toxic protein	Major basic protein	Toxic to parasites and mammalian cells Triggers histamine release from mast cells
	Eosinophil cationic protein	Ribonuclease Toxic to parasites Neurotoxin
	Eosinophil-derived neurotoxin	Neurotoxin
Cytokine	IL-4, IL-13, IL-3, GM-CSF	Amplify eosinophil production by bone marrow Eosinophil activation
	TGF-α, TGF-β	Epithelial proliferation Myofibroblast formation
Chemokine	CXCL8 (IL-8)	Promotes influx of leukocytes
Lipid mediator	Leukotrienes C4, D4, E4	Smooth muscle contraction Increase vascular permeability Increase mucus secretion Bronchoconstriction
	Platelet-activating factor	Attracts leukocytes Amplifies production of lipid mediators Activates neutrophils, eosinophils, and platelets

responses, eosinophils can contribute to airway tissue remodeling. In allergic tissue reactions, eosinophils may accumulate in large numbers, and the continued presence of eosinophils is characteristic of chronic allergic inflammation, and they may be major contributors to tissue damage.

Because their inappropriate activation is harmful to the host, the activation and degranulation of eosinophils is strictly regulated, The first level of control acts on the production of eosinophils by the bone marrow. Few eosinophils are produced in the absence of infection or other immune stimulation. But when T_H2 cells are activated, the cytokines they produce, such as IL-5 and GM-CSF, increase the production of eosinophils in the bone marrow and their release into the circulation. However, transgenic animals overexpressing IL-5 have increased numbers of eosinophils (**eosinophilia**) in the circulation but not in their tissues, indicating that the migration of eosinophils from the circulation into tissues is regulated separately by a second set of controls.

The key molecule regulating the entry of eosinophils into tissues is the chemokine receptor CCR3. CCR3 is highly expressed on eosinophils and is also expressed on basophils, mast cells, and T_H2 cells. CCR3 is quite promiscuous and binds several CC chemokines. Three CC chemokines have been named **eotaxins** because of their specificity for eosinophils—CCL11 (eotaxin 1), CCL24 (eotaxin 2), and CCL26 (eotaxin 3)—and each binds to CCR3. In addition, the CC chemokines CCL5, CCL7, and CCL13 also bind CCR3 and will induce eosinophil chemotaxis and activation. Identical or similar chemokines stimulate mast cells and basophils. For example, eotaxins attract basophils and cause their degranulation. T_H2 cells also express CCR3 and will migrate toward eotaxins.

Basophils are also present at the site of an inflammatory reaction. Growth factors for basophils are very similar to those for eosinophils; they include IL-3,

IL-5, and GM-CSF. There is evidence for reciprocal control of the maturation of the stem-cell population into basophils or eosinophils. For example, TGF-β in the presence of IL-3 suppresses eosinophil differentiation and enhances that of basophils. Basophils are normally present in very low numbers in the circulation and seem to have a similar role to that of eosinophils in defense against pathogens. Like eosinophils, they are recruited to the sites of IgE-mediated allergic reactions. Basophils express high-affinity FcεRI on their cell surfaces and so have IgE bound. On activation by antigen binding to IgE or by cytokines, they release histamine from their granules and also produce IL-4 and IL-13.

Eosinophils, mast cells, and basophils can interact with each other. Eosinophil degranulation releases **major basic protein** (see Fig. 14.10), which in turn causes the degranulation of mast cells and basophils. This effect is augmented by any of the cytokines that affect eosinophil and basophil growth, differentiation, and activation, such as IL-3, IL-5, and GM-CSF.

14-8 IgE-mediated allergic reactions have a rapid onset but can also lead to chronic responses.

Under laboratory conditions, the clinical response of a sensitized individual to challenge by intradermal allergen or inhalation of allergen can be divided into an 'immediate reaction' and a 'late-phase reaction' (**Fig. 14.11**). The immediate reaction is due to IgE-mediated mast-cell activation and starts within seconds of allergen exposure. It is the result of the actions of histamine, prostaglandins, and other preformed or rapidly synthesized mediators released by mast cells. These mediators cause a rapid increase in vascular permeability,

Fig. 14.11 Allergic reactions in response to test antigens can be divided into an immediate response and a late-phase response. Left panel: The response to an inhaled antigen can be divided into early and late responses. An asthmatic response in the lungs with narrowing of the airways caused by the constriction of bronchial smooth muscle and development of edema can be measured as a fall in the peak expiratory flow rate (PEFR). PEFR is a person's maximum ability to breathe out air and is a measure of the flow of air through the bronchi of the lungs. The immediate response peaks within minutes after antigen inhalation and then subsides, returning to near-baseline PEFR. Six to eight hours after antigen challenge, there can be a late-phase response that also results in a fall in the PEFR. The immediate response is caused by the direct effects on blood vessels, nerves, and smooth muscle of rapidly metabolized mediators such as histamine and lipid mediators released by mast cells. The late-phase response is caused by the continued production of these mediators, by the production of vasoactive compounds that dilate blood vessels, and by recruitment of lymphocytes and myeloid cells, which together lead to the production of edema. Right panel: A wheal-and-flare allergic reaction develops within a minute or two of intradermal injection of antigen and lasts for up to 30–60 minutes. The more widespread edematous response characteristic of the late phase develops approximately 6 hours later and can persist for up to 2 or 3 days. The photograph shows an intradermal skin challenge with allergen resulting in a wheal-and-flare (early-phase) reaction observed 15 minutes after allergen challenge (left) and a late-phase reaction occurring 6 hours after challenge (right). The allergen was grass pollen extract.

resulting in visible edema and reddening of the skin (in a skin response) and airway narrowing as result of edema and the constriction of smooth muscle (in an airway response). In the skin, histamine acting on H_1 receptors on local blood vessels causes an immediate increase in vascular permeability, which leads to extravasation of fluid and edema. Histamine also acts on H_1 receptors on local nerve endings, leading to reflex vasodilation of cutaneous blood vessels and local reddening of the skin. The resulting skin lesion is called a **wheal-and-flare reaction** (see Fig. 14.11, right panel).

Whether or not a **late-phase reaction** occurs depends on allergen dose and on aspects of the cellular immune activation that are difficult to quantify. At doses of intradermally administered allergen that are deemed safe for skin testing of subjects with allergic asthma, for example, a late reaction occurs in about 50% of individuals who show an immediate response (see Fig. 14.11, right panel). The late reaction peaks between 3 and 9 hours after antigen challenge, and in skin tests it becomes obvious as a much increased area and degree of edema that can persist for 24 hours or longer. The late-phase reaction is caused by the continued synthesis and release of inflammatory mediators by mast cells, especially vasoactive mediators such as calcitonin gene–related peptide (CGRP) and vascular endothelial growth factor (VEGF), which cause vasodilation and vascular leakage that result in edema and the recruitment of eosinophils, basophils, monocytes, and lymphocytes. The importance of this cellular influx is shown by the ability of glucocorticoid medications to block the late-phase response through their inhibition of cell recruitment, whereas glucocorticoids do not block the immediate response. A late-phase reaction can also occur after aerosol exposure to allergen and is characterized by a second phase of airway narrowing with sustained edema and cellular infiltration into the peribronchial spaces.

In individuals with a clinical history of allergic disease, allergists use the immediate response to help assess and confirm sensitization and to determine which allergens are responsible. Minute amounts of potential allergens are introduced into the skin by a skin prick—one site for each allergen—and if the individual is sensitive to any of the allergens tested, a wheal-and-flare reaction will occur at the site within a few minutes (see Fig. 14.11, right panel). Although the reaction after the administration of such small amounts of allergen is usually very localized, there is a small risk of inducing anaphylaxis. Another standard test for allergy is to measure the circulating concentration of IgE antibody specific for a particular allergen in an ELISA (see Appendix I, Section A-4).

IgE-mediated allergic diseases can cause chronic allergic inflammation with serious long-term consequences, such as chronic asthma. In long-standing asthma, for example, the cytokines and vasoactive mediators such as CGRP and VEGF result in persistent edema and narrowing of the airways. This can also lead to **airway tissue remodeling**, which changes the bronchial tissue via smooth muscle hypertrophy (an increase in the size of the muscle cells) and hyperplasia (an increase in the number of cells), subepithelial deposition of collagen, and often goblet-cell hyperplasia.

The clinical symptoms produced by an IgE-mediated allergic reaction depend on several variables: the dose of allergen, the amount of allergen-specific IgE present, the route by which the allergen is introduced, and probably some underlying defect in barrier function in the particular tissue or organ affected. The outcomes produced by different combinations of allergen dose and route of entry are summarized in **Fig. 14.12**. When exposure to allergen in a sensitized individual triggers an allergic reaction, both the immediate and the chronic effects are focused at the site at which mast-cell degranulation occurs, and they involve the recruitment of many soluble and cellular components of effector pathways.

Connective tissue mast cells (MC_CT)		Mucosal mast cells (MC_T)	
Route of allergen entry			
Intravenous	Subcutaneous	Inhalation	Ingestion

Mast-cell activation

| Widespread release of histamine, which acts on blood vessels to increase permeability, leading to hives (low dose, micrograms or less) or anaphylactic shock (medium to high dose, milligrams to grams) | Local release of histamine causes wheal-and-flare reaction. Airborne or topical allergens penetrating skin can also be a cause of atopic eczema | Allergic rhinitis (upper airway), caused by increased mucus production and nasal irritation. Asthma (lower airway) due to contraction of bronchial smooth muscle and increased mucus secretion | Contraction of intestinal smooth muscle induces vomiting. Outflow of fluid into gut causes diarrhea. Antigen diffuses into blood vessels and is widely disseminated, causing urticaria (hives), anaphylaxis, or atopic eczema |

Fig. 14.12 The route of administration of allergen determines the type of IgE-mediated allergic reaction that results. There are two main anatomic distributions of mast cells: those associated with vascularized connective tissues and called connective tissue mast cells (MC_CT) and those found in submucosal layers of the gut and respiratory tract and called mucosal mast cells (MC_T). In an allergic individual, all of these mast cells are coated through their cell-surface Fcε receptors with IgE directed against specific allergens. The response to an allergen then depends on which mast cells are activated. Allergen in the bloodstream (intravenous) activates connective tissue mast cells throughout the body, resulting in the systemic release of histamine and other mediators. Entry of allergen through the skin activates local connective tissue mast cells, leading to a local inflammatory reaction. After an experimental skin prick with allergen or a bite from an insect to which the individual is sensitized, this manifests as a wheal-and-flare reaction. In atopic individuals, airborne or topically applied allergens that penetrate the skin may lead to atopic eczema. Inhaled allergen that penetrates respiratory mucosal epithelia activates mainly mucosal mast cells, causing increased secretion of mucus by the mucosal epithelium and irritation in the nasal mucosa, leading to allergic rhinitis—or to asthma if constriction of smooth muscle in the lower airways occurs. Ingested allergen penetrates the gut epithelium, causing vomiting due to intestinal smooth muscle contraction and diarrhea due to outflow of fluid across the gut epithelium. Food allergens can also be disseminated in the bloodstream, causing widespread urticaria (hives) when the allergen reaches the skin, or they may cause eczema.

14-9 Allergen introduced into the bloodstream can cause anaphylaxis and urticaria.

If allergen is introduced directly into the bloodstream, for example, by a bee or wasp sting, or is rapidly absorbed into the bloodstream from the gut in a sensitized individual, connective tissue mast cells associated with blood vessels throughout the body can become immediately activated, resulting in a widespread release of histamine and other mediators that causes the systemic reaction called anaphylaxis. The symptoms of a systemic allergic reaction can range in severity from mild **urticaria** (hives) to fatal **anaphylactic shock** (see Fig. 14.12, first and fourth panels).

Acute urticaria is a response to foreign allergens that are delivered to the skin via the systemic blood circulation. Activation of mast cells in the skin by allergen causes them to release histamine, which in turn causes itchy, red swellings all over the body—a disseminated version of the wheal-and-flare reaction. Acute urticaria is commonly caused by an IgE-mediated reaction against an allergen. In some patients, treatment with omalizumab (a therapeutic monoclonal anti-IgE antibody) leads to resolution of hives, demonstrating a role for IgE in these individuals, even though the antigen that elicited the IgE often cannot be identified. There is also an autoimmune disorder of chronic urticaria that persists or recurs over long periods of time. This can be caused by autoantibodies against the α chain of FcεRI or against IgE itself, which can directly trigger mast-cell degranulation.

In anaphylactic shock, a widespread increase in vascular permeability and smooth muscle contraction results from a massive release of histamine and other mediators, such as leukotrienes, derived from mast cells and basophils. The consequences are a catastrophic reduction of blood pressure, culminating in hypotensive shock (a condition in which low blood pressure leads to inadequate supply of blood to vital organs, often leading to death), and constriction of the airways, culminating in respiratory failure. The most common causes of anaphylaxis are allergic reactions to wasp and bee stings, ingested or injected medications, or allergic responses to foods in sensitized individuals. For example, anaphylaxis in individuals allergic to peanuts is relatively common. Severe anaphylactic shock can be rapidly fatal if untreated but can usually be controlled by the immediate injection of epinephrine, which causes relaxation of airway smooth muscles via stimulation of β-adrenergic receptors, and reverses the life-threatening cardiovascular effects via stimulation of α-adrenergic receptors.

Systemic allergic reactions can occur after repeated treatment with many classes of drugs, notably penicillin and related drugs. Allergic reaction to penicillin by injection can cause anaphylaxis and even result in death, while administration of oral penicillin to an allergic individual can cause anaphylaxis, but the reaction is usually less severe than that caused by injection. One of the reasons that penicillin is particularly prone to inducing allergic reactions is that it acts as a hapten (see Appendix I, Section A-1); it is a small molecule with a highly reactive β-lactam ring that is crucial for its antibacterial activity. This ring reacts with amino groups on host proteins to form covalent conjugates. Thus, when administered, penicillin can form conjugates with self proteins; it can be recognized as foreign by T cells by modifying self peptides and by B cells as a hapten. Most people treated with intravenous penicillin develop IgG antibodies against the drug, but these usually cause no symptoms. But in some individuals, IgE antibody is produced against the penicillin hapten. When penicillin is injected intravenously into these individuals, penicillin-modified proteins can cross-link IgE molecules on tissue mast cells and circulating basophils and cause anaphylaxis. Great care should be taken to avoid giving a drug to patients with a past history of allergy to that drug or to a close structural relative.

As is true for individuals with sensitivity to inhalant allergens, patients with a past history of anaphylactic-type reactions to penicillin or other β-lactam antibiotics can be evaluated by skin-prick testing. A positive skin test, which can occur when the antigen is delivered subcutaneously (see Fig. 14.12, second panel), is manifested by the formation of a wheal-and-flare reaction at the site of the test and can be associated with a substantial risk of developing an anaphylactic reaction during treatment with therapeutic doses of the drug.

14-10 Allergen inhalation is associated with the development of rhinitis and asthma.

The respiratory tract is an important route of allergen entry (see Fig. 14.12, third panels). Many atopic people react to airborne allergens with an IgE-mediated allergic reaction known as **allergic rhinitis**. This results from the activation of mucosal mast cells beneath the nasal epithelium caused by allergens that have diffused across the mucous membranes of the nasal passages. Allergic rhinitis is characterized by intense itching and sneezing; local edema leading to blocked nasal passages; a nasal discharge, which is typically rich in eosinophils; and irritation of the nasal mucosa as a result of histamine release. A similar reaction to airborne allergens deposited on the conjunctiva of the eye is called **allergic conjunctivitis**. Allergic rhinitis and conjunctivitis are commonly caused by environmental allergens that are present only during certain seasons of the year. For example, hay fever (known clinically as **seasonal allergic rhinoconjunctivitis**) is caused by a variety of allergens, including certain grass and tree pollens. Symptoms in the late summer or autumn are commonly caused by weed pollen, such as that of ragweed, or the spores of fungi such as *Alternaria*. Ubiquitous allergens such as Fel d 1 in cat dander, Der p 1 in the feces of house dust mites, and Bla g 1 in cockroaches can be a cause of year-round, or perennial, allergic rhinoconjunctivitis.

A more serious IgE-mediated respiratory disease is **allergic asthma**, which is triggered by allergen-induced activation of submucosal mast cells in the lower airways. This can lead within seconds to bronchial constriction and an increased secretion of fluid and mucus into the airways, making breathing more difficult by trapping inhaled air in the lungs. People with allergic asthma usually need treatment, and severe asthmatic attacks can be life threatening. The same allergens that cause allergic rhinitis and conjunctivitis commonly cause asthma attacks. For example, respiratory arrest caused by severe attacks of asthma in the summer or autumn has been associated with the inhalation of *Alternaria* spores.

Chronic allergen exposure leads to an important feature of asthma; namely, chronic inflammation of the airways, which is characterized by the continued presence of increased numbers of pathologic lymphocytes, eosinophils, neutrophils, basophils, and other leukocytes (**Fig. 14.13**). The concerted actions of these cells cause airway hyperreactivity and remodeling—a thickening of the airway walls due to hyperplasia and hypertrophy of the smooth muscle layer, with the eventual development of fibrosis. Fibrotic remodeling leads to a permanent narrowing of the airways and is responsible for many of the clinical manifestations of chronic allergic asthma. In chronic asthmatics, a general hyperreactivity of the airways to non-immunological stimuli such as perfumes or volatile irritants also often develops.

A rare but dramatic manifestation of chronic allergic inflammation is the formation of **Charcot–Leyden crystals** (CLCs) in inflamed tissues such as nasal passages (**Fig. 14.14**). CLCs form from crystallization of a highly abundant protein, galectin-10, which is produced by eosinophils and which presumably accumulates in tissues over time from the death of eosinophils in chronically inflamed tissues. Importantly, the crystalline form of galectin-10 is itself inherently inflammatory, possibly due to the direct activation of the NLRP3 inflammasome (see Section 3-11). This effect acts in a positive feedback loop that helps to perpetuate the chronically inflamed allergic state. Recently, a novel therapeutic approach was described in which monoclonal antibodies that recognize monomeric galectin-10 are able to dissolve CLCs and may be useful in reversing chronic allergic inflammation.

Individuals with asthma can vary greatly in their responsiveness to therapies, in the nature of their airway inflammatory cell infiltrates, and in inflammatory mediators present in the airways. Different patterns of asthma have been

Fig. 14.13 Histologic evidence of chronic inflammation in the airways of an asthmatic individual. Panel a shows a section through a bronchus of an individual who died of asthma; there is almost total occlusion of the airway by a mucus plug, seen as the circular bluish area in the airway. In panel b, a close-up view of the bronchial wall shows injury to the epithelium lining the bronchus, accompanied by a dense inflammatory infiltrate, evident from the dense areas with numerous dark nuclei of various granulocytes. Although not discernible at this magnification, the infiltrate includes eosinophils, neutrophils, and lymphocytes.

Allergic Asthma

Charcot–Leyden crystals and eosinophils are abundantly found in an airway mucus plug of an individual with allergic bronchopulmonary aspergillosis

Charcot–Leyden crystals purified from an individual and used for X-ray structure determination

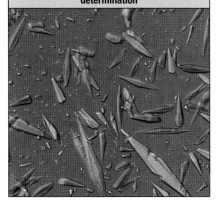

Fig. 14.14 Charcot-Leyden crystals of galectin-10 made by eosinophils contribute to chronic allergic inflammation. Top panel: Severe allergic rhinitis is characterized by eosinophils and in some cases by crystals formed from the abundant protein galectin-10 produced by eosinophils, as visible in this tissue section stained with hematoxylin and eosin. These crystals become an irritant that helps to perpetuate chronic rhinitis, likely through activation of the NLRP3 inflammasome. Bottom panel: Crystals of galectin-10 were purified directly from individuals and used to determine their molecular structure. Monoclonal antibodies that bind to galectin-10 and block crystal formation can be used to dissolve crystals and may be useful in treating this condition.

called asthma 'endotypes.' Because different endotypes may result from different underlying disorders, it may be beneficial to consider an individual's endotype when selecting a therapy. The most common endotype is allergic asthma, but other endotypes include exercise-induced asthma, neutrophil-predominant (as opposed to eosinophil-predominant) asthma, and steroid-resistant severe asthma. The fundamental driver in allergic asthma is thought to be pathologically activated T_H2 cells, and eosinophils and basophils are prominent in the inflammatory infiltrates in the lungs. In severe, steroid-resistant asthma, T_H17 cells appear to play a larger role, and neutrophils are prominent in the inflammatory infiltrates. T_H17 cells also appear to be major inducers of the asthmatic syndrome allergic bronchopulmonary aspergillosis (ABPA).

In allergic asthma, allergens cause activation of mast cells leading to mast-cell mediator release and may also stimulate the airway epithelium directly through TLRs and other damage receptors to release IL-25 and IL-33, which activate submucosal ILC2 cells, which in turn release IL-4, IL-5, IL-9, and IL-13. Bronchial epithelial cells can produce the chemokines CCL5 and CCL11, which bind to CCR3 expressed on T_H2 cells, eosinophils, and basophils, further enhancing the response. Airway remodeling is induced in part by the production of TGF-β. A major feature of chronic allergic asthma is goblet-cell metaplasia, which is the differentiation of epithelial cells into goblet cells, and a consequent increase in mucus secretion, which occurs in response to T_H2-derived cytokines such as IL-9 and IL-13.

A disease resembling human asthma develops in mice deficient in Tbet, a transcription factor that is required for T_H1 differentiation (see Section 9-15). These mice have T-cell responses that are skewed toward the T_H2 phenotype and develop airway inflammation involving lymphocytes and eosinophils (**Fig. 14.15**). They also develop nonspecific airway hyperreactivity to non-immunological stimuli, similar to what is seen in human asthma. These changes occur in the absence of any exogenous inflammatory stimulus and show that, in extreme circumstances, a genetic imbalance toward T_H2 responses can cause allergic disease.

Chronic inflammation in asthma seems to be perpetuated even in the apparent absence of ongoing exposure to the inciting allergen. The airways become characteristically hyperreactive, and factors other than antigen can trigger asthma attacks. Asthmatics characteristically show hyperresponsiveness to environmental chemical irritants such as cigarette smoke and sulfur dioxide. Viral agents, especially rhinovirus, or, to a lesser extent, bacterial respiratory tract infections can also exacerbate the disease. Both irritant agents and the infectious agents can induce IL-25 and IL-33 release from airway epithelial cells, leading to activation of ILC2 cells and exacerbation of the chronic asthmatic inflammation. The significance of viral augmentation of the asthmatic response is evident from the fact that rhinovirus infection is one of the main causes of hospitalizations for asthma and is associated with the majority of deaths from asthma.

14-11 Allergy to particular foods causes systemic reactions as well as symptoms limited to the gut.

Adverse reactions to particular foods are common, but only some are due to an immune reaction. 'Food allergy' can be classified into IgE-mediated allergic reactions, non-IgE-mediated food allergy (celiac disease, discussed in Section 14-16), idiosyncrasies, and food intolerance. Idiosyncrasies are abnormal responses to particular foods whose cause is unknown but which can provoke symptoms resembling those of an allergic response. Food intolerances are non-immune adverse reactions due mainly to metabolic deficits, such as intolerance of cow's milk due to the inability to digest lactose.

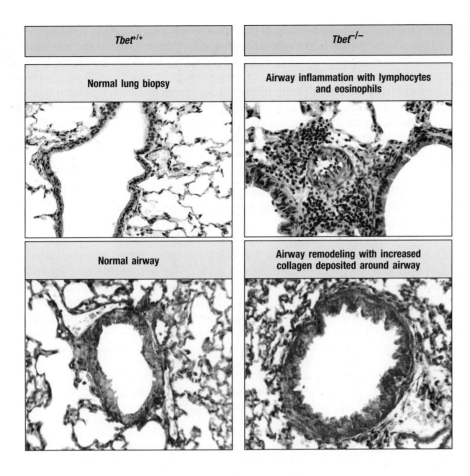

Fig. 14.15 **Mice lacking the transcription factor Tbet develop allergic airway inflammation and T-cell responses polarized toward T$_H$2.** Tbet binds to the promoter of the gene encoding IL-2 and is present in T$_H$1 but not T$_H$2 cells. Mice with a gene-targeted deletion of Tbet (*Tbet*$^{-/-}$) manifest impaired T$_H$1 responses and show spontaneous differentiation of T$_H$2 cells and development of an asthma-like phenotype in the lungs. Left panels: Lung and airways in normal mice. Right panels: Tbet-deficient mice show lung inflammation, with lymphocytes and eosinophils around the airway and blood vessels (top) and airway remodeling with increased collagen around the airway (bottom).

IgE-mediated food allergies affect about 1–4% of American and European adults and are slightly more frequent in children (around 5%). About 25% of food allergy in children is due to peanuts, and peanut allergy is increasing in incidence. **Figure 14.16** lists risk factors for developing IgE-mediated food allergy. IgE-mediated food allergy can manifest itself in a variety of ways, ranging from a swelling of the lips and oral tissue on contact with the allergen to gastrointestinal cramping, diarrhea, or vomiting. Local gastrointestinal symptoms are due to activation of mucosal mast cells, leading to transepithelial fluid loss and smooth muscle contractions. Food allergens that subsequently reach the bloodstream can lead to urticaria, asthma, and, in the most severe cases, systemic anaphylaxis that can lead to cardiovascular collapse (see Section 14-9).

Certain foods, most importantly peanuts, tree nuts, and shellfish, are particularly associated with severe anaphylaxis. Around 150 deaths occur each year in the United States as a result of a severe allergic reaction to food, with peanut and tree nut allergies accounting for most of the deaths. Peanut allergy is a significant public health problem, especially in schools, where children may be unwittingly exposed to peanuts, which are present in many foods. Recent studies offer hope for reducing the incidence of severe food allergy. In one study, infants with severe eczema who were at high risk for developing peanut allergy were randomly assigned either to be fed peanuts regularly, starting between ages 4 and 11 months, or to be on a peanut-avoidance diet for 5 years. At the age of 5, the children who had consumed peanuts showed more than a threefold reduction in the frequency of peanut allergy; the reduction was associated with decreased production of peanut-specific IgE. This suggests deliberate introduction into the diet of allergen at the appropriate time to at-risk individuals may suppress the development of food allergy.

Risk factors for the development of food allergy
Immature mucosal immune system
Early introduction of solid food
Hereditary increase in mucosal permeability
IgA deficiency or delayed IgA production
Inadequate colonization of the intestinal immune system by commensal flora
Birth by cesarean section
Genetically determined bias toward a T$_H$2 environment
Polymorphisms of T$_H$2 cytokine or IgE receptor genes
Impaired enteric nervous system
Immune alterations (e.g., low levels of TGF-β)
Gastrointestinal infections

Fig. 14.16 **Risk factors for the development of food allergy.**

One of the characteristic features of food allergens is a high degree of resistance to digestion by pepsin in the stomach. This allows them to reach the mucosal surface of the small intestine as intact allergens. Cases of IgE-mediated food allergies arising in small numbers of previously unaffected adults who were taking antacids or proton-pump inhibitors for ulcers or acid reflux have been proposed to be due to impaired digestion of potential allergens in the less acidic stomach conditions produced by these medications. However, the ability to undergo digestion seems to be relevant for some, but not all, food allergens and is not a basis to predict the allergenicity of a food.

14-12 IgE-mediated allergic disease can be treated by inhibiting effector pathways or by desensitization to restore biological tolerance.

Most of the existing drugs that are used to treat allergic disease either treat only the symptoms—examples of such drugs are antihistamines and β-agonists—or are general anti-inflammatory or immunosuppressive drugs such as the corticosteroids (**Fig. 14.17**). Treatment is largely palliative, rather than curative, and the drugs often need to be taken throughout life.

Fig. 14.17 Approaches to the treatment of allergic disease. Examples of treatments in current clinical use for allergic reactions are listed in the top half of the table, with approaches under investigation listed below. mAb, monoclonal antibody against monomeric galectin-10.

Treatments for allergic disease		
Target	**Mechanism of treatment**	**Specific approach**
In clinical use		
Mediator action	Inhibit effects of mediators on specific receptors Inhibit synthesis of specific mediators	Antihistamines, β-agonists Leukotriene receptor blockers Lipoxygenase inhibitors
Chronic inflammatory reactions	General anti-inflammatory effects	Corticosteroids
T$_H$2 response	Induction of regulatory T cells	Desensitization therapy by injections of specific antigen
IgE binding to mast cell	Bind to IgE Fc region and prevent IgE binding to Fc receptors on mast cells	Anti-IgE antibodies (omalizumab)
Proposed or under investigation		
T$_H$2 activation	Induction of regulatory T cells	Injection of specific antigen peptides Administration of cytokines, e.g., IFN-γ, IL-10, IL-12, TGF-β Use of adjuvants such as CpG oligodeoxynucleotides to stimulate T$_H$1 response
Activation of B cell to produce IgE	Block co-stimulation Inhibit T$_H$2 cytokines	Inhibit CD40L Inhibit IL-4 or IL-13
Mast-cell activation	Inhibit effects of IgE binding to mast cell	Blockade of IgE receptor
Eosinophil-dependent inflammation	Block cytokine and chemokine receptors that mediate eosinophil recruitment and activation	Inhibit IL-5 Block CCR3
Charcot–Leyden crystals	Dissolution of crystal by mAb	Antibody to galectin-10

Anaphylactic reactions are treated with epinephrine, which stimulates the re-formation of endothelial tight junctions, promotes the relaxation of constricted bronchial smooth muscle, and stimulates the heart. Antihistamines that block the action of histamine at the H_1 receptor reduce symptoms in allergic rhinoconjunctivitis and IgE-triggered urticaria. In urticaria, for example, the relevant H_1 receptors include those on blood vessels and unmyelinated nerve fibers in the skin. Anticholinergic drugs, such as atropine, bronchodilate constricted airways and reduce respiratory secretions. Antileukotriene drugs act as antagonists of leukotriene receptors on smooth muscle, endothelial cells, and mucous-gland cells, and are also used to relieve the symptoms of allergic rhinoconjunctivitis and asthma. Inhaled bronchodilators that act on β-adrenergic receptors to relax constricted muscle relieve acute asthma attacks. In chronic allergic disease it is extremely important to treat and prevent the chronic inflammatory injury to tissues, and regular use of inhaled corticosteroids is recommended in persistent asthma to help suppress inflammation. Topical corticosteroids are used to suppress the chronic inflammatory changes seen in eczema.

Another type of allergy-suppressive therapy is the blockade of IgE function by using monoclonal anti-IgE antibodies. An example of this is omalizumab, which binds the Fc portion of IgE at the same site that binds FcεRI on basophils and mast cells. The portion of the Fc domain of IgE that binds to the low-affinity IgE receptor (FcεRII) that is expressed on a variety of leukocytes other than basophils and mast cells is different from the domain that binds the high-affinity FcεRI. Omalizumab blocks binding of IgE to the low-affinity receptor as well as to FcεRI. Prevention of binding of IgE to its receptors on basophils results in down-regulation of these receptors on these cells, making them less easily activated by exposure to allergens. The antibody is administered by subcutaneous injection once every 2–4 weeks and is highly effective for individuals with chronic urticaria and also appears to be effective in individuals with severe chronic asthma. Of special interest is that in studies of children with moderate to severe asthma who were treated for 4 years with omalizumab, most remained symptom free without any anti-asthma treatment, suggesting that the anti-IgE therapy modified the natural history of the disease.

Another, more routinely used approach that aims to permanently eliminate the allergic response is **allergen desensitization**. This form of immunotherapy aims to restore the patient's ability to tolerate exposure to the allergen. Patients are desensitized by injection with escalating doses of allergen, starting with tiny amounts. The mechanism by which desensitization occurs is not definitively established, but for most successfully desensitized patients, the procedure results in a change in the antibody response from one dominated by IgE to one dominated by an IgG. The exact mechanisms for this immunoregulatory effect are still obscure but may involve the induction of T_{reg} cells. Nonetheless, the procedure is associated with a reduction in the numbers of inflammatory cells at the site of the allergic reaction. Despite the extremely small doses of allergen used for desensitization, some patients can experience an IgE-mediated allergic response, including bronchospasms, and many physicians believe that this procedure is contraindicated in individuals with severe asthma. For patients who experience resolution of their allergy symptoms during allergen immunotherapy, weekly or every-other-week injections are continued for 3 years, and then the therapy is discontinued. In approximately half of patients treated in this fashion, symptoms do not recur after cessation of the injections.

When a patient is allergic to a drug that is essential for treatment of a disease (such as an antibiotic, insulin, or a chemotherapeutic agent), it is often possible to achieve a state of temporary **acute desensitization** by treating the patient with progressively increasing doses of the drug, starting at a very low dose that causes no allergic symptoms and increasing the dose every half hour until the therapeutic dose is reached. It is common for patients undergoing drug desensitization to manifest mild to moderate allergic symptoms (itching, urticaria, mild wheezing) at some time during the procedure. If this occurs, the physician reduces the dose to the previous tolerated dose and then advances the dose again. This procedure is thought to lead to subclinical activation of mast cells and basophils that have been sensitized with IgE against the drug, inducing them to gradually release their intracellular mediators at a rate that does not cause severe symptoms; eventually, all of the cell-bound IgE is consumed by this process, leaving insufficient IgE available to cause an allergic reaction when subsequent therapeutic doses are administered. In order to maintain the desensitized state, the patient must receive daily therapeutic doses of the drug. If treatment is interrupted, then newly formed mast cells and basophils can be charged with newly secreted drug-specific IgE and can accumulate at levels sufficient to yield a new anaphylactic reaction.

A further approach to the treatment of allergic disease may be to block the recruitment of eosinophils to sites of allergic inflammation. The eotaxin receptor CCR3 is a potential target in this context. In experimental animals, the production of eosinophils in bone marrow and their exit into the circulation is reduced by blocking IL-5 action. Anti-IL-5 antibody (mepolizumab) is beneficial in treating patients who have **hypereosinophilic syndrome**, in which chronic overproduction of eosinophils causes severe organ damage. Clinical trials of anti-IL-5 treatment of asthma, however, show that, in practice, any beneficial effect is likely to be limited to a small subset of asthma patients who have prednisone-dependent eosinophilic asthma; in these patients, IL-5 blockade seems to reduce the number of asthma attacks when the corticosteroid dose is reduced.

Summary.

The allergic response to innocuous antigens reflects the pathophysiological aspects of a defensive immune response whose physiological role is to protect against helminth parasites. It is triggered by the binding of antigen to IgE antibodies that are bound to the high-affinity IgE receptor FcεRI on mast cells and basophils. Mast cells are strategically distributed beneath the mucosal surfaces of the body and in connective tissue. Antigen cross-linking the IgE on the surface of mast cells causes them to release large amounts of inflammatory mediators. The resulting inflammation can be divided into early events that are characterized by short-lived mediators, such as histamine, and later events that involve leukotrienes, cytokines, and chemokines, which recruit and activate eosinophils, basophils, and other leukocytes. This response can evolve into chronic inflammation, which is characterized by the presence of effector T cells and eosinophils and is most clearly seen in chronic allergic asthma.

Non-IgE-mediated allergic diseases.

In this part of the chapter we focus on immunological hypersensitivity responses involving IgG antibodies and type 1 or type 3 immune responses that involve antigen-specific T_H1 or T_H17 cells or CD8 T cells. These effector arms of the immune response occasionally react with noninfectious antigens to produce acute or chronic allergic reactions. Although the mechanisms initiating the various forms of hypersensitivity are different, much of the pathology is due to the same immunological effector mechanisms.

14-13 Non-IgE-dependent drug-induced hypersensitivity reactions in susceptible individuals occur by binding of the drug to the surface of circulating blood cells.

Antibody-mediated destruction of red blood cells (hemolytic anemia) or platelets (thrombocytopenia) can be caused by some drugs, including the β-lactam antibiotics penicillin and cephalosporin. Drug-induced hemolytic anemia (DIHA) is a very rare condition and in the Gell and Coombs classification is a type II hypersensitivity reaction, typically mediated by IgG or IgM and complement. In these reactions, the drug binds covalently to the cell surface and is a target for anti-drug antibodies that cause destruction of the cell. The anti-drug antibodies are made in only a minority of people, and it is not clear why these individuals make them. The cell-bound antibody triggers the clearance of the cell from the circulation, predominantly by tissue macrophages in the spleen, which bear Fcγ receptors.

14-14 Systemic disease caused by immune-complex formation can follow the administration of large quantities of poorly catabolized antigens.

Hypersensitivity reactions can arise after treatment with soluble antigens such as animal antisera. The pathology is caused by the deposition of antigen:antibody aggregates, or **immune complexes**, in particular tissues and sites. Immune complexes are generated in all antibody responses, but their pathogenic potential is determined, in part, by their size and by the amount, affinity, and isotype of the responding antibody. Larger aggregates fix complement and are readily cleared from the circulation by the mononuclear phagocyte system. However, the small complexes that form when antigen is in excess tend to be deposited in blood vessel walls. There they can ligate Fc receptors on leukocytes, leading to leukocyte activation and tissue injury.

A local hypersensitivity reaction called an **Arthus reaction** (Fig. 14.18) can be triggered in the skin of sensitized individuals who possess IgG antibodies

| Locally injected antigen in immune individual with IgG antibody | Local immune-complex formation activates complement. C5a binds to and sensitizes the mast cell to respond to immune complexes | Activation of FcγRIII on mast cells induces their degranulation | Local inflammation, increased fluid and protein release, phagocytosis, and blood vessel occlusion |

C5a

1–2 hours

Fig. 14.18 The deposition of immune complexes in tissues causes a local inflammatory response known as an Arthus reaction. In individuals who have already made IgG antibody against an antigen, the same antigen injected into the skin forms immune complexes with IgG antibody that has diffused out of the capillaries. Because the dose of antigen is low, the immune complexes are formed only close to the site of injection, where they activate mast cells bearing Fcγ receptors (FcγRIII). The immune complex induces activation of complement, and the complement component C5a contributes to sensitizing the mast cell to respond to immune complexes. As a result of mast-cell activation, inflammatory cells invade the site, and blood vessel permeability and blood flow are increased. Platelets also accumulate inside the vessel at the site, ultimately leading to vessel occlusion. If the reaction is severe, all these changes can lead to tissue necrosis.

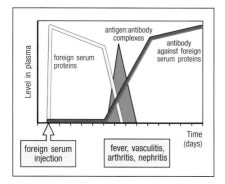

Fig. 14.19 Serum sickness is a classic example of a transient immune complex–mediated syndrome. An injection of a foreign protein, such as horse antitoxin, leads to an anti-horse serum antibody response. These antibodies form immune complexes with the circulating foreign proteins. The complexes are deposited in small blood vessels and activate complement and phagocytes, inducing fever and inflammatory lesions in blood vessels in the skin and connective tissues (vasculitis), in the kidney (nephritis), and in joints (arthritis). All these effects are transient and resolve when the foreign protein is cleared.

Drug-Induced Serum Sickness

against the sensitizing antigen. When antigen is injected into the skin, circulating IgG antibody that has diffused into the skin forms immune complexes with the antigen locally and so in the Gell and Coombs classification is a type III hypersensitivity reaction. The immune complexes bind Fc receptors such as FcγRIII on mast cells and other leukocytes, generating a local inflammatory response and increased vascular permeability. Fluid and cells, especially neutrophils, enter from local blood vessels. The immune complexes also activate complement, generating complement fragment C5a, which activates C5a receptors on leukocytes to recruit them to the site of inflammation (see Section 2-13).

A systemic type III hypersensitivity reaction known as **serum sickness** can result from the injection of large quantities of a poorly catabolized foreign antigen. This illness was so named because it frequently followed the administration of therapeutic horse antiserum. In the pre-antibiotic era, antiserum made by immunizing horses with *Streptococcus pneumoniae* was used to treat pneumococcal pneumonia; the specific anti-pneumococcal antibodies in the horse serum would help the patient to clear the infection. In much the same way, **antivenin** (serum from sheep or horses immunized with snake venoms) is still used today as a source of neutralizing antibodies to treat people suffering from the bites of poisonous snakes.

Serum sickness occurs 7–10 days after the injection of horse serum, an interval that corresponds to the time required to produce an IgG-switched primary immune response against the foreign horse serum antigens (**Fig. 14.19**). The onset of disease occurs when these antibodies form immune complexes with their antigens, activate complement, and bind Fc receptors on leukocytes throughout the body, which in turn cause tissue damage. The clinical features of serum sickness are chills, fever, rash, arthritis, and sometimes glomerulonephritis (inflammation of the glomeruli of the kidneys). Formation of immune complexes causes clearance of the foreign antigen, so serum sickness is usually a self-limiting disease. Urticaria is a prominent feature of the rash, implying a role for histamine derived from mast-cell degranulation. In this case, the mast-cell degranulation is triggered by the ligation of cell-surface FcγRIII by IgG-containing immune complexes and by the anaphylatoxins C3a and C5a released due to complement activation by these complexes. With the increasing clinical use of humanized monoclonal antibodies, serum sickness is rare, but it can occur if the monoclonal antibody was not successfully humanized and the patient produces a reaction against it. However, symptoms are generally mild, resulting mainly in more rapid clearance of the therapeutic antibody from the circulation, thereby reducing its therapeutic effects.

Pathological immune-complex deposition is seen in other situations in which antigen persists. For example, when an adaptive antibody response fails to clear the infecting pathogen, as occurs in subacute bacterial endocarditis or chronic viral hepatitis, the replicating pathogen continually generates new antigen in the presence of a persistent antibody response, with the consequent formation of abundant immune complexes. These are deposited within small blood vessels and result in injury in many tissues and organs, including the skin, kidneys, and nerves.

Immune-complex disease also occurs when inhaled allergens provoke IgG rather than IgE antibody responses, perhaps because they are present at relatively high levels in the air. When a person is reexposed to high doses of such allergens, immune complexes form in the walls of alveoli in the lungs. This leads to the accumulation of fluid, protein, and cells in the alveolar wall, slowing blood–air exchange of O_2 and CO_2 and compromising lung function. This type of reaction is more likely to occur in occupations such as farming, in which there is repeated exposure to hay dust or mold spores, and the resulting disease is known as **farmer's lung**. If exposure to antigen is sustained, the lining of the lungs can be permanently damaged.

14-15 Hypersensitivity reactions can be mediated by T$_H$1 cells and cytotoxic CD8 T cells.

Here we consider the hypersensitivity diseases caused by T$_H$1 and cytotoxic CD8 T cells (**Fig. 14.20**). Unlike the immediate hypersensitivity reactions, which are mediated by antibodies, **cellular hypersensitivity reactions** such as **delayed-type hypersensitivity (DTH)** reactions are mediated by antigen-specific effector T cells; in the Gell and Coombs classification, these are type IV hypersensitivity reactions. These cells function in hypersensitivity in essentially the same way as when they respond to a pathogen, and the responses can be transferred between experimental animals by purified T cells or cloned T-cell lines.

The prototypic DTH hypersensitivity reaction is the **Mantoux test**, the standard tuberculin test to determine if an individual has been infected previously with *Mycobacterium tuberculosis*. In the Mantoux test, the subject is injected intradermally with small amounts of tuberculin, an extract of peptides and carbohydrates derived from *M. tuberculosis*. In people who have been infected by the *M. tuberculosis* bacterium or immunized with BCG (bacillus Calmette–Guérin, a live-attenuated vaccine form of *Mycobacterium bovis*), a local T cell–mediated inflammatory reaction evolves over 24–72 hours. The response is caused by T$_H$1 cells, which enter the site of antigen injection, recognize complexes of peptide:MHC class II molecules on antigen-presenting cells, and release inflammatory cytokines such as IFN-γ, TNF-α, and lymphotoxin (LT). These cytokines stimulate the expression of adhesion molecules on endothelium and increase local blood vessel permeability, allowing plasma and accessory cells to enter the site, thus causing a visible swelling (**Fig. 14.21**). Each of these phases takes several hours and so the fully developed response only appears 24–72 hours after challenge. The cytokines produced by the activated T$_H$1 cells and their actions are shown in **Fig. 14.22**.

Very similar reactions are observed in **allergic contact dermatitis** (also called contact hypersensitivity), which is an immune-mediated local inflammatory

Cellular hypersensitivity reactions are mediated by antigen-specific effector T cells		
Syndrome	**Antigen**	**Consequence**
Delayed-type hypersensitivity	Proteins: Insect venom Mycobacterial proteins (tuberculin, lepromin)	Local skin swelling: Erythema Induration Cellular infiltrate Dermatitis
Contact hypersensitivity	Haptens: Pentadecacatechol (poison ivy) DNFB Small metal ions: Nickel Chromate	Local epidermal reaction: Erythema Cellular infiltrate Vesicles Intraepidermal abscesses
Gluten-sensitive enteropathy (celiac disease)	α-Gliadin	Villous atrophy in small bowel Malabsorption

Fig. 14.20 Cellular hypersensitivity reactions. These responses are mediated by T cells and require 3–5 days or more to develop. They can be grouped into three syndromes, according to the route by which antigen passes into the body. In delayed-type hypersensitivity the antigen is injected into the skin; in contact hypersensitivity it is absorbed into the skin; and in gluten-sensitive enteropathy it is absorbed by the gut. In contact hypersensitivity, vesicles commonly form. They represent accumulations of fluid in small blisterlike lesions at the level of the basement membrane between the dermis and epidermis. Their formation at this location is probably the result of antigen penetrating the epidermis, accumulating at the basement membrane, and inducing a local inflammatory response with edema fluid. DNFB (dinitrofluorobenzene) is a sensitizing agent that can cause contact hypersensitivity.

Fig. 14.21 The stages of a delayed-type hypersensitivity reaction. The first phase involves uptake, processing, and presentation of the antigen by local antigen-presenting cells. In the second phase, T$_H$1 cells that have been primed by a previous exposure to the antigen migrate into the site of injection and become activated. Because these specific cells are rare, and because there is little inflammation to attract cells into the site, it can take several hours for a T cell of the correct specificity to arrive. These cells release mediators that activate local endothelial cells, which recruit an inflammatory-cell infiltrate dominated by macrophages and cause the accumulation of fluid, serum proteins, and more leukocytes, thus producing a visible lesion.

reaction in the skin caused by direct skin contact with certain antigens. Allergic contact dermatitis can be caused by the activation of CD4 or CD8 T cells, depending on the pathway by which the antigen is processed. Typically the antigens are highly reactive small molecules that penetrate intact skin, especially if they cause itching that leads to scratching and its consequent injury to the skin barrier. These chemicals then react with self proteins, creating haptenated proteins that can be processed for presentation as modified peptides bound to MHC molecules and recognized by T cells as foreign antigens.

As with other allergic responses, there are two phases to allergic contact dermatitis: sensitization and elicitation. During the sensitization phase,

Fig. 14.22 The delayed-type hypersensitivity response is directed by chemokines and cytokines released by antigen-stimulated T$_H$1 cells. Antigen in the local tissues is internalized and processed by antigen-presenting cells and presented on MHC class II molecules. Antigen-specific T$_H$1 cells that recognize the antigen:MHC complexes locally at the site of antigen injection release chemokines and cytokines that recruit macrophages and other leukocytes to the site. Antigen presentation by the newly recruited macrophages then amplifies the response. T cells can also affect local blood vessels through the release of TNF-α and lymphotoxin (LT) and stimulate the production of macrophages through the release of IL-3 and GM-CSF. T$_H$1 cells activate macrophages through the release of IFN-γ and TNF-α and kill macrophages and other sensitive cells through the cell-surface expression of the Fas ligand.

| Contact-sensitizing agent penetrates the skin and binds to self proteins, which are taken up by dendritic cells and Langerhans cells | Self peptides haptenated with the contact-sensitizing agent are presented to T_H1 cells, which secrete IFN-γ and other cytokines | Activated keratinocytes secrete cytokines such as IL-1 and TNF-α and chemokines such as CXCL8, CXCL11, and CXCL9 | The products of keratinocytes and T_H1 cells activate macrophages to secrete mediators of inflammation |

Fig. 14.23 Elicitation of a delayed-type hypersensitivity response to a contact-sensitizing agent. A contact-sensitizing agent is a small, highly reactive molecule that can penetrate intact skin. It binds covalently as a hapten to a variety of endogenous proteins, altering their structures so they become antigenic. These modified proteins are internalized, processed by Langerhans cells (the major antigen-presenting cells of skin), and presented to effector T_H1 cells (which were primed in lymph nodes as a result of prior antigen exposure). The activated T_H1 cells then secrete cytokines such as IFN-γ that stimulate keratinocytes to secrete additional cytokines and chemokines, which in turn attract monocytes and induce their maturation into activated tissue macrophages, further contributing to inflammatory lesions like those caused by poison ivy (see Fig. 14.24). NO, nitric oxide.

Langerhans cells in the epidermis and dendritic cells in the dermis take up and process antigen and migrate to regional lymph nodes, where they activate T cells (see Fig. 9.17). These eventually leave the lymph node and localize in the dermis as tissue-resident memory T cells. In the elicitation phase, a subsequent exposure to the sensitizing chemical leads to antigen presentation to these T cells, inducing the release of cytokines such as IFN-γ and IL-17. This stimulates the keratinocytes of the epidermis to release IL-1, IL-6, TNF-α, GM-CSF, the chemokine CXCL8, and the interferon-inducible chemokines CXCL11 (IP-9), CXCL10 (IP-10), and CXCL9 (Mig, a monokine induced by IFN-γ). These cytokines and chemokines enhance the inflammatory response by inducing the migration of monocytes into the lesion and their maturation into macrophages and by attracting more T cells (**Fig. 14.23**).

The rash produced by contact with the **poison ivy** plant (**Fig. 14.24**) is a common example of allergic contact dermatitis in the United States and is caused by a CD8 T-cell response to urushiol oil (a mixture of pentadecacatechols) in the plant. These chemicals are lipid-soluble and so can cross the cell membrane and attach to intracellular proteins, which are processed and presented on the cell surface by MHC class I molecules. CD8 T cells recognizing the peptides cause damage either by killing the eliciting cell or by secreting cytokines such as IFN-γ. Common clinical features of allergic contact dermatitis are erythema of the affected skin; development of a dermal and epidermal infiltrate consisting of monocytes, macrophages, lymphocytes, scant neutrophils, and mast cells; formation of intraepidermal abscesses; and vesicles (blisterlike collections of edema fluid between the dermis and epidermis).

Some insect proteins and metals can elicit a delayed-type hypersensitivity response. One example of this in the skin is a severe reaction to mosquito bites. Instead of a small itchy bump, people allergic to proteins in mosquito saliva can develop an immediate hypersensitivity reaction such as urticaria and swelling or, much more rarely, anaphylactic shock (see Section 14-9). Some allergic individuals subsequently develop a delayed reaction (consisting of a late-phase response) that can include profound swelling that can involve an entire limb. The divalent cation nickel can alter the conformation or peptide binding of MHC class II molecules and provoke a T-cell response. Sensitization

Fig. 14.24 Blistering skin lesions on the hand of an individual with allergic contact dermatitis caused by poison ivy.

Contact Sensitivity to Poison Ivy

to nickel is widespread as a result of prolonged contact with nickel-containing items such as jewelry, buttons, and clothing fasteners. Some countries now have standards that specify that such products must have non-nickel coatings in an attempt to reduce the prevalence of nickel allergy.

14-16 Celiac disease has features of both an allergic response and autoimmunity.

Celiac Disease

Celiac disease is a chronic condition of the upper small intestine caused by an immune response directed at gluten, a complex of proteins present in wheat, oats, and barley. Elimination of gluten from the diet restores normal gut function, but to date no approach for desensitization to gluten has been developed, so gluten ingestion must be avoided throughout life. The pathology of celiac disease is characterized by the loss of the slender, fingerlike villi formed by the intestinal epithelium (a condition termed villous atrophy), together with an increase in the size of the sites in which epithelial cells are renewed (crypt hyperplasia) (**Fig. 14.25**). These pathological changes result in the loss of the mature epithelial cells that cover the villi and normally absorb and digest food and are accompanied by severe inflammation of the intestinal wall, with increased numbers of T cells, macrophages, and plasma cells in the lamina propria, as well as increased numbers of lymphocytes in the epithelial layer. Gluten seems to be the only food component that provokes intestinal inflammation in this way, a property that reflects gluten's ability to stimulate both innate and specific immune responses in genetically susceptible individuals. The incidence of celiac disease has increased fourfold in the past 60 years, correlating with changes in baking practice that include adding large amounts of extra gluten to dough to decrease the time required for the dough to rise and to improve the texture.

Celiac disease shows an extremely strong genetic predisposition, with more than 95% of individuals expressing the HLA-DQ2 class II MHC allele. In

Fig. 14.25 The pathological features of celiac disease. Left panel: The surface of the normal small intestine is folded into fingerlike villi, which provide an extensive surface for nutrient absorption. Right panel: The local immune response against the food protein α-gliadin, a prominent component of wheat, oat, and barley gluten, leads to massive infiltration of the lamina propria (in the deeper, inner portion of the villi) by CD4 T cells, plasma cells, macrophages, and smaller numbers of other leukocytes, ultimately leading to destruction of the villi. In parallel, there is lengthening and increased mitotic activity in the underlying crypts, where new epithelial cells are produced. Because the villi contain all the mature epithelial cells that digest and absorb foodstuffs, their loss can result in life-threatening malabsorption and diarrhea.

Normal jejunum

Celiac jejunum

monozygotic twins, if one twin develops it, there is an 80% probability that the other will, but only a 10% concordance is observed in dizygotic twins. Nevertheless, most individuals expressing HLA-DQ2 do not develop celiac disease despite the almost universal presence of gluten in the Western diet. Thus, other genetic or environmental factors must make important contributions to susceptibility. Normally, food proteins induce oral tolerance, but it is unknown why this mechanism breaks down in people with celiac disease. The incidence of celiac disease is especially high in individuals with trisomy 21 (Down syndrome), approximately sixfold higher than in the normal population, underscoring the impact of genetic factors on disease prevalence.

Most evidence indicates that celiac disease requires the aberrant priming of IFN-γ–producing CD4 T cells by antigenic peptides present in α-gliadin, one of the major proteins in gluten. It is generally accepted that only a limited number of peptides can provoke an immune response leading to celiac disease. This is likely due to the unique structure of the peptide-binding groove of the HLA-DQ2 molecule. The key step in the immune recognition of α-gliadin is the deamidation of its peptides by the enzyme tissue transglutaminase (tTG), which converts selected glutamine residues to negatively charged glutamic acid. Only peptides containing negatively charged residues in certain positions bind strongly to HLA-DQ2, and thus the transamination reaction promotes the formation of peptide:HLA-DQ2 complexes, which can activate antigen-specific CD4 T cells (**Fig. 14.26**). Activated gliadin-specific CD4 T cells accumulate in the lamina propria, producing IFN-γ, a cytokine that when present in this location leads to intestinal inflammation.

Celiac disease is entirely dependent on the presence of the foreign antigen, gluten. It is not associated with a specific immune response against self antigens in the intestinal epithelium. Thus, celiac disease is not a classical autoimmune disease. But it does have some features of autoimmunity. Autoantibodies

| Peptides naturally produced from gluten do not bind to MHC class II molecules | An enzyme, tissue transglutaminase (tTG), modifies the peptides so they now can be processed and bind to the MHC class II molecules | The bound peptide activates gluten-specific CD4 T cells | The activated T cells can kill mucosal epithelial cells by binding Fas. They also secrete IFN-γ, which activates the epithelial cell to produce cytokines and chemokines that recruit other inflammatory cells |

Fig. 14.26 Molecular basis of immune recognition of gluten in celiac disease. After the digestion of gluten by gut digestive enzymes, deamidation of epitopes by tissue transglutaminase renders the gluten more susceptible to being readily processed by local antigen-presenting cells, ultimately leading to its binding to HLA-DQ molecules and priming of the immune system.

Gluten peptides activate mucosal epithelial cells to express MIC molecules	Intraepithelial lymphocytes (IELs) express NKG2D, which binds to MIC molecules and activates the IELs to kill the epithelial cell

IL-1 MIC
IL-1R
CD8 T cell (IEL)
NKG2D

Fig. 14.27 The activation of cytotoxic T cells by the innate immune system in celiac disease. Gluten peptides can induce the expression of the MHC class Ib molecules MIC-A and MIC-B on gut epithelial cells and the synthesis and release of IL-1 from these cells. Intraepithelial lymphocytes (IELs), many of which are cytotoxic CD8 T cells, recognize the MIC proteins via the receptor NKG2D, which, together with the co-stimulator IL-1, activates the IELs to kill the MIC-bearing cells, leading to destruction of the gut epithelium.

against tissue transglutaminase are found in all individuals with celiac disease, but there is no evidence that they contribute directly to tissue damage. Indeed, the presence of serum IgA antibodies against this enzyme is used as a sensitive and specific test for the disease. Notably, no tTG-specific T cells have been found, but gluten-reactive T cells may provide help to tTG-reactive B cells that capture gluten in a complex with transglutaminase.

The gluten protein also seems to have several properties that contribute to pathogenesis. As well as its relative resistance to digestion, there is mounting evidence that some gliadin-derived peptides stimulate the innate immune system by inducing the release of IL-15 by intestinal epithelial cells. This process is antigen-nonspecific and involves peptides that cannot be bound by HLA-DQ2 molecules or recognized by CD4 T cells. IL-15 release leads to the activation of dendritic cells in the lamina propria, as well as the up-regulation of nonclassical MHC class Ib molecules MIC-A and MIC-B expression by epithelial cells (see Section 6-17). CD8 T cells in the mucosal epithelium can be activated via their NKG2D receptors, which recognize MIC-A, and they can kill MIC-A–expressing epithelial cells via these same NKG2D receptors (**Fig. 14.27**). Triggering of these innate immune responses by α-gliadin may create some intestinal damage on its own and also induce some of the co-stimulatory events necessary for initiating an antigen-specific CD4 T-cell response to other parts of the α-gliadin molecule. The ability of gluten to stimulate both innate and adaptive immune responses may thus explain its unique ability to induce celiac disease.

Summary.

Hypersensitivity reactions include several non-IgE-mediated conditions that reflect normal immune mechanisms that are inappropriately directed against innocuous antigens or inflammatory stimuli. These include both immediate and delayed-type reactions. Immediate-type reactions are due to the binding of specific IgG antibodies to allergen-modified cell surfaces, as in drug-induced hemolytic anemia (that is, type II hypersensitivity reactions), or to the formation of immune complexes of antibodies bound to poorly catabolized antigens, as occurs in serum sickness (type III hypersensitivity reactions). Cellular hypersensitivity reactions mediated by T_H1 cells and cytotoxic T cells develop more slowly than immediate-type reactions (type IV hypersensitivity reactions). The T_H1-mediated hypersensitivity reaction in the skin provoked by mycobacterial tuberculin is used to diagnose previous exposure to *Mycobacterium tuberculosis*. The allergic reaction to poison ivy is due to the recognition and destruction by cytotoxic T cells of skin cells modified by a plant molecule and to cytotoxic T-cell cytokines. These T cell–mediated responses require the induced synthesis of effector molecules and develop over 1–10 days. Finally, celiac disease represents a response to the gluten protein and has features of both cell-mediated allergic reaction and autoimmune disease.

Summary to Chapter 14.

In susceptible individuals, immune responses to otherwise innocuous antigens can produce allergic reactions upon reexposure to the same antigen. Most allergic reactions involve the production of IgE antibody against common environmental allergens. Some people are intrinsically prone to making IgE antibodies against many allergens, and such people are said to be atopic. IgE production is driven by cytokines produced in the type 2 immune responses, with T_H2/ILC2 cytokines and chemokines predominant, although the genetic and environmental factors causing this response are largely still unknown. Nonetheless, the IgE produced in this response binds to the high-affinity IgE receptor FcεRI on mast cells and basophils, and subsequent encounter with the antigen sets the allergic response in motion. Specific effector T cells, mast cells, and eosinophils, in combination with T_H1 and T_H2 cytokines and chemokines, orchestrate chronic allergic inflammation, which is the major cause of the chronic morbidity of asthma. Failure to regulate these responses can occur at many levels of the immune system. Therapies to suppress allergic responses include blocking the effector pathways, with antihistamines for example, as well as elimination of circulating IgE using anti-IgE antibodies.

Discussion Questions

14.1 Explain the basis for the association between the IgE isotype antibody against an antigen and the triggering of an allergic reaction to that same antigen.

14.2 Using the typical example of a bee sting, describe the process leading to the rapid swelling at the site of injury. Describe how this process could lead to systemic shock and death.

14.3 Describe a way in which epithelial cells may promote the generation of an allergic response to an antigen.

14.4 In Netherton syndrome, what is the connection between a protease and the development of an allergic response?

14.5 Describe the mechanism underlying the rash caused by exposure to the poison ivy plant.

14.6 Celiac disease is caused by an immune response to gluten. In what way is celiac disease like an allergic response? In what ways is it like an autoimmune disease?

General references.

Fahy, J.V.: Type 2 inflammation in asthma—present in most, absent in many. *Nat. Rev. Immunol.* 2015, 15:57–65.

Gell, P.G.H., and Coombs, R.R.A.: *Clinical Aspects of Immunology*, 2nd ed. Oxford: Blackwell Scientific, 1968.

Holgate, S.T.: Innate and adaptive immune responses in asthma. *Nat. Med.* 2012, 18:673–683.

Johansson, S.G., Bieber, T., Dahl, R., Friedmann, P.S., Lanier, B.Q., Lockey, R.F., Motala, C., Ortega Martell, J.A., Platts-Mills, T.A., Ring, J., et al.: Revised nomenclature for allergy for global use: report of the Nomenclature Review Committee of the World Allergy Organization, October 2003. *J. Allergy Clin. Immunol.* 2004, 113:832–836.

Kay, A.B.: Allergy and allergic diseases. First of two parts. *N. Engl. J. Med.* 2001, 344:30–37.

Kay, A.B.: Allergy and allergic diseases. Second of two parts. *N. Engl. J. Med.* 2001, 344:109–113.

Valenta, R., Hochwallner, H., Linhart, B., and Pahr, S.: Food allergies: the basics. *Gastroenterology* 2015, 148:1120–1131.

Section references.

14-1 Sensitization involves class switching to IgE production on first contact with an allergen.

Akuthota, P., Wang, H., and Weller, P.F.: Eosinophils as antigen-presenting cells in allergic upper airway disease. *Curr. Opin. Allergy Clin. Immunol.* 2010, 10:14–19.

Berkowska, M.A., Heeringa, J.J., Hajdarbegovic, E., van der Burg, M., Thio, H.B., van Gahen, P.M., Boon, L., Orfao, A., van Dongen, J.J.M, and van Zelm, M.C.: Human IgE⁺B cells are derived from T cell-dependent and T cell-independent pathways. *J. Allergy Clin. Immunol.* 2014, 134:688–697.

Bieber, T.: The pro- and anti-inflammatory properties of human antigen-presenting cells expressing the high affinity receptor for IgE (FcεRI). *Immunobiology* 2007, 212:499–503.

Gold, M.J., Antignano, F., Halim, T.Y.F., Hirota, J.A., Blanchet, M.-R., Zaph, C., Takei, F., and McNagny, K.M.: Group 2 innate lymphoid cells facilitate sensitization to local, but not systemic, T_H2-inducing allergen exposures. *J. Allergy Clin. Immunol.* 2014, 133:1142–1148.

He, J.S., Narayanan, S., Subramaniam, S., Ho, W.Q., Lafaille, J.J., and Curotto de Lafaille, M.A.: Biology of IgE production: IgE cell differentiation and the memory of IgE responses. *Curr. Opin. Microbiol. Immunol.* 2015, 388:1–19.

Kumar, V.: Innate lymphoid cells: new paradigm in immunology of inflammation. *Immunol. Lett.* 2014, 157:23–37.

Mikhak, Z., and Luster, A.D.: The emergence of basophils as antigen-presenting cells in Th2 inflammatory responses. *J. Mol. Cell Biol.* 2009, 1:69–71.

Mirchandani, A.S., Salmond, R.J., and Liew, F.Y.: Interleukin-33 and the function of innate lymphoid cells. *Trends Immunol.* 2012, 33:389–396.

Platzer, B., Baker, K., Vera, M.P., Singer, K., Panduro, M., Lexmond, W.S., Turner, D., Vargas, S. O., Kinet, J.-P., Maurer, D., et al.: Dendritic cell-bound IgE functions to restrain allergic inflammation at mucosal sites. *Mucosal Immunol.* 2015, 8:516–532.

Spencer, L.A., and Weller, P.F.: Eosinophils and Th2 immunity: contemporary insights. *Immunol. Cell Biol.* 2010, 88:250–256.

Wu, L.C., and Zarrin, A.A.: The production and regulation of IgE by the immune system. *Nat. Rev. Immunol.* 2014, 14:247–259.

14-2 Although many types of antigens can cause allergic sensitization, proteases are common sensitizing agents.

Brown, S.J., and McLean, W.H.I.: One remarkable molecule: filaggrin. *J. Invest. Dermatol.* 2012, 132:751–762.

Furio, L., de Veer, S., Jaillet, M., Briot, A., Robin, A., Deraison, C., and Hovnanian, A.: Transgenic kallikrein 5 mice reproduce major cutaneous and systemic hallmarks of Netherton syndrome. *J. Exp. Med.* 2014, 211:499–513.

Grunstein, M.M., Veler, H., Shan, X., Larson, J., Grunstein, J.S., and Chuang, S.: Proasthmatic effects and mechanisms of action of the dust mite allergen, Der p 1, in airway smooth muscle. *J. Allergy Clin. Immunol.* 2005, 116:94–101.

Lambrecht, B.N., and Hammad, H.: Allergens and the airway epithelium response: gateway to allergic sensitization. *J. Allergy Clin. Immunol.* 2014, 134:499–507.

Larson, R.P., Comeau, M.R., and Ziegler, S.F.: **Cutting edge: allergen-specific CD4 T cells respond indirectly to thymic stromal lymphopoietin to promote allergic responses in the skin.** *J. Immunol.* 2013, **190**:4474–4477.

Serhan, N., Basso, L., Sibilano, R., Petitfils, C., Meixiong, J., Bonnart, C., Reber, L.L., Marichal, T., Starkl, P., Cenac, N., *et al.*: **House dust mites activate nociceptor-mast cell clusters to drive type 2 skin inflammation.** *Nat. Immunol.* 2019, **20**:1435–1443.

Shadmehr, D., Turkoz, A., Manivasagam, S., Yockey, L.J., Turkoz, M., and Kopan, R.: **Elevated epidermal thymic stromal lymphopoietin levels establish an antitumor environment in the skin.** *Cancer Cell.* 2012, **22**:494–505.

Sprecher, E., Tesfaye-Kedjela, A., Ratajczak, P., Bergman, R., and Richard, G.: **Deleterious mutations in SPINK5 in a patient with congenital ichthyosiform erythroderma: molecular testing as a helpful diagnostic tool for Netherton syndrome.** *Clin. Exp. Dermatol.* 2004, **29**:513–517.

Wan, H., Winton, H.L., Soeller, C., Tovey, E.R., Gruenert, D.C., Thompson, P.J., Stewart, G.A., Taylor, G.W., Garrod, D.R., Cannell, M.B., *et al.*: **Der p 1 facilitates transepithelial allergen delivery by disruption of tight junctions.** *J. Clin. Invest.* 1999, **104**:123–133.

14-3   Genetic factors contribute to the development of IgE-mediated allergic disease.

Cookson, W.: **The immunogenetics of asthma and eczema: a new focus on the epithelium.** *Nat. Rev. Immunol.* 2004, **4**:978–988.

Demenais, F., Margaritte-Jeannin, P., Barnes, K.C., Cookson, W.O.C., Altmüller, J., Ang, W., Barr, R.G., Beaty, T.H., Becker, A.B., Beilby, J., *et al.*: **Multiancestry association study identifies new asthma risk loci that colocalize with immune-cell enhancer marks.** *Nat. Genet.* 2018, **50**:42–53.

Illing, P.R., Vivian, J.P., Purcell, A.W., Rossjohn, J., and McCluskey J.: **Human leukocyte antigen-associated drug hypersensitivity.** *Curr. Opin. Immunol.* 2013, **25**:81–89.

Li, X., Howard, T.D., Zheng, S.L., Haselkorn, T., Peters, S.P., Meyers, D.A., and Bleecker, E.R.: **Genome-wide association study of asthma identifies RAD50-IL13 and HLA-DR/DQ regions.** *J. Allergy Clin. Immunol.* 2010, **125**:328–335.

Li, Z., Hawkins, G.A., Ampleford, E.J., Moore, W.C., Li, H., Hastie, A.T., Howard, T.D., Boushey H.A., Busse, W.W., Calhoun, W.J., *et al.*: **Genome-wide association study identifies T$_H$1 pathway genes associated with lung function in asthmatic patients.** *J. Allergy Clin. Immunol.* 2013, **132**:313–320.

Moffatt, M.F., Kabesch, M., Liang, L., Dixon, A.L., Strachan, D., Heath, S., Depner, M., von Berg, A., Bufe, A., Rietschel, E., *et al.*: **Genetic variants regulating ORMDL3 expression contribute to the risk of childhood asthma.** *Nature* 2007, **448**:470-473.

Morahan, G., Huang, D., Wu, M., Holt, B.J., White, G.P., Kendall, G.E., Sly, P.D., and Holt, P.G.: **Association of IL12B promoter polymorphism with severity of atopic and non-atopic asthma in children.** *Lancet* 2002, **360**:455–459.

Peiser, M.: **Role of Th17 cells in skin inflammation of allergic contact dermatitis.** *Clin. Dev. Immunol.* 2013, **2013**:261037. doi: 10.1155/2013/261037.

Simper, G.S., Hò, G.T., Celik, A.A., Huyton, T., Kuhn, J., Kunze-Schumacher, H., Blasczyk, R., and Bade-Döding, C.: **Carbamazepine-mediated adverse drug reactions: CBZ-10,11-epoxide but not carbamazepine induces the alteration of peptides presented by HLA-B*15:02.** *J. Immunol. Res.* 2018, **2018**:5086503.

Thyssen, J.P., Carlsen, B.C., Menné, T., Linneberg, A., Nielsen, N.H., Meldgaard, M., Szecsi, P.B., Stender, S., and Johansen, J.D.: **Filaggrin null-mutations increase the risk and persistence of hand eczema in subjects with atopic dermatitis: results from a general population study.** *Br. J. Dermatol.* 2010, **163**:115–120.

Van den Oord, R.A.H.M., and Sheikh, A.: **Filaggrin gene defects and risk of developing allergic sensitisation and allergic disorders: systematic review and meta-analysis.** *BMJ* 2009, **339**:b2433.

Van Eerdewegh, P., Little, R.D., Dupuis, J., Del Mastro, R.G., Falls, K., Simon, J., Torrey, D., Pandit, S., McKenny, J., Braunschweiger, K., *et al.*: **Association of the *ADAM33 gene with asthma and bronchial hyperresponsiveness.*** *Nature* 2002, **418**:426–430.

Weiss, S.T., Raby, B.A., and Rogers, A.: **Asthma genetics and genomics.** *Curr. Opin. Genet. Dev.* 2009, **19**:279–282.

Zwollo, P., Ehrlich-Kautzky, E., Scharf, S.J., Ansari, A.A., Erlich, H.A., and Marsh, D.G.: **Sequencing of HLA-D in responders and nonresponders to short ragweed allergen, Amb a V.** *Immunogenetics* 1991, **33**:141–151.

14-4   Environmental factors may interact with genetic susceptibility to cause allergic disease.

Culley, F.J., Pollott, J., and Openshaw, P.J.: **Age at first viral infection determines the pattern of T cell-mediated disease during reinfection in adulthood.** *J. Exp. Med.* 2002, **196**:1381–1386.

Dakhama, A., Park, J.W., Taube, C., Joetham, A., Balhorn, A., Miyahara, N., Takeda, K., and Gelfand, E.W.: **The enhancement or prevention of airway hyper-responsiveness during reinfection with respiratory syncytial virus is critically dependent on the age at first infection and IL-13 production.** *J. Immunol.* 2005, **175**:1876–1883.

Deshane, J., Zmijewski, J.W., Luther, R., Gaggar, A., Deshane, R., Lai, J.F., Xu, X., Spell, M., Estell, K., Weaver, C.T., *et al.*: **Free radical-producing myeloid-derived regulatory cells: potent activators and suppressors of lung inflammation and airway hyperresponsiveness.** *Mucosal Immunol.* 2011, **4**:503–518.

Fuchs, C., and von Mutius, E.: **Prenatal and childhood infections: implications for the development and treatment of childhood asthma.** *Lancet Respir. Med.* 2013, **1**:743–754.

Redd, S.C.: **Asthma in the United States: burden and current theories.** *Environ. Health Perspect.* 2002, **110**(suppl. 4):557–560.

Romieu, I., Ramirez-Aguilar, M., Sienra-Monge, J.J., Moreno-Macías, H., del Rio-Navarro, B.E., David, G., Marzec, J., Hernández-Avila, M., and London, S.: **GSTM1 and GSTP1 and respiratory health in asthmatic children exposed to ozone.** *Eur. Respir. J.* 2006, **28**:953–959.

Saxon, A., and Diaz-Sanchez, D.: **Air pollution and allergy: you are what you breathe.** *Nat. Immunol.* 2005, **6**:223–226.

Scheltema, N.M., Nibbelke, E.E., Pouw, J., Blanken, M.O., Rovers, M.M., Naaktgeboren, C.A., Mazur, N.I., Wildenbeest, J.G., van der Ent, C.K., and Bont, L.J.: **Respiratory syncytial virus prevention and asthma in healthy preterm infants: a randomised controlled trial.** *Lancet Respir. Med.* 2018, **6**:257–264.

Strachan, D.P.: **Hay fever, hygiene, and household size.** *BMJ* 1989, **299**:1259–1260.

van Tilburg Bernardes, E., and Arrietam, M.C.: **Hygiene hypothesis in asthma development: is hygiene to blame?** *Arch. Med. Res.* 2017, **48**:717–726.

von Mutius, E.: **Allergies, infections and the hygiene hypothesis—the epidemiologic evidence.** *Immunobiology* 2007, **212**:433–439.

14-5   Most IgE is cell-bound and engages effector mechanisms of the immune system by pathways different from those of other antibody isotypes.

Conner, E.R., and Saini, S.S.: **The immunoglobulin E receptor: expression and regulation.** *Curr. Allergy Asthma Rep.* 2005, **5**:191–196.

Gilfillan, A.M., and Tkaczyk, C.: **Integrated signalling pathways for mast-cell activation.** *Nat. Rev. Immunol.* 2006, **6**:218–230.

Mcglashan, D.W., Jr.: **IgE-dependent signalling as a therapeutic target for allergies.** *Trends Pharmacol. Sci.* 2012, **33**:502–509.

Suzuki, R., Scheffel, J., and Rivera, J.: **New insights on the signalling and function of the high-affinity receptor for IgE.** *Curr. Top. Microbiol. Immunol.* 2015, **388**:63–90.

Turner, H., and Kinetm J.P.: **Signalling through the high-affinity IgE receptor Fc epsilonRI.** *Nature* 1999, **402**:24–30.

14-6   Mast cells reside in tissues and orchestrate allergic reactions.

Gonzalez-Espinosa, C., Odom, S., Olivera, A., Hobson, J.P., Martinez, M.E., Oliveira-Dos-Santos, A., Barra, L., Spiegel, S., Penninger, J.M., and Rivera, J.: **Preferential signaling and induction of allergy-promoting lymphokines upon weak stimulation of the high affinity IgE receptor on mast cells.** *J. Exp. Med.* 2003, **197**:1453–1465.

Kitamura, Y., Oboki, K., and Ito, A.: Development of mast cells. *Proc. Jpn. Acad. Ser. B Phys. Biol. Sci.* 2007, **83**:164–174.

Krishnan, S., Mali, R.S., Koehler, K.R., Vemula, S., Chatterjee, A., Ghosh, J., Ramdas, B., Ma, P., Hashino, E., and Kapur, R.: Class I(A) PI3Kinase regulatory subunit, p85α, mediates mast cell development through regulation of growth and survival related genes. *PLoS ONE* 2012, **7**:e28979.

Metcalfe, D.: Mast cells and mastocytosis. *Blood* 2007, **112**:946–956.

Schwartz, L.B.: Diagnostic value of tryptase in anaphylaxis and mastocytosis. *Immunol. Allergy Clin. North Am.* 2006, **26**:451–463.

Smuda, C., and Bryce, P.J.: New development in the use of histamine and histamine receptors. *Curr. Allergy Asthma Rep.* 2011, **11**:94–100.

Taube, C., Miyahara, N., Ott, V., Swanson, B., Takeda, K., Loader, J., Shultz, L.D., Tager, A.M., Luster, A.D., Dakhama, A., *et al.*: The leukotriene B4 receptor (BLT1) is required for effector CD8+ T cell-mediated, mast cell-dependent airway hyperresponsiveness. *J. Immunol.* 2006, **176**: 3157–3164.

Thurmond, R.L.: The histamine H4 receptor: from orphan to the clinic. *Front. Pharmacol.* 2015, **6**:65.

14-7 Eosinophils and basophils cause inflammation and tissue damage in allergic reactions.

Blanchard, C., and Rothenberg, M.E.: Biology of the eosinophil. *Adv. Immunol.* 2009, **101**:81–121.

Hogan, S.P., Rosenberg, H.F., Moqbel, R., Phipps, S., Foster, P.S., Lacy, P., Kay, A.B., and Rothenberg, M.E.: Eosinophils: biological properties and role in health and disease. *Clin. Exp. Allergy* 2008, **38**:709–750.

Lee, J.J., Jacobsen, E.A., McGarry, M.P., Schleimer, R.P., and Lee, N.A.: Eosinophils in health and disease: the LIAR hypothesis. *Clin. Exp. Allergy* 2010, **40**:563–575.

MacGlashan, D., Jr., Gauvreau, G., and Schroeder, J.T.: Basophils in airway disease. *Curr. Allergy Asthma Rep.* 2002, **2**:126–132.

Ohnmacht, C., Schwartz, C., Panzer, M., Schiedewitz, I., Naumann, R., and Voehringer, D.: Basophils orchestrate chronic allergic dermatitis and protective immunity against helminths. *Immunity* 2010, **33**:364–374.

Schwartz, C., Eberle, J.U., and Voehringer, D.: Basophils in inflammation. *Eur. J. Pharmacol.* 2016, **778**:90–95. doi: 10.1016/j.ejphar.2015.04.049.

Tomankova, T., Kriegova, E., and Liu, M.: Chemokine receptors and their therapeutic opportunities in diseased lung: far beyond leukocyte trafficking. *Am. J. Physiol. Lung Cell. Mol. Physiol.* 2015, **308**:L603–L618.

14-8 IgE-mediated allergic reactions have a rapid onset but can also lead to chronic responses.

deShazo, R.D., and Kemp, S.F.: Allergic reactions to drugs and biologic agents. *JAMA* 1997, **278**:1895–1906.

Nabe, T., Ikedo, A., Hosokawa, F., Kishima, M., Fujii, M., Mizutani, N., Yoshino, S., Ishihara, K., Akiba, S., and Chaplin, D.D.: Regulatory role of antigen-induced interleukin-10, produced by CD4(+) T cells, in airway neutrophilia in a murine model for asthma. *Eur. J. Pharmacol.* 2012, **677**:154–162.

Pawankar, R., Hayashi, M., Yamanishi, S., and Igarashi, T.: The paradigm of cytokine networks in allergic airway inflammation. *Curr. Opin. Allergy Clin. Immunol.* 2015, **15**:27–32.

Taube, C., Duez, C., Cui, Z.H., Takeda, K., Rha, Y.H., Park, J.W., Balhorn, A., Donaldson, D.D., Dakhama, A., and Gelfand, E.W.: The role of IL-13 in established allergic airway disease. *J. Immunol.* 2002, **169**:6482–6489.

14-9 Allergen introduced into the bloodstream can cause anaphylaxis and urticaria.

Fernandez, M., Warbrick, E.V., Blanca, M., and Coleman, J.W.: Activation and hapten inhibition of mast cells sensitized with monoclonal IgE anti-penicillin antibodies: evidence for two-site recognition of the penicillin derived determinant. *Eur. J. Immunol.* 1995, **25**:2486–2491.

Fiebiger, E., Maurer, D., Holub, H., Reininger, B., Hartmann, G., Woisetschläger, M., Kinet, J.P., and Stingl, G.: Serum IgG autoantibodies directed against the alpha chain of Fc epsilon RI: a selective marker and pathogenetic factor for a distinct subset of chronic urticaria patients? *J. Clin. Invest.* 1995, **96**:2606–2612.

Finkelman, F.D., Rothenberg, M.E., Brandt, E.B., Morris, S.C., and Strait, R.T.: Molecular mechanisms of anaphylaxis: lessons from studies with murine models. *J. Allergy Clin. Immunol.* 2005, **115**:449–457.

Golden, D.B.: Anaphylaxis to insect stings. *Immunol. Allergy Clin. North Am.* 2015, **35**:287–302.

Sicherer, S.H., and Leung, D.Y.: Advances in allergic skin disease, anaphylaxis, and hypersensitivity reactions to foods, drugs, and insects in 2014. *J. Allergy Clin. Immunol.* 2015, **35**:357–367.

Weltzien, H.U., and Padovan, E.: Molecular features of penicillin allergy. *J. Invest. Dermatol.* 1998, **110**:203–206.

14-10 Allergen inhalation is associated with the development of rhinitis and asthma.

Bousquet, J., Jeffery, P.K., Busse, W.W., Johnson, M., and Vignola, A.M.: Asthma. From bronchoconstriction to airways inflammation and remodeling. *Am. J. Respir. Crit. Care Med.* 2000, **161**:1720–1745.

Boxall, C., Holgate, S.T., and Davies, D.E.: The contribution of transforming growth factor-β and epidermal growth factor signalling to airway remodelling in chronic asthma. *Eur. Respir. J.* 2006, **27**:208–229.

Finotto, S., Neurath, M.F., Glickman, J.N., Qin, S., Lehr, H.A., Green, F.H., Ackerman, K., Haley, K., Galle, P.R., Szabo, S.J., *et al.*: Development of spontaneous airway changes consistent with human asthma in mice lacking T-bet. *Science* 2002, **295**:336–338.

George, B.J., Reif, D.M., Gallagher, J.E., Williams-DeVane, C.R., Heidenfelder, B.L., Hudgens, E.E., Jones, W., Neas, L., Cohen Hubal, E.A., and Edwards, S.W.: Data-driven asthma endotypes defined from blood biomarker and gene expression data. *PLoS ONE* 2015, **10**:e0117445.

Gour, N., and Wills-Karp, M.: IL-4 and IL-13 signaling in allergic airway disease. *Cytokine* 2015, **75**:68–78.

Haselden, B.M., Kay, A.B., and Larche, M.: Immunoglobulin E-independent major histocompatibility complex-restricted T cell peptide epitope-induced late asthmatic reactions. *J. Exp. Med.* 1999, **189**:1885–1894.

Kuperman, D.A., Huang, X., Koth, L.L., Chang, G.H., Dolganov, G.M., Zhu, Z., Elias, J.A., Sheppard, D., and Erle, D.J.: Direct effects of interleukin-13 on epithelial cells cause airway hyperreactivity and mucus overproduction in asthma. *Nat. Med.* 2002, **8**:885–889.

Lotvall, J., Akdis, C.A., Bacharier, L.B., Bjermer, L., Casale, T.B., Custovic, A., Lemanske, R.F., Jr., Wardlaw, A.J., Wenzel, S.E., and Greenberger, P.A.: Asthma endotypes: a new approach to classification of disease entities within the asthma syndrome. *J. Allergy Clin. Immunol.* 2011, **127**:355–360.

Newcomb, D.C., and Peebles, R.S., Jr.: Th17-mediated inflammation in asthma. *Curr. Opin. Immunol.* 2013, **25**:755–760.

Peebles, R.S., Jr.: At the bedside: the emergence of group 2 innate lymphoid cells in human disease. *J. Leukoc. Biol.* 2015, **97**:469–475.

Persson, E.K., Verstraete, K., Heyndrickx, I., Gevaert, E., Aegerter, H., Percier, J.M., Deswarte, K., Verschueren, K.H.G., Dansercoer, A., Gras, D., *et al.*: Protein crystallization promotes type 2 immunity and is reversible by antibody treatment. *Science* 2019, **364**:eaaw4295. doi: 10.1126/science.aaw4295.

Yan, X., Chu, J.-H., Gomez, J., Koenigs, M., Holm, C., He, X., Perez, M.F., Zhao, H., Mane, S., Martinez, F.D., *et al.*: Non-invasive analysis of the sputum transcriptome discriminates clinical phenotypes of asthma. *Am. J. Respir. Crit. Care Med.* 2015, **191**:1116–1125.

14-11 Allergy to particular foods causes systemic reactions as well as symptoms limited to the gut.

Du Toit, G., Robert, G., Sayre, P.H., Bahnson, H.T., Radulovic, S., Santos, A.D., Brough, H.A., Phippard, D., Basting, M., Feeney, M., *et al.*: Randomized trial of peanut consumption in infants at risk for peanut allergy. *N. Engl. J. Med.* 2015, **372**:803–813.

Lee, L.A., and Burks, A.W.: Food allergies: prevalence, molecular characterization, and treatment/prevention strategies. *Annu. Rev. Nutr.* 2006, **26**:539–565.

Verhoeckx, K., Bøgh, K.L., Dupont, D., Egger, L., Gadermaier, G., Larré, C., Mackie, A., Menard, O., Adel-Patient, K., Picariello, G., *et al.*: The relevance of a digestibility evaluation in the allergenicity risk assessment of novel proteins. Opinion of a joint initiative of COST action ImpARAS and COST action INFOGEST. *Food Chem. Toxicol.* 2019, **129**:405–423.

14-12 IgE-mediated allergic disease can be treated by inhibiting effector pathways or by desensitization to restore biological tolerance.

Akdis, C.A., and Akdis, M.: Mechanisms of allergen-specific immunotherapy and immune tolerance to allergens. *World Allergy Organ. J.* 2015, **8**:17.

Dunn, R.M., and Wechsler, M.E.: Anti-interleukin therapy in asthma. *Clin. Pharmacol. Ther.* 2015, **97**:55–65.

Eckman, J.A., Sterba, P.M., Kelly, D., Alexander, V., Liu, M.C., Bochner, B.S., MacGlashan, D.W., and Saini, S.S.: Effects of omalizumab on basophil and mast cell responses using an intranasal cat allergen challenge. *J. Allergy Clin. Immunol.* 2010, **125**:889–895.

Haldar, P., Brightling, C.E., Hargadon, B., Gupta, S., Monteiro, W., Sousa, A., Marshall, R.P., Bradding, P., Green, R.H., Wardlaw A.J., *et al.*: Mepolizumab and exacerbations of refractory eosinophilic asthma. *N. Engl. J. Med.* 2009, **360**:973–984.

Lai, T., Wang, S., Xu, Z., Zhang, C., Zhao, Y., Hu, Y., Cao, C., Ying, S., Chen, Z., Li, W., *et al.*: Long-term efficacy and safety of omalizumab in patients with persistent uncontrolled allergic asthma: a systematic review and meta-analysis. *Sci. Rep.* 2015, **5**:8191.

Larche, M.: Mechanisms of peptide immunotherapy in allergic airways disease. *Ann. Am. Thorac. Soc.* 2014, **11**:S292–S296.

Nair, P., Pizzichini, M.M.M., Kjarsgaard, M., Inman, M.D., Efthimiadis, A., Pizzichini, E., Hargreave, F.E., and O'Byrne, P.M.: Mepolizumab for prednisone-dependent asthma with sputum eosinophilia. *N. Engl. J. Med.* 2009, **360**:985–993.

Peters-Golden, M., and Henderson, W.R., Jr.: The role of leukotrienes in allergic rhinitis. *Ann. Allergy Asthma Immunol.* 2005, **94**:609–618.

Roberts, G., Hurley, C., Turcanu, V., and Lack, G.: Grass pollen immunotherapy as an effective therapy for childhood seasonal allergic asthma. *J. Allergy Clin. Immunol.* 2006, **117**:263–268.

Zhu, D., Kepley, C.L., Zhang, K., Terada, T., Yamada, T., and Saxon, A.: A chimeric human–cat fusion protein blocks cat-induced allergy. *Nat. Med.* 2005, **11**:446–449.

14-13 Non-IgE-dependent drug-induced hypersensitivity reactions in susceptible individuals occur by binding of the drug to the surface of circulating blood cells.

Arndt, P.A.: Drug-induced immune hemolytic anemia: the last 30 years of changes. *Immunohematology* 2014, **30**:44–54.

Greinacher, A., Potzsch, B., Amiral, J., Dummel, V., Eichner, A., and Mueller Eckhardt, C.: Heparin-associated thrombocytopenia: isolation of the antibody and characterization of a multimolecular PF4–heparin complex as the major antigen. *Thromb. Haemost.* 1994, **71**:247–251.

Semple, J.W., and Freedman, J.: Autoimmune pathogenesis and autoimmune hemolytic anemia. *Semin. Hematol.* 2005, **42**:122–130.

14-14 Systemic disease caused by immune-complex formation can follow the administration of large quantities of poorly catabolized antigens.

Bielory, L., Gascon, P., Lawley, T.J., Young, N.S., and Frank, M.M.: Human serum sickness: a prospective analysis of 35 patients treated with equine anti-thymocyte globulin for bone marrow failure. *Medicine (Baltimore)* 1988, **67**:40–57.

Davies, K.A., Mathieson, P., Winearls, C.G., Rees, A.J., and Walport, M.J.: Serum sickness and acute renal failure after streptokinase therapy for myocardial infarction. *Clin. Exp. Immunol.* 1990, **80**:83–88.

Hansel, T.T., Kropshofer, H., Singer, T., Mitchell, J.A., and George, A.J.: The safety and side effects of monoclonal antibodies. *Nat. Rev. Drug Discov.* 2010, **9**:325–338.

Schifferli, J.A., Ng, Y.C., and Peters, D.K.: The role of complement and its receptor in the elimination of immune complexes. *N. Engl. J. Med.* 1986, **315**:488–495.

Schmidt, R.E., and Gessner, J.E.: Fc receptors and their interaction with complement in autoimmunity. *Immunol. Lett.* 2005, **100**:56–67.

Skokowa, J., Ali, S.R., Felda, O., Kumar, V., Konrad, S., Shushakova, N., Schmidt, R.E., Piekorz, R.P., Nurnberg, B., Spicher, K., *et al.*: Macrophages induce the inflammatory response in the pulmonary Arthus reaction through $G\alpha_{i2}$ activation that controls C5aR and Fc receptor cooperation. *J. Immunol.* 2005, **174**:3041–3050.

14-15 Hypersensitivity reactions can be mediated by T_H1 cells and cytotoxic CD8 T cells.

Fyhrquist, N., Lehto, E., and Lauerma, A.: New findings in allergic contact dermatitis. *Curr. Opin. Allergy Clin. Immunol.* 2014, **14**:430–435.

Kalish, R.S., Wood, J.A., and LaPorte, A.: Processing of urushiol (poison ivy) hapten by both endogenous and exogenous pathways for presentation to T cells *in vitro. J. Clin. Invest.* 1994, **93**:2039–2047.

Mark, B.J., and Slavin, R.G.: Allergic contact dermatitis. *Med. Clin. North Am.* 2006, **90**:169–185.

Muller, G., Saloga, J., Germann, T., Schuler, G., Knop, J., and Enk, A.H.: IL-12 as mediator and adjuvant for the induction of contact sensitivity *in vivo. J. Immunol.* 1995, **155**:4661–4668.

Schmidt, M., Raghavan, B., Müller, V., Vogl, T., Fejer, G., Tchaptchet, S., Keck, S., Kalis, C., Nielsen, P.J., Galanos, C., *et al.*: Crucial role for human Toll-like receptor 4 in the development of contact allergy to nickel. *Nat. Immunol.* 2010, **11**:814–819.

Vollmer, J., Weltzien, H.U., and Moulon, C.: TCR reactivity in human nickel allergy indicates contacts with complementarity-determining region 3 but excludes superantigen-like recognition. *J. Immunol.* 1999, **163**:2723–2731.

Wakabayashi, T., Hu, D.L., Tagawa, Y., Sekikawa, K., Iwakura, Y., Hanada, K., and Nakane, A.: IFN-gamma and TNF-alpha are involved in urushiol-induced contact hypersensitivity in mice. *Immunol. Cell Biol.* 2005, **83**:18–24.

14-16 Celiac disease has features of both an allergic response and autoimmunity.

Ciccocioppo, R., Di Sabatino, A., and Corazza, G.R.: The immune recognition of gluten in celiac disease. *Clin. Exp. Immunol.* 2005, **140**:408–416.

Green, P.H.R., Lebwohl, B., and Greywoode, R.: Celiac disease. *J. Allergy Clin. Immunol.* 2015, **135**:1099–1106.

Koning, F.: Celiac disease: caught between a rock and a hard place. *Gastroenterology* 2005, **129**:1294–1301.

Shan, L., Molberg, O., Parrot, I., Hausch, F., Filiz, F., Gray, G.M., Sollid, L.M., and Khosla, C.: Structural basis for gluten intolerance in celiac sprue. *Science* 2002, **297**:2275–2279.

van Bergen, J., Mulder, C.J., Mearin, M.L., and Koning, F.: Local communication among mucosal immune cells in patients with celiac disease. *Gastroenterology* 2015, **148**:1187–1194.

Autoimmunity and Transplantation

15

Chapter 14 described how environmental antigens can elicit allergic and atopic reactions. In contrast, this chapter will examine how self antigens can elicit immune responses against the body's own tissues. We will also describe how transplanted organs and even some commensal organisms can elicit undesirable immune responses. Responses to self antigens that lead to tissue damage and disease are broadly referred to as **autoimmunity**. Responses associated with the microbiota are called **xenoimmunity**, as these antigens are not encoded by the human genome, but we will consider these immune-mediated diseases as part of the spectrum of **autoimmune diseases**. Finally, the immune response to nonself antigens on transplanted organs is called an **alloimmune response**.

In Section 6-13, we introduced the basic features of alloreactive T cells. Such T cells from one individual react strongly to nonself MHC molecules because of both an inherent affinity of T-cell receptors to bind MHC molecules and the process of positive selection described in Chapter 8. Normal lymphocyte development generates a state of **self-tolerance**, in which an individual's immune system does not attack the normal tissues of the body. Autoimmunity represents a breakdown or failure of the mechanisms of self-tolerance. First, we will briefly review the mechanisms that regulate self-tolerance and see how these may fail. Then, we will describe several specific autoimmune diseases that illustrate various pathogenic mechanisms by which autoimmunity can damage the body. Next, we will discuss how genetic and environmental factors can predispose to or trigger autoimmunity. Finally, we will describe immune responses to the nonself tissue antigens that cause transplant rejection.

The making and breaking of self-tolerance.

Chapter 8 described the processes that generate the repertoire of B and T cells that form the adaptive immune system. For B cells, both deletion and the process of receptor editing contribute to the elimination of strongly self-reactive cells in the primary immune repertoire. For T cells, negative selection, as well as the development of T_{reg} cells, contribute to self-tolerance. Despite the operation of these mechanisms, some potentially self-reactive lymphocytes do populate the primary immune repertoire. Additional mechanisms act in the periphery of the body to keep these cells in check, but under some conditions, these can fail and allow autoimmunity to develop.

15-1 Multiple mechanisms normally contribute to prevent autoimmunity.

Chapter 8 described some of the mechanisms that contribute to the development of a self-tolerant repertoire of B and T lymphocytes (see Sections 8-7 and 8-20). After successful rearrangements in the various antigen receptor genes, B-cell or T-cell receptors are expressed on the surface of newly developing lymphocytes. Receptors that interact strongly with 'self' molecules expressed in the bone marrow or thymus can cause a change in a lymphocyte's development, affecting either the lymphocyte's survival or, in some cases, the receptor that is expressed. Strongly self-reactive T cells and B cells may be eliminated entirely, whereas some self-reactive B cells may undergo receptor editing to allow replacement with a non-self-reactive receptor. Newly formed lymphocytes are especially sensitive to inactivation or deletion by strong signals through their antigen receptors, while the same signals may activate a mature lymphocyte in the periphery. Such tolerance induced during lymphocyte development is known as **central tolerance**.

However, we know that these processes are not perfect and that lymphocytes with potentially self-reactive antigen receptors do populate the peripheral repertoire. The term **peripheral tolerance** is sometimes used to refer collectively to a number of mechanisms that control the potentially self-reactive lymphocytes in the peripheral repertoire. This term originated well before there was an understanding of the mechanisms that control self-reactive lymphocytes. Some of these mechanisms have been described in earlier chapters, and we will only briefly recount them here. First, the system of innate recognition receptors, such as TLRs, that recognize the presence of pathogens (see Chapter 3) help to establish a threshold for lymphocyte activation in the periphery. They do this by providing a 'danger' signal needed to induce co-stimulatory molecules that are required to fully activate immune responses (see Section 9-6). As such, antigen recognition in the absence of such signals (that is, in a non-immunogenic context) may not lead to lymphocyte activation, but rather may induce a nonresponsive (anergic) state in lymphocytes. Also, we now recognize the importance of the subset of CD4 T cells called regulatory T cells (T_{reg} cells), which can inhibit responses to self antigens (see Sections 9-15 and 9-17). Some self antigens are expressed in locations that are not normally accessible to surveillance by immune cells, where there is a physical barrier to access of the antigen, leading to 'immunological ignorance.' Also, some tissues act as so-called 'immune-privileged sites' by using mechanisms to actively suppress lymphocyte activation. The various components of self-tolerance and peripheral tolerance are listed in **Fig. 15.1**.

Fig. 15.1 Self-tolerance depends on the concerted action of a variety of mechanisms that operate at different sites and stages of development. The different ways in which the immune system prevents activation of and damage caused by autoreactive lymphocytes are listed, along with the specific mechanism and the site where such tolerance predominantly occurs.

Layers of self-tolerance		
Type of tolerance	**Mechanism**	**Site of action**
Central tolerance	Deletion Editing	Thymus (T cells) Bone marrow (B cells)
Antigen segregation	Physical barrier to self-antigen access to lymphoid system	Peripheral organs (e.g., thyroid, pancreas)
Peripheral anergy	Cellular inactivation by weak signaling without co-stimulus	Secondary lymphoid tissue
Regulatory T cells	Suppression by cytokines, intercellular signals	Secondary lymphoid tissue and sites of inflammation; multiple tissues in steady state
Functional deviation	Differentiation of regulatory T cells that limit inflammatory cytokine secretion	Secondary lymphoid tissue and sites of inflammation
Activation-induced cell death	Apoptosis	Secondary lymphoid tissue and sites of inflammation
Immunological ignorance	Low-affinity interaction in absence of co-activation	Peripheral organs
Immunologically privileged sites	TGF-β Fas	Brain, eye, testis, uterus (fetus)

Disease	Disease mechanism	Consequence	Prevalence
Psoriasis	Autoreactive T cells against skin-associated antigens	Inflammation of skin with formation of scaly patches or plaques	1 in 50
Rheumatoid arthritis	Autoreactive T cells, autoantibodies against antigens localized to joint synovium, and rheumatoid factor.	Joint inflammation and destruction causing arthritis	1 in 100
Graves' disease	Autoantibodies against the thyroid-stimulating hormone (TSH) receptor	Hyperthyroidism: overproduction of thyroid hormones	1 in 100
Hashimoto's thyroiditis	Autoantibodies and autoreactive T cells against thyroid antigens	Destruction of thyroid tissue leading to hypothyroidism: underproduction of thyroid hormones	1 in 200
Systemic lupus erythematosus	Autoantibodies and autoreactive T cells against DNA, chromatin proteins, and ubiquitous ribonucleoprotein antigens	Glomerulonephritis, vasculitis, rash	1 in 200
Sjögren's syndrome	Autoantibodies and autoreactive T cells against ribonucleoprotein antigens	Lymphocyte infiltration of exocrine glands, leading to dry eyes and/or dry mouth; other organs may be involved, leading to systemic disease	1 in 300
Crohn's disease	Autoreactive T cells against intestinal flora antigens	Intestinal inflammation and scarring	1 in 500
Multiple sclerosis	Autoreactive T cells against brain and spinal cord antigens	Formation of sclerotic plaques in brain and spinal cord with destruction of myelin sheaths surrounding nerve cell axons, leading to muscle weakness, ataxia, and other symptoms	1 in 700
Type 1 diabetes mellitus (insulin-dependent diabetes mellitus; IDDM)	Autoreactive T cells against pancreatic islet cell antigens	Destruction of pancreatic islet β cells leading to nonproduction of insulin	1 in 800

Fig. 15.2 Some common autoimmune diseases. The diseases listed are among the most common autoimmune diseases and will be used as examples in this chapter. They are listed in order of prevalence.

The concept of autoimmunity was first presented at the beginning of the 20th century by Paul Ehrlich, who described it as '*horror autotoxicus*.' Autoimmune responses resemble normal immune responses to pathogens in being activated by specific antigens, but in this case by self antigens, or **autoantigens**. Like normal immune responses, autoimmune responses involve the generation of effector T cells and the production of antibodies, but these are directed against self antigens, or autoantigens. Such antibodies are called **autoantibodies**. Collectively, autoimmune disorders may affect as much as 5% of the populations of the United States, but individual types of autoimmunity are relatively rare. **Figure 15.2** lists several of the more common autoimmune syndromes and illustrates the wide variety of effector mechanisms and tissue distributions that can arise.

We have already described one situation in which central tolerance fails (see Section 8-25). Many self antigens are expressed in the thymus by either thymic epithelial cells in the medulla or a CD8α⁺ subset of dendritic cells to allow for the deletion of T cells that strongly react. Some 'peripheral genes' expressed in a highly tissue-restricted manner, such as insulin, are also expressed in the thymus because of the action of the transcription factor AIRE expressed in the thymic medulla (see Fig. 8.30). Individuals with a defect in the gene *AIRE* exhibit a rare inherited form of autoimmunity—**APECED (autoimmune polyendocrinopathy–candidiasis–ectodermal dystrophy)**, also known as autoimmune polyglandular syndrome type I (APS-I). Individuals with APECED exhibit damage to multiple endocrine tissues, including insulin-producing pancreatic islets, and frequently acquire fungal infections, particularly candidiasis. Mice engineered to lack *AIRE* fail to express many peripheral genes in the thymus and develop a similar syndrome. The autoimmunity that accompanies AIRE deficiency takes time to develop and does not always affect all potential organ targets.

Autoimmune Polyendocrinopathy– Candidiasis–Ectodermal Dystrophy (APECED)

15-2 Lymphocytes that bind self antigens with relatively low affinity usually ignore them but in some circumstances become activated.

Another mechanism that prevents activation of potentially self-reactive lymphocytes is called **immunological ignorance**. This mechanism applies to lymphocytes that have a low affinity for self antigens and normally make no effector response against them. However, such 'ignorance' can be converted into an autoimmune response if the threshold for lymphocyte activation is sufficiently reduced; for example, by the induction of co-activating factors in antigen-presenting cells. This may occur during an infection, when naive T cells can encounter activated dendritic cells presenting the self antigen along with strong co-stimulatory signals and pro-inflammatory cytokines.

Immunological ignorance can also be broken when the autoantigen is also a ligand for a Toll-like receptor (TLR). These receptors recognize a variety of microbial-associated molecular patterns (see Section 3-5), but some such patterns can also be found among self molecules. For example, TLR-9 recognizes unmethylated CpG sequences in DNA. Normally much more common in bacterial than mammalian DNA, CpG sequences are enriched in mitochondrial DNA and in apoptotic mammalian cells. When extensive cell death occurs under conditions of inadequate clearance of apoptotic fragments, B cells with receptors that happen to bind chromatin components may internalize CpG sequences via their B-cell receptors. The internalized CpG can activate the intracellular TLR-9 (see Fig. 3.11), thereby activating the previously ignorant B cell (**Fig. 15.3**) and leading to the production of anti-chromatin autoantibodies. These B cells may also act as antigen-presenting cells for autoreactive T cells. Ribonucleoprotein complexes containing uridine-rich RNA have similarly been shown to activate naive B cells through binding by TLR-7 or TLR-8. Autoantibodies against DNA, chromatin, and ribonucleoproteins are produced in the autoimmune disease **systemic lupus erythematosus (SLE)**, and this appears to be one mechanism by which self-reactive B cells are stimulated to produce them.

Ignorant lymphocytes may also become activated by a change in the availability or form of self antigens. Antigens that are normally intracellular and not encountered by lymphocytes may be released as a result of tissue injury or inflammation. These antigens can then activate ignorant T and B cells, leading to autoimmunity. This can occur after myocardial infarction, when an autoimmune response is detectable some days after the release of cardiac antigens. Such reactions are typically transient and cease when the autoantigens have been removed; however, when clearance mechanisms are inadequate, they can continue, causing clinical autoimmune disease.

Fig. 15.3 Self antigens that are recognized by Toll-like receptors can activate autoreactive B cells by providing co-stimulation. B cells that have a low affinity for DNA can escape deletion in the bone marrow and persist in the periphery but are not normally activated. Under some conditions and in genetically susceptible individuals, the concentration of DNA may increase, leading to the ligation of enough B-cell receptors to activate these B cells. When this occurs, B cells signal through their receptor (left panel). This will also result in the uptake of DNA (center panel) and its delivery to an endosomal compartment (right panel), where it may be recognized by TLR-9. DNA that is enriched in unmethylated CpG DNA sequences present in microbial DNA normally allows TLR-9 to distinguish pathogens from self. But unmethylated CpG DNA sequences are also enriched in mitochondrial DNA and can arise from apoptotic mammalian cells, which can be sufficient to activate TLR-9. This pathway can promote the activation of the DNA-specific B cells and lead to the production of autoantibodies against DNA.

B cells with specificity for DNA bind soluble fragments of DNA, sending a signal through the B-cell receptor

The cross-linked B-cell receptor is internalized with the bound DNA molecule

GC-rich fragments from the internalized DNA bind to TLR-9 in an endosomal compartment, sending a co-stimulatory signal

Additionally, some autoantigens are present in great quantity but are usually in a non-immunogenic form. IgG is a good example, as there are large quantities of it in blood and extracellular fluids. B cells specific for the IgG constant region are not usually activated because IgG is monomeric and cannot cross-link the B-cell receptor. However, when immune complexes form after infection or immunization, enough IgG is in multivalent form to evoke a response from otherwise ignorant B cells. The anti-IgG autoantibody they produce is called **rheumatoid factor** because it is often present in rheumatoid arthritis. Again, this response is normally short-lived, as long as the immune complexes are cleared rapidly.

Systemic Lupus Erythematosus

Rheumatoid Arthritis

15-3 Antigens in immunologically privileged sites do not induce immune attack but can serve as targets.

Foreign tissue grafts placed in some body sites do not elicit immune responses. For instance, grafts placed in the brain and anterior chamber of the eye do not induce rejection. Such locations are termed **immunologically privileged sites** (**Fig. 15.4**). It was originally believed that immunological privilege arose from the failure of antigens to leave privileged sites and induce immune responses. Subsequent studies have shown that antigens do leave these sites and interact with T cells. However, instead of eliciting an effector immune response, they induce a tolerogenic response that does not injure the tissue.

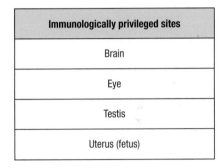

Immunologically privileged sites
Brain
Eye
Testis
Uterus (fetus)

Fig. 15.4 Some sites in the body are immunologically privileged. Tissue grafts placed in these sites often last indefinitely, and antigens placed in these sites do not elicit destructive immune responses.

Immunologically privileged sites seem to be unusual in three ways. First, communication between the privileged site and the body is atypical in that extracellular fluid does not pass through conventional lymphatics, although proteins placed in these sites do leave and can have immunological effects. Privileged sites are generally surrounded by tissue barriers that exclude naive lymphocytes. The brain, for example, is guarded by the blood–brain barrier. Second, soluble factors that affect the course of an immune response are produced in privileged sites. The anti-inflammatory transforming growth factor-β (TGF-β) seems to be particularly important in this regard. Under homeostatic conditions, antigens recognized in concert with TGF-β tend to induce T_{reg} responses, rather than pro-inflammatory T_H17 responses, which are induced by TGF-β in the presence of IL-6 (see Section 9-15). Third, the expression of Fas ligand in immunologically privileged sites may provide a further level of protection by inducing the apoptosis of Fas-bearing effector lymphocytes that enter these sites (see Section 11-16).

Paradoxically, antigens sequestered in immunologically privileged sites are often targets of autoimmune attack; for example, brain and spinal cord autoantigens such as myelin basic protein are targeted in the autoimmune disease **multiple sclerosis**, a chronic inflammatory demyelinating disease of the central nervous system (see Fig. 15.2). Thus, the tolerance normally shown to these antigens cannot be due to previous deletion of the self-reactive T cells. In **experimental autoimmune encephalomyelitis (EAE)**, a mouse model for multiple sclerosis, mice become diseased only when they are immunized with myelin antigens and adjuvants, which cause infiltration of the central nervous system with antigen-specific T_H17 and T_H1 cells that induce a local inflammatory response that damages nerve tissue. This result also emphasizes that autoimmunity can be provoked by inducing a specific adaptive immune response to self antigens. But in humans, autoimmunity usually arises spontaneously, and the events that initiate the immune response to self are largely unknown. Some strains of mice also exhibit spontaneous autoimmunity, but the genetic basis of the disease is known to be multigenic and is still an active area of research.

Thus, some antigens expressed in immunologically privileged sites induce neither tolerance nor lymphocyte activation in normal circumstances, but if autoreactive lymphocytes are activated elsewhere, these autoantigens can

Fig. 15.5 Damage to an immunologically privileged site can induce an autoimmune response. In the disease sympathetic ophthalmia, trauma to one eye releases the sequestered eye antigens into the surrounding tissues, making them accessible to T cells (left panel). Antigens that localize to lymph nodes can activate effector cells and induce an immune response (middle panel). These lymphocytes can then attack the traumatized eye and also infiltrate and attack the healthy eye (right panel). Thus, although the sequestered antigens do not induce a response by themselves, if a response is induced elsewhere they can serve as targets for attack.

| Trauma to one eye results in the release of sequestered intraocular protein antigens | Released intraocular antigen is carried to lymph nodes and activates T cells | Effector T cells return via bloodstream and encounter antigen in both eyes |

become targets for autoimmune attack. Likely, T cells specific for antigens sequestered in immunologically privileged sites are in a state of immunological ignorance. Further evidence comes from the eye disease **sympathetic ophthalmia** (Fig. 15.5). If one eye is ruptured by a blow or other trauma, an autoimmune response to eye proteins can occur, although this happens only rarely. Once the response is induced, it often attacks both eyes. Immunosuppression—and, rarely, removal of the damaged eye, the source of antigen—is required to preserve vision in the undamaged eye.

Unsurprisingly, effector T cells can enter immunologically privileged sites when such sites become infected by some pathogen. Effector T cells can enter most tissues after activation (see Chapter 11), but the accumulation of these cells is seen only when antigen is recognized in the site, triggering the production of cytokines that alter tissue barriers.

15-4 Autoimmune responses can be controlled at various stages by regulatory T cells.

Tolerance due to regulatory lymphocytes is distinguished from other forms of self-tolerance by the fact that T_{reg} cells have the potential to suppress self-reactive lymphocytes that recognize antigens different from those recognized by the T_{reg} cell (Fig. 15.6). This type of tolerance is known as **regulatory tolerance**. The key feature of regulatory tolerance is that regulatory cells can suppress autoreactive lymphocytes that recognize a variety of different self antigens, as long as the antigens are from the same tissue or are presented by the same antigen-presenting cell.

As discussed in Chapter 9, two general types of regulatory T cells have been defined experimentally. 'Natural' T_{reg} (nT_{reg}) cells are programmed in the thymus to express the transcription factor FoxP3 in response to self antigens. When activated by the same antigens in peripheral tissues, nT_{reg} cells inhibit other self-reactive T cells that recognize antigens in the same tissue to prevent their differentiation into effector T cells or prevent their effector

Regulatory tolerance	
T cell specific for self antigen recognized in thymus becomes a natural regulatory T (nT_{reg}) cell	T cell specific for self or commensal microbiota antigen recognized in presence of TGF-β becomes an induced regulatory T (iT_{reg}) cell

Thymus | Periphery

Cytokines (IL-10 and TGF-β) produced by T_{reg} cells inhibit other self-reactive T cells

Periphery

Fig. 15.6 Tolerance mediated by regulatory T cells can inhibit multiple autoreactive T cells that all recognize antigens from the same tissue. Specialized autoreactive natural regulatory T (nT_{reg}) cells develop in the thymus in response to stimulation by self antigens that is too weak to cause deletion but is greater than required for simple positive selection (upper left panel). Regulatory T cells can also be induced (iT_{reg} cells) from naive self-reactive T cells in the periphery if the naive T cell recognizes its antigen and is activated in the presence of the cytokine TGF-β (upper right panel). nT_{reg} and iT_{reg} cells are able to inhibit other self-reactive T cells (lower panel), in part by secretion of inhibiting cytokines such as IL-10 and TGF-β that inhibit all surrounding autoreactive T cells, regardless of their precise autoantigen specificity.

function. 'Induced' T_{reg} (iT_{reg}) cells also express FoxP3 but develop in peripheral immune tissues in response to antigens recognized in the presence of TGF-β but in the absence of pro-inflammatory cytokines. Giving animals large amounts of self antigen orally, which induces so-called **oral tolerance** (see Section 12-7), can sometimes lead to unresponsiveness to these antigens when given by other routes and can prevent autoimmune disease. Oral tolerance is routinely generated to antigens such as food antigens and is accompanied by the generation of iT_{reg} cells in the gut-draining mesenteric lymph nodes. These cells are able to suppress immune responses to the given antigen in the gut.

A protective role for FoxP3-expressing T_{reg} cells has been demonstrated in several autoimmune syndromes in mice, including diabetes, EAE, SLE, and inflammation of the large intestine, or colon (colitis). Experiments in mouse models of these diseases have established that $FoxP3^+$ T_{reg} cells actively suppress disease in the normal immune system, as depletion of these cells results in multi-organ autoimmune disease. T_{reg} cells have also been shown to prevent or ameliorate other immunopathologic syndromes, such as graft-versus-host disease and graft rejection, which are described later in this chapter.

FoxP3-expressing T_{reg} cells are not the only type of regulatory lymphocyte that has been identified. For example, FoxP3-negative regulatory T cells characterized by their production of IL-10 are enriched in the intestinal tissues, where they may suppress inflammatory bowel disease (IBD) through an IL-10–dependent mechanism. The developmental origins of these cells are not currently understood. Almost every type of lymphocyte has been shown to display regulatory activity in some circumstance. Even B cells can regulate experimentally induced autoimmune syndromes, including collagen-induced arthritis (CIA) and EAE. This activity is probably mediated in a similar way to that of regulatory CD4 T cells, with the secretion of cytokines that inhibit proliferation and differentiation of effector T cells.

In addition to the extrinsic regulation of autoreactive T and B cells by regulatory cells, lymphocytes have intrinsic proliferation and survival limits that can help restrict autoimmune as well as normal responses (see Section 11-16). This is illustrated by the development of spontaneous autoimmunity that is caused by mutations in pathways that control apoptosis, such as the Bcl-2 pathway or the Fas pathway (see Section 9-21); mutations in these pathways lead to spontaneous autoimmunity. This form of autoimmunity provides evidence that autoreactive cells are normally generated but are then eliminated by apoptosis. This seems to be an important mechanism for both T- and B-cell tolerance.

Summary.

Self-reactive lymphocytes always exist in the natural immune repertoire but are not often activated due to several different mechanisms. Under various conditions, self-reactive lymphocytes become activated by autoantigens and, if activation persists, can cause autoimmune diseases. The various tolerance mechanisms normally work together to prevent autoimmunity (see Fig. 15.1), but failure of these mechanisms can lead to a variety of different diseases (see Fig. 15.2). Central tolerance relies on eliminating overtly autoreactive cells during lymphocyte development in the thymus and bone marrow. Central tolerance also involves the generation of 'natural' (or 'thymic') T_{reg} cells that suppress autoimmune responses after exiting the thymus. Mechanisms of peripheral tolerance, such as anergy and deletion, or the extrathymic production of 'induced' (or 'peripheral') T_{reg} cells, complement these central tolerance mechanisms for antigens that are not expressed in the thymus or bone marrow. Tissue barriers and immune-privileged sites also control autoimmune responses by restricting access to antigens and by providing a tolerogenic environment through external apoptosis-inducing signals, such as those mediated by Fas. Weak self-reactivity in lymphocytes does not result in deletion, as this may too severely limit the immune repertoire and impair responses to pathogens. Instead, weakly self-reactive cells are normally suppressed in the periphery by the absence of danger signals that induce the necessary co-stimulatory molecules and by T_{reg} cells of related tissue specificity.

Autoimmune diseases and pathogenic mechanisms.

In this part of the chapter, we describe some common clinical autoimmune syndromes, along with the mechanisms by which self-reactive lymphocytes can cause tissue damage. The mechanisms of pathogenesis resemble in many ways those that target invading pathogens. Damage by autoantibodies, mediated through the complement and Fc receptor systems, has an important role in some diseases, such as SLE. Similarly, self-reactive cytotoxic T cells can destroy tissues in the same way they would eliminate virus-infected cells; this is one way by which pancreatic β cells are destroyed in diabetes. However, unlike most pathogens, self proteins are not typically eliminated, so that, with rare exceptions—such as the islet cells in the pancreas—the response persists chronically. Some pathogenic mechanisms are unique to autoimmunity, such as antibodies against cell-surface receptors that affect their function, as in myasthenia gravis.

15-5 Autoimmunity can be classified into either organ-specific or systemic disease.

From a clinical perspective, it is useful to classify autoimmunity into two major patterns: 'organ-specific' autoimmune diseases restricted to specific organs, and 'systemic' autoimmune diseases that affect many tissues of the body. Examples of both kinds are listed in **Fig. 15.7**. Both kinds of disease tend to become chronic because most autoantigens persist in the body. Even when the response completely destroys the target tissue, as in **type 1 diabetes mellitus**, where the insulin-producing pancreatic β cells are eliminated and the autoimmune response abates, the consequences are nonetheless chronic. Some autoimmune diseases seem to be dominated by the pathogenic effects of a particular immune effector pathway, either autoantibodies or effector T cells. However, both of these pathways often contribute to the overall pathogenesis.

In organ-specific diseases, autoantigens from one or a few organs are targeted, and disease is limited to those organs. Examples include **Hashimoto's thyroiditis** and **Graves' disease**, which both predominantly affect the thyroid gland, and type 1 diabetes mellitus, which is caused by immune attack on insulin-producing pancreatic β cells. Examples of systemic autoimmune disease are SLE and primary **Sjögren's syndrome**, in which tissues as diverse as the skin, kidneys, and brain may all be affected (see Fig. 15.7).

The autoantigens recognized in these two categories of disease are themselves organ-specific and systemic, respectively. Thus, Graves' disease is characterized by the production of antibodies against the thyroid-stimulating hormone (TSH) receptor, Hashimoto's thyroiditis by antibodies against thyroid peroxidase, and type 1 diabetes mellitus by anti-insulin antibodies. By contrast, SLE is characterized by the presence of antibodies against antigens that are ubiquitous and abundant in every cell of the body, such as chromatin and the proteins of the pre-mRNA splicing machinery—the spliceosome complex.

Organ-specific autoimmune diseases
Type 1 diabetes mellitus
Goodpasture's syndrome
Multiple sclerosis Crohn's disease Psoriasis
Graves' disease Hashimoto's thyroiditis Autoimmune hemolytic anemia Autoimmune Addison's disease Vitiligo Myasthenia gravis

Systemic autoimmune diseases
Rheumatoid arthritis
Scleroderma
Systemic lupus erythematosus Primary Sjögren's syndrome Polymyositis

Fig. 15.7 Some common autoimmune diseases classified according to their 'organ-specific' or 'systemic' nature. Diseases that tend to occur in clusters are grouped in single boxes. Clustering is defined as more than one disease affecting a single individual or different members of a family. Not all autoimmune diseases can be classified according to this scheme. For example, autoimmune hemolytic anemia can occur in isolation or in association with systemic lupus erythematosus.

A strict separation of diseases into organ-specific and systemic categories does break down to some extent, however, because not all autoimmune diseases can be usefully classified in this manner. For example, autoimmune hemolytic anemia, in which red blood cells are destroyed, sometimes occurs as a solitary entity and could be classified as an organ-specific disease. In other circumstances it can occur in conjunction with SLE as part of a systemic autoimmune disease.

A prevalent variant of chronic inflammatory disease is **inflammatory bowel disease (IBD)**, which includes two main clinical entities: **Crohn's disease** (discussed later in this chapter) and **ulcerative colitis**. We discuss IBD in this chapter because it has many features of an autoimmune disease, even though it is not primarily targeted against self-tissue antigens. Instead, the targets of the dysregulated immune response in IBD are antigens derived from the commensal microbiota resident in the intestines. Strictly speaking, therefore, IBD is an outlier among autoimmune diseases in that the immune response is not directed against 'self' antigens; rather, it is directed against microbial antigens of the resident, or 'self,' microbiota. Nevertheless, features of immune tolerance breakdown are also seen in IBD, and, as with the organ-specific autoimmune diseases, the tissue destruction wrought by the aberrant immune response is primarily localized to a single organ—the intestines.

15-6 Multiple components of the immune system are typically recruited in autoimmune disease.

Understanding which parts of the immune system mediate different autoimmune syndromes can be useful in determining the disease etiology and in developing therapies. For example, in **myasthenia gravis**, it is the autoantibodies produced against the acetylcholine receptor that cause disease by blocking receptor function at the neuromuscular junction, resulting in muscle weakness. In other autoimmune conditions, antibodies in the form of immune complexes are deposited in tissues and cause tissue damage as a consequence of the inflammation that results from complement activation (see Section 2-14) and ligation of Fc receptors on inflammatory cells (see Section 10-20).

Relatively common autoimmune diseases in which effector T cells seem to be the main destructive agents include type 1 diabetes mellitus, psoriasis, IBD, and multiple sclerosis. In these diseases, T cells recognize self peptides or peptides derived from the commensal microbiota that are complexed with self MHC molecules. The damage in such diseases is caused by T cells recruiting and activating myeloid cells of the innate immune system to cause local inflammation or by direct T-cell damage to tissue cells.

The ability to transfer disease from a diseased individual to a healthy one by transferring autoantibodies and/or self-reactive T cells both confirms that the disease is autoimmune in nature and proves the involvement of the transferred material in the pathological process. In myasthenia gravis, serum from affected individuals can transfer symptoms to animal recipients, thus proving the pathogenic role of the anti-acetylcholine autoantibodies (**Fig. 15.8**).

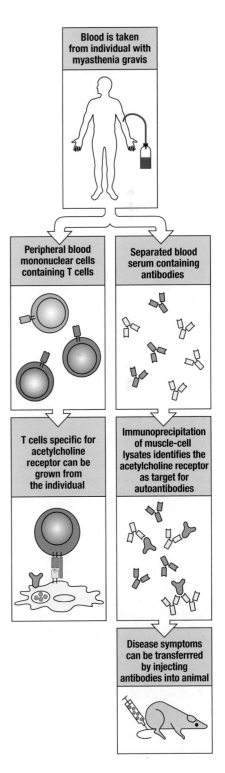

Fig. 15.8 Identification of autoantibodies that can transfer disease in individuals with myasthenia gravis. Autoantibodies from the serum of individuals with myasthenia gravis immunoprecipitate the acetylcholine receptor from lysates of skeletal muscle cells (right-hand panels). Because the antibodies can bind to both the murine and the human acetylcholine receptor, they can transfer disease when injected into mice (bottom panel). This experiment demonstrates that the antibodies are pathogenic. However, to be able to produce antibodies, the same individuals should have CD4 T cells that respond to a peptide derived from the acetylcholine receptor. To detect them, T cells from individuals with myasthenia gravis are isolated and grown in the presence of the acetylcholine receptor plus antigen-presenting cells of the correct MHC type (left-hand panels). T cells specific for epitopes of the acetylcholine receptor are stimulated to proliferate and can thus be detected.

Fig. 15.9 T cells specific for myelin basic protein mediate inflammation of the brain in experimental autoimmune encephalomyelitis (EAE). Disease is induced by injecting mice with isolated spinal cord homogenized in Freund's complete adjuvant. This generates an inflammatory reaction in the brain that produces a progressive paralysis, first affecting the tail and hind limbs and progressing to forelimb paralysis and eventual death. One autoantigen identified in the spinal cord homogenate is myelin basic protein (MBP). Immunization with MBP alone in Freund's complete adjuvant can also cause these disease symptoms. Inflammation of the brain and paralysis are mediated by T_H1 and T_H17 cells specific for MBP. Production of GM-CSF and recruitment of myeloid cells contributes to disease. Cloned MBP-specific T_H1 cells can transfer symptoms of EAE to naive recipients provided that the recipients carry the correct MHC allele. Other purified components of the myelin sheath can also induce the symptoms of EAE, so there is more than one autoantigen in this disease.

Similarly, in the animal model disease EAE, T cells from affected animals can transfer disease to normal animals (**Fig. 15.9**).

Pregnancy can demonstrate a role for antibodies in disease, because IgG antibodies, but not T cells, can cross the placenta (see Section 10-17). The autoantibodies produced in several autoimmune diseases can cross the placenta and into the fetus and neonate (**Fig. 15.10**). For example, in Graves' disease, autoantibodies produced against the mother's thyroid-stimulating hormone (TSH) receptor can pass into the fetal circulation to produce disease in the neonate (**Fig. 15.11**). The symptoms of disease in the newborn infant typically disappear rapidly as the maternal antibody is catabolized, but in some cases the antibodies cause organ injury before they are removed. In SLE or Sjögren's syndrome, damage to the conducting tissue of the heart can occur in babies. Antibody clearance can be accelerated by exchange of the infant's blood or plasma (plasmapheresis), although this is not useful after permanent injury has occurred.

Fig. 15.10 Some autoimmune diseases can be transferred across the placenta by pathogenic IgG autoantibodies. These diseases are caused mostly by autoantibodies against cell-surface or tissue-matrix molecules. This suggests an important factor determining whether an autoantibody that crosses the placenta causes disease in the fetus or newborn baby is the accessibility of the antigen to the autoantibody. Autoimmune congenital heart block is caused by fibrosis of the developing cardiac conducting tissue, which expresses abundant Ro antigen. Ro protein is a constituent of an intracellular small cytoplasmic ribonucleoprotein, but it is unclear whether or not it is expressed at the cell surface of cardiac conducting tissue to act as a target for autoimmune tissue injury. Nevertheless, autoantibody binding leads to tissue damage and results in slowing of the heart rate (bradycardia). TSH, thyroid-stimulating hormone.

Autoimmune diseases transferred across the placenta to the fetus and newborn infant		
Disease	**Autoantibody**	**Symptom**
Myasthenia gravis	Anti-acetylcholine receptor	Muscle weakness
Graves' disease	Anti-TSH receptor	Hyperthyroidism
Thrombocytopenic purpura	Anti-platelet antibodies	Bruising and hemorrhage
Neonatal lupus rash and/or congenital heart block	Anti-Ro antibodies Anti-La antibodies	Photosensitive rash and/or bradycardia
Pemphigus vulgaris	Anti-desmoglein-3	Blistering rash

| Patient with Graves' disease makes anti-TSHR antibodies | Transfer of antibodies across placenta into the fetus | Newborn infant also suffers from Graves' disease | Plasmapheresis removes maternal anti-TSHR antibodies and cures the disease |

Fig. 15.11 Antibody-mediated autoimmune diseases can appear in the infants of affected mothers as a consequence of transplacental antibody transfer. In pregnant women, IgG antibodies cross the placenta and accumulate in the fetus before birth (see Fig. 10.30). Babies born to mothers with IgG-mediated autoimmune disease therefore frequently show symptoms similar to those of the mother in the first few weeks of life. Fortunately, there is little lasting damage because the symptoms disappear along with the maternal antibody. In Graves' disease, the symptoms are caused by antibodies against the thyroid-stimulating hormone receptor (TSHR). Children of mothers making thyroid-stimulating antibody are born with hyperthyroidism. These symptoms usually disappear as the maternal antibodies are eventually degraded but can be corrected by replacing the plasma with normal plasma (plasmapheresis), thus removing the maternal antibody.

Figure 15.12 lists a selection of autoimmune diseases, along with the parts of the immune response that contribute to their pathogenesis. These examples illustrate that disease may engage multiple effector pathways, but that not all may act to drive disease. Similar to immune responses to pathogens, autoimmune diseases may involve T, B, and innate immune cells. Indeed, innate immune cells—particularly phagocytic myeloid cells—mediate tissue damage in most autoimmune diseases.

15-7 Chronic autoimmune disease develops through positive feedback from inflammation, inability to clear the self antigen, and a broadening of the autoimmune response.

In general, autoimmune diseases are characterized by an early activation phase with the involvement of only a few autoantigens, followed by a chronic stage. Also, many self antigens are present at a relative excess compared with the amount of antigens associated with pathogens. The persistence of self antigens may produce a chronic response, which may cause the release of more autoantigens as a result of tissue damage. This effect also breaks a restraint on autoimmunity known as 'sequestration,' by which many self antigens are

Autoimmune diseases involve all aspects of the immune response			
Disease	**T cells**	**B cells**	**Antibody**
Systemic lupus erythematosus	Pathogenic Help for antibody	Present antigen to T cells	Pathogenic
Type 1 diabetes mellitus	Pathogenic	Present antigen to T cells	Present, but role unclear
Myasthenia gravis	Help for antibody	Antibody secretion	Pathogenic
Multiple sclerosis	Pathogenic	Present antigen to T cells	Present, but role unclear

Fig. 15.12 Autoimmune diseases involve all aspects of the immune response. Although some autoimmune diseases have traditionally been thought to be mediated by B cells or T cells, it is useful to consider that, typically, all aspects of the immune system have a role. For four important autoimmune diseases, the figure lists the roles of T cells, B cells, and antibody. In some diseases, such as SLE, T cells can have multiple roles such as helping B cells to make autoantibody and directly promoting tissue damage. B cells can have either of two roles—presenting autoantigens to stimulate T cells and secreting pathogenic autoantibodies.

Circulating B cell binds self antigens released from injured cells	B cell is activated by a T cell specific for self peptide	B cells differentiate into plasma cells, secreting large amounts of self antigen-specific antibody	At sites of injury, self antigen-specific antibody initiates an inflammatory response, causing more cell injury	More B cells bind self antigens, amplifying the cycle of tissue damage

Fig. 15.13 Autoantibody-mediated inflammation can lead to the release of autoantigens from damaged tissues, which in turn promotes further activation of autoreactive B cells. Autoantigens, particularly intracellular ones that are targets in SLE, stimulate B cells only when released from dying cells (first panel). The result is the activation of autoreactive T and B cells (second panel) and the eventual secretion of autoantibodies (third panel). These autoantibodies can mediate tissue damage through a variety of effector functions resulting in further cell death (fourth panel). These additional autoantigens released form a positive feedback loop that recruits and activates additional autoreactive B cells (fifth panel).

normally kept apart from the immune system. Chronic responses also attract nonspecific effector cells, such as macrophages and neutrophils, which can release cytokines and chemokines from injured tissues, thus further propagating a self-destructive process (**Fig. 15.13**).

As an autoimmune response progresses, additional clones of lymphocytes are recruited that are reactive to new epitopes of the original autoantigen, as well as to new autoantigens. This phenomenon, known as **epitope spreading**, can occur in several ways. Self antigens that have already induced autoantibodies can be captured and processed by B cells more efficiently for presentation to T cells. Some peptide epitopes that were previously not presented to T cells, called **cryptic epitopes**, may become processed and presented, and then induce additional autoreactive T cells, which may further provide help to any B cells presenting these peptides, enhancing a greater variety of autoantibodies. Further, by binding and internalizing specific antigen via their B-cell receptor, B cells will also internalize any other molecules closely associated with that antigen. By this route, B cells can act as antigen-presenting cells for peptides derived from antigens completely different from the original autoantigen that initiated the autoimmune reaction.

Epitope spreading is illustrated in SLE, in which autoantibodies are eventually produced against both the DNA and protein components of chromatin (**Fig. 15.14**). The initial autoreactive B cells that are specific for DNA can capture histone proteins, another component of chromatin, and thereby process and present peptide epitopes to T cells. This serves to recruit T cells specific for such epitopes into the autoimmune response. In turn, these T cells provide help not only to the original DNA-specific B cells but also to histone-specific B cells, resulting in the production of both anti-DNA and anti-histone antibodies.

Pemphigus Vulgaris

Epitope spreading is also linked to the progression of the autoimmune disease **pemphigus vulgaris**, characterized by severe blistering of the skin and mucosal membranes. This disease is caused by autoantibodies against desmogleins, a type of cadherin present in cell junctions (desmosomes) that holds cells of the epidermis together (**Fig. 15.15**). Binding of autoantibodies to the extracellular domains of these adhesion molecules causes dissociation of the junctions and dissolution of the affected tissue. Pemphigus vulgaris usually starts

Fig. 15.14 Epitope spreading occurs when B cells specific for various components of a complex antigen are stimulated by an autoreactive helper T cell of a single specificity. In individuals with SLE, an ever-broadening immune response is made against nucleoprotein antigens such as nucleosomes, which consist of histones and DNA and are released from dying and disintegrating cells. The upper panel shows how the emergence of a single clone of autoreactive CD4 T cells can lead to a diverse B-cell response to nucleosome components. The T cell in the center is specific for a particular peptide (red) from the linker histone H1, which is present on the surface of the nucleosome. The B cells at the top are specific for epitopes on the surface of a nucleosome, on histone H1 (left side) and DNA (right side), and thus bind and endocytose intact nucleosomes, process the constituents, and present the H1 peptide to the helper T cell. These B cells will be activated to make antibodies, which in the case of the DNA-specific B cell will be anti-DNA antibodies. The B cell at the bottom right is specific for an epitope on histone H2, which is hidden inside the intact nucleosome and is thus inaccessible to the B-cell receptor. This B cell does not bind the nucleosome and does not become activated by the H1-specific helper T cell. A B cell specific for another type of nucleoprotein particle, the ribosome (which is composed of RNA and specific ribosomal proteins), will not bind nucleosomes (bottom left) and will not be activated by the T cell. In reality, a T cell interacts with one B cell at a time, but different members of the same T-cell clone will interact with B cells of different specificity. The lower panel shows the broadening of the T-cell response to the nucleosome. The H1-specific B cell in the center has processed an intact nucleosome and is presenting a variety of nucleosome-derived peptide antigens on its MHC class II molecules. This B cell can activate a T cell specific for any of these peptide antigens, which will include those from the internal histones H2, H3, and H4 as well as those from H1. This H1-specific B cell will not activate T cells specific for peptide antigens of ribosomes because ribosomes do not contain histones.

CD4 T cells specific for one epitope of a macromolecular complex can provide help to B cells specific for other accessible epitopes of the complex

A B cell that internalizes a macromolecular complex can present antigens to T cells specific for any one of the proteins of the complex

with lesions in the oral and genital mucosa; only later does the skin become involved. In the mucosal stage, autoantibodies are directed against only certain epitopes on desmoglein Dsg-3, which seem unable to cause skin blistering. But epitope spreading leads to antibodies against additional regions of Dsg-3 that can cause deep skin blistering and against regions of another desmoglein, Dsg-1, which is more abundant in the epidermis. Dsg-1 is also the autoantigen in a less severe variant of the disease, pemphigus foliaceus. In that disease, the autoantibodies first produced against Dsg-1 cause no damage, and disease appears only after autoantibodies are made against epitopes on parts of the protein involved in the adhesion of epidermal cells.

15-8 Both antibody and effector T cells can cause tissue damage in autoimmune disease.

Historically, the mechanisms of tissue injury in autoimmunity have been classified according to the scheme of 'hypersensitivity' reactions defined by Gell and Coombs in the early 1960s, which we introduced at the beginning of Chapter 14. It is now possible to classify autoimmune diseases using a more modern understanding of immune mechanisms, as illustrated in **Fig. 15.16** for several common autoimmune diseases. The dominant effector mechanisms used to clear various types of pathogens are also the ones that become dysregulated in autoimmunity. It is the mechanism by which the antigen-bearing tissues are damaged that determines the nature of the pathology and clinical expression of the disease.

Type 2 immune responses mediated by IgE (previously referred to as type I hypersensitivity) typically cause allergic or atopic inflammatory disease (see Chapter 14) and are not a major component in most forms of autoimmunity. By contrast, antibody-mediated tissue damage, caused either by direct recognition of cell surfaces or extracellular matrix (type II hypersensitivity) or by immune-complex deposition in tissues (type III hypersensitivity), appears to be linked to dysregulated type 3 (T_H17) or type 1 (T_H1) immunity or to T cell–independent generation of IgM-producing B cells. Such diseases can be either organ-specific or systemic, because antibodies can damage specific cell or tissue types (for example, autoimmune thyroiditis), or alternately can result from

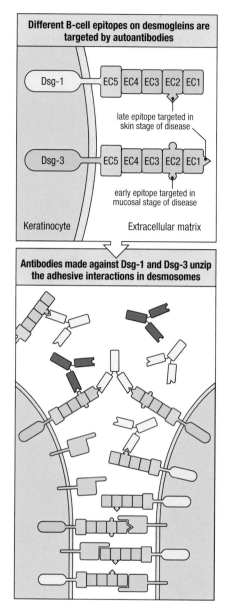

Different B-cell epitopes on desmogleins are targeted by autoantibodies

late epitope targeted in skin stage of disease

early epitope targeted in mucosal stage of disease

Keratinocyte   Extracellular matrix

Antibodies made against Dsg-1 and Dsg-3 unzip the adhesive interactions in desmosomes

Fig. 15.15 Pemphigus vulgaris is a skin-blistering disease caused by autoantibodies specific for desmoglein. Desmogleins are adhesion molecules in the cell junctions that hold keratinocytes together. They are cell-surface proteins with five extracellular domains (EC1–EC5; upper panel). Early in the autoimmune response, antibodies are made against the EC5 domain of shed desmoglein-3 (Dsg-3) but do not cause disease. However, in time, intramolecular and intermolecular epitope spreading occurs, and IgG antibodies are made against the EC1 and EC2 domains of Dsg-3 and Dsg-1. These autoantibodies can inhibit adhesion of desmoglein in desmosomes (lower panel) and thereby interfere with the physiological adhesive interactions of desmoglein that are necessary for maintaining skin integrity. Consequently, the antibodies cause the outer layers of the skin to separate, producing blisters.

Some common autoimmune diseases classified by immunopathogenic mechanism		
Syndrome	**Autoantigen**	**Consequence**
Antibody against cell-surface or matrix antigens		
Autoimmune hemolytic anemia	Rh blood group antigens, I antigen	Destruction of red blood cells by complement and FcR⁺ phagocytes, anemia
Autoimmune thrombocytopenic purpura	Platelet integrin GpIIb:IIIa	Abnormal bleeding
Goodpasture's syndrome	Noncollagenous domain of basement membrane collagen type IV	Glomerulonephritis, pulmonary hemorrhage
Pemphigus vulgaris	Epidermal cadherin	Blistering of skin
Acute rheumatic fever	Streptococcal cell-wall antigens. Antibodies cross-react with cardiac muscle	Arthritis, myocarditis, late scarring of heart valves
Immune-complex disease		
Mixed essential cryoglobulinemia	Rheumatoid factor IgG complexes (with or without hepatitis C antigens)	Systemic vasculitis
Rheumatoid arthritis	Rheumatoid factor IgG complexes	Arthritis
T cell-mediated disease		
Type 1 diabetes mellitus	Pancreatic β-cell antigen	β-cell destruction
Rheumatoid arthritis	Unknown synovial joint antigen	Joint inflammation and destruction
Multiple sclerosis	Myelin basic protein, proteolipid protein, myelin oligodendrocyte glycoprotein	Brain and spinal cord invasion by CD4 T cells, muscle weakness, and other neurological symptoms
Crohn's disease	Antigens of intestinal microbiota	Regional intestinal inflammation and scarring
Psoriasis	Unknown skin antigens	Inflammation of skin with formation of plaques

Fig. 15.16 Mechanisms of tissue damage in autoimmune diseases. Autoimmune diseases can be grouped according to the predominant type of immune response and the mechanism by which it damages tissues. In many autoimmune diseases, several immunopathogenic mechanisms operate in parallel. This is illustrated here for rheumatoid arthritis, which appears in more than one category of immunopathogenic mechanism.

immune complexes that are deposited in specific vascular beds (for example, rheumatoid arthritis). In some forms of autoimmunity, such as SLE, autoantibodies cause damage by both of these mechanisms. Finally, several organ-specific autoimmune diseases are due to a type 1 immune response in which T_H1 cells and/or cytotoxic T cells directly cause tissue damage (type IV hypersensitivity; for example, type 1 diabetes mellitus); alternatively, some such diseases are due to a type 3 immune response in which T_H17 cells promote inflammation at barrier tissues (for example, psoriasis or Crohn's disease).

In most autoimmune diseases, however, several mechanisms of pathogenesis operate. Thus, helper T cells are almost always required for the production of pathogenic autoantibodies. Reciprocally, B cells often have an important role in the maximal activation of T cells that mediate tissue damage or help autoantibody production. In type 1 diabetes mellitus and rheumatoid arthritis, for example, both T cell–mediated and antibody-mediated pathways cause tissue injury. SLE is an example of autoimmunity that was previously thought to be mediated solely by antibodies and immune complexes but is now known to have a component of T cell–mediated pathogenesis. Moreover, in virtually all autoimmune diseases, innate immune cells contribute to inflammation and antibody-mediated or T cell–mediated tissue injury.

15-9 Autoantibodies against blood cells promote their destruction.

IgG or IgM responses against antigens located on the surface of blood cells lead to their rapid destruction, as occurs in **autoimmune hemolytic anemia**. Red-cell destruction can occur in two ways (**Fig. 15.17**). First, the IgG or IgM antibody bound to red cells can interact with Fc or complement receptors, respectively, on cells of the mononuclear–macrophage phagocytic system, particularly in the spleen, leading to red-cell clearance from the circulation. Alternatively, the autoantibody-sensitized red blood cells can be lysed by formation of the membrane-attack complex of complement. In **autoimmune thrombocytopenic purpura**, autoantibodies against the GpIIb:IIIa fibrinogen receptor or other platelet-specific surface antigens can cause thrombocytopenia (a depletion of platelets), which can in turn cause hemorrhage.

Lysis of nucleated cells by complement is less common because these cells are better defended by complement-regulatory proteins, which protect cells against immune attack by interfering with the activation of complement components (see Section 2-16). Nevertheless, circulating nucleated cells targeted by autoantibodies are still destroyed by cells of the mononuclear phagocytic system or NK cells via antibody-dependent cell-mediated cytotoxicity (ADCC). Autoantibodies against neutrophils, for example, cause neutropenia, which increases susceptibility to infection with pyogenic bacteria. In all these cases, accelerated clearance of autoantibody-sensitized cells is the cause of their depletion. One therapeutic approach to this type of autoimmunity is removal of the spleen, the organ in which the main clearance of red cells, platelets, and leukocytes occurs. Another is the administration of large quantities of nonspecific IgG (termed IVIG, for intravenous immunoglobulin), which among other mechanisms inhibits the Fc receptor–mediated uptake of antibody-coated cells and activates inhibitory Fc receptors to suppress production of inflammatory mediators by myeloid cells.

15-10 The fixation of sublytic doses of complement to cells in tissues stimulates a powerful inflammatory response.

The binding of IgG and IgM antibodies to cells in tissues causes inflammatory injury by a variety of mechanisms. One of these is the fixation of complement. Although nucleated cells are relatively resistant to lysis by complement, the assembly of sublytic amounts of the membrane-attack complex on their surface provides a powerful activating stimulus. Depending on the cell type, this interaction can cause cytokine release, a respiratory burst, or the mobilization

Fig. 15.17 Antibodies can destroy red blood cells by clearance and by lysis. In autoimmune hemolytic anemias, red blood cells (erythrocytes) coated with IgG autoantibodies against a cell-surface antigen (upper panel) are rapidly cleared from the circulation by uptake by Fc receptor–bearing macrophages located primarily in the spleen (lower left panel). Erythrocytes coated with IgM autoantibodies fix C3 and are cleared by CR1-bearing macrophages. The binding of certain rare autoantibodies that fix complement extremely efficiently causes the formation of the membrane-attack complex on the red cells, leading to intravascular hemolysis (lower right panel).

Autoimmune
Hemolytic Anemia

of membrane phospholipids to generate arachidonic acid—the precursor of prostaglandins and leukotrienes, lipid mediators of inflammation.

Most cells in tissues are fixed in place, and innate and adaptive immune cells are attracted to them by chemoattractant molecules. One such molecule is the complement fragment C5a, which is released as a result of complement activation triggered by autoantibody binding. Other chemoattractants, such as leukotriene B4, can be released by the autoantibody-targeted cells. Inflammatory leukocytes are further activated by binding to autoantibody Fc regions and fixed complement C3 fragments on cells. Tissue injury can result from the products of the activated leukocytes and by ADCC mediated by NK cells (see Section 10-23). A probable example of this type of autoimmunity is Hashimoto's thyroiditis, in which autoantibodies against tissue-specific antigens are found at extremely high levels for prolonged periods. Direct T cell–mediated cytotoxicity, which we discuss later, is probably also important in this disease.

15-11 Autoantibodies against receptors cause disease by stimulating or blocking receptor function.

Autoimmune disease can occur when autoantibody binds a cell-surface receptor. Antibody binding to a receptor can either stimulate the receptor or block stimulation by the natural ligand. In Graves' disease, autoantibodies against the thyroid-stimulating hormone (TSH) receptor on thyroid cells stimulate excessive production of thyroid hormone. The production of thyroid hormone is normally controlled by feedback regulation; high levels of thyroid hormone inhibit the release of TSH by the pituitary. In Graves' disease, feedback inhibition fails because the autoantibody continues to stimulate the TSH receptor in the absence of TSH, and the individual produces chronically elevated levels of thyroid hormone ('hyperthyroidism'; Fig. 15.18).

Fig. 15.18 Feedback regulation of thyroid hormone production is disrupted in Graves' disease. Graves' disease is caused by autoantibodies specific for the receptor for thyroid-stimulating hormone (TSH). Normally, thyroid hormones are produced in response to TSH and limit their own production by inhibiting the production of TSH by the pituitary gland (left panels). In Graves' disease, the autoantibodies are agonists for the TSH receptor expressed in the thyroid gland and therefore directly stimulate the production of thyroid hormones (right panels). The thyroid hormones inhibit TSH production in the normal way but do not affect production of the autoantibody; the excessive thyroid hormone production induced in this way causes hyperthyroidism.

The pituitary gland secretes thyroid-stimulating hormone (TSH), which acts on the thyroid to induce the release of thyroid hormones

Autoimmune B cell makes antibodies against TSH receptor that also stimulate thyroid hormone production

Thyroid hormones act on the hypothalamus and the pituitary to shut down production of TSH, suppressing further thyroid hormone synthesis (feedback suppression)

Thyroid hormones shut down TSH production but have no effect on autoantibody production, which continues to cause excessive thyroid hormone production

Fig. 15.19 Autoantibodies inhibit receptor function in myasthenia gravis. In normal circumstances, acetylcholine released from stimulated motor neurons at the neuromuscular junction binds to acetylcholine receptors expressed on skeletal muscle cells, triggering muscle contraction (upper panel). Myasthenia gravis is caused by autoantibodies against the α subunit of the receptor for acetylcholine. These autoantibodies bind to the receptor without activating it and also cause the receptor to be internalized and degraded (lower panel). As the number of receptors on the muscle is decreased, the muscle becomes less responsive to acetylcholine, causing weakness.

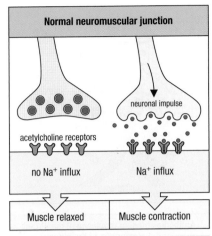

In myasthenia gravis, autoantibodies against the α chain of the nicotinic acetylcholine receptor present at neuromuscular junctions in skeletal muscle cells can block stimulation of muscle contraction. The antibodies are believed to drive internalization and degradation of the receptor (**Fig. 15.19**). Individuals with myasthenia gravis develop potentially fatal progressive weakness as a result of their disease. Diseases caused by autoantibodies that act as agonists or antagonists on cell-surface receptors are listed in **Fig. 15.20**.

15-12 Autoantibodies against extracellular antigens cause inflammatory injury.

Antibody responses to extracellular matrix molecules are infrequent but can be very damaging. In **Goodpasture's syndrome**, antibodies are formed against the α_3 chain of basement membrane collagen (type IV collagen). These antibodies bind to the basement membranes of renal glomeruli (**Fig. 15.21**) and, in some cases, to the basement membranes of pulmonary alveoli, causing a rapidly fatal disease if untreated. The autoantibodies bound to basement membrane ligate Fcγ receptors on innate effector cells, such as monocytes and neutrophils, leading to their activation. These cells, in turn, release chemokines that attract a further influx of monocytes and neutrophils into glomeruli, causing severe tissue injury. The autoantibodies also cause a local activation of complement, which amplifies tissue injury.

Immune complexes are produced when there is an antibody response to a soluble antigen. Normally, such complexes cause little tissue damage because they are cleared efficiently by red blood cells that bear complement receptors and by phagocytes of the mononuclear phagocytic system that have both complement and Fc receptors. This clearance system can, however, fail in circumstances where the production of immune complexes exceeds the capacity of the normal clearance mechanisms or when there are deficiencies in normal clearance mechanisms. An example of the former is serum sickness (see Section 14-14), which is caused by the injection of large amounts of serum proteins or by small-molecule drugs binding to serum proteins and acting as

Drug-Induced Serum Sickness

Fig. 15.20 Autoimmune diseases caused by autoantibodies against cell-surface receptors. These antibodies produce different effects depending on whether they are agonists (which stimulate the receptor) or antagonists (which inhibit it). Note that different autoantibodies against the insulin receptor can either stimulate or inhibit signaling.

Diseases mediated by antibodies against cell-surface receptors				
Syndrome	**Antigen**	**Antibody**	**Consequence**	**Target cell**
Graves' disease	Thyroid-stimulating hormone receptor	Agonist	Hyperthyroidism	Thyroid epithelial cell
Myasthenia gravis	Acetylcholine receptor	Antagonist	Progressive muscle weakness	Muscle
Insulin-resistant diabetes	Insulin receptor	Antagonist	Hyperglycemia, ketoacidosis	All cells
Hypoglycemia	Insulin receptor	Agonist	Hypoglycemia	All cells
Chronic urticaria	Receptor-bound IgE or IgE receptor	Agonist	Persistent itchy rash	Mast cells

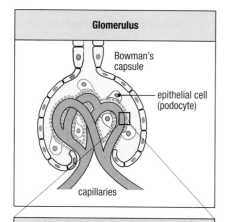

Glomerulus

Bowman's capsule

epithelial cell (podocyte)

capillaries

Antibodies binding to basement membrane of the glomerulus of the kidney activate complement and recruit neutrophils and monocytes

fenestrae of endothelial cell

glomerular basement membrane

foot processes of podocytes

Fig. 15.21 Autoantibodies reacting with glomerular basement membrane cause the inflammatory glomerular disease known as Goodpasture's syndrome. Upper two panels: The autoantibody binds to type IV collagen within the basement membrane of the glomerular capillaries, causing complement activation and recruitment and activation of neutrophils and monocytes. Third panel: In this biopsy from a kidney of an individual with Goodpasture's syndrome, the glomerulus is stained for IgG deposition by immunofluorescence (green) showing the antibody to be deposited in a linear fashion along the glomerular basement membrane. Bottom panel: Silver staining of a section through a renal glomerulus shows that the glomerulus capillaries (G) are compressed by the formation of a crescent (C), composed of proliferating epithelial cells and an influx of neutrophils (N) and monocytes (M), that have filled the urinary (Bowman's) space surrounding the glomerular capillaries.

haptens. Serum sickness is a transient disease, lasting until the immune complexes have been cleared. Similarly, normal clearance mechanisms can be overwhelmed in chronic infections, such as bacterial endocarditis, in which the immune response to bacteria lodged on a cardiac valve is incapable of clearing the infection. The persistent release of bacterial antigens from the valve infection in the presence of a strong antibacterial antibody response causes widespread immune-complex injury to small blood vessels in organs such as the kidney and the skin. Other chronic infections, such as hepatitis C infection, can lead to the production of cryoglobulins and the condition **mixed essential cryoglobulinemia**, in which immune complexes are deposited in joints and tissues. Alternatively, there can be inherited impairment of mechanisms that contribute to normal clearance of immune complexes; such impairment may be caused by reduced expression of or functional defects in specific components of either complement or its receptors or by reduced expression of or functional defects in Fc receptors, each of which occurs in subsets of people with SLE.

Indeed, SLE can result from either the overproduction or the defective clearance of immune complexes, or both, at multiple levels (**Fig. 15.22**). In this disease, there is chronic IgG antibody production directed at ubiquitous self antigens present in nucleated cells, leading to a wide range of autoantibodies against common cellular constituents. The main antigens are three types of intracellular nucleoprotein particles—the nucleosome subunits of chromatin, the spliceosome, and a small cytoplasmic ribonucleoprotein complex containing two proteins known as Ro and La (named after the first two letters of the surnames of the two individuals in whom autoantibodies against these proteins were discovered). For these autoantigens to participate in immune-complex formation, they must become extracellular. The autoantigens of SLE are exposed on dead and dying cells released from injured tissues.

In SLE, large quantities of antigen are available, so large amounts of small immune complexes are produced continually and are deposited in the walls of small blood vessels in the renal glomerular basement membrane, joints, and other organs (**Fig. 15.23**). This leads to the activation of phagocytic cells through their Fc receptors. A hereditary deficiency of some complement proteins, specifically those for C1q, C2, and C4, is strongly associated with the development of SLE in humans. C1q, C2, and C4 are early components in the classical complement pathway, which is important in antibody-mediated clearance of apoptotic cells and immune complexes (see Chapter 2). If apoptotic cells and immune complexes are not cleared, the chance that their antigens will activate low-affinity self-reactive lymphocytes in the periphery is increased. The consequent tissue damage releases more nucleoprotein complexes, which in turn form more immune complexes. During this process, autoreactive T cells also become activated, although much less is known about their specificity. Animal models for SLE cannot be initiated without the help of T cells, and T cells can also be directly pathogenic, forming part of the cellular infiltrates in the skin and kidney. As discussed in the next section, T cells contribute to autoimmune disease in two ways: by helping B cells make antibodies, analogous to a normal

Fig. 15.22 Defective clearance of nucleic acid–containing immune complexes activates overproduction of BAFF and type I interferons that can cause SLE. In SLE, antibody:nucleic acid immune complexes, containing ssRNA or dsDNA from dead cells, are bound by FcγRIIA (green rods) on plasmacytoid dendritic cells. The Fc receptor–bound ssRNA and dsRNA are delivered to endosomes, where they activate TLR-7 and TLR-9, respectively, to induce IFN-α production (upper panel). IFN-α increases BAFF production by monocytes and dendritic cells, and BAFF interacts with receptors on B cells. Excess BAFF can increase autoreactive B-cell survival, leading to increased autoantibody production (lower panel).

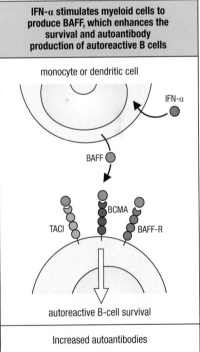

T-dependent immune response, and by direct effector functions as they infiltrate and destroy target tissues.

15-13 T cells specific for self antigens can cause direct tissue injury and sustain autoantibody responses.

Traditionally, it has been more difficult to demonstrate the existence of autoreactive T cells than to show the presence of autoantibodies for a number of reasons. First, autoreactive human T cells cannot transfer disease to experimental animals because T-cell recognition is MHC-restricted. Second, autoantibodies can be used to stain self tissues to reveal distribution of the autoantigen, whereas T cells cannot be used in the same way. However, the use of fluorophore-labeled peptide:MHC tetramers (see Appendix I, Section A-24) to stain antigen-specific T cells for flow cytometry provides a means to both identify and track autoreactive T cells *in vivo* in autoimmune diseases. Furthermore, there is already strong evidence for the involvement of autoreactive T cells in many autoimmune diseases. In type 1 diabetes mellitus, for example, the insulin-producing β cells of the pancreatic islets are selectively destroyed by cytotoxic T cells. This is borne out by the finding that in the rare cases in which persons with diabetes were transplanted with half a pancreas from an identical twin donor, the β cells in the grafted tissue were rapidly and selectively destroyed by the recipient's T cells. Recurrence of disease can be prevented by the immunosuppressive drug cyclosporin A (see Chapter 16), which inhibits T-cell activation.

Autoantigens recognized by CD4 T cells can be identified by adding cells or tissues containing autoantigens to cultures of blood mononuclear cells and testing for recognition by CD4 cells derived from an autoimmune individual. If the autoantigen is present, it should be effectively recognized by autoreactive CD4 T cells. The identification of autoantigenic peptides is particularly difficult in autoimmune diseases in which CD8 T cells have a role, because autoantigens recognized by CD8 T cells are not effectively presented in such cultures. Peptides presented by MHC class I molecules must usually be made by the target cells themselves (see Chapter 6); intact cells of target tissue from the individual must therefore be used to study autoreactive CD8 T cells that cause tissue damage. Conversely, the pathogenesis of the disease can itself give clues to the identity of the antigen in some CD8 T cell–mediated diseases. For example, in type 1 diabetes mellitus, the insulin-producing β cells seem to be specifically targeted and destroyed by CD8 T cells (**Fig. 15.24**). This suggests a protein unique to β cells is the source of the peptide recognized by the pathogenic CD8 T cells. Studies in the NOD (non-obese diabetic) mouse model of type 1 diabetes mellitus have shown that peptides from insulin itself are recognized by pathogenic CD8 T cells, confirming insulin as one of the principal autoantigens in this model of diabetes.

Multiple sclerosis (MS) is a T cell–mediated neurological disease caused by a destructive immune response against central nervous system myelin antigens, including myelin basic protein (MBP; not to be confused with *major basic protein*), proteolipid protein (PLP), and myelin oligodendrocyte

Multiple Sclerosis

Fig. 15.23 Deposition of immune complexes in the renal glomeruli causes renal failure in systemic lupus erythematosus (SLE). Panel a: A microscopic section stained with hematoxylin and eosin shows a renal glomerulus from an individual with SLE. The deposition of immune complexes has caused thickening of the glomerular basement membrane that appears as the clear 'canals' running through the glomerulus.

Panel b: A similar section stained with fluorescently labeled anti-immunoglobulin, revealing immunoglobulin deposits in the basement membrane. Panel c: The immune complexes are seen under the electron microscope as dense protein deposits between the glomerular basement membrane and the renal epithelial cells. Polymorphonuclear neutrophilic leukocytes are also present, attracted by the deposited immune complexes.

glycoprotein (MOG) (**Fig. 15.25**). MS takes its name from the hard (sclerotic) lesions, or plaques, that develop in the white matter of the central nervous system. These lesions show dissolution of the myelin sheath that normally surrounds nerve-cell axons, along with inflammatory infiltrates of lymphocytes and macrophages, particularly surrounding blood vessels. People with MS may develop a variety of neurological symptoms, including muscle weakness, ataxia, blindness, and paralysis. Normally, few lymphocytes cross the blood–brain barrier, but if this barrier breaks down, activated CD4 T cells specific for myelin antigens and expressing $\alpha_4\beta_1$ integrin can bind vascular cell adhesion molecules (VCAMs) on activated endothelium (see Section 11-4), enabling the T cells to migrate out of the blood vessel. There they reencounter their specific autoantigen presented by MHC class II molecules on infiltrating macrophages or microglial cells (phagocytic macrophage-like cells resident in the central nervous system). Inflammation causes increased vascular permeability, and the site becomes heavily infiltrated by T_H17 and T_H1 effector CD4 T cells, which produce IL-17, IFN-γ, and GMCSF. Cytokines and chemokines produced by these effector T cells in turn recruit and activate myeloid cells that exacerbate inflammation, resulting in further recruitment of T cells, B cells, and innate immune cells to the lesion. Autoreactive B cells produce autoantibodies against myelin antigens with help from T cells. These combined activities lead to demyelination and interference with neuronal function.

Fig. 15.24 Destruction of pancreatic β cells in type 1 diabetes mellitus indicates that the autoantigen is produced in β cells and recognized on their surface. In type 1 diabetes mellitus, insulin-producing β cells in the pancreatic islets of Langerhans are destroyed, but other islet cell types (α and δ) are spared.

The islets of Langerhans contain several cell types secreting distinct hormones. Each cell expresses different tissue-specific proteins

In type 1 diabetes mellitus, an effector T cell recognizes peptides from a β cell–specific protein and kills the β cell

Glucagon and somatostatin are still produced by the α and δ cells, but no insulin can be made

Fig. 15.25 The pathogenesis of multiple sclerosis (MS). The initiating trigger of MS remains unknown, but its pathophysiology is more clear. At sites of inflammation, activated T cells autoreactive for brain antigens can cross the blood–brain barrier and enter the brain, where they reencounter their antigens on microglial cells and secrete cytokines such as GM-CSF and IFN-γ. The production of cytokines by T cells and macrophages further increases inflammation and recruits additional cells and blood proteins (such as complement) into the affected site. The individual roles of these components in demyelination and loss of neuronal function are still not well understood. CNS, central nervous system.

The clinical course of MS both mirrors what is seen in other autoimmune diseases and also displays how the tissue specificity of such conditions affects their progression. Most people with MS experience a disease course characterized by acute attacks (relapse) followed by a reduction in disease activity (remission) that may last for months or years. This relapsing–remitting course is characteristic of many autoimmune diseases in terms of both the symptoms individuals experience and the degree of immune-cell infiltration into the affected organ. Not only are the triggers of relapses not always clear, but also the events leading to spontaneous disease remission—even when the auto-antigen is still present in the organ—remain to be discovered. Furthermore, the relapsing–remitting nature of diseases such as MS makes conducting clinical trials around these disorders especially difficult, as they must be performed over relatively long periods of time to ensure a therapy is effective in preventing relapses and disability.

Ultimately, often after decades, most people with MS change from a relapsing–remitting disease course to 'secondary progressive' MS. In this phase they begin to undergo a steady neurological decline without overt periods of remission, and for many people their disease becomes less responsive to the therapies that effectively target the adaptive immune system in relapsing–remitting MS, although the reasons for this are unclear.

Rheumatoid arthritis (RA) is a chronic disease characterized by inflammation of the synovium (the thin lining of a joint). As disease progresses, the inflamed synovium invades and damages the cartilage; this is followed by bone erosion (**Fig. 15.26**), leading to chronic pain, loss of function, and disability. RA was first considered an autoimmune disease driven by B cells producing anti-IgG autoantibodies called rheumatoid factor (see Section 15-2). However, the identification of rheumatoid factor in some healthy individuals, and its absence in some individuals with rheumatoid arthritis, suggested that more complex mechanisms orchestrate this pathology. The discovery that RA has an association with particular class II HLA-DR genes of the MHC suggested that T cells are also involved in the pathogenesis of this disease. In RA, as in MS, most data from humans and mouse models indicate that, at least early in disease development, autoreactive T_H17 cells become activated. Autoreactive

Rheumatoid
Arthritis

Fig. 15.26 The pathogenesis of rheumatoid arthritis.
Inflammation of the synovial membrane, initiated by some unknown trigger, attracts autoreactive lymphocytes and macrophages to the inflamed tissue. Autoreactive effector CD4 T cells activate macrophages, and pro-inflammatory cytokines such as IL-1, IL-6, IL-17, and TNF-α are produced. Fibroblasts activated by cytokines produce matrix metalloproteinases (MMPs), which contribute to tissue destruction. The TNF family cytokine RANK ligand (RANKL), expressed by T cells and fibroblasts in the inflamed joint, is the primary activator of bone-destroying osteoclasts. Antibodies against several joint proteins are also produced (not shown), but their role in pathogenesis is uncertain.

T cells provide help to B cells to produce arthritogenic antibodies. The activated T_H17 cells also produce cytokines that recruit neutrophils and monocytes/macrophages, which, along with endothelial cells and synovial fibroblasts, are stimulated to produce more pro-inflammatory cytokines such as TNF-α, IL-1, or chemokines (CXCL8, CCL2), and finally matrix metalloproteinases, which are responsible for tissue destruction. IL-17A, which has been found in high concentrations in the synovium and synovial fluid of people with RA, can induce expression of the ligand for receptor activator of NFκB (RANKL), which stimulates the differentiation of osteoclast precursors into mature osteoclasts that resorb bone in affected joints. Although we do not yet know how RA starts, mouse models have shown that both T cells and B cells are needed to initiate disease. Notably, interrupting this complex cascade at multiple levels—including therapeutic antibodies against cytokines (TNF-α), B cells, and T-cell activation—have all been successful in treating the symptoms of the disease.

Studies of the targets of autoantibodies in RA have yielded insights into how this disease develops and have also identified a more global mechanism by which self proteins may be seen as foreign in other autoimmune conditions. During inflammation, the amino acid arginine can be converted into citrulline, and this change may result in structural alterations of the self protein that cause the immune system to now view it as nonself (**Fig. 15.27**). Experimental models have shown that antibodies against these altered proteins can be pathogenic, and diagnostic tests for anti-citrullinated protein antibodies (ACPAs) are highly specific for RA. Notably, smoking—long known as the most important environmental risk factor for RA development—has been associated with APCAs in individuals with HLA risk alleles, suggesting that

The enzyme PAD converts positively charged arginine residues to neutral citrulline residues

Loss of surface charges makes the protein more susceptible to proteolytic degradation

Peptides with citrulline residues are presented by HLA class II to CD4 T cells

Fig. 15.27 The enzyme peptidyl arginine deiminase converts the arginine residues of tissue proteins to citrulline. In tissues stressed by wounds or infection, peptidyl arginine deiminase (PAD) activity is induced. By converting arginine residues to citrulline, PAD destabilizes proteins and makes them more susceptible to degradation. This also introduces novel B-cell and T-cell epitopes into tissue proteins that can stimulate an autoimmune response.

this tolerance-breaking mechanism may be an important node in the gene–environment interactions that lead to autoimmunity. Finally, other post-translational modifications (oxidation, glycosylation) of self proteins in the periphery have now been shown to stimulate T- and B-cell responses in other autoimmune diseases.

Summary.

Autoimmune diseases can be broadly classified into those that affect a specific organ and those that affect tissues throughout the body. Organ-specific autoimmune diseases include type 1 diabetes mellitus, multiple sclerosis, Graves' disease, and Crohn's disease. In each case the effector functions target autoantigens that are restricted to particular organs—insulin-producing β cells of the pancreas (type 1 diabetes mellitus), the myelin sheathing on axons in the central nervous system (multiple sclerosis), and the thyroid-stimulating hormone receptor (Graves' disease)—or, in the case of Crohn's disease, components of the intestinal microbiota. In contrast, systemic diseases such as systemic lupus erythematosus (SLE) cause inflammation in multiple tissues because their autoantigens, which include chromatin and ribonucleoproteins, are found in most cells of the body. In some organ-specific diseases, immune destruction of the target tissue and the unique self antigens it expresses leads to cessation of autoimmune activity, but systemic diseases tend to be chronically active if untreated, because their autoantigens cannot be cleared.

Another way of classifying autoimmune diseases is according to the effector functions that are most important in pathogenesis. Autoimmune diseases are mediated by autoreactive lymphocytes and their soluble products, pro-inflammatory cytokines, and autoantibodies responsible for inflammation and tissue injury. A few autoimmune diseases are caused by antibodies that bind to cell-surface receptors, causing either excess activity or inhibition of receptor function. In some diseases, transplacental passage of IgG autoantibodies can cause disease in the fetus and neonate. T cells can be involved directly in inflammation or cellular destruction, and they are typically required to initiate and sustain an autoantibody response. Similarly, B cells are important antigen-presenting cells for sustaining autoantigen-specific T-cell responses and causing epitope spreading. It is becoming clear, however, that many diseases once thought to be mediated solely by one effector function actually involve several. In this way, autoimmune diseases resemble pathogen-directed immune responses, which typically elicit the activities of multiple effectors—adaptive and innate. In spite of our knowledge of the mechanisms of tissue damage and the therapeutic approaches that this information has engendered, it remains to be determined how autoimmune responses are induced.

The genetic and environmental basis of autoimmunity.

Given the complex mechanisms that exist to prevent autoimmunity, it is not surprising that autoimmune diseases are the result of multiple factors, both genetic and environmental. We first discuss the genetic basis of autoimmunity, attempting to understand how genetic defects can perturb various tolerance mechanisms. Genetic defects alone are not, however, always sufficient to cause autoimmune disease. Environmental factors also play a part, although these factors are poorly understood. As we shall see, genetic and environmental factors together can overcome tolerance mechanisms and result in disease.

15-14 Autoimmune diseases have a strong genetic component.

It is increasingly clear that susceptibility to acquiring autoimmune diseases has a strong genetic component. Some autoimmune diseases, including type 1 diabetes mellitus, run in families, and most convincingly, if one identical (monozygotic) twin is affected, the other twin is quite likely to be affected as well, whereas concordance of disease is much less in nonidentical (dizygotic) twins. Not surprisingly, a number of autoimmune-like symptoms can be generated in mice by targeted mutations in genes that encode proteins that clear antigen or antigen:antibody complexes or that encode cytokines, co-receptors, co-stimulatory molecules, or proteins involved in apoptosis (**Fig. 15.28**). It is easy to speculate how alteration in such genes could contribute to autoimmunity, but in most cases a precise explanation is missing. Notably, results from experimental systems do not ensure that similar autoimmune diseases are caused by mutations in the same genes in humans.

In humans, genetic susceptibility to autoimmune disorders has been assessed recently by large-scale **genome-wide association studies (GWASs)**, which we introduced in Section 14-3. These studies look for a correlation between disease frequency and genetic variants, usually **single-nucleotide polymorphisms,** or **SNPs**. Such studies typically involve thousands of people with a given autoimmune disease diagnosis and healthy controls in order to identify highly significant associations. **Figure 15.29** shows a 'Manhattan' plot for a GWAS analyzing SNPs associated with Crohn's disease. Resembling a skyscraper skyline, these graphs show strength of association of all genetic loci with a particular disease, specifically plotting the p value of the association as a function of the genomic coordinate. Each dot represents one SNP. Hundreds of significant variants have been identified for multiple autoimmune diseases, suggesting that genetic susceptibility to autoimmune disease in humans may be due to a combination of susceptibility alleles at multiple loci.

GWASs have suggested that allelic variation in certain immune pathways may be common to different forms of autoimmunity. For example, type 1 diabetes mellitus, Graves' disease, Hashimoto's thyroiditis, rheumatoid arthritis, and multiple sclerosis all show genetic association with the *CTLA4* locus on chromosome 2. CTLA-4 is expressed on the surface of activated T cells and is an inhibitory receptor for B7 co-stimulatory molecules (see Section 9-17). But it remains unclear how the allelic variations identified by these SNPs contribute directly to autoimmunity. The majority of risk-associated SNPs (>80%) are not contained within exons that encode proteins, but are typically found kilobases away from immunologically relevant genes in intragenic regions that presumably influence the timing or level of gene expression. **Figure 15.30** illustrates how various candidate genes collected from different GWASs may influence the effector mechanisms of eight different autoimmune diseases that exhibit characteristics of T_H1 or T_H17 response. This figure illustrates that candidate genes may impact different steps in each of these pathways, may act in either dendritic cells or T cells, and may contribute to more than one disease, in some cases as many as seven different diseases.

15-15 Monogenic defects of immune tolerance.

While many autoimmune diseases are associated with multiple SNPs, there are several monogenic autoimmune diseases in which one mutant allele confers a very high risk of disease to the individual (**Fig. 15.31**). Such variants are typically rare and have a low overall impact on the population but are of great interest because they identify important pathways normally required to prevent development of autoimmune responses. Monogenic autoimmune disease was first observed in mutant mice in which the inheritance of

Proposed mechanism	Murine models	Disease phenotype	Human gene affected	Disease phenotype
Antigen clearance and presentation	C1q knockout	Lupus-like	*C1QA*	Lupus-like
	C4 knockout		*C2, C4*	
			Mannose-binding lectin	
	AIRE knockout	Multi-organ autoimmunity resembling APECED	*AIRE*	APECED
	Mer knockout	Lupus-like		
Signaling	SHP-1 knockout	Lupus-like		
	Lyn knockout			
	CD22 knockout			
	CD45 E613R point mutation			
	B cells deficient in all Src family kinases (triple knockout)			
	FcγRIIB knockout (inhibitory signaling molecule)		*FCGR2A*	Lupus
Co-stimulatory molecules	CTLA-4 knockout (blocks inhibitory signal)	Lymphocyte infiltration into organs		
	PD-1 knockout (blocks inhibitory signal)	Lupus-like		
	BAFF overexpression (transgenic mouse)			
Apoptosis	Fas knockout (*lpr*)	Lupus-like with lymphocyte infiltrates	*FAS* and *FASL* mutations (ALPS)	Lupus-like with lymphocyte infiltrates
	FasL knockout (*gld*)			
	Bcl-2 overexpression (transgenic mouse)	Lupus-like		
	Pten heterozygous deficiency			
T_{reg} development/ function	*scurfy* mouse	Multi-organ autoimmunity	*FOXP3*	IPEX
	Foxp3 knockout			

Fig. 15.28 Categories of genetic defects that lead to autoimmune syndromes. Many genes have been identified in which mutations predispose to autoimmunity in humans and in animal models. These are best understood by the type of process affected by the genetic defect. Such genes or the related protein are listed in the table according to the immune process they perform. Some of these genes have been identified in both mice and humans. In other cases, different genes affecting the same mechanism are implicated in mice and humans. ALPS, autoimmune lymphoproliferative syndrome; IPEX, immune dysregulation, polyendocrinopathy, enteropathy, X-linked.

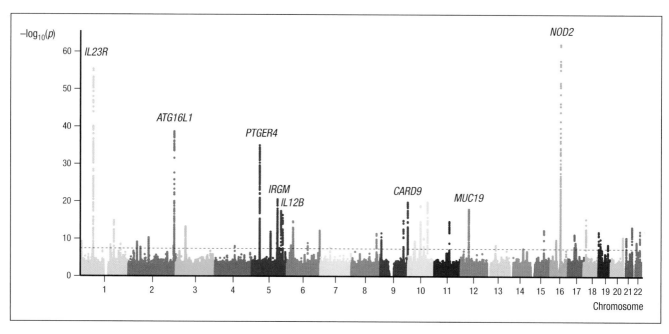

Fig. 15.29 Manhattan plot depicting risk alleles from genome-wide association studies (GWASs) of Crohn's disease. The plot highlights several gene loci identified by analyses of single-nucleotide polymorphisms (SNPs) as being associated with Crohn's disease. Each dot represents an individual SNP. The height of a dot reflects the statistical significance of the association. The horizontal position of a dot represents its genomic location. The dotted line indicates the threshold for significant associations (5×10^{-8}).

an autoimmune syndrome followed a pattern consistent with a single-gene defect. Such alleles are often recessive or X-linked. For example, the disease APECED described in Section 15-1 is a recessive autoimmune disease caused by a defect in the gene *AIRE*.

Two monogenic autoimmune syndromes have been linked to defects in regulatory T cells. The X-linked recessive autoimmune syndrome **IPEX (immune dysregulation, polyendocrinopathy, enteropathy, X-linked)** is typically caused by missense mutations in the gene encoding the transcription factor FoxP3, which is key in the differentiation and function of some types of T_{reg} cells (see Section 9-15). This disease is characterized by severe allergic inflammation, autoimmune polyendocrinopathy, secretory diarrhea, hemolytic anemia, and thrombocytopenia and usually leads to early death. Despite mutation of the gene *FOXP3*, the number of FoxP3$^+$ T_{reg} cells in the blood of individuals with IPEX is comparable to the number in healthy individuals; however, the suppressive function normally displayed by these cells is impaired. A spontaneous frameshift mutation in the mouse gene *Foxp3* (the *scurfy* mutation) that results in loss of the DNA-binding domain of FoxP3 or complete knockout of *Foxp3* leads to an analogous systemic autoimmune disease, in this case associated with the absence of FoxP3$^+$ T_{reg} cells.

Autoimmunity caused by defective development and survival of T_{reg} cells also results from mutation of the gene *IL2RA*, which encodes CD25, the high-affinity chain of the IL-2 receptor complex that is constitutively expressed by T_{reg} cells (see Section 9-10). Because deficiency of CD25 affects the development and function of effector T cells as well, in addition to autoimmunity, persons affected by this mutation suffer multiple immunological deficiencies and susceptibility to infections. These findings further confirm the importance of T_{reg} cells in the regulation of the immune system.

An interesting case of a monogenic autoimmune disease is **autoimmune lymphoproliferative syndrome (ALPS)**, a systemic autoimmune syndrome caused by mutations in the gene encoding Fas. Fas is normally present on the surface of

Immune Dysregulation, Polyendocrinopathy, Enteropathy, X-linked Syndrome

Autoimmune Lymphoproliferative Syndrome (ALPS)

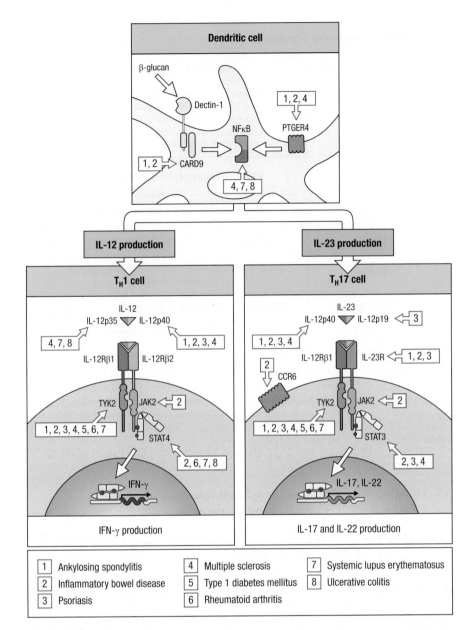

Fig. 15.30 Associations of components of the IL-12R and IL-23R response pathways with autoimmune diseases. Multiple components of the interleukin-12 receptor (IL-12R) and IL-23 receptor (IL-23R) response pathways show significant genome-wide associations with a broad range of immune-mediated diseases; that is, these components map within genomic intervals that are associated with the respective disease in genome-wide association studies. Although this figure shows these components in the conventional context of T helper 1 (T$_H$1) and T$_H$17 lymphocytes, it is now recognized that they are widely expressed in innate lymphoid cells, and the specific cell type may vary from phenotype to phenotype.

activated T and B cells, and when ligated by Fas ligand, it signals the Fas-bearing cell to undergo apoptosis (see Section 11-16). In this way it functions to limit the extent of immune responses. Mutations that eliminate or inactivate Fas lead in humans to a massive accumulation of lymphocytes, especially T cells, and in mice to the production of large quantities of pathogenic autoantibodies and a disease that resembles SLE. A mutation leading to this autoimmune syndrome was first observed in the MRL mouse strain and named *lpr*, for lymphoproliferation; it was subsequently identified as a mutation in *Fas*. The study of human individuals with the rare autoimmune lymphoproliferative syndrome, which is similar to the syndrome in the MRL/*lpr* mice, led to the identification of *FAS* as the mutant gene responsible for most of these cases (see Fig. 15.31).

Single-gene traits associated with autoimmunity			
Gene	**Human disease**	**Mouse mutant or knockout**	**Mechanism of autoimmunity**
AIRE	APECED (APS-I)	Knockout	Decreased expression of self antigens in the thymus, resulting in defective negative selection of self-reactive T cells
CTLA4	Association with Graves' disease, type 1 diabetes mellitus, and others	Knockout	Failure of T-cell anergy and reduced activation threshold of self-reactive T cells
FOXP3	IPEX	Knockout and mutation (*scurfy*)	Decreased function of CD4 CD25 regulatory T cells
FAS	ALPS	*lpr/lpr; gld/gld* mutants	Failure of apoptotic death of self-reactive B and T cells
C1q	SLE	Knockout	Defective clearance of immune complexes and apoptotic cells
ATG16L1	IBD	Hypomorph	Defective autophagy/clearance of bacteria by innate cells in intestines
IL10RA, IL10RB	IBD	Knockout	Defective IL-10 signaling; impaired anti-inflammatory response
INS	Type 1 diabetes mellitus	None	Decreased expression of insulin in thymus; impaired negative selection

Fig. 15.31 Single-gene traits associated with autoimmunity.
Listed are examples of monogenic disorders that cause autoimmunity in humans. Mice with targeted deletions (knockout) or spontaneous mutations (for example, *lpr/lpr*) in homologous genes have similar disease characteristics and are useful models for the study of the pathogenic basis for these disorders. APECED, autoimmune polyendocrinopathy–candidiasis–ectodermal dystrophy; APS-I, autoimmune polyglandular syndrome type I; IPEX, immune dysregulation, polyendocrinopathy, enteropathy, X-linked syndrome; ALPS, autoimmune lymphoproliferative syndrome. The *lpr* mutation in mice affects the gene for Fas, whereas the *gld* mutation affects the gene for FasL.

15-16 MHC genes have an important role in controlling susceptibility to autoimmune disease.

The genetic loci most consistently associated with susceptibility to autoimmune disease are certain MHC genotypes, particularly MHC class II alleles (**Fig. 15.32**). Recall from Section 6-11 that the MHC genes are highly polymorphic and have hundreds of different allelic variants. This association is identified by comparing the frequencies of various MHC alleles in individuals having a disease with the frequencies in the normal population. For example, HLA-DR3 and HLA-DR4 alleles are much more prevalent in individuals with type 1 diabetes mellitus than in the general population (**Fig. 15.33**). Similar analysis shows that the MHC class II allele HLA-DR2 has a dominant protective effect: individuals carrying HLA-DR2, even in association with one of the susceptibility alleles, rarely develop diabetes. It has also been shown that two siblings affected with the same autoimmune disease are far more likely than expected to share the same MHC haplotypes (**Fig. 15.34**). As HLA genotyping has become more exact through DNA sequencing, disease associations originally discovered by serotyping have been defined more precisely. For example, the association between type 1 diabetes mellitus and the DR3 and DR4 alleles is now known to be due to their tight genetic linkage to DQβ alleles that confer susceptibility to the disease. Indeed, susceptibility is most closely associated with polymorphisms at a particular position in the DQβ amino acid sequence that affect the peptide-binding cleft of MHC class II (**Fig. 15.35**). The diabetes-prone NOD strain of mice also has a serine residue polymorphism at that same position in the homologous mouse MHC class II molecule, known as I-A^{g7}.

The association of MHC genotype with autoimmune disease may result from allelic variants having different abilities to bind antigenic self peptides,

HLA- and gender-associated risk for autoimmune disease			
Disease	HLA allele	Relative risk	Sex ratio (♀: ♂)
Ankylosing spondylitis	B27	87.4	0.3
Type 1 diabetes mellitus	DQ2 and DQ8	~25	~1
Goodpasture's syndrome	DR2	15.9	~1
Pemphigus vulgaris	DR4	14.4	~1
Autoimmune uveitis	B27	10	<0.5
Psoriasis vulgaris	CW6	7	~1
Systemic lupus erythematosus	DR3	5.8	10–20
Addison's disease	DR3	5	~13
Multiple sclerosis	DR2	4.8	10
Rheumatoid arthritis	DR4	4.2	3
Graves' disease	DR3	3.7	4–5
Hashimoto's thyroiditis	DR5	3.2	4–5
Myasthenia gravis	DR3	2.5	~1
Type 1 diabetes mellitus	DQ6	0.02	~1

Fig. 15.32 Associations of HLA and sex with susceptibility to autoimmune disease. The 'relative risk' for an HLA allele in an autoimmune disease is calculated by comparing the observed number of individuals carrying the HLA allele with the number that would be expected, given the prevalence of the HLA allele in the general population. For type 1 diabetes mellitus (insulin-dependent diabetes mellitus), the association is in fact with the HLA-DQ gene, which is tightly linked to the DR genes but is not detectable by serotyping. Some diseases show a significant bias in the sex ratio; this is taken to imply that sex hormones are involved in pathogenesis. Consistent with this association, the difference in the sex ratio in these diseases is greatest between menarche and menopause, when levels of such hormones are highest.

consistent with the involvement of T cells in particular diseases. In diabetes, for example, there are associations with both MHC class I and MHC class II alleles, consistent with the finding that both CD8 and CD4 T cells mediate the autoimmune response. Evidence suggests that this explanation applies to the activation of insulin peptide–reactive T cells in the NOD strain of mice. An alternative hypothesis proposes that self peptides associated with certain MHC molecules may drive the positive selection of developing thymocytes that are specific for particular autoantigens. Such autoantigenic peptides might be expressed at too low a level or bind too poorly to MHC molecules to drive thymic negative selection but might be present at a sufficient level or bind strongly enough to drive positive selection.

15-17 Genetic variants that impair innate immune responses can predispose to T cell–mediated chronic inflammatory disease.

Section 15-5 introduced Crohn's disease (CD) as one of two major types of inflammatory bowel disease. CD is thought to result from abnormal hyper-responsiveness of CD4 T cells to antigens of the commensal gut microbiota

Fig. 15.33 Population studies show association of susceptibility to type 1 diabetes mellitus with HLA genotype. The HLA genotypes (determined by serotyping) of individuals with diabetes (lower panel) are not representative of those found in the general population (upper panel). Almost all individuals with diabetes express HLA-DR3 and/or HLA-DR4, and HLA-DR3/DR4 heterozygosity is greatly overrepresented in diabetics compared with controls. These alleles are linked tightly to HLA-DQ alleles that confer susceptibility to type 1 diabetes mellitus. By contrast, HLA-DR2 protects against the development of diabetes and is found only extremely rarely in individuals with diabetes. The small letter 'x' represents any allele other than DR2, DR3, or DR4.

Fig. 15.34 Family studies show strong linkage of susceptibility to type 1 diabetes mellitus with HLA genotype. In families in which two or more siblings have type 1 diabetes mellitus, it is possible to compare the HLA genotypes of affected siblings. Affected siblings share two HLA haplotypes much more frequently than would be expected if the HLA genotype did not influence disease susceptibility.

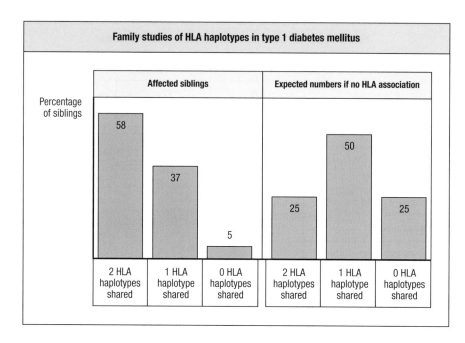

Family studies of HLA haplotypes in type 1 diabetes mellitus

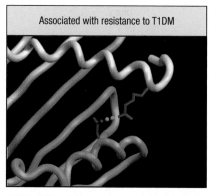

Position 57 of the DQβ chain affects susceptibility to type 1 diabetes mellitus

rather than to true self antigens. Dysregulation of T_H17 and T_H1 cells is thought to be pathogenic. Individuals with CD have episodes of severe inflammation that commonly affect the terminal ileum, with or without involvement of the colon—hence the alternative name 'regional ileitis' for this disease—but any part of the gastrointestinal tract can be involved. The disease is characterized by chronic inflammation and granulomatous lesions in the mucosa and submucosa of the intestine. Disease may result from a failure of mucosal innate immune mechanisms to sequester luminal bacteria from the adaptive immune system, from T cell–intrinsic defects that cause heightened effector responses, or from failure of T_{reg} cells to suppress microbiota-reactive T_H17 and T_H1 cells (**Fig. 15.36**).

Genetic analysis of people with CD and their families has identified a growing list of disease-susceptibility genes (see Fig. 15.29). One of the earliest to be identified was *NOD2* (also known as *CARD15*), which is expressed predominantly in monocytes, dendritic cells, and the Paneth cells of the small intestine and is involved in recognition of microbial antigens as part of the innate immune response (see Section 3-8). Mutations and rare polymorphic variants in NOD2 are strongly associated with CD. Mutations in the same gene are also the cause of a dominantly inherited granulomatous disease named **Blau syndrome**, in which granulomas typically develop in the skin, eyes, and joints. Whereas CD results from a loss of function of NOD2, it is thought that Blau syndrome results from a gain of function.

Fig. 15.35 Amino acid changes in the sequence of an MHC class II protein correlate with susceptibility to and protection from diabetes. The HLA-DQβ$_1$ chain contains an aspartic acid (Asp) residue at position 57 in most people. In Caucasoid populations, individuals with type 1 diabetes mellitus (T1DM) more often have valine, serine, or alanine at this position instead, as well as other differences. Asp57, shown in red on the backbone structure of the DQβ chain in the top panel, forms a salt bridge (shown in green in the center panel) to an arginine residue (shown in pink) in the adjacent α chain (gray). The change to an uncharged residue (for example, alanine, shown in yellow in the bottom panel) disrupts this salt bridge, altering the stability of the DQ molecule. The non-obese diabetic (NOD) strain of mice, which develops spontaneous diabetes, has a similar substitution of serine for the aspartic acid at position 57 of the homologous I-Aβ chain, and NOD mice transgenic for β chains with Asp57 have a marked reduction in diabetes incidence.

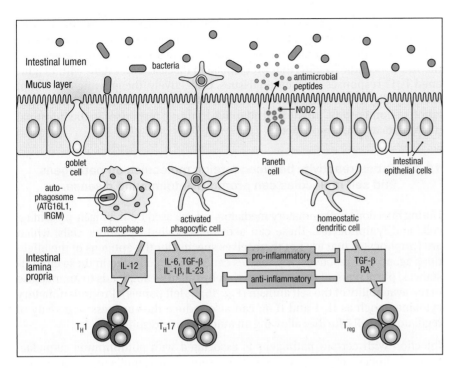

Fig. 15.36 Crohn's disease results from a breakdown of the homeostatic mechanisms that normally limit inflammatory responses to gut microbiota. The innate and adaptive immune systems normally cooperate to limit inflammatory responses to intestinal bacteria through a combination of mechanisms: a mucus layer produced by goblet cells; tight junctions between the intestinal epithelial cells; antimicrobial peptides released from epithelial cells and Paneth cells; and induction of T_{reg} cells that inhibit effector CD4 T-cell development and promote the production of IgA antibodies that are transported into the intestinal lumen, where they inhibit translocation of intestinal bacteria (not shown). In individuals with impaired homeostatic mechanisms, dysregulated T_H1- and T_H17-cell responses to the intestinal microbiota can result, generating disease-causing chronic inflammation. Crohn's disease susceptibility genes of innate immunity include *NOD2* and the autophagy genes *ATG16L1* and *IRGM*. A major susceptibility gene that affects adaptive immune cells is *IL23R*, which is expressed by T_H17 cells (see also Fig. 15.30). RA, retinoic acid.

ANIMATION 15.1

NOD2 is an intracellular receptor for the muramyl dipeptide derived from bacterial peptidoglycan, and its stimulation activates the transcription factor NFκB and the expression of genes encoding pro-inflammatory cytokines and chemokines (see Section 3-10 and Fig. 12.38). In Paneth cells—specialized intestinal epithelial cells in the base of the small intestinal crypts—activation of NOD2 stimulates the release of granules containing antimicrobial peptides that help sequester commensal bacteria to the intestinal lumen, away from the adaptive immune system. Mutant forms of NOD2 that have lost this function limit this innate antibacterial response, thereby predisposing the individual to heightened effector CD4 T-cell responses to the commensal microbiota and consequent chronic intestinal inflammation (see Sections 3-10 and 12-17).

Crohn's Disease

In addition to NOD2, other deficiencies in innate immunity have been identified in people with CD, including defective CXCL8 production and neutrophil accumulation, which can synergize with NOD2 defects to promote intestinal inflammation. Thus, compound defects in innate immunity and the regulation of inflammation may act synergistically to promote immunopathology in CD. Other candidate genes for CD may be linked to impaired innate immune functions (see Fig. 15.29). Defects in two genes (*ATG16L1* and *IRGM*) that contribute to autophagy have been linked to CD, suggesting that clearance of phagocytosed bacteria might be impaired, and thus predispose to chronic intestinal inflammation (see Section 6-6).

	Mechanism	
Mechanism	Disruption of cell or tissue barrier	Molecular mimicry
Effect	Release of sequestered self antigen; activation of nontolerized cells	Production of cross-reactive antibodies or T cells
Example	Sympathetic ophthalmia	Rheumatic fever Reactive arthritis Lyme arthritis

Fig. 15.37 Infectious agents could break self-tolerance in several different ways. Left panels: Some antigens are sequestered from the circulation, either behind a tissue barrier or retained within a cell. An infection can disrupt tissue barriers and damage cells, exposing hidden antigens to the immune system. Right panels: Molecular mimicry might result in infectious agents inducing either T- or B-cell responses that can cross-react with self antigens.

While defects in important pathways of the innate immune system contribute to CD, genes that regulate the adaptive immune response have also been associated with susceptibility. Most notably, there are variants of the gene for the IL-23 receptor (*IL23R*) that predispose to disease, consistent with heightened T_H17 responses in diseased tissues. Collectively, the growing number of susceptibility genes that confer increased risk for CD point to abnormal regulation of homeostatic innate and adaptive immune responses to the intestinal microbiota as a common factor.

15-18 Cross-reactivity between foreign molecules on pathogens and self molecules can promote autoimmune disease.

During infections, inflammatory mediators are released from antigen-presenting cells and lymphocytes. These can activate so-called bystander cells, which are lymphocytes that are not themselves specific for the antigens of the infectious agent. Self-reactive lymphocytes can become activated in these circumstances, particularly if tissue destruction by the infection leads to an increase in the availability of the self antigen (**Fig. 15.37**, left panels). Pro-inflammatory cytokines, such as IL-1 and IL-6, can also reduce the suppressive activity of regulatory T cells, further allowing an autoimmune response.

Infection with certain pathogens is associated with autoimmune sequelae. Some pathogens express antigens that resemble host molecules, a phenomenon called **molecular mimicry**. In such cases, antibodies produced against a pathogen epitope may cross-react with a self molecule (see Fig. 15.37, right panels). Such structures do not necessarily have to be identical: it is sufficient that they be similar enough to be recognized by the same antibody. Molecular mimicry may also activate autoreactive T cells and result in an attack on self tissues if a processed peptide from a pathogen antigen is similar to a host peptide. A model system to demonstrate molecular mimicry has been generated by using transgenic mice expressing a viral antigen in the pancreas. Normally, there is no response to this virus-derived 'self' antigen, but upon infection with the virus that was the source of the transgenic antigen, mice develop diabetes, because the virus activates T cells that are cross-reactive with the 'self' viral antigen (**Fig. 15.38**).

Some examples of autoimmune syndromes thought to involve molecular mimicry are the **rheumatic fever** that sometimes follows streptococcal infection and the reactive arthritis that can occur after enteric infection. Once self-reactive lymphocytes have been activated by such a mechanism, their effector

Fig. 15.38 Virus infection can break tolerance to a transgenic viral protein expressed in pancreatic β cells. Mice made transgenic for the lymphocytic choriomeningitis virus (LCMV) nucleoprotein under the control of the rat insulin promoter express the nucleoprotein in their pancreatic β cells but do not respond to this protein and therefore do not develop an autoimmune diabetes. However, if the transgenic mice are infected with LCMV, a potent antiviral cytotoxic T-cell response is elicited, and this kills the β cells, leading to diabetes. It is thought that infectious agents can sometimes elicit T-cell responses that cross-react with self peptides (a process known as molecular mimicry) and that this could cause autoimmune disease in a similar way.

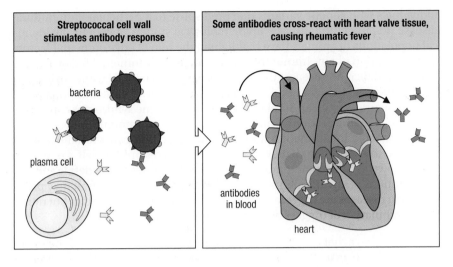

| Streptococcal cell wall stimulates antibody response | Some antibodies cross-react with heart valve tissue, causing rheumatic fever |

bacteria

plasma cell

antibodies in blood

heart

Fig. 15.39 Antibodies against streptococcal cell-wall antigens cross-react with antigens on heart tissue. The immune response to the bacteria produces antibodies against various epitopes of the bacterial cell surface. Some of these antibodies (yellow) cross-react with the heart valves, whereas others (blue) do not. An epitope in the heart (orange) is structurally similar but not identical to a bacterial epitope (red).

functions can destroy tissues. Autoimmunity of this type is sometimes transient and remits when the inciting pathogen is eliminated. This is the case in the autoimmune hemolytic anemia that follows *Mycoplasma* infection. The anemia ensues when antibodies against the pathogen cross-react with an antigen on red blood cells, leading to hemolysis (see Section 15-9). The autoantibodies disappear when the individual recovers from the infection. Sometimes, however, the autoimmunity persists well beyond the initial infection. This is true in some cases of rheumatic fever (**Fig. 15.39**), which occasionally follows a sore throat, scarlet fever, or local skin infections (impetigo) caused by *Streptococcus pyogenes*. The similarity of epitopes on streptococcal antigens to self epitopes leads to antibody-mediated, and possibly T cell–mediated, damage to a variety of tissues, including heart valves and the kidney. Although the tissue injury is typically transient, especially with antibiotic treatment, it can become chronic. Similarly, Lyme disease, an infection with the spirochete *Borrelia burgdorferi*, can be followed by late-developing autoimmunity (Lyme arthritis). In this case, the mechanism is not entirely clear, but it is likely to involve cross-reactivity of pathogen and host components, leading to autoimmunity.

Finally, certain external causative agents can result in human autoimmunity, specifically certain drugs that can elicit autoimmune reactions in a small proportion of individuals. Procainamide, a drug used to treat heart arrhythmias, is notable for inducing autoantibodies similar to those in SLE, although these are rarely pathogenic. Several drugs are associated with the development of autoimmune hemolytic anemia, in which autoantibodies against surface components of red blood cells attack and destroy these cells (see Section 15-9). Toxins in the environment can also cause autoimmunity. When heavy metals, such as gold or mercury, are administered to susceptible strains of mice, a predictable autoimmune syndrome, including the production of autoantibodies, ensues. The extent to which heavy metals promote autoimmunity in humans is unclear, but the animal models show that environmental factors such as toxins could have roles in certain syndromes. The mechanisms by which drugs and toxins cause autoimmunity are uncertain. Some drugs are thought to react chemically with self proteins and form derivatives that the immune system recognizes as foreign. The immune response to these haptenated self proteins can lead to inflammation, complement deposition, destruction of tissue, and finally immune responses to the original self proteins.

Autoimmune
Hemolytic Anemia

Summary.

The specific causes of most autoimmune diseases are not known. Genetic risk factors, including particular alleles of MHC class II molecules and polymorphisms or mutations of other genes, have been identified, but many individuals with genetic variants that predispose to a particular autoimmune disease do not get the disease. Epidemiological studies of genetically identical populations of animals have highlighted the role of environmental factors in the initiation of autoimmunity, but although environmental factors have a strong influence on disease, they are not well understood. Some toxins and drugs are known to cause autoimmunity, but their role in the common autoimmune diseases is unclear. Similarly, some autoimmune syndromes can follow viral or bacterial infections. Pathogens can promote autoimmunity by causing nonspecific inflammation and tissue damage and can sometimes elicit responses to self proteins if they express molecules resembling self, a phenomenon known as molecular mimicry. More research is needed to define specific contributions of environmental factors to autoimmune diseases. It may prove that most diseases are triggered not by a single environmental factor but rather by a combination of triggers or even random events.

Responses to alloantigens and transplant rejection.

Although organ transplantation is now a common and important medical therapy, immune rejection of transplants remains a major impediment. Rejection is primarily caused by immune responses to proteins expressed by the graft. These proteins, which vary between individuals and are perceived as foreign by the recipient, are called alloantigens. Section 6-13 introduced the basis of the alloreactive T-cell response to the polymorphic MHC molecules, which almost always trigger a response against the grafted organ. Matching the MHC type of the donor and the recipient increases the success rate of grafts, but perfect matching of all MHC loci is possible only when donor and recipient are closely related, and even in these cases, genetic differences at other loci can still trigger rejection, although less severely. Nevertheless, advances in immunosuppression and transplantation medicine now mean that the precise matching of tissues for transplantation is no longer the major factor in graft survival. In blood transfusion, the earliest and most common tissue transplant, MHC matching is not necessary for routine transfusions, because red blood cells and platelets express small amounts of MHC class I molecules and do not express MHC class II molecules; thus, they are not usually T-cell targets. However, antibodies made against platelet MHC class I molecules can be a problem when repeated transfusions of platelets are required. Blood must be matched for ABO and Rh blood group antigens to avoid the rapid destruction of mismatched red blood cells by antibodies in the recipient (see Appendix I, Sections A-6 and A-7), but because there are only four major ABO types and two Rh types, this is a relatively easy form of tissue matching.

In this part of the chapter, we examine the immune response to tissue grafts and also ask why such responses do not reject the one foreign tissue graft that is tolerated routinely—the mammalian fetus.

15-19 Transplant rejection is mediated primarily by T-cell responses to MHC molecules.

The basic rules of tissue grafting were first elucidated by skin transplantation between inbred strains of mice. Skin can be grafted with 100% success between different sites on the same animal or person (an **autograft**) or between genetically identical animals or people (a **syngeneic graft**). However, when skin is grafted between unrelated or **allogeneic** individuals (an **allograft**), the graft initially survives but is then rejected about 10–13 days after grafting (**Fig. 15.40**). This response is called an **acute rejection**, and it depends on a T-cell response,

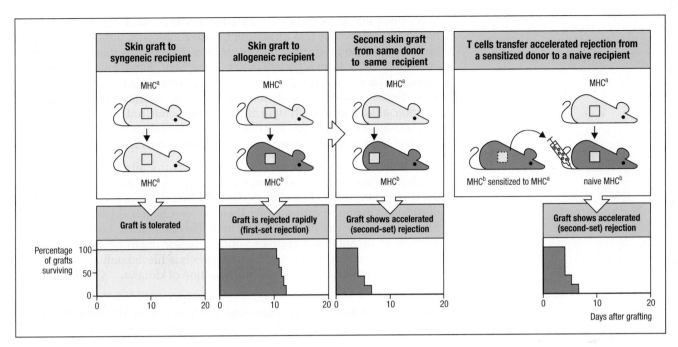

Fig. 15.40 Skin graft rejection is the result of a T cell–mediated anti-graft response. Grafts that are syngeneic are permanently accepted (first panels), but grafts differing at the MHC are rejected about 10–13 days after grafting (first-set rejection, second panels). When a mouse is grafted for a second time with skin from the same donor, it rejects the second graft faster (third panels). This is called a second-set rejection, and the accelerated response is MHC-specific; skin from a second donor of the same MHC type is rejected equally fast, whereas skin from an MHC-different donor is rejected in a first-set pattern (not shown). Naive mice that are given T cells from a sensitized donor behave as if they had already been grafted (final panels).

because skin grafted onto *nude* mice, which lack T cells, is not rejected. The ability to reject skin can be restored to *nude* mice by the adoptive transfer of normal T cells.

When a recipient that has previously rejected a graft (called first-set rejection) is regrafted with skin from the same donor, the second graft is rejected more rapidly (6–8 days) in an **accelerated rejection** (see Fig. 15.40). Skin from a third-party donor grafted onto the same recipient at the same time does not show this faster response but follows a first-set rejection course. The rapid course of second-set rejection can also be transferred to new recipients by T cells from the initial recipient, showing that second-set rejection is caused by a memory-type response (see Chapter 11) from clonally expanded and primed T cells specific for the donor skin.

Adaptive immune responses to a graft's foreign proteins are the major barrier to effective tissue transplantation. These responses can be mediated by CD8 or CD4 T cells, or both. Antigens that differ between members of the same species are known as **alloantigens**, and an immune response against such antigens is known as an **alloreactive** response. When donor and recipient express different MHC alleles, the host will mount an alloreactive immune response against the graft's nonself allogeneic MHC molecules. In most tissues these are predominantly MHC class I antigens. Once a recipient has rejected a graft of a particular MHC type, any further graft bearing the same nonself MHC will be rapidly rejected in a second response. As described in Section 6-13, the frequency of T cells specific for any nonself MHC molecule is relatively high, making allogeneic MHC molecules a potent trigger for graft rejection. Indeed, the MHC was originally so named because of its central role in graft rejection.

Once it became clear that nonself MHC molecules were a major trigger of graft rejection, a considerable amount of effort was put into MHC matching of recipient and donor. Today, with advances in immunosuppression, MHC matching has become less important for most allografts, although it remains important for bone marrow transplantation, for reasons that are discussed in Section 15-25. Even a perfect match at the MHC locus, known as the HLA (human leukocyte antigen) locus in humans, does not prevent rejection reactions. Grafts between HLA-identical siblings will invariably incite a rejection reaction, albeit more slowly than an unmatched graft, unless donor and recipient are identical twins. This reaction is the result of allelic differences between antigens from non-MHC proteins that also vary between individuals.

Thus, unless donor and recipient are identical twins, all graft recipients must be given immunosuppressive drugs chronically to prevent rejection. Indeed, the current success of clinical transplantation of solid organs is more the result of advances in immunosuppressive therapy (see Chapter 16) than of improved tissue matching. The limited supply of cadaveric organs, coupled with the urgency of identifying a recipient once a donor organ becomes available, means that accurate matching of tissue types is achieved only rarely, with the notable exception of matched-sibling donation of kidneys.

15-20 Rejection of MHC-identical grafts is caused by peptides from other alloantigens bound to graft MHC molecules.

When donor and recipient are identical at the MHC locus but differ at other genetic loci, graft rejection is not as rapid, but left unchecked it will still destroy the graft (**Fig. 15.41**). This is the reason that grafts between HLA-identical siblings (but not identical twins) would be rejected without immunosuppressive treatment. MHC class I and class II molecules bind and present a large selection of peptides derived from self proteins made in the cell, and if these proteins are polymorphic, then different peptides will be produced from them in different members of a species. Such proteins can also be recognized as **minor histocompatibility antigens** (**Fig. 15.42**). One set of proteins that induce minor histocompatibility responses is encoded on the male Y chromosome. Responses induced by these proteins are known collectively as H-Y. Because Y chromosome–specific genes are not expressed in females, females generate H-Y responses against male cells. However, male anti-female responses do not occur, because both sexes express X-chromosome genes. One H-Y antigen has

Fig. 15.41 Even complete matching at the MHC locus does not ensure graft survival. Although syngeneic grafts are not rejected (left panels), MHC-identical grafts from donors can differ at other loci (minor H antigen loci) that can generate peptides presented by the syngeneic MHC that are recognized as foreign by the recipient. This can lead to the graft being rejected (right panels), albeit more slowly than MHC-disparate grafts (center panels).

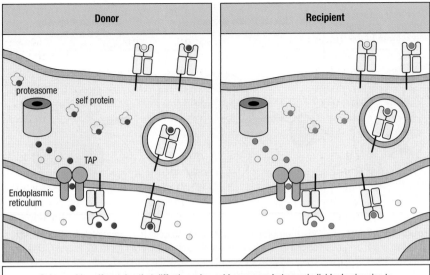

Polymorphic self proteins that differ in amino acid sequence between individuals give rise to minor H antigen differences between donor and recipient

Fig. 15.42 Minor H antigens are peptides derived from polymorphic cellular proteins bound to MHC class I molecules. Self proteins are routinely digested by proteasomes within the cell's cytosol, and peptides derived from them are delivered to the endoplasmic reticulum, where they are loaded onto MHC class I molecules and delivered to the cell surface. If a polymorphic protein differs between the graft donor (shown in red on the left) and the recipient (shown in blue on the right), it can give rise to an antigenic peptide (red on the donor cell) that can be recognized by the recipient's T cells as nonself and elicit an immune response, even when the donor and host have identical MHC alleles (shown as yellow). Such antigens are called minor histocompatibility (H) antigens.

been identified in mice and humans as peptides from a protein encoded by the gene *Smcy*. An X-chromosome homolog of *Smcy* (or *Kdm5d*), called *Smcx* (or *Kdm5c*), does not contain these peptide sequences, which are therefore expressed uniquely in males. Most minor histocompatibility antigens are encoded by autosomal genes, and their identity is largely unknown, although an increasing number have now been identified at the genetic level.

The response to minor histocompatibility antigens is in many ways analogous to the response to viral infection. However, whereas an antiviral response eliminates only infected cells, a large fraction of cells in the graft expresses minor histocompatibility antigens, and thus the graft is destroyed in the response against these antigens. Given the virtual certainty of mismatches in minor histocompatibility antigens between two individuals, and the potency of the reactions they incite, it is understandable that successful transplantation requires the use of powerful immunosuppressive drugs.

15-21 Alloreactive T cells reject transplanted organs by direct and indirect allorecognition.

For naive alloreactive T cells to become activated and acquire effector activities that cause organ rejection requires that they contact antigen-presenting cells expressing the allogeneic MHC and co-stimulatory molecules. Transplanted organs carry immune cells of donor origin, including tissue-resident dendritic cells and other antigen-presenting cells. These cells have been called passenger leukocytes. Until recently, it was presumed that passenger leukocytes were responsible for the direct activation of host alloreactive T cells, mediated by migration of the passenger leukocytes from the graft into secondary lymphoid tissues of the recipient. Because the lymphatic drainage of solid organ allografts is interrupted by transplantation, migration of donor antigen-presenting cells was initially thought to occur via the blood, and not the lymphatics. The alloreactive effector T cells activated in the lymph nodes or spleen would then circulate to the graft and mediate an immune attack (**Fig. 15.43**). In support of this **direct allorecognition** pathway (**Fig. 15.44**, upper panel) is the observation that the depletion of antigen-presenting cells from grafted tissue, carried out by treatment with antibodies or by prolonged incubation, can prolong graft survival. However, in experimental systems, it has been observed that only a small number of donor antigen-presenting cells reach secondary lymphoid

Fig. 15.43 Acute rejection of a kidney graft through the direct pathway of allorecognition. Donor dendritic cells in the graft (or exosomes that they secrete) carry complexes of donor HLA molecules and donor peptides on their surfaces via the blood to secondary lymphoid organs (in this case, a lymph node). In the case of exosomes, their membrane can be inserted directly into the membrane of host dendritic cells and presented to T cells (not shown). The recipient's alloreactive T cells (both CD8 and CD4) are activated by direct allorecognition (that is, with donor peptides bound to donor MHC). The effector T cells then travel in the blood to the grafted organ and attack cells that display the donor peptide:HLA molecule complexes for which the T cells are specific.

organs. Recently, a second route to activating host T cells via direct allorecognition has been observed and is based on the secretion of exosomes from donor antigen-presenting cells present in the graft. Exosomes are membrane-bound extracellular vesicles produced by the endocytic compartment of cells and are secreted by a budding process from the cell membrane. Exosomes secreted by donor antigen-presenting cells contain the allogeneic MHC of the donor and can circulate in the blood. By a reverse process, exosomes can be taken up by host dendritic cells in secondary lymphoid organs and incorporated directly into their plasma membrane, allowing direct presentation of allogeneic MHC to host alloreactive T cells. While this route has been demonstrated in experimental systems, it is still an area of active research, and the individual contributions of these two pathways to transplant rejection are still somewhat unclear.

A second mechanism of allograft recognition leading to graft rejection is the uptake of allogeneic proteins by the recipient's own antigen-presenting cells and their presentation to T cells by self MHC molecules. This is known as **indirect allorecognition** (see Fig. 15.44, lower panel). Peptides derived from both the foreign MHC molecules themselves and minor histocompatibility antigens can be presented by indirect allorecognition.

Direct allorecognition is thought to be largely responsible for acute rejection, especially when MHC mismatches mean that the frequency of directly alloreactive recipient T cells is high. Furthermore, a direct cytotoxic T-cell attack on graft cells can be made only by T cells that recognize the graft MHC molecules directly. Nonetheless, T cells with specificity for alloantigens presented on self MHC can contribute to graft rejection by activating macrophages, which cause tissue injury and fibrosis. T cells with indirect allospecificity are

Fig. 15.44 Direct and indirect pathways of allorecognition contribute to graft rejection. In direct allorecognition (upper panel), T-cell receptors of alloreactive CD4 and CD8 T cells in the recipient immediately recognize the allogeneic HLA class I and class II allotypes on a donor dendritic cell (donor DC). In indirect allorecognition (lower panel), antigens from donor cells are processed and presented to peptide-specific T cells by the recipient's dendritic cells (recipient DC), which can be delivered by membrane vesicles such as exosomes. These antigens include peptides derived from the minor H antigens (green) and from allogeneic HLA class I and class II allotypes (yellow), both of which are presented by the recipient's HLA molecules (orange). Presentation by HLA class II molecules to CD4 T cells (blue) is shown here, but peptides can also be presented by recipient HLA class I molecules to CD8 T cells (not shown).

also likely to be important in the development of an antibody response to a graft. Antibodies produced against nonself antigens from the same species are known as **alloantibodies**.

15-22 Antibodies that react with endothelium cause hyperacute graft rejection.

Antibody responses are an important potential cause of graft rejection. Preexisting alloantibodies against blood group antigens and polymorphic MHC antigens can cause rapid rejection of transplanted organs in a complement-dependent reaction that can occur within minutes of transplantation. This type of reaction is known as **hyperacute graft rejection**. Most grafts that are transplanted routinely in clinical medicine are vascularized organ grafts linked directly to the recipient's circulation. In some cases the recipient may have preexisting antibodies against donor graft antigens. Antibodies of the ABO type can bind to all tissues, not just red blood cells. In addition, antibodies against other antigens can be produced in response to a previous transplant or a blood transfusion. All such preexisting antibodies can cause rapid rejection of vascularized grafts because they react with antigens on the vascular endothelial cells of the graft and initiate the complement and blood-clotting cascades. The vessels of the graft become blocked, or thrombosed, causing its rapid destruction. Such grafts become engorged and purple-colored from hemorrhaged blood, which becomes deoxygenated (**Fig. 15.45**). This problem can be avoided by ABO matching and **cross-matching** donor and recipient. Cross-matching involves determining whether the recipient has antibodies that react with the white blood cells of the donor. Antibodies of this type, when found, have hitherto been considered a serious contraindication to transplantation of most solid organs, because in the absence of any treatment they lead to near-certain hyperacute rejection.

For reasons that are incompletely understood, some transplanted organs, particularly the liver, are less susceptible to this type of injury and can be transplanted despite ABO incompatibilities. In addition, the presence of donor-specific MHC alloantibodies and a positive cross-match are no longer considered an absolute contraindication for transplantation, as treatment with intravenous immunoglobulin has been successful in a proportion of people in whom antibodies against the donor tissue were already present.

A similar problem prevents routine use of animal organs—**xenografts**—in transplantation. If xenografts could be used, it would circumvent a limitation in organ replacement therapy: the shortage of donor organs. Pigs have been suggested as a source of organs for xenografting, but most humans have antibodies that react with a ubiquitous cell-surface carbohydrate antigen (galactose-α-1,3-galactose; α-Gal) of other mammalian species, including pigs. When pig xenografts are placed in humans, these antibodies trigger hyperacute rejection by binding graft endothelial cells and initiating complement and clotting cascades. The problem of hyperacute rejection is exacerbated in xenografts because complement-regulatory proteins such as CD59, DAF (CD55), and MCP (CD46) (see Sections 2-10 and 2-17) work less efficiently across a species barrier. A recent step toward xenotransplantation has been the development of transgenic pigs expressing human DAF as well as pigs that lack α-Gal. These approaches might one day reduce or eliminate hyperacute rejection in xenotransplantation.

15-23 Late failure of transplanted organs is caused by chronic injury to the graft.

The success of immunosuppression means that about 90% of cadaveric kidney grafts are still functioning a year after transplantation. There has, however, been little improvement in rates of long-term graft survival: the half-life for

Fig. 15.45 Preexisting antibody against donor graft antigens can cause hyperacute graft rejection. Prior to transplantation, some recipients have made antibodies that react with donor ABO or HLA class I antigens. When the donor organ is grafted into such a recipient, these antibodies bind to the vascular endothelium in the graft, initiating the complement and clotting cascades. Blood vessels in the graft become obstructed by clots and leak, causing hemorrhage of blood into the graft. The graft becomes engorged, turns purple from the presence of deoxygenated blood, and dies.

Fig. 15.46 Chronic rejection in the blood vessels of a transplanted kidney. Left panel: Chronic rejection is initiated by the interaction of anti-HLA class I alloantibodies with blood vessels of the transplanted organ. Antibodies bound to endothelial cells recruit Fc receptor–bearing monocytes and neutrophils. Right panel: Accumulating damage leads to thickening of the internal elastic lamina and to infiltration of the underlying intima with smooth muscle cells, macrophages, granulocytes, alloreactive T cells, and antibodies. The net effect is to narrow the lumen of the blood vessel and create a chronic inflammation that intensifies tissue remodeling. Eventually the vessel becomes obstructed, ischemic, and fibrotic.

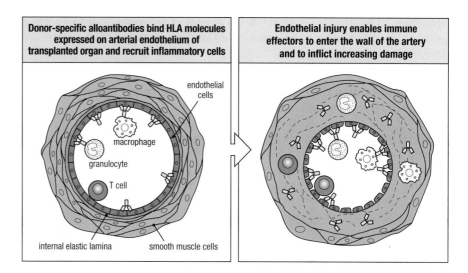

functional survival of renal allografts remains about 8 years. Although traditionally the late failure of a transplanted organ has been termed **chronic rejection**, it is typically difficult to determine whether the cause of chronic allograft injury involves specific immune alloreactivity, nonimmune injury, or both.

The pattern of chronic injury to transplanted organs is variable, depending on the tissue. A major component of late failure of vascularized transplanted organs is a chronic reaction called **chronic allograft vasculopathy**, which is a prominent cause of injury in heart and kidney allografts. This is characterized by concentric arteriosclerosis of graft blood vessels, which leads to hypoperfusion of the graft and its eventual fibrosis and atrophy (**Fig. 15.46**). Multiple mechanisms may contribute to this form of vascular injury, although the major cause is thought to be recurring, subclinical acute rejection events, whether due to the development of allospecific antibodies reactive to the vascular endothelium of the graft (so-called donor-specific antibodies) or to allograft-reactive effector T cells, or both. Some forms of immunosuppressive therapy (for example, calcineurin inhibitors such as cyclosporin A) also cause vascular injury, although this is typically more limited to very small arteries and causes a different pattern of injury, referred to as arteriolar hyalinosis, which is marked by proteinaceous deposits that narrow the vascular lumen. In transplanted livers, chronic rejection is associated with loss of bile ducts, the so-called vanishing bile duct syndrome, whereas in transplanted lungs, the major cause of late organ failure is accumulation of scar tissue in the bronchioles, termed bronchiolitis obliterans. Alloreactive responses can occur months to years after transplantation and may be associated with gradual loss of graft function that is hard to detect clinically.

Other important causes of chronic graft dysfunction include ischemia–reperfusion injury, which can promote sterile inflammatory signals at the time of grafting because of the restoration of blood flow after a period of poor perfusion of the organ to be transplanted; viral infections that emerge as a result of immunosuppression; and recurrence of the same disease in the allograft that destroyed the original organ. Irrespective of etiology, chronic allograft injury is typically irreversible and progressive, ultimately leading to complete failure of allograft function.

15-24 A variety of organs are transplanted routinely in clinical medicine.

Three major advances have made it possible to use organ transplantation routinely in the clinic. First, surgical techniques for performing organ replacement have advanced to the point where such surgeries are now relatively

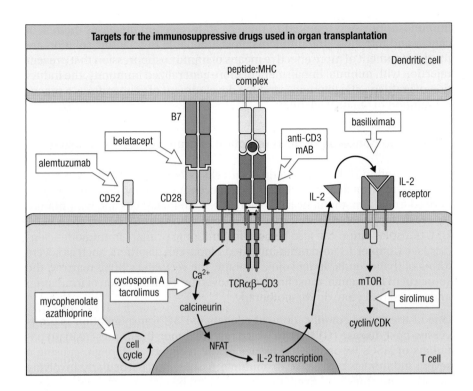

Targets for the immunosuppressive drugs used in organ transplantation

Fig. 15.47 Immunosuppressive drugs act at different stages in the activation of alloreactive T cells. The diagram illustrates the site of action of various immunosuppressive drugs. Rabbit anti-thymocyte globulin (Thymoglobulin) and anti-CD52 monoclonal antibody (alemtuzumab) are used to deplete T cells and other leukocytes before transplantation. Anti-CD3 monoclonal antibody (mAb) blocks signaling by the T-cell receptor complex. Cyclosporin A and tacrolimus inhibit calcineurin and prevent the translocation of nuclear factor of activated T cells (NFAT) to the nucleus. The CTLA-4–Fc fusion protein belatacept binds B7 and blocks co-stimulation of T cells by CD28. Basiliximab is an anti-CD25 antibody that binds to the high-affinity IL-2 receptor and prevents IL-2 signaling. Sirolimus interferes with activation of the mTOR cascade, which is required for differentiation of effector T cells. Azathioprine and mycophenolate inhibit the replication and proliferation of activated T cells.

routine in most major medical centers. Second, networks of transplantation centers have been organized to procure healthy organs that become available from cadaveric donors. Third, the use of powerful immunosuppressive drugs that inhibit T-cell activation, thereby limiting the development of anti-allograft effector T cells and antibodies, has markedly increased graft survival rates (**Fig. 15.47**). Five year survival rates for frequently transplanted organs or tissues and allografts between 2002 and 2007 are listed in **Fig. 15.48**, and these rates continue to improve. The most frequently transplanted solid organ is the kidney, the organ first successfully transplanted between identical twins in the 1950s; the half-life of survival of transplanted kidneys is now close to 8 years. These improvements stem from increased use of living donors and paired donors; better diagnosis of antibody-mediated rejection; improved treatment, such as anti-CD20 antibody (rituximab), which suppresses B cells; and plasma exchange therapy. Transplantation of the cornea is even more common than kidney transplantation; this tissue is a special case because it is not vascularized, and corneal grafts between unrelated people are usually successful without immunosuppression.

Many problems other than graft rejection are associated with organ transplantation. First, donor organs are difficult to obtain. Second, the disease that destroyed the transplant recipient's organ might also destroy the graft, as in the destruction of pancreatic β cells in autoimmune diabetes. Third, the

Fig. 15.48 Organs and tissues commonly transplanted in clinical medicine. The numbers of organ and tissue grafts performed in the United States in 2014 are shown. HSC, hematopoietic stem cells (includes bone marrow, peripheral blood HSCs, and cord blood transplants).*Number of grafts includes multiple organ grafts (for example, kidney and pancreas, or heart and lung). For solid organs, 5-year survival of the transplanted graft is based on transplants performed between 2002 and 2007. Data from the United Network for Organ Sharing.†Kidney survival listed (81.4%) is for kidneys from living donors; 5-year survival for cadaveric donor transplants is 69.1%.‡Pancreas survival listed (53.4%) is when transplanted alone; 5-year survival when transplanted with a kidney is 73.5%.§Includes autologous and allogeneic transplants.‖Successful HSC engraftment is assessed within weeks of transplant, not years. Nearly all solid organ grafts (for example, kidney, heart) require long-term immunosuppression.

Tissue transplanted	No. of grafts in USA (2014)*	5-year graft survival
Kidney	17,815	81.4%†
Liver	6729	68.3%
Heart	2679	74.0%
Pancreas	954	53.4%‡
Lung	1949	50.6%
Intestine	139	~48.4%
Cornea	~45,000	~70%
HSC transplants	~20,000§	>80%‖

immunosuppression required to prevent graft rejection increases the risk of cancer and infection. The problems most amenable to scientific solution are the development of more effective means of immunosuppression that prevent rejection with minimal impairment of more generalized immunity, the induction of graft-specific tolerance, and the development of xenografts as a practical solution to organ availability.

15-25 The converse of graft rejection is graft-versus-host disease.

Transplantation of hematopoietic stem cells (HSCs) from peripheral blood, bone marrow, or fetal cord blood is a successful therapy for some tumors derived from hematopoietic cells, such as certain leukemias and lymphomas. By replacing genetically defective stem cells with normal donor stem cells, HSC transplantation can also be used to cure some primary immunodeficiencies (see Chapter 13) and other inherited blood-cell disorders, such as severe forms of thalassemia. In leukemia therapy, the recipient's bone marrow, the source of the leukemia, must first be destroyed by a combination of irradiation and aggressive cytotoxic chemotherapy.

Graft-Versus-Host Disease

One of the major complications of allogeneic HSC transplantation is **graft-versus-host disease (GVHD)**, in which mature donor T cells present in preparations of HSCs recognize the tissues of the recipient as foreign, causing a severe inflammatory disease in multiple tissues, but particularly involving the skin, intestines, and liver and characterized by rashes, diarrhea, and liver dysfunction (**Fig. 15.49**). Because the consequences of GVHD are particularly aggressive when there is a mismatch of MHC class I or class II antigens, HLA matching between donor and recipient is more critical than in solid organ transplantation. Most transplants are therefore undertaken only when the donor and recipient are HLA-matched siblings or, less frequently, when there is an HLA-matched unrelated donor. Therefore, GVHD mostly occurs in the context of disparities between minor histocompatibility antigens, so immunosuppression must be used in every HSC transplant.

The presence of alloreactive donor T cells can be demonstrated experimentally by the **mixed lymphocyte reaction (MLR)**, in which lymphocytes from a potential donor are mixed with irradiated lymphocytes from the recipient. Naive donor T cells that recognize alloantigens on the recipient lymphocytes will proliferate or kill the recipient target cells, although the test does not accurately quantify alloreactive T cells. A more accurate test is a version of the limiting-dilution assay (see Appendix I, Section A-21), which precisely counts the frequency of alloreactive T cells.

Although GVHD is harmful to the recipient of an HSC transplant, it can have beneficial effects that are crucial to the success of the therapy. Much

Fig. 15.49 Graft-versus-host disease occurs when donor T cells in the graft attack the recipient's tissues. After bone marrow transplantation (left panel), any mature donor CD4 and CD8 T cells present in the graft that are alloreactive to the recipient's HLA allotypes become activated by encountering dendritic cells in secondary lymphoid tissues (middle panel). These donor-derived effector T cells move into the circulation and preferentially enter and attack tissues of the graft recipient (right panel), particularly epithelial cells of the skin, intestines, and liver that have been damaged by the conditioning regimen of chemotherapy and irradiation prior to transplantation.

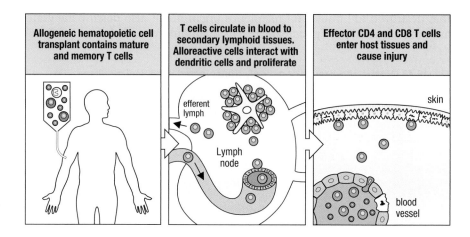

of the therapeutic effect of HSC transplantation for leukemia can be due to a **graft-versus-leukemia effect**, in which the donor T cells in the allogeneic preparations of HSCs recognize minor histocompatibility antigens expressed by the leukemic cells and kill the leukemic cells. One of the treatment options for suppressing the development of GVHD is the elimination of mature T cells from the preparations of donor HSCs *in vitro* before transplantation, thereby removing alloreactive T cells. Those T cells that subsequently mature from the donor marrow *in vivo* in the recipient are tolerant to the recipient's antigens. Although the elimination of GVHD has benefits for the patient, there is an increased risk of leukemic relapse, which provides strong evidence in support of the graft-versus-leukemia effect.

T_{reg} cells also participate in transplantation of allogeneic HSCs. In mice, depletion of $CD25^+$ T_{reg} cells in either the recipient or the HSC graft before transplantation accelerated the onset of GVHD and subsequent death, while supplementing the graft with T_{reg} cells delayed or even prevented death from GVHD. Also, treatment with a low dose of IL-2, which is thought to preferentially expand T_{reg} cells, has shown positive effects in preventing GVHD. Similar observations have been made in experimental mouse models of solid organ transplantation, where the transfer of either naturally occurring or induced T_{reg} cells significantly delayed allograft rejection. These experiments suggest that enriching or generating T_{reg} cells in preparations of donor HSCs might provide a possible therapy for GVHD in the future.

Immunodeficiency is another complication of donor T-cell depletion. Because most of the recipient's T cells are destroyed by the combination of chemotherapy and irradiation used to treat the recipient before transplant, donor T cells are the major source for reconstituting a mature T-cell repertoire early after transplant. This is particularly true in adults, who have poor residual thymic function and therefore a limited ability to repopulate their T-cell repertoire from T-cell precursors. Thus, if too many T cells are depleted from the graft, transplant recipients experience, and can die from, opportunistic infections. The need to balance the beneficial effects of the graft-versus-leukemia effect and immunocompetence with the adverse effects of GVHD caused by donor T cells has spawned much research. One particularly promising approach is to prevent donor T cells from reacting with recipient antigens that they could meet shortly after the transplant. This is accomplished by depleting the recipient's antigen-presenting cells. Here, the donor T cells are not activated during the initial inflammation that accompanies the transplant, and thereafter they do not promote GVHD. However, it is unclear whether there would be a graft-versus-leukemia effect in this context.

15-26 The fetus is an allograft that is tolerated repeatedly.

All of the transplants discussed so far are the result of advances in modern medicine. However, one 'foreign' tissue that is repeatedly grafted and tolerated is the mammalian fetus. The fetus carries paternal MHC and minor histocompatibility antigens that differ from those of the mother (**Fig. 15.50**), and yet a mother can successfully bear many children expressing the same nonself proteins derived from the father. The mysterious lack of fetal rejection has consistently puzzled immunologists, and no comprehensive explanation has yet emerged. One problem is that acceptance of the fetal allograft is so much the norm that it is difficult to study the mechanism that prevents rejection; if the mechanism for rejecting the fetus is rarely activated, how can one analyze the mechanisms that control it?

The mechanisms contributing to 'fetomaternal tolerance' are likely multifactorial and redundant. Although it has been proposed that the fetus is simply not recognized as foreign, women who have borne children often make antibodies

Fig. 15.50 The fetus is an allograft that is not rejected. With very few exceptions, the mother and father in human families have different HLA types (top panel). When the woman becomes pregnant, she carries for 9 months a fetus that expresses one HLA haplotype of maternal origin (pink) and one HLA haplotype of paternal origin (blue) (bottom panel). Although the paternal HLA class I and class II molecules expressed by the fetus are alloantigens against which the mother's immune system has the potential to respond, the fetus does not provoke such a response during pregnancy and is protected from preexisting alloreactive antibodies or T cells. Even when the mother bears several children to the same father, no sign of immunological rejection is seen.

directed against the father's MHC and red blood cell antigens. However, the placenta, which is a fetus-derived tissue, seems to sequester the fetus from the mother's T cells. The outer layer of the placenta—the interface between fetal and maternal tissues—is the trophoblast. This does not express MHC class II molecules and expresses only low levels and a restricted subset of MHC class I molecules, making it resistant to direct alloantigen recognition by maternal T cells. Tissues lacking MHC class I expression are, however, vulnerable to attack by NK cells (see Section 3-25). The trophoblast might be protected from attack by NK cells by the expression of a nonclassical and minimally polymorphic HLA class I molecule, HLA-G, which has been shown to inhibit killing by NK cells.

The placenta may also inhibit the mother's T cells by an active mechanism of nutrient depletion. The enzyme indoleamine 2,3-dioxygenase (IDO) is expressed at a high level by cells at the maternal–fetal interface. This enzyme depletes the essential amino acid tryptophan at this site, and T cells starved of tryptophan show reduced responsiveness. Inhibition of IDO in pregnant mice, using the inhibitor 1-methyltryptophan, causes rapid rejection of allogeneic, but not syngeneic, fetuses.

The cytokine milieu at the maternal–fetal interface also contributes to fetal tolerance. Both the uterine epithelium and the trophoblast secrete TGF-β and IL-10. This combination of cytokines suppresses the development of effector T cells in favor of induced T_{reg} (iT_{reg}) cells (see Section 9-14). Regulatory T cells are increased during pregnancy, including iT_{reg} cells in the placenta. These cells are important for suppressing responses to the fetus in mice, as iT_{reg} deficiency promotes fetal resorption—the equivalent of spontaneous abortion in humans—as does induction of T_H1-inducing cytokines (for example, IFN-γ and IL-12). Provocatively, a regulatory element that controls FoxP3 expression in iT_{reg} cells, but is not required for FoxP3 expression by natural T_{reg} (nT_{reg}) cells, has been found only in placental mammals. This suggests iT_{reg} cells might have evolved to play an important role in maternal–fetal tolerance. Finally, stromal cells of the specialized maternal uterine tissue that directly interfaces with the placenta— the decidua—appear to repress the local expression of key T cell–attracting chemokines. Collectively, then, both maternal and fetal factors contribute to the formation of an immunologically privileged site akin to other sites of local immune suppression that allow prolonged acceptance of tissue grafts, such as the eye (see Section 15-3).

Summary.

Clinical transplantation is now a common medical therapy that has been made possible by MHC matching, immunosuppressive drugs, and advances in surgical techniques. However, even accurate MHC matching does not prevent graft rejection, because other genetic differences between host and donor, such as minor histocompatibility antigens, can result in allogeneic responses that are based on indirect allorecognition. Because of the current inability to specifically suppress the response to the graft without compromising host defense, most transplants require generalized immunosuppression of the recipient that can increase the risk of cancer and infection. The fetus is a natural allograft that must be accepted for the species to survive. A number of mechanisms contribute to regulation of the maternal immune tolerance to the fetus, including contributions by innate cells, particularly NK cells. A better understanding of tolerance to the fetus could ultimately provide insights for inducing specific allograft tolerance in transplantation.

Summary to Chapter 15.

Ideally, the effector functions of the immune system would be targeted only to foreign pathogens and never to self tissues. There are several layers of mechanisms that act to control the production and activation of self-reactive lymphocytes, but these sometimes break down. For a chronic disease to occur, it seems that multiple layers of tolerance must fail together. These layers begin with central tolerance in the bone marrow and thymus to generate a repertoire that has been screened to remove lymphocytes with strong self-reactivity. Other mechanisms act in the periphery to control those lymphocytes that escape this screening process, including anergy or induction of apoptosis, immunological ignorance and immune-privileged sites, cytokine deviation, and regulatory T cells.

Autoimmune diseases can be classified in several ways, such as by being tissue-specific or systemic or by the predominant effector mechanisms in play. Genetic predisposition has an important role in determining which individuals will develop an autoimmune disease. Monogenic autoimmune diseases often have a clear mechanism that is based on the importance of a single gene product in maintaining tolerance. For other diseases, multiple allelic variants have been identified, but in most cases, the precise mechanism of collective action remains unclear. Environmental factors play a significant role, as even identical twins are not always both affected by the same autoimmune disease. Influences from the environment include infections, toxins, and perhaps unknown events. The effector mechanisms operating in autoimmune diseases are the same as those employed in responses to pathogens. Although the details vary from disease to disease, both antibody and T cells can be involved, and often in the same disease.

The study of the rules of skin transplantation in mice was a major factor in understanding the rules of the normal immune responses, leading to the identification of the major histocompatibility antigens that control the response to nonself transplanted organs and tissues. Transplantation has brought on syndromes of rejection that are in many ways similar to autoimmune disease, but the targets are either major or minor histocompatibility antigens. T cells are the main effectors in graft rejection and graft-versus-host disease, although antibodies can also contribute.

For each of the undesirable responses discussed here, the question is how to control the response without adversely affecting protective immunity to infection. The answer may lie in a more complete understanding of the regulation of the immune response, especially the suppressive mechanisms important in tolerance. The deliberate control of the immune response is examined further in Chapter 16.

Discussion Questions

15.1 What kind of evidence supports the idea that a genetic predisposition contributes to the development of autoimmune diseases? For the association of certain MHC alleles with autoimmune diseases, what kind of mechanisms might explain this tendency?

15.2 Discuss the evidence that environmental conditions or infectious history may play a role in the development of autoimmunity. Give an experimental example of one infectious trigger. What examples are known in humans?

15.3 A number of different candidate genes have allelic variants that are associated with various autoimmune diseases. Describe the different ways in which these genes can contribute to perturbing the normal immune response to promote autoimmunity.

15.4 In some diseases, the immune system not only damages the target tissue but also produces systemic symptoms related to the physiology of that tissue. Give some examples of these effects.

15.5 Explain the differences in mechanisms among acute rejection, chronic rejection, and hyperacute rejection.

15.6 In some transplant situations, the recipient may have preexisting antibodies that react with the donor tissues. Give an explanation for the presence of these antibodies, and describe their possible specificity.

15.7 In a transplant situation, the allogeneic MHC molecules expressed by donor dendritic cells may be responsible for the activation of alloreactive T cells that recognize the transplanted organ by direct allorecognition. As this priming step is thought to take place in the lymph nodes or spleen, describe two routes that allow donor MHC molecules to become located in those sites.

15.8 Minor histocompatibility antigens can also be targets of T cells in a transplant situation. Describe the similarities and differences between direct allorecognition of MHC molecules and indirect allorecognition of minor histocompatibility antigens.

15.9 (a) Describe how a fetus is protected from an immune response from the mother. (b) Newborns of mothers that have certain autoimmune diseases may exhibit symptoms of the same diseases. Describe how this can occur and the possible treatments to prevent it. (c) Not all types of autoimmune diseases in the mother can affect the neonate. Explain why.

Section references.

15-1   Multiple mechanisms normally contribute to prevent autoimmunity.

Ehrlich, P., and Morgenroth, J.: **On haemolysins**, in Himmelweit, F. (ed): *The Collected Papers of Paul Ehrlich*. London: Pergamon, 1957: 246–255.

Goodnow, C.C., Sprent, J., Fazekas de St Groth, B., and Vinuesa, C.G.: **Cellular and genetic mechanisms of self tolerance and autoimmunity**. *Nature* 2005, **435**:590–597.

Hogquist, K.A., Baldwin, T.A., and Jameson, S.C.: **Central tolerance: learning self-control in the thymus**. *Nat. Rev. Immunol.* 2005, **5**:772–782.

Janeway, C.A., Jr.: **The immune system evolved to discriminate infectious nonself from noninfectious self**. *Immunol. Today* 1992, **13**:11–16.

Kappler, J.W., Roehm, N., and Marrack, P.: **T cell tolerance by clonal elimination in the thymus**. *Cell* 1987, **49**:273–280.

Kyewski, B., and Klein, L.: **A central role for central tolerance**. *Annu. Rev. Immunol.* 2006, **24**:571–606.

Mathis, D., and Benoist, C.: **Aire**. *Annu. Rev. Immunol.* 2009, **27**:287–312.

Matzinger, P.: **The danger model: a renewed sense of self**. *Science* 2002, **296**:301–305.

Nemazee, D.A., and Burki, K.: **Clonal deletion of B lymphocytes in a transgenic mouse bearing anti-MHC class-I antibody genes**. *Nature* 1989, **337**:562–566.

15-2   Lymphocytes that bind self antigens with relatively low affinity usually ignore them but in some circumstances become activated.

Hannum, L.G., Ni, D., Haberman, A.M., Weigert, M.G., and Shlomchik, M.J.: **A disease-related RF autoantibody is not tolerized in a normal mouse: implications for the origins of autoantibodies in autoimmune disease**. *J. Exp. Med.* 1996, **184**:1269–1278.

Kurts, C., Sutherland, R.M., Davey, G., Li, M., Lew, A.M., Blanas, E., Carbone, F.R., Miller, J.F., and Heath, W.R.: **CD8 T cell ignorance or tolerance to islet antigens depends on antigen dose**. *Proc. Natl. Acad. Sci. USA* 1999, **96**:12703–12707.

Marshak-Rothstein, A.: **Toll-like receptors in systemic autoimmune disease**. *Nat. Rev. Immunol.* 2006, **6**:823–835.

Shlomchik, M.J.: **Sites and stages of autoreactive B cell activation and regulation**. *Immunity* 2008, **28**:18–28.

Walport, M.J.: **Lupus, DNase and defective disposal of cellular debris**. *Nat. Genet.* 2000, **25**:135–136.

15-3   Antigens in immunologically privileged sites do not induce immune attack but can serve as targets.

Chang. G.C., and Young, L.H.: **Sympathetic ophthalmia**. *Semin. Ophthalmol.* 2011, **26**:316–320.

Croxford, A.L., Lanzinger, M., Hartmann, F.J., Schreiner, B., Mair, F., Pelczar, P., Clausen, B.E., Jung, S., Greter, M., and Becher, B.: **The cytokine GM-CSF drives the inflammatory signature of CCR2+ monocytes and licenses autoimmunity**. *Immunity* 2015, **43**:502–514.

Forrester, J.V., Xu, H., Lambe, T., and Cornall, R.: **Immune privilege or privileged immunity?** *Mucosal Immunol.* 2008, **1**:372–381.

Glatigny, S., and Bettelli, E.: **Experimental autoimmune encephalomyelitis (EAE) as animal models of multiple sclerosis (MS)**. *Cold Spring Harb. Perspect. Med.* 2018, **8**:a028977.

Mellor, A.L., and Munn, D.H.: **Creating immune privilege: active local suppression that benefits friends, but protects foes**. *Nat. Rev. Immunol.* 2008, **8**:74–80.

Simpson, E.: **A historical perspective on immunological privilege**. *Immunol. Rev.* 2006, **213**:12–22.

15-4   Autoimmune responses can be controlled at various stages by regulatory T cells.

Dasgupta, S., Dasgupta, S., and Bandyopadhyay, M.: **Regulatory B cells in infection, inflammation, and autoimmunity**. *Cell. Immunol.* 2020, **352**:104076.

Fillatreau, S., Sweenie, C.H., McGeachy, M.J., Gray, D., and Anderton, S.M.: **B cells regulate autoimmunity by provision of IL-10**. *Nat. Immunol.* 2002, **3**:944–950.

Fontenot, J.D., and Rudensky, A.Y.: A well adapted regulatory contrivance: regulatory T cell development and the forkhead family transcription factor Foxp3. *Nat. Immunol.* 2005, 6:331–337.

Izcue, A., Coombes, J.L., and Powrie, F.: Regulatory lymphocytes and intestinal inflammation. *Annu. Rev. Immunol.* 2009, 27:313–338.

Mayer, L., and Shao, L.: Therapeutic potential of oral tolerance. *Nat. Rev. Immunol.* 2004, 4:407–419.

Maynard, C.L., and Weaver, C.T.: Diversity in the contribution of interleukin-10 to T-cell-mediated immune regulation. *Immunol. Rev.* 2008, 226:219–233.

Sakaguchi, S.: Naturally arising CD4+ regulatory T cells for immunologic self-tolerance and negative control of immune responses. *Annu. Rev. Immunol.* 2004, 22:531–562.

15-5   Autoimmunity can be classified into either organ-specific or systemic disease.

Davidson, A., and Diamond, B.: Autoimmune diseases. *N. Engl. J. Med.* 2001, 345:340–350.

D'Cruz, D.P., Khamashta, M.A., and Hughes, G.R.V.: Systemic lupus erythematosus. *Lancet* 2007, 369:587–596.

Marrack, P., Kappler, J., and Kotzin, B.L.: Autoimmune disease: why and where it occurs. *Nat. Med.* 2001, 7:899–905.

Parisis, D., Chivasso, C., Perret, J., Soyfoo, M.S., and Delporte, C.: Current state of knowledge on primary Sjögren's syndrome, an autoimmune exocrinopathy. *J. Clin. Med.* 2020, 9:2299.

15-6   Multiple components of the immune system are typically recruited in autoimmune disease.

Firestein, G.S.: Evolving concepts of rheumatoid arthritis. *Nature* 2003, 423:356–361.

Lehuen, A., Diana, J., Zaccone, P., and Cooke, A.: Immune cell crosstalk in type 1 diabetes. *Nat. Rev. Immunol.* 2010, 10:501–513.

Shlomchik, M.J., and Madaio, M.P.: The role of antibodies and B cells in the pathogenesis of lupus nephritis. *Springer Semin. Immunopathol.* 2003, 24:363–375.

15-7   Chronic autoimmune disease develops through positive feedback from inflammation, inability to clear the self antigen, and a broadening of the autoimmune response.

Marshak-Rothstein, A.: Toll-like receptors in systemic autoimmune disease. *Nat. Rev. Immunol.* 2006, 6:823–835.

Nagata, S., Hanayama, R., and Kawane, K.: Autoimmunity and the clearance of dead cells. *Cell* 2010, 140:619–630.

Salato, V.K., Hacker-Foegen, M.K., Lazarova, Z., Fairley, J.A., and Lin, M.S.: Role of intramolecular epitope spreading in pemphigus vulgaris. *Clin. Immunol.* 2005, 116:54–64.

Steinman, L.: A few autoreactive cells in an autoimmune infiltrate control a vast population of nonspecific cells: a tale of smart bombs and the infantry. *Proc. Natl. Acad. Sci. USA* 1996, 93:2253–2256.

Vanderlugt, C.L., and Miller, S.D.: Epitope spreading in immune-mediated diseases: implications for immunotherapy. *Nat. Rev. Immunol.* 2002, 2:85–95.

15-8   Both antibody and effector T cells can cause tissue damage in autoimmune disease.

Naparstek, Y., and Plotz, P.H.: The role of autoantibodies in autoimmune disease. *Annu. Rev. Immunol.* 1993, 11:79–104.

Vlahakos, D., Foster, M.H., Ucci, A.A., Barrett, K.J., Datta, S.K., and Madaio, M.P.: Murine monoclonal anti-DNA antibodies penetrate cells, bind to nuclei, and induce glomerular proliferation and proteinuria *in vivo*. *J. Am. Soc. Nephrol.* 1992, 2:1345–1354.

15-9   Autoantibodies against blood cells promote their destruction.

Beardsley, D.S., and Ertem, M.: Platelet autoantibodies in immune thrombocytopenic purpura. *Transfus. Sci.* 1998, 19:237–244.

Clynes, R., and Ravetch, J.V.: Cytotoxic antibodies trigger inflammation through Fc receptors. *Immunity* 1995, 3:21–26.

Domen, R.E.: An overview of immune hemolytic anemias. *Cleve. Clin. J. Med.* 1998, 65:89–99.

15-10   The fixation of sublytic doses of complement to cells in tissues stimulates a powerful inflammatory response.

Brandt, J., Pippin, J., Schulze, M., Hansch, G.M., Alpers, C.E., Johnson, R.J., Gordon, K., and Couser, W.G.: Role of the complement membrane attack complex (C5b-9) in mediating experimental mesangioproliferative glomerulonephritis. *Kidney Int.* 1996, 49:335–343.

Hansch, G.M.: The complement attack phase: control of lysis and non-lethal effects of C5b-9. *Immunopharmacology* 1992, 24:107–117.

15-11   Autoantibodies against receptors cause disease by stimulating or blocking receptor function.

Bahn, R.S., and Heufelder, A.E.: Pathogenesis of Graves' ophthalmopathy. *N. Engl. J. Med.* 1993, 329:1468–1475.

Drachman, D.B.: Myasthenia gravis. *N. Engl. J. Med.* 1994, 330:1797–1810.

Vincent, A., Lily, O., and Palace, J.: Pathogenic autoantibodies to neuronal proteins in neurological disorders. *J. Neuroimmunol.* 1999, 100:169–180.

15-12   Autoantibodies against extracellular antigens cause inflammatory injury.

Casciola-Rosen, L.A., Anhalt, G., and Rosen, A.: Autoantigens targeted in systemic lupus erythematosus are clustered in two populations of surface structures on apoptotic keratinocytes. *J. Exp. Med.* 1994, 179:1317–1330.

Clynes, R., Dumitru, C., and Ravetch, J.V.: Uncoupling of immune complex formation and kidney damage in autoimmune glomerulonephritis. *Science* 1998, 279:1052–1054.

Kotzin, B.L.: Systemic lupus erythematosus. *Cell* 1996, 85:303–306.

Lee, R.W., and D'Cruz, D.P.: Pulmonary renal vasculitis syndromes. *Autoimmun. Rev.* 2010, 9:657–660.

Mackay, M., Stanevsky, A., Wang, T., Aranow, C., Li, M., Koenig, S., Ravetch, J.V., and Diamond, B.: Selective dysregulation of the FcγIIB receptor on memory B cells in SLE. *J. Exp. Med.* 2006, 203:2157–2164.

Xiang, Z., Cutler, A.J., Brownlie, R.J., Fairfax, K., Lawlor, K.E., Severinson, E., Walker, E.U., Manz, R.A., Tarlinton, D.M., and Smith, K.G.: FcγRIIb controls bone marrow plasma cell persistence and apoptosis. *Nat. Immunol.* 2007, 8:419–429.

15-13   T cells specific for self antigens can cause direct tissue injury and sustain autoantibody responses.

Feldmann, M., and Steinman, L.: Design of effective immunotherapy for human autoimmunity. *Nature* 2005, 435:612–619.

Frohman, E.M., Racke, M.K., and Raine, C.S.: Multiple sclerosis—the plaque and its pathogenesis. *N. Engl. J. Med.* 2006, 354:942–955.

Klareskog, L., Stolt, P., Lundberg, K., Källberg, H., Bengtsson, C., Grunewald, J., Rönnelid, J., Erlandsson Harris, H., Ulfgren, A.K., Rantapää-Dahlqvist, S., et al.: A new model for an etiology of rheumatoid arthritis: smoking may trigger HLA–DR (shared epitope)–restricted immune reactions to autoantigens modified by citrullination. *Arthritis Rheum.* 2006, 54:38–46.

Lassmann, H., van Horssen, J., and Mahad, D.: Progressive multiple sclerosis: pathology and pathogenesis. *Nat. Rev. Neurol.* 2012, 8:647–656.

Ransohoff, R.M., and Engelhardt, B.: The anatomical and cellular basis of immune surveillance in the central nervous system. *Nat. Rev. Immunol.* 2012, 12:623–635.

Zamvil, S., Nelson, P., Trotter, J., Mitchell, D., Knobler, R., Fritz, R., and Steinman, L.: T-cell clones specific for myelin basic protein induce chronic relapsing paralysis and demyelination. *Nature* 1985, **317**:355–358.

15-14 Autoimmune diseases have a strong genetic component.

Duerr, R.H., Taylor, K.D., Brant, S.R., Rioux, J.D., Silverberg, M.S., Daly, M.J., Steinhart, A.H., Abraham, C., Regueiro, M., Griffiths, A., *et al.*: A genome-wide association study identifies IL23R as an inflammatory bowel disease gene. *Science* 2006, **314**:1461–1463.

Farh, K.K.-H., Marson, A., Zhu, J., Kleinewietfeld, M., Housley, W.J., Beik, S., Shoresh, N., Whitton, H., Ryan, R.J.H., Shishkin, A.A. *et al.*: Genetic and epigenetic fine mapping of causal autoimmune disease variants. *Nature* 2014, **518**:337–343.

Fernando, M.M.A., Stevens, C.R., Walsh, E.C., De Jager, P.L., Goyette, P., Plenge, R.M., Vyse, T.J., and Rioux, J.D.: Defining the role of the MHC in autoimmunity: a review and pooled analysis. *PLoS Genet.* 2008, **4**:e1000024.

Gregersen, P.K.: Pathways to gene identification in rheumatoid arthritis: PTPN22 and beyond. *Immunol. Rev.* 2005, **204**:74–86.

Parkes, M., Cortes, A., Van Heel, D.A., and Brown, M.A.: Genetic insights into common pathways and complex relationships among immune-mediated diseases. *Nat. Rev. Genet.* 2013, **14**:661–673.

Vijayakrishnan, L., Slavik, J.M., Illés, Z., Greenwald, R.J., Rainbow, D., Greve, B., Peterson, L.B., Hafler, D.A., Freeman, G.J., Sharpe, A.H., *et al.*: An autoimmune disease-associated CTLA-4 splice variant lacking the B7 binding domain signals negatively in T cells. *Immunity* 2004, **20**:563–575.

Wakeland, E.K., Liu, K., Graham, R.R., and Behrens, T.W.: Delineating the genetic basis of systemic lupus erythematosus. *Immunity* 2001, **15**:397–408.

Xavier, R.J., and Rioux, J.D.: Genome-wide association studies: a new window into immune-mediated diseases. *Nat. Rev. Immunol.* 2008, **8**:631–643.

15-15 Monogenic defects of immune tolerance.

Anderson, M.S., Venanzi, E.S., Chen, Z., Berzins, S.P., Benoist, C., and Mathis, D.: The cellular mechanism of Aire control of T cell tolerance. *Immunity* 2005, **23**:227–239.

Bacchetta, R., Passerini, L., Gambineri, E., Dai, M., Allan, S.E., Perroni, L., Dagna-Bricarelli, F., Sartirana, C., Matthes-Martin, S., Lawitschka, A., *et al.*: Defective regulatory and effector T cell functions in patients with FOXP3 mutations. *J. Clin. Invest.* 2006, **116**:1713–1722.

Ueda, H., Howson, J.M., Esposito, L., Heward, J., Snook, H., Chamberlain, G., Rainbow, D.B., Hunter, K.M., Smith, A.N., DiGenova, G., *et al.*: Association of the T-cell regulatory gene CTLA4 with susceptibility to autoimmune disease. *Nature* 2003, **423**:506–511.

Wildin, R.S., Ramsdell, F., Peake, J., Faravelli, F., Casanova, J.L., Buist, N., Levy-Lahad, E., Mazzella, M., Goulet, O., Perroni, L., *et al.*: X-linked neonatal diabetes mellitus, enteropathy and endocrinopathy syndrome is the human equivalent of mouse scurfy. *Nat. Genet.* 2001, **27**:18–20.

15-16 MHC genes have an important role in controlling susceptibility to autoimmune disease.

Fernando, M.M.A., Stevens, C.R., Walsh, E.C., De Jager, P.L., Goyette, P., Plenge, R.M., Vyse, T.J., and Rioux, J.D.: Defining the role of the MHC in autoimmunity: a review and pooled analysis. *PLoS Genet.* 2008, **4**:e1000024.

McDevitt, H.O.: Discovering the role of the major histocompatibility complex in the immune response. *Annu. Rev. Immunol.* 2000, **18**:1–17.

Stadinski, B.D., Zhang, L., Crawford, F., Marrack, P., Eisenbarth, G.S., and Kappler, J.W.: Diabetogenic T cells recognize insulin bound to IAg7 in an unexpected, weakly binding register. *Proc. Natl. Acad. Sci. USA* 2010, **107**:10978–10983.

15-17 Genetic variants that impair innate immune responses can predispose to T cell–mediated chronic inflammatory disease.

Cadwell, K., Liu, J.Y., Brown, S.L., Miyoshi, H., Loh, J., Lennerz, J.K., Kishi, C., Kc, W., Carrero, J.A., Hunt, S., *et al.*: A key role for autophagy and the autophagy gene Atg16l1 in mouse and human intestinal Paneth cells. *Nature* 2008, **456**:259–263.

Eckmann, L., and Karin, M.: NOD2 and Crohn's disease: loss or gain of function? *Immunity* 2005, **22**:661–667.

Xavier, R.J., and Podolsky, D.K.: Unravelling the pathogenesis of inflammatory bowel disease. *Nature* 2007, **448**:427–434.

15-18 Cross-reactivity between foreign molecules on pathogens and self molecules can promote autoimmune disease.

Bach, J.F.; The hygiene hypothesis in autoimmunity: the role of pathogens and commensals. *Nat. Rev. Immunol.* 2018, **18**:105–120.

Barnaba, V., and Sinigaglia, F.: Molecular mimicry and T cell-mediated autoimmune disease. *J. Exp. Med.* 1997, **185**:1529–1531.

Rose, N.R.: Infection, mimics, and autoimmune disease. *J. Clin. Invest.* 2001, **107**:943–944.

Rose, N.R., Herskowitz, A., Neumann, D.A., and Neu, N.: Autoimmune myocarditis: a paradigm of post-infection autoimmune disease. *Immunol. Today* 1988, **9**:117–120.

Sfriso, P., Ghirardello, A., Botsios, C., Tonon, M., Zen, M., Bassi, N., Bassetto, F., and Doria, A.: Infections and autoimmunity: the multifaceted relationship. *J. Leukoc. Biol.* 2010, **87**:385–395.

15-19 Transplant rejection is mediated primarily by T-cell responses to MHC molecules.

Cornell, L.D., Smith, R.N., and Colvin, R.B.: Kidney transplantation: mechanisms of rejection and acceptance. *Annu. Rev. Pathol.* 2008, **3**:189–220.

Macdonald, W.A., Chen, Z., Gras, S., Archbold, J.K., Tynan, F.E., Clements, C.S., Bharadwaj, M., Kjer-Nielsen, L., Saunders, P.M., Wilce, M.C.J., *et al.*: T cell allorecognition via molecular mimicry. *Immunity* 2009, **31**:897–908.

Macedo, C., Orkis, E.A., Popescu, I., Elinoff, B.D., Zeevi, A., Shapiro, R., Lakkis, F.G., and Metes, D.: Contribution of naive and memory T-cell populations to the human alloimmune response. *Am. J. Transplant.* 2009, **9**:2057–2066.

Opelz, G., and Wujciak, T.: The influence of HLA compatibility on graft survival after heart transplantation. The Collaborative Transplant Study. *N. Engl. J. Med.* 1994, **330**:816–819.

Wood, K.J., and Goto, R.: Mechanisms of rejection: current perspectives. *Transplantation.* 2012, **93**:1–10.

15-20 Rejection of MHC-identical grafts is caused by peptides from other alloantigens bound to graft MHC molecules.

Agulnik, A.I, Longepied, G., Ty, M.T., Bishop, C.E., and Mitchell, M.: Mouse H-Y encoding Smcy gene and its X chromosomal homolog Smcx. *Mamm. Genome* 1999, **10**:926–929.

den Haan, J.M., Meadows, L.M., Wang, W., Pool, J., Blokland, E., Bishop, T.L., Reinhardus, C., Shabanowitz, J., Offringa, R., Hunt, D.F., *et al.*: The minor histocompatibility antigen HA-1: a diallelic gene with a single amino acid polymorphism. *Science* 1998, **279**:1054–1057.

Dierselhuis, M., and Goulmy, E.: The relevance of minor histocompatibility antigens in solid organ transplantation. *Curr. Opin. Organ Transplant.* 2009, **14**:419–425.

Mutis, T., Gillespie, G., Schrama, E., Falkenburg, J.H., Moss, P., and Goulmy, E.: Tetrameric HLA class I-minor histocompatibility antigen peptide complexes demonstrate minor histocompatibility antigen-specific cytotoxic T lymphocytes in patients with graft-versus-host disease. *Nat. Med.* 1999, **5**:839–842.

15-21 Alloreactive T cells reject transplanted organs by direct and indirect allorecognition.

Jiang, S., Herrera, O., and Lechler, R.I.: New spectrum of allorecognition pathways: implications for graft rejection and transplantation tolerance. *Curr. Opin. Immunol.* 2004, **16**:550–557.

Lakkis, F.G., Arakelov, A., Konieczny, B.T., and Inoue, Y.: Immunologic ignorance of vascularized organ transplants in the absence of secondary lymphoid tissue. *Nat. Med.* 2000, **6**:686–688.

Liu, Q., Rojas-Canales, D.M., Divito. S.J., Shufesky, W.J., Stolz, D.B., Erdos, G., Sullivan, M.L.G., Gibson, G.A., Watkins, S.C., Larregina, A.T., and Morelli, A.E.: **Donor dendritic cell-derived exosomes promote allograft-targeting immune response.** *J. Clin. Invest.* 2016, **126**:2805–2820.

Safinia, N., Afzali, B., Atalar, K., Lombardi, G., and Lechler, R.I.: **T-cell alloimmunity and chronic allograft dysfunction.** *Kidney Int.* 2010, **78**(suppl. 119):S2–S12.

15-22   Antibodies that react with endothelium cause hyperacute graft rejection.

Griesemer, A., Yamada, K., and Sykes, M.: **Xenotransplantation: immunological hurdles and progress toward tolerance.** *Immunol. Rev.* 2014, **258**:241–258.

Montgomery, R.A., Cozzi, E., West, L.J., and Warren, D.S.: **Humoral immunity and antibody-mediated rejection in solid organ transplantation.** *Semin. Immunol.* 2011, **23**:224–234.

Williams, G.M., Hume, D.M., Hudson, R.P., Jr., Morris, P.J., Kano, K., and Milgrom, F.: **'Hyperacute' renal-homograft rejection in man.** *N. Engl. J. Med.* 1968, **279**:611–618.

15-23   Late failure of transplanted organs is caused by chronic injury to the graft.

Libby, P., and Pober, J.S.: **Chronic rejection.** *Immunity* 2001, **14**:387–397.

Smith, R.N., and Colvin, R.B.: **Chronic alloantibody mediated rejection.** *Semin. Immunol.* 2012, **24**:115–121.

15-24   A variety of organs are transplanted routinely in clinical medicine.

Alamartine, E., and Maillard, N.: **Therapeutic plasma exchange in nephrology. Where it applies?** *Transfus. Apher. Sci.* 2019, **58**:262–265.

Ekser, B., Ezzelarab, M., Hara, H., van der Windt, D.J., Wijkstrom, M., Bottino, R., Trucco, M., and Cooper, D.K.C.: **Clinical xenotransplantation: the next medical revolution?** *Lancet* 2012, **379**:672–683.

Lechler, R.I., Sykes, M., Thomson, A.W., and Turka, L.A.: **Organ transplantation—how much of the promise has been realized?** *Nat. Med.* 2005, **11**:605–613.

Ricordi, C., and Strom, T.B.: **Clinical islet transplantation: advances and immunological challenges.** *Nat. Rev. Immunol.* 2004, **4**:259–268.

Sood, P., and Hariharan, S.: **Anti-CD20 blocker rituximab in kidney transplantation.** *Transplantation* 2018, **102**:44–58.

15-25   The converse of graft rejection is graft-versus-host disease.

Blazar, B.R., Murphy, W.J., and Abedi, M.: **Advances in graft-versus-host disease biology and therapy.** *Nat. Rev. Immunol.* 2012, **12**:443–458.

Ferrer, I.R., Hester, J., Bushell, A., and Wood, K.J.: **Induction of transplantation tolerance through regulatory cells: from mice to men.** *Immunol. Rev.* 2014, **258**:102–116.

Jeon, Y.W., Lim, J.Y., Im, K.I., Kim, N., Nam, Y.S., Song, Y.J., and Cho, S.G.: **Enhancement of graft-versus-host disease control efficacy by adoptive transfer of type 1 regulatory T cells in bone marrow transplant model.** *Stem Cells Dev.* 2019, **28**:129–140.

Matsuoka, K.I.: **Low-dose interleukin-2 as a modulator of Treg homeostasis after HSCT: current understanding and future perspectives.** *Int. J. Hematol.* 2018, **107**:130–137.

Shlomchik, W.D.: **Graft-versus-host disease.** *Nat. Rev. Immunol.* 2007, **7**:340–352.

Tang, Q., and Bluestone, J.A.: **Regulatory T-cell therapy in transplantation: moving to the clinic.** *Cold Spring Harb. Perspect. Med.* 2013, **3**:1–15.

Qin, S., Cobbold, S.P., Pope, H., Elliott, J., Kioussis, D., Davies, J., and Waldmann, H.: **"Infectious" transplantation tolerance.** *Science* 1993, **259**:974–977.

15-26   The fetus is an allograft that is tolerated repeatedly.

Erlebacher, A.: **Mechanisms of T cell tolerance towards the allogeneic fetus.** *Nat. Rev. Immunol.* 2013, **13**:23–33.

Samstein, R.M., Josefowicz, S.Z., Arvey, A., Treuting, P.M., and Rudensky A.Y.: **Extrathymic generation of regulatory T cells in placental mammals mitigates maternal-fetal conflict.** *Cell* 2012, **150**:29–38.

Manipulation of the Immune Response

16

At the time of this writing, the global COVID-19 (coronavirus disease-2019) pandemic provides a daily reminder of the practical importance of the field of immunology. The efforts to generate a vaccine against severe acute respiratory syndrome coronavirus 2 (SARS-CoV-2) illustrate the advances in modern vaccine design but also reveal the great challenges to vaccine development and deployment. In this chapter, we consider ways to manipulate the immune system to induce protection against pathogens and against tumors as well. We will also discuss ways to suppress unwanted immune responses, as seen with autoimmunity, allergy, and graft rejection, using conventional drugs and new 'biologic' agents.

The intentional manipulation of the immune response dates back more than 500 years to the use of variolation in China as a measure to protect against smallpox. Following Edward Jenner's experiments with cowpox vaccination in 1796, numerous vaccines and antisera against other infectious agents had been developed by the late 1800s. Many vaccines are now routinely deployed and have brought many diseases under control. It is worth commenting that many important vaccines still in use were developed before the 'modern' era of molecular immunology. More recently, techniques of molecular biology have allowed the development of biological therapeutics, or 'biologics,' which are engineered forms of natural products, such as hormones, cytokines, and monoclonal antibodies, or derivatives of these, such as engineered fusion proteins. Such products can exert extraordinary specificity; many have been used for decades, such as the hormone insulin for type 1 diabetes mellitus, but recent advances have introduced a broad array of new biologics with very precise actions on the immune system. Long-standing efforts to use the power and specificity of adaptive immunity against tumors have resulted in major advances; biologics that target regulatory pathways have made a significant impact in clinical medicine. Along with these advances has come the identification of conventional pharmaceutical agents—typically inhibitors—that allow some control over unwanted immune reactions, and they remain an important component of clinical medicine. The categories of agents used to manipulate immune responses are listed in **Fig. 16.1**. This chapter will discuss these approaches, beginning with a discussion of vaccines against infectious diseases. We will then present more recent advances in the treatment of tumors, including the use of biologics and cell-based therapies. Finally, we discuss the use of biologics and pharmaceutical agents in clinical practice to relieve unwanted immune responses.

Fighting infectious diseases with vaccination.

Improvements in sanitation and widespread vaccination introduced over the past 100 years have markedly decreased deaths caused by infectious diseases, and yet these remain major causes of death worldwide. Modern immunology itself grew from the success of Edward Jenner's and Louis Pasteur's vaccines against smallpox and chicken cholera, respectively, and its greatest triumph has been the global eradication of smallpox, announced by the World Health Organization (WHO) in 1980. The global campaign by the WHO to eradicate

Agents used to manipulate immune responses	
Type	**Example**
Radiation	
Small molecules	
Drugs	Sirolimus (rapamycin)
Adjuvants	Alum
Macromolecules	
Hormones	Cortisol
Cytokines	Interferon-α
Antibodies	Rituximab (anti-CD20 antibody)
Fusion proteins	Abatacept (CTLA-4–Ig)
DNA vaccines	(Experimental)
Subunit vaccines	Hepatitis B vaccine
Conjugate vaccines	Hib (*Haemophilus influenzae* type b) vaccine
Cells and organisms	
Inactivated vaccines	IPV (inactivated poliovirus vaccine)
Live attenuated vaccines	MMR (measles, mumps, rubella) vaccine
Adoptive cell transfer	CAR (chimeric antigen receptor) T cells
Heterologous bone marrow transplant	

Fig. 16.1 Categories of immunomodulating agents.

polio began in 1988 and has led to elimination of the endemic wild virus in all but two countries, and the spread of the mutated oral vaccine viral strains is limited to only about 20 others. With the recent progress in basic immunology, particularly in the area of innate immunity, there is hope that vaccines for other major infectious diseases, including malaria, tuberculosis, and HIV, are within reach.

The goal of vaccination is the generation of long-lasting and protective immunity. Indeed, a single infection by a pathogen is often (but not always) sufficient to generate long-lasting protective immunity. Recognition of this effect was recorded more than 2000 years ago in accounts of the Peloponnesian War, during which two successive outbreaks of plague struck Athens. The Greek historian Thucydides noted that people who had survived infection during the first outbreak were not susceptible to infection during the second. Perhaps this recognition was what prompted the practice of **variolation** against smallpox, in which a small amount of dried material from a smallpox pustule of an infected individual was used to produce a mild infection in an uninfected individual that was then followed by long-lasting protection against reinfection. Smallpox itself has been recognized in medical literature for more than 1000 years; variolation seems to have been practiced in India and China many centuries before its introduction into the West (sometime in the 1400s to 1500s), and its practice was familiar to Jenner. However, infection after variolation was not always mild: fatal smallpox occurred in about 3% of cases, and this rate of complication would clearly not meet modern criteria of drug safety. It appears there was some recognition that milkmaids exposed to a bovine virus similar to smallpox—cowpox—seemed to be protected from smallpox infection, and there is even one historical account suggesting that cowpox inoculation had been tried before Jenner. However, Jenner's achievement was not simply the realization that infection with cowpox would provide protective immunity against smallpox in humans without the risk of significant disease, but also its experimental proof by the intentional subsequent variolation of people whom he had previously vaccinated. He named the process **vaccination** (from *vacca*, Latin for 'cow'), and Pasteur, in his honor, extended the term to the stimulation of protection against other infectious agents. Humans are not a natural host of cowpox, which establishes only a brief and limited subcutaneous infection. But the cowpox virus contains antigens that stimulate an immune response that cross-reacts with smallpox antigens and thereby confers protection against the human disease. Since the early 20th century, the virus used to vaccinate against smallpox has been vaccinia virus, which is related to both cowpox and smallpox, but whose origin is obscure.

As we will see, many current vaccines offer protection by inducing the formation of neutralizing antibodies. However, that statement contains a hidden tautology; pathogens for which current vaccines are effective may also be pathogens for which antibodies are sufficient for protection. For several major pathogens—malaria, tuberculosis, and HIV—even a robust antibody response is not sufficient to be fully protective. The elimination of these pathogens requires additional effector activities, such as the generation of strong and durable cell-mediated immunity, which are not efficiently generated by current vaccine technologies. These are the issues that face modern vaccine scientists.

16-1 Vaccines can be based on attenuated pathogens or material from killed organisms.

Vaccine development in the early part of the 20th century followed two empirical approaches. The first was the search for **attenuated** organisms (that is, those with reduced pathogenicity), which would stimulate protective immunity but not cause disease. This approach continues into the present with the design of genetically attenuated pathogens in which desirable mutations are introduced into the organism by recombinant DNA technologies. This idea is being applied to important pathogens, such as malaria, for which vaccines are currently unavailable, and may be important in the future for designing vaccines for influenza and HIV.

The second approach was the development of vaccines that were based on killed organisms and, subsequently, on purified components of organisms that would be as effective as live whole organisms. Killed vaccines were desirable because live vaccines, including vaccinia, have the risk of causing lethal systemic infection in immunosuppressed people or mutating and gaining the ability to spread or cause more virulent disease. Use of killed organisms as vaccines led to the development of conjugate vaccines composed of a mixture of purified antigens, as described below for *Haemophilus influenzae* (see Section 16-7). This evolution continues with the use of 'reverse immunogenetics' (see Section 16-12) to identify candidate peptide antigens for T cells and with strategies to use ligands that activate Toll-like receptors (TLRs) or other innate sensors as adjuvants to enhance responses to simple antigens.

Immunization based on these approaches is now considered so safe and so important that most states in the United States require all children to be immunized against several potentially deadly diseases (**Fig. 16.2**). These include the viral diseases measles, mumps, and polio, for which live-attenuated vaccines are used, and the bacterial diseases tetanus (caused by *Clostridium tetani*), diphtheria (caused by *Corynebacterium diphtheriae*), and whooping cough (caused by *Bordetella pertussis*), for which vaccines composed of inactivated toxins, or **toxoids**, prepared from the respective bacteria are used. More recently, a vaccine has become available against *Haemophilus influenzae* type b (Hib), one of the causative agents of meningitis, as well as two vaccines for childhood diarrhea caused by rotaviruses, and, as described in Section 16-20, a vaccine for preventing HPV infection for protection against cervical cancer. Most vaccines are given to children within the first year of life. The vaccines against measles, mumps, and rubella (MMR), against chickenpox (varicella), and against influenza, when recommended, are usually given between the ages of 1 and 2 years.

There still are many important infectious diseases for which we lack effective vaccines (**Fig. 16.3**). In some cases, natural infection with the pathogen does not seem to generate protective immunity, allowing for recurrent or chronic infections. In infections of this type, which include malaria, tuberculosis, and HIV, the antibodies that are produced are insufficient to prevent reinfection and to eliminate the pathogen or provide full immunity. Instead, these infections rely more on cell-mediated immunity to limit the pathogen. So it is not the absence of an antibody response to the pathogen that is the problem, but rather that this response does not clear the pathogen, eliminate pathogenesis, or prevent reinfection.

For vaccines that are used effectively in developed countries, such as that against measles, technical and economic problems can prevent widespread use in developing countries, where mortality from the diseases may still be significant. For example, the costs of storage and deployment can be significant barriers to the use of existing vaccines in poorer countries. Therefore, vaccine development remains an important goal of immunology. The latter half of the 20th century saw a shift to approaches that are based on molecular understanding of microbial pathogenicity, of the nature of protective host responses, and of the regulation of effective T- and B-lymphocyte responses.

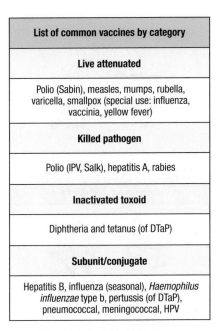

List of common vaccines by category
Live attenuated
Polio (Sabin), measles, mumps, rubella, varicella, smallpox (special use: influenza, vaccinia, yellow fever)
Killed pathogen
Polio (IPV, Salk), hepatitis A, rabies
Inactivated toxoid
Diphtheria and tetanus (of DTaP)
Subunit/conjugate
Hepatitis B, influenza (seasonal), *Haemophilus influenzae* type b, pertussis (of DTaP), pneumococcal, meningococcal, HPV

Fig. 16.2 List of common vaccines by category.

Some infections for which effective vaccines are not yet available	
Disease	**Estimated annual mortality**
Malaria	618,248
Schistosomiasis	21,797
Intestinal worm infestation	3,304
Tuberculosis	934,879
Diarrheal disease	1,497,724
Respiratory infections	3,060,837
HIV/AIDS	1,533,760

Fig. 16.3 Diseases for which effective vaccines are still needed. Mortality data are the most recent estimated figures available (2014).

Neutralization

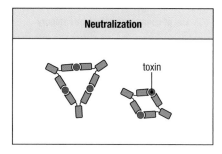

toxin

Antibodies against adhesins block colonization and uptake

Opsonization

Macrophage   bacterium

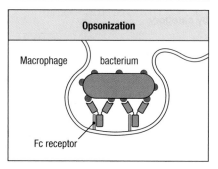

Fc receptor

Antibody blocks binding to virus receptor and can also block fusion event

Fig. 16.4 Mechanisms of protection by antibodies. Antibodies induced by vaccines provide protection in several ways. Antibodies may neutralize toxins produced by pathogens and prevent the damage that they cause (top panel). Antibodies against bacteria can prevent infection of cells by blocking their colonization and uptake into cells (second panel) and also can enhance the destruction of bacteria through opsonization by macrophages and neutrophils (third panel). Antibodies can neutralize viruses by binding to viral proteins that mediate cellular binding and uptake through fusion of the viral and cell membranes (bottom panel) and by mediating their destruction by complement lysis, opsonization, and phagocytosis (not shown).

16-2 Most effective vaccines generate antibodies that prevent damage caused by toxins or that neutralize pathogens and stop infection.

Although the requirements for generating protective immunity vary with the nature of the infecting organism, many effective vaccines currently work by inducing antibodies against the pathogen or its products (**Fig. 16.4**) For many pathogens, including extracellular organisms and viruses, antibodies can provide protective immunity. This is not the case for all pathogens, unfortunately. Protection against some pathogens may require additional cell-mediated immune responses such as those mediated by CD8 T cells.

In some cases, effective protective immunity against microorganisms requires preexisting antibody at the time of infection. Preexisting antibody can be required to prevent the damage caused by certain pathogens or toxins they produce, as illustrated by vaccines against tetanus and diphtheria. In these infections, the clinical manifestations are primarily caused by extremely powerful exotoxins (see Fig. 10.31). Preexisting antibody against the exotoxin is necessary to prevent the actions of these toxins. Indeed, the tetanus exotoxin is so powerful that the tiny amount that can cause disease may be insufficient to lead to a protective immune response; consequently, even survivors of tetanus require vaccination to be protected against the risk of subsequent attack.

In other cases, preexisting antibodies can protect by preventing infection for a second time by the same pathogen, as in the case of certain viral infections. While CD8 T cells are able to kill cells that are already infected by virus, preexisting antibodies are able to prevent the infection of cells. This action is called **neutralization**. The ability of an antibody to neutralize a pathogen may depend on its affinity, its isotype subclass, complement, and the activity of phagocytic cells. For example, preexisting antibodies are required to protect against the poliovirus, which infects critical host cells very soon after entering the body. This infection is not easily controlled by T lymphocytes once intracellular infection has been established. Vaccines against seasonal influenza virus provide protection in this same manner, by inducing antibodies that reduce the chance of a second infection by the same strain of influenza. For many viruses, antibodies produced by an infection or by vaccination can neutralize the virus and prevent further spread of infection, but this is not always the case. In HIV infection, despite the generation of antibodies that can bind to surface viral epitopes, most of these antibodies fail to neutralize the virus. In addition, HIV has many different strains, or clades, and most vaccines based on HIV proteins do not induce antibodies that neutralize all clades, presenting a challenge for effective vaccine design. Recent work has identified broadly neutralizing antibodies that can recognize multiple HIV clades and bind to conserved regions of the HIV envelope protein that are unlikely to mutate away under negative selection *in vivo*. One interesting vaccine strategy aims to design antigens that induce antibodies specifically against such conserved epitopes, thus inducing a natural broadly neutralizing antibody response (see Section 13-35 and Fig. 13.36).

Antibodies produced against infectious agents usually are directed at multiple epitopes, and only some of these antibodies, if any, confer protection. The antigen epitopes recognized by T cells can affect the nature of the antibody response. In Section 10-2, we described **linked recognition**, in which antigen-specific B cells and T cells provide mutually activating signals, leading to affinity maturation and isotype switching that may be required for neutralization. Linked recognition requires that B cells present an appropriate peptide epitope to T cells, and typically this epitope is contained within the region of the protein epitope recognized by the B cell. This requirement must be considered in modern vaccine design. Indeed, the predominant antigen epitope recognized by T cells after vaccination with respiratory syncytial virus induces a vigorous inflammatory response but fails to elicit neutralizing antibodies and thus causes pathology without protection.

16-3 Effective vaccines must induce long-lasting protection while being safe and inexpensive.

A successful vaccine must possess several features in addition to its ability to provoke a protective immune response (Fig. 16.5). First, it must be safe. Vaccines must be given to huge numbers of people, relatively few of whom are likely to die of, or sometimes even catch, the disease that the vaccine is designed to prevent. This means even a low level of toxicity is unacceptable. Second, the vaccine must be able to produce protective immunity in a very high proportion of the people to whom it is given. Third, particularly in poorer countries where it is impracticable to give regular 'booster' vaccinations to dispersed rural populations, a successful vaccine must generate long-lived immunological memory. This means the vaccine must prime both B and T lymphocytes. Fourth, vaccines must be very cheap if they are to be administered to large populations. Vaccines are one of the most cost-effective measures in health care, but this benefit is eroded as the cost per dose rises.

Another benefit of an effective vaccination program is the '**herd immunity**' that it confers on the general population. By lowering the number of susceptible members in the population, vaccination decreases the natural reservoir of infected individuals in that population and so reduces the probability of transmission of infection. Thus, even unvaccinated individuals will be provided with some degree of protection because their chance of encountering the pathogen is decreased. However, the effect of such herd immunity is seen only at relatively high levels of vaccination within a population; for mumps, the necessary level is estimated to be around 80%, and below this level sporadic epidemics can occur. This is illustrated by a marked increase in mumps in the United Kingdom in 2004 to 2005 in young adults as a result of the variable use in the mid-1990s of a measles/rubella vaccine rather than the combined MMR, as the combined vaccine was in short supply at that time.

Finally, as we discuss in detail later, a vaccine must be perceived by the general population as being safe, so that it will be adopted by sufficient numbers of people to protect susceptible individuals and achieve herd immunity.

Features of effective vaccines	
Safe	Vaccine must not itself cause illness or death
Protective	Vaccine must protect against illness resulting from exposure to live pathogen
Gives sustained protection	Protection against illness must last for several years
Induces neutralizing antibody	Some pathogens (such as polio virus) infect cells that cannot be replaced (e.g., neurons). Neutralizing antibody is essential to prevent infection of such cells
Induces protective T cells	Some pathogens, particularly intracellular, are more effectively dealt with by cell-mediated responses
Practical considerations	Low cost per dose Biological stability Ease of administration Few side-effects
Perceived as safe	The perception of whether a vaccine is safe will influence the adoption by the public

Fig. 16.5 **There are several criteria for an effective vaccine.**

16-4 Live-attenuated viral vaccines are usually more potent than 'killed' vaccines.

Most antiviral vaccines currently in use consist of either live-attenuated viruses or inactivated viruses (see Fig. 16.2). Inactivated, or 'killed,' viral vaccines consist of viruses treated so that they are unable to infect and replicate within host cells. Because peptides from the viral antigens are not produced within host cells, CD8 T-cell responses rely solely on cross-presentation of the antigenic protein material given with the killed vaccine. As a consequence, CD8 T-cell responses are less strongly induced with killed-virus vaccines than with live-attenuated vaccines, but with killed-virus vaccines, CD8 T cells are not required to eliminate a vaccine-derived viral infection. Live-attenuated viral vaccines are generally far more potent, because they activate cytotoxic CD8 T cells as well as CD4 T cells that help to shape the antibody response for the vaccine's subsequent protective effect. Cytotoxic CD8 T cells provide protection while infection by the virus itself is under way and, if maintained, may contribute to protective memory. Attenuated live viral vaccines include the routine childhood vaccines in use for polio, measles, mumps, rubella, and varicella (see Fig. 16.2). Other attenuated live viral vaccines that are licensed for special circumstances or for use in high-risk populations include influenza, poxvirus (vaccinia), and yellow fever virus.

Traditionally, attenuation is achieved by growing the virus in cultured cells. In this process, a series of mutations accumulate in the viral genome. Viruses are

Fig. 16.6 Viruses are traditionally attenuated by selecting for growth in nonhuman cells. To produce an attenuated virus, the virus must first be isolated by growing it in cultured human cells. The adaptation to growth in cultured human cells can cause some attenuation in itself; the rubella vaccine, for example, was made in this way. In general, however, the virus is then adapted to growth in cells of a different species, until it grows only poorly in human cells. The adaptation is a result of mutation, usually a combination of several point mutations. It is usually difficult to tell which of the mutations in the genome of an attenuated viral stock are critical to attenuation. An attenuated virus will grow poorly in the human host and will therefore produce immunity but not disease.

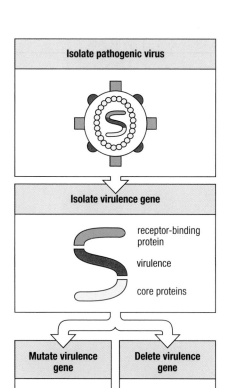

usually selected for preferential growth in nonhuman cells and, in the course of selection, become less able to grow in human cells (**Fig. 16.6**). Because these attenuated strains replicate poorly in human hosts, they induce immunity but not disease. Although attenuated virus strains contain multiple mutations in genes encoding several of their proteins, it might be possible for a pathogenic virus strain to reemerge by a further series of mutations. For example, the type 3 Sabin polio vaccine strain differs from a wild-type progenitor strain at only 10 of 7429 nucleotides. On extremely rare occasions, reversion of the vaccine to a neurovirulent strain can occur, causing paralytic disease in the unfortunate recipient.

Live-attenuated viral vaccines can also pose particular risks to immunodeficient recipients, in whom they often behave as virulent opportunistic infections. Immunodeficient infants who are vaccinated with live-attenuated poliovirus before their inherited immunoglobulin deficiencies have been diagnosed are at risk because they cannot clear the virus from their gut, and there is therefore an increased chance that mutations associated with the continuing uncontrolled replication of the virus in the gut will revert the virus to a virulent form and lead to fatal paralytic disease.

16-5 Live-attenuated viral vaccines can be made safer by the use of recombinant DNA technology.

While an empirical approach to attenuation is still in use, recombinant DNA technology provides additional ways to attenuate viruses for use as vaccines. In one approach, *de novo* attenuation of a virus could be achieved by mutating or deleting specific genes required for viral virulence (**Fig. 16.7**). This approach might be useful in developing live influenza vaccines. As described in Chapter 13, the influenza virus can reinfect the same host several times,

Fig. 16.7 Attenuation can be achieved more rapidly and reliably with recombinant DNA techniques. If a gene that is required for virulence but not for growth or immunogenicity can be identified in the virus, this gene can multiply either mutated (left lower panel) or deleted from the genome (right lower panel) by using recombinant DNA techniques. This procedure creates an avirulent (nonpathogenic) virus that can be used as a vaccine. The mutations in the virulence gene are usually large, so that it is very difficult for the virus to revert to the wild type.

because it undergoes antigenic shift and thus predominantly escapes the original immune response. The weak protection conferred by previous infections with a different influenza subtype is called **heterosubtypic immunity** and is observed in adults but not in children. The current approach to vaccination against influenza is to use a killed-virus vaccine that is reformulated annually on the basis of the prevalent strains of virus. The vaccine is moderately effective, reducing mortality in elderly people and illness in healthy adults. The ideal influenza vaccine would be an attenuated live organism that matched the prevalent virus strain. This could be created by first introducing a series of attenuating mutations into the gene encoding a viral polymerase protein, PB2. The mutated gene segment from the attenuated virus could then be substituted for the wild-type gene in a virus carrying the relevant **hemagglutinin** and **neuraminidase** antigen variants of the current epidemic or pandemic strain. Alternatively, broadly neutralizing antibodies that block the receptor-binding domain of the hemagglutinin can be generated in humans and could be used as a universal vaccine. Public attention has recently been directed toward the possibility of a flu pandemic caused by the **H5N1 avian flu** strain. This strain can be passed between birds and humans and is associated with a high mortality rate; however, a pandemic would occur only if human-to-human transmission could occur. A live-attenuated vaccine would be used only if a pandemic occurred, because to give it beforehand would introduce new influenza virus genes that might recombine with existing influenza viruses.

In some countries, polio infections are increasing because of the spread of certain vaccine strains of poliovirus, particularly type 2 oral vaccine. This so-called **circulating vaccine-derived poliovirus (cVDPV)** is caused by reversion mutations in the vaccine strain that enhance its replication. Once such a reversion mutation occurs in a vaccinated individual, it can spread by the usual fecal–oral route as with wild-type poliovirus, thus allowing it to spread within unvaccinated populations. Recombinant DNA technology is being applied in this setting to create new vaccine strains that cannot undergo such reversion mutations. For example, the type 2 Sabin vaccine strain had desirable mutations that reduced the stability of an RNA stem–loop structure in the 5′ untranslated region (5′ UTR), called domain V (*domV*), which reduced viral replication compared to that of wild polio strains. However, it was possible for the stem–loop's stability to be restored, and thus for viral replication to be increased, with only a single base-pair mutation. Such changes are called 'gatekeeper' mutations, because they increase the chance that the vaccine strain may acquire other mutations that increase viral virulence. A candidate vaccine has been made with a *domV* sequence such that no single nucleotide mutation can enhance stem–loop stability, thus reducing the chance for gatekeeper mutations to occur (**Fig. 16.8**). This vaccine is being tested by the World Health Organization in countries where cVDPV is present.

16-6 Vaccines against bacteria or parasites can be developed using nonpathogenic or disabled bacteria or genetically attenuated parasites (GAPs).

The most important example of an attenuated bacterial vaccine is the bacillus Calmette-Guérin (BCG) vaccine, which is quite effective at protecting against serious disseminated tuberculosis in children but is not protective against adult pulmonary tuberculosis. The current BCG vaccine, which remains the most widely used vaccine in the world, was obtained from a pathogenic isolate of *Mycobacterium bovis* and passaged in a laboratory at the beginning of the 20th century. Since then, several genetically diverse strains of BCG have evolved. The level of protection afforded by the BCG vaccine is extremely variable, ranging from none in some countries, such as Malawi, to 50–80% in the United Kingdom.

Fig. 16.8 Engineering a stable poliovirus vaccine strain that is resistant to reversion to neurovirulence. Top panel: The poliovirus genome encodes several capsid proteins (capsid) and several nonstructural proteins involved in protein processing and replication. Protein translation of the poliovirus positive-strand RNA genome is carried out by ribosomes that initiate at an internal ribosomal entry site, or IRES, formed in part by an RNA stem–loop called domain V (*domV*). Left panel: A major determinant of attenuation of the type 2 oral Sabin live viral vaccines is a mutation, 481G of wild polio to 481A (red), in *domV* of the vaccine strain. This mutation reduces stem–loop stability, impairing IRES function and reducing the virulence of the vaccine virus. However, in the original type 2 oral Sabin vaccines, stem–loop stability can be regained by a single nucleotide mutation back to 481G in *domV*, increasing the neurovirulence of revertant viruses. Right panel: In an engineered vaccine, S15, the *domV* stem–loop is redesigned to reduce its stability by the introduction of many alternative changes (shown in red), while keeping the original 481G nucleotide (red) of the wild polio sequence. By spreading the instability of the stem–loop over many nucleotide changes, no single nucleotide mutation can cause a full stabilization of the stem–loop, thus reducing the chance of reversion of the vaccine to a virulent form. OPV, oral polio vaccine.

Considering that tuberculosis remains one of the biggest killers worldwide, there is an urgent need for a new vaccine. Two recombinant BCG (rBCG) vaccines intended to prevent infection in unexposed individuals recently passed Phase I clinical trials. One was engineered to overexpress an immunodominant antigen of *M. tuberculosis*, to engender greater specificity toward the human pathogen. A second expresses the pore-forming protein listeriolysin from *Listeria monocytogenes* to induce the passage of BCG antigens from phagosomes into the cytoplasm and allow cross-presentation (see Section 6-5) on MHC class I molecules, thereby stimulating BCG-specific cytotoxic T cells.

A similar approach is being used to generate new vaccines for malaria. Analysis of different stages of *Plasmodium falciparum*, the major cause of fatal malaria, identified genes that are selectively expressed in sporozoites within the mosquito's salivary gland, where they first become infectious for human hepatocytes. Deletion of two such genes from the *P. falciparum* genome rendered sporozoites incapable of establishing a blood-stage infection in mice, yet capable of inducing an immune response that protected mice from subsequent infection by wild-type *P. falciparum*. This protection was dependent on CD8 T cells, and to some extent on IFN-γ, indicating that cell-mediated immunity is important for protection against this parasite (**Fig. 16.9**). This highlights once again the importance of being able to generate vaccines that are capable of inducing strong cell-mediated immunity.

16-7 Conjugate vaccines rely on linked recognition between T and B cells.

Many bacteria have an outer capsule composed of polysaccharides that are species- and type-specific for particular strains of the bacterium. Such bacteria include *Neisseria meningitidis* (meningococcus), *Streptococcus pneumoniae*

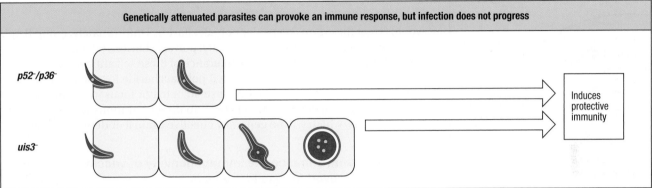

Fig. 16.9 Genetically attenuated parasites can be engineered as live vaccines to provide protective immunity. Top panel: Wild-type *Plasmodium* sporozoites transmitted through the bite of an infected mosquito enter the bloodstream and are carried to the liver, where they infect hepatocytes. Each sporozoite multiplies in the liver, killing the infected cell and releasing thousands of merozoites, the next stage in infection. Bottom panel: In mice immunized with sporozoites with targeted disruption of key genes [for example, *p52* and *p36* (*p52⁻/p36⁻*) or *uis3* (*uis3⁻*)], the sporozoites circulate in the bloodstream and mimic an early infection but cannot establish a productive infection in the liver. The mice do, however, produce an immune response against the sporozoites and are protected against a subsequent infection by wild-type sporozoites.

(pneumococcus), and *Haemophilus influenzae*. The most effective defense against these microorganisms is opsonization of the polysaccharide coat with antibody. The aim of vaccination for these organisms is therefore to elicit antibodies against the polysaccharide capsules of the bacteria. However, effective acellular vaccines cannot be made from a single isolated constituent of a microorganism, because generation of an effective antibody response requires the participation of several types of cells, and this fact has led to the development of **conjugate vaccines** (**Fig. 16.10**).

Capsular polysaccharides can be harvested from bacterial growth medium and, because they are T cell–independent antigens (see Section 10-1), they can be used on their own as vaccines. However, young children under the age of 2 years cannot make good T cell–independent antibody responses and cannot be vaccinated effectively with polysaccharide (PS) vaccines. An efficient way of overcoming this problem is to conjugate bacterial polysaccharides chemically to protein carriers (see Fig. 16.10). This carrier protein provides peptides that can be recognized by antigen-specific T cells, thus converting a T cell–independent response into a T cell–dependent antipolysaccharide antibody response. Using this approach, various conjugate vaccines have been developed against *H. influenzae* type b, an important cause of serious childhood chest infections and meningitis, and against *N. meningitidis* serogroup C, an important cause of meningitis, and these are now widely applied. The success of the latter vaccine in the United Kingdom is illustrated in **Fig. 16.11**, which shows that the incidence of meningitis C has been markedly reduced in comparison with meningitis B, against which there is currently no vaccine. Endemic meningitis B is due to diverse serogroup B strains, so an ideal vaccine

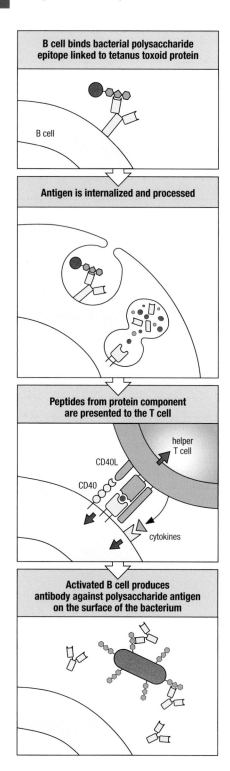

B cell binds bacterial polysaccharide epitope linked to tetanus toxoid protein

B cell

Antigen is internalized and processed

Peptides from protein component are presented to the T cell

helper T cell

CD40L

CD40

cytokines

Activated B cell produces antibody against polysaccharide antigen on the surface of the bacterium

Fig. 16.10 Conjugate vaccines take advantage of linked recognition to boost B-cell responses against polysaccharide antigens. The Hib vaccine against *Haemophilus influenzae* type b is a conjugate of bacterial polysaccharide and the tetanus toxoid protein. The B cell recognizes and binds the polysaccharide, internalizes and degrades the whole conjugate, and then displays toxoid-derived peptides on surface MHC class II molecules. Then, the helper T cells generated in response to earlier vaccination against the toxoid recognize the peptide:MHC complex on the B-cell surface, and this recognition by the T-cell receptor delivers a signal (red arrow) that leads to expression of surface CD40 ligand (CD40L) and the production of cytokines by the T cell. CD40L on the T cell then can engage CD40 on the B cells, and this interaction produces signals downstream of CD40 (red arrows). These, together with signals from cytokine receptors, activate the B cell to produce antibody to antipolysaccharide. This antibody can then protect against infection with *H. influenzae* type b.

would target the group B capsular polysaccharide. Unfortunately, group B polysaccharide is identical to some polysialyl polysaccharides on human cells and is poorly immunogenic because of tolerance of these self antigens. Some strategies to chemically modify the group B polysaccharide for use in a conjugate vaccine have been considered, but, instead, a major focus in group B meningococcal vaccine development has been to direct immunity against noncapsular antigens, which will be generally effective against endemic disease.

16-8 Adjuvants enhance the immunogenicity of vaccines, but few are approved for use in humans.

Vaccines that are based on peptides or purified proteins require additional components to mimic how real infections activate immunity. Such components of a vaccine are known as **adjuvants**, which are defined as substances that enhance the immunogenicity of antigens (see Appendix I, Section A-1). For example, tetanus toxoid is not immunogenic in the absence of adjuvants, and so tetanus toxoid vaccines contain inorganic aluminum salts (**alum**) in the form of noncrystalline gels that bind polyvalently to the toxoid by ionic interactions. Pertussis toxin has adjuvant properties in its own right and, when given mixed as a toxoid with tetanus and diphtheria toxoids, it not only protects against whooping cough but also acts as an additional adjuvant for the other two toxoids. This mixture makes up the DTaP triple vaccine given to infants in the first year of life.

The antigenic components and adjuvants in a vaccine are not approved for use on their own; they are approved only in the context of the specific vaccine in which they are formulated. At present, there are relatively few adjuvants approved by the U.S. Food and Drug Administration (FDA) for use in human vaccines marketed in the United States (**Fig. 16-12**). Alum is the common name for certain inorganic aluminum salts, of which aluminum hydroxide and aluminum phosphate are most frequently used as adjuvants. Monophosphoryl lipid A (MPL) is combined with alum for use in Cervarix, a vaccine against human papilloma virus isotypes 16 and 18, which are associated with a risk for cervical cancer, although this vaccine is no longer marketed in the United States. In Europe, in addition to the alum adjuvants, an oil (squalene)-in-water emulsion called **MF-59** is used as an adjuvant in a formulation of influenza vaccine and was approved for this use by the FDA in 2020. Alum seems to act as an adjuvant by stimulating one of the innate immune system's bacterial sensor mechanisms, **NLRP3**, thus activating the inflammasome and the inflammatory reactions that are a prerequisite for an effective adaptive immune response.

Several other adjuvants are widely used experimentally in animals but are not approved for use in humans. Many of these are sterile constituents of bacteria, particularly their cell walls. **Freund's complete adjuvant** is an oil-in-water emulsion containing killed mycobacteria. The peptidoglycan muramyl dipeptide and the glycolipid trehalose dimycolate (TDM) found in mycobacterial

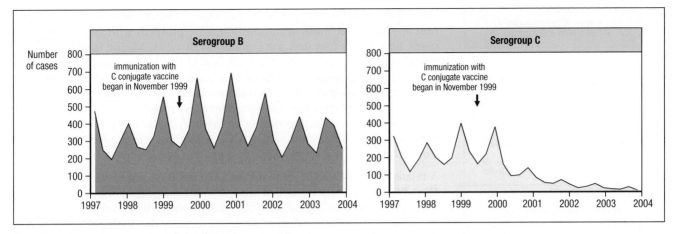

Fig. 16.11 The effect of vaccination against group *C Neisseria meningitidis* (meningococcus) on the number of cases of group B and group C meningococcal disease in England and Wales. Meningococcal infection affects roughly 5 in 100,000 people a year in the United Kingdom, with groups B and C meningococci accounting for almost all the cases. Before the introduction of the meningitis C vaccine, group C disease was the second most common cause of meningococcal disease, accounting for about 40% of cases. Group C disease now accounts for less than 10% of cases, with group B disease accounting for more than 80% of cases. After the introduction of the vaccine, there was a significant decrease in the number of laboratory-confirmed cases of group C disease in all age groups. The impact was greatest in the immunized groups, with reductions of more than 90% in these groups. An impact has also been seen in the unimmunized age groups, with a reduction of about 70%, suggesting that this vaccine has had a herd immunity effect.

cell walls contain much of the adjuvant activity of the whole killed organism. Other bacterial adjuvants include killed *Bordetella pertussis*, bacterial polysaccharides, bacterial heat-shock proteins, and bacterial DNA. Many of these adjuvants cause quite marked inflammation and are not suitable for use in vaccines for humans.

Many adjuvants seem to work by triggering viral and bacterial sensor pathways, such as the TLR and NOD-like receptor families expressed by various innate immune cells, such as dendritic cells that activate naive T cells (see Chapter 3). The TLR-4 agonist **lipopolysaccharide (LPS)** has adjuvant effects, but its use is limited by its toxicity. Small amounts of injected LPS can induce a state of shock and systemic inflammation that mimics Gram-negative sepsis, raising the question whether its adjuvant effect can be separated from its toxic effects. Monophosphoryl lipid A, an LPS derivative and TLR-4 ligand, partly achieves this by retaining adjuvant effects but being associated with much lower toxicity than that of LPS. Both unmethylated CpG dinucleotides, which activate TLR-9, and **imiquimod**, a small-molecule drug that acts as a TLR-7 agonist, can provide adjuvant activity experimentally, but neither is approved as an adjuvant in human vaccines.

16-9 Protective immunity can be induced by RNA- and DNA-based vaccination.

When bacterial plasmids were used to express proteins *in vivo* for gene therapy, some were found to stimulate an immune response. Later, it was found that DNA encoding a viral immunogen, when injected intramuscularly in mice, induced antibody responses and cytotoxic T cells that could protect against subsequent infection from the live virus. This response does not seem to damage the muscle tissue, is safe and effective, and, because it uses only a single microbial gene or a stretch of DNA encoding sets of antigenic peptides, does not carry the risk of active infection. This procedure, termed **DNA vaccination**, can be carried out in various ways. In one approach, DNA coated onto minute metal particles is administered by a 'gene gun,' so that particles penetrate the skin and potentially some underlying muscle, but other approaches, such as

Adjuvants used in FDA-approved vaccines	
Adjuvant	**Vaccine**
Alum (various aluminum salts)	Diphtheria/tetanus/ whooping cough Pneumococcal conjugate vaccine
Aluminum hydroxide	Cervarix
D,L-alpha-tocopherol (vitamin E) and squalene	H5N1 influenza vaccine
Squalene and water emulsion	Fluad (seasonal influenza vaccine)
CpG 1018 (synthetic DNA)	Hepatitis vaccine (Heplisav-B)
Quillaja saponaria (lipid from evergreen tree)	Shingrix (shingles vaccine for elderly)

Fig. 16.12 Adjuvants used in FDA-approved vaccines. Adjuvants are not individually approved for use in the same way as conventional drugs. Rather, adjuvants are tested in combination with specific vaccines and are approved for use in that configuration.

mRNA synthesized encoding SARS-CoV-2 viral spike protein

spike protein SARS-CoV-2

lipid carrier

mRNA encoding spike protein

mRNA injected intramuscularly

Viral spike protein synthesized within transfected muscle cells

Immune response to viral spike protein produces neutralizing antibodies

Fig. 16.13 RNA-based vaccines are being developed for COVID-19. Until 2020, there were no approved vaccines based on mRNA. The COVID-19 pandemic and the urgency for a vaccine has led to design and clinical testing of at least two RNA-based vaccines directed against the SARS-CoV-2 viral spike protein. In some configurations, mRNA produced *in vitro* is encapsulated in a lipid-based carrier and injected intramuscularly. Fusion of the lipid carrier with muscle cells releases the mRNA into the cells' cytoplasm, where it directs the translation of the spike protein, inducing an immune response and resulting in antibody response against the spike protein.

electroporation, are also possible. Because of DNA's stability, DNA vaccination is suitable for mass immunization. One problem with DNA-based vaccines, however, is that they are comparatively weak. Mixing in plasmids that encode cytokines such as IL-12, IL-23, or GM-CSF makes immunization with genes encoding protective antigens much more effective. In DNA vaccination, the antigen is produced by cells that are directly transfected, such as skin or muscle, but CD8 T-cell activation requires cross-presentation of the antigen by dendritic cells. Current approaches are identifying how best to transfect DNA into these dendritic-cell populations. DNA vaccines are being tested in human trials for malaria, influenza, HIV infection, and breast cancer.

A related approach to vaccine design involves RNA-based vaccines. As with DNA-based vaccines, the idea of using RNA to express the antigens in a vaccine is not new and dates back at least 20 years. However, this platform for vaccination has received a great deal of attention recently due to the COVID-19 pandemic. As of this writing, at least two RNA-based vaccines against SARS-CoV-2 have succeeded in clinical trials and are authorized for use in the general population. Like DNA-based vaccines, RNA vaccines are introduced into muscle cells, which then produce the encoded proteins. While inflammation caused by this process may serve as an adjuvant, the lipids selected to encapsulate the RNA also appear to exert a direct adjuvant effect, by activation of an inflammasome pathway, to enhance production of antibodies against the encoded proteins. The antigens encoded by the RNA vaccines against SARS-CoV-2 are forms of the coronavirus spike protein, which is bound to the viral membrane and serves to bind to host cellular receptors to initiate infection (**Fig. 16.13**). The receptor for this spike protein is the human angiotensin-converting enzyme 2 (ACE2), a membrane protein expressed by lung epithelial cells among others. The purpose of such vaccines is to induce antibodies capable of binding the spike protein, thus both neutralizing the virus and preventing cellular infection. Whether these vaccines will induce efficient T cell–mediated immunity is not yet clear. Recent analysis of convalescent COVID-19 patients suggests that the majority of T-cell epitopes against SARS-CoV-2 are derived from proteins other than the spike protein, such as nucleocapsid N protein or ORF1ab, the largest protein made by the virus. Compared to DNA vaccination and other conventional vaccines, RNA vaccines have the drawback of needing to be stored at very low temperatures from their production to the time of use, due to their relative instability, thus increasing the cost of their delivery.

16-10 The route of vaccination is an important determinant of success.

The ideal vaccination induces host defense at the point of entry of the infectious agent. Stimulation of mucosal immunity is therefore an important goal for vaccination against the many organisms that enter through mucosal surfaces. Still, most vaccines are given by injection, even though this route has several disadvantages. Injections are painful and unpopular, reducing vaccine uptake, and they are expensive, requiring needles, syringes, and a trained injector. Mass vaccination by injection is laborious. There is also the immunological drawback that injection may not be the most effective way of stimulating an appropriate immune response because it does not mimic the usual route of entry of the majority of pathogens against which vaccination is directed.

Many important pathogens infect mucosal surfaces or enter the body through mucosal surfaces. Examples include respiratory microorganisms such as *B. pertussis*, rhinoviruses, and influenza viruses, as well as enteric microorganisms such as *Vibrio cholerae*, *Salmonella enterica* serovar Typhi, enteropathogenic *Escherichia coli*, and *Shigella*. Likewise, infection with *Salmonella* stimulates a powerful mucosal and systemic immune response. The intranasally administered live-attenuated vaccine against influenza virus induces mucosal antibodies, which are more effective than systemic antibodies in the control of upper respiratory tract infection. However, the systemic antibodies induced by injection are effective in controlling lower respiratory tract disease, which is responsible for the severe morbidity and mortality due to this disease. Thus, a realistic goal of any pandemic influenza vaccine is to prevent the lower respiratory tract disease but accept the fact that mild illness may not be prevented.

The power of mucosal vaccination is illustrated by the effectiveness of live-attenuated polio vaccines. The Sabin oral polio vaccine consists of three attenuated poliovirus strains that are highly immunogenic. As we described in Section 16-5, these vaccine strains can be transmitted from one individual to another by the fecal–oral route by contamination of public swimming pools or other failures of hygiene, just as poliovirus itself is transmitted.

16-11 *Bordetella pertussis* vaccination illustrates the importance of the perceived safety of a vaccine.

The public perception of a vaccine's safety can influence its eventual effectiveness. The history of vaccination against the bacterium that causes whooping cough, *Bordetella pertussis*, illustrates not only the challenges of developing an effective vaccine but also the public appeal of acellular conjugate vaccines over attenuated live organisms. At the beginning of the 20th century, whooping cough killed about 0.5% of American children under the age of 5 years. In the early 1930s, a trial of a killed, whole bacterial cell vaccine on the Faroe Islands provided evidence of a protective effect. In the United States, systematic use of a whole-cell pertussis vaccine in combination with diphtheria and tetanus toxoids (the DTaP vaccine) during the 1940s resulted in a decline in the annual infection rate from 200 to fewer than 2 cases per 100,000 of the population. The first vaccination with DTaP was typically given at the age of 3 months.

Whole-cell pertussis vaccine causes side effects, typically redness, pain, and swelling at the site of the injection; less commonly, vaccination is followed by high temperature and persistent crying. Very rarely, fits and temporary sleepiness or a floppy unresponsive state ensue. During the 1970s, widespread concern developed after several anecdotal observations that encephalitis leading to irreversible brain damage might very rarely follow pertussis vaccination. In Japan, in 1972, about 85% of children were given the pertussis vaccine, and fewer than 300 cases of whooping cough and no deaths were reported. However, as a result of two deaths after vaccination in Japan in 1975, the use of DTaP was temporarily suspended and then reintroduced with the first vaccination at 2 years of age rather than at 3 months. In 1979, there were about 13,000 cases of whooping cough and 41 deaths. The possibility that pertussis vaccine very rarely causes severe brain damage has been studied extensively, and expert consensus is that pertussis vaccine is not a primary cause of brain injury. There is no doubt that there is greater morbidity from whooping cough than from the vaccine.

The perception that whole-cell pertussis vaccination might be unsafe provided a powerful incentive to develop safer pertussis vaccines. The natural immune response to *B. pertussis* infection induced antibodies against four components of the bacterium—pertussis toxin, filamentous hemagglutinin, pertactin, and fimbrial antigens. Immunization of mice with these antigens in purified form protected them against challenge with pertussis. This has led to the development of **acellular pertussis vaccines**, which contain purified pertussis toxoid; that is, toxin inactivated by chemical treatment, for example with hydrogen peroxide or formaldehyde, or more recently by genetic engineering of the toxin. Some pertussis vaccines also contain filamentous hemagglutinin, pertactin, and/or fimbrial antigens, either alone or in any combination of the three. Current evidence shows that these vaccines are probably as effective as whole-cell pertussis vaccine while lacking its common minor side effects. The acellular vaccine is more expensive, however, thus restricting its use in poorer countries, and there is continuing interest and current work to improve new live-attenuated pertussis vaccines.

The history of pertussis vaccination illustrates that, first and foremost, vaccines must be extremely safe and free of side effects; second, the public and the medical profession must perceive the vaccine to be safe; and third, careful study of the nature of the protective immune response can lead to acellular vaccines that are as effective as whole-cell vaccines but also safer. Still, public concerns about vaccination remain high. Unwarranted fears of a link between the combined live-attenuated MMR vaccine and autism saw the uptake of MMR vaccine in England fall from a peak of 92% of children in 1995–1996 to 84% in 2001–2002. Small clustered outbreaks of measles and mumps in London since 2002 illustrate the importance of maintaining high uptake of vaccine to maintain herd immunity.

16-12 Peptide-based vaccines can elicit protective immunity, but they require adjuvants and must be targeted to the appropriate cells and cell compartment to be effective.

Another vaccine strategy relies on identifying the T-cell peptide epitopes that stimulate protective immunity. These can be identified by testing overlapping peptides from immunogenic proteins for their ability to stimulate protective immunity or by predicting candidate peptide epitopes on the basis of the genome sequence of the pathogen. The latter approach has been applied to malaria by using the complete sequence of the *Plasmodium falciparum* genome. The starting point was the association between the human MHC class I molecule HLA-B53 and resistance to cerebral malaria, a relatively infrequent, but usually fatal, complication of infection by *P. falciparum*. It was thought that HLA-B53 might protect against cerebral malaria because it could present peptides that are particularly good at activating naive cytotoxic T lymphocytes. Peptides eluted from HLA-B53 frequently contain a proline as the second of their nine amino acids. On the basis of this information, reverse genetic analysis identified candidate protective peptides from four proteins of *P. falciparum* expressed in the early phase of hepatocyte infection—an important phase of infection to target in an effective immune response. One of the candidate peptides, from liver-stage antigen-1, has been shown to be recognized by cytotoxic T cells when bound to HLA-B53 and may be a useful peptide for use in vaccination.

Peptide-based vaccines have several drawbacks. First, a particular peptide may not bind to all the MHC molecules present in the population. Because humans are highly polymorphic in the MHC, a large panel of protective peptides would be needed for coverage of most individuals. Second, some direct exchange of short peptides on MHC molecules can occur without physiological antigen processing. Loading of antigenic peptides onto MHC molecules on cells other than dendritic cells may not stimulate immunity and may induce tolerance instead. Third, exogenous proteins and peptides delivered by a synthetic vaccine are efficiently processed for presentation by MHC class II molecules but require 'cross-presentation' in specific types of dendritic cells to be loaded onto MHC class I molecules (see Section 6-5). Directing peptide-based vaccines to cross-presenting dendritic cells may be required to enhance vaccine efficacy.

Recent peptide-based vaccines have already shown promise in human clinical trials. Individuals with established vulvar intraepithelial neoplasia, an early form of vulvar cancer caused by human papilloma virus (HPV), were treated with a vaccine consisting of long peptides covering the entire length of two oncoproteins of HPV-16—E6 and E7—and delivered in an oil-in-water emulsion as adjuvant. By using very long peptides, around 100 amino acids in length, multiple candidate peptide epitopes can be delivered that may also be presented by different MHC alleles. These peptides seem to be too long for direct exchange with peptides on cell surfaces and require processing by dendritic cells in order to be loaded onto MHC class I molecules. This vaccine induced complete clinical remission in one-quarter of the recipients, and about half of the treated patients showed significant clinical responses that correlated with *in vitro* evidence of enhanced cell-mediated immunity.

16-13 Vaccination and checkpoint blockade may be useful in controlling existing chronic infections.

There are many chronic diseases in which infection persists because of a failure of the immune system to eliminate disease. Such infections can be divided into two groups: those in which there is an obvious immune response that fails to eliminate the organism, and those that seem to be invisible to the immune system and evoke a barely detectable immune response.

In the first category, the immune response is often partly responsible for the pathogenic effects. Infection by the helminth *Schistosoma mansoni* is associated with a powerful T_H2-type response, characterized by high levels of IgE, circulating and tissue eosinophilia, and a harmful fibrotic response to schistosome ova in the liver, leading to hepatic fibrosis. Other common parasites, such as *Plasmodium* and *Leishmania* species, cause damage because they are not eliminated effectively by the immune response. The mycobacterial agents of tuberculosis and leprosy cause a persistent intracellular infection; a T_H1 response helps to contain these infections but also causes granuloma formation and tissue necrosis (see Fig. 11.13).

Among viruses, hepatitis B and hepatitis C infections are commonly followed by a persistent viral burden and hepatic injury, resulting in eventual death from hepatitis or from hepatocellular carcinoma. Infection with HIV, as we have seen in Chapter 13, also persists despite an ongoing immune response.

In the second category of chronic infection, which is predominantly viral, the immune response fails to clear the infection because of the relative invisibility of the infectious agent to the immune system. A good example is herpes simplex virus type 2, which is transmitted venereally, becomes latent in nerve tissue, and causes genital herpes, which is frequently recurrent. The invisibility of this virus seems to be caused by a viral protein, ICP-47, which binds to the TAP complex (see Section 6-3) and inhibits peptide transport into the endoplasmic reticulum in infected cells. Thus, viral peptides are not presented to the immune system by MHC class I molecules. A similar example in this category of chronic infection is genital warts, caused by certain papilloma viruses that evoke very little immune response, particularly a cell-mediated response. As discussed earlier, the results of a recent clinical trial showed that use of long-peptide vaccines against HPV-16 was effective in increasing the strength of cell-mediated immune responses to viral antigens and in reducing or eliminating precancerous lesions associated with the HPV infection (see Section 16-12). These results suggest that vaccines that enhance the T cell–mediated responses to other pathogens may be similarly effective.

Summary.

Vaccination is arguably the greatest success of immunology, having eradicated or virtually eliminated several human diseases. It is the single most successful manipulation of the immune system so far, because it takes advantage of the immune system's natural specificity and inducibility. But important human infectious diseases remain that lack effective vaccines. Most effective vaccines are based on attenuated live microorganisms, but such vaccines carry some risk and are potentially lethal to immunosuppressed or immunodeficient individuals. The live-attenuated polio vaccines can undergo revertant mutations that can enhance their virulence, but new molecular engineering is being applied to reduce the frequency of these events. New techniques are also being developed to generate genetically attenuated pathogens for use as vaccines, particularly for malaria and tuberculosis. Many bacterial vaccines are based on components of the microorganism, including components of the toxins that it produces. Protective responses to carbohydrate antigens, which in very young children do not provoke lasting immunity, can be enhanced by conjugation of the carbohydrate to a protein. Vaccines based on DNA, RNA, and very long peptides are just emerging from the experimental stage and are beginning to be tested in humans. In particular, RNA-based vaccines were developed during 2020 for use against COVID-19. A vaccine's immunogenicity often depends on adjuvants that can help, directly or indirectly, to activate antigen-presenting cells that are necessary for the initiation of immune responses. Adjuvants activate these cells by engaging the innate immune system and providing ligands for TLRs and other innate sensors on antigen-presenting cells.

Using the immune response to attack tumors.

Cancer is one of the leading causes of death in industrialized nations, the others being heart disease and stroke, and chronic respiratory diseases. As treatments for infectious diseases and cardiovascular diseases improve, and average life expectancy increases, cancer may become the most common fatal disease in these countries. Cancers are caused by the uncontrolled growth of the progeny of transformed cells. A major problem in treating cancer is controlling **metastasis**, or the spread of cancerous cells from one part of the body to unconnected parts. Curing cancer therefore requires that all the malignant cells be removed or destroyed without killing the patient. An attractive way of achieving this would be to induce an immune response against the tumor that would discriminate between tumor cells and their normal-cell counterparts, as vaccination induces a immune response that selectively targets only a particular pathogen. Immunological approaches to cancer treatment have been considered for more than a century. However, the remarkable progress over the past two decades in large part has resulted from the application of biologics—such as antibodies or cytokines—and their application to regulation of the adaptive immune response.

16-14 The development of transplantable tumors in mice led to the discovery of protective immune responses to tumors.

The finding that tumors could be induced in mice after treatment with chemical carcinogens or irradiation, coupled with the development of inbred strains of mice, made it possible to undertake the key experiments that led to the discovery of immune responses to tumors. These tumors could be transplanted between mice. The experimental study of tumor rejection has generally been based on such tumors. If they bear MHC molecules foreign to the mice into which they are transplanted, the tumor cells are readily recognized and destroyed by the immune system, a fact that was exploited to develop the first MHC-congenic strains of mice. Specific immunity to tumors must therefore be studied within inbred strains, so that host and tumor can be matched for their MHC type.

In mice, transplantable tumors exhibit a variable pattern of growth when injected into syngeneic recipients. Most tumors grow progressively and eventually kill the host. However, if mice are injected with irradiated tumor cells that cannot grow, they are frequently protected against subsequent injection with a normally lethal dose of viable cells from the same tumor (**Fig. 16.14**). There seems to be a spectrum of immunogenicity among transplantable tumors: injections of irradiated tumor cells seem to induce varying degrees of protective immunity against a challenge injection of viable tumor cells at a distant site. These protective effects are not seen in T cell–deficient mice but can be conferred by adoptive transfer of T cells from immune mice, showing the need for T cells to mediate these effects.

These observations indicate that the tumors express antigens that can become targets of a tumor-specific T-cell response that rejects the tumor. These **tumor-rejection antigens** are expressed by experimentally induced murine tumors (in which they are often termed tumor-specific transplantation antigens) and are usually specific for an individual tumor. Thus, immunization with irradiated tumor cells from one tumor usually protects a syngeneic mouse from challenge with live cells from that same tumor, but not from challenge with a different syngeneic tumor (see Fig. 16.14).

16-15 Tumors are 'edited' by the immune system as they evolve and can escape rejection in many ways.

Paul Ehrlich, who received the 1908 Nobel Prize for his work in immunology, was perhaps the first to propose that the immune system could be used to treat established tumors, suggesting that the molecules we call antibodies might be used to deliver toxins to cancer cells. In the 1950s, Frank Macfarlane Burnet, recipient of the 1960 Nobel Prize, and Lewis Thomas formulated the '**immune surveillance**' hypothesis, according to which cells of the immune system would detect and destroy tumor cells. Since then, it has become clear that the relationship between the immune system and cancer is considerably more complex, and this hypothesis has been modified to consider three phases of interactions between the immune system and a tumor. Many tumors are characterized by a loss of genome stability, in which not only is growth regulation disturbed, but so are the processes that ensure the faithful replication of the genome during cell division. Because of this, many tumors acquire mutations in proteins that may be recognized as 'foreign' by the immune system. Also, tumors can express ligands for NK-cell receptors such as NKG2D, which normally indicate cellular stress or infection (see Figure 6.26). For these reasons, early tumors may be recognized by innate cells, such as NK cells, and by T cells that react to '**neoantigens**,' or **neoepitopes**—antigens created by mutations. At this stage, the immune system may recognize and destroy potential tumor cells. This is the '**elimination phase**,' which was the phenomenon previously referred to as immune surveillance (**Fig. 16.15**). If elimination is not completely successful, what follows is an '**equilibrium phase**,' in which the proliferation of tumor cells causes additional changes or mutations. The selection pressure imposed by the immune system influences which of these new tumor cells can survive and which will be eliminated. During the equilibrium phase, a process known as **cancer immunoediting** continually shapes the properties of the tumor cells that survive. In the final '**escape phase**,' tumor cells that have acquired the ability to elude the attention of the immune system and grow unimpeded become clinically detectable.

Experimental evidence that these processes influence the development of certain types of tumors is based on observations of tumor growth in mice that have various targeted gene deletions or have been treated with antibodies to inhibit particular components of immunity. For example, mice lacking perforin, part of the killing mechanism of NK cells and cytotoxic CD8 T cells (see Section 9-22), show an increased frequency of lymphomas—tumors of the lymphoid system. Also, the frequency of fibrosarcomas induced by the

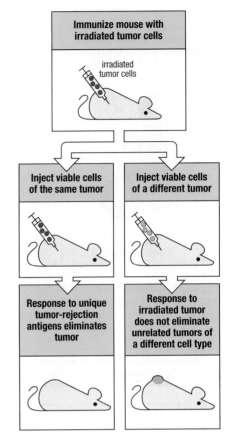

Fig. 16.14 Tumor-rejection antigens are specific to individual tumors. Mice immunized with irradiated tumor cells and challenged with viable cells of the same tumor can, in some cases, reject a lethal dose of that tumor (left panels). This is the result of an immune response to tumor-rejection antigens. If the immunized mice are challenged with viable cells of a different tumor, there is no protection and the mice die (right panels).

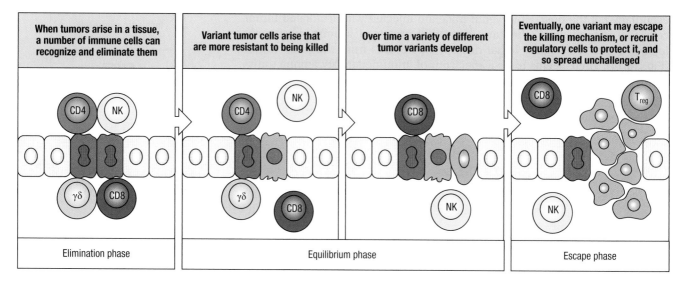

Fig. 16.15 Malignant cells can be controlled by immune surveillance. Some types of tumor cells are recognized by a variety of immune-system cells, which can eliminate them (left panel). If the tumor cells are not completely eliminated, variants occur that eventually escape the immune system and proliferate to form a tumor.

Fig. 16.16 Immune surveillance by lymphocytes reduces MCA-induced tumor formation. The idea that immune surveillance might protect against tumors is quite old, but direct experimental evidence of this process is relatively recent. This research relied on strains of mice engineered to lack lymphocytes or specific immune signaling pathways. In the experiment shown here, mice deficient in the gene *Rag2* (red line), and thus lacking T and B cells, were prospectively compared with wild-type mice (blue line) of the same genetic background for the rate of development of fibrosarcomas after treatment with the carcinogen methylcholanthrene (MCA). The absence of adaptive immunity was seen to cause an increased frequency in tumor formation.

chemical carcinogen methylcholanthrene (MCA) is greater in mice lacking the RAG-2 protein, which is necessary for the development of T cells and B cells (**Fig. 16.16**). MCA-induced tumor frequency is further increased in mice lacking both RAG-2 and STAT1, the latter a transcription factor that mediates signaling by receptors for IFN-γ and IFN-α/β. Mice lacking T lymphocytes expressing $\gamma\delta$ receptors show markedly increased susceptibility to skin tumors induced by the topical application of carcinogens, illustrating a role for intraepithelial $\gamma\delta$ T cells (see Section 6-20) in surveying and killing abnormal epithelial cells. Studies of the various effector cells of the immune system show that $\gamma\delta$ T cells are a major source of IFN-γ, which may explain their importance in the removal of cancer cells.

According to the immunoediting hypothesis, those tumor cells that survive the equilibrium phase have acquired additional changes, such as mutations during the equilibrium phase, that prevent their elimination by the immune system. In an immunocompetent individual, the equilibrium phase of the immune response continually removes tumor cells, delaying tumor growth; if the immune system is compromised, the equilibrium phase quickly turns into an escape phase, as no tumor cells at all are removed. An excellent clinical example of the presence of tumor cells in the equilibrium phase is the occurrence of cancer in recipients of organ transplants. One study reported the development of melanoma between 1 and 2 years after transplantation in two individuals who had received kidneys from the same donor, a woman who had been successfully treated for malignant melanoma 16 years before her death. Presumably, melanoma cells, which are known to spread easily to other organs, were present in the donor kidneys at the time of transplantation but were in equilibrium phase with the immune system. If so, this would indicate that the melanoma cells had not been completely eliminated by the immunocompetent immune system of the donor, but instead had simply been held in check. Because the recipients' immune systems were immunosuppressed to prevent graft rejection, the melanoma cells were released from equilibrium and began to divide rapidly and spread to other parts of the body.

Another situation in which the suppression of immunity can lead to tumor development is in **post-transplant lymphoproliferative disorder**, which can occur when patients are immunosuppressed after, for example, solid organ transplantation. It usually takes the form of a B-cell expansion driven by Epstein–Barr virus (EBV) in which the B cells can undergo mutations and

Mechanisms by which tumors avoid immune recognition				
Low immunogenicity	**Tumor treated as self antigen**	**Antigenic modulation**	**Tumor-induced immune suppression**	**Tumor-induced privileged site**
No peptide:MHC ligand No adhesion molecules No co-stimulatory molecules	Tumor antigens taken up and presented by APCs in absence of co-stimulation tolerize T cells	T cells may eliminate tumors expressing immunogenic antigens, but not tumors that have lost such antigens	Factors (e.g.,TGF-β, IL-10, IDO) secreted by tumor cells inhibit T cells directly. Expression of PD-L1 by tumors	Factors secreted by tumor cells create a physical barrier to the immune system

Fig. 16.17 Tumors can avoid immune recognition in a variety of ways. First panel: Tumors can have low immunogenicity. Tumors may lack antigens recognized by T cells, may have lost one or more MHC molecules, or may express inhibitory molecules that repress T-cell function, such as programmed death ligand-1 (PD-L1). Second panel: Tumor-specific antigens may be cross-presented by dendritic cells without co-stimulatory signals, inducing a tolerant state in T cells. Third panel: Tumors can initially express antigens to which the immune system responds. Such tumors may be eliminated.

The genetic instability of tumors allows antigenic change, part of an equilibrium phase, during which tumor cells lacking immunogenic antigens can expand. Fourth panel: Tumors often produce molecules, such as TGF-β, IL-10, indoleamine 2,3-dioxygenase (IDO), and PD-L1, that suppress immune responses directly or recruit regulatory T cells that can secrete immunosuppressive cytokines. Fifth panel: Tumor cells can secrete molecules such as collagen that form a physical barrier around the tumor, preventing lymphocyte access.

become malignant. Here, antiviral immunity functions as a form of cancer immunosurveillance, as it normally eliminates the EBV that leads to B-cell transformation.

Tumors can avoid stimulating an immune response or can evade it when it occurs by means of numerous mechanisms, which are summarized in **Fig. 16.17**. Spontaneous tumors may initially lack mutations that produce new tumor-specific antigens that elicit T-cell responses (see Fig. 16.17, first panel). Lack of co-stimulatory signals expressed by the antigen-presenting cells (APCs) presenting neoantigens to T cells may cause a failed response, or lead to tolerance (see Fig. 16.17, second panel). How long such tumors are treated as 'self' is unclear. Recent sequencing of entire tumor genomes reveals that mutations may generate as many as 10–15 unique antigenic peptides that could be recognized as 'foreign' by T cells. In addition, cellular transformation is frequently associated with induction of MHC class Ib proteins (such as ULBPs, MIC-A and MIC-B) that are ligands for NKG2D, thus allowing tumor recognition by NK cells (see Section 6-17). But cancer cells tend to be genetically unstable, so that clones that are not recognized by an immune response may be able to escape elimination.

Some tumors, such as colon and cervical cancers, lose the expression of a particular MHC class I molecule, perhaps through immune selection by T cells specific for a peptide presented by that MHC class I molecule (see Fig. 16.17, third panel). In experimental studies, when a tumor loses expression of all MHC class I molecules, it can no longer be recognized by cytotoxic T cells, although it might become susceptible to NK cells (**Fig. 16.18**). Tumors that lose only one MHC class I molecule might be able to avoid recognition by specific cytotoxic CD8 T cells while still remaining resistant to NK cells, conferring a selective advantage *in vivo*.

Acute Infectious Mononucleosis

Fig. 16.18 Tumors that lose expression of all MHC class I molecules as a mechanism of escape from immune surveillance are more susceptible to being killed by NK cells. Regression of transplanted tumors is largely due to the actions of cytotoxic T lymphocytes (CTLs), which recognize novel peptides bound to MHC class I antigens on the surface of the cell (left panels). NK cells have inhibitory receptors that bind MHC class I molecules, so variants of the tumor that have low levels of MHC class I, although less sensitive to cytotoxic CD8 T cells, become susceptible to NK cells (center panels). Although *nude* mice lack T cells, they have higher than normal levels of NK cells, and so tumors that are sensitive to NK cells grow less well in *nude* mice than in normal mice. Transfection with MHC class I genes can restore both resistance to NK cells and susceptibility to cytotoxic CD8 T cells (right panels).

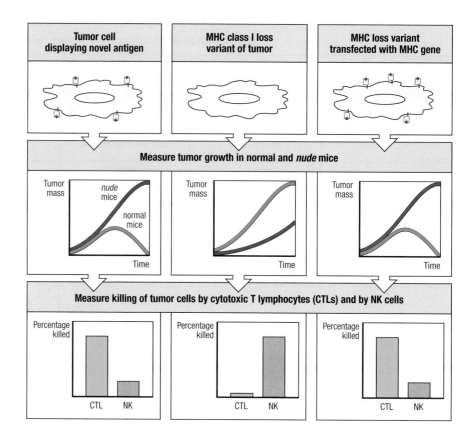

Tumors also seem to be able to evade immune attack by creating a microenvironment that is generally immunosuppressive (see Fig. 16.17, fourth panel). Many tumors make immunosuppressive cytokines. Transforming growth factor-β (TGF-β) was first identified in the culture supernatant of a tumor (hence its name), and, as we have seen, it tends to suppress the inflammatory T-cell responses and cell-mediated immunity that are needed to control tumor growth. Recall that TGF-β promotes the development of peripheral regulatory T cells (pT$_{reg}$ cells; see Section 9-15), which have been found in a variety of cancers and might expand specifically in response to tumor antigens. In mouse models, removal of T$_{reg}$ cells increases resistance to cancer, whereas their transfer into a T$_{reg}$-negative recipient allows cancer cells to proliferate.

The microenvironments of some tumors also contain populations of myeloid cells, collectively called **myeloid-derived suppressor cells (MDSCs)**, which can inhibit T-cell activation within the tumor. MDSCs may be heterogeneous, comprising both monocytic and polymorphonuclear cells, and are still incompletely characterized. Several tumors of different tissue origins, such as melanoma, ovarian carcinoma, and B-cell lymphoma, have also been shown to produce the immunosuppressive cytokine IL-10, which can reduce dendritic-cell activity and inhibit T-cell activation.

Tumors can express cell-surface proteins that directly inhibit immune responses (see Fig. 16.17, fourth panel). For example, some tumors express **programmed death ligand-1 (PD-L1)**, a B7 family member and ligand for the inhibitory receptor **PD-1** expressed by activated T cells (see Section 7-25). Tumors can also produce enzymes that suppress local immune responses. The enzyme **indoleamine 2,3-dioxygenase (IDO)** catabolizes tryptophan, an essential amino acid, in order to produce the immunosuppressive metabolite kynurenine. IDO seems to function in maintaining a balance between immune responses and tolerance during infections, but it can be induced during the equilibrium phase of tumor development. Finally, tumor cells can produce materials such as collagen, creating a physical barrier to interaction with cells of the immune system (see Fig. 16.17, last panel).

16-16 Tumor-rejection antigens can be recognized by T cells and form the basis of immunotherapies.

Several categories of tumor-rejection antigens can be distinguished (Fig. 16.19). One category of tumor-rejection antigens comprises peptides derived from tumor-cell proteins presented by MHC molecules to T cells. Some peptides of this category can also be present on normal tissues yet become the targets of a tumor-specific T-cell response. For example, immunotherapy in people with melanoma can produce vitiligo, an autoimmune destruction of pigmented cells in healthy skin. Other peptides in this category may become **tumor-specific antigens** as a result of gene mutations or rearrangements that alter specific amino acid residues and produce a peptide epitope for T cells that are already able to bind to MHC class I molecules or that allow mutant peptides to bind *de novo* to MHC class I molecules. Such neoantigens, or neoepitopes, are newly immunogenic versions of normal proteins and may evoke a new T-cell response against the tumor. In B- and T-cell tumors, which are derived from single clones of lymphocytes, a special class of tumor-specific antigen comprises the unique rearranged antigen receptor expressed by the clone. However, not all mutated peptides may be properly processed or be able to associate with MHC molecules and thus ensure that they stimulate an effective response.

Potential tumor-rejection antigens have a variety of origins			
Class of antigen	**Antigen**	**Nature of antigen**	**Tumor type**
Tumor-specific mutated oncogene or tumor suppressor gene	Cyclin-dependent kinase 4	Cell-cycle regulator	Melanoma
	β-Catenin	Relay in signal transduction pathway	Melanoma
	Caspase 8	Regulator of apoptosis	Squamous-cell carcinoma
	Surface Ig/idiotype	Specific antibody after gene rearrangements in B-cell clone	Lymphoma
Cancer-testis antigens	MAGE-1 MAGE-3 NY-ESO-1	Normal testicular proteins	Melanoma Breast Glioma
Differentiation	Tyrosinase	Enzyme in pathway of melanin synthesis	Melanoma
Abnormal gene expression	HER-2/neu	Receptor tyrosine kinase	Breast Ovary
	WT1	Transcription factor	Leukemia
Abnormal post-translational modification	MUC-1	Underglycosylated mucin	Breast Pancreas
Abnormal post-transcriptional modification	NA17	Retention of introns in the mRNA	Melanoma
Oncoviral protein	HPV type 16, E6 and E7 proteins	Viral transforming gene products	Cervical carcinoma

Fig. 16.19 Proteins selectively expressed in human tumors are candidate tumor-rejection antigens. The molecules listed here represent the various categories of tumor-rejection antigens. For surface Ig, 'idiotype' refers to the unique protein structure of the particular antibody clone expressed by the lymphoma cells. These molecules have been shown to be recognized by cytotoxic T lymphocytes raised from patients with the tumor type listed.

A second category of tumor-rejection antigens is the **cancer-testis antigens**. These are proteins encoded by genes that are normally expressed only in male germ cells in the testis. Male germ cells do not express MHC molecules, and therefore peptides from these molecules are not normally presented to T lymphocytes. Tumor cells can show widespread abnormalities of gene expression, including the activation of genes encoding cancer-testis antigens, such as the **melanoma-associated antigens (MAGEs)** (see Fig. 16.19). When expressed by tumor cells, peptides derived from these 'germ-cell' proteins can now be presented to T cells by MHC class I molecules. Therefore, these proteins are effectively tumor-specific in their expression as antigens. Perhaps the cancer-testis antigen best characterized immunologically is **NY-ESO-1** (New York esophageal squamous-cell carcinoma-1), which is highly immunogenic and is expressed by a variety of human tumors, including melanomas.

A third category of tumor-rejection antigens is the class of **differentiation antigens** encoded by genes that are expressed only in particular types of tissues. Examples of these are the differentiation antigens expressed in melanocytes and melanoma cells, which include several proteins in the pathways that produce the black pigment melanin, and the CD19 antigen expressed by B cells. A fourth category of tumor-rejection antigens consists of antigens that are strongly overexpressed in tumor cells compared with their normal counterparts. An example is **HER-2/neu** (also known as c-Erb-2), which is a receptor tyrosine kinase homologous to the epidermal growth factor receptor. HER-2/neu is overexpressed in many adenocarcinomas, including breast and ovarian cancers, where it is associated with a poor clinical prognosis. CD8 T lymphocytes have been found infiltrating solid tumors overexpressing HER-2/neu but are not capable of destroying such tumors *in vivo*. A fifth category of tumor-rejection antigens consists of molecules that display abnormal post-translational modifications. An example is underglycosylated mucin, MUC-1, which is expressed by several tumors, including breast and pancreatic cancers. A sixth category of tumor-rejection antigens consists of novel proteins that are generated when one or more introns are retained in the mRNA transcribed from a gene, which occurs in melanoma. A seventh category of tumor-rejection antigens comprises proteins encoded by viral oncogenes. These oncoviral proteins can have a critical role in the oncogenic process, and because they are foreign, they can evoke a T-cell response. Examples are the human papilloma virus type 16 proteins E6 and E7, which are expressed in cervical carcinoma (see Section 16-20).

In melanoma, tumor-specific antigens were discovered by culturing irradiated tumor cells with autologous lymphocytes, a technique known as the mixed lymphocyte–tumor cell culture. From such cultures, cytotoxic T cells were identified that were reactive against melanoma peptides and would kill tumor cells bearing the relevant tumor-specific antigen. Such studies have revealed that melanomas carry at least five different antigens that can be recognized by cytotoxic T lymphocytes. It seems that cytotoxic T lymphocytes reactive against melanoma antigens are not effective *in vivo*, perhaps due to deficient priming and insufficient effector function or to downstream resistance mechanisms. However, melanoma-specific T cells can be isolated from peripheral blood, lymph nodes, or directly from lymphocytes infiltrating the tumor and propagated *in vitro*. These T cells do not recognize the products of mutant proto-oncogenes or tumor suppressor genes, but instead recognize antigens derived from the protein products of other mutant genes or from normal proteins that are now displayed on tumor cells at levels detectable by T cells for the first time. Cancer-testis antigens such as the MAGEs discussed earlier probably represent early developmental antigens reexpressed in the process of tumorigenesis. Only a minority of people with melanoma have T cells reactive to the MAGEs, indicating that these antigens either are not expressed or are not immunogenic in most cases.

The most common melanoma antigens are peptides from the enzyme **tyrosinase** or from three other proteins—gp100, MART1, and gp75. These are differentiation antigens specific to the melanocyte lineage. It is likely that overexpression of these antigens in tumor cells leads to an abnormally high density of specific peptide:MHC complexes, and it is this that makes them immunogenic. Tumor-rejection antigens are usually presented as peptides by MHC class I molecules, but tyrosinase can also stimulate CD4 T-cell responses in some melanoma patients, likely presented by MHC class II molecules. Both CD8 and CD4 T cells are likely to be important in achieving immunological control of tumors. CD8 cells can kill the tumor cells directly, while CD4 T cells have a role in promoting the activation of cytotoxic CD8 T cells by helping to fully activate antigen-presenting cells, usually dendritic cells, that prime CD8 T cells. CD4 T cells may also kill tumor cells by means of the cytokines that they secrete, such as TNF-α.

Other potential tumor-rejection antigens include the products of mutated cellular oncogenes or tumor suppressors, such as Ras and p53, and also fusion proteins, such as the **Bcr–Abl tyrosine kinase** that results from the chromosomal translocation, t(9;22), found in chronic myeloid leukemia (CML). When present on CML cells, the HLA class I molecule HLA-A*0301 can display a peptide derived from the fusion site between Bcr and Abl. This peptide was detected by a powerful technique known as 'reverse immunogenetics,' in which endogenous peptides were eluted from the MHC binding groove, and their sequence was determined by highly sensitive mass spectrometry. This technique has identified HLA-bound peptides from other tumor antigens, such as the MART1 and gp100 tumor antigens of melanomas, as well as candidate peptide sequences for vaccination against infectious diseases.

T cells specific for the Bcr–Abl fusion peptide can be identified in peripheral blood from individuals with CML by using tetramers of HLA-A*0301 carrying the peptide as specific ligands for the antigen-specific T-cell receptor. Cytotoxic T lymphocytes specific for this and other tumor antigens can be selected *in vitro* by using peptides derived from the mutated or fused portions of these oncogenic proteins; these cytotoxic T cells are able to recognize and kill tumor cells.

After a bone marrow transplant to treat CML, mature lymphocytes from the bone marrow donor infused into the patient can help to eliminate any residual tumor. This technique is known as **donor lymphocyte infusion (DLI)**. At present, it is not clear to what extent the clinical response is due to a graft-versus-host effect, in which the donor lymphocytes are responding to general alloantigens expressed on the leukemia cells (see Section 15-25), or whether a specific antileukemic response is important. It is encouraging that it has been possible to separate T lymphocytes *in vitro* that mediate either a graft-versus-host effect or a graft-versus-leukemia effect. The ability to prime the donor cells against leukemia-specific peptides offers the prospect of enhancing the antileukemic effect while minimizing the risk of graft-versus-host disease.

16-17 Checkpoint blockade can augment immune responses to existing tumors.

Various approaches to harnessing the immune system to treat tumors have been tried. Some have aimed at making the tumor itself more immunogenic by inducing the expression of co-stimulatory molecules on tumor cells and using these cells to activate tumor-specific naive T cells. Similarly, tumor cells have been transfected with the gene encoding cytokines, such as granulocyte–macrophage colony-stimulating factor (GM-CSF), in an attempt to induce the maturation of tumor-proximal monocytes into monocyte-derived dendritic cells. Once these cells have differentiated and capture antigens from the tumor, it was hoped they would migrate to the local lymph nodes and activate tumor-specific T cells. No approved therapies have yet emerged from these approaches.

A different approach to cancer immunotherapy is to block the normal inhibitory signals that regulate lymphocytes, called **checkpoint blockade**. Immune responses are controlled by several positive and negative immunological checkpoints. A positive checkpoint for T cells is controlled by the co-stimulatory receptors, such as CD28 and members of the TNF receptor superfamily, such as CD27 and 4-1BB. These activating receptors are stimulated by engagement of their ligands expressed by antigen-presenting cells such as dendritic cells. Negative immunological checkpoints are provided by inhibitory receptors such as CTLA-4 and PD-1. CTLA-4 imposes a critical checkpoint for potentially autoreactive T cells by binding to B7 molecules on dendritic cells and effectively providing a negative signal that must be overcome by other signals before T cells can become activated. Blocking CTLA-4 with antibodies may therefore lower the threshold for T-cell activation. Some evidence also indicates that anti-CTLA-4 antibodies may augment immune responses by eliminating regulatory T cells, which constitutively express a high level of CTLA-4 on their surface. Whatever the mechanism, the absence of this checkpoint causes self-reactive T cells that are normally held in check to become activated and to produce a multi-tissue autoimmune reaction, as seen in CTLA-4–deficient mice.

Checkpoint blockade based on the anti-CTLA-4 antibody **ipilimumab** has now been shown to be effective in treating metastatic melanoma and was approved by the FDA for this indication in 2015. Patients with metastatic melanoma who were treated with ipilimumab showed an increase in the number and activity of T cells recognizing NY-ESO-1, a cancer-testis antigen expressed by melanoma. Overall, only about 15% of recipients exhibited a response to ipilimumab, but the treatment appeared to induce long-term remission in some responding patients. One side effect of ipilimumab in these patients seemed to be an increased risk of autoimmune phenomena, in line with the role of CTLA-4 in maintaining tolerance of self-reactive T cells.

Another checkpoint involves the inhibitory receptor PD-1 and its ligands PD-L1 and PD-L2 (**Fig. 16.20**). PD-L1 is expressed on a wide variety of human tumors; in renal-cell carcinoma, PD-L1 expression is associated with a poor prognosis. In mice, transfection of the gene encoding PD-L1 into tumor cells increased their growth *in vivo* and reduced their susceptibility to lysis by cytotoxic T cells. These effects were reversed by an antibody against PD-L1. In humans, the anti-PD-1 antibody **pembrolizumab** has been shown to be effective in previously treated melanoma patients, giving a nearly 30% response rate. It is FDA-approved for use in treatment of several types of cancers, including melanoma, a particular form of lung cancer, certain squamous-cell cancers of the head and neck, and others, usually in combination with other types of treatments, and the indications continue to broaden. Another anti-PD-1 antibody, **nivolumab**, is also approved for treatment of metastatic melanoma and is being considered for use in treatment of Hodgkin's lymphoma. Because PD-1 is an inhibitory receptor, it is important that the antibodies used in this therapy act only to block the interaction of PD-1 with its ligands and do not trigger PD-1 signaling in T cells, which would inhibit their responses rather than activate them. Checkpoint blockade using antibodies to PD-L1 has been

Fig. 16.20 Checkpoint blockade enhances ongoing T-cell responses to tumors expressing ligands for inhibitory receptors. Some, but not all, tumors express ligands for PD-1, such as PD-L1 or PD-L2. Left panels: T cells reacting to tumors without PD-1 ligands do not encounter the inhibitory signal from PD-1 and may deliver their cytotoxic action when recognizing tumor-specific antigens. In contrast, tumors expressing PD-1 ligands can repress T cells and be protected from cytotoxicity. Right panels: For tumors expressing PD-1 ligands, checkpoint blockade can be achieved by antagonistic antibodies against PD-1 or against the ligand, PD-L1 in this case.

FDA-approved for various indications. The PD-L1 antibody atezolizumab was approved in 2015 for treating metastatic urothelial cancer that failed to respond to prior chemotherapy, and the PD-L1 antibody avelumab was approved for treatment of an aggressive form of neuroendocrine skin cancer, Merkel-cell carcinoma.

Checkpoint blockade relies on activation of the patient's own immune system against tumors, and so its effects are not immediately evident. The delay between the initiation of treatment and clinical response presented a challenge in evaluating clinical responses to this therapy. Guidelines for evaluating clinical responses were previously based on the immediate effects of chemotherapeutic drugs or radiation, whereas checkpoint blockade requires more time for reversing immune inhibition and expanding tumor-specific T cells, which then exert their effects within the tumor. Once such issues were considered, it became possible to design clinical trials that could document the effects of checkpoint blockade used in combination with traditional anticancer therapies. For their contributions to the discovery of checkpoint blockade, James P. Allison and Tasuku Honjo received the 2018 Nobel Prize in Physiology or Medicine. Checkpoint blockade is an extremely active area of translational research, and the clinical landscape continues to change rapidly.

16-18 T cells expressing chimeric antigen receptors are an effective treatment in some leukemias.

Adoptive T-cell therapy involves *ex vivo* expansion of tumor-specific T cells to large numbers and the infusion of those T cells into patients. Cells are expanded *in vitro* by various methods, such as treatment with IL-2, anti-CD3 antibodies, and allogeneic antigen-presenting cells, to provide a co-stimulatory signal. Adoptive T-cell therapy is more effective when the patient is immunosuppressed before treatment and IL-2 is then administered systemically. Another approach that has elicited much interest is the use of retroviral vectors to transfer tumor-specific T-cell receptor (TCR) genes into a patient's T cells before reinfusion. This can have long-lasting effects as a result of the ability of T cells to become memory cells, and there is no requirement for histocompatibility because the transfused cells are derived from the patient.

T cells are harvested from the blood of a patient with a B-cell tumor

A retrovirus encoding an anti-CD19 CAR infects T cells that are activated with antibodies to CD3 and CD28

Infected T cells express an anti-CD19 CAR

T cells are infused into patient to mediate antitumor activity

Anti-CD19 CAR chimeric receptor

Fig. 16.21 Chimeric antigen receptors (CARs) expressed in T cells can confer antitumor specificity to lymphocytes. Bottom panel: A chimeric antigen receptor, CART-19, is composed of an extracellular single-chain antibody that binds to CD19, which is fused to intracellular signaling domains from 4-1BB and the CD3ζ chain. Top row of panels: A lentivirus, a type of retrovirus, is used to express the gene encoding CART-19 in the T cells harvested from a patient diagnosed with acute lymphocytic leukemia (ALL). After *in vitro* activation and expansion, the transfected CART-19 cells are infused into the patient and exert cytotoxic actions against CD19-expressing tumor cells as well as nontransformed B cells.

Another form of adoptive immunotherapy also uses a viral vector to introduce genes into a patient's T cells but involves expressing a novel type of receptor, known as a **chimeric antigen receptor (CAR)**. As we introduced in Section 7-27, CARs are fusion receptors containing extracellular antigen-specific domains fused to intracellular domains that provide signals for activation and co-stimulation. These receptors are introduced stably into T cells using lentiviral or retroviral vectors to produce so-called CARL T cells. This approach differs from conventional adoptive T-cell therapies, as use of a CAR allows the T cell's target specificity to be almost any molecule recognizable by an antibody (or other receptors), rather than use of a TCR that recognizes a specific peptide:MHC complex. This approach has been used to target CD19 as a tumor-rejection antigen in treating acute lymphocytic leukemia (ALL), an aggressive cancer of transformed B cells (**Fig. 16.21**). The CAR used in this case had an extracellular domain of an antibody that recognizes human CD19. The intracellular domain had three ITAMs from the ζ chain of the T-cell receptor CD3 complex (see Chapter 7) fused with a co-stimulation domain from 4-1BB, a member of the TNF receptor superfamily. These CART-19 transduced T cells were expanded *in vitro* and transferred into a patient. The results of this case combined with others have demonstrated that CD8 T cells expressing CART-19 (see Fig. 16.21) are effective at achieving complete clinical remissions in many individuals with ALL. This approach is not without its side effects, however, as it also eliminates normal B cells in patients, and they therefore require treatment with intravenous immunoglobulin (IVIG). This cell-based therapy is an example of 'personalized medicine' because it requires the modification of each patient's T cells, which are expanded and introduced back only into that same individual. This treatment was approved by the FDA in 2017, under the trade name **Kymriah**, for the treatment of certain adults with diffuse large B-cell lymphoma who have either relapsed or who were refractory to conventional therapy altogether.

16-19 Monoclonal antibodies against tumor antigens, alone or linked to toxins, can control tumor growth.

A tumor-specific antigen must be expressed on the tumor's cell surface to allow a monoclonal antibody to direct the activity of a cytotoxic cell, toxin, or radioactive nuclide to the tumor cell (**Fig. 16.22**). Some of the cell-surface molecules

Fig. 16.22 Monoclonal antibodies that recognize tumor-specific antigens have been used to help eliminate tumors. Tumor-specific antibodies of the correct isotypes can lyse tumor cells by recruiting effector cells such as NK cells and activating them via their Fc receptors (left panels). Another strategy has been to couple the antibody to a powerful toxin (center panels). When the antibody binds to the tumor cell and is endocytosed, the toxin is released from the antibody and can kill the tumor cell. If the antibody is coupled to a radioisotope (right panels), binding of the antibody to a tumor cell will deliver a dose of radiation sufficient to kill the tumor cell. In addition, nearby tumor cells could also receive a lethal radiation dose, even though they do not bind the antibody. Antibody fragments have started to replace whole antibodies for coupling to toxins or radioisotopes.

targeted in clinical trials are shown in **Fig. 16.23**, and some of these treatments have now been licensed. The monoclonal antibody **trastuzumab** (Herceptin) was approved in 1998 for treatment of patients whose breast cancer is positive for the receptor human epidermal growth factor receptor 2, also called HER-2/neu. This receptor is overexpressed in about one-quarter of individuals with breast cancer and is associated with a poor prognosis. Herceptin is thought to act by blocking the binding of the natural ligand to this receptor and by down-regulating the level of expression of the receptor. The effects of this antibody can be enhanced when it is combined with conventional chemotherapy. Experiments in mice suggest that some of trastuzumab's antitumor effects may also involve antibody-dependent cell-mediated cytotoxicity (ADCC) or the induction of antitumor T-cell responses. A monoclonal antibody that has yielded excellent results in the treatment of non-Hodgkin's B-cell lymphoma is the anti-CD20 antibody **rituximab**, which triggers the apoptosis of B cells upon binding to CD20 on their surface (see Section 16-28). ADCC may be another

Fig. 16.23 Examples of tumor antigens that have been targeted by monoclonal antibodies in therapeutic trials. CEA, carcinoembryonic antigen. Idiotype, the specific antibody structure expressed by the lymphoma.

Tumor tissue origin	Type of antigen	Antigen	Tumor type
Lymphoma/ leukemia	Differentiation antigen	CD5 Idiotype CD52 (Campath-1H)	T-cell lymphoma B-cell lymphoma T- and B-cell lymphoma/ leukemia
	B-cell signaling receptor	CD20	Non-Hodgkin's B-cell lymphoma
Solid tumors	Cell-surface antigens Glycoprotein Carbohydrate	CEA, mucin-1 Lewis^Y CA-125	Epithelial tumors (breast, colon, lung) Epithelial tumors Ovarian carcinoma
	Growth factor receptors	Epidermal growth factor receptor HER-2/neu IL-2 receptor Vascular endothelial growth factor (VEGF)	Lung, breast, and head and neck tumors Breast, ovarian tumors T- and B-cell tumors Colon cancer Lung, prostate, breast
	Stromal extracellular antigen	FAP-α Tenascin Metalloproteinases	Epithelial tumors Glioblastoma multiforme Epithelial tumors

mechanism by which rituximab acts, as its clinical efficacy has been linked to polymorphisms in activating Fc receptors.

However, monoclonal antibodies may be inefficient in killing tumor cells after binding, may not efficiently penetrate into tumors, and may be inactivated by abundant soluble antigens. The efficiency in killing tumor cells can be enhanced by linking the antibody to a toxin, producing a reagent called an **immunotoxin** (see Fig. 16.22): two favored toxins are ricin A chain and *Pseudomonas* toxin. The antibody must be internalized to allow cleavage of the toxin from the antibody in the endocytic compartment, permitting the freed toxin chain to penetrate and kill the cell. Toxins coupled to native antibodies have had limited success in cancer therapy. However, molecules can be engineered as a single chain to contain only the antibody variable region, or fragment (Fv), while retaining the ability to bind an antigen. Such single-chain Fv molecules may show promise in the design of an immunotoxin. An example of a successful immunotoxin is a recombinant Fv anti-CD22 antibody fused to a fragment of *Pseudomonas* toxin called **moxetumomab pasudotox-tdfk (Lumoxiti)**, which induced complete remissions in two-thirds of a group of people with a type of B-cell leukemia known as hairy-cell leukemia in whom the disease was resistant to conventional chemotherapy. This treatment was approved by the FDA in 2018, under the trade name Lumoxiti, for this indication in those with relapsed or refractory disease.

Monoclonal antibodies can also be conjugated to chemotherapeutic drugs or to radioisotopes. In the case of a drug-linked antibody, the binding of the antibody to a cell-surface antigen concentrates the drug to the site of the tumor. After internalization, the drug is released in the endosomes and exerts its cytostatic or cytotoxic effect. For example, the antibody trastuzumab has been linked to the cytotoxic agent mertansine, a drug that inhibits the assembly of microtubules, in a conjugate called **T-DM1**. Because HER-2 is overexpressed only in cancer cells, T-DM1 selectively delivers the toxin specifically to tumor cells. Another drug–antibody conjugate, brentuximab vedotin, links an anti-CD30 antibody with a different microtubule inhibitor and is approved for certain forms of relapsed lymphomas.

A variation on this approach is to link an antibody to an enzyme that metabolizes a nontoxic pro-drug to the active cytotoxic drug, a technique known as **antibody-directed enzyme/pro-drug therapy (ADEPT)**. With this technique, a small amount of enzyme localized by the antibody can generate much larger amounts of active cytotoxic drug in the immediate vicinity of tumor cells. Monoclonal antibodies linked to radioisotopes (see Fig. 16.22) have been successful in treatment of refractory B-cell lymphoma by using anti-CD20 antibodies linked to yttrium-90 (ibritumomab tiuxetan). These approaches have the advantage of also killing neighboring tumor cells, because the released drug or radioactive emissions can affect cells adjacent to those that bind the antibody. Monoclonal antibodies coupled to γ-emitting radioisotopes have also been used successfully to image tumors for the purposes of diagnosis and monitoring of tumor spread.

16-20 Enhancing the immune response to tumors by vaccination holds promise for cancer prevention and therapy.

Another approach to cancer immunotherapy is based on the idea that tumors are intrinsically poorly immunogenic, and that a vaccine may supply the missing immunogenicity. Some cancers are associated with viral infections, and vaccines that prevent these infections can reduce cancer risk. Human papilloma virus (HPV) is such a virus, and infections with two HPV strains, HPV-16 and HPV-18, are associated with 70% of cervical cancers. A major breakthrough in anticancer therapy occurred in 2005 with the completion of a clinical trial involving 12,167 women who tested a vaccine against HPV. This trial showed that a recombinant vaccine against HPV was 100% effective in preventing cervical cancer caused by HPV-16 and HPV-18.

The vaccine most likely prevents infection of cervical epithelium by HPV by inducing anti-HPV antibodies (**Fig. 16.24**). Although the 2005 trial involving 12,167 women showed the potential of vaccines to prevent cancer, attempts to use vaccines to treat existing tumors—called **therapeutic vaccination**—have been less effective. In the case of HPV, certain types of vaccines that have increased immunogenicity for eliciting T-cell responses are beginning to show effectiveness in treating existing intraepithelial neoplasia caused by the virus. Similarly, the majority of liver cancers are associated with chronic hepatitis caused by several viruses. The vaccine against hepatitis B can reduce primary liver cancer that is due to this virus, although the vaccine will not protect against cancers caused by infections by other viruses such as hepatitis C.

Vaccines based on tumor antigens, in principle, could provide a basis for T cell–mediated cancer immunotherapy, but they are difficult to develop. While the relevant antigens are known for HPV, the relevant neoantigens for most spontaneous tumors would require a sequence analysis to identify potential candidates, and these would not be the same in different patients' tumors. Further, the suitability of the epitopes would depend on the individual's particular MHC alleles. Practically, tumor vaccines may require a range of tumor antigens and might be effective only when the tumor burden is low, such as after surgery and chemotherapy.

The sources of antigens for cell-based cancer vaccines are the individual patients' tumors removed at surgery. These vaccines are prepared by mixing either irradiated tumor cells or tumor extracts with killed bacteria such as bacillus Calmette–Guérin (BCG) or *Corynebacterium parvum*, which act as adjuvants to enhance the immunogenicity of the tumor antigens (see Appendix I, Section A-1). Vaccination using BCG adjuvants has had variable results in the past, but renewed interest is based on recent appreciation of their interaction with Toll-like receptors (TLRs). Stimulation of TLR-4 by BCG and other ligands has been tested against melanoma and other solid tumors. CpG DNA, which binds to TLR-9, has also been used to increase the immunogenicity of cancer vaccines. In cases where candidate tumor-rejection antigens have been identified (for example, in melanomas), experimental vaccination strategies have included the use of whole proteins; peptide vaccines based on sequences recognized by cytotoxic T lymphocytes and helper T lymphocytes (either administered alone or presented by the patient's own dendritic cells); and recombinant viruses encoding these peptide epitopes. One cell-based cancer vaccine, **sipuleucel-T (Provenge)**, was approved in 2010 for treatment of metastatic prostate cancer. In this therapy, a patient's monocytes are extracted from peripheral blood and cultured with a fusion protein containing the antigen **prostatic acid phosphatase (PAP)**, which is expressed by most prostate cancers, and the cytokine granulocyte–macrophage colony-stimulating factor (GM-CSF), which induces monocytes to undergo maturation to monocyte-derived dendritic cells. The resulting cells are reinfused into the patient in the hope of inducing an immune response specific to the PAP antigen. This treatment reduced the risk of death by 22% and improved survival by about 4 months relative to a placebo group. However, this approach has not had the same clinical impact as other therapies, such as checkpoint blockade.

Summary.

Some tumors elicit specific immune responses that suppress or modify their growth. Tumors evade or suppress these responses in several ways, passing through various stages of a process known as immunological editing. Understanding how the immune system promotes and prevents cancer growth has led to new therapies now deployed in the clinic. Checkpoint

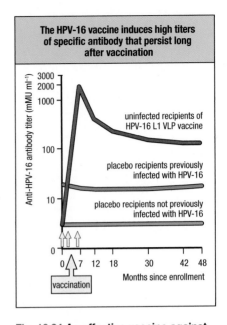

The HPV-16 vaccine induces high titers of specific antibody that persist long after vaccination

uninfected recipients of HPV-16 L1 VLP vaccine

placebo recipients previously infected with HPV-16

placebo recipients not previously infected with HPV-16

vaccination

Months since enrollment

Fig. 16.24 An effective vaccine against human papilloma virus (HPV) induces antibodies that protect against HPV infection. Serotype 16 of HPV (HPV-16) is highly associated with the development of cervical cancer. In a clinical trial, 755 healthy uninfected women were immunized with a vaccine generated from highly purified noninfectious 'viruslike particles' (VLPs) consisting of the capsid protein L1 of HPV-16 and formulated with an alum adjuvant (in this case, aluminum hydroxyphosphate sulfate). In comparison with the very low titers of antibody in placebo-treated uninfected women (green line) or in women previously infected with HPV who received placebo (blue line), the women treated with the viruslike particle vaccine (red line) developed high titers of antibody against the L1 capsid protein. None of these immunized women subsequently became infected by HPV-16. An anti-HPV vaccine marketed as Gardasil is now available and recommended for use in girls and young women as a protection from cervical cancer caused by HPV serotypes 6, 11, 16, and 18. mMU, milli-Merck units.

blockade strategies for CTLA-4 and PD-1 have been approved for treating melanoma, and related strategies are being developed for other biologic targets to stimulate antitumor immune responses or block inhibitory mechanisms that suppress such responses. The possibility of eradicating cervical cancer has been brought closer by an effective vaccine against the specific HPV strains associated with cancer that prevents infection. CAR T cells engineered to recognize CD19 expressed on B cells can be an effective treatment for acute lymphocytic leukemia. Monoclonal antibodies can be used for tumor immunotherapy, including an anti-CD20 antibody used to treat B-cell lymphoma and anti-HER-2/neu for treatment of certain types of breast cancers. Attempts are also being made to develop vaccines incorporating antigens from a patient's tumor in order to generate effective cytotoxic and helper T-cell responses. One vaccine using monocyte-derived dendritic cells has been approved for treatment of prostate cancer. A current trend in cancer therapy has been to incorporate immunotherapy with other traditional anticancer treatments to take advantage of the specificity and power of the immune system.

Treatment of unwanted immune responses.

Unwanted immune responses occur in many settings, such as autoimmune disease, transplant rejection, and allergy, which present different therapeutic challenges. The goal of treatment in all cases is to prevent tissue damage and disruption of tissue function. Some unwanted immune responses can be anticipated in advance, as with tissue transplantation, so that preventive measures may be taken. Other unwanted responses may be undetectable until after they become established, as is the case with autoimmune diseases or allergic reactions. The relative difficulty of suppressing established immune responses is seen in animal models of autoimmunity, in which treatments that could have prevented induction of the disease are usually unable to halt it once it is established.

Conventional immunosuppressive drugs—meaning natural or synthetic small-molecule compounds—can be divided into several different categories (**Fig. 16.25**). There are the powerful anti-inflammatory drugs of the corticosteroid family, such as prednisone; cytotoxic drugs, such as azathioprine and cyclophosphamide; and noncytotoxic fungal and bacterial derivatives,

Fig. 16.25 Conventional immunosuppressive drugs in clinical use.

Conventional immunosuppressive drugs in clinical use	
Immunosuppressive drug	**Mechanism of action**
Corticosteroids	Inhibit inflammation; inhibit many targets including cytokine production by macrophages
Azathioprine, cyclophosphamide, mycophenolate	Inhibit proliferation of lymphocytes by interfering with DNA synthesis
Cyclosporin A, tacrolimus (FK506)	Inhibit the calcineurin-dependent activation of NFAT; block IL-2 production by T cells and proliferation by T cells
Rapamycin (sirolimus)	Inhibits proliferation of effector T cells by blocking Rictor-dependent mTOR activation
Fingolimod (FTY720)	Blocks lymphocyte trafficking out of lymphoid tissues by interfering with signaling by the sphingosine 1-phosphate receptor
Jakinibs	Inhibit the Janus kinases (JAKs) that mediate the signaling of various cytokine receptors

such as cyclosporin A, tacrolimus (FK506 or fujimycin), and rapamycin (sirolimus), which inhibit intracellular signaling pathways within T lymphocytes. A relatively new drug, **fingolimod**, interferes with signaling by the sphingosine 1-phosphate receptor that controls the egress of B and T cells from lymphoid organs, thus preventing effector lymphocytes from reaching peripheral tissues. Most of these drugs exert broad inhibition of the immune system and suppress helpful as well as harmful responses. Opportunistic infection is therefore a common complication of immunosuppressive drug therapy. A recently developed class of drugs called **JAK inhibitors**, or '**jakinibs**,' are kinase inhibitors that block signaling by a variety of cytokine receptors and provide somewhat greater selectivity in the form of inhibition.

Besides conventional small-molecule drugs, there are now many biopharmaceuticals—or **biologics**—that can be used to manipulate the immune response. The most immediate way of inhibiting a particular part of the immune response is by using antibodies that act on specific proteins expressed on or secreted by immune cells. Monoclonal antibodies directed against cytokines, such as the drug **infliximab** (anti-TNF-α) used in the treatment of rheumatoid arthritis, can neutralize local excesses of cytokines or chemokines or target natural cellular regulatory mechanisms to inhibit unwanted immune responses. Proteins other than antibodies are also in use to control immune responses, an example being **abatacept**, a fusion protein consisting of the Fc region of an immunoglobulin fused to the extracellular domain of CTLA-4. Abatacept reduces co-stimulation of T cells by binding to B7 molecules and blocking their interactions with CD28. It is currently used to treat rheumatoid arthritis in individuals who fail to respond to anti-TNF-α therapy.

16-21 Corticosteroids are powerful anti-inflammatory drugs that alter the transcription of many genes.

Corticosteroid drugs are powerful anti-inflammatory and immunosuppressive agents that are used widely to attenuate the harmful effects of autoimmune or allergic immune responses (see Chapters 14 and 15), as well as responses against transplanted organs. **Corticosteroids** are derivatives of the glucocorticoid family of steroid hormones that play a crucial role in maintaining the body's homeostasis; one of the most widely used is **prednisone**, a synthetic version of the hormone cortisol. Corticosteroids cross the cell's plasma membrane and bind to intracellular receptors of the nuclear receptor family. Activated glucocorticoid receptors are transported to the nucleus, where they bind to DNA and regulate a large number of genes expressed in leukocytes. The response to steroid therapy is complex, given the large number of genes regulated in leukocytes and in other tissues. With respect to immunosuppression, corticosteroids exert multiple anti-inflammatory effects, which are briefly summarized in Fig. 16.26.

Corticosteroids target the pro-inflammatory functions of monocytes and macrophages and reduce the number of CD4 T cells. They can induce the expression of certain anti-inflammatory genes, such as *AnxaI*, which encodes a protein inhibitor of phospholipase A$_2$ and thereby prevents this enzyme from generating pro-inflammatory **prostaglandins** and **leukotrienes** (see Section 3-3 and Section 14-6). Conversely, corticosteroids can also suppress the expression of pro-inflammatory genes, including those encoding the cytokines IL-1β and TNF-α.

The therapeutic effects of corticosteroid drugs are due to their presence at much higher concentrations than the natural concentration of glucocorticoid hormones, causing exaggerated responses with both toxic and beneficial effects. Adverse effects include fluid retention, weight gain, diabetes, bone mineral loss, and thinning of the skin, requiring a careful balance to

Corticosteroid therapy	
Effect on	**Physiological effects**
↓ IL-1, TNF-α, GM-CSF ↓ IL-3, IL-4, IL-5, CXCL8	↓ Inflammation caused by cytokines
↓ NOS	↓ NO
↓ Phospholipase A$_2$ ↓ Cyclooxygenase-2 ↑ Annexin-1	↓ Prostaglandins ↓ Leukotrienes
↓ Adhesion molecules	Reduced emigration of leukocytes from vessels
↑ Endonucleases	Induction of apoptosis in lymphocytes and eosinophils

Fig. 16.26 Anti-inflammatory effects of corticosteroid therapy. Corticosteroids regulate the expression of many genes, with a net anti-inflammatory effect. First, they reduce the production of inflammatory mediators, including cytokines, prostaglandins, and nitric oxide (NO). Second, they inhibit inflammatory-cell migration to sites of inflammation by inhibiting the expression of adhesion molecules. Third, corticosteroids promote the death of leukocytes by apoptosis. The layers of complexity are illustrated by the actions of annexin-1 (originally identified as a factor induced by corticosteroids and named lipocortin), which has been shown to participate in all of the effects of corticosteroids listed on the right. NOS, NO synthase.

be maintained between beneficial and harmful effects. These drugs can also decrease in effectiveness over time. Despite these drawbacks, inhaled corticosteroids have proven highly beneficial in the treatment of chronic asthma (see Section 14-12). In the treatment of autoimmunity or allograft rejection, in which high doses of oral corticosteroids are needed to be effective, they are most often administered in combination with other immunosuppressant drugs to keep the corticosteroid dose and side effects to a minimum. These other drugs include cytotoxic agents that act as immunosuppressants by killing rapidly dividing lymphocytes and drugs that more specifically target lymphocyte signaling pathways.

16-22 Cytotoxic drugs cause immunosuppression by killing dividing cells and have serious side effects.

The three cytotoxic drugs most commonly used as immunosuppressants are **azathioprine**, **cyclophosphamide**, and **mycophenolate**. These drugs interfere with DNA synthesis, and their major pharmacological action is on tissues in which cells are continually dividing. Developed originally to treat cancer, these drugs were found to be immunosuppressive after observations that they were cytotoxic to dividing lymphocytes. Azathioprine also interferes with CD28 co-stimulation in T cells, thus promoting T-cell apoptosis (see Section 7-22). The use of these compounds is, however, limited by their toxic effects on all tissues in which cells are dividing, such as the skin, gut lining, and bone marrow. Effects include decreased immune function, as well as anemia, leukopenia, thrombocytopenia, damage to intestinal epithelium, hair loss, and fetal death or injury. Because of their toxicity, these drugs are used at high doses only when the aim is to eliminate all dividing lymphocytes, as in the treatment of lymphoma and leukemia; in these cases, treated patients require subsequent bone marrow transplantation to restore their hematopoietic function. When used to treat unwanted immune responses such as autoimmune conditions, they are used at lower doses and in combination with other drugs such as corticosteroids.

Azathioprine is converted *in vivo* to the purine analog 6-thioguanine (6-TG), which is metabolized to 6-thioinosinic acid. Competing with inosine monophosphate, 6-thioinosinic acid blocks the *de novo* synthesis of adenosine monophosphate and guanosine monophosphate, thus inhibiting DNA synthesis. 6-TG is also incorporated into the DNA in place of guanine, and accumulation of 6-TG increases the DNA's sensitivity to mutations induced by the ultraviolet radiation in sunlight. Thus, patients treated with azathioprine have the long-term side effect of increased risk of skin cancer. Azathioprine also generates 6-thioguanine triphosphate (6-thio-GTP), which in T cells binds to the small GTPase Rac1 in place of GTP and suppresses its activity. Signaling from CD28 co-stimulation requires Rac1, and T cells therefore do not receive the anti-apoptotic signals from co-stimulation and instead undergo apoptosis. **Mycophenolate mofetil**, the 2-morpholinoethyl ester of mycophenolic acid, is the newest addition to the family of cytotoxic immunosuppressive drugs; it works in a similar fashion as azathioprine. It is metabolized to mycophenolic acid, which inhibits the enzyme inosine monophosphate dehydrogenase, thus blocking the *de novo* synthesis of guanosine monophosphate.

Azathioprine and mycophenolate are less toxic than cyclophosphamide, which is metabolized to phosphoramide mustard, which alkylates DNA. Cyclophosphamide is a member of the nitrogen mustard family of compounds, which were originally developed as chemical weapons. It has a range of highly toxic effects including inflammation of and hemorrhage from the bladder, known as hemorrhagic cystitis, and induction of bladder neoplasia.

16-23 Cyclosporin A, tacrolimus, and rapamycin are effective immunosuppressive agents that interfere with various T-cell signaling pathways.

Three noncytotoxic alternatives to the cytotoxic drugs are available as immunosuppressants and are widely used to treat transplant recipients. These are **cyclosporin A**, **tacrolimus** (previously known as **FK506**), and **rapamycin** (also known as **sirolimus**). Cyclosporin A is a cyclic decapeptide derived from a soil fungus found in Norway, *Tolypocladium inflatum*. Tacrolimus is a macrolide compound from the filamentous bacterium *Streptomyces tsukubaensis*, found in Japan; macrolides are compounds that contain a many-membered lactone ring to which is attached one or more deoxysugars. Rapamycin, another macrolide, is derived from *Streptomyces hygroscopicus*, found on Easter Island ('Rapa Nui' in Polynesian—hence the name of the drug). All three compounds exert their pharmacological effects by binding to members of a family of intracellular proteins known as the **immunophilins**, forming complexes that interfere with signaling pathways important for the clonal expansion of lymphocytes.

ANIMATION 16.1

As explained in Section 7-14, cyclosporin A and tacrolimus block T-cell proliferation by inhibiting the phosphatase activity of the Ca^{2+}-activated protein phosphatase **calcineurin**, which is required for the activation of the transcription factor NFAT. Both drugs reduce the expression of several cytokine genes that are normally induced upon T-cell activation (**Fig. 16.27**), including the gene encoding interleukin-2 (IL-2), which is an important factor for regulating T cells (see Section 9-15). Cyclosporin A and tacrolimus inhibit T-cell proliferation in response to either specific antigens or allogeneic cells and are used extensively in medical practice to prevent the rejection of allogeneic organ grafts. Although the major immunosuppressive effects of both drugs are probably the result of inhibition of T-cell proliferation, they also act on other cells and have a large variety of other immunological effects (see Fig. 16.27).

These two drugs inhibit calcineurin by first binding to an immunophilin molecule; cyclosporin A binds to the **cyclophilins**, and tacrolimus binds to the **FK-binding proteins (FKBPs)**. Immunophilins are peptidyl-prolyl *cis–trans* isomerases, but their isomerase activity is not relevant to the immunosuppressive activity of the drugs that bind them. Rather, the immunophilin:drug complexes bind to calcineurin and inhibit its phosphatase activity. In a normal immune response, the increase in intracellular calcium ions in response to T-cell receptor signaling activates the calcium-binding protein calmodulin; calmodulin then activates calcineurin (see Fig. 7.19). Binding of the

Immunological effects of cyclosporin A and tacrolimus	
Cell type	**Effects**
T lymphocyte	Reduced expression of IL-2, IL-3, IL-4, GM-CSF, TNF-α Reduced proliferation after decreased IL-2 production Reduced Ca^{2+}-dependent exocytosis of granule-associated serine esterases Inhibition of antigen-driven apoptosis
B lymphocyte	Inhibition of proliferation secondary to reduced cytokine production by T lymphocytes Inhibition of proliferation after ligation of surface immunoglobulin Induction of apoptosis after B-cell activation
Granulocyte	Reduced Ca^{2+}-dependent exocytosis of granule-associated serine esterases

Fig. 16.27 Cyclosporin A and tacrolimus inhibit lymphocyte function and some granulocyte responses.

With calcium bound to it, calmodulin can activate the enzyme calcineurin to dephosphorylate NFAT, which can then enter the nucleus to stimulate IL-2 transcription

The binding of cyclosporin A to an immunophilin creates a complex that inhibits calcineurin activation by calmodulin, thus preventing the dephosphorylation of NFAT

Fig. 16.28 Cyclosporin A and tacrolimus inhibit T-cell activation by interfering with the serine/threonine-specific phosphatase calcineurin. Top panel: Signaling via T-cell receptor–associated tyrosine kinases leads to opening of calcium release–activated calcium (CRAC) channels in the plasma membrane. This increases the concentration of Ca^{2+} in the cytoplasm and promotes calcium binding to the regulatory protein calmodulin (see Fig. 7.19). Calmodulin is activated by binding Ca^{2+} and can then target many downstream effector proteins such as the phosphatase calcineurin. Binding by calmodulin activates calcineurin to dephosphorylate the transcription factor NFAT (see Section 7-14), which then enters the nucleus and transcribes genes that are required for T-cell activation to progress. Bottom panel: When cyclosporin A or tacrolimus or both are present, they form complexes with their immunophilin targets, cyclophilin and FK-binding protein, respectively. These complexes bind to calcineurin, preventing it from becoming activated by calmodulin, and thereby preventing the dephosphorylation of NFAT.

immunophilin:drug complex to calcineurin prevents the latter's activation by calmodulin. Thus, the bound calcineurin is unable to dephosphorylate and activate NFAT (**Fig. 16.28**). Calcineurin is found in other cells besides T cells, but its levels in T cells are much lower than in other tissues. T cells are therefore particularly susceptible to the inhibitory effects of these drugs.

Cyclosporin A and tacrolimus are effective immunosuppressants but can inhibit all immune responses indiscriminately. This problem can be controlled by carefully varying the dose of drug given during the course of a response. During organ transplantation, for example, high doses are required during the time of grafting, but once the graft is established, the dose can be decreased to allow for protective immune responses while maintaining suppression of a response against the grafted tissue. Maintaining this balance requires careful monitoring of the patient. These drugs also have effects on many different tissues and thus can have broad side effects, such as injury to kidney tubule epithelial cells. Finally, treatment with these drugs is relatively expensive, because they are complex natural products that must be taken for long periods. Nevertheless, at present they are the immunosuppressants of choice in clinical transplantation, and they are also being tested in a variety of autoimmune diseases, especially those that, like graft rejection, are mediated by T cells.

Rapamycin has a different mechanism of action from either cyclosporin A or tacrolimus. Like tacrolimus, rapamycin binds to the FKBP family member of the immunophilins, but the rapamycin:immunophilin complex does not inhibit calcineurin activity. Instead, it inhibits a serine/threonine kinase known as **mTOR (mammalian target of rapamycin)**, which is involved in regulating cell growth and proliferation (see Section 7-17). The mTOR pathway can be activated by different upstream signaling pathways, including the Ras–MAPK pathway and the PI 3-kinase pathway. These pathways activate the kinase **Akt**, which phosphorylates and inactivates a regulatory complex called the tuberous sclerosis complex (**TSC**) (see Fig. 7-24). The non-phosphorylated TSC is active and normally acts as an inhibitor of the small GTPase **Rheb**. But after Akt phosphorylates TSC, Rheb becomes free to activate mTOR (see Fig. 7.24). Two distinct mTOR complexes can be formed, called **mTORC1** and **mTORC2**. These are controlled by two regulatory proteins called **Raptor** and **Rictor**, respectively, and which activate different downstream cellular pathways of mTOR (**Fig. 16.29**). The rapamycin:FKBP complex selectively inhibits the Raptor-dependent pathway (see Fig. 16.29), which markedly reduces T-cell proliferation, arrests cells in the G$_1$ phase of the cell cycle, and promotes apoptosis. Rapamycin inhibits lymphocyte proliferation driven by growth factors such as IL-2, IL-4, and IL-6, and selectively reduces the outgrowth of effector T cells while apparently enhancing the formation of memory T cells.

Although not directly acting on T-cell activation, one recently introduced drug regulates the migration of effector cells to the sites of a graft or of autoimmune disease. In Section 9-5, we described how emigration of lymphocytes out of the lymphoid tissues requires recognition of the lipid molecule

Fig. 16.29 Rapamycin inhibits cell growth and proliferation by selectively blocking activation of the kinase mTOR by Raptor. Rapamycin binds FK-binding protein (FKBP), the same immunophilin protein that binds to tacrolimus (FK506). The rapamycin:FKBP complex does not inhibit calcineurin, but instead blocks one of two complexes that activate mTOR, a large kinase that regulates many metabolic pathways. mTOR is activated downstream of various growth factor signaling pathways and becomes associated with either of two proteins, Raptor (regulatory-associated protein of mTOR) or Rictor (rapamycin-insensitive companion of mTOR). The complex with Raptor, mTORC1, promotes cell proliferation, translation of proteins, and autophagy, and the complex with Rictor, mTORC2, influences cell adhesion and migration by controlling the actin cytoskeleton. The rapamycin:FKBP complex acts to inhibit the Raptor-associated mTORC1, and thereby selectively reduces cell growth and proliferation.

sphingosine 1-phosphate (S1P) by the G protein–coupled receptor S1PR1. Fingolimod (FTY720), a sphingosine 1-phosphate analog, causes the retention of effector lymphocytes in lymphoid organs, thus preventing these cells from mediating their effector activities in target tissues. Fingolimod was approved in 2010 for treatment of the autoimmune disease multiple sclerosis and has shown promise in the treatment of kidney graft rejection and asthma.

16-24 JAK inhibitors can be used to treat autoimmune and inflammatory diseases.

Cytokines activate many aspects of the immune response. Many cytokine receptors use **Janus kinases (JAKs)** in their signal transduction (see Section 3-16), but they use different combinations of JAK proteins (**Fig. 16.30**). The four JAK family members, Jak1, Jak2, Jak3, and Tyk2, bind and phosphorylate the cytoplasmic regions of cytokine receptors and initiate the activation of different STAT transcription factors. Selective JAK inhibitors have been developed over the past decade that can block the kinase activity of one or more members of this family. Because different JAKs binds to different cytokine receptors, JAK inhibitors, or 'jakinibs,' can exert potentially specific effects on the quality of T-cell development.

The development of selective JAK inhibitors has advanced rapidly over the past several years, and there are currently eight drugs of this class approved in various countries for use in treating various inflammatory diseases (**Fig. 16.31**). For example, **tofacitinib** inhibits Jak3, interfering with signaling by IL-2 and IL-4, and somewhat more weakly Jak1, interfering with signaling by IL-6. Tofacitinib is approved for treatment of rheumatoid arthritis. **Ruxolitinib** inhibits Jak1 and Jak2 and has been approved for treating myelofibrosis, an abnormal proliferation of bone marrow progenitor cells that causes fibrosis. Jakinibs have been developed that selectively inhibit Jak1, including upadacitinib, which was recently approved by the FDA for the treatment of rheumatoid arthritis.

16-25 Antibodies against cell-surface molecules can be used to eliminate lymphocyte subsets or to inhibit lymphocyte function.

All the drugs discussed so far exert a general inhibition on immune responses and can have severe side effects, but antibodies can act in a more specific manner and with less direct toxicity. The initial therapeutic use of antibodies extends back to the late 1800s with the development of equine sera for treatment of diphtheria and tetanus. Today, intravenous immunoglobulin (IVIG), a collection of polyvalent IgG antibodies pooled from many blood donors, is still widely used as a treatment for various primary and acquired immune deficiencies. It is also used in some acute infections, where it likely works by neutralizing certain pathogens or their toxins. Finally, IVIG is also used to treat

Cytokine receptors and JAKs	
Cytokine	**JAKs used by receptors**
EPO, TPO, GH, GM-CSF, IL-3, IL-5	Jak2
IL-6, IFN-γ	Jak1 + Jak2
IL-2, IL-4, IL-7, IL-9, IL-15, IL-21	Jak1 + Jak3
IFN-α/β, type III interferons (IFN-γ)	Jak1 + Tyk2
IL-12, IL-23	Jak2 + Tyk2

Fig. 16.30 Cytokine receptors and the Janus kinases (JAKs) they use. EPO, erythropoietin; TPO, thrombopoietin; GH, growth hormone; GM-CSF, granulocyte–macrophage colony-stimulating factor.

Drug-Induced Serum Sickness

JAK inhibitors approved for use in autoimmune conditions		
Jakinib	**JAKs targeted**	**Indication**
Ruxolitinib	Jak1/Jak2	Myelofibrosis, polycythemia vera
Tofacitinib	Jak1/Jak3	Rheumatoid arthritis, psoriatic arthritis
Oclacitinib	Jak1	Pruritus, atopic dermatitis (dogs)
Baricitinib	Jak1/Jak2	Rheumatoid arthritis
Fedratinib	Jak2	Myelofibrosis
Upadacitinib	Jak1	Rheumatoid arthritis
Filgotinib	Jak1	Rheumatoid arthritis (EU/Japan)
Peficitinib	Jak3	Rheumatoid arthritis (Japan)

Fig. 16.31 Several JAK inhibitors are approved for use in autoimmune conditions. Shown are the targeted Janus kinases (JAKs) and the approved clinical indication for each drug. Some are approved only in the European Union (EU) or Japan, as indicated.

certain autoimmune and inflammatory diseases, such as immune thrombocytopenia and Kawasaki disease. In these cases, IVIG exerts an immunomodulatory effect that seems to operate through interactions with inhibitory Fc receptors that inhibit immune-cell activation.

The relatively recent expansion in the use of antibodies as therapeutic agents has extended their use beyond simply targeting pathogens to acting on components of the immune system itself. For example, the potential of antibodies to eliminate unwanted lymphocytes is demonstrated by **anti-lymphocyte globulin**, a preparation of polyclonal immunoglobulin from rabbits (and previously horses) immunized with human lymphocytes, which has been used for many years to treat episodes of acute graft rejection. Anti-lymphocyte globulin does not, however, discriminate between useful lymphocytes and those responsible for the unwanted responses and therefore leads to global immunosuppression. Foreign immunoglobulins are also highly antigenic in humans, and the large doses of anti-lymphocyte globulin used in therapy often cause a condition called **serum sickness**, resulting from the formation of immune complexes of the animal immunoglobulin and human antibodies against it (see Section 14-14).

Anti-lymphocyte globulin is nevertheless still used to treat acute rejection, and this has stimulated the quest for monoclonal antibodies (see Appendix I, Section A-8) that would achieve more specifically targeted effects. One such antibody is **alemtuzumab** (marketed as Campath-1H), which is directed at the cell-surface protein CD52 expressed by most lymphocytes. It has actions similar to those of anti-lymphocyte globulin, causing long-standing lymphopenia. It is also used to eliminate cancer cells in the treatment of chronic lymphocytic leukemia.

Immunosuppressive monoclonal antibodies act by one of two general mechanisms. Some, such as alemtuzumab, trigger the destruction of lymphocytes *in vivo* and are referred to as **depleting antibodies**, whereas others are **nondepleting** and act by blocking the function of their target protein without killing the cell that bears it. Depleting monoclonal IgG antibodies bind to lymphocytes and target them to macrophages and NK cells, which bear Fc receptors and kill the lymphocytes by phagocytosis or ADCC, respectively. Complement-mediated lysis may also play a part in lymphocyte destruction.

16-26 Antibodies can be engineered to reduce their immunogenicity in humans.

A major impediment to therapy with monoclonal antibodies in humans has been that these antibodies are most readily made by immunizing nonhuman species, such as the mouse, to generate antibodies of the desired specificity (see Appendix I, Section A-8). Humans may develop an antibody response against such nonhuman antibodies, because aggregated forms of foreign antibodies can be immunogenic. Such a reaction not only interferes with the therapeutic actions of the antibodies but also leads to allergic reactions and, if treatment is continued, may result in **anaphylaxis** (see Section 14-1). Once a patient has made a response to an antibody, it can no longer be used for treatment. In principle, this problem can be avoided by making antibodies that are not recognized as foreign by the human immune system, a process called **humanization**.

Various approaches have been tried to humanize antibodies. The variable regions encoding the antigen-recognition determinants from a murine antibody can be spliced onto the Fc regions of human IgG by gene manipulation. Antibodies of this type are called chimeric antibodies. However, this approach leaves regions within the murine variable regions that could potentially induce immune responses (**Fig. 16.32**). Genetically engineered mice that harbor human immunoglobulin genes inserted into their immunoglobulin

-omab

light chain

heavy chain

Fully mouse

-ximab

Chimeric

-zumab

Humanized

-umab

Fully human

Fig. 16.32 Monoclonal antibodies used to treat human diseases can be engineered to decrease immunogenicity but maintain their antigen specificity. Antibodies that are derived fully from mice, named with the suffix -*omab*, are immunogenic in humans. This causes patients to generate antibodies against them, limiting their usefulness over time. This immunogenicity can be reduced by making chimeric antibodies in which the V regions from the mouse are spliced onto human antibody constant regions; such antibodies are named with the suffix -*ximab*. Humanization is the process of splicing in just the complementarity-determining regions from the mouse antibody, further reducing immunogenicity; humanized antibodies are named with the suffix -*zumab*. New techniques allow fully human (-*umab*) monoclonal antibodies to be derived, which are the least immunogenic type of antibody currently used for treating humans.

locus represent one way that human antibodies may be obtained from the immunization of mice. Newer methods are aimed at generating fully human monoclonal antibodies directly from human cells through the use of viral transformation of human primary B-cell lines or antibody-secreting plasmablasts or by generating human B-cell hybridomas.

Monoclonal antibodies belong to a new class of therapeutic compounds called biologics, which includes other natural proteins such as anti-lymphocyte globulin, cytokines, protein fragments, and even whole cells, the latter used, for example, in the adoptive transfer of T cells in cancer immunotherapy. Many monoclonal antibodies have been, or are in the process of being, approved for clinical use by the FDA (**Fig. 16.33**). A systematic naming process identifies the type of antibody. Murine monoclonal antibodies are designated by the suffix **-omab**, except for muromonab (originally called OKT3), a murine antibody against CD3, which was named before the nomenclature was established. Chimeric antibodies in which the entire variable region is spliced into human constant regions have the suffix **-ximab**, such as basiliximab, an anti-CD25 (anti-IL-2Rα) antibody approved for the treatment of transplantation rejection. Humanized antibodies in which the murine hypervariable regions have been spliced into a human antibody have the suffix **-zumab**, as in alemtuzumab and **natalizumab** (Tysabri). The latter is directed against the α4 integrin subunit and is used to treat multiple sclerosis and Crohn's disease. Antibodies derived entirely from human sequences have the suffix **-umab**, as in adalimumab, an antibody derived from phage display (see Appendix I, Section A-9) that binds TNF-α; it is used to treat several autoimmune diseases.

16-27 Monoclonal antibodies can be used to prevent allograft rejection.

Antibodies specific for various physiological targets are being used or are under investigation to prevent the rejection of transplanted organs by inhibiting the development of harmful inflammatory and cytotoxic responses. For example, alemtuzumab, discussed in Section 16-25, is licensed for the treatment of certain leukemias but is also used in both solid organ and bone marrow transplantation. In solid organ transplantation, alemtuzumab may be given to the recipient around the time of transplantation to remove mature

Fig. 16.33 Monoclonal antibodies developed for immunotherapy. A substantial fraction of pharmaceuticals currently under development are antibodies, and additions to this list, current as of this writing, are under development and in clinical trials. BLyS, B-lymphocyte stimulator, also known as BAFF (B-cell activating factor).

Monoclonal antibodies developed for immunotherapy			
Generic name	**Specificity**	**Mechanism of action**	**Approved indication**
Rituximab	Anti-CD20	Eliminates B cells	Non-Hodgkin's lymphoma
Alemtuzumab (Campath-1H)	Anti-CD52	Eliminates lymphocytes	Chronic lymphocytic leukemia
Muromonab (OKT3)	Anti-CD3	Inhibits T-cell activation	Kidney transplantation
Daclizumab	Anti-IL-2Rα	Reduces T-cell activation	
Basiliximab	Anti-IL-2Rα	Reduces T-cell activation	
Infliximab	Anti-TNF-α	Inhibit inflammation induced by TNF-α	Crohn's disease
Certolizumab	Anti-TNF-α		Rheumatoid arthritis
Adalimumab	Anti-TNF-α		
Golimumab	Anti-TNF-α		
Tocilizumab	Anti-IL-6R	Blocks inflammation induced by IL-6 signaling	
Canakinumab	Anti-IL-1β	Blocks inflammation caused by IL-1	Muckle–Wells syndrome
Denosumab	Anti-RANKL	Inhibits activation of osteoclasts by RANKL	Bone loss
Ustekinumab	Anti-IL-12/23	Inhibits inflammation caused by IL-12 and IL-23	Psoriasis
Efalizumab	Anti-CD11a (α$_L$ integrin subunit)	Block lymphocyte trafficking	Psoriasis (withdrawn from use in United States and European Union)
Natalizumab	Anti-α$_4$ integrin		Multiple sclerosis
Omalizumab	Anti-IgE	Removes IgE antibody	Chronic asthma
Belimumab	Anti-BLyS (BAFF)	Reduces B-cell responses	Systemic lupus erythematosus (pending approval)
Ipilimumab	Anti-CTLA-4	Increases CD4 T-cell responses	Metastatic melanoma
Raxibacumab	Anti-*Bacillus anthracis* protective antigen (the cell-binding moiety of anthrax toxin)	Prevents action of anthrax toxins	Anthrax infection (pending approval)

T lymphocytes from the circulation. In bone marrow transplantation, alemtuzumab can be used *in vitro* to deplete donor bone marrow of mature T cells before its infusion into a recipient or used *in vivo* to treat the recipient after infusion. Elimination of mature T cells from donor bone marrow is very effective at reducing the incidence of graft-versus-host disease (see Section 15-25). In this disease, the T lymphocytes in the donor bone marrow recognize the recipient as foreign and mount a damaging response, causing rashes, diarrhea, and hepatitis, which can occasionally be fatal. Bone marrow transplantation is also used as a treatment for leukemia, as T cells in the graft can have a so-called graft-versus-leukemia effect where they recognize the leukemic cells as foreign and destroy them. It was originally thought that elimination of mature donor T cells during such procedures would be disadvantageous, as the antileukemic action of the donor T cells could be lost, but this seems to not be the case when alemtuzumab is used as the depleting agent.

Graft-Versus-Host Disease

Specific antibodies directed against T cells have been used to treat episodes of graft rejection that occur after transplantation. The murine antibody **muromonab** (OKT3) targets the CD3 complex and leads to T-cell immunosuppression by inhibiting signaling through the T-cell receptor. It has been used clinically in solid organ transplantation but is often associated with a dangerous side effect, namely, the stimulation of pro-inflammatory cytokine release, and its use is declining. This cytokine release is related to muromonab's intact Fc region, which can activate Fc receptors via cross-linking and activate the cells that bear these receptors. In an antibody against the CD3? chain called teplizumab, or OKT3γ1 Ala-Ala, the amino acids 234 and 235 in the human IgG1 Fc region have been changed to alanines, and this antibody no longer stimulates cytokine release.

Two other antibodies, **daclizumab** and **basiliximab**, approved for treating kidney transplant rejection, are directed against CD25 (a subunit of the IL-2 receptor), reducing T-cell activation, presumably by blocking the growth-promoting signals delivered by IL-2.

A primate model of kidney transplant rejection showed promising effects for a humanized monoclonal antibody against the **CD40 ligand** expressed by T cells (see Section 9-20). A possible mechanism of protection by this antibody is blockade of the activation of dendritic cells by helper T cells that recognize donor antigens. Only preliminary studies of anti-CD40 ligand antibodies have been performed in humans. One antibody was associated with thromboembolic complications and was withdrawn; a different anti-CD40 ligand antibody was administered to patients with the autoimmune disease systemic lupus erythematosus (SLE) without significant complications, but also with little evidence of efficacy.

In experimental models, monoclonal antibodies against other targets have also had some success in preventing graft rejection, including nondepleting antibodies that bind the CD4 co-receptor or the co-stimulatory receptor CD28 on lymphocytes. Similarly, abatacept, a soluble recombinant CTLA-4–Ig fusion protein that binds to the co-stimulatory B7 molecules on antigen-presenting cells and prevents their interaction with CD28 on T cells, is approved for the treatment of rheumatoid arthritis.

Systemic Lupus Erythematosus

Rheumatoid Arthritis

16-28 Depletion of autoreactive lymphocytes can treat autoimmune disease.

In addition to their use in preventing transplantation rejection, monoclonal antibodies can be used to treat certain autoimmune diseases, and in the next few sections we discuss the different immune mechanisms targeted. Here we will discuss the use of depleting and nondepleting antibodies to remove lymphocytes nonspecifically. The anti-CD20 monoclonal antibody rituximab was originally developed to treat B-cell lymphomas but has also been tried in treating certain autoimmune diseases. By ligating CD20, rituximab (Rituxan; MabThera) transduces a signal that induces lymphocyte apoptosis and depletes B cells for several months. Certain autoimmune diseases are believed to involve autoantibody-mediated pathogenesis. There is evidence for the efficacy of rituximab in some individuals with autoimmune hemolytic anemia, SLE, rheumatoid arthritis, or type II mixed cryoglobulinemia, all of which have autoantibodies as a part of their clinical presentation. Although CD20 is not expressed on antibody-producing plasma cells, their B-cell precursors are targeted by anti-CD20, resulting in a substantial reduction in the short-lived, but not the long-lived, plasma-cell population.

Alemtuzumab, discussed earlier as a treatment for leukemia and in transplant rejection, has shown some beneficial effect in studies of small numbers of people with multiple sclerosis. However, immediately after its infusion, most multiple sclerosis patients suffered a frightening, although fortunately brief, flare-up of their illness, illustrating another potential complication of antibody therapy. Alemtuzumab was acting as intended, killing cells by complement- and Fc-dependent mechanisms. However, it also stimulated the release of cytokines, including TNF-α, IFN-γ, and IL-6, which transiently block nerve conduction in nerve fibers previously affected by demyelination. This caused the transient but dramatic exacerbation of symptoms. Nevertheless, alemtuzumab may be useful at early stages of the disease, when the inflammatory response is maximal, but this has yet to be determined.

Treatment of rheumatoid arthritis and multiple sclerosis with anti-CD4 antibodies has been tried, but with disappointing results. In controlled studies, the antibodies showed only small therapeutic effects but caused depletion of T lymphocytes from peripheral blood for more than 6 years after treatment. The likely explanation for the failure seems to be that these antibodies failed to delete already primed CD4 T cells secreting pro-inflammatory cytokines, and may thus have missed their target. This cautionary tale shows that it is possible to deplete large numbers of lymphocytes and yet completely fail to kill the cells that matter.

16-29 Biologics that block TNF-α, IL-1, or IL-6 can alleviate autoimmune diseases.

Anti-inflammatory therapy can attempt to eliminate an autoimmune response altogether, as with immunosuppressive drugs or depleting antibodies, or try to reduce the tissue injury caused by the immune response. This second category of treatment is called **immunomodulatory therapy** and is illustrated by the use of conventional anti-inflammatory agents such as aspirin, nonsteroidal anti-inflammatory drugs, or low-dose corticosteroids. A newer avenue of immunomodulatory therapy using biologics is illustrated by several FDA-approved antibodies that block the activity of powerful pro-inflammatory cytokines such as TNF-α, IL-1, and IL-6.

Rheumatoid Arthritis

Multiple Sclerosis

Crohn's Disease

Anti-TNF therapy was the first specific biological therapeutic to enter the clinic. Anti-TNF-α antibodies induced striking remissions in rheumatoid arthritis (**Fig. 16.34**) and reduced inflammation in Crohn's disease, an inflammatory bowel disease (see Section 15-5). Two types of established biologics are used to antagonize TNF-α in clinical practice. The first type comprises the anti-TNF-α antibodies, such as infliximab and adalimumab, which bind to TNF-α and block its activity. The second type is a recombinant human TNF receptor (TNFR) subunit p75–Fc fusion protein called **etanercept**, which also binds TNF-α, neutralizing its activity. These are extremely potent anti-inflammatory agents, and the number of diseases in which they have been shown to be effective is growing as further clinical trials are performed. In addition to rheumatoid arthritis, the rheumatic diseases **ankylosing spondylitis**, **psoriatic arthropathy**, and juvenile idiopathic arthritis (other than the systemic-onset subset) respond well to blockade of TNF-α, and this treatment is now routine in many cases.

An illustration of the importance of TNF-α in defending against infection is the observation that TNF-α blockade carries a small but increased risk of serious infections, including tuberculosis (see Section 3-20). Anti-TNF-α therapy has not been successful in all diseases. TNF-α blockade as a treatment for **experimental autoimmune encephalomyelitis (EAE)**, a mouse model of multiple sclerosis, led to amelioration of the disease, but in human patients with

Fig. 16.34 Anti-inflammatory effects of anti-TNF-α therapy in rheumatoid arthritis. The clinical course of 24 patients was followed for 4 weeks after treatment with either a placebo or a monoclonal antibody against TNF-α at a dose of 10 mg kg⁻¹. The antibody therapy was associated with a reduction in both subjective and objective parameters of disease activity (as measured by pain score and swollen-joint count, respectively) and in the systemic inflammatory acute-phase response, measured as a fall in the concentration of the acute-phase C-reactive protein (CRP).

multiple sclerosis treated with anti-TNF-α, relapses became more frequent, possibly because of an increase in T-cell activation.

Antibodies and recombinant proteins against the pro-inflammatory cytokine IL-1 and its receptor have not proved as effective as TNF-α blockade for treating rheumatoid arthritis in humans, despite being equally powerful in animal models of arthritis. An antibody against the cytokine IL-1 has been licensed for clinical use against the hereditary autoinflammatory disease Muckle–Wells syndrome (see Section 13-18), and blockade of the IL-1β receptor by the recombinant protein **anakinra** (Kineret) has also proven useful in adults with moderate to severe rheumatoid arthritis.

Another cytokine antagonist in clinical use is the humanized antibody **tocilizumab**; by virtue of being directed against the IL-6 receptor, it blocks the effects of the pro-inflammatory cytokine IL-6. This seems to be as effective as anti-TNF-α in individuals with rheumatoid arthritis and also shows promise in treating systemic-onset juvenile idiopathic arthritis, an autoinflammatory condition.

Interferon-β (Avonex) is used to treat diseases of viral origin on the basis of its ability to enhance immunity, but it is also effective in treating multiple sclerosis, attenuating its course and severity and reducing the occurrence of relapses. Until recently, it was unclear how IFN-β could reduce rather than enhance immunity. In Section 3-11, we described the inflammasome, in which innate sensors of the NLR family activate caspase 1 to cleave the IL-1 pro-protein into the active form of the cytokine (see Fig. 3.20). We now know that IFN-β acts at two levels to reduce IL-1 production. It inhibits the activity of the NALP3 (NLRP3) and NLRP1 inflammasomes and also reduces expression of the IL-1 pro-protein, reducing the substrate available to caspase 1. Thus, IFN-β limits the production of a powerful pro-inflammatory cytokine, which may explain its observed effects on the symptoms of multiple sclerosis.

Hereditary Periodic
Fever Syndromes

Systemic Juvenile
Idiopathic Arthritis

16-30 Biologics can block cell migration to sites of inflammation and reduce immune responses.

Effector lymphocytes expressing the **integrin α₄β₁** (VLA-4) bind to VCAM-1 on endothelium in the central nervous system, while those expressing **integrin α₄β₇** (lamina propria–associated molecule 1) bind to MAdCAM-1 on the endothelium in the gut. The humanized monoclonal antibody **natalizumab** is

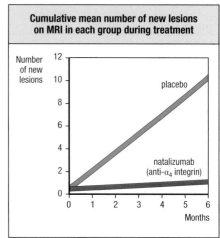

Fig. 16.35 Treatment with an anti-α₄ integrin humanized monoclonal antibody reduces relapses in multiple sclerosis. Left panel: Interaction between $\alpha_4\beta_1$ integrin (VLA-4) on lymphocytes, monocytes, and macrophages and VCAM-1 expressed on endothelial cells permits the adhesion of these cells to brain endothelium. This facilitates the migration of these cells into the plaques of inflammation in multiple sclerosis. Center panel: The monoclonal antibody natalizumab (blue) binds to the α_4 chain of the integrin and blocks adhesive interactions between lymphocytes, monocytes, and macrophages and VCAM-1 on endothelial cells, thus preventing the cells from entering the tissue and exacerbating the inflammation. The future of this treatment is unclear because of the development of a rare infection as a side effect (see the text). Right panel: The number of new lesions detected on magnetic resonance imaging (MRI) of the brain is greatly reduced in patients treated with natalizumab compared with those treated with placebo.

specific for the α_4 integrin subunit and binds both VLA-4 and $\alpha_4\beta_7$, preventing their interaction with their ligands (**Fig. 16.35**). This antibody has shown therapeutic benefit in placebo-controlled trials in individuals with Crohn's disease and those with multiple sclerosis. The early signs that this treatment could be successful illustrate the fact that disease depends on the continuing emigration of lymphocytes, monocytes, and macrophages from the circulation into the tissues of the brain in multiple sclerosis, and into the gut wall in Crohn's disease. However, blockade of $\alpha_4\beta_1$ integrin is not specific and, like anti-TNF therapy, could lead to reduced defense against infection. Rarely, patients treated with natalizumab have developed **progressive multifocal leukoencephalopathy (PML)**, an opportunistic infection caused by the JC virus, a very common and normally harmless virus. This led to the temporary withdrawal of natalizumab from the market in 2005, but in June 2006 it was again allowed to be prescribed for multiple sclerosis and for Crohn's disease.

A similar problem with multifocal leukoencephalopathy led to the 2009 withdrawal from the market in the United States and Europe of another anti-integrin antibody, efalizumab; this drug targets the α_L subunit (CD11a) and had shown promise in treating **psoriasis**, an inflammatory skin disease driven primarily by T cells that produce pro-inflammatory cytokines.

16-31 Blockade of co-stimulatory pathways that activate lymphocytes can be used to treat autoimmune disease.

Blocking co-stimulatory pathways, as noted earlier in connection with the prevention of transplantation rejection (see Section 16-27), has also been applied to autoimmune diseases. For example, CTLA-4–Ig (abatacept) blocks the interaction of the B7 expressed by antigen-presenting cells with the CD28 expressed by T cells. This drug is approved for the treatment of rheumatoid arthritis and also seems to be beneficial in treating psoriasis. When CTLA-4–Ig was given to individuals with psoriasis, there was an improvement in the psoriatic rash and histological evidence of loss of activation of keratinocytes, T cells, and dendritic cells within the damaged skin.

Another co-stimulatory pathway that has been targeted in psoriasis is the interaction between the adhesion molecule CD2 on T cells and CD58 (LFA-3) on antigen-presenting cells. A recombinant CD58–IgG1 fusion protein, called **alefacept** (Amevive), inhibits the interaction between CD2 and CD58 and is now a routine and effective treatment for psoriasis. Although memory T cells are targeted by this therapy, responses to vaccination such as anti-tetanus remain intact.

16-32 Some commonly used drugs have immunomodulatory properties.

Certain existing medications, such as the statins and angiotensin-converting enzyme (ACE) inhibitors widely used in the prevention and treatment of cardiovascular disease, can also modulate the immune response in experimental animals. **Statins** are very widely prescribed drugs that block the enzyme **3-hydroxy-3-methylglutaryl-coenzyme A (HMG-CoA) reductase**, thereby reducing cholesterol levels. They also reduce the increased level of expression of MHC class II molecules in some autoimmune diseases. These effects may be due to an alteration in the cholesterol content of membranes, thereby influencing lymphocyte signaling. In animal models, these drugs also seem to cause T cells to switch from a more pathogenic T_H1 response to a more protective T_H2 response, although whether this occurs in humans is not clear.

The hormone vitamin D_3, essential for bone and mineral homeostasis, also exerts immunomodulatory effects. It decreases IL-12 production by dendritic cells and leads to a decrease in IL-2 and IFN-γ production by CD4 T cells. Protective effects have been demonstrated in a variety of animal models of autoimmunity, such as EAE (see Section 15-3) and diabetes, as well as in transplantation. The major drawback of vitamin D_3 is that its immunomodulatory effects are seen only at dosages that would lead to hypercalcemia and bone resorption in humans. There is a major search under way for structural analogs of vitamin D_3 that retain the immunomodulatory effects but do not cause hypercalcemia.

 Multiple Sclerosis

16-33 Controlled administration of antigen can be used to manipulate the nature of an antigen-specific response.

In some diseases, the target antigen of an unwanted immune response can be identified. It can be possible, then, to use the antigen itself, rather than drugs or antibodies, to treat the disease, because the manner of antigen presentation can alter the immune response and reduce or eliminate its pathogenic features. As discussed in Section 14-12, this principle has been applied with some success to the treatment of allergies caused by an IgE response to very low doses of antigen. Repeated treatment of allergic individuals with increasing doses of allergen seems to divert the allergic response to one dominated by T cells that favor the production of IgG and IgA antibodies from B cells. These antibodies are thought to desensitize the patient by binding the small amounts of allergen normally encountered and preventing it from binding to IgE.

There has been considerable interest in using peptide antigens to suppress pathogenic responses in T cell–mediated autoimmune disease. The type of CD4 T-cell response induced by a peptide depends on the way in which it is presented to the immune system (see Section 9-14). For instance, peptides given orally tend to induce regulatory T cells through production of TGF-β but do not induce T_H1 cells or systemic antibody production (see Section 12-7). Experiments in animals indicate that oral antigens can protect against induced autoimmune disease. Diseases resembling multiple sclerosis or rheumatoid arthritis can be induced in mice by the injection of myelin basic protein

(MBP) or type II collagen, respectively, in Freund's complete adjuvant (see Section 16-8). Oral administration of MBP or type II collagen inhibits the development of these diseases in animals, but oral administration of the whole protein in individuals with multiple sclerosis or rheumatoid arthritis has had marginal therapeutic effects. Similarly, no protective effect was found in a large study that examined whether giving low-dose parenteral insulin could delay the onset of diabetes in people at high risk of developing the disease.

Other approaches using antigen to shift the autoimmune T-cell response to a less damaging T_H2 response have been more effective in humans. The peptide drug glatiramer acetate (Copaxone) is approved for treating multiple sclerosis, in which it may reduce relapse rates by up to 30%. It is a polymer consisting of the four amino acids glutamic acid, alanine, tyrosine, and lysine in ratios that mimic their composition in MBP, and it induces a T_H2-type protective response. A more refined strategy uses **altered peptide ligands (APLs)**, in which amino acid substitutions have been made in specific amino acids at the T-cell receptor contact positions of an antigenic peptide. APLs can be designed to act as partial agonists or antagonists or to induce regulatory T cells. But despite the success of APLs in treating EAE in mice, a trial of these peptides for multiple sclerosis in some patients led to exacerbated disease or to allergic reaction associated with a vigorous T_H2 response, and so their value in humans remains to be seen.

Summary.

Treatments for unwanted immune responses, such as graft rejection, autoimmunity, or allergic reactions, include conventional drugs—anti-inflammatory, cytotoxic, and immunosuppressive drugs and JAK inhibitors—as well as biologic agents such as monoclonal antibodies and immunomodulatory proteins. Anti-inflammatory drugs, of which the most potent are the corticosteroids, have a broad spectrum of actions and a wide range of toxic side effects. Their dose must be carefully controlled, and they are normally used in combination with either cytotoxic or immunosuppressive drugs. The cytotoxic drugs kill dividing cells and prevent lymphocyte proliferation but suppress all immune responses indiscriminately and also kill other types of dividing cells. The immunosuppressive drugs, such as cyclosporin A and rapamycin, interfere in specific signaling pathways and are generally less toxic but are more expensive and still suppress the immune response somewhat indiscriminately.

Several types of biologic agents are now established in the clinic for treating transplant rejection and autoimmune diseases (**Fig. 16.36**). Many monoclonal antibodies approved for human use deplete lymphocytes either generally or selectively, or inhibit lymphocyte activation through receptor blockade, or prevent lymphocyte migration into tissues. Immunomodulatory agents also include monoclonal antibodies or fusion proteins that inhibit the inflammatory actions of TNF-α, a notable success for immunotherapy.

Summary to Chapter 16.

Arguably, the greatest achievement of immunology has been the development of vaccines to control or prevent the threat of infectious diseases. The global COVID-19 pandemic has brought this aspect of immunology's contributions to the forefront, as new technologies have been rapidly applied on the basis of a deep understanding of the mechanisms of protective immunity. The current armamentarium of therapeutic technologies is vast, ranging from rather old approaches that used live but attenuated virus strains, through an array of subunit and conjugate vaccines, to the newly developed and rapidly deployable mRNA-based vaccines that hold the promise of keeping up with quickly evolving viral variants. Even today, the original oral Sabin vaccines are undergoing

Therapeutic agents used to treat human autoimmune diseases				
Target	**Therapeutic agent**	**Disease**	**Disease outcome**	**Disadvantages**
Integrins	$\alpha_4\beta_1$ integrin–specific monoclonal antibody (mAb)	Relapsing/remitting multiple sclerosis (MS) Rheumatoid arthritis (RA) Inflammatory bowel disease	Reduction in relapse rate; delay in disease progression	Increased risk of infection; progressive multifocal encephalopathy
B cells	CD20-specific mAb	RA Systemic lupus erythematosus (SLE) MS	Improvement in arthritis, possibly in SLE	Increased risk of infection
HMG-coenzyme A reductase	Statins	MS	Reduction in disease activity	Hepatotoxicity; rhabdomyolysis
T cells	CD3-specific mAb	Type 1 diabetes mellitus	Reduced insulin use	Increased risk of infection
	CTLA-4–immunoglobulin fusion protein	RA Psoriasis MS	Improvement in arthritis	
Cytokines	TNF-specific mAb and soluble TNFR fusion protein	RA Crohn's disease Psoriatic arthritis Ankylosing spondylitis	Improvement in disability; joint repair in arthritis	Increased risk of tuberculosis and other infections; slight increase in risk of lymphoma
	IL-1 receptor antagonist	RA	Improves disability	Low efficacy
	IL-15–specific mAb	RA	May improve disability	Increased risk of opportunistic infection
	IL-6 receptor–specific mAb	RA	Decreased disease activity	Increased risk of opportunistic infection
	Type I interferons	Relapsing/remitting MS	Reduction in relapse rate	Liver toxicity; influenza-like syndrome is common

Fig. 16.36 Therapeutic agents for human autoimmunity. The immunosuppressive agents listed in Fig 16.33 can act in one of three general ways. First (red), they can act by depleting cells from inflammatory sites, causing global cell-specific depletion, or by blocking integrin interactions, thereby inhibiting lymphocyte trafficking. Second (blue), agents may block specific cellular interactions or inhibit various co-stimulatory pathways. Third (green), agents may target the terminal effector mechanisms, such as by neutralizing various pro-inflammatory cytokines.

modernization with molecular design aimed at reducing their potential for reversion, a feature that still challenges the goal of global polio eradication. A future challenge in immunology is to control the immune system so that unwanted immune responses can be suppressed and desirable responses elicited. Current methods of suppressing unwanted responses rely heavily on drugs that suppress adaptive immunity indiscriminately and are thus inherently flawed. We have seen in this book that the immune system can suppress its own responses in an antigen-specific manner and that, by studying these endogenous regulatory events, it has been possible to devise strategies to manipulate specific responses while sparing general immune competence. New treatments, including many monoclonal antibodies and new classes of drugs, such as the jakinibs, have emerged as clinically important therapies to selectively suppress the responses that lead to allergy, autoimmunity, or the rejection of grafted organs. Similarly, as we understand more about tumors and infectious agents, better strategies to mobilize the immune system against cancer and infection are becoming possible. To achieve all this, we need to learn more about the induction of immunity and the biology of the immune system and to apply what we have learned to human disease.

Discussion Questions

16.1 The earliest vaccines developed were live pathogens, such as cowpox variolation and the live-attenuated oral Sabin vaccines for polio. Compare vaccination using live-attenuated pathogens to vaccination using killed or conjugate vaccines.

16.2 The live oral Sabin vaccines for polio were generated during a time when characterization of the mutations responsible for attenuation was not possible, and yet they were tested and used without such knowledge. Discuss the issues that affect the development of a live-attenuated vaccine for COVID-19 using such approaches today.

16.3 What are the benefits and/or drawbacks in using solely the SARS-CoV-2 spike protein as an antigen in vaccines against COVID-19?

16.4 Discuss the importance of herd immunity. Should vaccination against important pathogens such as polio or SARS-CoV-2 be mandatory?

16.5 In cancer treatment, what types of clinical issues must be considered when evaluating the efficacy of checkpoint blockade therapies compared to that of conventional cytotoxic drug therapies? If the tumor continues to be viable 1 week after checkpoint blockade, has the treatment necessarily failed?

16.6 Antibodies against PD-1 were available long before PD-1 checkpoint blockade was recognized as an effective treatment for cancers in mice. What properties of an antibody against an inhibitory receptor are required for it to be useful in checkpoint blockade? What other information might be required?

16.7 Explain how the drug cyclosporin A can still exert effects selectively on T cells, even though the immunophilin to which it binds is ubiquitous and is expressed at even higher levels by other tissues.

16.8 Rapamycin inhibits mTORC1 and supresses the emergence of effector T cells. How could it be potentially useful in augmenting the action of a vaccine?

16.9 Anti-TNF-α antibodies are useful in treating rheumatoid arthritis. What is the downside of this therapy?

General references.

Feldmann, M.: **Translating molecular insights in autoimmunity into effective therapy.** *Annu. Rev. Immunol.* 2009, **27**:1–27.

Kappe, S.H., Vaughan, A.M., Boddey, J.A., and Cowman, A.F.: **That was then but this is now: malaria research in the time of an eradication agenda.** *Science* 2010, **328**:862–866.

Kaufmann, S.H.: **Future vaccination strategies against tuberculosis: thinking outside the box.** *Immunity* 2010, **33**:567–577.

Korman, A.J., Peggs, K.S., and Allison, J.P.: **Checkpoint blockade in cancer immunotherapy.** *Adv. Immunol.* 2006, **90**:297–339.

Maus, M.V., Fraietta, J.A., Levine, B.L., Kalos, M., Zhao, Y., and June, C.H.: **Adoptive immunotherapy for cancer or viruses.** *Annu. Rev. Immunol.* 2014, **32**:189–225.

Plotkin, S.A., Orenstein, W.A., Offit, P.A., and Edwards, K.M.: *Plotkin's Vaccines*, 7th ed. Philadelphia: Elsevier, 2018.

Section references.

16-1   Vaccines can be based on attenuated pathogens or material from killed organisms.

Anderson, R.M., Donnelly, C.A., and Gupta, S.: **Vaccine design, evaluation, and community-based use for antigenically variable infectious agents.** *Lancet* 1997, **350**:1466–1470.

Dermer, P., Lee, C., Eggert, J., and Few, B.: **A history of neonatal group B streptococcus with its related morbidity and mortality rates in the United States.** *J. Pediatr. Nurs.* 2004, **19**:357–363.

Rabinovich, N.R., McInnes, P., Klein, D.L., and Hall, B.F.: **Vaccine technologies: view to the future.** *Science* 1994, **265**:1401–1404.

16-2   Most effective vaccines generate antibodies that prevent damage caused by toxins or that neutralize pathogens and stop infection.

Caskey, M., Klein, F., and Nussenzweig, M.C.: **Broadly neutralizing anti-HIV-1 monoclonal antibodies in the clinic.** *Nat. Med.* 2019, **25**:547–553.

Kapikian, A.Z., Mitchell, R.H., Chanock, R.M., Shvedoff, R.A., and Stewart, C.E.: **An epidemiologic study of altered clinical reactivity to respiratory syncytial (RS) virus infection in children previously vaccinated with an inactivated RS virus vaccine.** *Am. J. Epidemiol.* 1969, **89**:405–421.

Levine, M.M., and Levine, O.S.: **Influence of disease burden, public perception, and other factors on new vaccine development, implementation, and continued use.** *Lancet* 1997, **350**:1386–1392.

Mouque, H., Scheid, J.F., Zoller, M.J., Krogsgaard, M., Ott, R.G., Shukair, S., Artyomov, M.N., Pietzsch, J., Connors, M., Pereyra, F., *et al.*: **Polyreactivity increases the apparent affinity of anti-HIV antibodies by heteroligation.** *Nature* 2010, **467**:591–595.

Nichol, K.L., Lind, A., Margolis, K.L., Murdoch, M., McFadden, R., Hauge, M., Palese, P., and Garcia-Sastre, A.: **Influenza vaccines: present and future.** *J. Clin. Invest.* 2002, **110**:9–13.

Steichen. J.M., Kulp, D.W., Tokatlian, T., Escolano, A., Dosenovic, P., Stanfield, R.L., McCoy, L.E., Ozorowski, G., Hu, X., and Kalyuzhniy, O.: **HIV vaccine design to target germline precursors of glycan-dependent broadly neutralizing antibodies.** *Immunity* 2016, **45**:483-496.

Varga, S.M., Wang, X., Welsh, R.M., and Braciale, T.J.: **Immunopathology in RSV infection is mediated by a discrete oligoclonal subset of antigen-specific CD4(+) T cells.** *Immunity* 2001, **15**:637–646.

16-3   Effective vaccines must induce long-lasting protection while being safe and inexpensive.

Gupta, R.K., Best, J., and MacMahon, E.: **Mumps and the UK epidemic 2005.** *BMJ* 2005, **330**:1132–1135.

Hviid, A., Rubin, S., and Mühlemann, K.: **Mumps.** *Lancet* 2008, **371**:932–944.

Magnan, S., and Drake, M.: **The effectiveness of vaccination against influenza in healthy, working adults.** *N. Engl. J. Med.* 1995, **333**:889–893.

16-4   Live-attenuated viral vaccines are usually more potent than 'killed' vaccines.

Murphy, B.R., and Collins, P.L.: **Live-attenuated virus vaccines for respiratory syncytial and parainfluenza viruses: applications of reverse genetics.** *J. Clin. Invest.* 2002, **110**:21–27.

Nomoto, A., Omata, T., Toyoda, H., Kuge, S., Horie, H., Kataoka, Y., Genba, Y., Nakano, Y., and Imura, N.: Complete nucleotide sequence of the attenuated poliovirus Sabin 1 strain genome. *Proc. Natl. Acad. Sci. USA* 1982, **79**:5793–5797.

Stanway, G., Cann, A.J., Hauptmann, R., Mountford, R.C., Clarke, L.D., Reeve, P., Minor, P.D., Schild, G.C., and Almond, J.W.: Nucleic acid sequence of the region of the genome encoding capsid protein VP1 of neurovirulent and attenuated type 3 polioviruses. *Eur. J. Biochem.* 1983, **135**:529–533.

Subbarao, K., Murphy, B.R., and Fauci, A.S.: Development of effective vaccines against pandemic influenza. *Immunity* 2006, **24**:5–9.

Whittle, J.R., Wheatley, A.K., Wu, L., Lingwood, D., Kanekiyo, M., Ma, S.S., Narpala, S.R., Yassine, H.M., Frank, G.M., Yewdell, J.W., *et al.*: Flow cytometry reveals that H5N1 vaccination elicits cross-reactive stem-directed antibodies from multiple Ig heavy-chain lineages. *J. Virol.* 2014, **88**:4047–4057.

16-5 Live-attenuated viral vaccines can be made safer by the use of recombinant DNA technology.

Grode, L., Seiler, P., Baumann, S., Hess, J., Brinkmann, V., Nasser Eddine, A., Mann, P., Goosmann, C., Bandermann, S., Smith, D., *et al.*: Increased vaccine efficacy against tuberculosis of recombinant *Mycobacterium bovis* bacille Calmette–Guérin mutants that secrete listeriolysin. *J. Clin. Invest.* 2005, **115**:2472–2479.

Mueller, S.N., Langley, W.A., Carnero, E., García-Sastre, A., and Ahmed, R.: Immunization with live attenuated influenza viruses that express altered NS1 proteins results in potent and protective memory CD8+ T-cell responses. *J. Virol.* 2010, **84**:1847–1855.

Pena, L., Vincent, A.L., Ye, J., Ciacci-Zanella, J.R., Angel, M., Lorusso, A., Gauger, P.C., Janke, B.H., Loving, C.L., and Perez, D.R.: Modifications in the polymerase genes of a swine-like triple-reassortant influenza virus to generate live attenuated vaccines against 2009 pandemic H1N1 viruses. *J. Virol.* 2011, **85**:456–469.

Van Damme, P., De Coster. I., Bandyopadhyay, A.S., Revets, H., Withanage, K., De Smedt, P., Suykens, L., Oberste, M.S., Weldon, W.C., and Costa-Clemens, S.A.: The safety and immunogenicity of two novel live attenuated monovalent (serotype 2) oral poliovirus vaccines in healthy adults: a double-blind, single-centre phase 1 study. *Lancet* 2019, **394**:148–158.

Yeh, M.T., Bujaki, E., Dolan, P.T., Smith, M., Wahid, R., Konz, J., Weiner, A.J., Bandyopadhyay, A.S., Van Damme. P., De Coster, I., *et. al.*: Engineering the live-attenuated polio vaccine to prevent reversion to virulence. *Cell Host Microbe* 2020, **27**:736–751.

16-6 Vaccines against bacteria or parasites can be developed using nonpathogenic or disabled bacteria or genetically attenuated parasites (GAPs).

Grode, L., Seiler, P., Baumann, S., Hess, J., Brinkmann, V., Nasser Eddine, A., Mann, P., Goosmann, C., Bandermann, S., Smith, D., *et al.*: Increased vaccine efficacy against tuberculosis of recombinant *Mycobacterium bovis* bacille Calmette–Guérin mutants that secrete listeriolysin. *J. Clin. Invest.* 2005, **115**:2472–2479.

Guleria, I., Teitelbaum, R., McAdam, R.A., Kalpana, G., Jacobs, W.R., Jr., and Bloom, B.R.: Auxotrophic vaccines for tuberculosis. *Nat. Med.* 1996, **2**:334–337.

Labaied, M., Harupa, A., Dumpit, R.F., Coppens, I., Mikolajczak, S.A., and Kappe, S.H.: *Plasmodium yoelii* sporozoites with simultaneous deletion of P52 and P36 are completely attenuated and confer sterile immunity against infection. *Infect. Immun.* 2007, **75**:3758–3768.

Martin, C.: The dream of a vaccine against tuberculosis; new vaccines improving or replacing BCG? *Eur. Respir. J.* 2005, **26**:162–167.

Nieuwenhuizen, N.E., Kulkarni, P.S., Shaligram, U., Cotton, M.F., Rentsch, C.A., Eisele, B., Grode, L., and Kaufmann, S.H.E.: The recombinant bacille Calmette-Guérin vaccine VPM1002: ready for clinical efficacy testing. *Front. Immunol.* 2017, **8**:1147.

Thaiss, C.A., and Kaufmann, S.H.: Toward novel vaccines against tuberculosis: current hopes and obstacles. *Yale J. Biol. Med.* 2010, **83**:209–215.

Vaughan, A.M., Wang, R., and Kappe, S.H.: Genetically engineered, attenuated whole-cell vaccine approaches for malaria. *Hum. Vaccin.* 2010, **6**:1–8.

16-7 Conjugate vaccines rely on linked recognition between T and B cells.

Berry, D.S., Lynn, F., Lee, C.H., Frasch, C.E., and Bash, M.C.: Effect of O acetylation of *Neisseria meningitidis* serogroup A capsular polysaccharide on development of functional immune responses. *Infect. Immun.* 2002, **70**:3707–3713.

Bröker, M., Dull, P.M., Rappuoli, R., and Costantino, P.: Chemistry of a new investigational quadrivalent meningococcal conjugate vaccine that is immunogenic at all ages. *Vaccine* 2009, **27**:5574–5580.

Levine, O.S., Knoll, M.D., Jones, A., Walker, D.G., Risko, N., and Gilani, Z.: Global status of *Haemophilus influenzae* type b and pneumococcal conjugate vaccines: evidence, policies, and introductions. *Curr. Opin. Infect. Dis.* 2010, **23**:236–241.

Peltola, H., Kilpi, T., and Anttila, M.: Rapid disappearance of *Haemophilus influenzae* type b meningitis after routine childhood immunisation with conjugate vaccines. *Lancet* 1992, **340**:592–594.

Rappuoli, R.: Conjugates and reverse vaccinology to eliminate bacterial meningitis. *Vaccine* 2001, **19**:2319–2322.

16-8 Adjuvants enhance the immunogenicity of vaccines, but few are approved for use in humans.

Coffman, R.L., Sher, A., and Seder, R.A.: Vaccine adjuvants: putting innate immunity to work. *Immunity* 2010, **33**:492–503.

Eisenbarth, S.C., Colegio, O.R., O'Connor, W., Sutterwala, F.S., and Flavell, R.A.: Crucial role for the Nalp3 inflammasome in the immunostimulatory properties of aluminium adjuvants. *Nature* 2008, **453**:1122–1126.

Hartmann, G., Weiner, G.J., and Krieg, A.M.: CpG DNA: a potent signal for growth, activation, and maturation of human dendritic cells. *Proc. Natl. Acad. Sci. USA* 1999, **96**:9305–9310.

Palucka, K., Banchereau, J., and Mellman, I.: Designing vaccines based on biology of human dendritic cell subsets. *Immunity* 2010, **33**:464–478.

Persing, D.H., Coler, R.N., Lacy, M.J., Johnson, D.A., Baldridge, J.R., Hershberg, R.M., and Reed, S.G.: Taking toll: lipid A mimetics as adjuvants and immunomodulators. *Trends Microbiol.* 2002, **10**:S32–S37.

Pulendran, B.: Modulating vaccine responses with dendritic cells and Toll-like receptors. *Immunol. Rev.* 2004, **199**:227–250.

Takeda, K., Kaisho, T., and Akira, S.: Toll-like receptors. *Annu. Rev. Immunol.* 2003, **21**:335–376.

16-9 Protective immunity can be induced by RNA- and DNA-based vaccination.

Donnelly, J.J., Ulmer, J.B., Shiver, J.W., and Liu, M.A.: DNA vaccines. *Annu. Rev. Immunol.* 1997, **15**:617–648.

Ferretti, A.P., Kula, T., Wang, Y., Nguyen, D.M.V., Weinheimer, A., Dunlap, G.S., Xu, Q., Nabilsi, N., Perullo, C.R., Cristofaro, A.W., *et al.*: Unbiased screens show CD8 + T cells of COVID-19 patients recognize shared epitopes in SARS-CoV-2 that largely reside outside the spike protein. *Immunity* 2020, **53**:1095–1107.e3. doi: 10.1016/j.immuni.2020.10.006.

Gurunathan, S., Klinman, D.M., and Seder, R.A.: DNA vaccines: immunology, application, and optimization. *Annu. Rev. Immunol.* 2000, **18**:927–974.

Heiser, A., Coleman, D., Dannull, J., Yancey, D., Maurice, M.A., Lallas, C.D., Dahm, P., Niedzwiecki, D., Gilboa, E., and Vieweg, J.: Autologous dendritic cells transfected with prostate-specific antigen RNA stimulate CTL responses against metastatic prostate tumors. *J. Clin. Invest.* 2002, **109**:409–417.

Li, L., Kim, S., Herndon, J.M., Goedegebuure, P., Belt, B.A., Satpathy, A.T., Fleming, T.P., Hansen, T.H., Murphy, K.M., and Gillanders, W.E.: Cross-dressed CD8α+/CD103+ dendritic cells prime CD8+ T cells following vaccination. *Proc. Natl. Acad. Sci. USA* 2012, **109**:12716–12721.

Nchinda, G., Kuroiwa, J., Oks, M., Trumpfheller, C., Park, C.G., Huang, Y., Hannaman, D., Schlesinger, S.J., Mizenina, O., Nussenzweig, M.C., *et al.*: The efficacy of DNA vaccination is enhanced in mice by targeting the encoded protein to dendritic cells. *J. Clin. Invest.* 2008, **118**:1427–1436.

Wolff, J.A., and Budker, V.: The mechanism of naked DNA uptake and expression. *Adv. Genet.* 2005, **54**:3–20.

16-10 The route of vaccination is an important determinant of success.

Amorij, J.P., Hinrichs, W.Lj., Frijlink, H.W., Wilschut, J.C., and Huckriede, A.: Needle-free influenza vaccination. *Lancet Infect. Dis.* 2010, **10**:699–711.

Belyakov, I.M., and Ahlers, J.D.: What role does the route of immunization play in the generation of protective immunity against mucosal pathogens? *J. Immunol.* 2009, **183**:6883–6892.

Douce, G., Fontana, M., Pizza, M., Rappuoli, R., and Dougan, G.: Intranasal immunogenicity and adjuvanticity of site-directed mutant derivatives of cholera toxin. *Infect. Immun.* 1997, **65**:2821–2828.

Dougan, G., Ghaem-Maghami, M., Pickard, D., Frankel, G., Douce, G., Clare, S., Dunstan, S., and Simmons, C.: The immune responses to bacterial antigens encountered in vivo at mucosal surfaces. *Philos. Trans. R. Soc. Lond. B Biol. Sci.* 2000, **355**:705–712.

Eriksson, K., and Holmgren, J.: Recent advances in mucosal vaccines and adjuvants. *Curr. Opin. Immunol.* 2002, **14**:666–672.

16-11 *Bordetella pertussis* vaccination illustrates the importance of the perceived safety of a vaccine.

Decker, M.D., and Edwards, K.M.: Acellular pertussis vaccines. *Pediatr. Clin. North Am.* 2000, **47**:309–335.

Jahnmatz, M., Richert, L., Al-Tawil, N., Storsaeter, J., Colin, C., Bauduin, C., Thalen. M., Solovay, K., Rubin, K., Mielcarek, N., *et al.*: Safety and immunogenicity of the live attenuated intranasal pertussis vaccine BPZE1: a phase 1b, double-blind, randomised, placebo-controlled dose-escalation study. *Lancet Infect. Dis.* 2020, **20**:1290–1301.

Madsen, K.M., Hviid, A., Vestergaard, M., Schendel, D., Wohlfahrt, J., Thorsen, P., Olsen, J., and Melbye, M.: A population-based study of measles, mumps, and rubella vaccination and autism. *N. Engl. J. Med.* 2002, **347**:1477–1482.

Mortimer, E.A.: Pertussis vaccines, in Plotkin, S.A., and Mortimer, E.A. (eds): *Vaccines*, 2nd ed. Philadelphia: W.B. Saunders, 1994.

Poland, G.A.: Acellular pertussis vaccines: new vaccines for an old disease. *Lancet* 1996, **347**:209–210.

16-12 Peptide-based vaccines can elicit protective immunity, but they require adjuvants and must be targeted to the appropriate cells and cell compartment to be effective.

Alonso, P.L., Sacarlal, J., Aponte, J.J., Leach, A., Macete, E., Aide, P., Sigauque, B., Milman, J., Mandomando, I., Bassat, Q., *et al.*: Duration of protection with RTS, S/AS02A malaria vaccine in prevention of *Plasmodium falciparum* disease in Mozambican children: single-blind extended follow-up of a randomised controlled trial. *Lancet* 2005, **366**:2012–2018.

Berzofsky, J.A.: Epitope selection and design of synthetic vaccines. Molecular approaches to enhancing immunogenicity and cross-reactivity of engineered vaccines. *Ann. N.Y. Acad. Sci.* 1993, **690**:256–264.

Davenport, M.P., and Hill, A.V.: Reverse immunogenetics: from HLA-disease associations to vaccine candidates. *Mol. Med. Today* 1996, **2**:38–45.

Hill, A.V.: Pre-erythrocytic malaria vaccines: towards greater efficacy. *Nat. Rev. Immunol.* 2006, **6**:21–32.

Hoffman, S.L., Rogers, W.O., Carucci, D.J., and Venter, J.C.: From genomics to vaccines: malaria as a model system. *Nat. Med.* 1998, **4**:1351–1353.

Ottenhoff, T.H., Doherty, T.M., Dissel, J.T., Bang, P., Lingnau, K., Kromann, I., and Andersen, P.: First in humans: a new molecularly defined vaccine shows excellent safety and strong induction of long-lived *Mycobacterium tuberculosis*-specific Th1-cell like responses. *Hum. Vaccin.* 2010, **6**: 1007–1015.

Zwaveling, S., Ferreira Mota, S.C., Nouta, J., Johnson, M., Lipford, G.B., Offringa, R., van der Burg, S.H., and Melief, C.J.: Established human papillomavirus type 16-expressing tumors are effectively eradicated following vaccination with long peptides. *J. Immunol.* 2002, **169**:350–358.

16-13 Vaccination and checkpoint blockade may be useful in controlling existing chronic infections.

Chang, K.C., Burnham, C.A., Compton, S.M., Raschem D.P., Mazuski, R.J., McDonough, J.S., Unsinger, J., Korman, A.J., Green, J.M., and Hotchkiss, R.S.: Blockade of the negative co-stimulatory molecules PD-1 and CTLA-4 improves survival in primary and secondary fungal sepsis. *Crit Care.* 2013, **17**:R85.

Hill, A., Jugovic, P., York, I., Russ, G., Bennink, J., Yewdell, J., Ploegh, H., and Johnson, D.: Herpes simplex virus turns off the TAP to evade host immunity. *Nature* 1995, **375**:411–415.

Khamesipour, A.: Therapeutic vaccines for leishmaniasis. *Expert Opin. Biol. Ther.* 2014, **14**:1641–1649.

Nagill, R., and Kaur, S.: Vaccine candidates for leishmaniasis: a review. *Int. Immunopharmacol.* 2011, **11**:1464–1488.

Plebanski, M., Proudfoot, O., Pouniotis, D., Coppel, R.L., Apostolopoulos, V., and Flannery, G.: Immunogenetics and the design of *Plasmodium falciparum* vaccines for use in malaria-endemic populations. *J. Clin. Invest.* 2002, **110**: 295–301.

Reiner, S.L., and Locksley, R.M.: The regulation of immunity to *Leishmania major.* *Annu. Rev. Immunol.* 1995, **13**:151–177.

Stanford, J.L.: The history and future of vaccination and immunotherapy for leprosy. *Trop. Geogr. Med.* 1994, **46**:93–107.

16-14 The development of transplantable tumors in mice led to the discovery of protective immune responses to tumors.

Jaffee, E.M., and Pardoll, D.M.: Murine tumor antigens: is it worth the search? *Curr. Opin. Immunol.* 1996, **8**:622–627.

Klein, G.: Tumor-specific transplantation antigens: G. H. A. Clowes memorial lecture. *Cancer Res.* 1968, **28**:625–635.

Klein, G.: The strange road to the tumor-specific transplantation antigens (TSTAs). *Cancer Immun.* 2001, **1**:6.

16-15 Tumors are 'edited' by the immune system as they evolve and can escape rejection in many ways.

Dunn, G.P., Old, L.J., and Schreiber, R.D.: The immunobiology of cancer immunosurveillance and immunoediting. *Immunity* 2004, **21**:137–148.

Gajewski, T.F., Meng, Y., Blank, C., Brown, I., Kacha, A., Kline, J., and Harlin, H.: Immune resistance orchestrated by the tumor microenvironment. *Immunol. Rev.* 2006, **213**:131–145.

Girardi, M., Oppenheim, D.E., Steele, C.R., Lewis, J.M., Glusac, E., Filler, R., Hobby, P., Sutton, B., Tigelaar, R.E., and Hayday, A.C.: Regulation of cutaneous malignancy by γδ T cells. *Science* 2001, **294**:605–609.

Kloor, M., Becker, C., Benner, A., Woerner, S.M., Gebert, J., Ferrone, S., and von Knebel Doeberitz, M.: Immunoselective pressure and human leukocyte antigen class I antigen machinery defects in microsatellite unstable colorectal cancers. *Cancer Res.* 2005, **65**:6418–6424.

Koblish, H.K., Hansbury, M.J., Bowman, K.J., Yang, G., Neilan, C.L., Haley, P.J., Burn, T.C., Waeltz, P., Sparks, R.B., Yue, E.W., *et al.*: Hydroxyamidine inhibitors of indoleamine-2,3-dioxygenase potently suppress systemic tryptophan catabolism and the growth of IDO-expressing tumors. *Mol. Cancer. Ther.* 2010, **9**:489–498.

Koebel, C.M., Vermi, W., Swann, J.B., Zerafa, N., Rodig, S.J., Old, L.J., Smyth, M.J., and Schreiber, R.D.: Adaptive immunity maintains occult cancer in an equilibrium state. *Nature* 2007, **450**:903–907.

Koopman, L.A., Corver, W.E., van der Slik, A.R., Giphart, M.J., and Fleuren, G.J.: Multiple genetic alterations cause frequent and heterogeneous human histocompatibility leukocyte antigen class I loss in cervical cancer. *J. Exp. Med.* 2000, **191**:961–976.

Munn, D.H., and Mellor, A.L.: Indoleamine 2,3-dioxygenase and tumor-induced tolerance. *J. Clin. Invest.* 2007, **117**:1147–1154.

Ochsenbein, A.F., Sierro, S., Odermatt, B., Pericin, M., Karrer, U., Hermans, J., Hemmi, S., Hengartner, H., and Zinkernagel, R.M.: Roles of tumour localization, second signals and cross priming in cytotoxic T-cell induction. *Nature* 2001, 411:1058–1064.

Peggs, K.S., Quezada, S.A., and Allison, J.P.: Cell intrinsic mechanisms of T-cell inhibition and application to cancer therapy. *Immunol. Rev.* 2008, 224:141–165.

Peranzoni, E., Zilio, S., Marigo, I., Dolcetti, L., Zanovello, P., Mandruzzato, S., and Bronte, V.: Myeloid-derived suppressor cell heterogeneity and subset definition. *Curr. Opin. Immunol.* 2010, 22:238–244.

Schreiber, R.D., Old. L.J., and Smyth, M.J.: Cancer immunoediting: integrating immunity's roles in cancer suppression and promotion. *Science* 2011, 331:1565–1570.

Shankaran, V., Ikeda, H., Bruce, A.T., White, J.M., Swanson, P.E., Old, L.J., and Schreiber, R.D.: IFN-γ and lymphocytes prevent primary tumour development and shape tumour immunogenicity. *Nature* 2001, 410:1107–1111.

Shroff, R., and Rees, L.: The post-transplant lymphoproliferative disorder—a literature review. *Pediatr. Nephrol.* 2004, 19:369–377.

Wang, H.Y., Lee, D.A., Peng, G., Guo, Z., Li, Y., Kiniwa, Y., Shevach, E.M., and Wang, R.F.: Tumor-specific human CD4+ regulatory T cells and their ligands: implications for immunotherapy. *Immunity* 2004, 20:107–118.

16-16 Tumor-rejection antigens can be recognized by T cells and form the basis of immunotherapies.

Clark, R.E., Dodi, I.A., Hill, S.C., Lill, J.R., Aubert, G., Macintyre, A.R., Rojas, J., Bourdon, A., Bonner, P.L., Wang, L., *et al.*: Direct evidence that leukemic cells present HLA-associated immunogenic peptides derived from the BCR-ABL b3a2 fusion protein. *Blood* 2001, 98:2887–2893.

Comoli, P., Pedrazzoli, P., Maccario, R., Basso, S., Carminati, O., Labirio, M., Schiavo, R., Secondino, S., Frasson, C., Perotti, C., *et al.*: Cell therapy of stage IV nasopharyngeal carcinoma with autologous Epstein–Barr virus-targeted cytotoxic T lymphocytes. *J. Clin. Oncol.* 2005, 23:8942–8949.

Disis, M.L., Knutson, K.L., McNeel, D.G., Davis, D., and Schiffman, K.: Clinical translation of peptide-based vaccine trials: the HER-2/neu model. *Crit. Rev. Immunol.* 2001, 21:263–273.

Dudley, M.E., Wunderlich, J.R., Yang, J.C., Sherry, R.M., Topalian, S.L., Restifo, N.P., Royal, R.E., Kammula, U., White, D.E., Mavroukakis, S.A., *et al.*: Adoptive cell transfer therapy following non-myeloablative but lymphodepleting chemotherapy for the treatment of patients with refractory metastatic melanoma. *J. Clin. Oncol.* 2005, 23:2346–2357.

Matsushita, H., Vesely, M.D., Koboldt, D.C., Rickert, C.G., Uppaluri, R., Magrini, V.J., Arthur, C.D., White, J.M., Chen, Y.S., Shea, L.K., *et al.*: Cancer exome analysis reveals a T-cell-dependent mechanism of cancer immunoediting. *Nature* 2012, 482:400–404.

Michalek, J., Collins, R.H., Durrani, H.P., Vaclavkova, P., Ruff, L.E., Douek, D.C., and Vitetta, E.S.: Definitive separation of graft-versus-leukemia- and graft-versus-host-specific CD4+ T cells by virtue of their receptor β loci sequences. *Proc. Natl. Acad. Sci. USA* 2003, 100:1180–1184.

Morris, E.C., Tsallios, A., Bendle, G.M., Xue, S.A., and Stauss, H.J.: A critical role of T cell antigen receptor-transduced MHC class I-restricted helper T cells in tumor protection. *Proc. Natl. Acad. Sci. USA* 2005, 102:7934–7939.

Schultz, E.S., Schuler-Thurner, B., Stroobant, V., Jenne, L., Berger, T.G., Thielemanns, K., van der Bruggen, P., and Schuler, G.: Functional analysis of tumor-specific Th cell responses detected in melanoma patients after dendritic cell-based immunotherapy. *J. Immunol.* 2004, 172:1304–1310.

16-17 Checkpoint blockade can augment immune responses to existing tumors.

Ansell, S.M., Lesokhin, A.M., Borrello, I., Halwani, A., Scott, E.C., Gutierrez, M., Schuster, S.J., Millenson, M.M., Cattry, D., Freeman, G.J., *et al.*: PD-1 blockade with nivolumab in relapsed or refractory Hodgkin's lymphoma. *N. Engl. J. Med.* 2015, 372:311–319.

Bendandi, M., Gocke, C.D., Kobrin, C.B., Benko, F.A., Sternas, L.A., Pennington, R., Watson, T.M., Reynolds, C.W., Gause, B.L., Duffey, P.L., *et al.*: Complete molecular remissions induced by patient-specific vaccination plus granulocyte-monocyte colony-stimulating factor against lymphoma. *Nat. Med.* 1999, 5:1171–1177.

Egen, J.G., Kuhns, M.S., and Allison, J.P.: CTLA-4: new insights into its biological function and use in tumor immunotherapy. *Nat. Immunol.* 2002, 3:611–618.

Hamid, O., Robert, C., Daud, A., Hodi, F.S., Hwu, W.J., Kefford, R., Wolchok, J.D., Hersey, P., Joseph, R.W., Weber, J.S., *et al.*: Safety and tumor responses with lambrolizumab (anti-PD-1) in melanoma. *N. Engl. J. Med.* 2013, 369:134–144.

Hodi, F.S., O'Day, S.J., McDermott, D.F., Weber, R.W., Sosman, J.A., Haanen, J.B., Gonzalez, R., Robert, C., Schadendorf, D., Hassel, J.C., *et al.*: Improved survival with ipilimumab in patients with metastatic melanoma. *N. Engl. J. Med* 2010; 363:711–723

Li, Y., Hellstrom, K.E., Newby, S.A., and Chen, L.: Costimulation by CD48 and B7–1 induces immunity against poorly immunogenic tumors. *J. Exp. Med.* 1996, 183:639–644.

Phan, G.Q., Yang, J.C., Sherry, R.M., Hwu, P., Topalian, S.L., Schwartzentruber, D.J., Restifo, N.P., Haworth, L.R., Seipp, C.A., Freezer, L.J., *et al.*: Cancer regression and autoimmunity induced by cytotoxic T lymphocyte-associated antigen 4 blockade in patients with metastatic melanoma. *Proc. Natl. Acad. Sci. USA* 2003, 100:8372–8377.

Yuan, J., Gnjatic, S., Li, H., Powel, S., Gallardo, H.F., Ritter, E., Ku, G.Y., Jungbluth, A.A., Segal, N.H., Rasalan, T.S., *et al.*: CTLA-4 blockade enhances polyfunctional NY-ESO-1 specific T cell responses in metastatic melanoma patients with clinical benefit. *Proc. Natl. Acad. Sci. USA* 2008, 105:20410–20415.

16-18 T cells expressing chimeric antigen receptors are an effective treatment in some leukemias.

Grupp, S.A., Kalos, M., Barrett, D., Aplenc, R., Porter, D.L., Rheingold, S.R., Teachey, D.T., Chew, A., Hauck, B., Wright, J.F., *et al.*: Chimeric antigen receptor-modified T cells for acute lymphoid leukemia. *N. Engl. J. Med.* 2013, 368:1509–1518.

June, C.H.: Remote controlled CARs: towards a safer therapy for leukemia. *Cancer Immunol. Res.* 2016, 4:643.

June, C.H., and Sadelain, M.: Chimeric antigen receptor therapy. *N. Engl. J. Med.* 2018, 379:64–73.

Lim, W.A., and June, C.H.: The principles of engineering immune cells to treat cancer. *Cell* 2017, 168:724–740.

Maus, M.V., and June, C.H.: Making better chimeric antigen receptors for adoptive T-cell therapy. *Clin. Cancer Res.* 2016, 22:1875–1884.

Stromnes, I.M., Schmitt, T.M., Chapuis, A.G., Hingorani, S.R., and Greenberg, P.D.: Re-adapting T cells for cancer therapy: from mouse models to clinical trials. *Immunol. Rev.* 2014, 257:145–164.

16-19 Monoclonal antibodies against tumor antigens, alone or linked to toxins, can control tumor growth.

Bradley, A.M., Devine, M., and DeRemer, D.: Brentuximab vedotin: an anti-CD30 antibody-drug conjugate. *Am. J. Health Syst. Pharm.* 2013, 70:589–597.

Hortobagyi, G.N.: Trastuzumab in the treatment of breast cancer. *N. Engl. J. Med.* 2005, 353:1734–1736.

Kreitman, R.J., Wilson, W.H., Bergeron, K., Raggio, M., Stetler-Stevenson, M., FitzGerald, D.J., and Pastan, I.: Efficacy of the anti-CD22 recombinant immunotoxin BL22 in chemotherapy-resistant hairy-cell leukemia. *N. Engl. J. Med.* 2001, 345:241–247.

Park, S., Jiang, Z., Mortenson, E.D., Deng, L., Radkevich-Brown, O., Yang, X., Sattar, H., Wang, Y., Brown, N.K., Greene, M., *et al.*: The therapeutic effect of anti-HER2/neu antibody depends on both innate and adaptive immunity. *Cancer Cell* 2010, 18:160–170.

Tol, J., and Punt, C.J.: Monoclonal antibodies in the treatment of metastatic colorectal cancer: a review. *Clin. Ther.* 2010, 32:437–453.

Veeramani, S., Wang, S.Y., Dahle, C., Blackwell, S., Jacobus, L., Knutson, T., Button, A., Link, B.K., and Weiner, G.J.: Rituximab infusion induces NK activation in lymphoma patients with the high-affinity CD16 polymorphism. *Blood* 2011, 118:3347–3349.

Verma, S., Miles, D., Gianni, L., Krop, I.E., Welslau, M., Baselga, J., Pegram, M., Oh, D.Y., Diéras, V., Guardino, E., *et al.*: Trastuzumab emtansine for HER2-positive advanced breast cancer. *N. Engl. J. Med.* 2012, **367**:1783–1791.

Weiner, L.M., Dhodapkar, M.V., and Ferrone, S.: Monoclonal antibodies for cancer immunotherapy. *Lancet* 2009, **373**:1033–1040.

Weng, W.K., and Levy, R.: Genetic polymorphism of the inhibitory IgG Fc receptor FcgammaRIIb is not associated with clinical outcome in patients with follicular lymphoma treated with rituximab. *Leuk. Lymphoma* 2009, **50**:723–727.

16-20 Enhancing the immune response to tumors by vaccination holds promise for cancer prevention and therapy.

Kantoff, P.W., Higano, C.S., Shore, N.D., Berger, E.R., Small, E.J., Penson, D.F., Redfern, C.H., Ferrari, A.C., Dreicer, R., Sims, R.B., *et al.*: Sipuleucel-T immunotherapy for castration-resistant prostate cancer. *N. Engl. J. Med.* 2010, **363**:411–422.

Kenter, G.G., Welters, M.J., Valentijn, A.R., Lowik, M.J., Berends-van der Meer, D.M., Vloon, A.P., Essahsah, F., Fathers, L.M., Offringa, R., Drijfhout, J.W., *et al.*: Vaccination against HPV-16 oncoproteins for vulvar intraepithelial neoplasia. *N. Engl. J. Med.* 2009, **361**:1838–1847.

Mao, C., Koutsky, L.A., Ault, K.A., Wheeler, C.M., Brown, D.R., Wiley, D.J., Alvarez, F.B., Bautista, O.M., Jansen, K.U., and Barr, E.: Efficacy of human papillomavirus-16 vaccine to prevent cervical intraepithelial neoplasia: a randomized controlled trial. *Obstet. Gynecol.* 2006, **107**:18–27.

Palucka, K., Ueno, H., Fay, J., and Bancherau, J.: Dendritic cells and immunity against cancer. *J. Intern. Med.* 2011, **269**:64–73.

Vambutas, A., DeVoti, J., Nouri, M., Drijfhout, J.W., Lipford, G.B., Bonagura, V.R., van der Burg, S.H., and Melief, C.J.: Therapeutic vaccination with papillomavirus E6 and E7 long peptides results in the control of both established virus-induced lesions and latently infected sites in a pre-clinical cottontail rabbit papillomavirus model. *Vaccine* 2005, **23**:5271–5280.

16-21 Corticosteroids are powerful anti-inflammatory drugs that alter the transcription of many genes.

Barnes, P.J.: Glucocorticosteroids: current and future directions. *Br. J. Pharmacol.* 2011, **163**:29–43.

Kampa, M., and Castanas, E.: Membrane steroid receptor signaling in normal and neoplastic cells. *Mol. Cell. Endocrinol.* 2006, **246**:76–82.

Löwenberg, M., Verhaar, A.P., van den Brink, G.R., and Hommes, D.W.: Glucocorticoid signaling: a nongenomic mechanism for T-cell immunosuppression. *Trends Mol. Med.* 2007, **13**:158–163.

Rhen, T., and Cidlowski, J.A.: Antiinflammatory action of glucocorticoids—new mechanisms for old drugs. *N. Engl. J. Med.* 2005, **353**:1711–1723.

16-22 Cytotoxic drugs cause immunosuppression by killing dividing cells and have serious side effects.

Aarbakke, J., Janka-Schaub, G., and Elion, G.B.: Thiopurine biology and pharmacology. *Trends Pharmacol. Sci.* 1997, **18**:3–7.

Allison, A.C., and Eugui, E.M.: Mechanisms of action of mycophenolate mofetil in preventing acute and chronic allograft rejection. *Transplantation* 2005, **802**(suppl.):S181–S190.

O'Donovan, P., Perrett, C.M., Zhang, X., Montaner, B., Xu, Y.Z., Harwood, C.A., McGregor, J.M., Walker, S.L., Hanaoka, F., and Karran, P.: Azathioprine and UVA light generate mutagenic oxidative DNA damage. *Science* 2005, **309**:1871–1874.

Taylor, A.L., Watson, C.J., and Bradley, J.A.: Immunosuppressive agents in solid organ transplantation: mechanisms of action and therapeutic efficacy. *Crit. Rev. Oncol. Hematol.* 2005, **56**:23–46.

Zhu, L.P., Cupps, T.R., Whalen, G., and Fauci, A.S.: Selective effects of cyclophosphamide therapy on activation, proliferation, and differentiation of human B cells. *J. Clin. Invest.* 1987, **79**:1082–1090.

16-23 Cyclosporin A, tacrolimus, and rapamycin are effective immunosuppressive agents that interfere with various T-cell signaling pathways.

Araki, K., Turner, A.P., Shaffer, V.O., Gangappa, S., Keller, S.A., Bachmann, M.F., Larsen, C.P., and Ahmed, R.: mTOR regulates memory CD8 T-cell differentiation. *Nature* 2009, **460**:108–112.

Battaglia, M., Stabilini, A., and Roncarolo, M.G.: Rapamycin selectively expands CD4+CD25+FoxP3+ regulatory T cells. *Blood* 2005, **105**:4743–4748.

Bierer, B.E., Mattila, P.S., Standaert, R.F., Herzenberg, L.A., Burakoff, S.J., Crabtree, G., and Schreiber, S.L.: Two distinct signal transmission pathways in T lymphocytes are inhibited by complexes formed between an immunophilin and either FK506 or rapamycin. *Proc. Natl. Acad. Sci. USA* 1990, **87**:9231–9235.

Crabtree, G.R.: Generic signals and specific outcomes: signaling through Ca^{2+}, calcineurin, and NF-AT. *Cell* 1999, **96**:611–614.

Crespo, J.L., and Hall, M.N.: Elucidating TOR signaling and rapamycin action: lessons from *Saccharomyces cerevisiae*. *Microbiol. Mol. Biol. Rev.* 2002, **66**:579–591.

Fleischmann, R., Kremer, J., Cush, J., Schulze-Koops, H., Connell, C.A., Bradley, J.D., Gruben, D., Wallenstein, G.V., Zwillich, S.H., Kanik, K.S., *et al.*: Placebo-controlled trial of tofacitinib monotherapy in rheumatoid arthritis. *N. Engl. J. Med.* 2012, **367**:495–507.

16-24 JAK inhibitors can be used to treat autoimmune and inflammatory diseases.

Gadina, M., Chisolm, D.A., Philips, R.L., McInness, I.B., Changelian, P.S., and O'Shea J.J.: Translating JAKs to jakinibs. *J. Immunol.* 2020, **204**:2011–2020.

Kontzias, A., Kotlyar, A., Laurence, A., Changelian, P., and O'Shea, J.J.: Jakinibs: a new class of kinase inhibitors in cancer and autoimmune disease. *Curr. Opin. Pharmacol.* 2012, **12**:464–470.

Pesu, M., Laurence, A., Kishore, N., Zwillich, S.H., Chan, G., and O'Shea, J.J.: Therapeutic targeting of Janus kinases. *Immunol. Rev.* 2008, **223**:132–142.

16-25 Antibodies against cell-surface molecules can be used to eliminate lymphocyte subsets or to inhibit lymphocyte function.

Graca, L., Le Moine, A., Cobbold, S.P., and Waldmann, H.: Antibody-induced transplantation tolerance: the role of dominant regulation. *Immunol. Res.* 2003, **28**:181–191.

Nagelkerke, S.Q, and Kuijpers, T.W.: Immunomodulation by IVIg and the role of Fc-gamma receptors: classic mechanisms of action after all? *Front. Immunol.* 2015, **5**:674.

Nagelkerke, S.Q., Dekkers, G., Kustiawan, I., van de Bovenkamp, F.S., Geissler, J., Plomp, R., Wuhrer, M., Vidarsson, G., Rispens, T., van den Berg, T.K., *et al*: Inhibition of FcγR-mediated phagocytosis by IVIg is independent of IgG-Fc sialylation and FcγRIIb in human macrophages. *Blood* 2014, **124**:3709–3718.

Waldmann, H., and Hale, G.: CAMPATH: from concept to clinic. *Philos. Trans. R. Soc. Lond. B Biol. Sci.* 2005, **360**:1707–1711.

16-26 Antibodies can be engineered to reduce their immunogenicity in humans.

Kim, S.J., Park, Y., and Hong, H.J.: Antibody engineering for the development of therapeutic antibodies. *Mol. Cell* 2005, **20**:17–29.

Liu, X.Y., Pop, L.M., and Vitetta, E.S.: Engineering therapeutic monoclonal antibodies. *Immunol. Rev.* 2008, **222**:9–27.

Smith, K., Garman, L., Wrammert, J., Zheng, N.Y., Capra, J.D., Ahmed, R., and Wilson, P.C.: Rapid generation of fully human monoclonal antibodies specific to a vaccinating antigen. *Nat. Protoc.* 2009, **4**:372–384.

Traggiai, E., Becker, S., Subbarao, K., Kolesnikova, L., Uematsu, Y., Gismondo, M.R., Murphy, B.R., Rappuoli, R., and Lanzavecchia, A.: An efficient method to make human monoclonal antibodies from memory B cells: potent neutralization of SARS coronavirus. *Nat. Med.* 2004, **10**:871–875.

Winter, G., Griffiths, A.D., Hawkins, R.E., and Hoogenboom, H.R.: Making anti-bodies by phage display technology. *Annu. Rev. Immunol.* 1994, **12**:433–455.

16-27   Monoclonal antibodies can be used to prevent allograft rejection.

Kirk, A.D., Burkly, L.C., Batty, D.S., Baumgartner, R.E., Berning, J.D., Buchanan, K., Fechner, J.H., Jr., Germond, R.L., Kampen, R.L., Patterson, N.B., *et al.*: Treatment with humanized monoclonal antibody against CD154 prevents acute renal allograft rejection in nonhuman primates. *Nat. Med.* 1999, **5**:686–693.

Li, X.C., Strom, T.B., Turka, L.A., and Wells, A.D.: T-cell death and transplanta-tion tolerance. *Immunity* 2001, **14**:407–416.

Londrigan, S.L., Sutherland, R.M., Brady, J.L., Carrington, E.M., Cowan, P.J., d'Apice, A.J., O'Connell, P.J., Zhan, Y., and Lew, A.M.: In situ protection against islet allograft rejection by CTLA4Ig transduction. *Transplantation* 2010, **90**:951–957.

Masharani, U.B., and Becker, J.: Teplizumab therapy for type 1 diabetes. *Expert Opin. Biol. Ther.* 2010, **10**:459–465.

Pham, P.T., Lipshutz, G.S., Pham, P.T., Kawahji, J., Singer, J.S., and Pham, P.C.: The evolving role of alemtuzumab (Campath-1H) in renal transplantation. *Drug Des. Devel. Ther.* 2009, **3**:41–49.

Sageshima, J., Ciancio, G., Chen, L., and Burke, G.W.: Anti-interleukin-2 receptor antibodies—basiliximab and daclizumab—for the prevention of acute rejection in renal transplantation. *Biologics* 2009, **3**:319–336.

16-28   Depletion of autoreactive lymphocytes can treat autoimmune disease.

Coiffier, B., Lepage, E., Briere, J., Herbrecht, R., Tilly, H., Bouabdallah, R., Morel, P., Van Den Neste, E., Salles, G., Gaulard, P., *et al.*: CHOP chemotherapy plus ritux-imab compared with CHOP alone in elderly patients with diffuse large-B-cell lymphoma. *N. Engl. J. Med.* 2002, **346**:235–242.

Coles, A., Deans, J., and Compston, A.: Campath-1H treatment of multiple sclerosis: lessons from the bedside for the bench. *Clin. Neurol. Neurosurg.* 2004, **106**:270–274.

Edwards, J.C., Leandro, M.J., and Cambridge, G.: B lymphocyte depletion in rheumatoid arthritis: targeting of CD20. *Curr. Dir. Autoimmun.* 2005, **8**: 175–192.

Yazawa, N., Hamaguchi, Y., Poe, J.C., and Tedder, T.F.: Immunotherapy using unconjugated CD19 monoclonal antibodies in animal models for B lympho-cyte malignancies and autoimmune disease. *Proc. Natl. Acad. Sci. USA* 2005, **102**:15178–15783.

Zaja, F., De Vita, S., Mazzaro, C., Sacco, S., Damiani, D., De Marchi, G., Michelutti, A., Baccarani, M., Fanin, R., and Ferraccioli, G.: Efficacy and safety of rituximab in type II mixed cryoglobulinemia. *Blood* 2003, **101**:3827–3834.

16-29   Biologics that block TNF-α, IL-1, or IL-6 can alleviate autoimmune diseases.

Guarda, G., Braun, M., Staehli, F., Tardivel, A., Mattmann, C., Förster, I., Farlik, M., Decker, T., Du Pasquier, R.A., Romero, P., *et al.*: Type I interferon inhibits inter-leukin-1 production and inflammasome activation. *Immunity* 2011, **34**:213–223.

Feldmann, M., and Maini, R.N.: Lasker Clinical Medical Research Award. TNF defined as a therapeutic target for rheumatoid arthritis and other autoimmune diseases. *Nat. Med.* 2003, **9**:1245–1250.

Hallegua, D.S., and Weisman, M.H.: Potential therapeutic uses of interleukin 1 receptor antagonists in human diseases. *Ann. Rheum. Dis.* 2002, **61**:960–967.

Karanikolas, G., Charalambopoulos, D., Vaiopoulos, G., Andrianakos, A., Rapti, A., Karras, D., Kaskani, E., and Sfikakis, P.P.: Adjunctive anakinra in patients with active rheumatoid arthritis despite methotrexate, or leflunomide, or cyclospor-in-A monotherapy: a 48-week, comparative, prospective study. *Rheumatology* 2008, **47**:1384–1388.

Mackay, C.R.: New avenues for anti-inflammatory therapy. *Nat. Med.* 2002, **8**:117–118.

16-30   Biologics can block cell migration to sites of inflammation and reduce immune responses.

Boster, A.L., Nicholas, J.A., Topalli, I., Kisanuki, Y.Y., Pei, W., Morgan-Followell, B., Kirsch, C.F., Racke, M.K., and Pitt, D.: Lessons learned from fatal progressive multifocal leukoencephalopathy in a patient with multiple sclerosis treated with natalizumab. *JAMA Neurol.* 2013, **70**:398–402.

Clifford, D.B., De Luca, A., Simpson, D.M., Arendt, G., Giovannoni, G., and Nath, A.: Natalizumab-associated progressive multifocal leukoencephalopathy in patients with multiple sclerosis: lessons from 28 cases. *Lancet Neurol.* 2010, **9**:438–446.

Cyster, J.G.: Chemokines, sphingosine-1-phosphate, and cell migration in secondary lymphoid organs. *Annu. Rev. Immunol.* 2005, **23**:127–159.

Idzko, M., Hammad, H., van Nimwegen, M., Kool, M., Muller, T., Soullie, T., Willart, M.A., Hijdra, D., Hoogsteden, H.C., and Lambrecht, B.N.: Local application of FTY720 to the lung abrogates experimental asthma by altering dendritic cell function. *J. Clin. Invest.* 2006, **116**:2935–2944.

Kappos, L., Radue, E.W., O'Connor, P., Polman, C., Hohlfeld, R., Calabresi, P., Selmaj, K., Agoropoulou, C., Leyk, M., Zhang-Auberson, L., *et al.*: A placebo-controlled trial of oral fingolimod in relapsing multiple sclerosis. *N. Engl. J. Med.* 2010, **362**:387–401.

Podolsky, D.K.: Selective adhesion-molecule therapy and inflammatory bowel disease—a tale of Janus? *N. Engl. J. Med.* 2005, **353**:1965–1968.

16-31   Blockade of co-stimulatory pathways that activate lymphocytes can be used to treat autoimmune disease.

Ellis, C.N., and Krueger, G.G.: Treatment of chronic plaque psoriasis by selective targeting of memory effector T lymphocytes. *N. Engl. J. Med.* 2001, **345**:248–255.

Fife, B.T., and Bluestone, J.A.: Control of peripheral T-cell tolerance and auto-immunity via the CTLA-4 and PD-1 pathways. *Immunol. Rev.* 2008, **224**:166–182.

Kraan, M.C., van Kuijk, A.W., Dinant, H.J., Goedkoop, A.Y., Smeets, T.J., de Rie, M.A., Dijkmans, B.A., Vaishnaw, A.K., Bos, J.D., and Tak, P.P.: Alefacept treatment in psoriatic arthritis: reduction of the effector T cell population in peripheral blood and synovial tissue is associated with improvement of clinical signs of arthritis. *Arthritis Rheum.* 2002, **46**:2776–2784.

Lowes, M.A., Chamian, F., Abello, M.V., Fuentes-Duculan, J., Lin, S.L., Nussbaum, R., Novitskaya, I., Carbonaro, H., Cardinale, I., Kikuchi, T., *et al.*: Increase in TNF-α and inducible nitric oxide synthase-expressing dendritic cells in psori-asis and reduction with efalizumab (anti-CD11a). *Proc. Natl. Acad. Sci. USA* 2005, **102**:19057–19062.

Menter, A.: The status of biologic therapies in the treatment of moderate to severe psoriasis. *Cutis* 2009, **84**:14–24.

16-32   Some commonly used drugs have immunomodulatory properties.

Baeke, F., Takiishi, T., Korf, H., Gysemans, C., and Mathieu, C.: Vitamin D: modulator of the immune system. *Curr. Opin. Pharmacol.* 2010, **10**:482–496.

Okwan-Duodu, D., Datta, V., Shen, X.Z., Goodridge, H.S., Bernstein, E.A., Fuchs, S., Liu, G.Y., and Bernstein, K.E.: Angiotensin-converting enzyme overexpression in mouse myelomonocytic cells augments resistance to *Listeria* and methicillin-resistant *Staphylococcus aureus. J. Biol. Chem.* 2010, **285**:39051–39060.

Ridker, P.M., Cannon, C.P., Morrow, D., Rifai, N., Rose, L.M., McCabe, C.H., Pfeffer, M.A., and Braunwald, E.: Pravastatin or Atorvastatin Evaluation and Infection Therapy-Thrombolysis in Myocardial Infarction 22 (PROVE IT-TIMI 22) Investigators: C-reactive protein levels and outcomes after statin therapy. *N. Engl. J. Med.* 2005, **352**:20–28.

Youssef, S., Stuve, O., Patarroyo, J.C., Ruiz, P.J., Radosevich, J.L., Hur, E.M., Bravo, M., Mitchell, D.J., Sobel, R.A., Steinman, L., *et al.*: The HMG-CoA reductase inhibitor, atorvastatin, promotes a Th2 bias and reverses paralysis in central nervous system autoimmune disease. *Nature* 2002, **420**:78–84.

16-33   Controlled administration of antigen can be used to manipulate the nature of an antigen-specific response.

Diabetes Prevention Trial: Type 1 Diabetes Study Group: **Effects of insulin in relatives of patients with type 1 diabetes mellitus.** *N. Engl. J. Med.* 2002, **346**:1685–1691.

Haselden, B.M., Kay, A.B., and Larché, M.: **Peptide-mediated immune responses in specific immunotherapy.** *Int. Arch. Allergy Immunol.* 2000, **122**:229–237.

Mowat, A.M., Parker, L.A., Beacock-Sharp, H., Millington, O.R., and Chirdo, F.: **Oral tolerance: overview and historical perspectives.** *Ann. N.Y. Acad. Sci.* 2004, **1029**:1–8.

Steinman, L., Utz, P.J., and Robinson, W.H.: **Suppression of autoimmunity via microbial mimics of altered peptide ligands.** *Curr. Top. Microbiol. Immunol.* 2005, **296**:55–63.

Weiner, H.L., da Cunha, A.P., Quintana, F., and Wu, H.: **Oral tolerance.** *Immunol. Rev.* 2011, **241**:241–259.

APPENDICES

Note: eAppendices II–IV are available on the Digital Landing Page for this book and in the ebook.

The Immunologist's Toolbox

A-1 Immunization.

Natural immune responses are normally directed at antigens borne by pathogenic microorganisms. The immune system can also be induced to respond to simple nonliving antigens, and experimental immunologists have focused on the responses to these simple antigens in developing our understanding of the immune response. The deliberate induction of an immune response is known as **immunization**. Experimental immunizations are routinely carried out by injecting the test antigen into the animal or human subject. The route, dose, and form in which antigen is administered can profoundly affect whether a response occurs and the type of response that is produced. The induction of protective immune responses against common microbial pathogens is often called vaccination, although this term originally referred to the induction of immune responses against smallpox by immunizing with the cross-reactive virus, vaccinia.

To determine whether an immune response has occurred and to follow its course, the immunized individual is monitored for the appearance of immune reactants. Immune responses to most antigens include soluble factors, such as cytokines and specific antibodies, and cellular responses, such as the generation of specific effector T cells. Monitoring the cytokine and antibody responses usually involves the analysis of relatively crude preparations of **antiserum** (plural: **antisera**). **Serum** is the fluid phase of clotted blood, which, if taken from an individual immunized against a particular antigen, is called antiserum. To study immune responses mediated by T cells, blood lymphocytes or cells from lymphoid organs such as the spleen are tested; T-cell responses are more commonly studied in experimental animals than in humans.

Antisera generated by immunization with even the simplest antigen will contain many different antibody molecules that bind to the immunogen in slightly

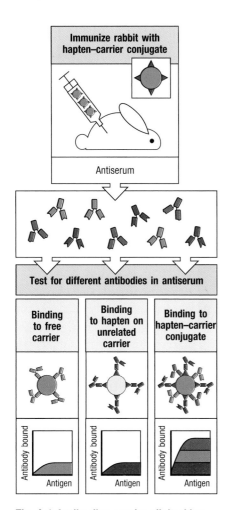

Fig. A.1 Antibodies can be elicited by small chemical groups called haptens only when the hapten is linked to an immunogenic protein carrier. After immunization with a hapten–carrier conjugate, three types of antibodies are produced. One set (blue) binds the carrier protein alone and is called carrier-specific. One set (red) binds to the hapten on any carrier or to free hapten in solution and is called hapten-specific. One set (purple) binds only the specific conjugate of hapten and carrier used for immunization, apparently binding to sites at which the hapten joins the carrier, and is called conjugate-specific. The amount of antibody of each type in this serum is shown schematically in the graphs at the bottom; note that the original antigen binds more antibody than the sum of anti-hapten and anti-carrier antibodies as a result of the additional binding of conjugate-specific antibody.

different ways. In addition, antisera contain many antibodies that do not bind at all to the immunizing antigen, because they were present in the individual prior to immunization. These nonspecific antibodies often lead to technical difficulties in using antisera for detecting an immunogen. To circumvent this problem, antibodies that bind to the immunogen can be purified by affinity chromatography using immobilized antigen (see Section A-3). Alternatively, these problems can be avoided by making monoclonal antibodies (see Section A-8).

Any substance that can elicit an immune response is said to be **immunogenic** and is called an **immunogen**. There is a clear operational distinction between an immunogen and an antigen. Immunogens are substances that elicit an adaptive immune response, whereas an antigen is defined as any substance that can bind to a specific antibody. All antigens therefore have the potential to elicit specific antibodies; however, not all antigens are immunogenic. An example of this distinction is evident when considering protein antigens. In spite of the fact that antibodies against proteins are of enormous utility in experimental biology and medicine, purified proteins are not generally immunogenic. This is because purified proteins lack microbial-associated molecular patterns (MAMPs), and therefore do not elicit an innate immune response. To provoke an immune response to a purified protein, the protein must be administered together with an adjuvant (discussed shortly).

Certain properties of antigens that favor the initiation of an adaptive immune response have been defined by studying antibody responses to simple natural proteins such as hen egg-white lysozyme, to synthetic polypeptide antigens, and to small organic molecules of simple structure. The study of antibody responses to small organic molecules, such as phenyl arsonates and nitrophenyls, was essential in defining early immunological principles. These molecules do not provoke antibodies when injected by themselves. However, antibodies can be raised against them if the molecule is attached covalently, by simple chemical reactions, to a protein carrier. Such small molecules were termed **haptens** (from the Greek *haptein*, 'to fasten') by the immunologist Karl Landsteiner, who first studied them in the early 20th century. He found that animals immunized with a hapten–carrier conjugate produced three distinct sets of antibodies (**Fig. A.1**). One set comprised hapten-specific antibodies that reacted with the same hapten on any carrier, as well as with free hapten. The second set of antibodies was specific for the carrier protein, as shown by their ability to bind both the hapten-modified and unmodified carrier protein. Finally, some antibodies reacted only with the specific conjugate of hapten and carrier used for immunization. Landsteiner's studies focused primarily on the antibody response to the hapten, as these small molecules could be synthesized in many closely related forms. He observed that antibodies raised against a particular hapten bind that hapten but, in general, fail to bind even very closely related chemical structures. The binding of haptens by anti-hapten antibodies has played an important part in defining the precision of antigen binding by antibody molecules. Anti-hapten antibodies are also important medically because they mediate allergic reactions to penicillin and other compounds that elicit antibody responses when they attach to self proteins (see Section 14-9).

The route by which antigen is administered affects both the magnitude and the type of response obtained. The most common routes by which antigen is introduced experimentally or as a vaccine into the body are as follows: into tissue by **subcutaneous (s.c.)** injection into the fatty layer just below the dermis or by **intradermal (i.d.)** or **intramuscular (i.m.)** injection; directly into the bloodstream by **intravenous (i.v.)** injection or transfusion; into the gastrointestinal tract by oral administration; and into the respiratory tract by **intranasal (i.n.)** administration or inhalation. Antigens may also be introduced into the peritoneal cavity by **intraperitoneal (i.p.)** injection.

Fig. A.2 The dose of antigen used in an initial immunization affects the primary and the secondary antibody response. The typical antigen dose–response curve shown here illustrates both the influence of dose on a primary antibody response (amounts of antibody produced expressed in arbitrary units) and the effect of the dose used for priming on a secondary antibody response elicited by a dose of antigen of 10^3 arbitrary mass units. Very low doses of antigen do not cause an immune response at all. Slightly higher doses seem to inhibit specific antibody production, an effect known as low-zone tolerance. Above these doses there is a steady increase in the response with antigen dose until an optimum response is reached; this response persists across a broad range of doses. Very high doses of antigen also inhibit immune responsiveness to a subsequent challenge, a phenomenon known as high-zone tolerance.

Antigens injected subcutaneously generally elicit strong responses, most probably because the antigen is taken up by resident dendritic cells in the skin and efficiently presented in local lymph nodes, and so this is the method most commonly used when the object of the experiment is to elicit specific antibodies or T cells against a given antigen. Antigens injected or transfused directly into the bloodstream tend to induce immune unresponsiveness or tolerance unless they bind to host cells or are in the form of aggregates that are readily taken up by antigen-presenting cells.

Antigen administration via the gastrointestinal tract is used mostly in the study of allergy. It has distinctive effects, frequently eliciting a local antibody response in the intestinal lamina propria, while producing a systemic state of tolerance that manifests as a diminished response to the same antigen if subsequently administered in immunogenic form elsewhere in the body (see Chapter 12). This 'split tolerance' may be important in avoiding allergy to antigens in food, because the local response prevents food antigens from entering the body, while the inhibition of systemic immunity helps to prevent the formation of IgE antibodies, which are the cause of such allergies (see Chapter 14).

The immune response to an antigen is also influenced by the dose of immunogen administered. Below a certain threshold dose, most proteins do not elicit any immune response. Above the threshold dose, there is a gradual increase in the response as the dose of antigen is increased, until a broad plateau level is reached, followed by a decline at very high antigen doses (**Fig. A.2**). In general, secondary and subsequent immune responses occur at lower antigen doses and achieve higher plateau values, which is a sign of immunological memory.

Most proteins are poorly immunogenic or non-immunogenic when administered by themselves. Strong adaptive immune responses to protein antigens almost always require that the antigen be injected in a mixture known as an adjuvant. An adjuvant is any substance that enhances the immunogenicity of substances mixed with it. Commonly used adjuvants are listed in **Fig. A.3**.

Adjuvants generally enhance immunogenicity in two different ways. First, adjuvants convert soluble protein antigens into particulate material, which is more readily ingested by phagocytic antigen-presenting cells such as macrophages and dendritic cells. For example, the antigen can be adsorbed on particles of the adjuvant (such as alum), be made particulate by emulsification in mineral oils, or be incorporated into the colloidal particles of immune stimulatory complexes (ISCOMs). Second, and more important, adjuvants contain pathogen-associated molecular patterns (PAMPs) that elicit a strong innate immune response. When taken up by phagocytic cells, the PAMPs in the adjuvant stimulate inflammatory cytokine production and induce the activation of the antigen-presenting cell. The activated antigen-presenting cells up-regulate abundant levels of co-stimulatory molecules that are important for activating T cells. Activated antigen-presenting cells also up-regulate high levels of MHC class I and class II proteins, plus many of the proteins important for efficient antigen processing and presentation (see Section 3-12). Because of the strong local inflammatory responses induced by adjuvants that contain PAMPs, most

Fig. A.3 Common adjuvants and their use. Adjuvants are mixed with the antigen and usually render it particulate, which helps to retain the antigen in the body and promotes uptake by macrophages. Most adjuvants include bacteria or bacterial components that stimulate macrophages and dendritic cells, aiding in the induction of the immune response. ISCOMs are small micelles of the detergent Quil A; when viral proteins are placed in these micelles, they apparently fuse with the antigen-presenting cell, allowing the antigen to enter the cytosol. Thus, the antigen-presenting cell can stimulate a response to the viral protein, much as a virus infecting these cells would stimulate an antiviral response. Vaccines designed to elicit responses to purified proteins often include compounds that stimulate pattern-recognition receptors, such as Toll-like receptors (TLRs), NOD-like receptors (NLRs), or C-type lectin receptors.

Adjuvants that enhance immune responses		
Adjuvant name	**Composition**	**Mechanism of action**
Freund's incomplete adjuvant	Oil-in-water emulsion	Delayed release of antigen; enhanced uptake by macrophages
Freund's complete adjuvant	Oil-in-water emulsion with dead mycobacteria that stimulate C-type lectin receptors	Delayed release of antigen; enhanced uptake by macrophages; induction of co-stimulators in macrophages
Freund's adjuvant with MDP	Oil-in-water emulsion with muramyl dipeptide (MDP), a constituent of mycobacteria that stimulates NOD-like receptors	Similar to Freund's complete adjuvant
Alum (aluminum hydroxide)	Aluminum hydroxide gel	Delayed release of antigen; enhanced macrophage uptake
Alum plus *Bordetella pertussis*	Aluminum hydroxide gel with killed *B. pertussis*	Delayed release of antigen; enhanced uptake by macrophages; induction of co-stimulators
Immune stimulatory complexes (ISCOMs)	Matrix of Quil A containing viral proteins	Delivers antigen to cytosol; allows induction of cytotoxic T cells
TLR agonists	Lipopolysaccharide, flagellin, lipopeptides, dsRNA, unmethylated DNA	Inflammatory cytokine production, induction of co-stimulators, enhanced antigen presentation to T cells
NOD-like receptor (NLR) agonists	Muramyl dipeptide (bacterial cell wall constituent)	Inflammatory cytokine production, induction of co-stimulators, enhanced antigen presentation to T cells
C-type lectin receptor agonists	Mycobacterial cell wall component trehalose-6,6′-dimycolate	Inflammatory cytokine production

of the adjuvants commonly used in experimental animals are not approved for use in humans.

Nevertheless, some human vaccines naturally contain microbial antigens that can also act as effective adjuvants. For example, purified constituents of the bacterium *Bordetella pertussis*, which is the causative agent of whooping cough, are used as both antigen and adjuvant in the triplex DTaP (diphtheria, pertussis, tetanus) vaccine. In addition, modified TLR ligands, such as monophosphoryl lipid A, a derivative of LPS, or poly(I):poly(C12U), a derivative of polyI:C, are currently included as components of several human vaccines.

A-2 Antibody responses.

B cells contribute to adaptive immunity by secreting antibodies, and the response of B cells to an injected immunogen is usually measured by analyzing the specific antibody produced in a **humoral immune response**. This is most conveniently achieved by assaying the antibody that accumulates in the fluid phase of whole blood, or **plasma**; such antibodies are known as circulating antibodies. Circulating antibody is usually measured by collecting blood, allowing it to clot, and then isolating the serum from the clotted blood. The amount and characteristics of the antibody in the resulting antiserum are then determined using the assays described later. Because assays for antibody were originally conducted using antisera from immune individuals, they are commonly referred to as **serological assays**, and the use of antibodies in such testing is often called **serology**.

The most important characteristics of an antibody response are the specificity, amount, isotype or class, and affinity of the antibodies produced. The **specificity** determines the ability of the antibody to distinguish the immunogen from other antigens. The amount of antibody can be determined in many different ways and is a function of the number of responding B cells, their rate of antibody synthesis, and the persistence of the antibody after production. The persistence of an antibody in the plasma and extracellular fluid bathing the tissues is determined mainly by its isotype or class (see Section 4-6 and Section 10-15); each isotype has a different half-life *in vivo*. The isotypic composition of an antibody response also determines the biological functions these antibodies can perform and the sites in which antibody will be found. Finally, the strength of binding of the antibody to its antigen in terms of a single antigen-binding site binding to a monovalent antigen is termed its **affinity**; the total binding strength of a molecule with more than one binding site is called its **avidity**. Binding strength is important: the higher the affinity of the antibody for its antigen, the less antibody is required to eliminate the antigen, because antibodies with higher affinity will bind at lower antigen concentrations. All these parameters of the humoral immune response help to determine the capacity of that response to protect the host from infection.

A-3   Affinity chromatography.

The specificity of antigen–antibody binding interactions can be exploited for the purification of a specific antigen from a complex mixture or alternatively for the purification of specific antibodies from antiserum containing a mixture of different antibodies. The technique employed is called **affinity chromatography (Fig. A.4)**. For purification of an antigen, antigen-specific antibodies are bound, often covalently, to small, chemically reactive beads, which are loaded into a column. The antigen mixture is allowed to pass over the beads. The specific antigen binds; all the other components in the mixture can then be washed away. The specific antigen is then eluted, typically by lowering the pH to 2.5 or raising it to greater than 11. Antibodies bind stably under physiological conditions of salt concentration, temperature, and pH, but the binding is reversible because the bonds are noncovalent. Affinity chromatography can also be used to purify antibodies from complex antisera by using beads coated with specific antigen. The technique is known as affinity chromatography because it separates molecules on the basis of their affinity for one another.

A-4   Radioimmunoassay (RIA), enzyme-linked immunosorbent assay (ELISA), and competitive inhibition assay.

Radioimmunoassay (RIA) and **enzyme-linked immunosorbent assay (ELISA)** are direct binding assays for antigen or antibody; both work on the same principle, but the means of detecting specific binding is different. Radioimmunoassays are commonly used to measure the levels of hormones in blood and tissue fluids, while ELISAs are frequently used in viral diagnostics; for example, in detecting cases of infection with the human immunodeficiency virus (HIV), which is the cause of AIDS. For both of these methods, one needs a pure preparation of a known antigen or antibody, or both, in order to standardize the assay. We will describe the assay that is used to determine the amount of a specific antigen in a sample; for instance, the amount of HIV p24 protein in a patient's serum. For this, a preparation of pure antibody specific for the antigen is required. One can also use RIA or ELISA to determine the amount of specific antibody in a mixture, such as serum; in this case, a preparation of pure antigen is needed as a starting point.

For the most sensitive determination of antigen concentration, an RIA is used. In this technique, pure antibody against the antigen is radioactively labeled,

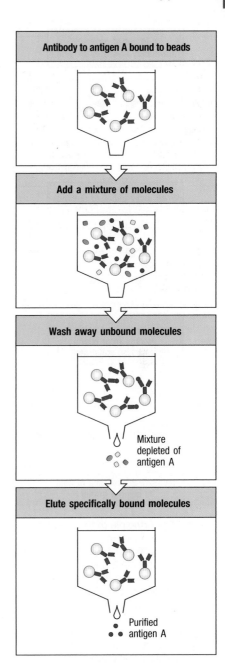

Fig. A.4 Affinity chromatography uses antigen–antibody binding to purify antigens or antibodies. To purify a specific antigen from a complex mixture of molecules, a monoclonal antibody is attached to an insoluble matrix, such as chromatography beads, and the mixture of molecules is passed over the matrix. The specific antibody binds the antigen of interest; other molecules are washed away. Specific antigen is then eluted by altering the pH, which can usually disrupt antibody–antigen bonds. Antibodies can be purified in the same way on beads coupled to antigen (not shown).

Within the figure:
- Antibody to antigen A bound to beads
- Add a mixture of molecules
- Wash away unbound molecules — Mixture depleted of antigen A
- Elute specifically bound molecules — Purified antigen A

Add anti-A antibody covalently linked to enzyme

Sample 1 (antigen A)   Sample 2 (antigen B)

Wash away unbound antibody

Enzyme makes colored product from added colorless substrate

Measure absorbance of light by colored product

Fig. A.5 The principle of the enzyme-linked immunosorbent assay (ELISA). To detect antigen A, purified antibody specific for antigen A is linked chemically to an enzyme. The samples to be tested are coated onto the surface of plastic wells, to which they bind nonspecifically; residual sticky sites on the plastic are blocked by adding irrelevant proteins (not shown). The labeled antibody is then added to the wells under conditions that prevent nonspecific binding, so that only binding to antigen A causes the labeled antibody to be retained on the surface. Unbound labeled antibody is removed from all wells by washing, and bound antibody is detected by an enzyme-dependent color-change reaction. This assay allows arrays of wells known as microtiter plates to be read in fiber-optic multichannel spectrometers, greatly speeding the assay. Modifications of this basic assay allow antibody or antigen in unknown samples to be measured as shown in Figs. A.6 and A.25.

usually with[125]I. For ELISA, a non-radioactive approach, an enzyme is linked chemically to the antibody. The unlabeled component, which in this case would be the solution containing an unknown amount of antigen, is attached to a solid support, such as the wells of a plastic multiwell plate, which will adsorb a certain amount of any protein. After this, the labeled antibody is added to the well and allowed to bind to the unlabeled antigen under conditions in which nonspecific adsorption is blocked, and any unbound antibody and other proteins are washed away. Antibody binding in RIA is measured directly in terms of the amount of radioactivity retained by the coated wells, whereas in ELISA the binding is detected by a reaction that converts a substrate into a reaction product of a different color (**Fig. A.5**). The color change can be read directly in the reaction tray, making data collection very easy and providing a quantitative measurement of reaction-product concentration; furthermore, ELISA also avoids the hazards of radioactivity. This makes ELISA the preferred method for most direct-binding assays. In a variation of this assay, labeled anti-immunoglobulin antibodies can also be used in RIA or ELISA as a second layer, after the binding of unlabeled antibody to unlabeled antigen-coated plates. The use of such a second layer amplifies the signal, because at least two molecules of the labeled anti-immunoglobulin antibody are able to bind to each unlabeled antibody. As mentioned above, RIA and ELISA can also be carried out in reverse when the goal is to determine the amount of antibody in a solution; in this case, unlabeled antibody is adhered to the plates, labeled antigen is added, and the amount of labeled antigen bound after washing is measured.

A modification of ELISA known as a **capture (or sandwich) ELISA** (or more generally as an **antigen-capture assay**) is commonly used to detect secreted products such as cytokines. Rather than the antigen being directly attached to a plastic plate, antigen-specific antibodies are bound to the plate. These are able to bind antigen with high affinity, and thus concentrate it on the surface of the plate, even with antigens that are present in very low concentrations in the initial mixture. A separate labeled antibody that recognizes a different epitope from that recognized by the immobilized first antibody is then used to detect the bound antigen.

These assays illustrate two crucial aspects of all serological assays. First, at least one of the reagents must be available in a pure, detectable form in order to obtain quantitative information. Second, there must be a means of separating the bound fraction of the labeled reagent from the unbound, free fraction so that the percentage of specific binding can be determined. Normally, this separation is achieved by having the unlabeled partner trapped on a solid support. Labeled molecules that do not bind can then be washed away, leaving just the labeled partner that has bound. In Fig. A.5, the unlabeled antigen is attached to the well, and the labeled antibody is trapped by binding to it. The separation of bound reagent from the free fraction is an essential step in every assay that uses antibodies.

RIA and ELISA do not allow one to measure directly the amount of antigen or antibody in a sample of unknown composition, because both depend on the binding of a pure labeled antigen or antibody. There are various ways around this problem, one of which is to use a **competitive inhibition assay**, as shown in **Fig. A.6**. In this type of assay, the presence and amount of a particular test antigen in a sample of unknown composition are determined by the ability of the antigen, if present, to compete with a known amount of that antigen, but in this case labeled, for binding to an antibody attached to a plastic well. To perform this assay, an antibody specific for the antigen is adhered to an assay plate well. A standard curve is determined using a known quantity of labeled antigen, which is mixed with increasing amounts of the same antigen, but unlabeled. As the unlabeled antigen concentration increases, the binding of the labeled antigen to the antibody will decrease. In separate assay wells, the labeled antigen is mixed with increasing amounts of the sample of unknown

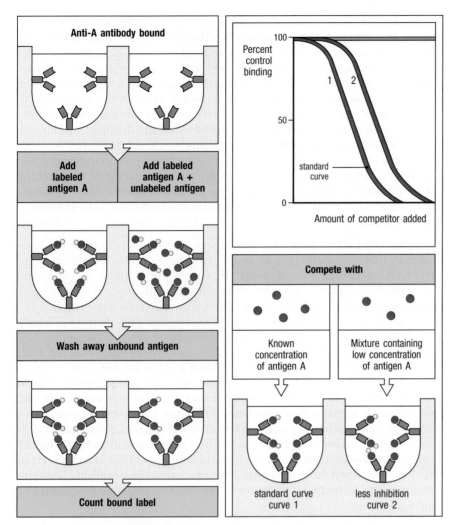

Fig. A.6 Competitive inhibition assay for antigen in samples of unknown composition. A fixed amount of unlabeled antibody is attached to a set of wells, and a standard reference preparation of a labeled antigen is bound to it. Unlabeled standard or test samples are then added in various amounts, and the displacement of labeled antigen is measured, generating characteristic inhibition curves. A standard curve is obtained by using known amounts of unlabeled antigen identical to those used for the labeled species, and comparison with this curve allows the amount of antigen in samples of unknown composition to be calculated. The green line on the graph represents a sample lacking any substance that reacts with anti-A antibodies.

composition, and the amount of labeled antigen bound to the antibody is measured to determine a binding curve for the test sample. A comparison of the two curves indicates the presence or absence of the antigen in the test sample and, if present, its concentration in the sample.

A-5 Multiplex bead assay for detection of cytokines, antibody responses, or antigens.

Another binding assay used to detect specific proteins in complex mixtures such as serum samples from humans or experimental animals is known as a **multiplex assay**. The term 'multiplex' refers to the fact multiple antigens or antibodies can simultaneously be detected and quantified in a single sample. This technique is often utilized to examine the levels of multiple cytokines or multiple antibodies when sample availability is limited, and therefore it is not feasible to measure each cytokine or antibody individually.

For this type of assay, small microspheres are differentially labeled with fluorescent dyes that can be distinguished on the basis of their distinct emission spectra. Each population of microspheres is labeled with a given fluorescent dye and is conjugated to antibodies specific for one antigen; for instance, a single cytokine. Up to 100 different populations of microspheres can be prepared, and then mixed together. This mixture is added to the sample to capture the antigens. Bound antigen is then detected using a second antibody for each antigen and which binds the antigen at a site distinct from the site bound by the first antibody that was conjugated to the microspheres. This second antibody is conjugated to a different fluorescent dye, and the magnitude of its fluorescence is a measure of the quantity of bound antigen. The machine that performs this multiplex analysis, the Luminex analyzer, then measures the amount of fluorescence associated with each differentially labeled microsphere population.

Multiplex bead assays have also been developed for analysis of serum antibodies by flow cytometry (see Section A-19). One example is the BioLegend LEGENDplex carboxyl bead assay, in which populations of beads are differentially labeled with the fluorochrome allophycocyanin (APC). Each population of beads is conjugated to a different antigen, and the beads are then mixed together in equimolar ratios. This mixture of beads is incubated with a serum sample. Antibodies present in the serum will bind to a bead in the mixture if the antibodies have specificity for the antigen conjugated to that bead. The unbound antibodies are washed away, and the beads are then incubated with biotinylated antibodies specific to human immunoglobulin, followed by streptavidin conjugated to a second fluorochrome, such as phycoerythrin (PE). After flow cytometry analysis, each population of beads can be resolved on the basis of different APC fluorescence intensities, and beads with bound human antibodies from the serum sample will show enhanced PE fluorescence. This assay has been developed as a sensitive measure of serum antibodies to SARS-CoV-2 to determine an individual's exposure to the virus responsible for COVID-19 (**Fig. A.7**).

A-6   Hemagglutination and blood typing.

The direct measurement of antibody binding to antigen is used in most quantitative serological assays. However, some important assays are based on the ability of antibody binding to alter the physical state of the antigen to which the antibody binds. These secondary interactions can be detected in a variety of ways. For instance, when the antigen is displayed on the surface of a large particle such as a bacterium, antibodies can cause the bacteria to clump, or **agglutinate**. The same principle applies to the reactions used in blood typing, only here the target antigens are on the surface of red blood cells, and the clumping reaction caused by antibodies against them is called **hemagglutination** (from the Greek *haima*, 'blood').

Hemagglutination is used to determine the **ABO blood group** of blood donors and transfusion recipients. Clumping or agglutination is induced by antibodies or agglutinins called anti-A or anti-B that bind to the A or B blood-group substances, respectively (**Fig. A.8**). These blood-group antigens are arrayed in many copies on the surface of the red blood cell, causing the cells to agglutinate when cross-linked by antibodies. Because hemagglutination involves the cross-linking of blood cells by the simultaneous binding of antibody molecules to identical antigens on different cells, this reaction also demonstrates that each antibody molecule must have at least two identical antigen-binding sites.

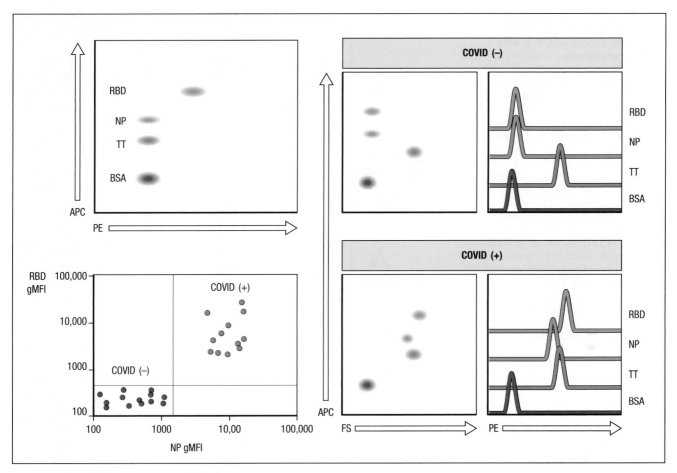

Fig. A.7. Multiplex bead assay for detection of human antibodies specific to SARS-CoV-2 spike protein and nucleoprotein. The BioLegend LEGENDplex carboxyl beads of different sizes and allophycocyanin (APC) fluorescence intensities were conjugated to bovine serum albumin (BSA), tetanus toxoid (TT), SARS-CoV-2 spike protein receptor-binding domain (RBD), and SARS-CoV-2 nucleoprotein (NP). Upper left panel: Flow cytometry analysis shows the levels of fluorescence and the forward scatter (FS; size) of the conjugated beads after mixing the four populations of beads together. Right panels: Serum samples from one healthy control individual [COVID (–)] and one individual previously infected with SARS-CoV-2 [COVID (+)] were incubated with the mixture of beads. Samples were washed and then incubated with biotinylated anti-human Ig followed by streptavidin conjugated to phycoerythrin (PE) and analyzed by flow cytometry. Plots on the left show the relative fluorescence intensities for PE versus APC, and histograms on the right show the PE fluorescence from the dot plots on the left. Lower left panel: Thirteen pre-COVID serum samples [COVID (–)] and 12 serum samples from patients that screened positive for SARS-CoV-2 [COVID (+)] were analyzed using the multiplex bead assay. The average and standard deviation for all negative samples was determined; the value of 3 times the standard deviation (3XSD) is indicated by the thin black lines. All positive samples are well above the cutoff, easily identifying the seropositive COVID-positive patients. gMFI, geometric mean fluorescence intensity. Data provided by Ross Kedl.

A-7   Coombs tests and the detection of rhesus incompatibility.

Coombs tests use anti-immunoglobulin antibodies to detect the antibodies that cause **hemolytic disease of the newborn,** or **erythroblastosis fetalis**. Anti-immunoglobulin antibodies were first developed by R. R. A. Coombs, and the test for this disease is still called the Coombs test. Hemolytic disease of the newborn occurs when a mother makes IgG antibodies specific for the **rhesus (or Rh) blood-group antigen** expressed on the red blood cells of her fetus. Rh-negative mothers make these antibodies when they are exposed at delivery to Rh-positive fetal red blood cells bearing the paternally inherited Rh antigen. During subsequent pregnancies, these anti-Rh antibodies are transported across the placenta to the fetus. The

Fig. A.8 Hemagglutination is used to type blood groups and match compatible donors and recipients for blood transfusion. Common gut bacteria bear antigens that are similar or identical to blood-group antigens, and these bacterial antigens will stimulate the formation of antibodies against blood-group antigens in individuals who do not bear the corresponding antigens on their own red blood cells (left column); thus, type O individuals, who lack A and B, have both anti-A and anti-B antibodies, whereas type AB individuals have neither. The pattern of agglutination of the red blood cells of a transfusion donor or recipient with anti-A and anti-B antibodies reveals the individual's ABO blood group. Before transfusion, the serum of the recipient is also tested for antibodies that agglutinate the red blood cells of the donor, and vice versa, a procedure called a cross-match, which may detect potentially harmful antibodies against other blood groups that are not part of the ABO system.

	Red blood cells from individuals of type			
	O	A	B	AB
	Express the carbohydrate structures			
Serum from individuals of type	R–GlcNAc–Gal | Fuc	R–GlcNAc–Gal–GalNAc | Fuc	R–GlcNAc–Gal | Fuc	R–GlcNAc–Gal–GalNAc | Fuc + R–GlcNAc–Gal–Gal | Fuc
O Anti-A and anti-B antibodies	No agglutination	Agglutination	Agglutination	Agglutination
A Anti-B antibodies	No agglutination	No agglutination	Agglutination	Agglutination
B Anti-A antibodies	No agglutination	Agglutination	No agglutination	Agglutination
AB No antibodies to A or B	No agglutination	No agglutination	No agglutination	No agglutination

normal process of transporting maternal IgG across the placenta is generally beneficial, as it protects newborn infants against infection. However, IgG anti-Rh antibodies coat the fetal red blood cells, which are then destroyed by phagocytic cells in the liver, causing a hemolytic anemia in the fetus and newborn infant.

Rh antigens are widely spaced on the red blood cell surface, and so the IgG anti-Rh antibodies do not bind in the correct conformation to fix complement and so do not cause lysis of red blood cells *in vitro*. Furthermore, for reasons that are not fully understood, antibodies against Rh antigens do not agglutinate red blood cells, unlike antibodies against the ABO blood-group antigens. Thus, detecting anti-Rh antibodies was difficult until anti-human immunoglobulin antibodies were developed. With these, maternal IgG antibodies bound to the fetal red blood cells can be detected after washing the cells to remove unbound immunoglobulin that is present in the fetal serum. Adding anti-human immunoglobulin antibodies against the washed fetal red blood cells agglutinates any cells to which maternal antibodies are bound. This is the **direct Coombs test** (**Fig. A.9**), so called because it directly detects antibody bound to the surface of the fetal red blood cells. An **indirect Coombs test** is used to detect non-agglutinating anti-Rh antibody in maternal serum: the serum is first incubated with Rh-positive red blood cells, which bind the anti-Rh antibody, after which the antibody-coated cells are washed to remove unbound immunoglobulin and are then agglutinated with anti-immunoglobulin antibody (see Fig. A.9). The indirect Coombs test allows Rh incompatibilities that might lead to hemolytic disease of the newborn to be detected, and this knowledge allows the disease to be prevented. The Coombs test is also commonly used to detect antibodies against drugs that bind to red blood cells and cause hemolytic anemia.

A-8   Monoclonal antibodies.

The antibodies generated in a natural immune response or after immunization in the laboratory are a mixture of molecules of different specificities and affinities. Some of this heterogeneity results from the production of antibodies that bind to different epitopes on the immunizing antigen, but even antibodies directed at a single antigenic determinant such as a hapten can be markedly heterogeneous, as shown by **isoelectric focusing**. In this technique, proteins are separated on the basis of their isoelectric point, the pH at which their net charge is zero. By electrophoresing proteins in a pH gradient for long enough, each molecule migrates along the pH gradient until it reaches the pH at which it is neutral and is thus concentrated (focused) at that point. When antiserum containing anti-hapten antibodies is treated in this way and then transferred to a solid support such as nitrocellulose paper, the anti-hapten antibodies can be detected by their ability to bind labeled hapten. The binding of antibodies of various isoelectric points to the hapten shows that even antibodies that bind the same antigenic determinant can be heterogeneous.

Antisera are valuable for many biological purposes, but they have certain inherent disadvantages that relate to the heterogeneity of the antibodies they contain. First, each antiserum is different from all other antisera, even if raised in a genetically identical animal by using the identical preparation of antigen and the same immunization protocol. Second, antisera can be produced in only limited volumes, and thus it is impossible to use the identical serological reagent in a long or complex series of experiments or clinical tests. Finally, even antibodies purified by affinity chromatography (see Section A-3) can include minor populations of antibodies that give unexpected cross-reactions, which confound the analysis of experiments. To avoid these problems, and to harness the full potential of antibodies, it was necessary to develop a way of making an unlimited supply of antibody molecules of homogeneous structure and known specificity. This has been achieved through the production of monoclonal antibodies from cultures of hybrid antibody-forming cells or, more recently, by genetic engineering.

Starting in the 1950s, biochemists in search of a homogeneous preparation of antibody that they could subject to detailed chemical analysis turned to proteins produced by individuals with multiple myeloma, a common tumor of plasma cells. It was known that antibodies are normally produced by plasma cells, and because this disease is associated with the presence of large amounts of a homogeneous gamma globulin called **myeloma protein** in a patient's serum, it seemed likely that myeloma proteins would serve as models for normal antibody molecules. Thus, much of the early knowledge of antibody structure came from studies on myeloma proteins. These studies showed that monoclonal antibodies could be obtained from immortalized plasma cells. However, the antigen specificity of most myeloma proteins was unknown, which limited their usefulness as objects of study or as immunological tools.

This problem was solved by Georges Köhler and César Milstein, who devised a technique for producing a homogeneous population of antibodies of known antigenic specificity. They did this by fusing spleen cells from an immunized mouse to cells of a mouse myeloma to produce hybrid cells that both proliferated indefinitely and secreted antibody specific for the antigen used to immunize the spleen-cell donor. The spleen cell provides the ability to make specific antibody, while the myeloma cell provides the ability to grow indefinitely in culture and secrete immunoglobulin continually. By using a myeloma-cell partner that produces no antibody proteins itself, the antibody produced by the hybrid cells comes only from the immune spleen-cell partner. After fusion, the hybrid cells are selected using drugs that kill the myeloma parental cell, while the unfused parental spleen cells have a limited life span and soon die, so that only hybrid myeloma-cell lines, or **hybridomas**, survive. Those hybridomas

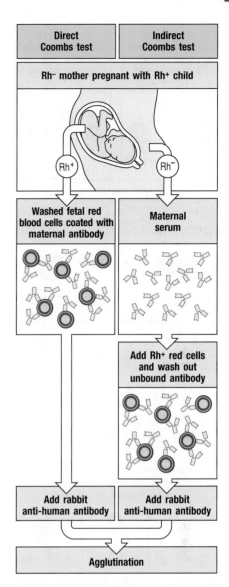

Fig. A.9 The Coombs direct and indirect anti-globulin tests for antibody against red blood cell antigens. An Rh⁻ mother of an Rh⁺ fetus can become immunized to fetal red blood cells that enter the maternal circulation at the time of delivery. In a subsequent pregnancy with an Rh⁺ fetus, IgG anti-Rh antibodies can cross the placenta and damage the fetal red blood cells. In contrast to anti-Rh antibodies, maternal anti-ABO antibodies are of the IgM isotype and cannot cross the placenta, and so do not cause harm. Anti-Rh antibodies do not agglutinate red blood cells, but their presence on the fetal red blood cell surface can be shown by washing away unbound immunoglobulin and then adding antibody against human immunoglobulin, which agglutinates the antibody-coated cells. Anti-Rh antibodies can be detected in the mother's serum in an indirect Coombs test; the serum is incubated with Rh⁺ red blood cells, and once the antibody has bound, the red blood cells are treated as in the direct Coombs test.

Spleen cells producing antibody from mouse immunized with antigen A

Myeloma cells (immortal) lacking antibody secretion and the enzyme HGPRT

Mix and fuse cells with PEG

Transfer to HAT medium

Immortal hybridomas proliferate; mortal spleen cells and unfused HGPRT⁻ myeloma cells die

Select hybridoma that makes antibody specific for antigen A

Clone selected hybridoma

Fig. A.10 The production of monoclonal antibodies. Mice are immunized with antigen A and given an intravenous booster immunization 3 days before they are sacrificed, in order to produce a large population of spleen cells secreting specific antibody. Spleen cells die after a few days in culture. To produce a continual source of antibody, they are fused with immortal myeloma cells by use of polyethylene glycol (PEG), resulting in a hybrid cell line called a hybridoma. The myeloma cells are selected beforehand to ensure that they are not secreting antibody themselves and that they lack the enzyme hypoxanthine-guanine phosphoribosyltransferase (HGPRT); without this enzyme, unfused myeloma cells are sensitive to the hypoxanthine–aminopterin–thymidine (HAT) medium, which is used to select hybrid cells. The HGPRT gene contributed by the spleen cell allows hybrid cells to survive in the HAT medium, and only hybrid cells can grow continually in culture, because of the malignant potential contributed by the myeloma cells combined with the finite life span of unfused spleen cells. Unfused myeloma cells and unfused spleen cells therefore die in the HAT medium, as shown here by cells with dark, irregular nuclei. Individual hybridomas are obtained by single-cell dilution and then screened for antibody production, and single clones that make antibody of the desired specificity can be isolated and grown. The cloned hybridoma cells are grown in bulk culture to produce large amounts of antibody. As each hybridoma is descended from a single cell, all the cells of a hybridoma cell line make the same antibody molecule, which is thus called a monoclonal antibody.

producing antibody of the desired specificity are then identified and cloned by regrowing the cultures from single cells (**Fig. A.10**). Because each hybridoma is a **clone** derived from fusion with a single B cell, all the antibody molecules it produces are identical in structure, including their antigen-binding site and isotype. Such antibodies are called **monoclonal antibodies**. This technology has revolutionized the use of antibodies by providing a limitless supply of antibody of a single and known specificity. Monoclonal antibodies are now used in most serological assays, as diagnostic probes, and as therapeutic agents. So far, efforts to use the same approach to make human monoclonal antibodies have met with limited success. 'Fully human' therapeutic monoclonal antibodies are currently made by using phage display technology (described in Section A-9), by using recombinant DNA technology to clone and express antibody genes from human plasma cells (see Section A-10), or by immunizing transgenic mice (see Section A-35) carrying human antibody genes.

A-9 Phage display libraries for antibody V-region production.

In a technique for producing antibody-like molecules, gene segments encoding the antigen-binding variable, or V, domains of antibodies are fused to genes encoding the coat protein of a bacteriophage. Bacteriophages containing such gene fusions are used to infect bacteria, and the resulting phage particles have coats that express the antibody-like fusion protein, with the antigen-binding domain displayed on the outside of the bacteriophages. A collection of recombinant phages, each displaying a different antigen-binding domain on the surface, is known as a **phage display library**. In much the same way that antibodies specific for a particular antigen can be isolated from a complex mixture by affinity chromatography (see Section A-3), phages expressing antigen-binding domains specific for a particular antigen can be isolated by selecting the phages in the library for binding to that antigen. The phage particles that bind are recovered and used to infect fresh bacteria. Each phage isolated in this way will produce a monoclonal antigen-binding particle analogous to a monoclonal antibody (**Fig. A.11**). The genes encoding the antigen-binding site, which are unique to each phage, can then be recovered from the phage DNA and used to construct genes for a complete antibody molecule by joining them to parts of immunoglobulin genes that encode the invariant parts of an antibody. When these reconstructed antibody genes are introduced into a suitable host-cell line, such as the non-antibody-producing myeloma cells used for hybridomas, the transfected cells can secrete antibodies with all the desirable characteristics of monoclonal antibodies produced from hybridomas.

| Isolate population of genes encoding antibody variable regions | Construct fusion protein of V region with a bacteriophage coat protein | Cloning a random population of variable regions gives rise to a mixture of bacteriophages—a phage display library | Select phages with desired V regions by specific binding to antigen |

Fig. A.11 The production of antibodies by genetic engineering. Short primers to consensus sequences in heavy- and light-chain variable (V) regions of immunoglobulin genes are used to generate a library of heavy- and light-chain V-region DNAs by the polymerase chain reaction (PCR), with spleen DNA as the starting material. These heavy- and light-chain V-region genes are cloned randomly into filamentous phages such that each phage expresses one heavy-chain and one light-chain V region as a surface fusion protein with antibody-like properties. The resulting phage display library is multiplied in bacteria, and the phages are then bound to a surface coated with antigen. The unbound phages are washed away; the bound phages are recovered, multiplied in bacteria, and again bound to antigen. After a few cycles, only specific high-affinity antigen-binding phages are left. These can be used like antibody molecules, or their V genes can be recovered and engineered into antibody genes to produce genetically engineered antibody molecules (not shown). This technology may replace the hybridoma technology for producing monoclonal antibodies and has the advantage that humans can be used as the source of DNA.

A-10 Generation of human monoclonal antibodies from vaccinated individuals.

In some cases, human monoclonal antibodies can be made by cloning the rearranged antibody heavy- and light-chain gene sequences from plasma cells isolated from vaccinated individuals. Based on the expression of cell-surface molecules such as CD27 and CD38, human plasma cells can be isolated from the peripheral blood of individuals who were immunized approximately 1 week earlier. Individual plasma cells are sorted into wells of microtiter plates, and the antibody heavy- and light-chain variable-region sequences are cloned from each cell by PCR. These sequences are then inserted into constructs that re-create the full-length antibody heavy- and light-chain genes, and the paired heavy- and light-chain vectors are introduced into an immortalized human cell line. Human cells are then screened to identify those secreting antibody proteins that bind to the immunizing antigen. These immortalized cells become a permanent source of the specific human antibody protein.

A-11 Microscopy and imaging using fluorescent dyes.

Because antibodies bind stably and specifically to their corresponding antigen, they are invaluable as probes for identifying a particular molecule in cells, tissues, or biological fluids. Antibody molecules can be used to locate their target molecules accurately in single cells or in tissue sections by a variety of different labeling techniques. When the antibody itself, or the anti-immunoglobulin antibody used to detect it, is labeled with a fluorescent dye (a fluorochrome or fluorophore) and then detected by microscopy, the technique is known as **immunofluorescence microscopy**. As in all serological techniques, the antibody binds stably to its antigen, allowing unbound antibody to be removed by thorough washing. Because antibodies against proteins recognize the surface features of the native, folded protein, the native structure of the protein being sought usually needs to be preserved, either by using only the most gentle chemical fixation techniques or by using frozen tissue sections that are fixed only after the antibody reaction has been performed. Some antibodies,

Excitation and emission wavelengths of some commonly used fluorochromes		
Probe	Excitation (nm)	Emission (nm)
R-phycoerythrin (PE)	480; 565	578
Fluorescein	495	519
PerCP	490	675
Texas Red	589	615
Rhodamine	550	573

Fig. A.12 Excitation and emission wavelengths for common fluorochromes.

however, bind proteins even if they are denatured, and such antibodies will bind specifically even to protein in fixed tissue sections.

The fluorescent dye can be covalently attached directly to the specific antibody; however, the bound antibody is more commonly detected by fluorescently labeled anti-immunoglobulin, a technique known as **indirect immunofluorescence**. The dyes chosen for immunofluorescence are excited by light of one wavelength, usually blue or green, and emit light of a different wavelength in the visible spectrum. The most commonly used fluorochromes are fluorescein, which emits green light; Texas Red and peridinin chlorophyll protein (PerCP), which emit red light; and rhodamine and phycoerythrin (PE), which emit orange-red light (**Fig. A.12**). By using selective filters, only the light coming from the fluorochrome used is detected in the fluorescence microscope (**Fig. A.13**). Although Albert Coons devised this technique to identify the plasma cell as the source of antibody, it can be used to detect the distribution of any protein. By attaching different dyes to different antibodies, the distribution of two or more molecules can be determined in the same cell or tissue section (see Fig. A.13).

The development of the **confocal fluorescent microscope**, which uses computer-aided techniques to produce ultrathin optical sections of a cell or tissue, gives very high resolution (sub-micrometer) fluorescence microscopy without the need for elaborate sample preparation. The light source for excitation (a laser) is focused onto a particular plane in the specimen, and the emitted light is refocused through a 'pinhole' so that only light from the desired plane reaches the detector, thus removing out-of-focus emissions from above or below the plane. This gives a sharper image than conventional fluorescence microscopy, and a three-dimensional picture can be built up from successive optical sections taken along the 'vertical' axis. Confocal microscopy can be used on fixed cells stained with fluorescently tagged antibodies or on living cells expressing proteins tagged with naturally fluorescent proteins. The first of these fluorescent proteins to come into wide use was green fluorescent protein (GFP), isolated from the jellyfish *Aequorea victoria*. The list of fluorescent proteins in routine use now includes those emitting red, blue, cyan, or yellow fluorescence. By using cells transfected with genes encoding different fusion

Fig. A.13 Immunofluorescence microscopy. Antibodies labeled with a fluorescent dye such as fluorescein (green triangle) are used to reveal the presence of their corresponding antigens in cells or tissues. The stained cells are examined using a microscope that exposes them to blue or green light to excite the fluorescent dye. The excited dye emits light at a characteristic wavelength, which is captured by viewing the sample through a selective filter. This technique is applied widely in biology to determine the location of molecules in cells and tissues. Different antigens can be detected in tissue sections by labeling antibodies with dyes of distinctive color. Here, antibodies against the protein glutamic acid decarboxylase (GAD) coupled to a green dye are shown to stain the β cells of pancreatic islets of Langerhans. The α cells do not make this enzyme and are labeled with antibodies against the hormone glucagon coupled with an orange fluorescent dye. GAD is an important antigen in type 1 diabetes mellitus, a disease in which the insulin-secreting β cells of the islets of Langerhans are destroyed by an immune attack on self tissues (see Chapter 15).

proteins, it has been possible to visualize the redistribution of T-cell receptors, co-receptors, adhesion molecules, and other signaling molecules, such as CD45, that takes place when a T cell makes contact with a target cell (see Fig. 9.40).

Confocal microscopy, however, can penetrate only around 80 μm into a tissue, and at the wavelengths typically used for excitation, the source light will soon bleach the fluorescent label and damage the specimen. This means the technique is not suitable for imaging a live specimen over a period of time sufficient, for example, to track the movements of cells in a tissue. The more recently developed technique of **two-photon scanning fluorescence microscopy** overcomes some of these limitations. In this technology, ultrashort pulses of laser light of much longer wavelength (and thus with photons of lower energy) are used for excitation, and two of these lower-energy photons arriving nearly simultaneously are required to excite the fluorophore. Excitation will therefore occur in only a very small region at the focus of the microscope, where the beam of light is most intense, and so fluorescence emission will be restricted to the plane of focus, producing a sharp, high-contrast image. The longer-wavelength light (typically in the near infrared) is also less damaging to living tissue than the blue and ultraviolet wavelengths typically used in confocal microscopy, and so imaging can be carried out over a longer period. More of the emitted light is collected than in confocal microscopy, and because single photons scattering within the tissue cannot cause fluorescence and consequent background haze, imaging to greater depths (several hundred micrometers) is possible. Like confocal microscopy, two-photon microscopy produces thin optical sections from which a three-dimensional image can be built up.

To track the movements of molecules or cells over time, confocal or two-photon microscopy is combined with **time-lapse video imaging** using sensitive digital cameras. In immunology, time-lapse two-photon fluorescence imaging has been particularly valuable for tracking the movements of individual T cells and B cells expressing fluorescent proteins in intact lymphoid organs and observing where they interact (see Chapter 10).

A-12 Immunoelectron microscopy.

Antibodies can be used to detect the intracellular location of structures or particular proteins at high resolution by electron microscopy, a technique known as immunoelectron microscopy. Antibodies against the required antigen are labeled with gold particles and then applied to ultrathin sections, which are then examined in the transmission electron microscope. Antibodies labeled with gold particles of different diameters enable two or more proteins to be studied simultaneously (see Fig. 6.12). The difficulty with this technique is in staining the ultrathin section adequately, because few molecules of antigen are present in each section.

A-13 Immunohistochemistry.

An alternative to immunofluorescence (see Section A-11) for detecting a protein in tissue sections is **immunohistochemistry**, in which the specific antibody is chemically coupled to an enzyme that converts a colorless substrate into a colored reaction product *in situ*. The localized deposition of the colored product where antibody has bound can be directly observed under a light microscope. The antibody binds stably to its antigen, allowing unbound antibody to be removed by thorough washing. This method of detecting bound antibody is analogous to ELISA (see Section A-4) and frequently uses the same coupled enzymes, the difference in detection being primarily that in immunohistochemistry the colored products are insoluble and precipitate at the site where they are formed. Horseradish peroxidase and alkaline phosphatase are the two enzymes most commonly used in these applications. Horseradish peroxidase oxidizes the substrate diaminobenzidine to produce a brown precipitate, while alkaline phosphatase can produce red or blue dyes depending on the substrates used; a common substrate is 5-bromo-4-chloro-3-indolyl phosphate plus nitroblue tetrazolium (BCIP/NBT), which gives rise to a dark blue or purple stain. As with immunofluorescence, the native structure of the protein being sought usually needs to be preserved so that it will be recognized by the antibody. Tissues are fixed by the most gentle chemical fixation techniques or frozen tissue sections are used that are fixed only after the antibody reaction has been performed.

A-14 Immunoprecipitation and co-immunoprecipitation.

To raise antibodies against membrane proteins and other cellular structures that are difficult to purify, mice are often immunized with whole cells or crude cell extracts. Antibodies against the individual molecules are then obtained by using these immunized mice to produce hybridomas making monoclonal antibodies (see Section A-8) that bind to the cell type used for immunization. To characterize the molecules identified by the antibodies, cells of the same type are labeled with radioisotopes and dissolved in nonionic detergents that disrupt cell membranes but do not interfere with antigen–antibody interactions. This allows the labeled protein to be isolated by binding to the antibody in a reaction known as **immunoprecipitation**. The antibody is usually attached to a solid support, such as the beads that are used in affinity chromatography (see Section A-3), or to Protein A, a protein derived from the cell wall of *Staphylococcus aureus* that binds tightly to the Fc region of IgG antibodies. Cells can be labeled in two main ways for immunoprecipitation analysis. All the proteins in a cell can be labeled metabolically by growing the cell in a medium containing radioactive amino acids that are then incorporated into cellular proteins (**Fig. A.14**). Alternatively, one can label only the cell-surface

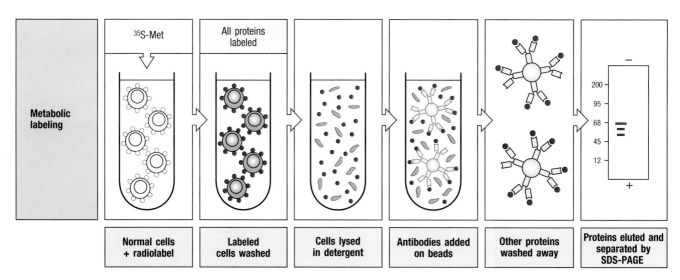

Fig. A.14 Cellular proteins reacting with an antibody can be characterized by immunoprecipitation of labeled cell lysates. All actively synthesized cellular proteins can be labeled metabolically by incubating cells with radioactive amino acids (shown here for methionine; ^{35}S-Met), or one can label just the cell-surface proteins by using radioactive iodine in a form that cannot cross the cell membrane or by a reaction with the small molecule biotin, detected by its reaction with labeled avidin (not shown). Cells are lysed with detergent, and individual, labeled, cell-associated proteins can be precipitated with a monoclonal antibody attached to beads. After unbound proteins have been washed away, the bound protein is eluted in the detergent sodium dodecyl sulfate (SDS), which dissociates it from the antibody and also coats the protein with a strong negative charge, allowing it to migrate according to its size in polyacrylamide gel electrophoresis (PAGE). The positions of the labeled proteins are determined by autoradiography using X-ray film. This technique of SDS-PAGE can be used to determine the molecular mass and subunit composition of a protein. Patterns of protein bands observed with metabolic labeling are usually more complex than those revealed by radioiodination, owing to the presence of precursor forms of the protein (right panel). The mature form of a surface protein can be identified as being the same size as that detected by surface iodination or biotinylation (not shown).

Fig. A.15 Two-dimensional gel electrophoresis of MHC class II molecules. Proteins in a human B-cell line expressing HLA-DR2 have been labeled metabolically (see Fig. A.14), precipitated with a monoclonal antibody against the human MHC class II molecule HLA-DR, and separated by isoelectric focusing (IEF) in one direction and SDS-PAGE in a second direction at right angles to the first (hence the term two-dimensional gel electrophoresis). This allows one to distinguish molecules of the same molecular mass on the basis of their charge. The separated proteins are detected by autoradiography. The MHC class II molecule is composed of two chains, α and β, labeled as HLA-DRA and HLA-DRB, respectively. Each chain is present in multiple isoforms that resolve into distinct spots upon isoelectric focusing. Three standard markers are included in the sample: 1, soybean trypsin inhibitor (TI); 2, actin; and 3, bovine serum albumin (BSA).

proteins by radioiodination under conditions that prevent iodine from crossing the plasma membrane and labeling proteins inside the cell or by a reaction that labels only cell-surface proteins with biotin, a small molecule that is detected readily by labeled avidin, a protein found in egg whites that binds biotin with very high affinity.

Once the labeled proteins have been isolated by the antibody, they can be characterized in several ways. The most common is polyacrylamide gel electrophoresis (PAGE) of the proteins after they have been dissociated from antibody in the strong ionic detergent sodium dodecyl sulfate (SDS), a technique generally abbreviated as **SDS-PAGE**. SDS binds relatively homogeneously to proteins, conferring a charge that allows the electrophoretic field to drive protein migration through the gel. The rate of migration is controlled mainly by protein size (see Fig. A.14). Proteins of differing charges can be separated using isoelectric focusing (see Section A-8). This technique can be combined with SDS-PAGE in a procedure known as **two-dimensional gel electrophoresis**, in which the immunoprecipitated protein is eluted in urea, a nonionic solubilizing agent, and run on an isoelectric focusing gel in a narrow tube of polyacrylamide. This first-dimensional isoelectric focusing gel is then placed across the top of an SDS-PAGE slab gel, which is then run vertically to separate the proteins by molecular weight (**Fig. A.15**). Two-dimensional gel electrophoresis is a powerful technique that allows many hundreds of proteins in a complex mixture to be distinguished from one another.

Immunoprecipitation and the related technique of immunoblotting (see Section A-15) are useful for determining the molecular mass and isoelectric point of a protein as well as its abundance, distribution, and whether, for example, it undergoes changes in molecular mass and isoelectric point as a result of processing within the cell.

Co-immunoprecipitation is an extension of the immunoprecipitation technique and is used to determine whether a given protein interacts physically with another given protein. Cell extracts containing the presumed interaction complex are first immunoprecipitated with antibody against one of the proteins. The material isolated by this means is then tested for the presence of the other protein by immunoblotting (see Section A-15) with a specific antibody against the second protein.

A-15 Immunoblotting (western blotting).

Like immunoprecipitation (see Section A-14), **immunoblotting** is used for identifying the presence of a given protein in a cell lysate, but it avoids the problem of having to label large quantities of cells with radioisotopes. Unlabeled cells are placed in detergent to solubilize all cell proteins, and the lysate is run on SDS-PAGE to separate the proteins (see Section A-14). The size-separated proteins are then transferred from the gel to a stable support such as a nitrocellulose membrane. Specific proteins are detected by treatment with antibodies able to react with SDS-solubilized proteins (mainly those that react with denatured sequences); the bound antibodies are revealed by anti-immunoglobulin

Fig. A.16 Western blotting is used to identify antibodies against the human immunodeficiency virus (HIV) in serum from infected individuals. The virus is dissociated into its constituent proteins by treatment with the detergent SDS, and its proteins are separated using SDS-PAGE. The separated proteins are transferred to a nitrocellulose sheet and reacted with the test serum. Anti-HIV antibodies in the serum bind to the various HIV proteins and are detected with enzyme-linked anti-human immunoglobulin, which deposits colored material from a colorless substrate. This general methodology will detect any combination of antibody and antigen and is used widely, although the denaturing effect of SDS means that the technique works most reliably with antibodies that recognize the antigen when it is denatured.

antibodies labeled with an enzyme. The term **western blotting** as a synonym for immunoblotting arose because the comparable technique for detecting specific DNA sequences is known as Southern blotting, after Edwin Southern, who devised it, which in turn provoked the name 'northern' for blots of size-separated RNA, and 'western' for blots of size-separated proteins. Western blots have many applications in basic research and clinical diagnosis. They are often used to test sera for the presence of antibodies against specific proteins; for example, to detect antibodies against different constituents of HIV (**Fig. A.16**).

A-16 Use of antibodies in the isolation and characterization of multiprotein complexes by mass spectrometry.

Many of the proteins that function in immune cells are components of multiprotein complexes. This is the case for cell-surface receptors, such as the T-cell and B-cell antigen receptors and most cytokine receptors, as well as intracellular proteins involved in signal transduction, gene expression, and cell death. Antibodies that bind to one member of such a complex can be used to identify the other members of the complex by a process of co-immunoprecipitation followed by Western blotting or **mass spectrometry**.

This technology can be used to identify protein complexes from primary immune cells that have been genetically engineered to express a small 8-amino-acid tag sequence, called Strep-tag, on the terminus of a single protein. This small peptide tag binds with extremely high affinity and specificity to a modified form of the streptavidin molecule often used to isolate biotinylated proteins. This modified streptavidin, called Strep-tactin, is tethered to an affinity resin. When cell lysates are passed over this resin, the tagged protein along with its binding partners are retained and can be eluted to process for mass spectrometry.

A mass spectrometer can provide extremely precise measurements of the masses of constituents in a preparation of molecules. To identify unknown proteins in a sample, such as that acquired by co-immunoprecipitation, the sample often is first subjected to one-dimensional SDS-PAGE or two-dimensional gel electrophoresis (see Section A-14) to separate the proteins in the complex for individual analysis. Gel slices are excised and treated with a proteolytic enzyme, such as trypsin, to digest the protein into a series of peptides that can be easily eluted from the gel. The peptide mixture is then introduced into the mass spectrometer, which ionizes the peptides, transfers them to the gas phase, and then separates them under high vacuum by subjecting them to a magnetic field. The separation is based on the mass-to-charge (m/z) ratio of each ion, and a detector collects information on the signal intensity for each ion and displays the data as a histogram (**Fig. A.17**). This histogram, usually referred to as a spectrum, can be compared with a database containing potential cleavage sites (for the proteolytic enzyme used) in all known protein sequences. Because of the precision of these measurements, and the information derived from multiple peptides composing the initial protein, the spectrum can often be unambiguously assigned to a unique protein in the database.

Fig. A.17 Characterization of multiprotein complexes by mass spectrometry. After immunoprecipitation of a multiprotein complex using antibodies specific for one component of the complex, the individual proteins are separated by gel electrophoresis. An individual band representing one protein is isolated and digested with a protease such as trypsin. The digested protein sample is injected into the mass spectrometer, which ionizes the peptides, transfers them to the gas phase, and then separates them on the basis of differences in their mass-to-charge (*m/z*) ratio by subjecting them under high vacuum to a magnetic field. A detector collects information on the signal intensity for each peptide ion and displays the information as a histogram. This histogram, usually referred to as a spectrum, is compared with a database containing potential cleavage sites for the proteolytic enzyme used in all known protein sequences, allowing for identification of the protein in the sample.

Modern multidimensional mass spectrometers allow peptide ions to be sequenced as well as analyzed by their mass. In these instruments, peptide ions separated in one sector are fragmented in a second sector by collision with other molecules (often an inert gas such as N_2), with the resultant fragments separated in a third section (**Fig. A.18**). Fragmentation occurs primarily in the peptide backbone, allowing the sequence of the peptide to be read directly from the mass spectrum of the mixture of fragments. In place of gel electrophoresis, a liquid chromatograph can be employed upstream of the mass analyzers (LC-MS/MS) to provide additional separation of peptides prior to mass separation and allow a very complex mixture of thousands of peptides to be

Fig. A.18 Determining the amino acid sequence of a peptide by multidimensional mass spectrometry (MS/MS). Multidimensional mass spectrometers consist of two mass spectrometers linked in tandem but with an interceding middle sector that fragments ions. In the first sector, the first mass spectrometer separates peptide ions, as shown in Fig. A.17. Each peptide ion from this first separation is then fragmented in the middle sector of the apparatus by collision with other molecules (often an inert gas such as N_2). Because fragmentation occurs primarily in the peptide backbone, a mixture of fragments is generated in which the fragments each differ by one amino acid residue. The resultant fragments are then separated in the second mass spectrometer, the final sector. The sequence of the peptide can be read directly from the second mass spectrum. The order of amino acid residues in the peptide can be deduced because of the exquisite precision of the measurements of each ion together with knowledge of the exact mass of each possible amino acid residue.

sequenced in a single run. It was this latter technique that played an essential role in the early studies that identified the repertoire of peptides bound to MHC molecules on the surface of antigen-presenting cells (see Chapter 6).

A-17 Isolation of peripheral blood lymphocytes by density-gradient fractionation.

The first step in studying lymphocytes is to isolate them so that their behavior can be analyzed *in vitro*. Human lymphocytes can be isolated most readily from peripheral blood by density centrifugation over a step gradient consisting of a mixture of the carbohydrate polymer Ficoll-Hypaque and the dense iodine-containing compound metrizamide. A step gradient is made by preparing a solution of Ficoll-Hypaque at a precise density (1.077 g/liter for human cells) and placing a layer of this solution at the bottom of a centrifuge tube. A sample of heparinized blood mixed with saline (heparin prevents clotting) is carefully layered on top of the Ficoll-Hypaque solution. After centrifugation for about 30 minutes, the components of the blood have separated on the basis of their densities. The upper layer contains the blood plasma and platelets, which remain in the top layer during the short centrifugation. Red blood cells and granulocytes have a higher density than the Ficoll-Hypaque solution and collect at the bottom of the tube. The population called **peripheral blood mononuclear cells (PBMCs)** collects at the interface between the blood and the Ficoll-Hypaque layers and consists mainly of lymphocytes and monocytes (**Fig. A.19**). Although this population is readily accessible, it is not necessarily representative of the lymphoid system, because only recirculating lymphocytes can be isolated from blood.

The 'normal' ranges in the numbers of the different types of white blood cells in blood and the normal ranges in concentrations of the various antibody classes are given in **Fig. A.20**.

A-18 Isolation of lymphocytes from tissues other than blood.

In experimental animals, and occasionally in humans, lymphocytes are isolated from lymphoid organs, such as spleen, thymus, bone marrow, lymph nodes, or mucosa-associated lymphoid tissue—in humans, most commonly the palatine tonsils (see Fig. 12.6). A specialized population of lymphocytes resides in surface epithelia; these cells are isolated by fractionating the epithelial layer after its detachment from the basement membrane. Finally, in situations where local immune responses are prominent, lymphocytes can be isolated from the site of the response itself. For example, in order to study the autoimmune reaction that is thought to be responsible for rheumatoid arthritis, an inflammatory response in joints, lymphocytes are isolated from the fluid aspirated from the inflamed joint space.

Fig. A.19 Peripheral blood mononuclear cells can be isolated from whole blood by Ficoll-Hypaque centrifugation. Diluted anticoagulated blood (left panel) is layered over Ficoll-Hypaque and centrifuged. Red blood cells and polymorphonuclear leukocytes or granulocytes are denser and travel through the Ficoll-Hypaque, while mononuclear cells consisting of lymphocytes together with some monocytes band over it and can be recovered at the interface of the two layers (right panel).

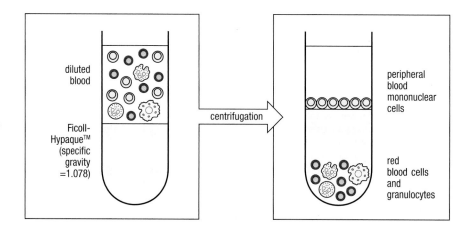

Evaluation of the cellular components of the human immune system in peripheral blood			
	B cells	**T cells**	**Phagocytes**
Normal numbers (x10⁹ per liter of blood)	Approximately 0.3	Total 1.0–2.5 CD4 0.5–1.6 CD8 0.3–0.9	Monocytes 0.15–0.6 Polymorphonuclear leukocytes: Neutrophils 3.00–5.5 Eosinophils 0.05–0.25 Basophils 0.02
Measurement of function *in vivo*	Serum Ig levels Specific antibody levels	Skin test	—
Measurement of function *in vitro*	Induced antibody production in response to pokeweed mitogen	T-cell proliferation in response to phytohemagglutinin or to tetanus toxoid	Phagocytosis Nitroblue tetrazolium uptake Intracellular killing of bacteria

Evaluation of the humoral components of the human immune system in peripheral blood					
	Immunoglobulins				**Complement**
Component	IgG	IgM	IgA	IgE	
Normal levels	600–1400 mg dl⁻¹	40–345 mg dl⁻¹	60–380 mg dl⁻¹	0–200 IU ml⁻¹	CH_{50} of 125–300 IU ml⁻¹

Fig. A.20 The major immune cells and humoral immune components of human blood. Human blood contains B cells, T cells, and myeloid cells, as well as high concentrations of antibodies and complement proteins. CH_{50} is a measurement of total complement activity in the serum and is based on a cell lysis assay.

Laser-capture microdissection is a technique used to isolate specific populations of cells from an intact tissue sample or histologic specimen after visualizing the cells by light microscopy. The cells of interest can be 'captured' by placing a polymer over the sample on the microscope slide and using an infrared laser to melt the polymer onto the sample in discrete locations. Once completed, the polymer–cell composite can be lifted, and DNA, RNA, or proteins can be isolated from the dissected cells (**Fig. A.21**). A variant of this approach makes use of an ultraviolet (UV) laser, rather than infrared. In this case, the UV laser acts as a molecular cutting tool and can be used to cut away or even ablate the unwanted portions of the tissue, leaving intact the area of interest.

A-19 Flow cytometry and FACS analysis.

An immensely powerful tool for defining and enumerating populations of immune cells is the flow cytometer, which detects and counts individual cells passing in a stream through a laser beam. A flow cytometer equipped to separate the identified cells is called a **fluorescence-activated cell sorter (FACS)**. These instruments are used to study the properties of cell subsets that are identified by using monoclonal antibodies against cell-surface or intracellular proteins. Individual cells within a mixed population are first labeled by treatment with specific monoclonal antibodies coupled to fluorescent dyes or by specific antibodies followed by fluorescently tagged anti-immunoglobulin antibodies. The mixture of labeled cells is then suspended in a much larger volume of saline and forced through a small nozzle, creating a fine stream of liquid composed of droplets, each containing a single cell. As each cell passes through a laser beam it scatters the laser light, and any dye molecules bound to the cell are excited and fluoresce. Sensitive photomultiplier tubes detect both the scattered light, which gives information about the size and granularity of the cell, and the fluorescence emissions, which give information about the binding of the labeled monoclonal antibodies and hence about the expression of cell-surface or intracellular proteins by each cell (**Fig. A.22**).

In the cell sorter, the signals passed back to the computer are used to generate an electric charge, which is passed from the nozzle through the liquid stream

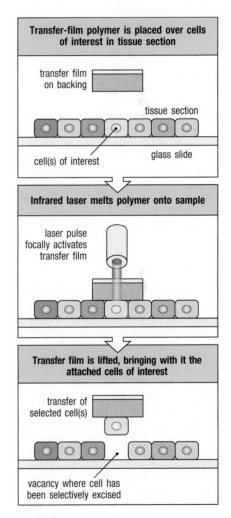

Transfer-film polymer is placed over cells of interest in tissue section

transfer film on backing

tissue section

cell(s) of interest — glass slide

Infrared laser melts polymer onto sample

laser pulse focally activates transfer film

Transfer film is lifted, bringing with it the attached cells of interest

transfer of selected cell(s)

vacancy where cell has been selectively excised

Fig. A.21 Laser-capture microdissection. Specific populations of cells from an intact tissue sample or histologic specimen can be isolated after visualizing the cells by light microscopy. A polymer called the transfer film is placed over the sample on the microscope slide, and an infrared laser is used to melt the polymer onto the sample in discrete locations. The polymer–cell composite is then lifted, and the cells of interest are isolated. DNA, RNA, or proteins can be prepared from the dissected cells.

Fig. A.22 Flow cytometers allow individual cells to be identified by their cell-surface antigens and to be sorted. Cells to be analyzed by flow cytometry are first labeled with fluorescent dyes (top panel). Direct labeling uses dye-coupled antibodies specific for cell-surface antigens (as shown here), while indirect labeling uses a dye-coupled immunoglobulin to detect unlabeled cell-bound antibody. The cells are forced through a nozzle in a single-cell stream that passes through a laser beam (second panel). Photomultiplier tubes (PMTs) detect the scattering of light, which is a sign of cell size and granularity, as well as emissions from the different fluorescent dyes. This information is analyzed by computer (CPU). By examining a large number of cells, the proportion of cells with a specific set of characteristics can be determined, and levels of expression of various molecules on these cells can be measured. The lower part of the figure shows how these data can be represented, the example in this case being the expression of two surface immunoglobulins, IgM and IgD, on a sample of B cells from a mouse spleen. The two immunoglobulins have been labeled with different-colored dyes. When the expression of just one type of molecule is to be analyzed (IgM or IgD), the data are usually displayed as a histogram, as in the left-hand panels. Histograms display the distribution of cells expressing a single measured parameter (for example, size, granularity, fluorescence intensity). When two or more parameters are measured for each cell (IgM and IgD), various types of two-dimensional plots can be used to display the data, as shown in the right-hand panel. All four plots represent the same data, and in each case, the horizontal axis represents intensity of IgM fluorescence, and the vertical axis represents the intensity of IgD fluorescence. Two-color plots provide more information than histograms; they allow recognition, for example, of cells that are 'bright' for both colors, 'dull' for one and bright for the other, dull for both, negative for both, and so on. For example, the cluster of dots in the extreme lower left portions of the plots represents cells that do not express either immunoglobulin and are mostly T cells. The standard dot plot (upper left) places a single dot for each cell whose fluorescence is measured. This format works well for identifying cells that lie outside the main groups but tends to saturate in areas containing a large number of cells of the same type. A second means of presenting these data is the color dot plot (lower left), which uses color density to indicate high-density areas. A contour plot (upper right) draws 5% 'probability' contours, with contour lines drawn to indicate each successive 5% of the population; this format provides the best monochrome visualization of regions of high and low density. The lower right plot is a 5% probability contour map, which also shows outlying cells as dots.

at the precise time that the stream breaks up into droplets, each containing no more than a single cell; droplets containing a charge can then be deflected from the main stream of droplets as they pass between plates of opposite charge, so that positively charged droplets are attracted to a negatively charged plate, and vice versa. Once deflected, droplets containing cells are collected in tubes. In this way, specific subpopulations of cells, distinguished by the binding of the labeled antibody, can be purified from a mixed population of cells.

Alternatively, to deplete a population of cells, the same fluorochrome can be used to label different antibodies directed at marker proteins expressed by the various undesired cell types. The cell sorter can be used to direct labeled cells to a waste channel, retaining only the unlabeled cells.

When cells are labeled with a single fluorescent antibody, the data from a flow cytometer are usually displayed in the form of a one-dimensional histogram of fluorescence intensity versus cell numbers. If two or more antibodies are used, each coupled to a different fluorescent dye, then the data are usually displayed in the form of a two-dimensional scatter diagram or as a contour diagram, where the fluorescence of one dye-labeled antibody is plotted against that of a second, with the result that a population of cells labeled with one antibody can be further subdivided by its labeling with the second antibody (see Fig. A.22). By examining large numbers of cells, flow cytometry can give quantitative data on the percentage of cells bearing different proteins, such as surface immuno-globulin, which characterizes B cells; the T-cell receptor–associated molecules known as CD3; and the CD4 and CD8 co-receptor proteins that distinguish the major T-cell subsets. Likewise, FACS analysis has been instrumental in defining stages in the early development of B and T cells. This technology also played a vital role in the early identification of AIDS as a disease in which T cells bearing CD4 are depleted selectively (see Chapter 13). Advances in FACS technology permit progressively more antibodies labeled with distinct fluores-cent dyes to be used at the same time. For experiments aimed at cell analy-sis, rather than cell sorting, machines with four lasers that can simultaneously measure 18 different fluorescent dyes are currently available. However, FACS analysis is constrained by the spectral properties of the fluorescent dyes used for coupling to antibodies, and this technology may have reached its limit.

An alternative to FACS is a technology based on detecting heavy-metal atoms that are coupled to antibodies. Cell populations labeled with heavy metal–coupled antibodies are analyzed on a machine called a CyTOF, which combines liquid fluidics with a mass spectrometer. As each cell is analyzed, the quantity of each heavy metal associated with that cell, and thus the abundance of the target of each antibody, is measured. In total, this technology is estimated to have the capability to measure 100 distinct heavy metals, greatly expanding the range of analysis that is currently possible by FACS. However, with this tech-nique, the cells are destroyed by the ionization process required for the mass spectrometry analysis, so the CyTOF cannot function as a cell sorter.

A-20 Lymphocyte isolation using antibody-coated magnetic beads.

Although FACS is superb for isolating small numbers of cells in pure form, mechanical means of separating cells are preferable when large numbers of lymphocytes must be prepared quickly. A powerful and efficient way of iso-lating lymphocyte populations is to couple paramagnetic beads to mono-clonal antibodies that recognize distinguishing cell-surface molecules. These antibody-coated beads are mixed with the cells to be separated and are run through a column containing material that attracts the paramagnetic beads when the column is placed in a strong magnetic field. Cells binding the mag-netically labeled antibodies are retained; cells lacking the appropriate surface molecule can be washed away (**Fig. A.23**). The retained cells are recovered by

Heterogeneous population of lymphocytes is mixed with antibodies coupled to paramagnetic particles or beads and poured over an iron wool mesh

When a magnetic field is applied, the coupled cells stick to the iron wool; unlabeled cells are washed out

The magnetic field is removed, releasing the coupled cells

Fig. A.23 Lymphocyte subpopulations can be separated physically by using antibodies coupled to paramagnetic particles or beads. A mouse monoclonal antibody specific for a particular cell-surface molecule is coupled to paramagnetic particles or beads. It is mixed with a heterogeneous population of lymphocytes and poured over an iron wool mesh in a column. A magnetic field is applied so that the antibody-bound cells stick to the iron wool while cells that have not bound antibody are washed out; these cells are said to be negatively selected for lack of the molecule in question. The bound cells are released by removing the magnetic field; they are said to be positively selected for presence of the antigen recognized by the antibody.

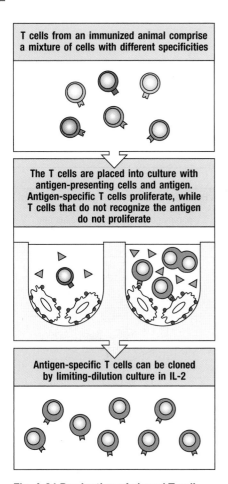

T cells from an immunized animal comprise a mixture of cells with different specificities

The T cells are placed into culture with antigen-presenting cells and antigen. Antigen-specific T cells proliferate, while T cells that do not recognize the antigen do not proliferate

Antigen-specific T cells can be cloned by limiting-dilution culture in IL-2

Fig. A.24 Production of cloned T-cell lines. T cells from an immunized donor, comprising a mixture of cells with different specificities, are activated with antigen and antigen-presenting cells. Single responding cells are cultured in the T-cell growth factor IL-2, which selectively stimulates the responding cells to proliferate. From these single cells, cloned lines specific for antigen are identified and can be propagated by culture with antigen, antigen-presenting cells, and IL-2.

removing the column from the magnetic field. In this case, the bound cells are positively selected for expression of the particular cell-surface molecule, while the unbound cells are negatively selected for its absence.

A-21 Isolation of homogeneous T-cell lines.

The analysis of specificity and effector function of T cells depends heavily on the study of monoclonal populations of T lymphocytes. These can be obtained in four distinct ways—T-cell hybrids, cloned T-cell lines, T-cell tumors, and limiting-dilution culture. By analogy with B-cell hybridomas (see Section A-8), normal T cells proliferating in response to specific antigen can be fused to malignant T-cell lymphoma lines to generate **T-cell hybrids**. The hybrids express the receptor of the normal T cell but proliferate indefinitely owing to the cancerous state of the lymphoma parent. T-cell hybrids can be cloned to yield a population of cells all having the same T-cell receptor. When stimulated by their specific antigen, these cells release cytokines such as the T-cell growth factor interleukin-2 (IL-2), and the production of cytokines is used as an assay to assess the antigen specificity of the T-cell hybrid.

T-cell hybrids are excellent tools for the analysis of T-cell specificity because they grow readily in suspension culture. However, they cannot be used to analyze the regulation of specific T-cell proliferation in response to antigen because they are continually dividing. T-cell hybrids also cannot be transferred into an animal to test for function *in vivo* because they would give rise to tumors. Functional analysis of T-cell hybrids is also confounded by the fact that the malignant partner cell affects their behavior in functional assays. Therefore, the regulation of T-cell growth and the effector functions of T cells must be studied using **T-cell clones**. These are clonal cell lines of a single T-cell type and antigen specificity, which are derived from cultures of heterogeneous T cells, called **T-cell lines**, whose growth is dependent on periodic restimulation with specific antigen and, frequently, on the addition of T-cell growth factors (**Fig. A.24**). T-cell clones also require periodic restimulation with antigen and are more tedious to grow than T-cell hybrids, but because their growth depends on specific antigen recognition, they maintain antigen specificity, which is often lost in T-cell hybrids. Cloned T-cell lines can be used for studies of effector function both *in vitro* and *in vivo*. In addition, the proliferation of T cells, a critical aspect of clonal selection, can be characterized only in cloned T-cell lines, where such growth is dependent on antigen recognition. Thus, both types of monoclonal T-cell lines, T-cell hybrids and antigen-dependent T-cell clones, have valuable applications in experimental studies.

Studies of human T cells have relied largely on T-cell clones because a suitable fusion partner for making T-cell hybrids has not been identified. However, a human T-cell lymphoma line, called Jurkat, has been characterized extensively because it secretes IL-2 when its antigen receptor is cross-linked with anti-receptor monoclonal antibodies. This simple assay system has yielded much information about signal transduction in T cells. One of the Jurkat cell line's most interesting features, shared with T-cell hybrids, is that it stops growing when its antigen receptor is cross-linked. This has allowed mutants lacking the receptor or having defects in signal transduction pathways to be selected simply by culturing the cells with anti-receptor antibody and selecting those that continue to grow. Thus, T-cell tumors, T-cell hybrids, and cloned T-cell lines all have valuable applications in experimental immunology.

A-22 ELISPOT assay.

A modification of the ELISA antigen-capture assay (see Section A-4), called the **ELISPOT assay**, is a powerful tool for measuring the frequency of T-cell responses and also provides information about the cytokines produced.

Fig. A.25 The frequency of cytokine-secreting T cells can be determined by the ELISPOT assay. The ELISPOT assay is a variant of ELISA in which antibodies bound to a plastic surface are used to capture cytokines secreted by individual T cells. Usually, cytokine-specific antibodies are bound to the surface of a plastic tissue-culture well, and the unbound antibodies are removed (top panel). Activated T cells are then added to the well and settle onto the antibody-coated surface (second panel). If a T cell is secreting the appropriate cytokine, this will then be captured by the antibody molecules on the plate surrounding the T cell (third panel). After a period of time the T cells are removed, and the presence of the specific cytokine is detected using an enzyme-labeled second antibody specific for the same cytokine. Where this antibody binds, a colored reaction product can be formed (fourth panel). Each T cell that originally secreted the cytokine gives rise to a single spot of color, hence the name of the assay. The results of such an ELISPOT assay for T cells secreting IFN-γ in response to different stimuli are shown in the last panel. In this example, T cells from an individual exposed to *Mycobacterium tuberculosis* were left unstimulated (left), stimulated with anti-CD3 antibody as a positive control (middle), or stimulated with purified protein derivative (PPD) isolated from *Mycobacterium tuberculosis* bacteria. As can be seen, there are more spots in the PPD-stimulated condition than in the unstimulated condition, a clear indication that the individual's T cells were previously exposed to *Mycobacterium tuberculosis* antigens.

Cytokine-specific antibodies are bound to the surface of a plastic well

Activated T cells are added to the well. These T cells are a mixture of cells with different effector functions

Cytokine secreted by some activated T cells is captured by the bound antibody

The captured cytokine is revealed by a second cytokine-specific antibody, which is coupled to an enzyme, giving rise to a spot of insoluble colored precipitate

No stimuli	Anti-CD3	PPD
4 spots	687 spots	22 spots

Populations of T cells are stimulated with the antigen of interest and are then allowed to settle onto a plastic plate coated with antibodies against the cytokine that is to be assayed (**Fig. A.25**). If an activated T cell is secreting that cytokine, the cytokine is captured by the antibody on the plastic plate. After a period of time the cells are removed, and a second antibody against the cytokine is added to the plate to reveal a circle ('spot') of bound cytokine surrounding the position of each activated T cell; it is these circles that give the ELISPOT assay its name. By counting each spot and knowing the number of T cells originally added to the plate, one can easily calculate the frequency of T cells secreting that particular cytokine. ELISPOT can also be used to detect specific antibody secretion by B cells, in this case by using antigen-coated surfaces to trap specific antibody and labeled anti-immunoglobulin to detect the bound antibody.

A-23 Identification of functional subsets of T cells based on cytokine production or transcription factor expression.

One problem with the detection of cytokine production on a single-cell level is that the cytokines are secreted by the T cells into the surrounding medium, and any association with the originating cell is lost. Three methods have been devised that allow the cytokine profile produced by individual cells to be determined. The first, that of **intracellular cytokine staining** (**Fig. A.26**), relies on the use of metabolic poisons that inhibit protein export from the cell. The cytokine thus accumulates within the endoplasmic reticulum and vesicular network of the cell. If the cells are subsequently fixed and rendered permeable by the use of mild detergents, antibodies can gain access to these intracellular compartments and detect the cytokine. The T cells can be stained for other markers simultaneously, and thus the frequency of IL-10–producing CD25+ CD4 T cells, for example, can be easily obtained.

A second method, which has the advantage that the cells being analyzed are not killed in the process, is called cytokine capture. This technique uses hybrid antibodies, in which the two separate heavy- and light-chain pairs from different antibodies are combined to give a mixed antibody molecule in which the two antigen-binding sites recognize different ligands (**Fig. A.27**). In the bispecific antibodies used to detect cytokine production, one of the antigen-binding sites is specific for a T-cell surface marker, while the other is specific for the cytokine in question. The bispecific antibody binds to the T cells through the binding site for the cell-surface marker, leaving the cytokine-binding site free. If that T cell is secreting the particular cytokine, the cytokine is captured by the bound antibody before it diffuses away from the surface of the cell. It can then be detected by adding to the cells a fluorochrome-labeled second antibody specific for the cytokine.

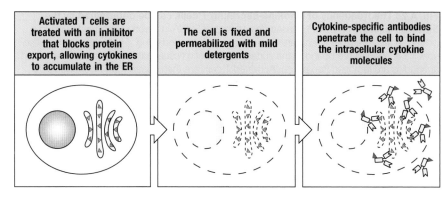

Fig. A.26 Cytokine-secreting cells can be identified by intracellular cytokine staining. Fluorochrome-labeled antibodies can be used to detect the cytokines secreted by activated T cells after the cytokine molecules have been allowed to accumulate inside the cell. The accumulation of cytokine molecules to a high enough concentration for efficient detection is achieved by treating the activated T cells with inhibitors of protein export. In such treated cells, proteins destined to be secreted are instead retained within the endoplasmic reticulum (ER; left panel). These treated cells are then fixed, to cross-link the proteins inside the cell and in the cell membranes, so that they are not lost when the cell is permeabilized by dissolving the cell membrane in a mild detergent (center panel). Fluorochrome-labeled antibodies can now enter the permeabilized cell and bind to the cytokines inside the cell (right panel). Cells labeled in this way can also be labeled with antibodies that bind to cell-surface proteins to determine which subsets of T cells are secreting particular cytokines.

A third method for identifying which T cells in a population produce a particular cytokine utilizes cytokine gene reporter mice. In these lines of mice, a cDNA clone encoding a readily detectable protein (the 'reporter' protein) is inserted into the 3′ untranslated region of the targeted cytokine gene downstream of a sequence known as an internal ribosome entry site (IRES). The IRES sequence allows translation of the reporter protein from the same mRNA as that encoding the cytokine; thus, the reporter protein is produced

Fig. A.27 Hybrid antibodies containing cell-specific and cytokine-specific binding sites can be used to assay cytokine secretion by living cells and to purify cells secreting particular cytokines. Hybrid antibodies can be made by mixing together heavy- and light-chain pairs from antibodies of different specificities; for example, an antibody against an MHC class I molecule and an antibody specific for a cytokine such as IL-4 (first panel). The hybrid antibodies are then added to a population of activated T cells and bind to each cell via the MHC class I binding arm (second panel). If some of the cells in the population are secreting the appropriate cytokine, IL-4, this is captured by the cytokine-specific arm of the hybrid antibody (third panel). The presence of the cytokine can then be revealed; for example, by using a fluorochrome-labeled second antibody specific for the same cytokine but binding to a different site from the one used by the hybrid antibody (last panel). The labeled cells are analyzed by flow cytometry or are isolated using a fluorescence-activated cell sorter (FACS). Alternatively, the second cytokine-specific antibody can be coupled to magnetic beads and the cytokine-producing cells isolated magnetically.

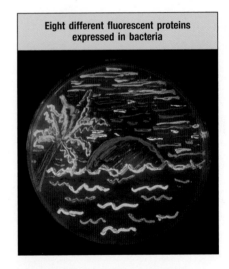

Fig. A.28 Cytokine-expressing cells can be tracked *in vivo* using cytokine gene knock-in reporter mice. To identify cells expressing a specific cytokine in intact animals, the locus encoding the cytokine is modified by homologous recombination (see Fig. A.45 and Section A-36). An internal ribosome entry site (IRES) and the gene for a fluorescent protein such as eGFP are inserted 3′ of the last exon of the cytokine gene, downstream of the cytokine protein stop codon and upstream of the mRNA transcription termination and polyadenylation signal [the poly(A) site]. The IRES element allows the ribosome to initiate translation of a second protein-coding sequence at an internal site on the mRNA. When the modified locus is transcribed and spliced to form the mature mRNA, both the intact cytokine protein and the fluorescent reporter protein (for example, eGFP) are produced from the same transcript. This allows the identification and characterization of cytokine-expressing cells, such as by flow cytometry, on the basis of the detection of eGFP.

only when the cytokine mRNA is expressed (**Fig. A.28**). Common reporter proteins for this application are fluorescent proteins, such as green fluorescent protein (GFP). In fact, the GFP commonly used for this purpose contains a point mutation that greatly improves its spectral properties for experimental purposes. This version of GFP is commonly referred to as 'enhanced GFP,' or 'eGFP' for short. eGFP can be detected by FACS or by fluorescent microscopy using the settings designed to detect the commonly used fluorescent dye FITC. Because of the broad utility of these fluorescent proteins, a host of GFP derivatives has been developed by genetic engineering of the original GFP protein. Each derivative has distinct fluorescent properties and therefore can be uniquely identified, allowing these proteins to be used in combination with each other to provide information about multiple cytokines at the same time (**Fig. A.29**).

Several of these techniques for measuring cytokine expression by T-cell subsets have been adapted to examine the transcription factors expressed by T cells and other lymphocytes, providing an alternative method for identifying functional lymphocyte subsets. In one approach, antibodies specific for lineage-defining transcription factors are used to label permeabilized cells. As was described earlier for the intracellular cytokine staining assay, the cells can then be examined by flow cytometry or immunofluorescence microscopy. In another approach, lines of reporter mice have been generated in which the gene locus encoding a transcription factor is modified to express a fluorescent protein, such as eGFP. For both of these approaches, the advantage of using transcription factors to identify lymphocyte subsets is that there is no need to stimulate the cells prior to antibody staining or to assess reporter protein expression, as lineage-defining transcription factors are constitutively expressed by the cells. Therefore, this latter approach is more widely used for the identification of T-cell and other lymphocyte subsets in intact tissues by microscopy.

Fig. A.29 Fluorescent proteins are available in a rainbow of colors. Derivatives of GFP and a red-fluorescent coral protein can generate eight different fluorescent colors. A beach scene is drawn with bacterial strains expressing each fluorescent protein.

A-24 Identification of T or B lymphocytes on the basis of antigen receptor specificity.

For many years, the ability to identify antigen-specific T cells directly through their receptor specificity eluded immunologists. Foreign antigen could not be used directly to identify T cells because, unlike B cells, T cells do not recognize antigen alone but rather the complexes of peptide fragments of antigen bound to self MHC molecules. Moreover, the affinity of interaction between the T-cell receptor and the peptide:MHC complex is in practice so low that attempts to label T cells with their specific peptide:MHC complexes routinely failed. The breakthrough in labeling antigen-specific T cells came with the idea of making multimers of the peptide:MHC complex, so as to increase the avidity of the interaction.

Peptides can be biotinylated using the bacterial enzyme BirA, which recognizes a specific amino acid sequence. Recombinant MHC molecules containing this target sequence are used to make peptide:MHC complexes, which are then biotinylated. Avidin, or its bacterial counterpart streptavidin, contains four sites that bind biotin with extremely high affinity. Mixing the biotinylated peptide:MHC complex with avidin or streptavidin results in the formation of a **peptide:MHC tetramer**—four specific peptide:MHC complexes bound to a single molecule of streptavidin (**Fig. A.30**). Routinely, the streptavidin moiety is labeled with a fluorochrome to allow detection of those T cells capable of binding the peptide:MHC tetramer. Similar methods have been developed to identify antigen-specific B cells. In this case, biotinylated antigen is bound to fluorochrome-conjugated streptavidin, creating tetramers of the antigen (see Fig. A.30).

Peptide:MHC tetramers have been used to identify populations of antigen-specific T cells in, for example, patients with acute Epstein–Barr virus infections (infectious mononucleosis), showing that up to 80% of the peripheral T cells in infected individuals can be specific for a single peptide:MHC complex. They have also been used to follow responses over timescales of years in individuals with HIV or cytomegalovirus infections. These reagents have also been important in identifying the cells responding, for example, to nonclassical MHC class I molecules such as HLA-E or HLA-G, in both cases showing that these nonclassical molecules are recognized by subsets of NK receptors. Studies identifying antigen-specific B cells have been instrumental in identifying autoreactive B cells in autoimmune individuals and in characterizing B-cell responses to vaccination. In many cases, particularly in studies of human memory T and B cells, the frequency of antigen-specific cells is very low (<1% of total peripheral blood lymphocytes). In these cases, cells are first incubated with the fluorochrome-conjugated peptide:MHC or antigen tetramers, followed by the addition of magnetic beads that bind to the fluorochrome. The antigen-specific T or B cell populations can then be enriched by passing the cells over a magnet. This enrichment step makes further characterization and/or sorting of the antigen-specific cells more reliable and efficient and is frequently used to sort cells for molecular analyses of their T-cell or B-cell receptor repertoires or their transcriptomes.

A-25 Biosensor assays for measuring the rates of association and dissociation of antigen receptors for their ligands.

Two important questions are always asked of any receptor–ligand interaction: What is the strength of binding, or affinity, of the interaction, and what are the rates of association and dissociation? These parameters are generally assessed using purified preparations of proteins. For receptors that are integral membrane proteins in their native state, soluble forms of the proteins are prepared, usually by truncating the proteins to eliminate their membrane-spanning

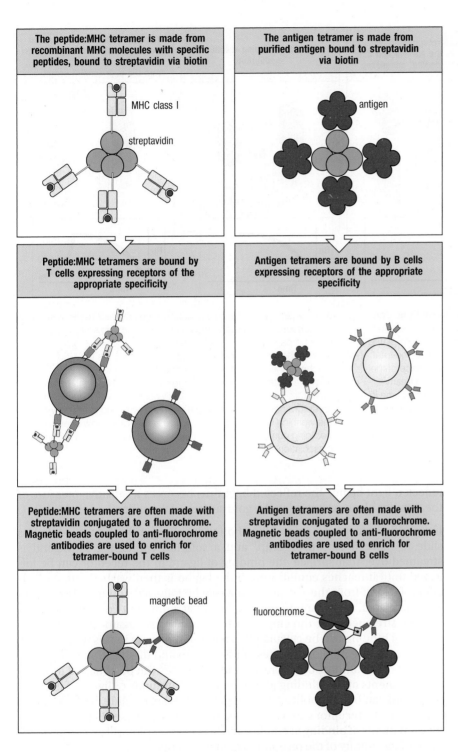

The peptide:MHC tetramer is made from recombinant MHC molecules with specific peptides, bound to streptavidin via biotin

MHC class I

streptavidin

Peptide:MHC tetramers are bound by T cells expressing receptors of the appropriate specificity

Peptide:MHC tetramers are often made with streptavidin conjugated to a fluorochrome. Magnetic beads coupled to anti-fluorochrome antibodies are used to enrich for tetramer-bound T cells

magnetic bead

The antigen tetramer is made from purified antigen bound to streptavidin via biotin

antigen

Antigen tetramers are bound by B cells expressing receptors of the appropriate specificity

Antigen tetramers are often made with streptavidin conjugated to a fluorochrome. Magnetic beads coupled to anti-fluorochrome antibodies are used to enrich for tetramer-bound B cells

fluorochrome

Fig. A.30 Peptide:MHC complexes coupled to streptavidin to form tetramers are able to stain antigen-specific T cells. A peptide:MHC tetramer is formed from recombinant refolded peptide:MHC complexes containing a single defined peptide epitope. MHC molecules that contain biotin can be chemically synthesized, but usually the recombinant MHC heavy chain is linked to a bacterial biotinylation sequence, a target for the *Escherichia coli* enzyme BirA, which is used to add a single biotin group to the MHC molecule. Streptavidin is a tetramer, each subunit having a single binding site for biotin; hence the streptavidin:peptide:MHC complex creates a tetramer of peptide:MHC complexes (top left panel). Although the affinity between the T-cell receptor and its peptide:MHC ligand is too low for a single complex to bind stably to a T cell, the tetramer makes a more avid interaction with multiple peptide:MHC complexes binding simultaneously and is able to bind to T cells whose receptors are specific for the particular peptide:MHC complex (middle left panel). Routinely, the streptavidin molecules are coupled to a fluorochrome, so that the binding to T cells can be monitored by flow cytometry. Additionally, anti-fluorochrome antibodies coupled to magnetic beads can be used to enrich for tetramer-binding T cells (bottom left panel), as shown in Figure A.23. A similar strategy is used to generate antigen tetramers by mixing biotinylated antigen together with streptavidin (top right panel). Antigen tetramers will be bound by B cells expressing receptors of the appropriate specificity (middle right panel). When antigen tetramers are made with fluorochrome-conjugated streptavidin, antigen-specific B cells can be monitored by flow cytometry or enriched after incubation with anti-fluorochrome antibodies coupled to magnetic beads (bottom right panel).

domains. With these purified proteins, binding rates can be measured by following the binding of ligands to receptors immobilized on gold-plated glass slides using a phenomenon known as **surface plasmon resonance (SPR)** to detect the binding (**Fig. A.31**). A full explanation of surface plasmon resonance is beyond the scope of this textbook, as it is based on advanced physical and quantum mechanical principles. In brief, it relies on the total internal reflection of a beam of light from the surface of a gold-coated glass slide. As the light is reflected, some of its energy excites electrons in the gold coating, and these excited electrons are affected by the electric field of any molecules binding to the surface of the gold coating. The more molecules that bind to the surface, the greater is the effect on the excited electrons, and this in turn affects the

| The ligand to be tested, in this case peptide:MHC complexes, is immobilized on a special gold-plated surface | Soluble T-cell receptors are allowed to flow over the surface and bind to the peptide:MHC complexes | Receptor binding reaches equilibrium | Unbound receptors are washed away; continued washing removes receptors as they dissociate from the peptide:MHC complexes |

Fig. A.31 Measurement of receptor–ligand interactions can be made in real time using a biosensor. Biosensors are able to measure the binding of molecules on the surface of gold-plated glass chips through the indirect effects of the binding on the total internal reflection of a beam of polarized light at the surface of the chip. Changes in the angle and intensity of the reflected beam are measured in 'resonance units' (Ru) and plotted against time in what is termed a 'sensorgram.' Depending on the exact nature of the receptor–ligand pair to be analyzed, either the receptor or the ligand can be immobilized on the surface of the chip. In the example shown, peptide:MHC complexes are immobilized on such a surface (first panel). T-cell receptors in solution are now allowed to flow over the surface and to bind to the immobilized peptide:MHC complexes (second panel). As the T-cell receptors bind, the sensorgram (insets) reflects the increasing amount of protein bound. As the binding reaches either saturation or equilibrium (third panel), the sensorgram shows a plateau, as no more protein binds. At this point, unbound receptors can be washed away. With continued washing, bound receptors now start to dissociate and are removed in the flow of the washing solution (last panel). The sensorgram now shows a declining curve, reflecting the rate at which receptor and ligand dissociation occurs.

reflected light beam. The reflected light thus becomes a sensitive measure of the number of atoms bound to the gold surface of the slide.

If a purified receptor is immobilized on the surface of the gold-coated glass slide to make a biosensor 'chip,' and a solution containing the ligand is streamed over that surface, the binding of ligand to the receptor can be followed until it reaches equilibrium. If the ligand is then washed out, dissociation of ligand from the receptor can easily be followed and the dissociation rate calculated. A new solution of the ligand at a different concentration can then be streamed over the chip and the binding once again measured. The affinity of binding can be calculated in a number of ways in this type of assay. Most simply, the ratio of the rates of association and dissociation will give an estimate of the affinity, but more accurate estimates can be obtained from the measurements of the binding at different concentrations of ligand. Similarly, the ligand can be immobilized on the gold-coated glass slide, and a solution containing the receptor can be streamed over the surface (see Fig. A.31). From measurements of binding at equilibrium, a Scatchard plot will give a measurement of the affinity of the receptor–ligand interaction.

A-26 Assays of lymphocyte proliferation.

To function in adaptive immunity, rare antigen-specific lymphocytes must proliferate extensively before they differentiate into functional effector cells in order to generate sufficient numbers of effector cells of a particular specificity. Thus, the analysis of induced lymphocyte proliferation is a central issue in their study. It is difficult, however, to detect the proliferation of normal lymphocytes in response to specific antigen because only a minute proportion of cells will be stimulated to divide. Great impetus was given to the field of lymphocyte culture by the finding that certain substances induce many or all lymphocytes of a given type to proliferate. These substances are referred to collectively as **polyclonal mitogens** because they induce mitosis in lymphocytes of many different specificities or clonal origins. T and B lymphocytes are stimulated by different polyclonal mitogens (**Fig. A.32**). Polyclonal mitogens seem to trigger essentially the same growth-response mechanisms as antigen. Lymphocytes normally exist as resting cells in the G_0 phase of the cell cycle. When stimulated with polyclonal mitogens, they rapidly enter the G_1 phase and progress through the cell cycle. In most studies, lymphocyte proliferation is most simply measured by the incorporation of ^{3}H-thymidine into DNA. This assay is used clinically for assessing the ability of lymphocytes from patients with suspected immunodeficiencies to proliferate in response to a nonspecific stimulus.

An alternative to the use of a radioisotope to measure lymphocyte proliferation is to use a fluorescent assay that can be performed by FACS. For this assay, the lymphocytes are incubated with a fluorescent dye such as carboxyfluorescein succinimidyl ester (CFSE). This dye enters the cell and, once in the cytosol, becomes covalently coupled to lysine residues on cellular proteins. Each time the cell divides, the amount of CFSE is cut in half, as each daughter cell inherits one-half of the CFSE-labeled proteins. When a population of dividing cells is analyzed by FACS, peaks of CFSE fluorescence can be detected, each of which represents cells that have undergone a fixed number of divisions (**Fig. A.33**). This assay is capable of detecting up to 7–8 cell divisions, after which CFSE fluorescence can no longer be measured.

Once lymphocyte culture had been optimized using the proliferative response to polyclonal mitogens as an assay, it became possible to detect antigen-specific T-cell proliferation in culture by measuring ^{3}H-thymidine uptake in response to an antigen to which the T-cell donor had previously been immunized (**Fig. A.34**). This is the assay most commonly used for assessing T-cell responses after immunization, but it reveals little about the functional capabilities of the responding T cells. These must be ascertained by functional assays, as outlined in Sections A-28 and A-29.

Mitogen	Responding cells
Phytohemagglutinin (PHA) (red kidney bean)	T cells
Concanavalin (ConA) (jack bean)	T cells
Pokeweed mitogen (PWM) (pokeweed)	T and B cells
Lipopolysaccharide (LPS) (*Escherichia coli*)	B cells (mouse)

Fig. A.32 Polyclonal mitogens, many of plant origin, stimulate lymphocyte proliferation in tissue culture. Many of these mitogens are used to test the ability of lymphocytes in human peripheral blood to proliferate.

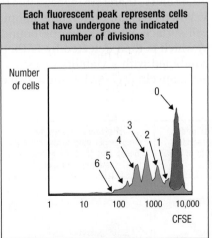

Fig. A.33 A flow cytometric assay based on CFSE dilution to measure cell proliferation. Cells are first incubated with a fluorescent dye such as carboxyfluorescein succinimidyl ester (CFSE). This dye enters the cell and, once in the cytosol, becomes covalently coupled to lysine residues on cellular proteins. Each time the cell divides, the amount of CFSE is diluted by one-half, as each daughter cell inherits one-half of the CFSE-labeled proteins. Cell division can then be analyzed by flow cytometry, where a histogram of CFSE fluorescence displays a series of peaks, each of which represents cells that have undergone a fixed number of divisions. Under optimal conditions, this assay is capable of detecting up to 7–8 cell divisions, after which CFSE fluorescence can no longer be measured.

Fig. A.34 Antigen-specific T-cell proliferation is used frequently as an assay for T-cell responses. T cells from mice or humans that have been immunized with an antigen (antigen A) proliferate when they are exposed to antigen A and antigen-presenting cells but not when cultured with unrelated antigens to which the hosts have not been immunized (antigen B). Proliferation can be measured by incorporation of ³H-thymidine into the DNA of actively dividing cells. Antigen-specific proliferation is a hallmark of specific CD4 T-cell immunity.

A-27 Measurements of apoptosis.

Apoptotic cells can be detected by a procedure known as **TUNEL (TdT-dependent dUTP–biotin nick-end labeling) staining**. In this technique, the 3′ ends of the DNA fragments generated in apoptotic cells are labeled with biotin-coupled uridine by using the enzyme terminal deoxynucleotidyl transferase (TdT). The biotin label is then detected with enzyme-tagged streptavidin, which binds to biotin. When the colorless substrate of the enzyme is added to a tissue section or cell culture, it produces a colored precipitate only in cells that have undergone apoptosis (**Fig. A.35**).

Additional methods are often used to detect apoptosis of cells in experimental animals. One simple method is to incubate cells with a fluorescently labeled preparation of the protein **annexin V**. This protein has a high affinity for a specific membrane phospholipid, phosphatidylserine (PS). In healthy cells, PS is found exclusively on the inner leaflet of the plasma membrane and is therefore inaccessible to extracellular incubation with annexin V. When cells are undergoing apoptosis, the PS is transported to the outer cell surface, where it can be bound by the fluorescently labeled annexin V, which is then detected by FACS (**Fig. A.36**). Annexin V staining is often combined with a viability dye such as propidium iodide (PI) or 7-amino-actinomycin D (7-AAD). These two dyes fluoresce when bound to DNA but

Fig. A.35 In the TUNEL assay, fragmented DNA is labeled by terminal deoxynucleotidyl transferase (TdT) to reveal apoptotic cells. When cells undergo programmed cell death, or apoptosis, their DNA becomes fragmented (first panel). The enzyme TdT is able to add nucleotides to the ends of DNA fragments; most commonly in this assay, biotin-labeled nucleotides (usually dUTP) are added (second panel). The biotinylated DNA can be detected by using streptavidin, which binds to biotin, coupled to enzymes that convert a colorless substrate into a colored insoluble product (third panel). Cells stained in this way can be detected by light microscopy, as shown in the photograph of apoptotic cells (stained red) in the thymic cortex.

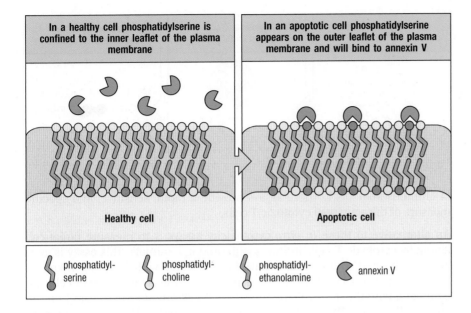

| phosphatidyl-serine | phosphatidyl-choline | phosphatidyl-ethanolamine | annexin V |

Fig. A.36 Detection of apoptotic cells with annexin V. In healthy cells, the membrane phospholipid phosphatidylserine is oriented with its polar headgroup facing the cytosolic face of the plasma membrane. When cells undergo apoptosis, the enzyme responsible for maintaining phosphatidylserine polarity, called flippase, is no longer active. As a result, phosphatidylserine becomes randomly oriented, with many molecules exposing their polar head groups on the extracellular face of the plasma membrane. The protein annexin V binds tightly to the exposed phosphatidylserine and, if fluorescently labeled, can be used to detect apoptotic cells by FACS.

are unable to enter viable or apoptotic cells prior to their loss of membrane integrity. Therefore, when combined with annexin V, cells in the early stages of apoptosis can be identified as annexin V–positive but PI/7-AAD–negative, whereas cells in the late stages of apoptosis are both annexin V–positive and PI/7-AAD–positive.

An additional assay that provides a sensitive means of detecting apoptotic cells by FACS analysis is based on the detection of activated caspase 3, a cysteine protease that functions in the execution phase of the apoptotic cell-death program. Caspase 3 is initially synthesized by cells in an inactive precursor form called a pro-caspase. When cells are undergoing apoptosis, pro-caspase 3 is cleaved into two subunits that dimerize to form the active enzyme. Antibodies have been generated that detect the active form of caspase 3, but not pro-caspase 3, and fluorescently coupled versions of these antibodies can be used to detect apoptotic cells that have been fixed and permeabilized (**Fig A.37**).

A-28 Assays for cytotoxic T cells.

Activated CD8 T cells generally kill any cells that display the specific peptide:MHC class I complex they recognize. Thus, CD8 T-cell function can be determined using the simplest and most rapid T-cell bioassay—the killing of a target cell by a cytotoxic T cell. This is usually detected in a ^{51}Cr-release assay. Live cells will take up, but do not spontaneously release, radioactively labeled sodium chromate, $Na_2{}^{51}CrO_4$. When these labeled cells are killed, the radioactive chromate is released, and its presence in the supernatant of mixtures of target cells and cytotoxic T cells can be measured (**Fig. A.38**). In a similar assay, proliferating target cells such as tumor cells can be labeled with ^{3}H-thymidine, which is incorporated into the replicating DNA. On attack by a cytotoxic T cell, the DNA of the target cells is rapidly fragmented and retained in the filtrate, while large, unfragmented DNA is collected on a filter, and one can measure either the release of these fragments or the retention of ^{3}H-thymidine

Fig. A.37 Detection of apoptotic cells by intracellular staining for active caspases. An early event in the apoptotic process is the release of cytochrome *c* from mitochondria. Cytochrome *c* binds to Apaf-1, leading to the cleavage of pro-caspase 9 into active caspase 9. Caspase 9 then cleaves pro-caspase 3 and pro-caspase 7 to yield their active forms, 'executioner' caspases that promote cell death. Antibodies that recognize the active caspase 3 or caspase 7, but not the pro-caspase forms of these enzymes, will detect permeabilized cells undergoing apoptosis.

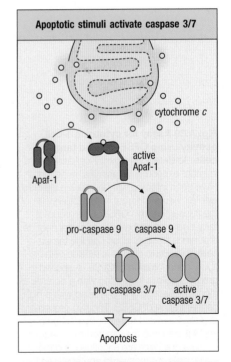

Apoptotic stimuli activate caspase 3/7

cytochrome *c*

Apaf-1   active Apaf-1

pro-caspase 9   caspase 9

pro-caspase 3/7   active caspase 3/7

Apoptosis

Specific antibody binds only to active caspase 3/7

Fig. A.38 Cytotoxic T-cell activity is often assessed by chromium release from labeled target cells. Target cells are labeled with radioactive chromium as $Na_2{}^{51}CrO_4$, washed to remove excess radioactivity, and exposed to cytotoxic T cells. Cell destruction is measured by the release of radioactive chromium into the medium, detectable within 4 hours of mixing target cells with T cells.

| Label target cells with $Na_2{}^{51}CrO_4$ | Add cytotoxic T cells to labeled target cells | Killed cells release radioactive chromium |

in chromosomal DNA. These assays provide a rapid, sensitive, and specific measure of the activity of cytotoxic T cells.

An alternative to these *in vitro* cytotoxicity assays is to measure target-cell killing by cytotoxic T cells in intact experimental animals. This assay is generally performed with mice that have been infected with a pathogen known to induce a strong cytotoxic T-cell response, such as a virus. Target cells are incubated with the antigenic peptide, which will bind to MHC class I on the target-cell surface. These cells are then incubated with a low concentration of the fluorescent dye CFSE (see Section A-26). A control population of cells that is not given the antigenic peptide is incubated with a high concentration of CFSE, allowing these cells to be distinguished from the antigen-bearing target cells. The two cell populations are mixed 1:1 and injected into the experimental animals. Four hours later, spleen cells are recovered from the animals and analyzed by FACS, allowing the specific target-cell lysis to be calculated from the ratio of the two CFSE-labeled cell populations (**Fig. A.39**).

A-29 Assays for CD4 T cells.

CD4 T-cell functions usually involve the activation rather than the killing of cells bearing specific antigen. The activating effects of CD4 T cells on B cells or macrophages are mediated in large part by cytokines, which are released by

Fig. A.39 Assay for cytotoxic T-cell activity using CFSE-labeled target cells. To detect cytotoxic T-cell activity in intact experimental animals, mice that have been infected with a virus are injected with a mixture of target cells labeled with the fluorescent dye CFSE. One group of target cells is incubated with a viral peptide that binds to MHC class I on the target cells; this group of cells is labeled with a low concentration of CFSE. A second group of cells is incubated with a control (nonviral) peptide and is labeled with a high concentration of CFSE. The two groups of cells are mixed together in a 1:1 ratio and injected into the infected mice. After 4 hours, the mice are sacrificed and the target cells are recovered and analyzed by flow cytometry. Examination of the ratio of the two target-cell populations provides a measure of specific lysis of viral peptide–coated target cells.

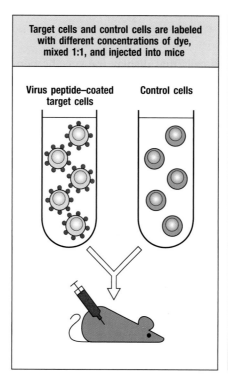

Target cells and control cells are labeled with different concentrations of dye, mixed 1:1, and injected into mice

Virus peptide–coated target cells   Control cells

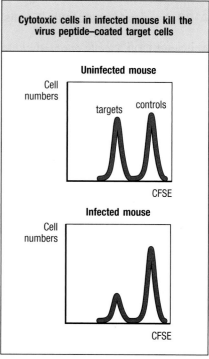

Cytotoxic cells in infected mouse kill the virus peptide–coated target cells

Uninfected mouse

Cell numbers

targets   controls

CFSE

Infected mouse

Cell numbers

CFSE

the T cell when it recognizes antigen. Thus, CD4 T-cell function is usually studied by measuring the type and amount of cytokine released. Because different effector T cells release different amounts and types of cytokines, one can learn about the effector potential of a T cell by measuring the proteins it produces.

Cytokines can be detected by their activity in biological assays of cell growth, where the cytokines serve either as growth factors or as growth inhibitors. A more specific assay is a modification of ELISA known as a capture or sandwich ELISA (see Section A-4). In this assay, the cytokine is characterized by its ability to act as a bridge between two monoclonal antibodies reacting with different epitopes on the cytokine molecule. Cytokine-secreting cells can also be detected by ELISPOT (see Section A-22).

Sandwich ELISA and ELISPOT avoid a major problem of cytokine bioassays; namely, the ability of different cytokines to stimulate the same response in a bioassay. Bioassays must always be confirmed by inhibition of the response with neutralizing monoclonal antibodies specific for the cytokine. Another way of identifying cells actively producing a given cytokine is to stain them with a fluorescently tagged anti-cytokine monoclonal antibody, and then identify and count them by FACS (see Section A-23).

A quite different approach to detecting cytokine production is to determine the presence and amount of the relevant cytokine mRNA in stimulated T cells. This can be done for single cells by *in situ* hybridization and for cell populations by the **reverse transcriptase–polymerase chain reaction (RT–PCR)**. Reverse transcriptase is an enzyme used by certain RNA viruses, such as HIV, to convert an RNA genome into a DNA copy, or complementary DNA (cDNA). In RT–PCR, mRNA is isolated from cells, and cDNA copies are made *in vitro* using reverse transcriptase. The desired cDNA is then selectively amplified by PCR by using sequence-specific primers. When the products of the reaction are subjected to electrophoresis on an agarose gel, the amplified DNA can be visualized as a band of a specific size. The amount of amplified cDNA sequence will be proportional to its representation in the mRNA; stimulated T cells actively producing a particular cytokine will produce large amounts of that particular mRNA and will thus give correspondingly large amounts of the selected cDNA on RT–PCR. The level of cytokine mRNA in the original tissue is usually determined by comparison with the outcome of RT–PCR on the mRNA produced by a so-called housekeeping gene expressed by all cells.

A-30 Transfer of protective immunity.

Protective immunity to a pathogen may involve humoral immunity, cell-mediated immunity, or both. For studies in experimental animals such as inbred mice, the nature of protective immunity can be determined by transferring serum or lymphoid cells from an immunized donor animal to an unimmunized syngeneic recipient (that is, a genetically identical animal of the same inbred strain). If protection against infection can be conferred by the transfer of serum, the immunity is provided by circulating antibodies and is called **humoral immunity**. Transfer of immunity by antiserum or purified antibodies provides immediate protection against many pathogens and against toxins such as those of tetanus and snake venom (**Fig. A.40**). However, although protection is immediate, it is temporary, lasting only so long as the transferred antibodies remain active in the recipient's body. This type of transfer is therefore called **passive immunization**, to distinguish it from **active immunization** with antigen, which can provide lasting immunity. A disadvantage of passive immunization is that the recipient may become immunized to the antiserum used to transfer immunity. Horse or sheep sera are the usual sources of anti-snake venoms used in humans, and repeated administration can lead either to serum sickness or if the recipient becomes allergic to the foreign serum, to anaphylaxis (see Section 14-1).

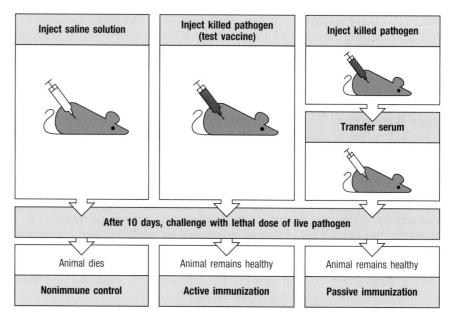

Inject saline solution	Inject killed pathogen (test vaccine)	Inject killed pathogen
		Transfer serum

After 10 days, challenge with lethal dose of live pathogen

Animal dies	Animal remains healthy	Animal remains healthy
Nonimmune control	**Active immunization**	**Passive immunization**

Fig. A.40 *In vivo* assay for the presence of protective immunity after vaccination in animals. Mice are injected with the test vaccine, such as a heat-killed pathogen, or a control such as saline solution. Different groups are then challenged with lethal or pathogenic doses of the test pathogen or with an unrelated pathogen as a specificity control (not shown). Unimmunized animals die or become severely infected (left panel). Successful vaccination is seen as specific protection of immunized mice against infection with the test pathogen. This is called active immunity, and the process is called active immunization (middle panel). If this immune protection can be transferred to a normal syngeneic recipient with serum from an immune donor, then immunity is mediated by antibodies; such immunity is called humoral immunity and the process is called passive immunization (right panel). If immunity can be transferred only by infusing lymphoid cells from the immune donor into a normal syngeneic recipient, then the immunity is called cell-mediated immunity and the transfer process is called adoptive transfer or adoptive immunization (not shown). Passive immunity is short-lived, because antibody is eventually catabolized, but adoptively transferred immunity is mediated by immune cells, which can survive and provide longer-lasting immunity.

Protection against many diseases cannot be transferred with serum but can be transferred by lymphoid cells from immunized donors. The transfer of lymphoid cells from an immune donor to a normal syngeneic recipient is called **adoptive transfer**, or **adoptive immunization**, and the immunity transferred is called **adoptive immunity**. Immunity that can be transferred only with lymphoid cells is called **cell-mediated immunity**. Such cell transfers must be between genetically identical donors and recipients, such as members of the same inbred strain of mouse, so that the donor lymphocytes are not rejected by the recipient and do not attack the recipient's tissues. Adoptive transfer of immunity is used clinically in humans in experimental approaches to cancer therapy or as an adjunct to bone marrow transplantation; in these cases, the patient's own T cells, or the T cells of the bone marrow donor, are given.

A-31 Adoptive transfer of lymphocytes.

Ionizing radiation from X-ray or gamma-ray sources kills lymphoid and other immune cells at doses that spare the other tissues of the body. This makes it possible to eliminate immune function in a recipient animal before attempting to restore immune function by adoptive transfer and allows the effect of the adoptively transferred cells to be studied in the absence of other lymphoid cells. James Gowans originally used this technique to prove the role of the lymphocyte in immune responses. He showed that all active immune responses could be transferred to irradiated recipients by small lymphocytes from immunized donors.

Fig. A.41 Adoptive transfer of congenically marked cells. Hematopoietic cells can be transferred between genetically identical (or nearly identical) mice. The transferred cells, usually a minority population in the recipient, are identified on the basis of expression of an allelic variant of an abundant cell-surface receptor. One common receptor used for this purpose is CD45, which has two alleles that can be distinguished by allele-specific antibodies. When cells from a CD45.1+ mouse are transferred into mice of the identical strain (save for their expression of CD45.2), the donor-cell population can easily be identified by antibody staining followed by flow cytometry or immunofluorescence microscopy.

One common use of adoptive transfer assays takes advantage of the availability of T-cell receptor or B-cell receptor transgenic mice (see Section A-35). In this case, the adoptively transferred lymphocytes are a homogeneous population with a fixed antigen specificity. These cells can be transferred into unmanipulated recipient animals of the same inbred strain without the need to deplete the host immune system, and their ability to respond to immunization or challenge by infection can be monitored. One advantage of this experimental strategy is that relatively small numbers of antigen-specific T cells or B cells can be transferred; after dilution by the recipient's lymphocyte population, the responses of these cells can be examined in the environment of a normal immune response carried out by the host's immune system. Commonly, the transferred cells are 'marked' with an allelic variant of an abundant cell-surface receptor, such as CD45 (**Fig. A.41**). When the donor lymphocytes express one allelic variant of CD45 and the recipient cells express a different variant, the transferred cells can easily be distinguished from the host cells by staining with an antibody that binds to one variant of CD45 but not the other. When two strains of mice are genetically identical with the exception of a single gene, they are said to be **congenic**. In the example above, the donor strain and the recipient strain are referred to as 'CD45 congenics'; it should be noted, however, that in the case where one strain is a T-cell receptor or B-cell receptor transgenic line, this terminology is not completely accurate, as the presence of the transgenic DNA as a genetic difference is conveniently ignored. Such adoptive transfer studies are a cornerstone in the study of the intact immune system. They have provided a rapid and convenient means of determining the effects of many gene deficiencies, such as those in cell-surface receptors, transcription factors, cytokines, and cell-survival or cell-death genes, on the ability of T cells or B cells to mount protective immune responses.

A-32 Assessment of lymphocyte tissue residency by parabiosis.

While many immune cells in the body are found circulating between the blood and the secondary lymphoid organs, some subsets home to tissue sites and persist in these locations as long-term tissue-resident cells. Mucosal surfaces, such as the skin, lung, and gastrointestinal tract, are particularly rich in tissue-resident immune cells. Often, as in studies of memory T-cell populations generated in response to infection, it is difficult to distinguish circulating T cells from tissue-resident T cells on the basis of flow cytometry analysis of surface markers. One approach to resolving the tissue-resident from the recirculating populations utilizes an experimental technique known as **parabiosis**. In this technique, two mice generally differing in the expression of a congenic marker are joined at the flanks by suturing skin from the two mice together (**Fig. A.42**). Approximately 2 weeks after this surgery, new vasculature is formed in the

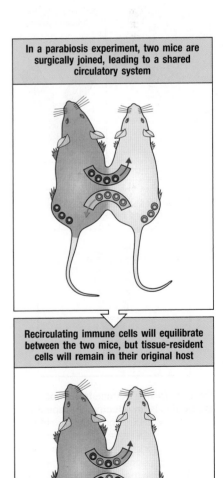

Fig. A.42 Parabiotic mice are used to assess recirculating versus tissue-resident hematopoietic cell populations. When two mice are surgically joined by the skin of their flanks, the vascular systems of the mice also join together. By 2–3 weeks after surgery, recirculating immune-cell populations equilibrate between the two animals, and the hematopoietic-cell populations in the blood become a mixture of the two types. If the mice carry congenic markers, the cells of each donor can be distinguished (shown as red versus blue cells). However, tissue-resident populations, such as tissue-resident memory T cells, do not equilibrate between the two conjoined mice and remain in the tissue of their origin.

skin, and the mice develop a joined circulatory system. Circulating cells in the blood will be a mixture of cells derived from the two mice. However, cells that reside in the tissues without recirculating in the blood will remain in their original host.

A-33 Hematopoietic stem-cell transfers.

All cells of hematopoietic origin can be eliminated by treatment with high doses of gamma radiation or X-rays, allowing replacement of the entire hematopoietic system, including lymphocytes, by transfusion of donor bone marrow or purified hematopoietic stem cells from another animal. The resulting animals are called **radiation bone marrow chimeras**, from the Greek word *chimera*, a mythical animal that had the head of a lion, the tail of a serpent, and the body of a goat. This technique is used experimentally to examine the development of immune-cell lineages, as opposed to their effector functions, and has been particularly important in studying T-cell development. Essentially the same technique is used in humans to replace the hematopoietic system when it fails, as in aplastic anemia or after nuclear accidents, or to eradicate the bone marrow and replace it with normal marrow in the treatment of certain cancers. In humans, bone marrow is the main source of hematopoietic stem cells, but they are increasingly being obtained from peripheral blood after the donor has been treated with hematopoietic growth factors, such as GM-CSF, or from umbilical cord blood, which is rich in such stem cells (see Chapter 15).

A-34 *In vivo* administration of antibodies.

Antibodies administered to intact experimental animals or to humans provide a potent means of manipulating the immune system. Depending on the target molecule recognized by the antibody, and the intrinsic properties of each antibody, *in vivo* antibody administration can either inhibit the function of the target molecule or, in some cases, lead to the elimination of a cell population that expresses the target molecule.

In animal models, antibodies targeting an individual cytokine have been used to inhibit that cytokine's function during an otherwise intact immune response. Experiments of this type provided some of the first evidence that the cytokine IL-12 provides an important signal in polarizing CD4$^+$ T cells into the T_H1 lineage after infection with an intracellular protozoan. This approach has also been used with great success in humans. One of the most common treatments for the inflammatory autoimmune disease rheumatoid arthritis (see Chapter 16) is the administration of an antibody that binds to the cytokine TNF-α; in this case, the inhibition of TNF-α activity provides patients with relief from the symptoms of joint inflammation. The great utility of this antibody therapy has led to the development of related strategies for inhibiting cytokine actions *in vivo*. One successful approach has been to create a hybrid protein that has the ligand-binding domain of the cytokine's receptor fused to the constant-region domains (Fc) of an antibody heavy chain (**Fig. A.43**). This Fc-fusion protein acquires the stability and long half-life of an antibody but has the binding properties of the cytokine receptor. When given *in vivo*, the Fc-fusion protein binds to the cytokine, thereby interfering with the cytokine's ability to stimulate its receptor on immune cells. As an example, the Fc-fusion protein containing the TNF-receptor ligand-binding domain has also been used as an effective treatment for patients with rheumatoid arthritis.

Antibody administration can also be used to augment the immune response by interfering with T-cell surface receptors, such as CTLA-4 or PD-1. When engaged by their ligands, these receptors normally function to down-regulate the immune response. From experiments in mice, antibodies that bind to and inhibit these receptors have been found to enhance immune responses to

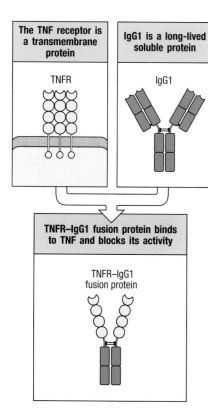

Fig. A.43 *In vivo* administration of antibodies is an effective therapeutic. The cytokine TNF-α contributes to chronic inflammation in a range of conditions, including rheumatoid arthritis, by binding to and triggering signaling of the TNF receptor (TNFR). To treat these conditions, a fusion protein consisting of the constant-region domains of human IgG1 is fused to the extracellular portion of the TNFR, creating a therapeutic known as etanercept. When administered to patients, this fusion protein is effective at binding TNF-α and preventing it from triggering TNFR signaling, thereby reducing inflammation.

tumors, leading in some cases to tumor eradication. Currently, these strategies are being tested in humans for a variety of tumor types, and the initial results have shown great promise.

In vivo administration of antibodies can also be used to deplete specific cell populations. The efficiency with which a given antibody functions for *in vivo* depletion is quite variable, as the mechanism relies on a process known as **antibody-dependent cell-mediated cytotoxicity (ADCC)** (see Section 10-23 and Fig. 10.42). When a cell is coated with antibodies, it becomes a target of natural killer (NK) cells that express the Fc receptor known as CD16, or FcγRIII. The cross-linking of FcγRIII induces the NK cell to kill the antibody-coated target cell. While FcγRIII is a receptor for IgG, it does not bind with equal affinity to all IgG subtypes; thus the efficiency of ADCC after administration of a given antibody is determined by its ability to cross-link FcγRIII and induce NK-cell killing. Common uses for this technique include the depletion of CD4$^+$ T cells with an antibody to CD4 or the depletion of CD8$^+$ T cells with an antibody to CD8. In human patients undergoing organ transplantation, T cells are transiently depleted by administering an antibody to the CD3 component of the T-cell receptor complex. This produces a severe, but temporary, state of immunosuppression during the early post-transplantation stages. As with all *in vivo* antibody-depletion regimens, the depleted cell population gradually returns as cells of that subset are replenished by ongoing lymphocyte development.

A-35 Transgenic mice.

The function of genes has traditionally been studied by observing the effects of spontaneous mutations in whole organisms and, more recently, by analyzing the effects of targeted mutations in cultured cells. The advent of gene cloning and *in vitro* mutagenesis now makes it possible to produce specific mutations in whole animals. Mice with extra copies or altered copies of a gene in their genome can be generated by **transgenesis**, which is now a well-established procedure. To produce **transgenic mice**, a cloned gene is introduced into the mouse genome by microinjection into the male pronucleus of a fertilized egg, which is then implanted into the uterus of a pseudopregnant female mouse. In some of the eggs, the injected DNA becomes integrated randomly into the genome, giving rise to a mouse that has an extra genetic element of known structure, the transgene (**Fig. A.44**).

This technique allows one to study the impact of a newly discovered gene on development, to identify the regulatory regions of a gene required for its normal tissue-specific expression, to determine the effects of its overexpression or its expression in inappropriate tissues, and to find out the impact of mutations on gene function. Transgenic mice have been particularly useful in studying the role of T-cell and B-cell receptors in lymphocyte development, as described in Chapter 8, and in providing a source of primary T and B lymphocytes of known antigen specificity for adoptive transfer studies (see Section A-31). This utility is largely due to the fact that expression of the transgene-encoded T-cell and B-cell receptors preempts the rearrangement and expression of the endogenous antigen receptor genes during T-cell and B-cell development, respectively, thereby generating homogeneous populations of cells bearing a unique antigen receptor of known specificity.

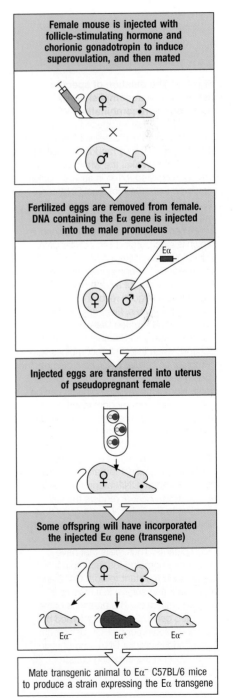

Fig. A.44 The function and expression of genes can be studied in vivo by using transgenic mice. DNA encoding a protein of interest, here the mouse MHC class II protein Eα, is purified and microinjected into the male pronuclei of fertilized eggs. The eggs are then implanted into pseudopregnant female mice. The resulting offspring are screened for the presence of the transgene in their cells, and positive mice are used as founders that transmit the transgene to their offspring, establishing a line of transgenic mice that carry one or more extra genes. The function of the Eα gene used here is tested by breeding the transgene into C57BL/6 mice that carry an inactivating mutation in their endogenous Eα gene.

A-36 Gene knockout by targeted disruption.

In many cases, the functions of a particular gene can be fully understood only if a mutant animal that does not express the gene can be obtained. Whereas genes used to be discovered through the identification of mutant phenotypes, it is now far more common to discover and isolate the normal gene and then determine its function by replacing it *in vivo* with a defective copy. This procedure is known as **gene knockout**, and it has been made possible by two developments: a powerful strategy to select for targeted mutation by homologous recombination, and the development of continually growing lines of **embryonic stem cells (ES cells)**. These are embryonic cells that, on implantation into a blastocyst, can give rise to all cell lineages in a chimeric mouse.

The technique of **gene targeting** takes advantage of the phenomenon known as **homologous recombination** (**Fig. A.45**). Cloned copies of the target gene are altered to make them nonfunctional and are then introduced into the ES cell, where they recombine with the homologous gene in the cell's genome, replacing the normal gene with a nonfunctional copy. Homologous recombination is a rare event in mammalian cells, and thus a powerful selection strategy is required to detect those cells in which it has occurred. Most commonly, the introduced gene construct has its sequence disrupted by an inserted antibiotic-resistance gene such as that for neomycin resistance (neo^r). If this construct undergoes homologous recombination with the endogenous copy of the gene, the endogenous gene is disrupted but the antibiotic-resistance gene remains functional, allowing cells that have incorporated the gene to be selected in culture for resistance to the neomycin-like drug G418. However, antibiotic resistance on its own shows only that the cells have taken up and integrated the neomycin-resistance gene. To be able to select for those cells

Fig. A.45 The deletion of specific genes can be accomplished by homologous recombination. When pieces of DNA are introduced into cells, they can integrate into cellular DNA in two different ways. If they randomly insert into sites of DNA breaks, the whole piece is usually integrated, often in several copies. However, extrachromosomal DNA can also undergo homologous recombination with the cellular copy of the gene, in which case only the central, homologous region is incorporated into cellular DNA. Inserting a selectable marker gene such as resistance to neomycin (neo^r) into the coding region of a gene does not prevent homologous recombination, and it achieves two goals. First, any cell that has integrated the injected DNA is protected from the neomycin-like antibiotic G418. Second, when the gene recombines with homologous cellular DNA, neo^r disrupts the coding sequence of the modified cellular gene. Homologous recombinants can be discriminated from random insertions if the gene encoding herpes simplex virus thymidine kinase (HSV-tk) is placed at one or both ends of the DNA construct, which is often known as a 'targeting construct' because it targets the cellular gene. In random DNA integrations, HSV-tk is retained. HSV-tk renders the cell sensitive to the antiviral agent ganciclovir. However, as HSV-tk is not homologous to the target DNA, it is lost from homologous recombinants. Thus, cells that have undergone homologous recombination are uniquely resistant to both G418 and ganciclovir and survive in a mixture of the two antibiotics. The presence of the disrupted gene has to be confirmed by Southern blotting or by PCR using primers in neo^r and in cellular DNA lying outside the region used in the targeting construct. By using two different resistance genes, one can disrupt the two cellular copies of a gene, making a deletion mutant (not shown).

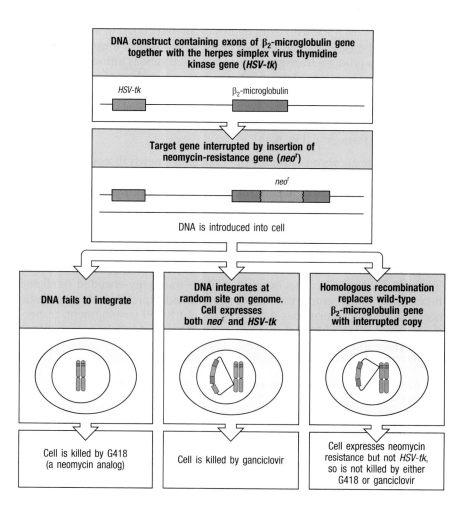

Fig. A.46 Gene knockout in embryonic stem cells enables mutant mice to be produced. Specific genes can be inactivated by homologous recombination in cultures of embryonic stem cells (ES cells). Homologous recombination is performed as described in Fig. A.45. In this example, the gene encoding β_2-microglobulin in ES cells is disrupted by homologous recombination with a targeting construct. Only a single copy of the gene needs to be disrupted. ES cells in which homologous recombination has taken place are injected into mouse blastocysts. If the mutant ES cells give rise to germ cells in the resulting chimeric mice (striped in the figure), the mutant gene can be transferred to their offspring. By breeding the mutant gene to homozygosity, offspring can be tested to determine if a mutant phenotype is generated. In this case, the homozygous mutant mice lack MHC class I molecules on their cells, because MHC class I molecules have to pair with β_2-microglobulin for surface expression. The β_2-microglobulin–deficient mice can then be bred with mice transgenic for subtler mutants of the deleted gene, allowing the effect of such mutants to be tested *in vivo*.

in which homologous recombination has occurred, the ends of the construct usually carry the thymidine kinase gene from the herpes simplex virus (*HSV-tk*). Cells that incorporate DNA randomly usually retain the entire DNA construct including *HSV-tk*, whereas homologous recombination between the construct and cellular DNA, the desired result, involves the exchange of homologous DNA sequences so that the nonhomologous *HSV-tk* genes at the ends of the construct are eliminated. Cells carrying *HSV-tk* are killed by the antiviral drug ganciclovir, and so cells with homologous recombinations have the unique feature of being resistant to both neomycin and ganciclovir, allowing them to be selected efficiently when these drugs are added to the cultures (see Fig. A.45).

To knock out a gene *in vivo*, it is necessary only to disrupt one copy of the cellular gene in an ES cell. These ES cells are then injected into a blastocyst, which is reimplanted into the uterus. The cells carrying the disrupted gene become incorporated into the developing embryo and contribute to all tissues of the resulting chimeric offspring, including those of the germline. The mutated gene can therefore be transmitted to some of the offspring of the original chimera, and further breeding to homozygosity of the mutant gene produces mice that completely lack the expression of that particular gene product (**Fig. A.46**). The effects of the absence of the gene's function can then be studied. In addition, the parts of the gene that are essential for its function can be identified by determining whether function can be restored by introducing different mutated copies of the gene back into the genome by transgenesis. The manipulation of the mouse genome by gene knockout and transgenesis has revolutionized our understanding of the role of individual genes in lymphocyte development and function.

Because the most commonly used ES cells are derived from a poorly characterized strain of mice known as strain 129, the analysis of the function of a gene knockout often requires extensive back-crossing to another strain. One can track the presence of the mutant copy of the gene by the presence of the gene *neo*[r]. After sufficient back-crossing, the mice are intercrossed to produce mutants on a stable genetic background.

A problem with gene knockouts arises when the function of the gene is essential for the survival of the animal; in such cases the gene is termed a **recessive lethal gene**, and homozygous animals cannot be produced. To study the function of such a gene, tissue-specific or developmentally regulated gene deletion can be employed. This strategy makes use of the DNA sequences and enzymes used by bacteriophage P1 to excise itself from a host cell's genome. Integrated bacteriophage P1 DNA is flanked by recombination signal sequences called *loxP* sites. A recombinase, Cre, recognizes these sites, cuts the DNA, and joins the two ends, thus excising the intervening DNA in the form of a circle. This mechanism can be adapted to allow the deletion of specific genes in a transgenic animal only in certain tissues or at certain times in development. First, *loxP* sites flanking a gene, or perhaps flanking just a single exon, are introduced

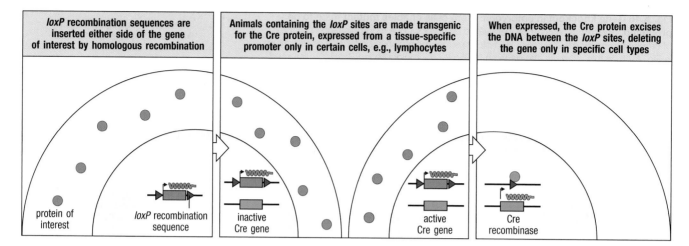

| loxP recombination sequences are inserted either side of the gene of interest by homologous recombination | Animals containing the loxP sites are made transgenic for the Cre protein, expressed from a tissue-specific promoter only in certain cells, e.g., lymphocytes | When expressed, the Cre protein excises the DNA between the loxP sites, deleting the gene only in specific cell types |

protein of interest   loxP recombination sequence   inactive Cre gene   active Cre gene   Cre recombinase

Fig. A.47 The P1 bacteriophage recombination system can be used to eliminate genes in particular cell lineages. The P1 bacteriophage protein Cre excises DNA that is bounded by recombination signal sequences called *loxP* sequences. These sequences can be introduced at either end of a gene by homologous recombination (left panel). Animals carrying genes flanked by *loxP* can also be made transgenic for the gene encoding the Cre protein, which is placed under the control of a tissue-specific promoter so that it is expressed only in certain cells or only at certain times during development (center panel). In the cells in which the Cre protein is expressed, it recognizes the *loxP* sequences and excises the DNA lying between them (right panel). Thus, individual genes can be deleted only in certain cell types or only at certain times. In this way, genes that are essential for the normal development of a mouse can be analyzed for their function in the developed animal and/or in specific cell types. Genes are shown as boxes, RNA as squiggles, and proteins as colored balls.

by homologous recombination (**Fig. A.47**). Usually, the introduction of these sequences into flanking or intronic DNA does not disrupt the normal function of the gene. Next, mice containing such *loxP* mutant genes are mated with mice made transgenic for Cre recombinase that has been placed under the control of a tissue-specific or inducible promoter. When the Cre recombinase is active, either in the appropriate tissue or when induced, it excises the DNA between the inserted *loxP* sites, thus inactivating the gene or exon. Thus, for example, using a T cell–specific promoter to drive expression of the Cre recombinase, a gene can be deleted only in T cells while remaining functional in all other cells of the animal. This extremely powerful genetic technique was used to demonstrate the importance of B-cell receptors in B-cell survival.

Recently, a new technology has been developed for inducing specific gene disruptions in mice; it is known as the CRISPR/Cas9 system. This technique is adapted from a bacterial system that uses an RNA-based strategy to generate double-strand DNA breaks in the genomes of invading pathogens or plasmids, a form of bacterial immunity. The Cas9 gene encodes an endonuclease; this has been modified for use in eukaryotic cells by incorporating a nuclear localization signal into the protein-coding sequence of the enzyme. To target mutations to a particular gene, a synthetic guide RNA is produced that incorporates a short sequence (~20 nucleotides) homologous to the gene being targeted along with sequences that bind the Cas9 enzyme. The guide RNA recruits Cas9 to the genomic location, where the endonuclease will produce a double-strand DNA break (**Fig. A.48**). When this break is repaired by the nonhomologous end-joining DNA repair pathway, small insertions or deletions are commonly introduced, leading to a disruption of the original sequence.

This powerful technique can be used to generate homozygous gene deficiencies in cultured cells and cell lines, but importantly, it can also be used as a single-step means of generating homozygous mutant mice. For this latter purpose, RNA molecules encoding Cas9 are mixed with guide RNAs and injected into single-cell mouse zygotes, using the same technique as that used to generate transgenic mouse lines (see Fig. A.44). Because of the efficiency of the CRISPR/Cas9 system, these embryos frequently harbor mutations on both alleles of the targeted gene. Thus, after transplantation of the embryos into

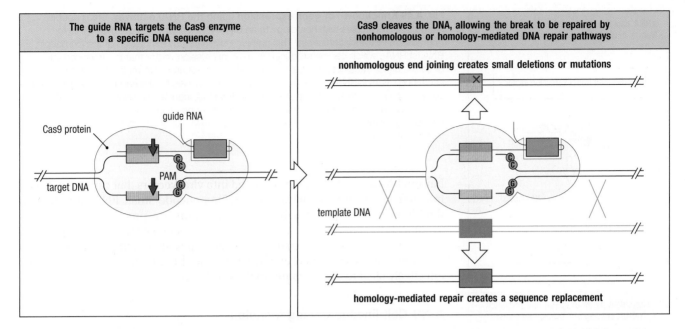

Fig. A.48 Genetic engineering using the bacterial CRISPR/Cas9 system. Genetic engineering can be targeted to a specific gene locus in cells by using two components, the bacterial Cas9 enzyme and a guide RNA (left panel). The guide RNA is a single-stranded RNA that contains two regions of sequence in tandem, the first with homology to the gene being targeted and a second recognized by the Cas9 enzyme. The guide RNA targets the enzyme to the homologous genomic region, promoting double-strand DNA cleavage by the Cas9 endonuclease 3–4 nucleotides upstream of the protospacer adjacent motif (PAM) sequence (right panel). The PAM sequence required by the Cas9 endonuclease is the dinucleotide GG (CC on the other strand). When the double-strand DNA break is repaired by the nonhomologous end-joining pathway, small deletions and/or point mutations are introduced into the target gene, often leading to loss of gene function. To induce a specific sequence replacement in the target gene, cells are provided with a template DNA, in addition to Cas9 and the guide RNA. This template is a double-strand DNA sequence homologous to the target gene but containing specific nucleotide changes. In the presence of this template, cells will repair the Cas9-mediated double-strand cleavage using homologous recombination, rather than nonhomologous end joining, thereby replacing the original sequence with the sequence provided in the template DNA.

foster mothers, the pups born from these embryos are already homozygous for the targeted gene, without the need for lengthy mouse breeding. A refinement of this technique has been developed that allows specific nucleotide changes to be introduced into the targeted gene, rather than the random changes resulting from nonhomologous end joining. This is accomplished by introducing a DNA oligonucleotide into the fertilized mouse zygotes along with the Cas9 and guide RNAs. The oligonucleotide contains the desired nucleotide changes flanked by sequences homologous to the targeted gene. When this oligonucleotide is present, the double-strand DNA break introduced by Cas9 is preferentially repaired by a homology-directed process that replaces the damaged DNA with the sequences from the oligonucleotide (see Fig. A.48).

A-37 Knockdown of gene expression by RNA interference (RNAi).

In some cases, the function of a gene can be assessed by reducing or even eliminating the expression of that gene in specific cells. This can be accomplished by harnessing a system known as RNA interference, or RNAi, that is present in many eukaryotic cell types. When small double-strand RNA molecules (referred to as small interfering RNAs, or siRNAs) are introduced into cells, the two RNA strands will be separated, and one will bind to an enzyme complex known as RISC (RNA-induced silencing complex). The bound siRNA targets the RISC to the mRNA to which it has homology, leading either to translation arrest or to degradation of the mRNA, and thus to silencing of the gene (**Fig. A.49**). For cells that are not easily transfected with siRNA molecules directly, such as primary lymphocytes and myeloid cells, gene silencing can be implemented by using recombinant viruses. In this case, genes encoding small

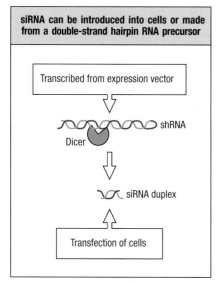

siRNA can be introduced into cells or made from a double-strand hairpin RNA precursor

Transcribed from expression vector

shRNA
Dicer

siRNA duplex

Transfection of cells

Fig. A.49 Knockdown of gene expression using the RNAi pathway. Small double-strand RNA molecules with homology to an mRNA transcript will target the mRNA for degradation or translation arrest. This pathway is initiated by expression of a short hairpin RNA (shRNA), which can be produced from an expression vector that is introduced into cells or by the direct transfection of cells with small double-strand RNA molecules called small interfering RNAs (siRNAs). shRNA molecules are processed by the enzyme Dicer to generate siRNA duplexes. The siRNA duplexes bind to the RNA-induced silencing complex (RISC), which separates the two RNA strands, retaining the noncoding strand of the siRNA. This noncoding strand targets the siRNA:RISC to the mRNA, leading to mRNA degradation or translation termination.

The siRNA binds to mRNA and promotes mRNA cleavage or translation arrest

RISC

RISC activation

siRNA-mediated target recognition

mRNA

mRNA cleavage

translation arrest

hairpin RNAs (shRNAs) are introduced into viral vectors that can be packaged into infectious viral particles. The shRNAs encode small RNAs that form a double-strand hairpin structure; these hairpins are processed by enzymes in the cell to generate the siRNAs needed for gene silencing (see Fig. A.49). Because many primary hematopoietic cell types are readily transduced with recombinant viruses, such as retroviruses and lentiviruses, shRNAs can be effectively used to silence genes in these cell types.

A-38 Cell-lineage tracing techniques

Studies of hematopoiesis and of immune responses *in vivo* pose challenges for the establishment of precise lineage relationships between precursor cells and their progeny. For example, in germinal centers where B cells undergo multiple rounds of somatic hypermutation, class switching, and proliferation, questions arise regarding the number of activated B-cell precursors that give rise to all of the B cells in a single germinal center. One approach to investigating this type of question is to irreversibly 'mark' the precursor cell, allowing identification of all its subsequent progeny, a process known as **lineage tracing**. In the example of germinal centers, the spatial localization of the cells is also essential information, necessitating analysis of lymphoid tissue sections by confocal microscopy. One popular method of lineage tracing for fluorescent microscopy is to utilize 'confetti' mice, also called 'brainbow' mice, the latter name referring to the original development of these mice for studies of neural development. Confetti mice carry a gene cassette encoding GFP and three variants of GFP, each of which emits in a different fluorescent wavelength (**Fig. A.50**). Upstream of the GFP genes is a strong promoter followed by a stop sequence that prevents transcription elongation; therefore, no GFP or GFP variant proteins are expressed from this cassette. Once the Cre enzyme is expressed, the *loxP* sites in the cassette (see Section A-36) are randomly chosen for recombination, leading to deletion or inversion of the intervening sequences, as shown in Figure A.50. Because each cell can utilize different *loxP* sites, the resulting population becomes a random mixture of cells expressing GFP, YFP, RFP, or CFP. If the cells carry the cassette on both alleles of the chromosome (that is, are homozygous), up to 10 different fluorescent signatures can be detected. If confetti mice are crossed to a line expressing Cre in all B cells, the pool of naive B cells would include a random mixture of fluorescent signatures. After immunization, germinal centers can be visualized by confocal microscopy to determine the likely number of precursors contributing to each germinal center.

Another approach to lineage tracing uses DNA bar codes to uniquely mark individual progenitor cells. For this method, a population of progenitor cells is transduced with a library of inheritable DNA bar-code sequences. Marked cells are then transferred into mice and allowed to mature and/or contribute to an immune response. Recovery of the transferred cells at later time points, often after immunization or infection, allows the identification of daughter cells that all derived from a single progenitor on the basis of the inheritance of the unique bar-code DNA sequence.

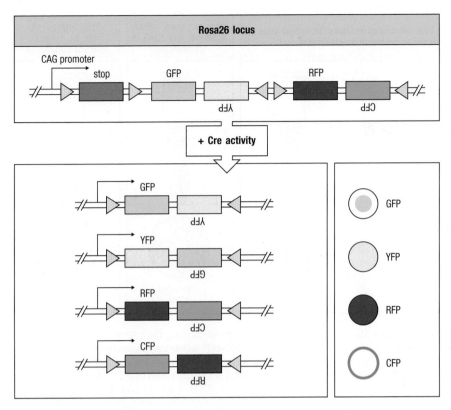

Fig. A.50 Cell-lineage tracing using multicolor fluorescent reporter mice. Confetti mice carry a gene cassette encoding four different variants of GFP [green (GFP), yellow (YFP), red (RFP), and cyan (CFP) fluorescent proteins], each of which emits in a different fluorescent wavelength (top panel). This cassette has been inserted into the Rosa26 locus, a site in the mouse genome that is highly permissive for gene expression in a wide array of cell types and tissues. The gene cassette has a strong promoter, called the CAG promoter, composed of elements from the cytomegalovirus early gene, the chicken β-actin gene, and the rabbit β-globin gene. A transcriptional 'stop' sequence prevents expression of any downstream genes. When Cre is induced in a cell lineage, this enzyme promotes recombination between two *loxP* elements (triangles). Depending on which *loxP* elements are chosen, deletions or inversions of sequences in the cassette can generate four different configurations, each of which expresses one of the GFP variants. Because individual cells in a lineage use different *loxP* elements, each cell and its progeny will be marked by expression of one variant. When the cassette is present in homozygous form, each copy recombines independently, creating up to 10 distinct fluorescent signals.

A-39 Single-cell analysis

Many questions about the immune system require analyses that assess differences between individual cells in a population. For several decades, this requirement has been met by flow cytometry techniques that use a panel of antibodies to assess the expression levels of specific proteins on a cell-by-cell basis. However, flow cytometry studies are limited to the detection of a modest number of proteins and, furthermore, require investigators to decide ahead of time which proteins to investigate. This restriction can largely be eliminated by unbiased approaches that assess mRNA expression profiles of each cell in a population. Collectively, these approaches are known as single-cell RNA-seq on the basis of their use of high-throughput parallel sequence analysis to determine the transcriptome (the totality of RNA molecules in the cell) of each single cell. One common platform for single-cell RNA-seq is the 10X Genomics Chromium System that separates single cells into GEMs (Gel Beads in Emulsion), generates cDNA from the mRNA molecules, tags each transcript with a cell-specific bar code, and then pools the cDNA to create libraries for parallel sequence analysis. Commonly, libraries are made with oligo-d(T)

Fig. A.51 To obtain information on the gene expression profile of single cells, a common approach uses the 10X Genomics Chromium System. This system starts with bar-coded gel beads that are each attached to oligonucleotides containing a PCR primer sequence, a bead-specific bar code, and an oligo-d(T) tail. The bar-code sequence differs for each bead in the mixture. Beads are mixed with cells at a high bead-to-cell ratio in a solution containing enzymes for cDNA synthesis. On average, each bead will associate with one or zero cells. Each bead (with or without a cell) along with some enzyme solution is encapsulated in an oil droplet. The enzymes then lyse the cell, allowing the mRNA molecules from the cell to bind to the oligo-d(T) sequences on the bead-associated oligonucleotides, and enzymes reverse transcribe the mRNA to generate cDNA, which is then amplified by PCR. When the oil is removed, a mixture of cDNA, each containing a bar-code tag denoting its cell of origin, is produced. After library preparation and deep sequencing, the sequence information is computationally analyzed to compile all sequences sharing a bar code, as a measure of the transcriptional profile of each individual cell.

primers, and so are used for 3′-end sequencing (**Fig. A.51**). Computational analysis then deconvolutes the sequence data to assign each transcript to its cell of origin, compiling the transcriptional profile of each single cell. While extremely powerful, the major disadvantage of this technology is that only 10–40% of the transcripts in any given cell are captured and sequenced. In general, low-abundance transcripts are at particular risk of being missed in these experiments.

An advance in single-cell RNA-seq approaches has been the addition of bar-coded antibodies to the library preparation process, a technique known as CITE-seq, short for Cellular Indexing of Transcriptomes and Epitopes by Sequencing (**Fig. A.52**). For this approach, cells are first incubated with antibodies that are covalently linked to a DNA bar-code sequence followed by a poly(A) tail. When single cells are isolated and prepared for 3′-end sequencing of cDNA, the bar codes from any cell-associated antibodies are included in the libraries and are linked to the cell-specific bar code. After library sequencing, the transcriptome information for each cell will be associated with protein expression data on the basis of the numbers of cell-specific reads for each antibody-linked bar code.

A population of cells is incubated with bar-coded antibodies. Single cells are then prepared for transcriptome analysis after encapsulation with bar-coded beads in oil droplets. Antibody-associated bar codes are tagged with the cell-specific bar code providing information about protein expression levels together with the gene-expression profile of each cell

Antibody binding, washing cells	Single-cell droplet encapsulation

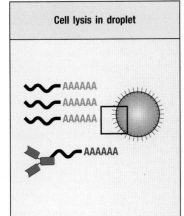

Cell lysis in droplet	mRNA and antibody-oligos hybridize to RT oligos and are indexed with cell bar code

Fig. A.52 Combination of protein expression with transcriptional profiles of single cells. A variation of the single-cell RNA-seq procedure provides information about the protein expression levels on each cell simultaneously with information about the cell's transcriptional profile. Prior to isolating single cells with bar-coded gel beads, the population of cells is incubated with a set of antibodies, each of which is linked to a bar-coded oligonucleotide that contains a 3′ poly(A) tail. Single cells encapsulated with beads will bring their bound antibodies into the reaction. The antibody-linked bar-coded oligonucleotides will be amplified along with the cell's cDNA and will acquire the cell-specific bar code from the bead. After library preparation and deep sequencing, the antibody bar codes associated with each cell can be identified by computational analysis. RT refers to reverse transcription.

Glossary

-omab   Suffix applied to fully murine monoclonal antibodies used for human therapies. (Chapter 16)

-umab   Suffix applied to fully human monoclonal antibodies used for human therapies. (Chapter 16)

-ximab   Suffix applied to chimeric (i.e., mouse/human) monoclonal antibodies used for human therapies. (Chapter 16)

-zumab   Suffix applied to humanized monoclonal antibodies used for human therapies. (Chapter 16)

2B4   A receptor belonging to the signaling lymphocyte activation molecule (SLAM) family expressed by NK cells, which binds to CD48, another SLAM receptor. These signal through SAP and Fyn to promote survival and proliferation. (Chapter 3)

12/23 rule   Phenomenon wherein two gene segments of an immunoglobulin or T-cell receptor can be joined only if one recognition signal sequence has a 12-base-pair spacer and the other has a 23-base-pair spacer. (Chapter 5)

19S regulatory caps   Multi-subunit component of the proteasome that functions to capture ubiquitinated proteins for degradation in the catalytic core. (Chapter 6)

20S catalytic core   Multi-subunit component of the proteasome that is responsible for protein degradation. (Chapter 6)

α-(1,3)-fucosyltransferase VII (FucT-VII)   An enzyme (glycosyltransferase) that adds fucose residues to core glycans displayed by different cell-surface proteoglycans on immune cells and endothelial cells to generate ligands that are recognized by the E-, P-, and L-selectins, which mediate cell rolling during the process of immune-cell extravasation from blood vessels. (Chapter 11)

$\alpha_4\beta_1$ (VLA-4, or CD49d:CD29)   *See* **integrins**. Properties of individual CD antigens can be found in eAppendix II. (Chapters 9, 11, 16)

$\alpha_4\beta_7$ *See* **integrin $\alpha_4\beta_7$**. (Chapters 9, 11, 16)

α_E integrin (CD103)   Alpha integrin molecule (ITGAE) that pairs with β_7 integrin to form the heterodimeric integrin, $\alpha_E\beta_7$, which binds the cellular adhesion molecule E-cadherin expressed by intestinal epithelial cells. Expressed by intraepithelial lymphocytes (IELs) and some dendritic cells associated with barrier tissues such as the intestines. Note that CD103 is often used to refer to the $\alpha_E\beta_7$ heterodimer despite strictly referring only to the α_E molecule. (Chapter 12)

$\alpha_E\beta_7$ Integrin heterodimer that recognizes E-cadherin expressed on intestinal epithelial cells. *See* α_E integrin **(CD103)**. (Chapter 12)

αβ heterodimer   The dimer of one α and one β chain that makes up the antigen-recognition portion of an αβ T-cell receptor. (Chapter 4)

αβ T-cell receptors   *See* **T-cell receptor**. (Chapter 4)

αβ T cells   T cells whose T-cell receptors are composed of rearranged TRA and TRB genes, typically recognizing peptide:MHC complexes but including NKT cells that recognize nonpeptide ligands expressed by nonclassical MHC class I–like proteins. (Chapter 6)

α-defensins   A class of antimicrobial peptides produced by neutrophils and the Paneth cells of the intestine. (Chapter 2)

α-galactosylceramide (α-GalCer)   An immunogenic glycolipid originally extracted from marine sponges but actually produced by various bacteria and which is a ligand presented by CD1 to invariant NKT (iNKT) cells. (Chapter 6)

abatacept   An Fc fusion protein that contains the CTLA-4 extracellular domain and used in treatment of rheumatoid arthritis to block co-stimulation of T cells by binding B7 molecules. (Chapter 16)

ABO blood group   Individuals in the human population vary in the expression of enzymes that modify carbohydrate antigens on the surfaces of red blood cells. Individuals with the A allele produce an enzyme that leads to carbohydrate structures distinct from those produced by the B allele–encoded enzyme. The O allele is a null allele and does not produce a functional glycosyltransferase. (Appendix I)

accelerated rejection   The more rapid rejection of a second graft after rejection of the first graft. It was one of the pieces of evidence that showed that graft rejection was due to an adaptive immune response. (Chapter 15)

accessory effector cells   Cells that aid in an adaptive immune response but are not involved in specific antigen recognition. They include phagocytes, neutrophils, mast cells, and NK cells. (Chapter 10)

acellular pertussis vaccines   A formulation of pertussis used for vaccination containing chemically inactivated antigens, including pertussis toxoid. (Chapter 16)

acquired immune deficiency syndrome (AIDS)   A disease caused by infection with the human immunodeficiency virus (HIV-1 or HIV-2). AIDS occurs when an infected individual has lost most of his or her CD4 T cells, so that infections with opportunistic pathogens occur. (Chapters 1, 13)

acquired immunodeficiency   *See* **secondary immunodeficiency**. (Chapter 13)

activating receptors   On NK cells, receptors whose stimulation results in activation of the cell's cytotoxic activity. (Chapter 3)

activation-induced cell death   A process by which autoreactive T cells are induced to die if they complete thymic maturation and migrate to the periphery. (Chapter 8)

activation-induced cytidine deaminase (AID)   Enzyme that initiates somatic hypermutation and isotype switching by deaminating DNA directly at cytosine in immunoglobulin V regions or switch regions. Loss of AID activity in patients leads to loss of both activities, causing hyper IgM and lack of affinity maturation. (Chapters 5, 10)

activation-induced cytidine deaminase deficiency (AID deficiency)   *See* **hyper IgM syndrome**. (Chapter 10)

activator protein 1 (AP-1)   A transcription factor formed as one of the outcomes of intracellular signaling by antigen receptors of lymphocytes. (Chapter 3)

active immunization   Immunization with antigen to provoke adaptive immunity. (Appendix I)

acute desensitization   An immunotherapeutic technique for rapidly inducing temporary tolerance to, for example, an essential drug such as insulin or penicillin in a person who is allergic to it. Also called rapid desensitization. When performed properly, it can produce symptoms of mild to moderate anaphylaxis. (Chapter 14)

acute phase   In reference to HIV infection, the period that occurs soon after a person becomes infected. It is characterized by an influenza-like illness, abundant virus in the blood, and a decrease in the number of circulating CD4 T cells. (Chapter 13)

acute-phase proteins　Proteins with innate immune function whose production is increased in the presence of an infection (the acute-phase response). They circulate in the blood and participate in early phases of host defense against infection. An example is mannose-binding lectin. (Chapter 3)

acute-phase response　A change in the proteins present in the blood that occurs during the early phases of an infection. It includes the production of acute-phase proteins, many of which are produced in the liver. (Chapters 2, 3)

acute rejection　The rejection of a tissue or organ graft from a genetically unrelated donor that occurs within 10–13 days of transplantation unless prevented by immunosuppressant treatment. (Chapter 15)

adaptive immunity　Immunity to infection conferred by an adaptive immune response. (Chapter 1)

adaptors　Nonenzymatic proteins that form physical links between members of a signaling pathway, particularly between a receptor and other signaling proteins. They recruit members of the signaling pathway into functional protein complexes. (Chapter 7)

ADCC　*See* **antibody-dependent cell-mediated cytotoxicity**. (Chapter 3)

adenoids　Paired mucosa-associated lymphoid tissue located in the nasal cavity. (Chapter 1)

adenosine deaminase (ADA) deficiency　An inherited defect characterized by nonproduction of the enzyme adenosine deaminase, which leads to the accumulation of toxic purine nucleosides and nucleotides in cells, resulting in the death of most developing lymphocytes within the thymus. It is a cause of severe combined immune deficiency. (Chapter 13)

adhesins　Cell-surface proteins on bacteria that enable them to bind to the surfaces of host cells. (Chapter 10)

adjuvant　Any substance that enhances the immune response to an antigen with which it is mixed. (Chapters 1, 3, 9, 16)

adoptive immunity　The immunity, or protection from infection, that is conferred on a recipient individual after transfer of lymphocytes from an immune donor. (Appendix I)

adoptive transfer (or **adoptive immunization**)　The transfer of immune cells from one individual to another individual. Usually performed using syngeneic mice. (Appendix I)

aerobic glycolysis　Originally described in tumor cells and referred to as the Warburg effect (after its discoverer, Otto Warburg), this is a form of glucose metabolism exhibited by activated lymphocytes preparing for rapid cell cycling, wherein glucose is converted into lactate instead of pyruvate to support biosynthesis of macromolecules. (Chapter 9)

afferent lymphatic vessels　Vessels of the lymphatic system that drain extracellular fluid from the tissues and carry antigen, macrophages, and dendritic cells from sites of infection to lymph nodes or other peripheral lymphoid organs. (Chapter 1)

affinity　The strength of binding of one molecule to another at a single site, such as the binding of a monovalent Fab fragment of antibody to a monovalent antigen. Cf. **avidity**. (Chapters 4, 5, Appendix I)

affinity chromatography　Purification of a specific antigen from a complex mixture using small beads coupled to antibodies that bind to the antigen. The mixture is mixed with the antibody-coated beads, and all nonbinding components in the original mixture can be washed away. (Appendix I)

affinity hypothesis　Hypothesis that proposes how the choice between negative selection and positive selection of T cells in the thymus is made, according to the strength of self-peptide:MHC binding by the T-cell receptor. Low-affinity interactions rescue the cell from death by neglect, leading to positive selection; high-affinity interactions induce apoptosis and thus negative selection. (Chapter 8)

affinity maturation　The increase in affinity of antibodies for their specific antigen as an adaptive immune response progresses. This phenomenon is particularly prominent in secondary and subsequent immunizations. (Chapters 1, 10)

agammaglobulinemia　An absence of antibodies in the blood. *See also* **X-linked agammaglobulinemia (XLA)**. (Chapter 13)

age-related macular degeneration (AMD)　A leading cause of blindness in the elderly, for which some single-nucleotide polymorphisms (SNPs) in the factor H genes confer an increased risk. (Chapter 2)

agglutination　The clumping together of particles in a solution. (Chapter 5, Appendix I)

agnathan paired receptors resembling Ag receptors (APARs)　Multigene family of genes containing immunoglobulin domains present in hagfish and lamprey that possibly represent ancestral predecessors of mammalian antigen receptors. (Chapter 5)

agnathans　A class of vertebrates comprising jawless fish lacking an adaptive immunity that is based on the RAG-mediated V(D)J recombination but possessing a distinct system of adaptive immunity that is based on somatically assembled VLRs. (Chapter 5)

agonist selection　A process by which T cells are positively selected in the thymus by their interaction with relatively high-affinity ligands. (Chapter 12)

AID　*See* **activation-induced cytidine deaminase**. (Chapter 10)

AIDS　*See* **acquired immune deficiency syndrome**. (Chapters 1, 13)

AIM2 (absent in melanoma 2)　A member of the PYHIN subfamily of the NLR (NOD-like receptor) family containing an N-terminal HIN domain. It activates caspase 1 in response to viral double-stranded DNA. (Chapter 3)

***AIRE* (autoimmune regulator)**　Gene encoding a protein (autoimmune regulator) that is involved in the expression of numerous genes by thymic medullary epithelial cells, enabling developing T cells to be exposed to self proteins characteristic of other tissues, thereby promoting tolerance to these proteins. Deficiency of AIRE leads to an autoimmune disease, APECED. (Chapter 8)

airway tissue remodeling　A thickening of the airway walls that occurs in chronic asthma due to hyperplasia and hypertrophy of the smooth muscle layer and mucus glands, with the eventual development of fibrosis. Often results in an irreversible decrease of lung function. (Chapter 14)

Akt　Serine/threonine kinase activated downstream of PI 3-kinase with numerous downstream targets involved in cell growth and survival, including activation of the mTOR pathways. (Chapter 16)

alefacept　Recombinant CD58–IgG1 fusion protein that blocks CD2 binding by CD58 and used in treatment of psoriasis. (Chapter 16)

alemtuzumab　Antibody to CD52 used for lymphocyte depletion, such as for T-cell depletion during bone marrow allografts used in treating chronic lymphoid leukemia. (Chapter 16)

allele　A variant form of a gene; many genes occur in several (or more) different forms within the general population. *See also* **heterozygous**, **homozygous**, **polymorphism**. (Chapters 4, 6)

allelic exclusion　In a heterozygous individual, the expression of only one of the two alternative alleles of a particular gene. In immunology, the term describes the restricted expression of the individual chains of the antigen receptor genes, such that each individual lymphocyte produces immunoglobulin or T-cell receptors of a single antigen specificity. (Chapter 8)

allergen　Any antigen that elicits an allergic reaction. (Chapter 14)

allergen desensitization　An immunotherapeutic technique that aims either to change an allergic immune response to a symptom-free non-allergic response or to develop immunological tolerance to an allergen that has been causing unpleasant clinical symptoms. The procedure involves exposing an allergic individual to increasing doses of allergen. (Chapter 14)

allergic asthma An allergic reaction to inhaled antigen, which causes constriction of the bronchi, increased production of airway mucus, and difficulty in breathing. (Chapter 14)

allergic conjunctivitis An allergic reaction involving the conjunctiva of the eye that occurs in sensitized individuals exposed to airborne allergens. It is usually manifested together with nasal allergy symptoms as allergic rhinoconjunctivitis, or hay fever. (Chapter 14)

allergic contact dermatitis A largely T cell–mediated immunological hypersensitivity reaction manifested by a skin rash at the site of contact with the allergen. Often the stimulus is a chemical agent, for example urushiol oil from the leaves of the poison ivy plant, which can haptenate normal host molecules to render them allergenic. (Chapter 14)

allergic reaction A specific response to an innocuous environmental antigen, or allergen, that is caused by sensitized B or T cells. Allergic reactions can be caused by various mechanisms, but the most common is the binding of allergen to IgE bound to mast cells, which causes the cells to release histamine and other biologically active molecules that cause the signs and symptoms of asthma, hay fever, and other common allergic responses. (Chapter 14)

allergic rhinitis An allergic reaction in the nasal mucosa that causes excess mucus production, nasal itching, and sneezing. (Chapter 14)

allergy The state in which a symptomatic immune reaction is made to a normally innocuous environmental antigen. It involves the interaction between the antigen and antibody or primed T cells produced by earlier exposure to the same antigen. (Chapter 1)

alloantibodies Antibodies produced against antigens from a genetically nonidentical member of the same species. (Chapter 15)

alloantigens Antigens from another genetically nonidentical member of the same species. (Chapter 15)

allogeneic Describes two individuals or two mouse strains that differ at genes in the MHC. The term can also be used for allelic differences at other loci. (Chapters 6, 15)

allograft A transplant of tissue from an allogeneic (genetically nonidentical) donor of the same species. Such grafts are invariably rejected unless the recipient is immunosuppressed. (Chapter 15)

allograft rejection The immunologically mediated rejection of grafted tissues or organs from a genetically nonidentical donor. It is due chiefly to recognition of nonself MHC molecules on the graft. (Chapter 1)

alloimmune response The general term for immune responses made by a host against the nonself antigens that are derived from transplanted organs. These responses can result from both direct and indirect allorecognition. (Chapter 15)

alloreaction, alloreactivity The recognition by T cells of MHC molecules other than self. Such responses are also called alloreactive responses. (Chapters 6, 15)

altered peptide ligands (APLs) Peptides in which amino acid substitutions have been made at the T-cell receptor contact positions of the peptides, which affects their binding to the receptor. (Chapter 16)

alternative pathway A form of complement activation that is initiated by spontaneous hydrolysis of C3 and which uses factor B and factor D to form the unique C3 convertase C3bBb. (Chapter 2)

alternative pathway C3 convertase The C3 convertase composed of C4b and C2a. This is also the C3 convertase of the classical complement pathway. (Chapter 2)

alternatively activated macrophages *See* **M2 macrophages**. (Chapter 11)

alum Inorganic aluminum salts (for example, aluminum phosphate and aluminum hydroxide); they act as adjuvants when mixed with antigens and are one of the few adjuvants permitted for use in humans. (Chapter 16)

alveolar macrophages Also referred to as 'dust cells'; resident macrophages within the pulmonary alveoli that are responsible for clearing inspired microbes and other particles. (Chapter 12)

amoeboid coelomocytes Phagocytic cells found in more primitive organisms (such as echinoderms and others) that carry out basic protective functions; these cells are a source of C3 homologs, thioester-containing proteins (TEPs), during infection by bacteria. (Chapter 2)

amorphic A type of genetic variation wherein the altered gene product lacks function. (Chapter 13)

amphipathic Describes molecules that have a positively charged (or hydrophilic) region separated from a hydrophobic region. (Chapter 2)

anakinra A recombinant IL-1 receptor antagonist (IL-1RA) that blocks IL-1 receptor activation and is used in treating rheumatoid arthritis. (Chapter 16)

anaphylactic shock *See* **anaphylaxis**. (Chapters 2, 14)

anaphylatoxins Pro-inflammatory complement fragments C5a and C3a released by cleavage during complement activation. They are recognized by specific receptors and recruit fluid and inflammatory cells to the site of their release. (Chapter 2)

anaphylaxis A rapid-onset and systemic allergic reaction to antigen; for example, to insect venom injected directly into the bloodstream or to foods such as peanuts. Severe systemic reactions can potentially be fatal due to circulatory collapse and suffocation from tracheal swelling. Anaphylaxis usually results from antigens binding to IgE bound by Fcε receptors on mast cells, leading to systemic release of inflammatory mediators. (Chapters 14, 16)

anchor residues Specific amino acid residues in antigenic peptides that determine peptide-binding specificity to MHC class I molecules. Anchor residues for MHC class II molecules exist but are less obvious than for MHC class I. (Chapter 4)

anergy A state of nonresponsiveness to antigen. People are said to be anergic when they cannot mount delayed-type hypersensitivity reactions to a test antigen, whereas T cells and B cells are said to be anergic when they cannot respond to their specific antigen under optimal conditions of stimulation. (Chapter 1)

angiotensin-converting enzyme 2 (ACE2) An ectoenzyme expressed on respiratory epithelial cells and other cells throughout the body that normally cleaves peptides, including the blood pressure regulator, angiotensin II. ACE2 is the host-cell entry receptor for SARS-CoV-2, bound by the receptor-binding domain (RBD) of the SARS-CoV-2 spike protein. (Chapter 12)

ankylosing spondylitis Inflammatory disease of the spine leading to vertebral fusion strongly associated with HLA-B27. (Chapter 16)

annexin V A protein that has high affinity for a plasma-membrane phospholipid, phosphatidylserine (PS). PS is normally present on the inner leaflet of the plasma membrane in healthy cells; however, cells undergoing apoptosis have PS on the outer cell surface. Addition of fluorescently labeled annexin V allows detection of the surface-exposed PS. (Appendix I)

antibody A protein that binds specifically to a particular substance—called its antigen. Each antibody molecule has a unique structure that enables it to bind specifically to its corresponding antigen, but all antibodies have the same overall structure and are known collectively as immunoglobulins. Antibodies are produced by differentiated B cells (plasma cells) in response to infection or immunization and bind to and neutralize pathogens or prepare them for uptake and destruction by phagocytes. (Chapters 1, 4)

antibody combining site *See* **antigen-binding site**. (Chapter 4)

antibody-dependent cell-mediated cytotoxicity (ADCC) The killing of antibody-coated target cells by cells with Fc receptors that recognize the constant region of the bound antibody. Most ADCC is mediated by NK cells that have the Fc receptor FcγRIII on their surface. (Chapters 3, 10, Appendix I)

antibody-directed enzyme/pro-drug therapy (ADEPT) Treatment in which an antibody is linked to an enzyme that metabolizes a nontoxic pro-drug to the active cytotoxic drug. (Chapter 16)

antibody repertoire The total variety of antibodies in the body of an individual. (Chapter 5)

antigen Any molecule that can bind specifically to an antibody or generate peptide fragments that are recognized by a T-cell receptor. (Chapters 1, 4)

antigen-binding site The site at the tip of each arm of an antibody that makes physical contact with the antigen and binds it noncovalently. The antigen specificity of the site is determined by its shape and the amino acids present. (Chapters 1, 4)

antigen-capture assay *See* **capture** (or **sandwich**) **ELISA**. (Appendix I)

antigenic determinant That portion of an antigenic molecule that is bound by the antigen-binding site of a given antibody or antigen receptor; it is also known as an epitope. (Chapters 1, 4)

antigenic drift The process by which influenza virus varies genetically in minor ways from year to year. Point mutations in viral genes cause small differences in the structure of the viral surface antigens. (Chapters 12, 13)

antigenic shift A radical change in the surface antigens of influenza virus, caused by reassortment of its segmented genome with that of another influenza virus, often from an animal. (Chapters 12, 13)

antigenic variation Alterations in surface antigens that occur in some pathogens (such as African trypanosomes) from one generation to another, which allows them to evade preexisting antibodies. (Chapter 13)

antigen presentation The display of antigen on the surface of a cell in the form of peptide fragments bound to MHC molecules. T cells recognize antigen when it is presented in this way. (Chapter 6)

antigen-presenting cells (APCs) Highly specialized cells that can process antigens and display their peptide fragments on the cell surface together with other, co-stimulatory, proteins required for activating naive T cells. The main antigen-presenting cells for naive T cells are dendritic cells, macrophages, and B cells. (Chapter 1)

antigen processing The intracellular degradation of foreign proteins into peptides that can bind to MHC molecules for presentation to T cells. All protein antigens must be processed into peptides before they can be presented by MHC molecules. (Chapter 6)

antigen receptor The cell-surface receptor by which lymphocytes recognize antigen. Each individual lymphocyte bears receptors of a single antigen specificity. (Chapter 1)

anti-lymphocyte globulin Antiserum raised in another species against human T cells. It is used in the temporary suppression of immune responses in transplantation. (Chapter 16)

antimicrobial enzymes Enzymes that kill microorganisms by their actions. An example is lysozyme, which digests bacterial cell walls. (Chapter 2)

antimicrobial peptides, antimicrobial proteins Amphipathic peptides or proteins secreted by epithelial cells and phagocytes that kill a variety of microbes nonspecifically, mainly by disrupting cell membranes. Antimicrobial peptides in humans include the defensins, the cathelicidins, the histatins, and RegIIIγ. (Chapters 1, 2)

antiserum (*pl.* **antisera**) The fluid component of clotted blood from an immune individual that contains antibodies against the antigen that was used for immunization. An antiserum contains a mixture of different antibodies that all bind the antigen, each of which has a different structure, its own epitope on the antigen, and its own set of cross-reactions. This heterogeneity makes each antiserum unique. (Appendix I)

antivenin Antibody raised against the venom of a poisonous snake or other organism and which can be used as an immediate treatment for the bite to neutralize the venom. (Chapters 10, 14)

aorta–gonad–mesonephros (AGM) An embryonic region in which hematopoietic cells arise during development. (Chapter 3)

AP-1 A heterodimeric transcription factor formed as one of the outcomes of intracellular signaling via the antigen receptors of lymphocytes and the TLRs of cells of innate immunity. Most often, it contains one Fos family member and one Jun family member. AP-1 mainly activates the expression of genes for cytokines and chemokines. (Chapter 7)

APECED *See* **autoimmune polyendocrinopathy–candidiasis–ectodermal dystrophy**. (Chapters 8, 13, 14)

APOBEC1 (apolipoprotein B mRNA editing catalytic polypeptide 1) An RNA-editing enzyme that deaminates cytidine to uracil in certain mRNAs, such as apolipoprotein B, and which is related to the enzyme AID involved in somatic hypermutation and isotype switching. (Chapter 10)

apoptosis A form of cell death common in the immune system, in which the cell activates an internal death program. It is characterized by nuclear DNA degradation, nuclear degeneration and condensation, and the rapid phagocytosis of cell remains. Proliferating lymphocytes experience high rates of apoptosis during their development and during immune responses. (Chapters 1, 9)

apoptosome A large, multimeric protein structure that forms in the process of apoptosis when cytochrome *c* is released from mitochondria and binds Apaf-1. A heptamer of cytochrome *c*–Apaf-1 heterodimers assembles into wheel-like structure that binds and activates pro-caspase 9, an initiator caspase, to initiate the caspase cascade. (Chapter 9)

appendix A gut-associated lymphoid tissue located at the beginning of the colon. (Chapters 1, 12)

APRIL A TNF family cytokine related to BAFF that binds the receptors TACI and BCMA on B cells to promote survival and regulate differentiation. (Chapter 10)

apurinic/apyrimidinic endonuclease-1 (APE1) A DNA repair endonuclease involved in class switch recombination. (Chapters 5, 10)

arginase-1 An enzyme that catalyzes the conversion of arginine to ornithine and urea in the last step of the urea cycle. This enzyme is highly expressed by, and is a marker for, M2 (alternatively activated) macrophages, where its degradation of arginine deprives NO synthase of its substrate for the generation of nitric oxide. The ornithine generated by this enzyme may also be directly toxic to helminths, and also stimulates smooth muscle contraction and contributes to the tissue repair response. (Chapter 11)

Artemis An endonuclease involved in the gene rearrangements that generate functional immunoglobulin and T-cell receptor genes. (Chapter 5)

Arthus reaction A local skin reaction that occurs when a sensitized individual with IgG antibodies against a particular antigen is challenged by injection of the antigen into the dermis. Antigen:IgG antibody immune complexes in the extracellular spaces in the dermis activate complement and phagocytic cells to produce a local inflammatory response. (Chapter 14)

aryl hydrocarbon receptor (AHR) A basic helix–loop–helix transcription factor that is activated by various aromatic ligands including, famously, dioxin. It functions in the normal activity of several types of immune cells including some ILCs and IELs. (Chapter 12)

ASC An adaptor protein containing pyrin and CARD domains involved in activating caspase 1 in the inflammasome. Also called PYCARD. (Chapter 3)

asymptomatic phase In reference to HIV infection, the period in which the infection is being partly held in check and no symptoms occur; it may last for many years. (Chapter 13)

ataxia telangiectasia A disease characterized by a staggering gait and multiple disorganized blood vessels and often accompanied by clinical immunodeficiency. It is caused by defects in the ATM protein, which is involved in DNA repair pathways that are also used in V(D)J recombination and class switch recombination. (Chapters 5, 10)

ATM A protein kinase that, when mutated, causes the disease ataxia telangiectasia. (Chapters 5, 10)

atopic march The clinical observation that it is common for children with atopic eczema to later develop allergic rhinitis and/or asthma. (Chapter 14)

atopy (adj. atopic) A genetically based increased tendency to produce IgE-mediated allergic reactions against innocuous substances. (Chapter 14)

ATP-binding cassette (ABC) A large family of proteins containing a particular domain for nucleotide binding that includes many transporters, such as TAP1 and TAP2, but also various NOD members. (Chapter 6)

attenuation The process by which human or animal pathogens are modified by growth in culture so that they can grow in their host and induce immunity without producing serious clinical disease. (Chapter 16)

atypical hemolytic uremic syndrome (aHUS) A condition characterized by damage to platelets and red blood cells and inflammation of the kidneys that is caused by uncontrolled complement activation in individuals with inherited deficiencies in complement-regulatory proteins. (Chapters 2, 13)

autoantibodies Antibodies specific for self antigens. (Chapter 15)

autoantigens A self antigen to which the immune system makes a response. (Chapter 15)

autocrine Describes a cytokine or other biologically active molecule acting on the cell that produces it. (Chapter 3)

autograft A graft of tissue from one site to another on the same individual. (Chapter 15)

autoimmune disease Disease in which the pathology is caused by adaptive immune responses to self antigens. (Chapters 1, 13, 14)

autoimmune hemolytic anemia A pathological condition with low levels of red blood cells (anemia), which is caused by autoantibodies that bind red blood cell surface antigens and target the red blood cell for destruction. (Chapter 15)

autoimmune lymphoproliferative syndrome (ALPS) An inherited syndrome in which a defect in the Fas gene leads to a failure in normal apoptosis, causing unregulated immune responses, including autoimmune responses. (Chapters 9, 11, 15)

autoimmune polyendocrinopathy–candidiasis–ectodermal dystrophy (APECED) A disease characterized by a loss of tolerance to self antigens, caused by a breakdown of negative selection in the thymus. It is due to defects in the gene AIRE, which encodes a transcriptional regulatory protein that enables many self antigens to be expressed by thymic medullary epithelial cells. Also called autoimmune polyglandular syndrome type I. (Chapters 8, 13, 14)

autoimmune polyglandular syndrome type I See **autoimmune polyendocrinopathy–candidiasis–ectodermal dystrophy**. (Chapter 8)

autoimmune thrombocytopenic purpura An autoimmune disease in which antibodies against platelets are made. Antibody binding to platelets causes them to be taken up by cells with Fc receptors and complement receptors, resulting in a decrease in platelet count that leads to purpura (bleeding). (Chapter 15)

autoimmunity Adaptive immunity specific for self antigens. (Chapter 15)

autoinflammatory diseases Diseases due to unregulated inflammation in the absence of infection; they can have a variety of causes, including inherited genetic defects. (Chapter 3)

autophagosome A double bilayer membrane structure that functions in macroautophagy by engulfing cytoplasmic contents and fusing with lysosomes. (Chapter 12)

autophagy The digestion and breakdown by a cell of its own organelles and proteins in lysosomes. It may be one route by which cytosolic proteins can be processed for presentation on MHC class II molecules. (Chapters 6, 12)

avidity The sum total of the strength of binding of two molecules or cells to one another at multiple sites. It is distinct from affinity, which is the strength of binding of one site on a molecule to its ligand. (Chapters 2, 4, Appendix I)

avoidance Mechanisms that prevent a host's exposure to microbes, such as anatomic barriers or particular behaviors. (Chapter 1)

azathioprine A powerful cytotoxic drug that is converted to its active form in vivo, which then kills rapidly proliferating cells, including proliferating lymphocytes; it is used as an immunosuppressant to treat autoimmune disease and in transplantation. (Chapter 16)

β1i (LMP2), β2i (MECL-1), β5i (LMP7) Alternative proteasome subunits that replace the constitutive catalytic subunits β1, β2, and β5 and which are induced by interferons and produce the immunoproteasome. (Chapter 6)

β2-microglobulin The light chain of the MHC class I proteins, encoded outside the MHC. It binds noncovalently to the heavy or α chain. (Chapter 4)

β5t Alternative proteasome subunit expressed by thymic epithelial cells that substitutes for β5 to produce the thymoproteasome involved in generating peptides encountered by thymocytes during development. (Chapter 6)

β-defensins Antimicrobial peptides made by virtually all multicellular organisms. In mammals they are produced by the epithelia of the respiratory and urogenital tracts, skin, and tongue. (Chapter 2)

β sandwich A secondary protein structure composed of two β sheets that fold such that one lies over the other, as in an immunoglobulin fold. (Chapter 4)

β sheet A secondary protein structure composed of β strands stabilized by noncovalent interactions between backbone amide and carbonyl groups. In 'parallel' β sheets, the adjacent strands run in the same direction; in 'antiparallel' β sheets, adjacent strands run in opposite directions. Immunoglobulin domains are made up of two antiparallel β sheets arranged in the form of a β barrel. (Chapter 4)

β strand A secondary protein structure in which the polypeptide backbone of several consecutive amino acids is arranged in a flat, or planar, conformation, and often illustrated as an arrow. (Chapter 4)

B-1 B cells A class of atypical, self-renewing B cells (also known as CD5 B cells) found mainly in the peritoneal and pleural cavities in adults and considered part of the innate rather than the adaptive immune system. They have a much less diverse antigen-receptor repertoire than conventional B cells and are the major source of natural antibody. (Chapters 8, 10)

B7.1 and B7.2 Cell-surface proteins on specialized antigen-presenting cells such as dendritic cells and which are the major co-stimulatory molecules for T cells. B7.1 (CD80) and B7.2 (CD86) are closely related members of the immunoglobulin superfamily, and both bind to the CD28 and CTLA-4 proteins on T cells. (Chapters 7, 9)

B and T lymphocyte attenuator (BTLA) An inhibitory CD28-related receptor expressed by B and T lymphocytes that interacts with the herpes virus entry molecule (HVEM). BTLA is a member of the TNF receptor family. (Chapter 7)

bacteria A vast kingdom of unicellular prokaryotic microorganisms, some species of which cause infectious diseases in humans and animals, while others make up most of the body's commensal microbiota. Disease-causing bacteria may live in the extracellular spaces or inside cells in vesicles or in the cytosol. (Chapter 1)

BAFF   Acronym for B-cell activating factor belonging to the TNF family, which binds the receptors BAFF-R and TACI to promote B cell survival. (Chapters 8, 10)

BAFF-R   Receptor for BAFF that can activate canonical and non-canonical NFκB signaling and promote survival of B cells. (Chapter 10)

bare lymphocyte syndrome (BLS)   *See* **MHC class I deficiency, MHC class II deficiency**. (Chapter 13)

base-excision repair   Type of DNA repair that can lead to mutation and which is involved in somatic hypermutation and class switching in B cells. (Chapter 10)

basiliximab   Antibody to human CD25 used to block IL-2 receptor signaling in T cells for treatment of rejection in renal transplantation. (Chapter 16)

basophil   Type of white blood cell containing granules that stain with basic dyes. It is thought to have a function similar to that of mast cells. (Chapters 1, 3)

BATF3   A transcription factor expressed in dendritic cells belonging to the AP1 family, which includes many other factors such as c-Jun and Fos. (Chapter 6)

BCAP   B-cell adaptor for PI 3-kinase (BCAP) is an adaptor that was recently found to link signaling by TLRs to activation of the PI 3-kinase and AKT pathway. (Chapter 3)

B cell, B lymphocyte   One of the two types of antigen-specific lymphocytes responsible for adaptive immune responses, the other being the T cells. The function of B cells is to produce antibodies. B cells are divided into two classes. Conventional B cells have highly diverse antigen receptors and are generated in the bone marrow throughout life, emerging to populate the blood and lymphoid tissues. B-1 cells have much less diverse antigen receptors and form a population of self-renewing B cells in the peritoneal and pleural cavities. (Chapter 1)

B-cell antigen receptor, B-cell receptor (BCR)   The cell-surface receptor on B cells for specific antigen. It is composed of a transmembrane immunoglobulin molecule (which recognizes antigen) associated with the invariant Igα and Igβ chains (which have a signaling function). On activation by antigen, B cells differentiate into plasma cells producing antibody molecules of the same antigen specificity as this receptor. (Chapters 1, 10)

B-cell co-receptor   A transmembrane signaling receptor on the B-cell surface composed of the proteins CD19, CD81, and CD21 (complement receptor 2), which binds complement fragments on bacterial antigens also bound by the B-cell receptor. Co-ligation of this complex with the B-cell receptor increases responsiveness to antigen by about 100-fold. (Chapter 7)

B-cell co-receptor complex   A transmembrane signaling receptor on the B-cell surface composed of the proteins CD19, CD81, and CD21 (complement receptor 2), which binds complement fragments on bacterial antigens also bound by the B-cell receptor. Co-ligation of this complex with the B-cell receptor increases responsiveness to antigen about 100-fold. (Chapter 10)

B-cell mitogens   Any substance that nonspecifically causes B cells to proliferate. (Chapter 10)

Bcl-2 family   Family of intracellular proteins that includes members that promote apoptosis (Bax, Bak, and Bok) and members that inhibit apoptosis (Bcl-2, Bcl-W, and Bcl-X$_L$). (Chapter 9)

Bcl-6   A transcriptional repressor that opposes differentiation of B cells into plasma cells. (Chapters 9, 10)

BCMA   Receptor of the TNFR superfamily that binds APRIL. (Chapter 10)

Bcr–Abl tyrosine kinase   Constitutively active tyrosine kinase fusion protein caused by a chromosomal translocation—the Philadelphia chromosome—between the *Bcr* and the *Abl* tyrosine kinase genes and which is associated with chronic myeloid leukemia. (Chapter 16)

BDCA-2 (blood dendritic cell antigen 2)   A C-type lectin expressed selectively as a receptor on the surface of human plasmacytoid dendritic cells. (Chapter 3)

Berlin patient   An American HIV patient, Timothy Ray Brown, who was treated in Berlin with a hematopoietic stem-cell (HSC) transplant from a donor deficient in a co-receptor for the virus (CCR5) for an unrelated illness (leukemia). He is believed to have been cured of HIV infection and is one of the only known patients in which the virus is thought to have been completely eliminated, a so-called 'sterilizing' cure. (Chapter 13)

biofilms   A consortium of microorganisms (typically bacteria) that are adherent to each other and a living (biotic) surface or nonliving (abiotic) surface by an extracellular matrix composed of DNA, polysaccharide, lipid, or protein polymers. The extracellular matrix allows the consortium to establish 'residence' in a favorable ecological niche and allows for shared metabolic resources between organisms. It also shields the consortium against certain threats, such as the immune system or antibiotics. (Chapter 13)

biologics   Medical treatments composed of natural proteins, such as antibodies and cytokines, and antisera or whole cells. (Chapter 16)

blast transformation   Morphological changes, including an increase in size, that occur in T and B cells activated by antigen or mitogens. (Chapter 9)

Blau syndrome   An inherited granulomatous disease caused by gain-of-function mutations in the NOD2 gene. (Chapters 3, 15)

BLIMP-1   A transcriptional repressor that promotes B-cell differentiation into plasma cells and suppresses proliferation, class switching, and affinity maturation. (Chapters 9, 10)

BLNK   B-cell linker protein. *See* **SLP-65**. (Chapter 7)

B lymphocytes (B cells)   *See* **B cells**. (Chapter 1)

bone marrow   The tissue where all the cellular elements of the blood—red blood cells, white blood cells, and platelets—are initially generated from hematopoietic stem cells. The bone marrow is also the site of further B-cell development in mammals and the source of stem cells that give rise to T cells on migration to the thymus. Thus, bone marrow transplantation can restore all the cellular elements of the blood, including the cells required for adaptive immune responses. (Chapter 1)

booster immunization   *See* **secondary immunization**. (Chapter 1)

bradykinin   A vasoactive peptide that is produced as a result of tissue damage and acts as an inflammatory mediator. (Chapter 3)

branching (or **asymmetric division**) **model of memory-cell development**   One of two general models of memory lymphocyte development that posits that memory and effector T (and B) cells arise from different daughter cells after the initial activation of naive T cells. *See also* **linear model of memory-cell development**. (Chapter 11)

broadly neutralizing antibodies   Antibodies that block viral infection by multiple strains. In reference to HIV, these are antibodies that block binding of the virus to CD4 and/or chemokine co-receptors. (Chapters 10, 13)

bronchus-associated lymphoid tissue (BALT)   Organized lymphoid tissue found in the bronchi in some animals. Adult humans do not normally have such organized lymphoid tissue in the respiratory tract, but it may be present in some infants and children. (Chapters 1, 12)

Bruton's tyrosine kinase (Btk)   A Tec family tyrosine kinase important in B-cell receptor signaling. Btk is mutated in the human immunodeficiency disease X-linked agammaglobulinemia. (Chapter 7)

Bruton's X-linked agammaglobulinemia   *See* **X-linked agammaglobulinemia**. (Chapters 8, 13)

BST2 (bone marrow stromal antigen 2)   Bone marrow stromal antigen 2, also called tetherin and CD317, is a type II integral membrane protein that functions as a viral restriction element trapping virions in the plasma membrane and inhibiting viral budding and which serves as a marker of plasmacytoid dendritic cells (pDCs), but is also expressed by B cells. (Chapter 3)

bursa of Fabricius   Lymphoid organ associated with the gut that is the site of B-cell development in chickens. (Chapters 1, 5, 12)

butyrate   A short-chain fatty acid produced abundantly by anaerobic digestion of carbohydrates in the intestine by commensals and which can influence host cells in several ways, acting as an energy source for enterocytes and as an inhibitor of histone deacetylases. (Chapter 12)

butyrophilin (BTN)   A subtype of surface membrane glycoprotein within the immunoglobulin superfamily comprising approximately 11 unique members, expressed on a variety of somatic tissues and composed of typically two extracellular immunoglobulin domains. (Chapters 6, 12)

C1 complex (C1)   Protein complex activated as the first step in the classical pathway of complement activation, composed of C1q bound to two molecules each of the proteases C1r and C1s. Binding of a pathogen or antibody to C1q activates C1r, which cleaves and activates C1s, which cleaves C4 and C2. (Chapter 2)

C1 inhibitor (C1INH)   An inhibitor protein for C1 that binds and inactivates C1r:C1s enzymatic activity. Deficiency in C1INH causes hereditary angioedema through production of vasoactive peptides that cause subcutaneous and laryngeal swelling. (Chapter 2)

C1q   A component of the C1 complex formed by a hexamer of trimers of a polypeptide with a globular domain that can bind bacterial surfaces or interact with Fc regions of antibodies and a carboxy-terminal collagen-like domain that mediates its assembly and association with C1r and C1s. (Chapter 2)

C1r   A serine protease that associates with C1q and C1s to help form the C1 complex. Its autocatalytic activity is triggered by conformational changes resulting from C1q binding to Fc or bacterial surfaces; C1r then cleaves C1s. (Chapter 2)

C1s   A serine protease that associates with C1q and C1r to help form the C1 complex. It is cleaved and activated by C1r and then functions to activate the downstream complement components 4 and 2 (C4 and C2). (Chapter 2)

C2   Complement protein of the classical and lectin pathways that is cleaved by the C1 complex to yield C2b and C2a. C2a is an active protease that forms part of the classical C3 convertase C4b2a. (Chapter 2)

C2a   The large fragment of C2 formed when C2 is cleaved by C1s. When bound to C4b, C2a is the serine protease of the C3 convertase (C4b2a) of the classical and the lectin pathways. (Chapter 2)

C3   Complement protein on which all complement activation pathways converge. C3 cleavage forms C3b, which can bind covalently to microbial surfaces, where it promotes destruction by phagocytes. (Chapter 2)

C3 convertase   Enzyme complex that cleaves C3 to C3b and C3a on the surface of a pathogen. The C3 convertase of the classical and lectin pathways is formed from membrane-bound C4b complexed with the protease C2a. The alternative pathway C3 convertase is formed from membrane-bound C3b complexed with the protease Bb. (Chapter 2)

C3a   *See* **anaphylatoxins**. (Chapter 2)

C3b   *See* **C3**. (Chapter 2)

C3bBb   The C3 convertase of the alternative pathway of complement activation. (Chapter 2)

C3b$_2$Bb   The C5 convertase of the alternative pathway of complement activation. (Chapter 2)

C3dg   Breakdown product of iC3b that remains attached to the microbial surface, where it can bind complement receptor 2 (CR2). (Chapter 2)

C3f   A small fragment of C3b that is removed by factor I and MCP to leave iC3b on the microbial surface. (Chapter 2)

C3 glomerulopathy   An inflammatory condition in the kidney in which C3b is abnormally deposited in the glomerulus leading to proteinuria and hematuria. It can be associated with autoantibodies, called nephritic factors, that can inhibit factor H, other complement-regulatory components, or that stabilize C3 convertase, leading to increased C3 deposition. (Chapter 2)

C3(H$_2$O)Bb   *See* **fluid-phase C3 convertase**. (Chapter 2)

C4   Complement protein of the classical and lectin pathways. C4 is cleaved by C1s to C4b, which forms part of the classical C3 convertase. (Chapter 2)

C4b-binding protein (C4BP)   A complement-regulatory protein that inactivates the classical pathway C3 convertase formed on host cells by displacing C2a from the C4b2a complex. C4BP binds C4b attached to host cells, but cannot bind C4b attached to pathogens. (Chapter 2)

C4b2a   C3 convertase of the classical and lectin pathways of complement activation. (Chapter 2)

C4b2a3b   C5 convertase of the classical and lectin pathways of complement activation. (Chapter 2)

C5 convertase   Enzyme complex that cleaves C5 to C5a and C5b. (Chapter 2)

C5a   *See* **anaphylatoxins**. (Chapter 2)

C5a receptor 1   A G protein–coupled receptor expressed by macrophages and activated by C5a that facilitates ingestion of opsonized bacteria bound to CR1. (Chapter 2)

C5a receptor 2   A nonsignaling surface receptor expressed by neutrophils and macrophages and which may act as a decoy receptor for C5a and thus regulate activity of the C5a receptor. (Chapter 2)

C5b   Fragment of C5 that initiates the formation of the membrane-attack complex (MAC). (Chapter 2)

C6, C7, C8, C9   Complement proteins that act with C5b to form the membrane-attack complex, producing a pore that leads to lysis of the target cell. (Chapter 2)

calcineurin   A cytosolic serine/threonine phosphatase with a crucial role in signaling via the T-cell receptor. The immunosuppressive drugs cyclosporin A and tacrolimus inactivate calcineurin, suppressing T-cell responses. (Chapters 7, 16)

calmodulin   Calcium-binding protein that is activated by binding Ca^{2+}; it is then able to bind to and regulate the activity of a wide variety of enzymes. (Chapter 7)

calnexin   A chaperone protein in the endoplasmic reticulum (ER) that binds to partly folded members of the immunoglobulin superfamily of proteins and retains them in the ER until folding is complete. (Chapter 6)

calprotectin   A complex of heterodimers of the antimicrobial peptides S100A8 and S100A9, which sequester zinc and manganese from microbes. Produced in abundance by neutrophils and in lesser amounts by macrophages and epithelial cells. (Chapters 2, 11)

calreticulin   A chaperone protein in the endoplasmic reticulum that, together with ERp57 and tapasin, forms the peptide-loading complex that loads peptides onto newly synthesized MHC class I molecules. (Chapter 6)

cancer immunoediting   A process that occurs during the development of a cancer when it is acquiring mutations that favor its survival and escape from immune responses, such that cancer cells with these mutations are selected for survival and growth. (Chapter 16)

cancer-testis antigens   Proteins expressed by cancer cells that are normally expressed only in male germ cells in the testis. (Chapter 16)

canonical NFκB pathway   This pathway relies on activation of the IκB kinase, or IKK, composed of IKKα, IKKβ, and IKKγ (NEMO). IKKβ phosphorylation by an upstream kinase, such as TAK1, activates IKK, which in turn phosphorylates IκB (inhibitor of κB), causing IκB degradation and release of the active NFκB p50:p65 heterodimer. (Chapter 10)

capping A process occurring in the nucleus in which the modified purine 7-methylguanosine is added to the 5′-phosphate of the first nucleotide of the RNA transcript. (Chapter 3)

capsular polysaccharides *See* **capsulated bacteria**. (Chapter 16)

capsulated bacteria Referring to bacteria surrounded by a polysaccharide shell that resists actions of phagocytes, resulting in pus formation at the site of infection. Also called pyogenic (pus-forming) bacteria. (Chapters 10, 16)

capture (or **sandwich**) **ELISA** An ELISA in which two antibodies recognizing different epitopes on the antigen are utilized. The first antibody is adhered to the assay plate well. The sample being tested is added, allowing antigen to bind. The bound antigen is detected with a second enzyme-linked antibody, followed by addition of substrate and measurement of the quantity of reaction product produced. This is also known as an antigen-capture assay. (Appendix I)

carboxypeptidase N (CPN) A metalloproteinase that inactivates C3a and C5a. CPN deficiency causes a condition of recurrent angioedema. (Chapter 2)

cardiolipin A lipid found in many bacteria and in the inner mitochondrial membrane that is a ligand recognized by some human $\gamma\delta$ T cells. (Chapter 6)

caspase 1 Also known as interleukin-1 converting enzyme (ICE), caspase 1 is a protease that becomes activated in the inflammasome response, and which then functions to process a variety of targets, such as the pro-forms of IL-1β and IL-18, and gasdermin D. (Chapter 3)

caspase 4, caspase 5 These human proteases are cytosolic sensors, counterparts to mouse caspase 11, that are activated by LPS and directly cleave and activate gasdermin D, leading to pyroptosis. (Chapter 3)

caspase 8 An initiator caspase activated by various receptors that activates the process of apoptosis. (Chapter 3)

caspase 11 This caspase is homologous to human caspase 4 and caspase 5. Its expression is induced by TLR signaling. Intracellular LPS can directly activate it, leading to pyroptosis. (Chapter 3)

caspase recruitment domain (CARD) A protein domain present in some receptor tails that can dimerize with other CARD-containing proteins, including caspases, thus recruiting them into signaling pathways. (Chapter 3)

caspases A family of cysteine proteases that cleave proteins at aspartic acid residues. They have important roles in apoptosis and in the processing of cytokine pro-polypeptides. (Chapter 3)

cathelicidins Family of antimicrobial peptides that in humans has one member. (Chapter 2)

cathelin A cathepsin L inhibitor. (Chapter 2)

cathepsins A family of proteases using cysteine at their active site and which frequently function in processing antigens taken into the vesicular pathway. (Chapter 6)

cation-pi interaction Chemical interaction between a cation (e.g., Na^+) and the pi-electron system of an aromatic moiety. (Chapter 4)

CC chemokines One of the two main classes of chemokines, distinguished by two adjacent cysteines (C) near the amino terminus. They have names CCL1, CCL2, etc. *See* eAppendix IV for a list of individual chemokines. (Chapter 3)

CCL19 Chemokine made by dendritic cells and stromal cells in T-cell zones of lymph nodes that binds CCR7 and functions to attract naive T cells. (Chapters 9, 10, 12)

CCL21 Chemokine made by dendritic cells and stromal cells in T-cell zones of lymph nodes that binds CCR7 and functions to attract naive T cells. (Chapters 9, 10, 12)

CCL25 (TECK) Chemokine made by small-intestinal epithelial cells that binds CCR9 to recruit gut-homing T and B cells. (Chapter 12)

CCL28 (MEC, mucosal epithelial chemokine) Chemokine made by colonic intestinal cells, salivary gland cells, and lactating mammary gland cells that binds CCR10 to recruit B lymphocytes producing IgA into these tissues. (Chapter 12)

CCR7 Chemokine receptor expressed by all naive T and B cells, and some memory T and B cells, such as central memory T cells, and which binds CCL19 and CCL21 made by dendritic cells and stromal cells in lymphoid tissues. (Chapters 9, 10, 12)

CCR9 Chemokine receptor expressed by dendritic cells, T cells, thymocytes, and some $\gamma\delta$ T cells that binds CCL25 and mediates recruitment of gut-homing cells. (Chapter 12)

CCR10 Chemokine receptor expressed by many cells that binds CCL27 and CCL28 and mediates intestinal recruitment of IgA-producing B lymphocytes. (Chapter 12)

CD1 Small family of MHC class I–like proteins that are not encoded in the MHC and can present glycolipid antigens to CD4 T cells. (Chapter 6)

CD3 complex The invariant proteins CD3γ, δ, and ε, and the dimeric ζ chains, which form the signaling complex of the T-cell receptor. Each of them contains one or more ITAM signaling motifs in their cytoplasmic tails. (Chapter 7)

CD4 The co-receptor for T-cell receptors that recognize peptide antigens bound to MHC class II molecules. It binds to the lateral face of the MHC molecule. (Chapters 1, 4)

CD8 The co-receptor for T-cell receptors that recognize peptide antigens bound to MHC class I molecules. It binds to the lateral face of the MHC molecule. (Chapters 1, 4)

CD8$\alpha\alpha$ Homodimer of CD8α molecule that is up-regulated on natural and peripheral IELs in the intestinal epithelium. Recognizes the nonclassical MHC molecule TL (thymus leukemia antigen) on intestinal epithelial cells, loss of which may trigger cytolytic NK-like activity of IELs. May also provide a survival signal for IELs. (Chapters 9, 12)

CD11b (α_M integrin) Integrin expressed by macrophages and some dendritic cells that functions with β2 integrin (CD18) as complement receptor 3 (CR3). (Chapter 9)

CD11c (α_X integrin) Integrin expressed at high levels by dendritic cells and at lower levels by some other myeloid cells that functions with β2 integrin (CD18) as both an adhesion molecule and complement receptor 4 (CR4). (Chapter 9)

CD19 *See* **B-cell co-receptor**. (Chapter 7)

CD21 Another name for complement receptor 2 (CR2). *See also* **B-cell co-receptor**. (Chapters 2, 7, 10)

CD22 An inhibitory receptor on B cells that binds sialic acid–modified glycoproteins commonly found on mammalian cells and contains an ITIM motif in its cytoplasmic tail. (Chapter 7)

CD23 The low-affinity Fc receptor for IgE. (Chapter 14)

CD24 A GPI-linked sialoprotein that is expressed by conventional dendritic cells. (Chapter 9)

CD25 Also known as IL-2 receptor α (IL-2Rα), this is the high-affinity component of the IL-2 receptor, which also includes IL-2Rβ and the common γ chain. It is up-regulated by activated T cells and is constitutively expressed by T_{reg} cells to confer responsiveness to IL-2. (Chapter 9)

CD27 A TNF receptor family protein constitutively expressed on naive T cells that binds CD70 on dendritic cells and delivers a potent co-stimulatory signal to T cells early in the activation process. (Chapter 11)

CD28 An activating receptor on T cells that binds to the B7 co-stimulatory molecules present on specialized antigen-presenting cells such as dendritic cells. CD28 is the major co-stimulatory receptor on naive T cells. (Chapters 7, 9)

CD31 A cell-adhesion molecule found both on lymphocytes and at endothelial cell junctions. CD31–CD31 interactions are thought to enable leukocytes to leave blood vessels and enter tissues. (Chapter 3)

CD35 *See* **CR1**. (Chapter 2)

CD40, CD40 ligand (CD40L) CD40 on B cells and CD40 ligand (CD40L, or CD154) on activated helper T cells are co-stimulatory molecules whose interaction is required for the proliferation and class switching of antigen-activated naive B cells. CD40 is also expressed by dendritic cells, and here the CD40–CD40L interaction provides co-stimulatory signals to naive T cells. (Chapters 10, 16)

CD40 ligand deficiency An immunodeficiency disease in which little or no IgG, IgE, or IgA antibody is produced and even IgM responses are deficient, but serum IgM levels are normal to high. It is due to a defect in the gene encoding CD40 ligand (CD154), which prevents class switching from occurring. Also known as X-linked hyper IgM syndrome, reflecting the location of the gene that encodes CD40L on the X chromosome and the phenotype of elevated IgM antibody relative to other immunoglobulins. (Chapters 11, 13)

CD44 Also known as phagocytic glycoprotein-1 (Pgp1), CD44 is a cell-surface glycoprotein expressed by naive lymphocytes and up-regulated on activated T cells. It is a receptor for hyaluronic acid and functions in cell–cell and cell–extracellular matrix adhesion. High expression of CD44 is used as a marker for effector and memory T cells. (Chapter 11)

CD45 A transmembrane tyrosine phosphatase found on all leukocytes. It is expressed in different isoforms on different cell types, including the different subtypes of T cells. Also called leukocyte common antigen, it is a generic marker for hematopoietically derived cells, with the exception of erythrocytes. (Chapters 3, 7)

CD45RA A full-length variant of CD45 that serves as a marker for naive human T cells. (Chapter 11)

CD45RO An alternatively spliced variant of CD45 that serves as a marker for memory T cells. (Chapter 11)

CD48 *See* **2B4**. (Chapter 3)

CD59, protectin Cell-surface protein that protects host cells from complement damage by blocking binding of C9 to the C5b678 complex, thus preventing MAC formation. (Chapter 2)

CD69 A cell-surface protein that is rapidly expressed by antigen-activated T cells. It acts to down-modulate the expression of the sphingosine 1-phosphate receptor 1 (S1PR1), thereby retaining activated T cells within T-cell zones of secondary lymphoid tissues as they divide and differentiate into effector T cells. (Chapter 9)

CD70 The ligand for CD27 that is expressed on activated dendritic cells and delivers a potent co-stimulatory signal to T cells early in the activation process. (Chapter 11)

CD81 *See* **B-cell co-receptor**. (Chapter 7)

CD84 *See* **SLAM**. (Chapter 10)

CD86 (B7-2) A transmembrane protein of the immunoglobulin superfamily that is expressed on antigen-presenting cells and binds to CD28 expressed by T cells. (Chapter 6)

CD94 A C-type lectin that is a subunit of the killer cell lectin-like receptors (KLRs) of NK cells. (Chapter 3)

CD103 Integrin $\alpha_E\beta_7$, a cell-surface marker on a subset of dendritic cells in the gastrointestinal tract that are involved in inducing tolerance to antigens from food and the commensal microbiota. Note that CD103 is often used to refer to the $\alpha_E\beta_7$ heterodimer despite strictly referring only to the α_E molecule. *See* α_E **integrin**. (Chapter 9)

CD127 Also known as IL-7 receptor α (IL-7Rα), which pairs with the common γ chain of the IL-2 receptor family to form the IL-7 receptor. It is expressed by naive T cells and a subset of memory T cells to support their survival. (Chapter 11)

cDC1 Type 1 conventional dendritic cell. A subset of conventional dendritic cell (cDC) that is specialized for the priming of CD8 T cells and for recruiting CD4 T-cell help for CD8 T-cell priming. These cDCs are responsible for cross-priming. (Chapter 9)

cDC2 Type 2 conventional dendritic cell. A subset of conventional dendritic cell (cDC) that is specialized for the priming of CD4 T cells. (Chapter 9)

celiac disease A chronic condition of the upper small intestine caused by an immune response directed at gluten, a complex of proteins present in wheat, oats, and barley. The gut wall becomes chronically inflamed, the villi are destroyed, and the gut's ability to absorb nutrients is compromised. (Chapters 12, 14)

cell-adhesion molecules Cell-surface proteins of several different types that mediate the binding of one cell to other cells or to extracellular matrix proteins. Integrins, selectins, and members of the immunoglobulin gene superfamily (such as ICAM-1) are among the cell-adhesion molecules important in the operation of the immune system. (Chapter 3)

cell-mediated immune responses An adaptive immune response in which antigen-specific effector T cells have the main role. The immunity to infection conferred by such a response is called cell-mediated immunity. A primary cell-mediated immune response is the T-cell response that occurs the first time a particular antigen is encountered. (Chapter 1)

cell-mediated immunity Immunity that can be transferred to a recipient individual by transfer of lymphocytes, but not by transfer of serum, from an immune donor. (Appendix I)

cellular hypersensitivity reactions A hypersensitivity reaction mediated largely by antigen-specific T lymphocytes. (Chapter 14)

cellular immunology The study of the cellular basis of immunity. (Chapter 1)

cellular tropism The host-cell types that are infected by a particular pathogen. (Chapter 12)

central lymphoid organs, central lymphoid tissues The sites of lymphocyte development; in humans, these are the bone marrow and thymus. B lymphocytes develop in bone marrow, whereas T lymphocytes develop within the thymus from bone marrow–derived progenitors. Also called the primary lymphoid organs and tissues. (Chapters 1, 8)

central memory T (T$_{CM}$) cells Memory lymphocytes that express CCR7 and recirculate between blood and secondary lymphoid tissues similarly to naive T cells. They require restimulation in secondary lymphoid tissues to become fully mature effector T cells. (Chapter 11)

central tolerance Immunological tolerance to self antigens that is established while lymphocytes are developing in central lymphoid organs. Cf. **peripheral tolerance**. (Chapters 8, 9, 15)

centroblasts Large, rapidly dividing activated B cells present in the dark zone of germinal centers in follicles of peripheral lymphoid organs. (Chapter 10)

centrocytes Small B cells that derive from centroblasts in the germinal centers of follicles in peripheral lymphoid organs; they populate the light zone of the germinal center. (Chapter 10)

cGAS (cyclic GAMP synthase) A cytosolic enzyme that is activated by double-stranded DNA to form cyclic guanosine monophosphate–adenosine monophosphate. *See* **cyclic dinucleotides (CDNs)**. (Chapter 3)

Charcot–Leyden crystals These result from the crystallization in tissues of the abundant protein galectin-10, which is abundantly produced by eosinophils. In chronic inflammation where eosinophils accumulate and die, this protein may acquire a crystalline form, which appears to be inherently inflammatory because of direct NLRP3 activation, thus producing positive feedback that may perpetuate the allergic state. (Chapter 14)

checkpoint blockade Approach to tumor therapy that attempts to interfere with the normal inhibitory signals that regulate lymphocytes. (Chapters 7, 13, 16)

checkpoint inhibitors Cancer therapeutics that target immune checkpoints to activate immune responses against cancers that have evaded immune attack by triggering immune checkpoints. (Chapter 9)

Chediak–Higashi syndrome A defect in phagocytic cell function caused by a defect in a protein involved in intracellular vesicle fusion. Lysosomes fail to fuse properly with phagosomes, and killing of ingested bacteria is impaired. (Chapter 13)

chemokines Small chemoattractant proteins that stimulate the migration and activation of cells, especially phagocytic cells and lymphocytes. Chemokines have a central role in inflammatory responses. Properties of individual chemokines are listed in eAppendix IV. (Chapters 1, 3)

chemotaxis Cellular movement occurring in response to chemical signals in the environment. (Chapter 3)

chimeric antigen receptor (CAR) Engineered fusion proteins composed of extracellular antigen-specific receptors (e.g., single-chain antibody) and intracellular signaling domains that activate and co-stimulate; expressed in T cells for use in cancer immunotherapy. (Chapter 16)

chronic allograft vasculopathy Chronic damage that can lead to late failure of transplanted organs. Arteriosclerosis of graft blood vessels leads to hypoperfusion of the graft and its eventual fibrosis and atrophy. (Chapter 15)

chronic granulomatous disease (CGD) An immunodeficiency in which multiple granulomas form as a result of defective elimination of bacteria by phagocytic cells. It is caused by defects in the NADPH oxidase system of enzymes that generate the superoxide radical involved in bacterial killing. (Chapters 3, 13)

chronic infantile neurologic cutaneous and articular syndrome (CINCA) An autoinflammatory disease that is due to defects in the gene *NLRP3*, which encodes one of the components of the inflammasome. (Chapter 13)

chronic rejection Late failure of a transplanted organ, which can be due to immunological or non-immunological causes. (Chapter 15)

CIIV (MHC class II vesicle) An early endocytic compartment containing MHC class II molecules in dendritic cells. (Chapter 6)

circulating vaccine-derived poliovirus (cVDPV) A form of poliovirus that arises from a mutation in the vaccine strain of poliovirus (frequently type 2 oral vaccine strain) that causes the reversion of the vaccine strain to acquire enhanced capacity for replication. This allows it to spread within unvaccinated populations. (Chapter 16)

class I cytokine receptors A group of receptors for the hematopoietin superfamily of cytokines. These include receptors using the common β chain for IL-2, IL-4, IL-7, IL-15, and IL-21, and a common β chain for GM-CSF, IL-3, and IL-5. (Chapter 3)

class II–associated invariant chain peptide (CLIP) A peptide of variable length cleaved from the invariant chain (Ii) by proteases. It remains associated with the MHC class II molecule in an unstable form until it is removed by the HLA-DM protein. (Chapter 6)

class II cytokine receptors A group of heterodimeric receptors for a family of cytokines that includes interferon (IFN)-α, IFN-β, IFN-γ, and IL-10.

classes The class of an antibody is defined by the type of heavy chain it contains. There are five main antibody classes: IgA, IgD, IgM, IgG, and IgE, containing heavy chains α, δ, μ, γ, and ε, respectively. The IgG class has several subclasses. *See also* **isotypes**. (Chapters 1, 4, 10)

classical C3 convertase The complex of activated complement components C4b2a, which cleaves C3 to C3b on pathogen surfaces in the classical pathway of complement activation. (Chapter 2)

classical MHC class I genes MHC class I genes whose proteins function by presenting peptide antigens for recognition by T cells. Cf. **nonclassical MHC class Ib genes**. (Chapter 5)

classical monocyte The major form of monocyte in circulation capable of recruitment to sites of inflammation and differentiation into macrophages. (Chapter 3)

classical pathway The complement-activation pathway that is initiated by C1 binding either directly to bacterial surfaces or to antibody bound to the bacteria, thus flagging the bacteria as foreign. *See also* **alternative pathway**, **lectin pathway**. (Chapters 2, 10)

classically activated macrophage *See* **M1 macrophages**. (Chapter 11)

class switching, class switch recombination A somatic gene recombination process in activated B cells that replaces one heavy-chain constant region with one of a different isotype, switching the isotype of antibodies from IgM to the production of IgG, IgA, or IgE. This affects the antibody effector functions but not their antigen specificity. Also known as isotype switching. Cf. **somatic hypermutation**. (Chapters 5, 10)

cleavage stimulation factor A multi-subunit protein complex involved in the modification of the 3′ end of pre-messenger RNA for the addition of the polyadenine (polyA) tail. (Chapter 5)

CLEC9A A cell-surface receptor expressed by type 1 conventional dendritic cells (cDC1) and which recognizes filamentous actin to enhance the uptake of dead cells, such as those killed during viral infections, thus contributing to antigen processing of viral proteins. (Chapter 6)

clonal contraction The phase of the T-cell infection response whereby most of the T-cell population dies via apoptosis, and the remaining 5–10% persists to seed a long-term memory T-cell population. (Chapters 9, 11)

clonal deletion The elimination of immature lymphocytes when they bind to self antigens, which produces tolerance to self as required by the clonal selection theory of adaptive immunity. Clonal deletion is the main mechanism of central tolerance and can also occur in peripheral tolerance. (Chapters 1, 8)

clonal expansion The proliferation of antigen-specific lymphocytes in response to antigenic stimulation that precedes their differentiation into effector cells. It is an essential step in adaptive immunity, allowing rare antigen-specific cells to increase in number so that they can effectively combat the pathogen that elicited the response. (Chapters 1, 9)

clonal selection theory The central paradigm of adaptive immunity. It states that adaptive immune responses derive from individual antigen-specific lymphocytes that are self-tolerant. These specific lymphocytes proliferate in response to antigen and differentiate into antigen-specific effector cells that eliminate the eliciting pathogen and into memory cells to sustain immunity. The theory was formulated by Frank Macfarlane Burnet and in earlier forms by Niels K. Jerne and David Talmage. (Chapter 1)

clone A population of cells all derived from the same progenitor cell. (Chapter 1, Appendix I)

clonotypic Describes a feature unique to members of a clone. For example, the distribution of antigen receptors in the lymphocyte population is said to be clonotypic, as the cells of a given clone all have identical antigen receptors. (Chapters 1, 4)

Clostridium difficile Gram-positive anaerobic toxogenic spore-forming bacterium frequently associated with severe colitis after treatment with certain broad-spectrum antibiotics. (Chapter 12)

club cells Columnar cells that are decorated with microvilli and are found in the small airways of the lungs, where they protect the bronchiolar epithelium through a variety of secretory molecules. (Chapter 12)

c-Maf A transcription factor acting in the development of T_{FH} cells. (Chapter 10)

coagulation system A collection of proteases and other proteins in the blood that trigger blood clotting when blood vessels are damaged. (Chapter 3)

coding joint DNA joint formed by the imprecise joining of a V gene segment to a DJ gene segment during recombination of the immunoglobulin or T-cell receptor genes. It is the joint retained in the rearranged gene. Cf. **signal joint**. (Chapter 5)

codominant Describes the situation in which the two alleles of a gene are expressed in roughly equal amounts in the heterozygote. Most genes show this property, including the highly polymorphic MHC genes. (Chapter 6)

co-immunoprecipitation An extension of the immunoprecipitation technique aimed at determining the proteins that physically interact with the target protein recognized by the immunoprecipitating antibody. *See also* **immunoprecipitation**. (Appendix I)

'cold' pyogenic infection Infection by pyogenic bacteria, such as *Staphylococcus aureus*, that elicits little or no inflammation in individuals with inherited deficiency of signaling molecules normally activated downstream of TLRs and IL-1 family receptors (e.g., MyD88 or IRAK4). (Chapter 13)

collectins A family of calcium-dependent sugar-binding proteins (lectins) containing collagen-like sequences. An example is mannose-binding lectin (MBL). (Chapter 2)

colonization resistance The ability of a healthy microbiota to resist incursion of new microbial species, including potential pathogens, thereby contributing to general host defense. Multiple mechanisms may be contributory, including nutrient competition and production of antimicrobial products. (Chapter 12)

combinatorial diversity The diversity among antigen receptors generated by combining separate units of genetic information, comprising two types. First, receptor gene segments are joined in many different combinations to generate diverse receptor chains; second, two different receptor chains (heavy and light in immunoglobulins; α and β, or γ and δ, in T-cell receptors) are combined to make the antigen-recognition site. (Chapters 1, 4, 5)

commensal bacteria *See* **commensal microbiota**. (Chapter 2)

commensal microbiota, commensal microorganisms Microorganisms (predominantly bacteria) that normally live harmlessly in symbiosis with their host (e.g., the gut bacteria in humans and other animals). Many commensals confer a positive benefit on their host in some way. (Chapters 1, 8)

common β chain ($β_c$) A transmembrane polypeptide (CD131) that is a common subunit for receptors of the cytokines IL-3, IL-5, and GM-CSF. (Chapter 3)

common γ chain ($γ_c$) A transmembrane polypeptide chain (CD132) that is common to a subgroup of cytokine receptors. (Chapter 3)

common lymphoid progenitor (CLP) Stem cell that can give rise to all the types of lymphocytes but is biased toward producing B cells. (Chapters 1, 3)

common mucosal immune system The mucosal immune system as a whole, the name reflecting the fact that lymphocytes that have been primed in one part of the mucosal system can recirculate as effector cells to other parts of the mucosal system. (Chapter 12)

common myeloid progenitor (CMP) Stem cell that can give rise to the myeloid cells of the immune system (the macrophages, granulocytes, mast cells, and dendritic cells of the innate immune system). This stem cell also gives rise to megakaryocytes and red blood cells. (Chapter 1)

common variable immunodeficiencies (CVIDs) Relatively common deficiencies in antibody production in which only one or a few isotypes are affected. CVIDs can be due to a variety of genetic defects. (Chapter 13)

competitive inhibition assay An assay to determine the presence as well as the amount of antigen in a sample of unknown composition. The assay is based on the ability of antigen in the sample, if present, to compete with a known amount of that antigen, but labeled, for binding to a specific antibody. (Appendix I)

complement A set of plasma proteins that act together as a defense against pathogens in extracellular spaces. The pathogen becomes coated with complement proteins that facilitate its removal by phagocytes and that can also kill certain pathogens directly. Activation of the complement system can be initiated in several different ways. *See* **classical pathway, alternative pathway, lectin pathway**. (Chapters 1, 2)

complement activation The activation of the normally inactive proteins of the complement system that occurs on infection. *See* **classical pathway, alternative pathway, lectin pathway**. (Chapters 1, 2, 10)

complement proteins *See* **C1, C2, C3,** etc. (Chapter 2)

complement receptors (CRs) Cell-surface proteins of various types that recognize and bind complement proteins that have become bound to an antigen such as a pathogen. Complement receptors on phagocytes enable them to identify and bind pathogens coated with complement proteins and to ingest and destroy them. *See* **CR1, CR2, CR3, CR4, CRIg,** and the **C1 complex**. (Chapters 1, 2)

complement-regulatory proteins Proteins that control complement activity and prevent complement from being activated on the surfaces of host cells. (Chapter 2)

complement system A set of plasma proteins that act together as a defense against pathogens in extracellular spaces. The pathogen becomes coated with complement proteins that facilitate its removal by phagocytes and which can also kill certain pathogens directly. Activation of the complement system can be initiated in several different ways. *See* **classical pathway, alternative pathway, lectin pathway**. (Chapter 2)

complementarity-determining regions (CDRs) Parts of the V domains of immunoglobulins and T-cell receptors that determine their antigen specificity and make contact with the specific ligand. The CDRs are the most variable part of the antigen receptor and contribute to the diversity of these proteins. There are three such regions (CDR1, CDR2, and CDR3) in each V domain. (Chapters 4, 5)

confocal fluorescent microscope A confocal microscope outfitted to capture fluorescent emission signals. Confocal microscopy provides enhanced image resolution over standard light microscopy by using a small, highly focused beam of light to produce images with reduced out-of-focus light interference. (Appendix I)

conformational epitope, discontinuous epitope Antigenic structure (epitope) on a protein antigen that is formed from several separate regions in the sequence of the protein brought together by protein folding. Antibodies that bind conformational epitopes bind only native folded proteins. (Chapter 4)

congenic Two individuals, usually mice, that are genetically identical at all loci with the exception of a single gene. (Appendix I)

conjugate vaccines Antibacterial vaccines made from bacterial capsular polysaccharides bound to proteins of known immunogenicity, such as tetanus toxoid. (Chapter 16)

constant Ig domains (C domains) Type of protein domain that makes up the constant regions of each chain of an immunoglobulin molecule. (Chapter 4)

constant region (C region) That part of an immunoglobulin or a T-cell receptor that is relatively constant in amino acid sequence between different molecules. Also known as the Fc region in antibodies. The constant region of an antibody determines its particular effector function. Cf. **variable region**. (Chapters 1, 4)

continuous epitope, linear epitope Antigenic structure (epitope) in a protein that is formed by a single small region of amino acid sequence.

Antibodies that bind continuous epitopes can bind to the denatured protein. The epitopes detected by T cells are continuous. (Chapter 4)

contraction phase   The period of the clonal lymphocyte response (T or B cell) that is marked by the rapid decline of daughter-cell numbers after pathogen clearance and decline in the antigenic load. (Chapter 11)

conventional (or **classical**) **dendritic cells (cDCs)**   The lineage of dendritic cells that mainly participates in antigen presentation to, and activation of, naive T cells. Cf. **plasmacytoid dendritic cells**. (Chapters 3, 9)

co-receptor   Cell-surface protein that increases the sensitivity of a receptor to its ligand by binding to associated ligands and participating in signaling. The antigen receptors on T cells and B cells act in conjunction with co-receptors, which are either CD4 or CD8 on T cells, and a co-receptor complex of three proteins, one of which is the complement receptor CR2, on B cells. (Chapters 1, 4)

coronavirus disease-2019 (COVID-19)   A respiratory illness caused by SARS-CoV-2, likely of zoonotic origin and responsible for the COVID-19 pandemic. (Chapter 12)

coronavirus spike protein (S)   The coronavirus surface protein that binds host-cell receptors to mediate viral entry. (Chapter 12)

cortex   The outer part of a tissue or organ; in lymph nodes it refers to the follicles, which are mainly populated by B cells. (Chapter 1)

corticosteroids   Family of drugs related to natural steroids such as cortisone. Corticosteroids can kill lymphocytes, especially developing thymocytes, inducing apoptotic cell death. They are medically useful anti-inflammatory and immunosuppressive agents. (Chapter 16)

co-stimulatory molecules   Cell-surface proteins on antigen-presenting cells that deliver co-stimulatory signals to naive T cells. Examples are the B7 molecules on dendritic cells, which are ligands for CD28 on naive T cells. (Chapters 1, 3)

co-stimulatory receptors   Cell-surface receptors on naive lymphocytes through which the cells receive signals additional to those received through the antigen receptor, and which are necessary for the full activation of the lymphocyte. Examples are CD30 and CD40 on B cells and CD27 and CD28 on T cells. (Chapters 3, 7)

CR1 (CD35)   A receptor expressed by phagocytic cells that binds to C3b. It stimulates phagocytosis and inhibits C3 convertase formation on host-cell surfaces. It also acts in conjunction with factor I to cleave C3b to its inactive derivative iC3b and thus prevent convertase formation. (Chapter 2)

CR2 (CD21)   Complement receptor that is part of the B-cell co-receptor complex. It binds to antigens coated with breakdown products of C3b, especially C3dg, and, by cross-linking the B-cell receptor, enhances sensitivity to antigen at least 100-fold. It is also the receptor used by the Epstein–Barr virus to infect B cells. (Chapter 2)

CR3 (CD11b:CD18)   Complement receptor 3. A β2 integrin that acts both as an adhesion molecule and as a complement receptor. CR3 on phagocytes binds iC3b, a breakdown product of C3b on pathogen surfaces, and stimulates phagocytosis. (Chapters 2, 3)

CR4 (CD11c:CD18)   A β2 integrin that acts both as an adhesion molecule and as a complement receptor. CR4 on phagocytes binds iC3b, a breakdown product of C3b on pathogen surfaces, and stimulates phagocytosis. (Chapters 2, 3)

CRAC channel   Channels in the lymphocyte plasma membrane that open to let calcium flow into the cell during the response of the cell to antigen. Channel opening is induced by release of calcium from the endoplasmic reticulum. (Chapter 7)

C-reactive protein   An acute-phase protein that binds to phosphocholine, a constituent of the surface C-polysaccharide of the bacterium *Streptococcus*

pneumoniae and of many other bacteria, thus opsonizing them for uptake by phagocytes. (Chapter 3)

CRIg (complement receptor of the immunoglobulin superfamily)   A complement receptor that binds to inactivated forms of C3b. (Chapters 2, 10)

Crohn's disease   Chronic inflammatory bowel disease thought to result from an abnormal overresponsiveness to the commensal gut microbiota. (Chapters 3, 12, 15)

cross-matching   A test used in blood typing and histocompatibility typing to determine whether donor and recipient have antibodies against each other's cells that might interfere with successful transfusion or grafting. (Chapter 15)

cross-presentation   The process by which extracellular proteins taken up by dendritic cells can give rise to peptides presented by MHC class I molecules. It enables antigens from extracellular sources to be presented by MHC class I molecules and activate CD8 T cells. (Chapters 6, 9)

cross-priming   Activation of CD8 T cells by dendritic cells in which the antigenic peptide presented by MHC class I molecules is derived from an exogenous protein (i.e., by cross-presentation) rather than produced within the dendritic cells directly. Cf. **direct presentation**. (Chapters 6, 9)

cryptdins   α-Defensins (antimicrobial peptides) made by the Paneth cells of the small intestine. (Chapter 2)

cryptic epitopes   Any epitope that cannot be recognized by a lymphocyte receptor until the antigen has been broken down and processed. (Chapter 15)

cryptopatches   Aggregates of lymphoid tissue in the gut wall that are thought to give rise to isolated lymphoid follicles. (Chapter 12)

CstF-64   Subunit of cleavage stimulation factor that favors polyadenylation at pA_1 leading to the secreted form of IgM. (Chapter 5)

cTECs   Epithelial cells of the thymic cortex responsible for expression of MHC class I and class II proteins bearing self peptides involved in the selection of αβ T cells. (Chapter 8)

C-terminal Src kinase (Csk)   A kinase that phosphorylates the C-terminal tyrosine of Src family kinases in lymphocytes, thus inactivating them. (Chapter 7)

CTLA-4   A high-affinity inhibitory receptor on T cells for B7 molecules; its binding inhibits T-cell activation. (Chapters 7, 9)

C-type lectins   Large class of carbohydrate-binding proteins that require Ca^{2+} for binding, including many that function in innate immunity. (Chapter 2)

cutaneous lymphocyte antigen (CLA)   A cell-surface molecule that is involved in lymphocyte homing to the skin in humans. (Chapter 11)

CVIDs   *See* **common variable immunodeficiencies**. (Chapter 13)

CX3CR1   Chemokine receptor expressed by monocytes, macrophages, NK cells, and activated T cells that binds CX3CL1 (fractalkine). (Chapter 12)

CXC chemokines   One of the two main classes of chemokines, distinguished by a Cys-X-Cys (CXC) motif near the amino terminus. They have names CXCL1, CXCL2, etc. See eAppendix IV for a list of individual chemokines. (Chapter 3)

CXCL12 (SDF-1)   Chemokine produced by stromal cells in the dark zone of the germinal center that binds CXCR4 expressed by centroblasts. (Chapter 10)

CXCL13   Chemokine produced in the follicle and the light zone of the germinal center that binds CXCR5 expressed on circulating B cells and centrocytes. (Chapters 9, 10, 12)

CXCR5   A chemokine receptor expressed by circulating B cells and activated T cells that binds the chemokine CXCL13 and directs cell migration into the follicle. (Chapters 9, 10, 12)

cyclic dinucleotides (CDNs)   Cyclic dimers of guanylate and/or adenylate monophosphate that are produced by various bacteria as second messengers and detected by STING. (Chapter 3)

cyclic guanosine monophosphate–adenosine monophosphate (cyclic GMP–AMP, or cGAMP) *See* **cyclic dinucleotides (CDNs)**. (Chapter 3)

cyclic neutropenia A dominantly inherited disease in which neutrophil numbers fluctuate from near normal to very low or absent, with an approximate cycle time of 21 days. This is in contrast to severe congenital neutropenia (SCN), in which the inherited defect results in persistently low neutrophil numbers. (Chapter 13)

cyclic reentry model An explanation of the behavior of B cells in lymphoid follicles, proposing that activated B cells in germinal centers lose and gain expression of the chemokine receptor CXCR4 and thus move from the light zone to the dark zone and back again under the influence of the chemokine CXCL12. (Chapter 10)

cyclophilins A family of prolyl isomerases that affect protein folding and also bind cyclosporin A to produce a complex that associates with calcineurin, preventing its activation by calmodulin. (Chapter 16)

cyclophosphamide A DNA-alkylating agent that is used as an immunosuppressive drug. It acts by killing rapidly dividing cells, including lymphocytes proliferating in response to antigen. (Chapter 16)

cyclosporin A (CsA) A powerful noncytotoxic immunosuppressive drug that inhibits signaling from the T-cell receptor, preventing T-cell activation and effector function. It binds to cyclophilin, and the complex formed binds to and inactivates the phosphatase calcineurin. (Chapters 7, 16)

cystic fibrosis Disease caused by defect in the CFTR gene, leading to abnormally thick mucus and causing serious recurrent infections of the lung. (Chapter 2)

cytidine deaminase activity (CDA) An enzymatic activity exhibited by AID-APOBEC family proteins of agnathan species that may mediate rearrangement and assembly of complete VLR genes. (Chapter 5)

cytokines Proteins made by a cell that affect the behavior of other cells, particularly immune cells. Cytokines made by lymphocytes are often called interleukins (abbreviated ILs). Cytokines and their receptors are listed in eAppendix III. Cf. **chemokines**. (Chapters 1, 3)

cytomegalovirus UL16 protein A nonessential glycoprotein of cytomegalovirus that is recognized by innate receptors expressed by NK cells. (Chapter 3)

cytosol One of several major compartments within cells containing elements such as the cytoskeleton and mitochondria and separated by membranes from distinct compartments such as the nucleus and vesicular system. (Chapter 6)

cytotoxic T cells, cytotoxic T lymphocytes (CTLs) T cells that can kill other cells, typically CD8 T cells defending against intracellular pathogens that live or reproduce in the cytosol, but in some cases also CD4 T cells. (Chapters 1, 6, 9)

daclizumab Antibody to human CD25 used to block IL-2 receptor signaling in T cells for treatment of rejection in renal transplantation. (Chapter 16)

DAG *See* **diacylglycerol**. (Chapters 6, 7)

damage-associated molecular patterns (DAMPs) *See* **pathogen-associated molecular patterns (PAMPs)**. (Chapter 3)

DAP10, DAP12 Signaling chains containing ITAMs that are associated with the tails of some activating receptors on NK cells. (Chapter 3)

dark zone A region of a germinal center enriched in rapidly dividing activated B cells. (Chapter 10)

DC-SIGN A lectin on the dendritic-cell surface that binds ICAM-3 with high affinity. (Chapter 9)

death domain A protein domain involved in protein–protein interactions with death domains in other proteins. The death domain was first identified in proteins involved in apoptosis. (Chapter 3)

death-inducing signaling complex (DISC) A multiprotein complex that is formed by signaling through members of the 'death receptor' family of apoptosis-inducing cellular receptors, such as Fas. It activates the caspase cascade to induce apoptosis. (Chapters 9, 11)

decay-accelerating factor (DAF or CD55) A cell-surface protein that protects cells from lysis by complement. Its absence causes the disease paroxysmal nocturnal hemoglobinuria. (Chapter 2)

Dectin-1 A phagocytic receptor on neutrophils and macrophages that recognizes β-(1,3)–linked glucans, which are common components of fungal cell walls. (Chapters 3, 9, 12)

defective ribosomal products (DRiPs) Peptides translated from introns in improperly spliced mRNAs, translations of frameshifts, or improperly folded proteins, which are recognized and tagged by ubiquitin for degradation by the proteasome. (Chapter 6)

defensins *See* **α-defensins, β-defensins**. (Chapter 2)

delayed-type hypersensitivity (DTH) A form of cell-mediated immunity elicited by antigen in the skin stimulating sensitized T_H1 CD4 lymphocytes and CD8 lymphocytes. It is called delayed-type hypersensitivity because the reaction appears hours to days after antigen is injected. Referred to as type IV hypersensitivity in the historic Gell and Coombs classification. (Chapters 11, 14)

dendritic cells Bone marrow–derived cells found in most tissues, including lymphoid tissues. There are two main functional subsets. Conventional dendritic cells take up antigen in peripheral tissues, are activated by contact with pathogens, and travel to the peripheral lymphoid organs, where they are the most potent stimulators of T-cell responses. Plasmacytoid dendritic cells can also take up and present antigen, but their main function in an infection is to produce large amounts of the antiviral interferons as a result of pathogen recognition through receptors such as TLRs. Both these types of dendritic cells are distinct from the follicular dendritic cell that presents antigen to B cells in lymphoid follicles. (Chapters 1, 3)

dendritic epidermal T cells (DETCs) A specialized class of γδ T cells found in the skin of mice and some other species, but not humans. They express $V_\gamma 5V_\delta 1$ and may interact with ligands such as Skint-1 expressed by keratinocytes. (Chapters 6, 8)

dephosphorylation The removal of a phosphate group from a molecule, usually a protein. (Chapter 7)

depleting antibodies Immunosuppressive monoclonal antibodies that trigger the destruction of lymphocytes *in vivo*. They are used for treating episodes of acute graft rejection. (Chapter 16)

Der p 1 A cysteine protease that is present in the feces of the house dust mite, *Dermatophagoides pteronyssinus*. Der p 1 induces an allergic reaction, likely through its ability to cleave the intercellular tight-junction protein occludin that is present in the airway mucosa. (Chapter 14)

diacyl and triacyl lipoproteins Ligands for the Toll-like receptors TLR-1–TLR-2 and TLR-2–TLR-6. (Chapter 3)

diacylglycerol (DAG) A lipid intracellular signaling molecule formed from membrane inositol phospholipids that are cleaved by the action of phospholipase C-γ after the activation of many different receptors. The diacylglycerol stays in the membrane and activates protein kinase C and RasGRP, which further propagate the signal. (Chapters 6, 7)

diapedesis The movement of blood cells, particularly leukocytes, from the blood across blood vessel walls into tissues. (Chapter 3)

differentiation antigens Referring to a category of genes with restricted expression patterns that can be targeted as antigens by immunotherapies in treatment of cancers. (Chapter 16)

DiGeorge syndrome Recessive genetic immunodeficiency disease in which there is a failure to develop thymic epithelium. Parathyroid glands are also absent, and there are anomalies in the large blood vessels. (Chapters 8, 13)

direct allorecognition   Host recognition of a grafted tissue that involves host T-cell recognition of donor antigen-presenting cells (APCs) directly without antigen processing by host APCs.   This may occur in the graft itself, or upon the migration of donor APCs from the graft to   regional lymph nodes, where they may activate host T cells. (Chapter 15)

direct Coombs test   This assay directly tests for antibodies bound to the surface of cells and is used to detect maternal anti-Rh IgG bound to fetal red blood cells. Anti-human immunoglobulin antibodies are mixed with the cells. If the red blood cells agglutinate, this indicates that they are coated with maternal antibodies. (Appendix I)

direct presentation   The process by which proteins produced within a given cell give rise to peptides presented by MHC class I molecules. This may refer to antigen-presenting cells, such as dendritic cells, or to nonimmune cells that will become the targets of cytotoxic T lymphocytes (CTLs). (Chapter 6)

dislocation   In reference to viral defense mechanisms, the degradation of newly synthesized MHC class I molecules by viral proteins. (Chapter 13)

disseminated intravascular coagulation (DIC)   Blood clotting occurring simultaneously in small vessels throughout the body in response to disseminated TNF-α, which leads to the massive consumption of clotting proteins, so that the individual's blood cannot clot appropriately. Seen in septic shock. (Chapter 3)

diversity gene segment, D_H gene segment   Short DNA sequences that form a join between the V and J gene segments in rearranged immunoglobulin heavy-chain genes and in T-cell receptor β- and δ-chain genes. *See* **gene segments**. (Chapter 5)

DN1, DN2, DN3, DN4   Stages in the development of CD4$^+$CD8$^+$ double-positive T cells in the thymus. Rearrangement of the TCR β-chain locus starts at DN2 and is completed by DN4. (Chapter 8)

DNA-dependent protein kinase (DNA-PK)   Protein kinase in the DNA repair pathway involved in the rearrangement of immunoglobulin and T-cell receptor genes. (Chapter 5)

DNA ligase IV   Enzyme responsible for joining the DNA ends to produce the coding joint during V(D)J recombination. (Chapter 5)

DNA transposons   Genetic elements encoding their own transposase that can insert themselves into and excise themselves from the DNA genomes of a host. (Chapter 5)

DNA vaccination   Vaccination by introduction into skin and muscle of DNA encoding the desired antigen; the expressed protein can then elicit antibody and T-cell responses. (Chapter 16)

donor lymphocyte infusion (DLI)   Transfer of mature lymphocytes (i.e., T cells) from donor into patient during bone marrow transplantation for cancer treatment to help eliminate residual tumor. (Chapter 16)

double-negative thymocytes   Immature T cells in the thymus that lack expression of the two co-receptors CD4 and CD8 and represent the progenitors to the remaining T cells developing in the thymus. In a normal thymus, these represent about 5% of thymocytes. (Chapter 8)

double-positive thymocytes   Immature T cells in the thymus that are characterized by expression of both the CD4 and the CD8 co-receptor proteins. They represent the majority (about 80%) of thymocytes and are the progenitors to the mature CD4 and CD8 T cells. (Chapter 8)

double-strand break repair (DSBR)   A nonhomologous end joining pathway of DNA repair used in the completion of isotype switching. (Chapter 5)

double-stranded RNA (dsRNA)   A chemical structure that is a replicative intermediate of many viruses and is recognized by TLR-3. (Chapter 3)

Down syndrome cell adhesion molecule (Dscam)   *See* **Dscam**.

DR4, DR5   Members of the TNFR superfamily expressed by many cell types and which can be activated by TRAIL to induce apoptosis. (Chapter 3)

draining lymph node   A lymph node downstream of a site of infection that receives antigens and microbes from the site via the lymphatic system. Draining lymph nodes often enlarge enormously during an immune response and can be palpated; they were originally called swollen glands. (Chapter 1)

Dscam   A member of the immunoglobulin superfamily that in insects is thought to opsonize invading bacteria and aid their engulfment by phagocytes. It can be made in a multiplicity of different forms as a result of alternative splicing. (Chapter 5)

dysbiosis   Altered balance of microbial species composing the microbiota resulting from a variety of causes (e.g., antibiotics, genetic disorders) and frequently associated with outgrowth of pathogenic organisms such as *Clostridium difficile*. (Chapter 12)

dysregulated self   Refers to changes that take place in infected or malignant cells that alter expression of various surface receptors that can be detected by the innate immune system. (Chapter 3)

E3 ligase   An enzymatic activity that directs the transfer of a ubiquitin molecule from an E2 ubiquitin-conjugating enzyme onto a specific protein target. (Chapters 6, 10)

early innate lymphoid progenitor (EILP)   A subset of progenitor cells arising from LMPPs.   EILPs give rise to the three lineages of innate lymphoid cells, ILC1 (including NK cells), ILC2, and ILC3. (Chapter 8)

early-onset sarcoidosis   Disease associated with activating NOD2 mutations characterized by inflammation in tissues such as liver. (Chapter 3)

early pro-B cell   *See* **pro-B cells**. (Chapter 8)

early thymic progenitor (ETP)   The major subset of progenitor cells that gives rise to T cells. (Chapter 8)

EBI2 (GPR183)   A chemokine receptor that binds oxysterols and regulates B-cell movement to the outer follicular and interfollicular regions during early phases of B-cell activation in lymphoid tissues. (Chapter 10)

edema   Swelling caused by the entry of fluid and cells from the blood into the tissues; it is one of the cardinal features of inflammation. (Chapter 3)

effector caspases   Intracellular proteases that are activated as a result of an apoptotic signal and mediate the cellular changes associated with apoptosis. To be distinguished from initiator caspases, which act upstream of effector caspases to initiate the caspase cascade. (Chapter 9)

effector CD4 T cells   The subset of differentiated effector T cells carrying the CD4 co-receptor molecule, which includes the T_H1, T_H2, T_H17, and regulatory T cells. (Chapter 6)

effector lymphocytes   The cells that differentiate from naive lymphocytes after initial activation by antigen and can then mediate the removal of pathogens from the body without further differentiation. They are distinct from memory lymphocytes, which must undergo further differentiation to become effector lymphocytes. (Chapter 1)

effector mechanisms   Those processes by which pathogens are destroyed and cleared from the body. Innate and adaptive immune responses use most of the same effector mechanisms to eliminate pathogens. (Chapter 1)

effector memory T (TEM) cells   Memory lymphocytes that recirculate between blood and peripheral tissues and are specialized for rapid maturation into effector T cells after restimulation with antigen in nonlymphoid tissues. (Chapter 11)

effector module   A collection of cell-mediated and humoral mechanisms that involve components of both the innate and adaptive immune systems. These mechanisms act together to achieve elimination of a particular category of pathogen. (Chapter 1)

effector regulatory T (eT_reg) cells T_reg cells that have received additional differentiative signals that cause them to migrate into peripheral tissues where they can regulate effector T-cell response. A signature cytokine of eT_reg cells is IL-10. (Chapters 9, 12)

effector T lymphocytes, effector T cells The T cells that perform the functions of an immune response (such as cell killing and cell activation) that clear the infectious agent from the body. There are several different subsets, each with a specific role in an immune response. (Chapters 1, 9)

efferocytosis The process of removal of apoptotic cells by phagocytes (from the Latin *effere*, meaning 'to take to the grave'). (Chapter 12)

electrostatic interaction Chemical interaction occurring between charged atoms, as in the charged amino acid side chains and an ion in a salt bridge. (Chapter 4)

elimination phase Stage of antitumor immune response that detects and eliminates cancer cells, also called immune surveillance. (Chapter 16)

ELISPOT assay A technique for enumerating lymphocytes in a population capable of secreting effector molecules, such as cytokines or antibodies. In the case of T cells, antibodies to a cytokine of interest are coated onto a plastic culture well, and activated T cells are allowed to settle on the plate. If a given T cell is secreting the cytokine of interest, the cytokine will be captured by the antibody on the plate and will be localized to a discrete spot. This spot of cytokine can be detected with a colorimetric assay and the number of spots on the plate counted. For B cells, this technique can be used to enumerate antibody-secreting cells in a population. (Appendix I)

elite controllers A subset of HIV-infected, long-term nonprogressors who have clinically undetectable levels of virus without antiretroviral therapy. (Chapter 13)

ELL2 A transcription elongation factor that favors the polyadenylation at pA_1 leading to the secreted form of IgM. (Chapter 5)

embryonic stem cells (ES cells) A continually growing cell line that can give rise to all cell lineages in a mouse after implantation into a developing mouse embryo at the blastocyst stage. (Appendix I)

endocrine Describes the action of a biologically active molecule such as a hormone or cytokine that is secreted by one tissue into the blood and acts on a distant tissue. Cf. **autocrine**, **paracrine**. (Chapter 3)

endogenous pyrogens Cytokines that can induce a rise in body temperature. (Chapter 3)

endoplasmic reticulum aminopeptidase associated with antigen processing (ERAAP) Also called ERAP1. Enzyme in the endoplasmic reticulum that trims polypeptides to a size at which they can bind to MHC class I molecules. (Chapter 6)

endoplasmic reticulum–associated protein degradation (ERAD) A system of enzymes in the endoplasmic reticulum that recognizes incompletely or misfolded proteins and ensures their eventual degradation. (Chapter 6)

endosteum The region in bone marrow adjacent to the inner surface of the bone; hematopoietic stem cells are initially located there. (Chapter 8)

endothelial activation The changes that occur in the endothelial walls of small blood vessels as a result of inflammation, such as increased permeability and the increased production of cell-adhesion molecules and cytokines. (Chapter 3)

endothelial cell Cell type that forms the endothelium, the epithelium of a blood vessel wall. (Chapter 1)

endothelial protein C receptor (EPCR) A nonclassical MHC class I protein induced on endothelial cells that can interact with the blood coagulation factor XIV (protein C) and can be recognized by some γδ T cells. (Chapter 6)

endothelium The epithelium that forms the walls of blood capillaries and the lining of larger blood vessels. (Chapter 1)

endotoxins Toxins derived from bacterial cell walls released by damaged cells. They can potently induce cytokine synthesis and in large amounts can cause a systemic reaction called septic shock or endotoxic shock. (Chapter 2)

enterocytes The cells that line the intestines. Also known as intestinal epithelial cells, or IECs. There are two general subtypes: absorptive (e.g., absorptive enterocyte) and secretory (e.g., Paneth cells), both of which differentiate from intestinal stem cells located in the base of the crypts of the small and large intestines. (Chapter 12)

enteroendocrine cells (EECs) A broad family of specialized intestinal epithelial cells (IECs) that produce hormones in response to a number of stimuli. EECs compose the largest collection of endocrine cells in humans. The secreted products of different types of EECs can act locally, via the bloodstream, or via the enteric nervous system to coordinate responses with other cells. (Chapter 12)

enzyme-linked immunosorbent assay (ELISA) An assay to measure quantities of a specific compound, such as a viral protein, in a complex mixture such as serum. The sample being tested is adhered to an assay plate well, and the antigen concentration in the sample is determined by binding an enzyme-linked antibody. The amount of bound antibody is determined by adding the enzyme's substrate and measuring the accumulation of a reaction product derived from the substrate. (Appendix I)

eosinophilia An abnormally large number of eosinophils in the blood. (Chapter 14)

eosinophil A type of white blood cell containing granules that stain with eosin. It is thought to be important chiefly in defense against parasitic infections but is also medically important as an effector cell in allergic reactions. (Chapters 1, 3)

eotaxins CC chemokines that act predominantly on eosinophils, including CCL11 (eotaxin 1), CCL24 (eotaxin 2), and CCL26 (eotaxin 3). (Chapter 14)

epitope A site on an antigen recognized by an antibody or an antigen receptor. T-cell epitopes are short peptides bound to MHC molecules. B-cell epitopes are typically structural motifs on the surface of the antigen. Also called an antigenic determinant. (Chapters 1, 4)

epitope spreading Increase in diversity of responses to autoantigens as the response persists, as a result of responses being made to epitopes other than the original one. (Chapter 15)

equilibrium phase Stage of antitumor immune response when immunoediting allows the immune response to continually shape the antigenic character of cancer cells. (Chapter 16)

ERAP1 *See* **endoplasmic reticulum aminopeptidase associated with antigen processing (ERAAP)**. (Chapter 6)

ERAP2 Enzyme in the endoplasmic reticulum in human cells that trims polypeptides to a size at which they can bind to MHC class I molecules. (Chapter 6)

Erk (extracellular signal-related kinase) A protein kinase that is the MAPK for one module of the T-cell receptor signaling pathway. Erk also functions in other receptors in other cell types. (Chapter 7)

ERp57 A chaperone protein involved in loading peptide onto MHC class I molecules in the endoplasmic reticulum. (Chapter 6)

error-prone 'translesion' DNA polymerases A DNA polymerase operates during DNA repair, such as Polη, which can repair a basic lesion by incorporating untemplated nucleotides into the newly formed DNA strand. (Chapter 10)

escape mutants Mutants of pathogens that are changed in such a way that they can evade the immune response against the original pathogen. (Chapter 13)

escape phase Final stage of antitumor immune response when immunoediting has removed the expression of antigenic targets such that the cancer cells are no loner detected by the immune system. (Chapter 16)

E-selectin   *See* **selectins**. (Chapter 3)

etanercept   Fc fusion protein containing the p75 subunit of the TNF receptor that neutralizes TNF-α and is used for treatment of rheumatoid arthritis and other inflammatory diseases. (Chapter 16)

eukaryotic initiation factor 3 (eIF3)   Multi-subunit complex that acts in formation of the 43S pre-initiation complex. It can bind IFN-induced protein with tetratricoid repeats (IFIT) proteins, which thereby suppress translation of viral proteins. (Chapter 3)

exogenous pyrogen   Any substance originating outside the body that can induce fever, such as the bacterial lipopolysaccharide LPS. Cf. **endogenous pyrogens**. (Chapter 3)

exotoxin   A protein toxin produced and secreted by a bacterium. (Chapter 2)

expansion phase   The period of the clonal lymphocyte response (T or B cell) that is initiated after antigen recognition, during which there is rapid cell division and a marked increase in the number of daughter cells of individual lymphocyte clones that can contribute to the adaptive immune response. (Chapter 11)

experimental autoimmune encephalomyelitis (EAE)   An inflammatory disease of the central nervous system that develops after mice are immunized with neural antigens in a strong adjuvant. (Chapters 15, 16)

extrachromosomal DNA   DNA not contained within chromosomes, such as the circular DNA produced by V(D)J recombination occurring between RSSs in the same chromosomal orientation and eventually lost from the cell. (Chapter 5)

extravasation   The movement of cells or fluid from within blood vessels into the surrounding tissues. (Chapter 3)

extrinsic (or death receptor) pathway of apoptosis   A pathway triggered by extracellular ligands binding to specific cell-surface receptors (death receptors) that signal the cell to undergo programmed cell death (apoptosis). (Chapters 9, 11)

Fab fragment   Antibody fragment composed of a single antigen-binding arm of an antibody without the Fc region, produced by cleavage of IgG by the enzyme papain. It contains the complete light chain plus the amino-terminal variable region and first constant region of the heavy chain, held together by an interchain disulfide bond. (Chapter 4)

F(ab′)$_2$ fragment   Antibody fragment composed of two linked antigen-binding arms (Fab fragments) without the Fc regions, produced by cleavage of IgG with the enzyme pepsin. (Chapter 4)

factor B   Protein in the alternative pathway of complement activation, in which it is cleaved to Ba and an active protease, Bb, the latter binding to C3b to form the alternative pathway C3 convertase, C3bBb. (Chapter 2)

factor D   A serine protease in the alternative pathway of complement activation, which cleaves factor B into Ba and Bb. (Chapter 2)

factor H   Complement-regulatory protein in plasma that binds C3b and competes with factor B to displace Bb from the convertase. It also acts in conjunction with factor I to cleave C3b to its inactive derivative iC3b and thus prevent convertase formation. (Chapter 2)

factor H binding protein (fHbp)   A protein produced by the pathogen *Neisseria meningitidis* that recruits factor H to its membrane, thereby inactivating C3b deposited on its surface, and evading destruction by complement. (Chapter 2)

factor I   Complement-regulatory protease in plasma that cleaves C3b to the inactive derivative iC3b, thus preventing the formation of a C3 convertase. (Chapter 2)

factor I deficiency   A genetically determined lack of the complement-regulatory protein factor I. This results in uncontrolled complement activation, so that complement proteins rapidly become depleted. Those with the deficiency suffer repeated bacterial infections, especially with ubiquitous pyogenic bacteria. (Chapters 2, 13)

factor P   Plasma protein released by activated neutrophils that stabilizes the C3 convertase C3bBb of the alternative pathway. Also known as properdin. (Chapter 2)

familial cold autoinflammatory syndrome (FCAS)   An episodic autoinflammatory disease caused by gain-of-function mutations in the genes *NLRP3* or *NLRP12*, encoding NLRP3 or NLRP12, respectively, members of the NOD-like receptor family and components of inflammasomes. The symptoms are caused by unregulated overproduction of inflammatory cytokines and are induced by exposure to cold. (Chapter 3)

familial cold autoinflammatory syndrome 1 (FCAS1)   A form of FCAS caused by gain-of-function mutations in *NLRP3*. (Chapter 13)

familial cold autoinflammatory syndrome 2 (FCAS2)   A form of FCAS caused by gain-of-function mutations in *NLRP12*. (Chapter 13)

familial hemophagocytic lymphohistiocytosis (FHL)   A family of progressive and potentially lethal inflammatory diseases caused by an inherited deficiency of one of several proteins involved in the formation or release of cytolytic granules. Large numbers of polyclonal CD8-positive T cells accumulate in lymphoid and other organs, and this is associated with activated macrophages that phagocytose blood cells, including erythrocytes and leukocytes. (Chapter 13)

familial Mediterranean fever (FMF)   A severe autoinflammatory disease, inherited as an autosomal recessive disorder. It is caused by mutation in the gene (*MEFV*) that encodes the protein Pyrin, which is expressed in granulocytes and monocytes. In individuals with this disorder, defective Pyrin is thought to spontaneously activate inflammasomes. (Chapter 13)

farmer's lung   A hypersensitivity disease caused by the interaction of IgG antibodies with large amounts of an inhaled antigen in the alveolar wall of the lung, causing alveolar wall inflammation and compromising respiratory gas exchange. (Chapter 14)

Fc fragment, Fc region   The carboxy-terminal halves of the two heavy chains of an IgG molecule disulfide-bonded to each other by the residual hinge region. It is produced by cleavage of IgG by papain. In the complete antibody this portion is often called the Fc region. (Chapters 1, 4)

Fc receptors   Family of cell-surface receptors that bind the Fc portions of different immunoglobulins: Fcγ receptors bind IgG, for example, and Fcε receptors bind IgE. (Chapters 1, 10)

FCAS   *See* **familial cold autoinflammatory syndrome**. (Chapter 3)

FcγRI (CD64)   Fc receptor highly expressed by monocytes and macrophages that has the highest affinity of the Fc receptors for IgG. (Chapter 12)

FcγRIIB   An inhibitory receptor on B cells that recognizes the Fc portion of IgG antibodies. FcγRIIB contains an ITIM motif in its cytoplasmic tail. (Chapter 7)

FcγRIII   Cell-surface receptor that binds the Fc portion of IgG molecules. Most Fcγ receptors bind only aggregated IgG, allowing them to discriminate bound antibody from free IgG. Expressed variously on phagocytes, B lymphocytes, NK cells, and follicular dendritic cells, the Fcγ receptors have a key role in humoral immunity, linking antibody binding to effector cell functions. (Chapter 7)

FcεRI   The high-affinity receptor for the Fc region of IgE. Expressed primarily on the surface of mast cells and basophils. When multivalent antigen interacts with IgE that is bound to FcεRI and cross-links nearby receptors, it causes activation of the receptor-bearing cell. (Chapter 14)

FcRn (neonatal Fc receptor)   A receptor that transports IgG from mother to fetus across the placenta and across other epithelia such as the epithelium of the gut. (Chapters 10, 12)

fecal microbiota transplantation (FMT)   The transfer of healthy donor stool (i.e., a healthy intestinal microbiota) to an individual with a damaged microbiota via colonoscopy, enema, nasoenteric tube, or capsules. FMT can be curative in treatment of some diseases, such as recurrent *C. difficile* infection caused by a broad-spectrum antibiotic, by engrafting a healthy microbiota that displaces a dysbiotic one. (Chapter 12)

FHL   *See* **familial hemophagocytic lymphohistiocytosis**. (Chapter 13)

fibrinogen-related proteins (FREPs)   Members of the immunoglobulin superfamily that are thought to have a role in innate immunity in the freshwater snail *Biomphalaria glabrata*. (Chapter 5)

fibroblast reticular cells (FRCs)   A lymph node stromal cell found in the T-cell zone of the lymph node cortex. FRCs create networks of collagen-rich reticular fibers that guide dendritic cells, T lymphocytes, and B lymphocytes in the lymphoid tissue. (Chapter 9)

ficolins   Carbohydrate-binding proteins that can initiate the lectin pathway of complement activation. They are members of the collectin family and bind to the *N*-acetylglucosamine present on the surface of some pathogens. (Chapter 2)

fingolimod   Small-molecule immunosuppressive drug that interferes with the actions of sphingosine, leading to retention of effector T cells in lymphoid organs. (Chapter 16)

FK506   *See* **tacrolimus**. (Chapters 7, 16)

FK-binding proteins (FKBPs)   Group of prolyl isomerases related to the cyclophilins and which bind the immunosuppressive drug tacrolimus (FK506). (Chapter 16)

flagellin   A protein that is the major constituent of the flagellum, the tail-like structure used in bacterial locomotion. TLR-5 recognizes intact flagellin protein that has dissociated from the flagellum. (Chapter 12)

fluid-phase C3 convertase   Short-lived alternative pathway C3 convertase, C3(H$_2$O)Bb, that is continually produced at a low level in the plasma that can initiate activation of the alternative pathway of complement activation. (Chapter 2)

fluorescence-activated cell sorter (FACS)   An instrument that assesses the presence of fluorescently tagged antibodies on each cell in a complex mixture using a laser that excites the fluorescent tags and detectors to measure the emission from each fluorochrome. The fluorescent signal derived from each cell can be used for analytical purposes or can be used to divert cells with a desired fluorescent signal into a collection tube for isolation. (Appendix I)

fMet-Leu-Phe (fMLF) receptor   A pattern-recognition receptor for the peptide fMet-Leu-Phe, which is specific to bacteria, on neutrophils and macrophages. fMet-Leu-Phe acts as a chemoattractant. (Chapter 3)

follicle-associated epithelium (FAE)   Specialized epithelium separating the lymphoid tissues of the gut wall from the intestinal lumen. As well as enterocytes it contains microfold cells, through which antigens enter the lymphoid organs from the gut. (Chapter 12)

follicles   An area of predominantly B cells in a peripheral lymphoid organ, such as a lymph node, which also contains follicular dendritic cells. (Chapter 1)

follicular B cells   The majority population of long-lived recirculating conventional B cells found in the blood, the spleen, and the lymph nodes. Also known as B-2 B cells. (Chapter 8)

follicular dendritic cell (FDC)   A cell type of uncertain origin in B-cell follicles of peripheral lymphoid organs that captures antigen:antibody complexes using non-internalized Fc receptors and presents them to B cells for internalization and processing during the germinal center reaction. (Chapters 9, 10)

FoxP3   A transcription factor that is a master regulator in the development and immune-inhibitory function of regulatory T cells. (Chapter 9)

fragment crystallizable region   *See* **Fc region**. (Chapter 1)

framework regions   Relatively invariant regions that provide a protein scaffold for the hypervariable regions in the V domains of immunoglobulins and T-cell receptors. (Chapter 4)

Freund's complete adjuvant   Emulsion of oil and water containing killed mycobacteria used to enhance immune responses to experimental antigens. (Chapter 16)

fungi   A kingdom of single-celled and multicellular eukaryotic organisms, including the yeasts and molds, that can cause a variety of diseases. Immunity to fungi is complex and involves both humoral and cell-mediated responses. (Chapter 1)

Fyn   *See* **Src family protein tyrosine kinases**. (Chapter 7)

γδ T cells   Subset of T lymphocytes bearing a T-cell receptor composed of the antigen-recognition chains, γ and δ, assembled in a γδ heterodimer. (Chapter 6)

γδ T-cell receptors   Antigen receptor carried by a subset of T lymphocytes that is distinct from the αβ T-cell receptor. It is composed of a γ and a δ chain, which are produced from genes that undergo gene rearrangement. (Chapter 4)

γ-glutamyl diaminopimelic acid (iE-DAP)   A product of degradation of the peptidoglycan of Gram-negative bacteria. It is sensed by NOD1. (Chapter 3)

GAPs   *See* **GTPase-activating proteins**. (Chapter 7)

gasdermin D   A cytosolic protein that undergoes proteolytic cleavage by caspases (caspase 1) and inserts into the plasma membrane, forming a pore. The pore is required for release of the active forms of IL-1β and IL-18 and also leads to a form of cell death called pyroptosis. (Chapter 3)

GATA3   Transcription factor that has multiple functions in hematopoietic and non-hematopoietic cells but is indispensable for the development of T$_H$2 cells and ILC2 cells. (Chapter 9)

GEFs   *See* **guanine nucleotide exchange factors**. (Chapters 3, 7)

GEM T cells   A subset of NKT cells that recognize the mycobacterial lipid antigen glucose monomycolate presented by CD1b and use a very restricted TCRα chain repertoire V$_α$1–2 and J$_α$9. (Chapter 6)

gene knockout   The experimental inactivation of a gene, generally in mice, by targeted mutation using homologous recombination. (Appendix I)

gene rearrangement   The process of somatic recombination of gene segments in the immunoglobulin and T-cell receptor genetic loci to produce a functional gene. This process generates the diversity found in immunoglobulin and T-cell receptor variable regions. (Chapter 5)

gene segments   Sets of short DNA sequences at the immunoglobulin and T-cell receptor loci that encode different regions of the variable domains of antigen receptors. Gene segments of each type are joined together by somatic recombination to form a complete variable-domain exon. There are three types of gene segments: V gene segments encode the first 95 amino acids, D gene segments (in heavy-chain and TCRα chain loci only) encode about 5 amino acids, and J gene segments encode the last 10–15 amino acids of the variable domain. There are multiple copies of each type of gene segment in the germline DNA, but only one of each type is joined together to form the variable domain. (Chapters 1, 5)

gene targeting   The experimental use of homologous recombination to generate specific mutations or deletions in a gene with the goal of generating a mouse line carrying the desired genetic alteration in all cells. (Appendix I)

genetic locus   The site of a gene on a chromosome. In the case of the genes for the immunoglobulin and T-cell receptor chains, the term locus refers to the complete collection of gene segments and C-region genes for the given chain. (Chapter 5)

genome-wide association studies (GWASs) Genetic association studies in the general population that look for a correlation between disease frequency and variant alleles by scanning the genomes of many people for the presence of informative single-nucleotide polymorphisms (SNPs). (Chapter 15)

germ-free mice Mice that are raised in the complete absence of intestinal and other microorganisms. Such mice have very depleted immune systems, but they can respond virtually normally to any specific antigen, provided it is mixed with a strong adjuvant. (Chapter 12)

germinal centers Sites of intense B-cell proliferation and differentiation that develop in lymphoid follicles during an adaptive immune response. Somatic hypermutation and class switching occur in germinal centers. (Chapters 1, 9, 10)

germline theory An excluded hypothesis that antibody diversity was encoded by a separate germline gene for each antibody, known not to be true for most vertebrates, although cartilaginous fishes do have some rearranged V regions in the germline. (Chapter 5)

glucosidase II (GlsII) An enzyme in the endoplasmic reticulum that acts to recognize and fully deglucosylate properly folded peptide:MHC class I complexes to release them from the peptide-loading complex and allow their transport to the Golgi apparatus and eventual expression on the cell surface. (Chapter 6)

gluten A type of protein found in certain common grains, including wheat, barley, and rye. In individuals with certain genetic risk factors, an aberrant immune response to gluten leads to inflammatory injury in the small intestine, causing celiac disease. (Chapter 12)

glycosylphosphatidylinositol (GPI) tail A glycolipid modification of proteins that can allow attachment to host membranes without the requirement of a transmembrane protein domain. (Chapter 2)

gnathostomes The class of jawed vertebrates comprising most fish and all mammals. These possess an adaptive immunity that is based on RAG-mediated V(D)J recombination. (Chapter 5)

gnotobiotic Reared in a controlled environment wherein microorganisms are either defined or absent. In the case of the latter, the organism so reared is referred to as germ-free. (Chapter 13)

gnotobiotic mice *See* germ-free mice. (Chapter 12)

goblet cell Specialized epithelial cell located in many sites throughout the body and responsible for mucus production; important in protection of the epithelium. (Chapter 12)

goblet cell–associated passages (GAPs) Route by which soluble antigens are transported across goblet cells in the intestinal tract. May be a principal route for the induction of oral tolerance. (Chapter 12)

Goodpasture's syndrome An autoimmune disease in which autoantibodies against type IV collagen (found in basement membranes) are produced, causing extensive inflammation in kidneys and lungs. (Chapter 15)

gout Disease caused by monosodium urate crystals deposited in the cartilaginous tissues of joints, causing inflammation. Urate crystals activate the NLRP3 inflammasome, which induces inflammatory cytokines. (Chapter 3)

G proteins Intracellular GTPases that act as molecular switches in signaling pathways. They bind GTP to induce their active conformation, which is lost when GTP is hydrolyzed to GDP. There are two kinds of G proteins: the heterotrimeric (α, β, γ subunits) receptor-associated G proteins, and the small G proteins, such as Ras and Raf, which act downstream of many transmembrane signaling events. (Chapter 3)

G protein–coupled receptors (GPCRs) A large class of seven-span transmembrane cell-surface receptors that associate with intracellular heterotrimeric G proteins after ligand binding and signal by activation of the G protein. Important examples are the chemokine receptors. (Chapters 2, 3)

G-quadruplex A structure formed from G-rich regions of DNA in which four guanine bases form a planar hydrogen-bonded network, or guanine tetrad, that can further stack on other guanine tetrads. G-quadruplexes processed from intronic switch region RNA may target AID back to the switch regions during isotype switching. (Chapter 10)

graft rejection *See* allograft rejection. (Chapter 1)

graft-versus-host disease (GVHD) An attack on the tissues of the recipient by mature T cells in a bone marrow graft from a nonidentical donor, which can cause a variety of symptoms; sometimes these are severe. (Chapters 13, 15)

graft-versus-leukemia effect A beneficial side-effect of bone marrow grafts given to treat leukemia, in which mature T cells in the graft recognize minor histocompatibility antigens or tumor-specific antigens on the recipient's leukemic cells and attack them. (Chapter 15)

Gram-negative bacteria Bacteria that fail to retain crystal violet stain after alcohol wash because of a thin peptidoglycan layer. (Chapter 2)

Gram-negative binding proteins (GNBPs) Proteins that act as the pathogen-recognition proteins in the Toll pathway of immune defense in *Drosophila*. (Chapter 3)

granulocyte–macrophage colony-stimulating factor (GM-CSF) A cytokine involved in the growth and differentiation of cells of the myeloid lineage, including dendritic cells, monocytes and tissue macrophages, and granulocytes. (Chapter 3)

granulocytes White blood cells with multilobed nuclei and cytoplasmic granules. They comprise the neutrophils, eosinophils, and basophils. Also known as polymorphonuclear leukocytes. (Chapter 1)

granuloma A site of chronic inflammation usually triggered by persistent infectious agents such as mycobacteria or by a nondegradable foreign body. Granulomas have a central area of macrophages, often fused into multinucleated giant cells, surrounded by T lymphocytes. (Chapter 11)

granulysin A cytolytic, pro-inflammatory protein released by cytotoxic immune cells. (Chapter 9)

granzymes Pro-apoptotic proteases released by cytotoxic T lymphocytes and natural killer cells. (Chapter 9)

Grass A serine protease of *Drosophila* that functions downstream of peptidoglycan-recognition proteins (PGRPs) and Gram-negative binding proteins (GNBPs) to initiate the proteolytic cascade leading to Toll activation. (Chapter 3)

Graves' disease An autoimmune disease in which antibodies against the thyroid-stimulating hormone receptor cause overproduction of thyroid hormone and thus hyperthyroidism. (Chapter 15)

Griscelli syndrome An inherited immunodeficiency disease that affects the pathway for secretion of lysosomes. It is caused by mutations in a small GTPase, Rab27a, which controls the movement of vesicles within cells. (Chapter 13)

group 1 ILCs (ILC1s) The subtype of innate lymphoid cells (ILCs) characterized by IFN-γ production. (Chapter 3)

group 2 ILCs (ILC2s) A subset of innate lymphoid cells characterized by production of IL-4, IL-5, and IL-13. (Chapter 3)

group 3 ILCs (ILC3s) A subset of innate lymphoid cells characterized by production of IL-17 and IL-22. (Chapter 3)

GTPase-activating proteins (GAPs) Regulatory proteins that accelerate the intrinsic GTPase activity of G proteins and thus facilitate the conversion of G proteins from the active (GTP-bound) state to the inactive (GDP-bound) state. (Chapter 7)

guanine nucleotide exchange factors (GEFs)   Proteins that can remove the bound GDP from G proteins, thus allowing GTP to bind and activate the G protein. (Chapters 3, 7)

gut-associated lymphoid tissue (GALT)   Lymphoid tissues associated with the gastrointestinal tract, comprising Peyer's patches, the appendix, and isolated lymphoid follicles found in the intestinal wall, where adaptive immune responses are initiated. (Chapters 1, 12)

GVHD   See **graft-versus-host disease**. (Chapters 13, 15)

H-2 locus, H-2 genes   The major histocompatibility complex of the mouse. Haplotypes are designated by a lowercase superscript, as in H-2^b. (Chapters 1, 6)

H-2DM   See **HLA-DM**. (Chapter 6)

H-2O   See **HLA-DO**. (Chapter 6)

H2-M3   A nonclassical MHC class Ib protein in mice that can bind and present peptides having an *N*-formylated amino terminus for recognition by CD8 T cells. (Chapter 6)

H5N1 avian flu   A highly pathogenic influenza subtype responsible for 'bird flu.' (Chapter 16)

haploinsufficient   Describes the situation in which the presence of only one normal allele of a gene is not sufficient for normal function. (Chapter 13)

hapten carrier effect   Antibody production against a small chemical group, the hapten, after its attachment to a carrier protein for which an immune response has been generated. (Chapter 10)

hapten   Any small molecule that can be recognized by a specific antibody but cannot by itself elicit an immune response. A hapten must be chemically linked to a protein molecule to elicit antibody and T-cell responses. (Chapter 4, Appendix I)

Hashimoto's thyroiditis   An autoimmune disease characterized by persistent high levels of antibody against thyroid-specific antigens. These antibodies recruit NK cells to the thyroid, leading to damage and inflammation. (Chapter 15)

heavy chain, H chain   One of the two types of protein chains in an immunoglobulin molecule, the other being called the light chain. There are several different classes, or isotypes, of heavy chain ($\alpha, \delta, \varepsilon, \gamma$, and μ), each of which confers a distinctive functional activity on the antibody molecule. Each immunoglobulin molecule contains two identical heavy chains. (Chapters 1, 4)

heavy-chain-only IgGs (hcIgGs)   Antibodies that are produced by some camelid species and composed of heavy-chain dimers without an associated light chain that retain antigen-binding capacity. (Chapter 4)

heavy-chain variable region (V$_H$)   Referring to the V region of the heavy chain of an immunoglobulin. (Chapter 5)

helper CD4 T cells, helper T cells   Effector CD4 T cells that stimulate or 'help' B cells to make antibody in response to antigenic challenge. T$_H$2, T$_H$1, and the T$_{FH}$ subsets of effector CD4 T cells can perform this function. (Chapter 1)

hemagglutination   The clumping of red blood cells, often caused by the binding of antibodies to target antigens on the surface of the cells. (Appendix I)

hemagglutinin   Substances that can cause hemagglutination, such as human antibodies that recognize the ABO blood group antigens on red blood cells, or the influenza virus hemagglutinin (H), a glycoprotein that functions in viral fusion with endosome membranes. (Chapters 10, 12, 16)

hematopoietic stem cells (HSCs)   Type of pluripotent (or multipotent) cell in the bone marrow that can give rise to all the different blood cell types. (Chapters 1, 8)

hematopoietin superfamily   Large family of structurally related cytokines that includes growth factors and many interleukins with roles in both adaptive and innate immunity. (Chapter 3)

hemochromatosis protein   A protein expressed by intestinal epithelial cells that regulates iron uptake and transport by interacting with the transferrin receptor to decrease its affinity for iron-loaded transferrin. (Chapter 6)

hemolytic disease of the newborn (erythroblastosis fetalis)   A severe form of Rh hemolytic disease in which maternal anti-Rh antibody enters the fetus and produces a hemolytic anemia so severe that the fetus has mainly immature erythroblasts in the peripheral blood. (Chapter 11, Appendix I)

hemophagocytic lymphohistiocytic (HLH) syndrome   A dysregulated expansion of CD8-positive lymphocytes that is associated with macrophage activation. The activated macrophages phagocytose blood cells, including erythrocytes and leukocytes. (Chapter 13)

hepatobiliary route   Route whereby mucosally produced dimeric IgA enters the portal veins in the lamina propria, is transported to the liver, and reaches the bile duct by transcytosis. This pathway is not of great significance in humans. (Chapter 12)

heptamer   The conserved seven-nucleotide DNA sequence in the recombination signal sequences (RSSs) flanking gene segments in the immunoglobulin and T-cell receptor loci. (Chapter 5)

HER-2/neu   A receptor tyrosine kinase overexpressed in many cancers, particularly breast cancer, that is the target of trastuzumab (Herceptin) used in its treatment. (Chapter 16)

herd immunity   Protection conferred to unvaccinated individuals in a population that is produced by vaccination of others and reduction in the natural reservoir for infection. (Chapter 16)

hereditary angioedema (HAE)   A genetic deficiency of the C1 inhibitor of the complement system. In the absence of C1 inhibitor, spontaneous activation of the complement system can cause diffuse fluid leakage from blood vessels, the most serious consequence of which is swelling of the larynx, leading to suffocation. (Chapters 2, 13)

hereditary hemochromatosis   A disease caused by defects in the HFE gene characterized by abnormally high retention of iron in the liver and other organs. (Chapter 6)

herpes virus entry molecule (HVEM)   See **B and T lymphocyte attenuator**. (Chapter 7)

herpes zoster   See **shingles**. (Chapter 13)

heterosubtypic immunity   Immune protection against a pathogen conferred by infection with a distinct strain, typically with reference to different influenza A serotypes. (Chapter 16)

heterotrimeric G proteins   See **G proteins**. (Chapter 3)

heterozygous   Describes individuals that have two different alleles of a given gene, one inherited from the mother and one from the father. (Chapter 6)

HFE   See **hemochromatosis protein**. (Chapter 6)

high endothelial cells, high endothelial venules (HEVs)   Specialized small venous blood vessels in lymphoid tissues. Lymphocytes migrate from the blood into lymphoid tissues by attaching to the high endothelial cells in the walls of the venules and squeezing between them. (Chapters 1, 9, 12)

hinge region   The flexible domain that joins the Fab arms to the Fc piece in an immunoglobulin. The flexibility of the hinge region in IgG and IgA molecules allows the Fab arms to adopt a wide range of angles, permitting binding to epitopes spaced variable distances apart. (Chapter 4)

HIP/PAP   An antimicrobial C-type lectin secreted by intestinal cells in humans. Also known as RegIIIα. (Chapter 2)

histamine   A vasoactive amine stored in mast-cell granules. Histamine released by antigen binding to IgE antibodies that are bound to mast cells causes the dilation of local blood vessels and the contraction of smooth muscle, producing some of the symptoms of IgE-mediated allergic reactions. Antihistamines are drugs that counter histamine action. (Chapter 14)

histatins   Antimicrobial peptides constitutively produced by the parotid, sublingual, and submandibular glands in the oral cavity. Active against pathogenic fungi such as *Cryptococcus neoformans* and *Candida albicans*. (Chapter 2)

HIV   *See* **human immunodeficiency virus**. (Chapter 13)

HLA   The genetic designation for the human MHC. Individual loci are designated by uppercase letters, as in HLA-A, and alleles are designated by numbers, as in HLA-A*0201. (Chapter 6)

HLA-DM   An invariant MHC protein resembling MHC class II in humans that is involved in loading peptides onto MHC class II molecules. A homologous protein in mice is called H-2M, or sometimes H2-DM. (Chapter 6)

HLA-DO   An invariant MHC class II molecule that binds HLA-DM, inhibiting the release of CLIP from MHC class II molecules in intracellular vesicles. A homologous protein in mice is called H-2O or H2-DO. (Chapter 6)

homeostatic chemokines   Chemokines that are produced at steady state to direct the localization of immune cells to lymphoid tissues. (Chapter 11)

homing   The direction of a lymphocyte into a particular tissue. (Chapter 9)

homing receptors   Receptors on lymphocytes for chemokines, cytokines, and adhesion molecules specific to particular tissues and which enable the lymphocyte to enter that tissue. (Chapter 11)

homologous recombination   A genetic process in which sequences in the DNA of a cell are replaced by similar, but not identical, sequences at the precise location of the original sequences. (Appendix I)

homozygous   Describes a genetic locus in an individual where the individual has two identical alleles of a given gene, inherited separately from each parent. (Chapter 6)

host-versus-graft disease (HVGD)   Another name for the allograft rejection reaction. The term is used mainly in relation to bone marrow transplantation when immune cells of the host recognize and destroy transplanted bone marrow or hematopoietic stem cells (HSCs). (Chapter 13)

human immunodeficiency virus (HIV)   The causative agent of the acquired immune deficiency syndrome (AIDS). HIV is a retrovirus of the lentivirus family that selectively infects macrophages and CD4 T cells, leading to their slow depletion, which eventually results in immunodeficiency. There are two major strains of the virus, HIV-1 and HIV-2, of which HIV-1 causes most disease worldwide. HIV-2 is endemic to West Africa but is spreading. (Chapter 13)

human leukocyte antigen (HLA)   *See* **HLA**. (Chapter 6)

humanization   The genetic engineering of mouse hypervariable loops of a desired specificity into otherwise human antibodies for use as therapeutic agents. Such antibodies are less likely to cause an immune response in people treated with them than are wholly mouse antibodies. (Chapter 16)

humoral   Referring to effector proteins in the blood or body fluids, such as antibodies in adaptive immunity or complement proteins in innate immunity. (Chapter 2)

humoral immunity, humoral immune response   Immunity due to proteins circulating in the blood, such as antibodies (in adaptive immunity) or complement (in innate immunity). Adaptive humoral immunity can be transferred to unimmunized recipients by the transfer of serum containing specific antibody. (Chapters 1, 10, Appendix I)

HVGD   *See* **host-versus-graft disease**. (Chapter 13)

hybridoma   Cells created by the fusion of two different parental cell types. Antibody-secreting hybridomas are generated by fusing a plasma cell with a non-antibody-secreting myeloma tumor cell to produce an immortalized antibody-secreting cell line. (Appendix I)

hydrophobic interaction   Chemical interaction occurring between nearby hydrophobic moieties typically excluding water molecules. (Chapter 4)

3-hydroxy-3-methylglutaryl-coenzyme A (HMG-CoA) reductase   Rate-limiting enzyme in the production of cholesterol and a target of cholesterol-lowering drugs such as the statins. (Chapter 16)

21-hydroxylase   An enzyme of nonimmune function but encoded in the MHC locus required for normal cortisol synthesis by the adrenal gland. (Chapter 6)

hygiene hypothesis   A hypothesis first proposed in 1989 that reduced exposure to ubiquitous environmental microorganisms was a cause of the increased frequency of patients with allergies observed over the course of the mid- to late-20th century. (Chapter 14)

hyper IgE syndrome (HIES)   Also called Job syndrome. A disease characterized by recurrent skin and pulmonary infections and high serum concentrations of IgE. (Chapter 13)

hyper IgM syndrome   A group of genetic diseases in which there is overproduction of IgM antibody, among other symptoms. They are due to defects in various genes for proteins involved in class switching such as CD40 ligand and the enzyme AID. *See* **activation-induced cytidine deaminase**; **CD40 ligand deficiency**. (Chapters 10, 13)

hyper IgM type 2 immunodeficiency   *See* **activation-induced cytidine deaminase**. (Chapter 10)

hyperacute graft rejection   Immediate rejection reaction caused by preformed natural antibodies that react against antigens on the transplanted organ. The antibodies bind to endothelium and trigger the blood-clotting cascade, leading to an engorged, ischemic graft and rapid death of the organ. (Chapter 15)

hypereosinophilic syndrome   Disease associated with an overproduction of eosinophils. (Chapter 14)

hypermorphic   A type of genetic variation wherein the affected wild-type gene is expressed at an increased level or its gene product has increased function. (Chapter 13)

hypervariable regions   *See* **complementarity-determining regions**. (Chapters 4, 5)

hypomorphic   A type of genetic variation wherein the affected gene has diminished, but not entirely lost, expression or the gene product has reduced, but not absent, function compared to wild type. (Chapter 13)

IκB   A cytoplasmic protein that constitutively associates with the NFκB homodimer, which is composed of p50 and p65 subunits. When IκB is phosphorylated by activated IKK (IκB kinase), IκB becomes degraded and allows the NFκB dimer to be released as an active transcription factor. (Chapter 3)

IκB kinase (IKK)   *See* **IKK**. (Chapter 3)

iC3b   Inactive complement fragment produced by cleavage of C3b. (Chapter 2)

ICAMs   ICAM-1, ICAM-2, ICAM-3. Cell-adhesion molecules of the immunoglobulin superfamily that bind to the leukocyte integrin CD11a:CD18 (LFA-1). They are crucial in the binding of lymphocytes and other leukocytes to antigen-presenting cells and endothelial cells. (Chapter 3)

ICOS (inducible co-stimulatory)   A CD28-related co-stimulatory receptor that is induced on activated T cells and can enhance T-cell responses. It binds a co-stimulatory ligand known as ICOSL (ICOS ligand), which is distinct from the B7 molecules. (Chapter 10)

ICOSL   *See* **ICOS**. (Chapter 10)

IFIT (IFN-induced protein with tetratricoid repeats)   A small family of host proteins induced by interferons that regulate protein translation during infection in part by interactions with eIF3. (Chapter 3)

IFIT1, IFIT2 IFN-induced protein with tetratricoid repeats (IFIT) 1 and 2 are proteins encoded by interferon-stimulated genes (ISGs) that regulate the translation of normally capped mRNAs and lead to reduced cellular proliferation. IFIT1 can also suppress translation of some viral RNAs that lack 2′-*O*-methylation (cap-0), such as Sindbis virus. In this way, IFIT1 and IFIT2 serve as restriction factors in certain viral infections. (Chapter 3)

IFITM (interferon-induced transmembrane protein) A small family of host transmembrane proteins induced by interferons that function in the cell's vesicular compartment to restrain various steps in viral replication. (Chapter 3)

IFITM1, IFITM3 Interferon-induced transmembrane protein (IFITM) 1 and 3 are proteins encoded by interferon-stimulated genes (ISGs) that interfere with membrane fusion between viral membranes and membranes of the lysosome (IFITM1) or endosome (IFITM3), and so serve as restriction factors in various viral infections. (Chapter 3)

IFN-α, IFN-β Antiviral cytokines produced by a wide variety of cells in response to infection by a virus, and which also help healthy cells resist viral infection. They act through the same receptor, which signals through a Janus-family tyrosine kinase. Also known as the type I interferons. (Chapter 3)

IFN-γ A cytokine of the interferon structural family produced by effector CD4 T$_H$1 cells, CD8 T cells, and NK cells. Its primary function is the activation of macrophages, and it acts through a different receptor from that of the type I interferons. (Chapters 1, 3)

IFN-γ–induced lysosomal thiol reductase (GILT) An enzyme present in the endosomal compartment of many antigen-presenting cells that denatures disulfide bonds to facilitate the degradation and processing of proteins. (Chapter 6)

IFN-λ Also called type III interferons, this family includes IL-28A, IL-28B, and IL-29, which bind a common receptor expressed by a limited set of epithelial tissues. (Chapters 3, 9)

IFN-λ receptor Heterodimeric receptor composed of a unique IL-28Rα subunit and the β subunit of the IL-10 receptor that recognizes IL-28A, IL-28B, and IL-29. (Chapter 3)

Igα, Igβ *See* **B-cell receptor**. (Chapter 7)

IgA Immunoglobulin class composed of α heavy chains that can occur in a monomeric and a polymeric (mainly dimeric) form. Polymeric IgA is the main antibody secreted by mucosal lymphoid tissues. (Chapter 4)

IgA deficiency The most common type of primary immunodeficiency. (Chapter 13)

IgD Immunoglobulin class composed of δ heavy chains that appears as surface immunoglobulin on mature B cells. (Chapter 4)

IgE Immunoglobulin class composed of ε heavy chains that acts in defense against parasite infections and in allergic reactions. (Chapters 4, 14)

IgG Immunoglobulin class composed of γ heavy chains that is the most abundant class of immunoglobulin in the plasma. (Chapter 4)

IgM Immunoglobulin class composed of μ heavy chains that is the first to appear on B cells and the first to be secreted. (Chapter 4)

IgM deficiency A rare genetic immunodeficiency characterized by selective low or absent IgM production with normal or elevated levels of IgG and IgA. (Chapter 13)

IgNAR *See* **immunoglobulin new antigen receptor**.

IgW Type of heavy-chain isotype present in cartilaginous fishes that is composed of six immunoglobulin domains. (Chapter 5)

IKK The IκB kinase, IKK, is a multi-subunit protein complex composed of IKKα, IKKβ, and IKKγ (the latter also known as NEMO). (Chapter 3)

IKKε A kinase that interacts with TBK1 (TANK-binding kinase 1) in the phosphorylation of IRF3 downstream of TLR-3 signaling. (Chapter 3)

IL-1 family One of four major families of cytokines, this family contains 11 cytokines that are structurally similar to IL-1α and are largely pro-inflammatory in function. (Chapter 3)

IL-1α, IL-1β Interleukin-1α and interleukin-1β are cytokines produced by activated macrophages that have many effects in the immune response, including the activation of vascular endothelium, activation of lymphocytes, and the induction of fever. IL-1β must be cleaved by caspase 1 before having biological activity, while IL-1α does not require cleavage. (Chapter 3)

IL-2Rα *See* **CD25**. (Chapter 9)

IL-4 *See* **interleukin (IL)**. (Chapter 9)

IL-5 *See* **interleukin (IL)**. (Chapter 9)

IL-6 Interleukin-6, a cytokine produced by activated macrophages and which has many effects, including lymphocyte activation, the stimulation of antibody production, and the induction of fever. (Chapters 3, 9)

IL-7Rα (CD127) *See* **CD127**. (Chapter 11)

IL-10 *See* **interleukin (IL)**. (Chapter 9)

IL-13 *See* **interleukin (IL)**. (Chapter 9)

IL-17A *See* **interleukin (IL)**. (Chapter 9)

IL-17F *See* **interleukin (IL)**. (Chapter 9)

IL-21 A cytokine produced by T cells (e.g., T$_{FH}$ cells) that activates STAT3 and promotes survival and proliferation, particularly of germinal center B cells. (Chapters 9, 10)

IL-22 *See* **interleukin (IL)**. (Chapter 9)

ILC1 A subset of innate lymphoid cells characterized by production of IFN-γ. (Chapters 1, 11)

ILC2 *See* **ILCs**. (Chapter 11)

ILC3 *See* **ILCs**. (Chapter 11)

ILCs (innate lymphoid cells) These are a class of innate immune cells having overlapping characteristics with T cells but lacking an antigen receptor. They arise in several groups, ILC1, ILC2, ILC3, and NK cells, which exhibit properties roughly similar to T$_H$1, T$_H$2, T$_H$17, and CD8 T cells. (Chapters 1, 3)

Imd (immunodeficiency) signaling pathway A defense against Gram-negative bacteria in insects that results in the production of antimicrobial peptides such as diptericin, attacin, and cecropin. (Chapter 3)

imiquimod Drug (Aldara) approved for treatment of basal-cell carcinoma, genital warts, and actinic keratoses known to activate TLR-7, although not approved as an adjuvant for vaccines. (Chapter 16)

immature B cells B cells that have rearranged a heavy- and a light-chain V-region gene and express surface IgM, but have not yet matured sufficiently to express surface IgD as well. (Chapter 8)

immature cDCs Conventional dendritic cells that have yet to be activated for antigenic priming of naive T cells. Immature cDCs typically are actively phagocytic but lack high expression of co-stimulatory molecules. (Chapter 9)

immediate hypersensitivity reactions Allergic reactions that occur within seconds to minutes of encounter with antigen, caused largely by activation of mast cells or basophils. (Chapters 11, 14)

immune complexes Complexes formed by the binding of antibody to its cognate antigen. Activated complement proteins, especially C3b, are often bound in immune complexes. Large immune complexes form when sufficient antibody is available to cross-link multivalent antigen; these are cleared by cells of the reticuloendothelial system that bear Fc receptors and complement receptors. Small, soluble immune complexes form when antigen is in excess; these can be deposited in small blood vessels and damage them. (Chapter 14)

immune effector modules   Sets of innate and adaptive immune cells whose responses are coordinated to focus host defense on different classes of pathogens. There are two broad classes of immune modules, cytotoxic and helper, the latter of which is further subdivided into types 1, 2, and 3, dedicated to the elimination of intracellular pathogens, helminths, and extracellular bacteria and fungi, respectively. Underpinning the orchestration of each module are ILCs and T lymphocytes that have shared transcriptional and effector programs: NK and cytotoxic CD8 T cells (cytotoxic module); ILC1 and T_H1 cells (type 1 module); ILC2 and T_H2 cells (type 2 module); and ILC3 and T_H17 cells (type 3 module). (Chapter 11)

immune evasion   Mechanisms used by pathogens to avoid detection and/or elimination by host immune defenses. (Chapters 2, 13)

immune synapse   The highly organized interface that develops between a T cell and the target cell it is in contact with, formed by T-cell receptors binding to antigen and cell-adhesion molecules binding to their counterparts on the two cells. Also known as the supramolecular activation complex (SMAC). (Chapter 7)

immune surveillance   The recognition, and in some cases the elimination, of tumor cells by the immune system before they become clinically detectable. (Chapter 16)

immune system   The tissues, cells, and molecules involved in innate immunity and adaptive immunity. (Chapter 1)

immunization   The deliberate induction of an immune response by exposing an individual to a specific antigen. Often called vaccination when used to induce a protective immune response to a microbial pathogen. (Appendix I)

immunodeficiency diseases   Any inherited or acquired disorder in which some aspect or aspects of host defense are absent or functionally defective. (Chapter 1)

immunodominant   Describes epitopes in an antigen that are preferentially recognized by T cells, such that T cells specific for those epitopes come to dominate the immune response. (Chapter 13)

immunoblotting   A technique in which proteins separated by SDS-PAGE are transferred from the acrylamide gel to a nylon or nitrocellulose membrane. A specific protein of interest is identified by incubating the membrane with an antibody to that protein, followed by an enzyme-linked anti-immunoglobulin antibody. Finally, the membrane is incubated with a colorless substrate, which is converted to a colored product on the membrane at the location of bound antibody. Also called western blotting. *See also* **SDS-PAGE**. (Appendix I)

immunoevasins   Viral proteins that prevent the appearance of peptide:MHC class I complexes on the infected cell, thus preventing the recognition of virus-infected cells by cytotoxic T cells. (Chapter 13)

immunofluorescence microscopy   Cells or tissue sections are incubated with fluorescently labeled antibodies to target molecules present in the cells or tissue. Binding of these antibodies is determined using a microscope that is outfitted to detect fluorescent dyes. (Appendix I)

immunogen   Any substance that can elicit an adaptive immune response. (Appendix I)

immunogenic   Elicitation of an adaptive immune response. (Chapter 1, Appendix I)

immunoglobulin (Ig)   The protein family to which antibodies and B-cell receptors belong. (Chapters 1, 4)

immunoglobulin A (IgA)   *See* **IgA**. (Chapter 4)

immunoglobulin D (IgD)   *See* **IgD**. (Chapter 4)

immunoglobulin domain, Ig domain   Protein domain first described in antibody molecules but present in many proteins. (Chapter 4)

immunoglobulin E (IgE)   *See* **IgE**. (Chapter 4)

immunoglobulin fold   The tertiary structure of an immunoglobulin domain, comprising a sandwich of two β sheets held together by a disulfide bond. (Chapters 4, 5)

immunoglobulin G (IgG)   *See* **IgG**. (Chapter 4)

immunoglobulin-like domain (Ig-like domain)   Protein domain structurally related to the immunoglobulin domain. (Chapter 4)

immunoglobulin-like proteins   Proteins containing one or more immunoglobulin-like domains, which are protein domains structurally similar to those of immunoglobulins. (Chapter 3)

immunoglobulin M (IgM)   *See* **IgM**. (Chapter 4)

immunoglobulin new antigen receptor (IgNAR)   A form of heavy-chain-only Ig molecule made by shark species. (Chapter 4)

immunoglobulin repertoire   The variety of antigen-specific immunoglobulins (antibodies and B-cell receptors) present in an individual. Also known as the antibody repertoire. (Chapter 5)

immunoglobulin superfamily   Large family of proteins with at least one Ig or Ig-like domain, many of which are involved in antigen recognition and cell–cell interaction in the immune system and other biological systems. (Chapter 4)

immunohistochemistry   Use of an enzyme-coupled antibody to detect a target antigen in cells or tissue samples. After antibody binding, the sample is incubated with a substrate that is converted from a colorless to a colored state by the coupled enzyme. Visualization of the colored reaction product indicates the location of the target antigen. (Appendix I)

immunological ignorance   A form of self-tolerance in which reactive lymphocytes and their target antigen are both detectable within an individual, yet no autoimmune attack occurs. (Chapter 15)

immunologically privileged sites   Certain sites in the body, such as the brain, that do not mount an immune response against tissue allografts. Immunological privilege can be due both to physical barriers to cell and antigen migration and to the presence of immunosuppressive cytokines. (Chapter 15)

immunological memory   The ability of the immune system to respond more rapidly and more effectively on a second encounter with an antigen. Immunological memory is specific for a particular antigen and is long-lived. (Chapters 1, 11)

immunological tolerance   *See* **tolerance**. (Chapter 1)

immunology   The study of all aspects of host defense against infection and also of the adverse consequences of immune responses. (Chapter 1)

immunomodulatory therapy   Treatments that seek to modify an immune response in a beneficial way; for example, to reduce or prevent an autoimmune or allergic response. (Chapter 16)

immunophilins   *See* **cyclophilins, FK-binding proteins**. (Chapter 16)

immunoprecipitation   A complex mixture, such as a cell lysate, is incubated with an antibody to a target antigen of interest. Antibody:antigen complexes are isolated by incubation with an anti-immunoglobulin antibody coupled to a solid matrix such as a latex bead. The latex beads are then separated from the remaining cell lysate. (Appendix I)

immunoproteasome   A form of proteasome found in cells exposed to interferons. It contains three subunits that are different from the normal proteasome. (Chapter 6)

immunoreceptor tyrosine-based activation motif (ITAM)   Sequence motifs in the signaling chains of receptors, such as antigen receptors on lymphocytes, that are the site of tyrosine phosphorylation after receptor activation, leading to recruitment of other signaling proteins. (Chapters 3, 7)

immunoreceptor tyrosine-based inhibition motif (ITIM)   Sequence motifs in the signaling chains of inhibitory receptors that are sites of tyrosine phosphorylation, leading to inhibitory signaling, such as through recruitment of phosphatases that remove phosphate groups added by tyrosine kinases. (Chapters 3, 7)

immunoreceptor tyrosine-based switch motif (ITSM)   A sequence motif present in the cytoplasmic tails of some inhibitory receptors. (Chapter 7)

immunotoxin   Antibodies that are chemically coupled to toxic proteins usually derived from plants or microbes. The antibody targets the toxin moiety to the required cells. (Chapter 16)

indirect allorecognition   Recognition of a grafted tissue that involves the uptake of allogeneic proteins from the donor tissue by the recipient's antigen-presenting cells, followed by antigen processing and presentation to T cells by self MHC molecules. (Chapter 15)

indirect Coombs test   This assay tests for anti-Rh antibody in maternal serum. The serum is mixed with Rh-positive red blood cells, followed by anti-human immunoglobulin antibodies. If the serum contains anti-Rh antibody, this antibody will bind to the Rh-positive cells, which will then be agglutinated by the addition of anti-human immunoglobulin antibodies. (Appendix I)

indirect immunofluorescence   Cells or tissue sections are incubated with antibodies to target molecules present in the cells or tissue. The samples are then incubated with a fluorescently labeled anti-immunoglobulin antibody specific for the first antibody. Binding of the second anti-immunoglobulin antibody is determined using a microscope that is outfitted to detect fluorescent dyes.   (Appendix I)

indoleamine 2,3-dioxygenase (IDO)   Enzyme expressed by immune cells and some tumors that catabolizes tryptophan into kynurenine metabolites that can have immunosuppressive functions. (Chapter 16)

infectious mononucleosis   The common form of infection with the Epstein–Barr virus. It consists of fever, malaise, and swollen lymph nodes. Also called glandular fever. (Chapter 13)

inflammasome   A pro-inflammatory protein complex that is formed after stimulation of the intracellular NOD-like receptors. Production of an active caspase in the complex processes cytokine proproteins into active cytokines. (Chapters 3, 12)

inflammation   General term for the local accumulation of fluid, plasma proteins, and white blood cells that is initiated by physical injury, infection, or a local immune response. (Chapters 1, 2)

inflammation-anergic macrophages   Macrophages in the homeostatic, noninflamed gastrointestinal mucosa that are hyporesponsive to inflammatory stimuli because of down-regulation of the LPS co-receptor CD14, IgA and IgG Fc receptors, and NFκB signaling molecules downstream of tonic TGF-β signaling. (Chapter 12)

inflammatory bowel disease (IBD)   General name for a set of inflammatory conditions in the gut, such as Crohn's disease and ulcerative colitis, that have an immunological component. (Chapters 12, 15)

inflammatory cells   Cells such as macrophages, neutrophils, and effector T$_H$1 lymphocytes that invade inflamed tissues and contribute to the inflammation. (Chapter 1)

inflammatory chemokines   Chemokines that are produced in response to infection or injury to direct the localization of immune cells to sites of inflammation. (Chapter 11)

inflammatory inducers   Chemical structures that indicate the presence of invading microbes or cellular damage, such as bacterial lipopolysaccharides, extracellular ATP, or urate crystals. (Chapter 1)

inflammatory mediators   Chemicals such as cytokines produced by immune cells that act on target cells to promote defense against microbes. (Chapter 1)

inflammatory monocytes   An activated form of monocytes producing a variety of pro-inflammatory cytokines. (Chapter 3)

inflammatory response   *See* **inflammation**. (Chapter 2)

infliximab   Chimeric antibody to TNF-α used in the treatment of inflammatory diseases, such as Crohn's disease and rheumatoid arthritis. (Chapter 16)

inherited immunodeficiency   *See* **primary immunodeficiency**. (Chapter 13)

inhibitory receptors   On NK cells, receptors whose stimulation results in suppression of the cell's cytotoxic activity. (Chapter 3)

initiator caspases   Proteases that promote apoptosis by cleaving and activating other caspases. (Chapter 9)

injectisome   Needle-like molecular complex employed by pathogenic bacteria to inject bacterial effector molecules into eukaryotic cells or other bacteria. (Chapters 12, 13)

iNKT cells   *See* **invariant NKT cells**. (Chapters 6, 8, 12)

innate immunity   The various innate resistance mechanisms that are encountered first by a pathogen, before adaptive immunity is induced, such as anatomical barriers, antimicrobial peptides, the complement system, and macrophages and neutrophils carrying nonspecific pathogen-recognition receptors. Innate immunity is present in all individuals at all times, does not increase with repeated exposure to a given pathogen, and discriminates between groups of similar pathogens, rather than responding to a particular pathogen. Cf. **adaptive immunity**. (Chapters 1, 2)

innate lymphoid cells (ILCs)   *See* **ILCs**. (Chapters 1, 3, 11)

innate recognition receptors   General term for a large group of proteins that recognize many different inflammatory inducers and that are encoded in the germline and do not need gene rearrangement in somatic cells to be expressed. (Chapter 1)

inositol 1,4,5-trisphosphate (IP$_3$)   A soluble second messenger produced by the cleavage of membrane inositol phospholipids by phospholipase C-γ. It acts on receptors in the endoplasmic reticulum membrane, resulting in the release of stored Ca^{2+} into the cytosol. (Chapter 7)

integrins   Heterodimeric cell-surface proteins involved in cell–cell and cell–matrix interactions. They are important in adhesive interactions between lymphocytes and antigen-presenting cells and in lymphocyte and leukocyte adherence to blood vessel walls and migration into tissues. (Chapter 3)

integrin α$_4$β$_1$ (VLA-4, or CD49d:CD29)   *See* **integrins**. (Chapter 16)

integrin α$_4$β$_7$ Integrin binding to VCAM-1, MAdCAM-1, and fibronectin and expressed by various cells, such as IELs, that traffic to intestinal lamina propria. Also called lamina propria–associated molecule 1. (Chapters 9, 16)

intercellular adhesion molecules (ICAMs)   *See* **ICAMs**. (Chapter 3)

interferon-α receptor (IFNAR)   This receptor recognizes IFN-α and IFN-β to activate STAT1 and STAT2 and induce expression of many ISGs. (Chapter 3)

interferon-γ   *See* **IFN-γ**. (Chapter 1)

interferon-induced transmembrane protein (IFITM)   *See* **IFITM**. (Chapter 3)

interferon-producing cells (IPCs)   *See* **plasmacytoid dendritic cells**. (Chapter 3)

interferon regulatory factor (IRF)   A family of nine transcription factors that regulate a variety of immune responses. For example, IRF3 and IRF7 are activated as a result of signaling from some TLRs. Several IRFs promote expression of the genes for type I interferons. (Chapter 3)

interferons (IFNs)   Several related families of cytokines originally named for their interference with viral replication. IFN-α and IFN-β are antiviral in their effects; IFN-γ has other roles in the immune system. (Chapter 3)

interferon-stimulated genes (ISGs)   A category of genes induced by interferons, which include many whose products promote innate defense against pathogens, such as oligoadenylate synthetase, PKR, and the Mx, IFIT, and IFITM proteins. (Chapter 3)

interleukin (IL)   A generic name for cytokines produced by leukocytes. The more general term cytokine is used in this book, but the term interleukin is used in the naming of specific cytokines such as IL-2. Some key interleukins are listed in the glossary under their abbreviated names; for example, IL-1β and IL-2. Cytokines are listed in eAppendix III. (Chapter 3)

intestinal stem cells (ISCs)   Multipotent adult stem cells located in the basal region of crypts in the large and small intestine. (Chapter 12)

intracellular cytokine staining   A technique for visualizing cells in a population capable of producing a cytokine of interest. Stimulated T cells are treated with a protein secretion inhibitor for several hours, then fixed and permeabilized. Cells are then incubated with a fluorescently tagged anti-cytokine antibody and analyzed by FACS. *See also* **fluorescence-activated cell sorter**. (Appendix I)

intradermal (i.d.)   Into the dermal layer of the skin. (Appendix I)

intraepithelial lymphocytes (IELs)   Lymphocytes present in the epithelium of mucosal surfaces such as the gut. They are predominantly T cells, and in the gut are predominantly CD8 T cells. (Chapter 12)

intramuscular (i.m.)   Into the muscle. (Appendix I)

intranasal (i.n.)   Introduced through the nose, often by inhalation. (Appendix I)

intraperitoneal (i.p.)   Within the peritoneal cavity (the site containing the abdominal organs). (Appendix I)

intrathymic dendritic cells   *See* **dendritic cells**. (Chapter 8)

intravenous (i.v.)   Into a vein. (Appendix I)

intrinsic (or mitochondrial) pathway of apoptosis   Signaling pathway that mediates apoptosis in response to noxious stimuli including UV irradiation, chemotherapeutic drugs, starvation, or lack of the growth factors required for survival. It is initiated by mitochondrial damage. (Chapters 9, 11)

invariant chain (Ii, CD74)   A polypeptide that binds in the peptide-binding cleft of newly synthesized MHC class II proteins in the endoplasmic reticulum and blocks other peptides from binding there. It is degraded in the endosome, allowing for loading of antigenic peptides there. (Chapters 4, 6)

invariant NKT (iNKT) cells   A type of innate-like lymphocyte that carries a T-cell receptor with an invariant α chain and a β chain of limited diversity that recognizes glycolipid antigens presented by CD1 MHC class Ib molecules. This cell type also carries the surface marker NK1.1, which is usually associated with NK cells. (Chapters 6, 8, 12)

IPEX (immune dysregulation, polyendocrinopathy, enteropathy, X-linked)   Immune dysregulation, polyendocrinopathy, enteropathy, X-linked syndrome. A very rare inherited condition in which CD4 CD25 regulatory T cells are lacking as a result of a mutation in the gene for the transcription factor FoxP3, leading to the development of autoimmunity. (Chapter 15)

ipilimumab   Antibody to human CTLA-4 used to treat melanoma, and first checkpoint blockade immunotherapy. (Chapter 16)

Ir (immune response) genes   An archaic term for genetic polymorphisms controlling the intensity of the immune response to a particular antigen, now known to result from allelic differences in MHC molecules, especially MHC class II molecules, that influence binding of particular peptides. (Chapter 6)

IRAK1, IRAK4   Protein kinases that are part of the intracellular signaling pathways leading from TLRs. (Chapter 3)

IRAK4 deficiency   An immunodeficiency characterized by recurrent bacterial infections, caused by inactivating mutations in the IRAK4 gene that result in a block in TLR signaling. (Chapter 3)

IRF9   A member of the IRF family of transcription factors that interacts with activated STAT1 and STAT2 to form the complex called ISGF3, which induces transcription of many ISGs. (Chapter 3)

ISGF3   *See* **IRF9**. (Chapter 3)

isoelectric focusing   An analytical technique that separates proteins on the basis of the pH at which their net charge is zero. A pH gradient is established within a matrix, such as a polyacrylamide gel, and subjected to an electric current. Proteins added to this matrix will migrate until they reach the pH at which they are electrically neutral. (Appendix I)

isoforms   Different forms of the same protein; for example, the different forms encoded by different alleles of the same gene. (Chapter 6)

isolated lymphoid follicles (ILFs)   A type of organized lymphoid tissue in the gut wall that is composed mainly of B cells. (Chapter 12)

isolation membrane   *See* **phagophore**. (Chapter 12)

isotype   The designation of an immunoglobulin chain with respect to the type of constant region it has. Light chains can be of either κ or λ isotype. Heavy chains can be of μ, δ, γ, α, or ε isotype. The different heavy-chain isotypes have different effector functions and determine the class and functional properties of antibodies (IgM, IgD, IgG, IgA, and IgE, respectively). (Chapters 1, 4, 10)

isotype switching   *See* **class switching**. (Chapter 10)

isotypic exclusion   Describes the use of one or other of the light-chain isotypes, κ or λ, by a given B cell or antibody. (Chapter 8)

JAK inhibitors ('jakinibs')   Small-molecule kinase inhibitors with relative selectivity for one or more of the Janus kinases. (Chapter 16)

Janus kinase (JAK) family, Janus kinases (JAKs)   Enzymes of the JAK–STAT intracellular signaling pathways that link many cytokine receptors with gene transcription in the nucleus. The kinases phosphorylate STAT proteins in the cytosol, which then move to the nucleus and activate a variety of genes. (Chapters 3, 16)

J chain   Small polypeptide chain made by B cells that attaches to polymeric immunoglobulins IgM and IgA by disulfide bonds and is essential for formation of the binding site for the polymeric immunoglobulin receptor. (Chapters 4, 12)

JNK   *See* **Jun kinase**. (Chapter 7)

Job syndrome   *See* **hyper IgE syndrome**. (Chapter 13)

joining gene segment, J gene segment   Short DNA sequences that encode the J regions of immunoglobulin and T-cell receptor variable domains. In a rearranged light-chain, TCRα, or TCRγ genes, the J gene segment is joined to a V gene segment. In a rearranged heavy-chain, TCRβ, or TCRδ locus, a J gene segment is joined to a D gene segment. (Chapter 5)

junctional diversity   The variability in sequence present in antigen-specific receptors that is created during the process of joining V, D, and J gene segments and which is due to imprecise joining and insertion of non-templated nucleotides at the joins between gene segments. (Chapters 1, 5)

Jun kinase (JNK)   A protein kinase that phosphorylates the transcription factor c-Jun, enabling it to bind to c-Fos to form the AP-1 transcription factor. (Chapter 7)

κ chain   One of the two classes or isotypes of immunoglobulin light chains. (Chapters 4, 5)

K63 linkages   In polyubiquitin chains, the covalent ligation of the lysine 63 amino group of one ubiquitin protein with the carboxy terminus of a second ubiquitin. This type of linkage is most associated with activation of signaling by formation of a scaffold recognized by signaling adaptors such as TAB1/2. (Chapter 3)

kallikreins   Proteases that can cleave desmosomes in the skin, leading to keratinocyte shedding and disturbed barrier function of the skin. (Chapter 14)

keratinocytes   Epithelial cells that produce keratin, which are the major cell type in the skin. (Chapter 12)

killer cell immunoglobulin-like receptors (KIRs)   Large family of receptors present on NK cells, through which the cells' cytotoxic activity is controlled. The family contains both activating and inhibitory receptors. (Chapters 3, 6)

killer cell lectin-like receptors (KLRs) Large family of receptors present on NK cells, through which the cells' cytotoxic activity is controlled. The family contains both activating and inhibitory receptors. (Chapter 3)

kinetic proofreading model A mathematical model for T-cell receptor signal initiation. The model posits a temporal lag between receptor–ligand binding and receptor signaling. When the duration of receptor binding is shorter than that needed to initiate signaling, the receptor and ligand disengage, and no downstream signal ensues. (Chapter 7)

kinin system An enzymatic cascade of plasma proteins that is triggered by tissue damage to produce several inflammatory mediators, including the vasoactive peptide bradykinin. (Chapter 3)

Kostmann's disease A form of severe congenital neutropenia, an inherited condition in which the neutrophil count is low. In Kostmann's disease, this is due to a deficiency of the mitochondrial protein HAX1, which leads to apoptosis of developing myeloid cells and persistent neutropenia. (Chapter 13)

Ku A DNA repair protein required for immunoglobulin and T-cell receptor gene rearrangement. (Chapter 5)

Kupffer cells Phagocytes lining the hepatic sinusoids; they remove debris and dying cells from the blood but are not known to elicit immune responses. (Chapter 3)

λ chain One of the two classes or isotypes of immunoglobulin light chains. (Chapters 4, 5)

λ5 *See* **surrogate light chain**. (Chapter 8)

lacteal A blind lymphatic capillary vessel that originates in the lamina propria of villi of the small intestine that ultimately delivers absorbed nutrients (especially lipids in the form of chylomicrons) to the draining lymph nodes. The vessels may also deliver antigens and immune cells to lymph nodes. (Chapter 12)

lamellar bodies Lipid-rich secretory organelles in keratinocytes and lung pneumocytes that release β-defensins into the extracellular space. (Chapter 2)

lamina propria A layer of connective tissue underlying a mucosal epithelium. It contains lymphocytes and other immune-system cells. (Chapter 1)

Langerhans cells A unique immune lineage with features of dendritic cells and monocyte-derived macrophages that resides in the epidermis but can migrate upon activation to lymph nodes and present antigens to T cells. (Chapters 6, 9, 12)

large pre-B cell Stage of B-cell development immediately after the pro-B cell, in which the cell expresses the pre-B-cell receptor and undergoes several rounds of division. (Chapter 8)

laser-capture microdissection A technique for isolating cells from a tissue using a microscope and a laser to capture the cells in a microscopic region of interest. (Appendix I)

LAT *See* **linker for activation of T cells**. (Chapter 7)

late-phase reaction Allergic reaction that occurs several hours after initial encounter with an antigen. Thought to be a manifestation of recruitment of multiple leukocyte subsets to the site of allergen exposure. (Chapter 14)

late pro-B cell Stage in B-cell development in which VH to DJH joining occurs. (Chapter 8)

latency A state in which a virus infects a cell but does not replicate. (Chapter 13)

Lck An Src family tyrosine kinase that associates with the cytoplasmic tails of CD4 and CD8 and phosphorylates the cytoplasmic tails of the T-cell receptor signaling chains, thus helping to activate signaling from the T-cell receptor complex once antigen has bound. (Chapters 4, 7)

lectin A carbohydrate-binding protein. (Chapter 2)

lectin pathway Complement-activation pathway that is triggered by mannose-binding lectin (MBL) or ficolins bound to bacteria. (Chapters 2, 10)

lentiviruses A group of retroviruses that include the human immunodeficiency virus, HIV-1. They cause disease after a long incubation period. (Chapter 13)

lethal factor protease An endopeptidase produced by *Bacillus anthracis* that cleaves NLRP1, inducing cell death within the infected cell, typically a macrophage. (Chapter 3)

leucine-rich repeat (LRR) Protein motif that is repeated in series to form, for example, the extracellular portions of Toll-like receptors. (Chapter 3)

leukocyte A white blood cell. Leukocytes include lymphocytes, polymorphonuclear leukocytes, and monocytes. (Chapter 1)

leukocyte adhesion deficiencies (LADs) A class of immunodeficiency diseases in which the ability of leukocytes to enter sites infected by extracellular pathogens is affected, impairing elimination of infection. There are several different causes, including a deficiency of the common β chain of the leukocyte integrins. (Chapters 3, 13)

leukocyte adhesion deficiency type 1 (LAD-1) Disease caused by defects in the production of integrin common β subunit CD18, a component of LFA-1 and other integrins needed for leukocyte adherence to blood endothelium. (Chapter 13)

leukocyte adhesion deficiency type 2 (LAD-2) Disease caused by defects in the production of sulfated sialyl-Lewis^X that prevent neutrophils from interacting with P-selectin and E-selectin, eliminating their ability to migrate properly to sites of infection. (Chapters 3, 13)

leukocyte adhesion deficiency type 3 (LAD-3) Disease caused by defects in the production of kindlin-3, a protein needed for the conversion of β integrins to their high-affinity binding state. High-affinity binding of integrins to their ligands on blood endothelium is required for leukocyte transmigration from the blood into tissues at sites of infection. (Chapter 13)

leukocyte functional antigens (LFAs) Cell-adhesion molecules on leukocytes that were initially defined using monoclonal antibodies. LFA-1 is a β2 integrin; LFA-2 (now usually called CD2) is a member of the immunoglobulin superfamily, as is LFA-3 (now called CD58). LFA-1 is particularly important in T-cell adhesion to endothelial cells and antigen-presenting cells. (Chapters 3, 9)

leukocyte receptor complex (LRC) A large cluster of immunoglobulin-like receptor genes that includes the killer cell immunoglobulin-like receptor (KIR) genes. (Chapter 3)

leukocytosis The presence of increased numbers of leukocytes in the blood. It is commonly seen in acute infection. (Chapter 3)

leukotrienes Lipid mediators of inflammation that are derived from arachidonic acid. They are produced by macrophages and other cells. (Chapters 3, 11, 16)

LFA-1 (CD11a:CD18, or α$_L$β$_2$) *See* **leukocyte functional antigens**. (Chapters 3, 9, 11)

LGP2 A member of the RLR family, it cooperates with RIG-I and MDA-5 in the recognition of viral RNA. (Chapter 3)

licensing The activation of a dendritic cell so that it is able to present antigen to naive T cells and activate them. (Chapter 9)

light chain, L chain The smaller of the two types of polypeptide chains that make up an immunoglobulin molecule. It consists of one V and one C domain and is disulfide-bonded to the heavy chain. There are two classes, or isotypes, of light chain, known as κ and λ, which are produced from separate genetic loci. (Chapters 1, 4)

light-chain variable region (V$_L$) Referring to the V region of the light chain of an immunoglobulin. (Chapter 5)

light zone A region of the germinal center enriched in B cells interacting with T follicular helper cells and antigen on follicular dendritic cells. (Chapter 10)

linear model of memory-cell development One of two general models of memory lymphocyte development that posits that memory T (and B) cells arise from fully differentiated effector cells. *See also* **branching** (or **asymmetric division**) **model of memory-cell development**. (Chapter 11)

lineage tracing The process of genetically marking a progenitor cell with the goal of tracing all of its subsequent progeny. (Appendix I)

lingual tonsils Paired masses of organized peripheral lymphoid tissue situated at the base of the tongue, in which adaptive immune responses can be initiated. They are part of the mucosal immune system. *See also* **palatine tonsils**. (Chapter 1)

linked recognition The rule that for a helper T cell to be able to activate a B cell, the epitopes recognized by the B cell and the helper T cell have to be derived from the same antigen (i.e., they must originally have been physically linked). (Chapters 10, 16)

linker for activation of T cells A cytoplasmic adaptor protein with several tyrosines that become phosphorylated by the tyrosine kinase ZAP-70. It helps to coordinate downstream signaling events in T-cell activation. (Chapter 7)

LIP10 A cleaved fragment of invariant chain retaining the transmembrane segments and which remains bound to MHC class II proteins and helps target the complex to the endosome. (Chapter 6)

LIP22 The initial cleaved fragment of invariant chain bound to MHC class II molecules. (Chapter 6)

lipocalin-2 An antimicrobial peptide produced in abundance by neutrophils and mucosal epithelial cells that inhibits bacterial and fungal growth by limiting availability of iron. (Chapter 11)

lipopeptide antigens A diverse set of antigens derived from microbial lipids typically presented by nonclassical MHC class Ib molecules such as CD1 molecules to invariant T-cell populations, including iNKT cells. (Chapter 6)

lipopolysaccharide (LPS) The surface lipopolysaccharide of Gram-negative bacteria, which stimulates TLR-4 on macrophages and dendritic cells. (Chapters 2, 3, 16)

lipoteichoic acids Components of bacterial cell walls that are recognized by Toll-like receptors. (Chapter 3)

listeriolysin O (LLO) A hemolysin secreted by the bacterium *Listeria monocytogenes* to disrupt endosomal membranes and allow bacterial entry into the cytosol of an infected cell. (Chapters 11, 12)

long-term nonprogressors HIV-infected individuals who mount an immune response that controls viral loads such that they do not progress to AIDS despite the absence of antiretroviral therapy. *See also* **elite controllers**. (Chapter 13)

LPS-binding protein Protein in blood and extracellular fluid that binds bacterial lipopolysaccharide (LPS) shed from bacteria. (Chapter 3)

L-selectin (CD62L) Adhesion molecule of the selectin family found on lymphocytes. L-selectin binds to CD34 and GlyCAM-1 on high endothelial venules to initiate the migration of naive lymphocytes into lymphoid tissue. (Chapters 9, 11, 12)

Ly49 receptors A family of C-type lectins expressed by mouse, but not human, NK cells. These can be either activating or inhibitory in function. (Chapter 3)

Ly49H *See* **Ly49 receptors**. (Chapter 3)

Ly108 *See* **SLAM**. (Chapter 10)

lymph The extracellular fluid that accumulates in tissues and is drained by lymphatic vessels that carry it through the lymphatic system to the thoracic duct, which returns it to the blood. (Chapter 1)

lymphatic system The system of lymph-carrying vessels and peripheral lymphoid tissues through which extracellular fluid from tissues passes before it is returned to the blood via the thoracic duct. (Chapter 1)

lymphatic vessels, lymphatics Thin-walled vessels that carry lymph. (Chapter 1)

lymph nodes A type of peripheral lymphoid organ present in many locations throughout the body where lymphatic vessels converge. (Chapter 1)

lymphoblast A lymphocyte that has enlarged after activation and has increased its rate of RNA and protein synthesis but is not yet fully differentiated. (Chapter 1)

lymphocyte A class of white blood cells that bear variable cell-surface receptors for antigen and are responsible for adaptive immune responses. There are two main types—B lymphocytes (B cells) and T lymphocytes (T cells)—which mediate humoral and cell-mediated immunity, respectively. On antigen recognition, a lymphocyte enlarges to form a lymphoblast and then proliferates and differentiates into an antigen-specific effector cell. (Chapter 1)

lymphocyte receptor repertoire All the highly variable antigen receptors carried by B and T lymphocytes. (Chapter 1)

lymphoid Describes tissues composed mainly of lymphocytes. (Chapter 1)

lymphoid–myeloid primed multipotent progenitors (LMPPs) Progenitor cells in the bone marrow that are no longer self-renewing stem cells, but are committed to producing lymphoid and myeloid cell lineages. (Chapter 8)

lymphoid organs Organized tissues characterized by very large numbers of lymphocytes interacting with a nonlymphoid stroma. The central, or primary, lymphoid organs, where lymphocytes are generated, are the thymus and bone marrow. The main peripheral, or secondary, lymphoid organs, in which adaptive immune responses are initiated, are the lymph nodes, spleen, and mucosa-associated lymphoid organs such as tonsils and Peyer's patches. (Chapter 1)

lymphoid tissue Tissue composed of large numbers of lymphocytes. (Chapter 1)

lymphoid tissue inducer (LTi) cells Cells of the blood lineage, which arise in the fetal liver and are carried in the blood to sites where they will form lymph nodes and other peripheral lymphoid organs. (Chapters 9, 12)

lymphoid tissue (LT)-resident cDCs Conventional dendritic cells that reside in the T-cell zones of secondary lymphoid tissues. (Chapter 9)

lymphopenia Abnormally low levels of lymphocytes in the blood. (Chapter 13)

lymphopoiesis The differentiation of lymphoid cells from a common lymphoid progenitor. (Chapter 8)

lymphotoxins (LTs) Cytokines of the tumor necrosis factor (TNF) family that are directly cytotoxic for some cells. They occur as trimers of LT-α chains (LT-α_3) and heterotrimers of LT-α and LT-β chains (LT-$\alpha_1\beta_2$). (Chapter 9)

lysogenic phase The phase of the viral life cycle in which the virus genome integrates into the host-cell genome but remains dormant, employing mechanisms to avoid destroying its cellular host. (Chapter 13)

lysozyme Antimicrobial enzyme that degrades bacterial cell walls. (Chapter 2)

lytic phase, productive phase The phase of the viral life cycle in which there is active viral replication followed by destruction of the infected host cell as the virus escapes to infect new target cells. (Chapter 13)

M1 macrophages The name sometimes given to 'classically' activated macrophages, which develop in the context of type 1 responses and have pro-inflammatory properties. (Chapter 11)

M2 macrophages The name sometimes given to 'alternatively' activated macrophages, which develop in the context of type 2 responses (e.g., parasite infection) and promote tissue remodeling and repair. (Chapter 11)

macrophages Large mononuclear phagocytic cells present in most tissues that have many functions; for example, scavenger cells, pathogen-recognition cells, and production of pro-inflammatory cytokines. Macrophages arise both embryonically and from bone marrow precursors throughout life. (Chapters 1, 3)

macropinocytosis A process in which large amounts of extracellular fluid are taken up into an intracellular vesicle. This is one way in which dendritic cells can take up a wide variety of antigens from their surroundings. (Chapters 1, 3, 9)

MAdCAM-1 Mucosal addressin cell-adhesion molecule-1. A mucosal addressin that is recognized by the lymphocyte surface proteins L-selectin and VLA-4, enabling the specific homing of lymphocytes to mucosal tissues. (Chapters 9, 11, 12)

MAIT cells *See* **mucosal associated invariant T cells**. (Chapter 6)

major basic protein Protein released by activated eosinophils that acts on mast cells and basophils to cause their degranulation. (Chapter 14)

major histocompatibility complex (MHC) A cluster of genes on human chromosome 6 that encodes a set of membrane glycoproteins called the MHC molecules. The MHC also encodes proteins involved in antigen processing and other aspects of host defense. The genes for the MHC molecules are the most polymorphic in the human genome, having large numbers of alleles at the various loci. (Chapters 1, 4)

MAL An adaptor protein that associates with MyD88 in signaling by TLR-2–TLR-1, TLR-2–TLR-6, and TLR-4. (Chapter 3)

mannose-binding lectin (MBL) Mannose-binding protein present in the blood. It can opsonize pathogens bearing mannose on their surfaces and can activate the complement system via the lectin pathway, an important part of innate immunity. (Chapter 2)

mannose receptor A receptor on macrophages that is specific for mannose-containing carbohydrates that occur on the surfaces of pathogens but not on host cells. (Chapter 3)

mantle zone A rim of B lymphocytes that surrounds lymphoid follicles. (Chapter 10)

MAp19 A non-enzymatically active splice variant encoded by the MASP-2 gene that can associate with mannose-binding lectin (MBL) and may regulate lectin pathway complement activation. (Chapter 2)

MAp44 A non-enzymatically active splice variant encoded by the MASP-1 gene that can associate with mannose-binding lectin (MBL) and may regulate lectin pathway complement activation. (Chapter 2)

MAP kinase (MAPK) *See* **mitogen-activated protein kinase**. (Chapter 7)

MARCO (macrophage receptor with a collagenous structure) *See* **scavenger receptor**. (Chapter 3)

marginal sinus A blood-filled vascular network that branches from the central arteriole and demarcates each area of white pulp in the spleen. (Chapters 9, 10)

marginal zone Area of lymphoid tissue lying at the border of the white pulp in the spleen. (Chapter 1)

marginal zone B cells A unique population of B cells found in the spleen marginal zones; they do not circulate and are distinguished from conventional B cells by a distinct set of surface proteins. (Chapters 1, 8, 9)

MASP-1, MASP-2, MASP-3 Serine proteases of the classical and lectin pathways of complement activation that bind to C1q, ficolins, and mannose-binding lectin, and function in their activation to cleave C4. (Chapter 2)

mass spectrometry A technique for measuring the mass-to-charge ratio of ions in a complex mixture. For instance, when a mixture of peptides is analyzed, a spectrum of separated peaks is generated. Each peak represents an ion, or peptide, with a distinct mass-to-charge ratio. The amino acid sequence of the peptide can often be inferred by the precisely measured mass-to-charge ratio of the peak. (Appendix I)

mast cell A large granule-rich cell found in connective tissues throughout the body, most abundantly in the submucosal tissues and the dermis. The granules store bioactive molecules including the vasoactive amine histamine, which are released on mast-cell activation. Mast cells are thought to be involved in defenses against parasites, and they have a crucial role in allergic reactions. (Chapters 1, 3, 10)

mastocytosis The overproduction of mast cells. (Chapter 10)

mature B cell B cell that expresses IgM and IgD on its surface and has gained the ability to respond to antigen. (Chapter 8)

mature cDCs Conventional dendritic cells that have been activated for antigenic priming of naive T cells, typically after recognition of pathogen-associated molecular patterns (PAMPs). Mature cDCs express high levels of co-stimulatory molecules, such as B7.1, and express high levels of MHC:peptide complexes but have down-regulated their antigen-processing capabilities. (Chapter 9)

MAVS (mitochondrial antiviral signaling protein) A CARD-containing adaptor protein attached to the outer mitochondrial membrane that signals downstream of RIG-I and MDA-5 to activate IRF3 and NFκB in response to viral infection. (Chapter 3)

MBL-associated serine proteases *See* **MASP-1, MASP-2, MASP-3**. (Chapter 2)

M cells Specialized epithelial cell type in the intestinal epithelium over Peyer's patches, through which antigens and pathogens enter from the gut. (Chapters 1, 9, 12)

MD-2 Accessory protein for TLR-4 activity. (Chapter 3)

MDA-5 (melanoma differentiation–associated 5, also helicard) This protein contains an RNA helicase–like domain similar to RIG-I and senses double-stranded RNA for detection of intracellular viral infections. (Chapter 3)

medulla The central or collecting point of an organ. The thymic medulla is the central area of each thymic lobe, rich in bone marrow–derived antigen-presenting cells and the cells of a distinctive medullary epithelium. The medulla of the lymph node is a site of macrophage and plasma-cell concentration through which the lymph flows on its way to the efferent lymphatics. (Chapter 8)

Mek1 A MAPK kinase in the Raf–Mek1–Erk signaling module, which is a part of a signaling pathway in lymphocytes leading to activation of the transcription factor AP-1. (Chapter 7)

melanoma-associated antigens (MAGEs) Heterogeneous group of proteins of diverse or unknown functions characterized by restricted expression limited to tumors (i.e., melanoma) or testis germ cells. (Chapter 16)

membrane-associated ring finger (C3HC4) 1, MARCH-1 An E3 ligase expressed in B cells, dendritic cells, and macrophages that induces the constitutive degradation of MHC class II molecules, regulating their steady-state expression. (Chapter 6)

membrane attack Effector pathway of complement that is based on formation of the membrane-attack complex (MAC). (Chapter 2)

membrane-attack complex (MAC) Protein complex composed of C5b to C9 that assembles a membrane-spanning hydrophilic pore on pathogen surfaces, causing cell lysis. (Chapter 2)

membrane cofactor of proteolysis (MCP or CD46) A complement-regulatory protein; a host-cell membrane protein that acts in conjunction with factor I to cleave C3b to its inactive derivative iC3b and thus prevent convertase formation. (Chapter 2)

membrane immunoglobulin (mIg)   Transmembrane immunoglobulin present on B cells; it is the B-cell receptor for antigen. (Chapter 1)

memory B cells   See **memory cells**. (Chapters 10, 11)

memory cells   B and T lymphocytes that mediate immunological memory. They are more sensitive to antigen than are naive lymphocytes and respond rapidly on reexposure to the antigen that originally induced them. (Chapters 1, 10, 11)

memory phase   The period of the clonal lymphocyte response (T or B cell) marked by the persistence of long-lived memory lymphocytes that emerge during the course of antigenic challenge. (Chapter 11)

memory T cells   See **memory cells**. (Chapter 11)

mesenteric lymph nodes   Lymph nodes located in the connective tissue (mesentery) that tethers the intestine to the rear wall of the abdomen. They drain the GALT. (Chapter 12)

metastasis   Spread of a tumor from its original location to distant organs of the body by traveling through the blood or lymphatics or by direct extension. (Chapter 16)

2'-O-methyltransferase (MTase)   An enzyme that transfers a methyl group to the 2' hydroxyl of the first and second ribose groups in mRNA. Viruses that acquire MTase can produce cap-1 and cap-2 on their transcripts and thereby evade restriction by IFIT1. (Chapter 3)

MF-59   A proprietary adjuvant based on squalene and water that is used in Europe, Canada, and the United States in conjunction with influenza vaccine. (Chapter 16)

MHC class I   See **MHC class I molecules**. (Chapters 1, 4)

MHC class I deficiency   An immunodeficiency disease in which MHC class I molecules are not present on the cell surface, usually as a result of an inherited deficiency of either TAP-1 or TAP-2. (Chapters 6, 13)

MHC class I molecules   Polymorphic cell-surface proteins encoded in the MHC locus and expressed on most cells. They present antigenic peptides generated in the cytosol to CD8 T cells and also bind the co-receptor CD8. (Chapters 1, 3, 4)

MHC class Ib molecules   Cell-surface receptors with structural homology to MHC class I molecules. Generally nonpolymorphic and able to present nonpeptide antigens to specialized subsets of T lymphocytes, such as γδ T cells, iNKT cells, and MAIT cells. (Chapter 4)

MHC class II   See **MHC class II molecules**. (Chapters 1, 4)

MHC class II compartment (MIIC)   The cellular vesicles in which MHC class II molecules accumulate, encounter HLA-DM, and bind antigenic peptides, before migrating to the surface of the cell. (Chapter 6)

MHC class II deficiency   A rare immunodeficiency disease in which MHC class II molecules are not present on cells as a result of various inherited defects. Individuals are severely immunodeficient and have few CD4 T cells. (Chapters 6, 13)

MHC class II molecules   Polymorphic cell-surface proteins encoded in the MHC locus and expressed primarily on specialized antigen-presenting cells. They present antigenic peptides derived from internalized extracellular pathogens to CD4 T cells and also bind the co-receptor CD4. (Chapters 1, 3, 4)

MHC class II transactivator (CIITA)   Protein that activates transcription of MHC class II genes. Defects in the CIITA gene are one cause of MHC class II deficiency. (Chapter 6)

MHC haplotype   A set of alleles in the MHC that is inherited unchanged (i.e., without recombination) from one parent. (Chapter 6)

MHC molecules   Highly polymorphic cell-surface proteins encoded by MHC class I and MHC class II genes involved in presentation of peptide antigens to T cells. They are also known as histocompatibility antigens. (Chapters 1, 4)

MHC restriction   The fact that a peptide antigen can only be recognized by a given T cell if it is bound to a particular self MHC molecule. MHC restriction is a consequence of events that occur during T-cell development. (Chapters 4, 6)

MIC-A, MIC-B   MHC class Ib proteins that are induced by stress, infection, or transformation in many cell types and are recognized by NKG2D. (Chapters 3, 6)

microbial glycolipids   Diverse class of antigens frequently presented by CD1 molecules to iNKT cells. (Chapter 6)

microbiome   The collection of genomes from all the microorganisms in an environment, such as the commensal microorganisms of the gut or skin. The term is to be contrasted with 'microbiota,' which refers to the collection of microorganisms themselves. See **commensal microorganisms**. (Chapters 1, 12)

microbiota   See **commensal microorganisms**. (Chapter 2)

microclusters   Assemblies of small numbers of T-cell receptors that may be involved in the initiation of T-cell receptor activation by antigen in naive T cells. (Chapter 7)

microfold cells   See **M cells**. (Chapters 1, 12)

microglial cell   An embryonically derived form of tissue macrophage in the central nervous system that is dependent on IL-34 for local self-renewal throughout life. (Chapter 3)

minor histocompatibility antigens   Peptides of polymorphic cellular proteins bound to MHC molecules that can lead to graft rejection when they are recognized by T cells. (Chapters 6, 15)

minor lymphocyte stimulating (Mls) antigens   An old term referring to non-MHC antigens responsible for unusually strong T-cell responses to cells from different strains of mice, now known to be superantigens encoded by endogenous retroviruses. (Chapter 6)

mismatch repair   A type of DNA repair that causes mutations and is involved in somatic hypermutation and class switching in B cells. (Chapter 10)

missing self   Refers to the loss of cell-surface molecules that engage with inhibitory receptors on NK cells, resulting in NK-cell activation. (Chapter 3)

mitogen-activated protein kinases (MAPKs)   A series of protein kinases that become phosphorylated and activated on cellular stimulation by a variety of ligands and lead to new gene expression by phosphorylating key transcription factors. The MAPKs are part of many signaling pathways, especially those leading to cell proliferation, and have different names in different organisms. (Chapters 3, 7)

mixed essential cryoglobulinemia   Disease due to the production of cryoglobulins (cold-precipitable immunoglobulins), sometimes in response to chronic infections such as hepatitis C, which can lead to the deposition of immune complexes in joints and tissues. (Chapter 15)

mixed lymphocyte reaction (MLR)   A test for histocompatibility in which lymphocytes from donor and recipient are cultured together. If the two people are histoincompatible, the recipient's T cells recognize the allogeneic MHC molecules on the cells of the donor as 'foreign' and proliferate. (Chapters 6, 15)

molecular mimicry   The similarity between some pathogen antigens and host antigens, such that antibodies and T cells produced against the former also react against host tissues. This similarity may be the cause of some autoimmunity. (Chapter 15)

monoclonal antibodies   Antibodies produced by a single clone of B lymphocytes, so that they are all identical. (Chapters 1, 4, Appendix I)

monocyte Type of white blood cell with a bean-shaped nucleus; it is a precursor of tissue macrophages. (Chapters 1, 3)

monocyte-derived DCs (MoDCs) Myeloid cells with dendritic morphology that are derived from circulating monocytes that are recruited into inflamed tissues. These cells can take up antigen and migrate to secondary lymphoid tissues where they deliver antigens to resident DCs for T-cell priming, but they are inefficient at naive T-cell priming themselves. (Chapter 9)

monogenic disorders Disorders that are caused by variations in a single gene. These disorders typically have a clear familial pattern of inheritance and can be dominant or recessive, or autosomal or sex-linked. (Chapter 13)

monoglucosylated glycan A protein modification consisting of a single attached glucosyl moiety indicating an incompletely folded protein within the endoplasmic reticulum. This modification of nascent MHC molecules is recognized by calreticulin to recruit incompletely loaded MHC class I proteins to the peptide-loading complex. (Chapter 6)

monomorphic Describes a gene that occurs in only one form. Cf. **polymorphic**. (Chapter 6)

motheaten A mutation in the SHP-1 protein phosphatase that impairs the function of some inhibitory receptors, such as Ly49, resulting in overactivation of various cells, including NK cells. Mice with this mutation have a 'motheaten' appearance because of chronic inflammation. (Chapter 3)

moxetumomab pasudotox-tdfk (Lumoxiti) An immunotoxin composed of an anti-CD22 variable region fused to a fragment of *Pseudomonas* toxin and used to treat a kind of B-cell leukemia, hairy-cell leukemia, in patients whose disease was resistant to chemotherapy. (Chapter 16)

MR1 (MHC-related protein 1) A 'nonclassical' MHC class Ib molecule that binds certain folic acid metabolites produced by bacteria for recognition by mucosal-associated invariant T (MAIT) cells. (Chapters 4, 6)

MSH2, MSH6 Mismatch repair proteins that detect uridine and recruit nucleases to remove the damaged and several adjacent nucleotides. (Chapter 10)

mTOR (mammalian target of rapamycin) A serine/threonine kinase that functions in regulating numerous aspects of cell metabolism and function in complex with regulatory proteins Raptor or Rictor. The Raptor:mTOR complex (mTORC1) is inhibited by the immunosuppressive drug rapamycin. (Chapters 7, 16)

mTORC1, mTORC2 Active complexes of mTOR formed with the regulatory proteins Raptor and Rictor, respectively. (Chapter 16)

MUC2 An oligomeric, mucus gel-forming protein in the colon, where it is secreted by epithelial goblet cells into the lumen of the large intestine to create a protective, lubricating barrier. (Chapter 12)

mucins Highly glycosylated cell-surface proteins. Mucin-like molecules are bound by L-selectin in lymphocyte homing. (Chapter 2)

Muckle–Wells syndrome An inherited episodic autoinflammatory disease caused by mutations in the gene encoding NLRP3, a component of the inflammasome. (Chapters 3, 13)

mucociliary escalator The system of cilia-transported mucus by which the airways of the respiratory system trap and transport particles toward the pharynx and out of the lungs. (Chapter 12)

mucosa-associated lymphoid tissue (MALT) Generic term for all organized lymphoid tissue found at mucosal surfaces, in which an adaptive immune response can be initiated. It comprises gut-associated lymphoid tissue (GALT), nasal-associated lymphoid tissue (NALT), and bronchus-associated lymphoid tissue (BALT) (when present). (Chapters 1, 9, 12)

mucosal-associated invariant T cells (MAIT cells) Primarily γδ T cells with limited diversity present in the mucosal immune system that respond to bacterially derived folate derivates presented by the nonclassical MHC class Ib molecule MR1. (Chapters 4, 12)

mucosal epithelia Mucus-coated epithelia lining the body's internal cavities that connect with the outside (such as the gut, airways, and vaginal tract). (Chapter 2)

mucosal immune system The immune system that protects internal mucosal surfaces (such as the linings of the gut, respiratory tract, and urogenital tracts), which are the site of entry for virtually all pathogens and other antigens. *See also* **mucosa-associated lymphoid tissue**. (Chapters 1, 12)

mucosal mast cells Specialized mast cells present in mucosa. They produce little histamine but large amounts of prostaglandins and leukotrienes. (Chapter 11)

mucosal tolerance The suppression of specific systemic immune responses to an antigen by the previous administration of the same antigen by a mucosal route. (Chapter 12)

mucus Sticky solution of proteins (mucins) secreted by goblet cells of internal epithelia, forming a protective layer on the epithelial surface. (Chapter 2)

multinucleated giant cells Large phagocytic cells that form at sites of chronic inflammation by the fusion of multiple monocytes or macrophages. These cells are often found as components of granulomas, such as those that develop in response to poorly eradicated infections (e.g., tuberculosis) or foreign bodies. (Chapter 11)

multiple sclerosis A neurological autoimmune disease characterized by focal demyelination in the central nervous system, lymphocytic infiltration in the brain, and a chronic progressive course. (Chapter 15)

multiplex assay An assay in which multiple antigens or antibodies can simultaneously be detected and quantified in a single sample. (Appendix I)

muramyl dipeptide (MDP) A component of the peptidoglycan of most bacteria that is recognized by the intracellular sensor NOD2. (Chapter 3)

muromonab A mouse antibody against human CD3 used to treat transplant rejection; this was the first monoclonal antibody approved as a drug in humans. (Chapter 16)

mutualism A symbiotic relationship between two organisms in which both benefit, such as the relationship between a human and its normal resident (commensal) gut microorganisms. (Chapter 12)

Mx (myxoma resistant) proteins Interferon-inducible proteins required for cellular resistance to influenza virus replication. (Chapter 3)

myasthenia gravis An autoimmune disease in which autoantibodies against the acetylcholine receptor on skeletal muscle cells cause a block in neuromuscular junctions, leading to progressive weakness and eventually death. (Chapter 15)

mycophenolate An inhibitor of the synthesis of guanosine monophosphate that acts as a cytotoxic immunosuppressive drug. It acts by killing rapidly dividing cells, including lymphocytes proliferating in response to antigen. (Chapter 16)

mycophenolate mofetil Pro-drug used in cancer treatment that is metabolized to mycophenolate, an inhibitor of inosine monophosphate dehydrogenase, thereby impairing guanosine monophosphate, and thus DNA, synthesis. (Chapter 16)

MyD88 An adaptor protein that functions in signaling by all TLR proteins except TLR-3. (Chapter 3)

myeloid Refers to the lineage of blood cells that includes all leukocytes except lymphocytes. (Chapter 1)

myeloid-derived suppressor cells (MDSCs) Cells in tumors that can inhibit T-cell activation within the tumor. (Chapter 16)

myeloma protein Individuals who have the disease multiple myeloma have a malignant expansion of plasma cells, all of which arose from a single cell, and therefore all secrete the same antibody protein. This antibody, known as myeloma protein, accumulates in large quantities in an affected individual's serum. (Appendix I)

myelomonocytic cells Innate immune cells derived from myelomonocytic bone marrow precursors, including neutrophils, basophils, eosinophils, monocytes, and dendritic cells. (Chapter 11)

NADPH oxidase Multicomponent enzyme complex that is assembled and activated in the phagolysosome membrane in stimulated phagocytes. It generates superoxide in an oxygen-requiring reaction called the respiratory burst. (Chapter 3)

NAIPs (NLR family, apoptosis inhibitory proteins) A family of NLR-containing proteins that serve as intracellular pattern-recognition receptors (PRRs). (Chapter 3)

NAIP2 An NLR protein that, together with NLRC4, recognizes the PrgJ protein of the *Salmonella enterica* ssp. *typhimurium* type III secretion system to activate an inflammasome pathway in response to infection. (Chapter 3)

NAIP5 An NLR protein that, together with NLRC4, recognizes intracellular flagellin to activate an inflammasome pathway in response to infection. (Chapter 3)

naive lymphocytes T cells or B cells that have undergone normal development in the thymus or the bone marrow but have not yet been activated by foreign (or self) antigens. (Chapter 1)

naive T cells Lymphocytes that have never encountered their specific antigen and thus have never responded to it, as distinct from effector and memory lymphocytes. (Chapter 9)

nasal- (or nasopharynx-) associated lymphoid tissue (NALT) Organized lymphoid tissues found in the upper respiratory tract. In humans, NALT consists of Waldeyer's ring, which includes the adenoids and palatine and lingual tonsils, plus other similarly organized lymphoid tissue located around the pharynx. It is part of the mucosal immune system. (Chapters 1, 12)

natalizumab Humanized antibody to α_4 integrin used to treat Crohn's disease and multiple sclerosis. It blocks the adhesion of lymphocytes to endothelium, impairing their migration into tissues. (Chapter 16)

natural antibodies Antibodies produced by the immune system in the apparent absence of any infection. They have a broad specificity for self and microbial antigens, can react with many pathogens, and can activate complement. (Chapter 2)

natural cytotoxicity receptors (NCRs) Activating receptors on NK cells that recognize infected cells and stimulate cell killing by the NK cell. (Chapter 3)

natural interferon-producing cells *See* **plasmacytoid dendritic cells**. (Chapter 3)

natural killer (NK) cell A type of ILC that is important in innate immunity to viruses and other intracellular pathogens and in antibody-dependent cell-mediated cytotoxicity (ADCC). NK cells express activating and inhibitory receptors but not the antigen-specific receptors of T or B cells. (Chapters 1, 3)

negative selection The process by which self-reactive thymocytes are deleted from the repertoire during T-cell development in the thymus. Autoreactive B cells undergo a similar process in bone marrow. (Chapter 8)

NEMO *See* **IKK**. (Chapters 3, 7)

NEMO deficiency *See* **X-linked hypohidrotic ectodermal dysplasia and immunodeficiency**. (Chapter 3)

neoantigen, neoepitope Type of tumor-rejection antigen created by mutations in protein that can be presented by self-MHC molecules to T cells. (Chapter 16)

neonatal Fc receptor (FcRn) *See* **FcRn**. (Chapter 12)

nephritic factor An autoantibody that leads to inflammation in the kidney by increasing C3 deposition. Nephritic factors may inhibit the activity of complement-regulatory proteins, such as factor H, or may stabilize the alternative pathway C3 convertase C3bBb. (Chapter 2)

neuraminidase An influenza virus protein that cleaves sialic acid from host cells to allow viral detachment; a common antigenic determinant and a target of antiviral neuraminidase inhibitors. (Chapters 12, 16)

neuroimmune interactions Interactions between components of the immune and nervous systems coordinated by chemical and electrophysiological signals. (Chapter 12)

neutralization Inhibition of the infectivity of a virus or the toxicity of a toxin molecule by the binding of antibodies. (Chapters 1, 10, 16)

neutralizing antibodies Antibodies that inhibit the infectivity of a virus or the toxicity of a toxin. (Chapter 10)

neutropenia Abnormally low levels of neutrophils in the blood. (Chapters 3, 13)

neutrophil The most numerous type of white blood cell in human peripheral blood. Neutrophils are phagocytic cells with a multilobed nucleus and granules that stain with neutral stains. They enter infected tissues and engulf and kill extracellular pathogens. (Chapters 1, 3)

neutrophil elastase Proteolytic enzyme stored in the granules of neutrophils that is involved in the processing of antimicrobial peptides. (Chapter 2)

neutrophil extracellular traps (NETs) A meshwork of nuclear chromatin that is released into the extracellular space by neutrophils undergoing apoptosis at sites of infection, serving as a scaffold that traps extracellular bacteria to enhance their phagocytosis by other phagocytes. (Chapter 3)

NFκB A heterodimeric transcription factor activated by the stimulation of Toll-like receptors and also by antigen receptor signaling composed of p50 and p65 subunits. (Chapter 3)

NFAT *See* **nuclear factor of activated T cells**. (Chapter 7)

Nfil3 A transcription factor important during the development of several types of immune cells including certain types of NK cells. (Chapter 3)

NHEJ *See* **nonhomologous end joining**. (Chapter 5)

nitric oxide (NO) A reactive molecular gas species produced by cells—particularly macrophages—during infection and which is toxic to bacteria and intracellular microbes. (Chapter 3)

nitric oxide radical The uncharged compound NO, having an unpaired electron conferring its high reactivity, formed in activated phagocytes by the action of inducible nitric oxide synthetase. (Chapter 3)

nivolumab Human anti-PD-1 antibody used for checkpoint blockade in treatment of metastatic melanoma. (Chapter 16)

NKG2 Family of C-type lectins that supply one of the subunits of the killer cell lectin-like receptors (KLRs) on NK cells. (Chapter 3)

NKG2D Activating C-type lectin receptor on NK cells, cytotoxic T cells, and $\gamma\delta$ T cells that recognizes the stress-response proteins MIC-A and MIC-B. (Chapter 3)

NK receptor complex (NKC) A cluster of genes that encode a family of receptors on NK cells. (Chapter 3)

NKT cell A subclass of $\alpha\beta$ T cells expressing surface receptors, such as NK1.1, that are more typical of NK cells. NKT cells recognize various nonpeptide ligands presented by nonclassical MHC class I–like proteins. (Chapter 6)

NLRC4 An NLR family member that cooperates with NAIP2 and NAIP5. (Chapter 3)

NLRP A group of 14 NOD-like receptor (NLR) proteins that contain a pyrin domain and function in the formation of a signaling complex called the inflammasome. (Chapter 3)

NLRP1 An NLR family member that assembles into an inflammasome that recruits and activates caspase 1. (Chapter 3)

NLRP3 A member of the family of intracellular NOD-like receptor proteins that have pyrin domains. It acts as a sensor of cellular damage and is part of the inflammasome. Sometimes called NALP3. (Chapters 3, 16)

N-nucleotides Non-templated nucleotides inserted by the enzyme terminal deoxynucleotidyl transferase into the junctions between gene segments of T-cell receptor and immunoglobulin heavy-chain V regions during gene segment joining. Translation of these N-regions markedly increases the diversity of these receptor chains. (Chapter 5)

nociceptors Various neuropeptide-producing sensory neurons that encode pain and are found in the skin. These cells can become stimulated by cysteine protease present in the feces of house dust mites to secrete substance P, which can activate nearby mast cells. (Chapter 14)

NOD A subgroup of NLR proteins that contain a CARD domain that is used for activation of downstream signaling. (Chapter 3)

NOD1, NOD2 Intracellular proteins of the NOD subfamily that contain a leucine-rich repeat (LRR) domain that binds components of bacterial cell walls to activate the NFκB pathway and initiate inflammatory responses. (Chapter 3)

NOD-like receptors (NLRs) Large family of proteins containing a nucleotide-binding and oligomerization domain (NOD) associated with various other domains, and whose general function is the detection of microbes and of cellular stress. (Chapters 1, 3, 12)

nonamer Conserved nine-nucleotide DNA sequence in the recombination signal sequences (RSSs) flanking gene segments in the immunoglobulin and T-cell receptor loci. (Chapter 5)

non-canonical NFκB pathway This pathway relies on activation of NIK (NFκB-inducing kinase) to induce proteolytic processing of the p100 precursor into p52, which forms an active transcription factor by associating with RelB. NIK is activated downstream of the receptors for various cytokines, such as lymphotoxin β. (Chapters 7, 10)

nonclassical MHC class Ib genes Genes encoded within the MHC whose proteins are related to the MHC class I molecules but are not highly polymorphic and present a restricted set of antigens. (Chapter 5)

nonclassical MHC class I proteins Proteins related to MHC class I molecules but are not highly polymorphic and present a restricted set of antigens.   (Chapter 6)

nonclassical MHC genes See **nonclassical MHC class Ib genes**. (Chapter 6)

nondepleting antibodies Immunosuppressive antibodies that block the function of target proteins on cells without causing the cells to be destroyed. (Chapter 16)

nonhomologous end joining (NHEJ) DNA repair pathway that directly ligates double-strand DNA breaks without use of a homologous template. (Chapter 5)

nonlymphoid tissue (NLT)-resident (or **migratory**) **cDCs** Conventional dendritic cells that reside in nonlymphoid tissues, particularly at barrier tissue sites, and migrate to T-cell zones of lymphoid organs in response to infection. (Chapter 9)

nonproductive rearrangements Rearrangements of T-cell receptor or immunoglobulin gene segments that cannot encode a protein because the coding sequences are in the wrong translational reading frame. (Chapter 5)

nonreceptor kinase Cytoplasmic protein kinases that associate with the intracellular tails of signaling receptors and help generate the signal but are not an intrinsic part of the receptor itself. (Chapter 7)

nuclear factor of activated T cells (NFAT) A family of transcription factors that are activated in response to increased cytoplasmic calcium after antigen receptor signaling in lymphocytes. (Chapter 7)

nucleotide-binding and oligomerization domain (NOD) A type of conserved domain originally recognized in ATP-binding cassette (ABC) transporters present in a large number of proteins, but which also mediates protein homo-oligomerization. (Chapters 3, 12)

nude A mutation in mice that results in hairlessness and defective formation of the thymic stroma, so that mice homozygous for this mutation have no mature T cells. (Chapters 8, 13)

NY-ESO-1 A particular highly immunogenic cancer-testis antigen expressed by many types of human tumors including melanoma. (Chapter 16)

occupational allergies An allergic reaction induced to an allergen to which someone is habitually exposed in their work. (Chapter 14)

odds ratio Represents the strength of association between the occurrence of a particular SNP and a phenotype, typically a disease. For example, an odds ratio of 10 for some specific SNP and asthma means that having that SNP confers 10 times the risk of having asthma over that of a person who has a common variant. (Chapter 14)

oligoadenylate synthetase Enzyme produced in response to stimulation of cells by interferon. It synthesizes unusual nucleotide polymers, which in turn activate a ribonuclease that degrades viral RNA. (Chapter 3)

Omenn syndrome A severe immunodeficiency disease characterized by defects in either of the *RAG* genes. Affected individuals make small amounts of functional RAG protein, allowing a small amount of V(D)J recombination. (Chapters 5, 13)

opportunistic pathogens Microorganisms that are unable to invade a healthy host, but can cause disease when there is compromise of host defenses, whether due to weakened immunity (e.g., chemotherapy or HIV/AIDS), alteration of the healthy microbiota (e.g., dysbiosis induced by antibiotic therapy), or breach of normal integrity of a barrier tissue (e.g., penetrating trauma). (Chapters 12, 13)

opsonization The coating of the surface of a pathogen by antibody and/or complement that makes it more easily ingested by phagocytes. (Chapters 1, 2, 10)

oral tolerance The suppression of specific systemic immune responses to an antigen by the prior administration of the same antigen by the oral (enteric) route. (Chapters 12, 15)

original antigenic sin The tendency of humans to make antibody responses to those epitopes shared between the first strain of a virus they encounter and subsequent related viruses, while ignoring other highly immunogenic epitopes on the second and subsequent viruses. (Chapter 11)

oxidative phosphorylation (OXPHOS) A highly efficient means of producing ATP in mitochondria from oxidative nutrients, such as pyruvate produced by glycolysis. In oxidative phosphorylation, a series of mitochondrial membrane–bound protein complexes catalyze oxidation–reduction reactions to generate a transmembrane electrical potential difference that ultimately drives ATP synthesis. (Chapter 9)

p50 See **NFκB**. (Chapter 3)

p65 See **NFκB**. (Chapter 3)

PA28 proteasome-activator complex A multi-subunit protein complex induced by interferon-γ and which takes the place of the 19S regulatory cap of the proteasome and increases the rate of peptides exiting from the proteasome catalytic core. (Chapter 6)

palatine tonsils   Paired masses of organized peripheral lymphoid tissues located on each side of the throat, and in which an adaptive immune response can be generated. They are part of the mucosal immune system. (Chapter 1)

Paneth cells   Specialized epithelial cells at the base of the crypts in the small intestine that secrete antimicrobial peptides. (Chapters 2, 12)

papain   A protease that cleaves the IgG antibody molecule on the amino-terminal side of disulfide linkages, producing two Fab fragments and one Fc fragment. (Chapter 4)

parabiosis   A technique in which two mice are surgically joined at the flanks by suturing skin from the two mice together. After 2 weeks, new blood vessels are formed in the skin, and the mice develop a shared circulatory system. Circulating cells in the blood of these mice will be a mixture of cells derived from the two conjoined partners. (Appendix I)

paracortical areas   The T-cell areas of lymph nodes. (Chapter 1)

paracrine   Describes a cytokine or other biologically active molecule acting on cells near to those that produce it. (Chapter 3)

parasites   Organisms that obtain sustenance from a live host. In immunology, it refers to worms and protozoa, the subject matter of parasitology. (Chapter 1)

paroxysmal nocturnal hemoglobinuria   A disease in which complement-regulatory proteins are defective, so that activation of complement binding to red blood cells leads to episodes of spontaneous hemolysis. (Chapters 2, 13)

passive immunization   The injection of antibody or immune serum into a naive recipient to provide specific immunological protection. Cf. **active immunization**. (Chapter 10, Appendix I)

pathogen   Microorganism that typically causes disease when it infects a host. (Chapters 1, 3)

pathogen-associated molecular patterns (PAMPs)   Molecules specifically associated with groups of pathogens that are recognized by cells of the innate immune system. (Chapters 1, 3)

pathogenesis   The origin or cause of the pathology of a disease. (Chapter 2)

pathogenic microorganism   Microorganism that typically causes disease when it infects a host. (Chapter 2)

patrolling monocyte   A form of circulating monocyte that adheres to and surveys the vascular endothelium, distinguished from classical monocytes by its low expression of Ly6C. (Chapter 3)

pattern-recognition receptors (PRRs)   Receptors of the innate immune system that recognize common molecular patterns on pathogen surfaces. (Chapters 1, 3)

PD-1 (programmed death-1)   A receptor on T cells that when bound by its ligands, PD-L1 and PD-L2, inhibits signaling from the antigen receptor. PD-1 contains an ITIM motif in its cytoplasmic tail. It is a target of cancer therapies aimed at stimulating T-cell responses to tumors. (Chapters 7, 16)

PD-L1 (programmed death ligand-1; B7-H1)   Transmembrane receptor that binds to the inhibitory receptor PD-1. PD-L1 is expressed on many cell types and is up-regulated by inflammatory cytokines. (Chapters 7, 16)

PD-L2 (programmed death ligand-2; B7-DC)   Transmembrane receptor that binds to the inhibitory receptor PD-1; mainly expressed on dendritic cells. (Chapter 7)

PECAM   *See* **CD31**. (Chapter 3)

pembrolizumab   Human anti-PD-1 antibody used for checkpoint blockade in treatment of metastatic melanoma. (Chapter 16)

pemphigus vulgaris   An autoimmune disease characterized by severe blistering of the skin and mucosal membranes. (Chapter 15)

pentameric IgM   Major form of the IgM antibodies produced by the action of J chain resulting in higher avidity for antigens. (Chapter 10)

pentraxin   A family of acute-phase proteins formed of five identical subunits, to which C-reactive protein and serum amyloid protein belong. (Chapter 3)

pepsin   A protease that cleaves several sites on the carboxy-terminal side of the disulfide linkages, producing the $F(ab')_2$ fragment and several fragments of the Fc region. (Chapter 4)

peptide-binding cleft, peptide-binding groove   The longitudinal cleft in the top surface of an MHC molecule into which the antigenic peptide is bound. (Chapter 4)

peptide editing   In the context of antigen processing and presentation, the removal of unstably bound peptides from MHC class II molecules by HLA-DM. (Chapter 6)

peptide-loading complex (PLC)   A protein complex in the endoplasmic reticulum that loads peptides onto MHC class I molecules. (Chapter 6)

peptide:MHC tetramer   Four specific peptide:MHC complexes bound to a single molecule of fluorescently labeled streptavidin, which is used to identify populations of antigen-specific T cells. (Appendix I)

peptidoglycan   A component of bacterial cell walls that is recognized by certain receptors of the innate immune system. (Chapter 2)

peptidoglycan-recognition proteins (PGRPs)   A family of *Drosophila* proteins that bind peptidoglycans from bacterial cell walls and serve to initiate the proteolytic cascade of the Toll pathway. (Chapter 3)

perforin   A cytolytic protein produced by cytotoxic T lymphocytes and natural killer cells. Perforin functions by binding to a target cell's plasma membrane and oligomerizing to form pores, which then allow pro-apoptotic granzymes to diffuse into the target cell. (Chapter 9)

periarteriolar lymphoid sheath (PALS)   Part of the inner region of the white pulp of the spleen; it contains mainly T cells. (Chapters 1, 9)

peripheral blood mononuclear cells (PBMCs)   The components of blood composed of mononucleated cells. This includes lymphocytes and monocytes, but excludes red blood cells and platelets, which have no nucleus, and excludes granulocytes (neutrophils, basophils, and eosinophils), which have multilobed nuclei. (Appendix I)

peripheral lymphoid organs, peripheral lymphoid tissues   The lymph nodes, spleen, and mucosa-associated lymphoid tissues, in which adaptive immune responses are induced, as opposed to the central lymphoid organs, in which lymphocytes develop. They are also called secondary lymphoid organs and tissues. (Chapters 1, 8)

peripheral tolerance   Tolerance acquired by mature lymphocytes in the peripheral tissues, as opposed to central tolerance, which is acquired by immature lymphocytes during their development. (Chapters 8, 12, 15)

Peyer's patches   Organized peripheral lymphoid organs under the epithelium in the small intestine, especially the ileum, and in which an adaptive immune response can be initiated. They contain lymphoid follicles and T-cell areas. They are part of the gut-associated lymphoid tissue (GALT). (Chapters 1, 9, 12)

phage display library   A collection of bacteriophages that have been engineered to express proteins of interest. Each bacteriophage expresses a single extra protein as a fusion of its surface-coat protein and therefore displays multiple copies of that extra protein on the bacteriophage surface. The collection of bacteriophages, each expressing a different extra protein on its surface, is known as a library. (Appendix I)

phagocyte oxidase   *See* **NADPH oxidase**. (Chapter 3)

phagocytic glycoprotein-1 (Pgp1)   *See* **CD44**. (Chapter 11)

phagocytosis   The internalization of particulate matter by cells by a process of engulfment, in which the cell membrane surrounds the material, eventually forming an intracellular vesicle (phagosome) containing the ingested material. (Chapters 2, 3)

phagolysosome   Intracellular vesicle formed by the fusion of a phagosome (containing ingested material) and a lysosome, and in which the ingested material is broken down. (Chapter 3)

phagophore   A crescent-shaped double-membrane cytoplasmic structure. (Chapter 12)

phagosome   Intracellular vesicle formed when particulate material is ingested by a phagocyte. (Chapter 3)

phosphatidylinositol 3-kinase (PI 3-kinase)   Enzyme involved in intracellular signaling pathways. It phosphorylates the membrane lipid phosphatidylinositol 4,5-bisphosphate (PIP$_2$) to form phosphatidylinositol 3,4,5-trisphosphate (PIP$_3$), which can recruit signaling proteins containing pleckstrin homology (PH) domains to the membrane. (Chapters 3, 7)

phosphatidylinositol kinases   Enzymes that phosphorylate the inositol headgroup on membrane lipids to produce phosphorylated derivatives that have a variety of functions in intracellular signaling. (Chapter 7)

phospholipase C-γ (PLC-γ)   Key enzyme in intracellular signaling pathways leading from many different receptors. It is activated by membrane recruitment and tyrosine phosphorylation after receptor ligation and cleaves membrane inositol phospholipids into inositol 1,4,5-trisphosphate (IP$_3$) and diacylglycerol. (Chapter 7)

phosphorylation   Addition of a phosphate group to a molecule, usually a protein, catalyzed by enzymes called kinases. (Chapter 7)

phycoerythrin (PE)   A light-harvesting protein pigment made by algae and used in conjunction with flow cytometry; it can also be recognized as a ligand by some γδ T-cell receptors. (Chapter 6)

pilin   An adhesin of *Neisseria gonorrhoeae* allowing attachment to and infection of epithelial cells of the urinary and reproductive tracts. (Chapter 10)

PIP$_2$ Phosphatidylinositol 4,5-bisphosphate, a membrane-associated phospholipid that is cleaved by phospholipase C-γ to give the signaling molecules diacylglycerol and inositol trisphosphate and is phosphorylated by PI 3-kinase to generate PIP$_3$. (Chapter 7)

PIP$_3$ Phosphatidylinositol 3,4,5-trisphosphate, a membrane-associated phospholipid that can recruit intracellular signaling molecules containing pleckstrin homology (PH) domains to the membrane. (Chapter 7)

PKR   Serine/threonine kinase activated by IFN-α and IFN-β. It phosphorylates the eukaryotic protein synthesis initiation factor eIF-2, inhibiting translation and thus contributing to the inhibition of viral replication. (Chapter 3)

plasma   The liquid component of whole blood. (Appendix I)

plasma cells   Terminally differentiated activated B lymphocytes. Plasma cells are the main antibody-secreting cells of the body. They are found in the medulla of the lymph nodes, in splenic red pulp, in bone marrow, and in mucosal tissues. (Chapters 1, 10)

plasmablasts   A B cell in a lymph node that already shows some features of a plasma cell. (Chapter 10)

plasmacytoid dendritic cells (pDCs)   A distinct lineage of dendritic cells that secrete large amounts of interferon on activation by pathogens and their products via receptors such as Toll-like receptors. Cf. **conventional dendritic cells**. (Chapters 3, 9)

platelet-activating factor (PAF)   A lipid mediator that activates the blood clotting cascade and several other components of the innate immune system. (Chapter 3)

pluripotent   Typically referring to the capacity of a progenitor cell to generate all possible lineages of an organ system. (Chapter 1)

P-nucleotides   Short palindromic nucleotide sequences formed between gene segments of the rearranged V-region gene generated by the asymmetric opening of the hairpin intermediate during RAG-mediated rearrangement. (Chapter 5)

poison ivy   This plant is a common cause of allergic contact dermatitis in the United States. The urushiol oil of this plant contains a mixture of pentadecacatechols that can cross cell membranes and attach to intracellular proteins. When modified peptides from these proteins are processed and presented by MHC class I molecules on the cell's surface, they may activate CD8 T cells that recognize the peptides and cause damage through killing and by cytokine secretion. (Chapter 14)

Polη   An error-prone 'translesion' DNA polymerase involved in repairing DNA damage caused by UV radiation and in somatic hypermutation. (Chapter 10)

polyclonal mitogens   Compounds that stimulate lymphocytes to undergo cell division regardless of the antigen specificity of the cells. (Appendix I)

polygenic   Containing several separate loci encoding proteins of identical function; applied to the MHC. Cf. **polymorphic**. (Chapter 6)

polymerase stalling   The halting of RNA polymerase during the transcription of a gene at locations within the gene locus, known to be a regulated process, and involved in mechanisms of isotype switching. (Chapter 10)

polymeric immunoglobulin receptor (pIgR)   The receptor for polymeric immunoglobulins IgA and IgM on basolateral surfaces of mucosal and glandular epithelial cells that transports IgA (or IgM) into secretions. (Chapters 10, 12)

polymorphic   Existing in a variety of different forms; applied to a gene, occurring in a variety of different alleles. (Chapters 1, 4, 6)

polymorphism   Applied to genes, variability at a gene locus in which all variants occur at a frequency greater than 1%. (Chapter 6)

polymorphonuclear leukocytes   *See* **granulocytes**. (Chapter 1)

polysaccharide capsule   A distinct structure in some bacteria—both Gram-negative and Gram-positive—that lies outside the cell membrane and cell wall and which can prevent direct phagocytosis by macrophages without the aid of antibody or complement. (Chapter 10)

polyubiquitin chains   Polymers of ubiquitin covalently linked from lysine residues within one ubiquitin monomer to the carboxy terminus of a second ubiquitin. (Chapter 3)

PorA   Outer membrane protein of *Neisseria meningitidis* that binds C4BP, thereby inactivating C3b deposited on its surface. (Chapter 2)

positive selection   A process occurring in the thymus in which only those developing T cells whose receptors can recognize antigens presented by self MHC molecules can mature. (Chapters 6, 8)

post-transplant lymphoproliferative disorder   B-cell expansion driven by Epstein–Barr virus (EBV) in which the B cells can undergo mutations and become malignant. This can occur when patients are immunosuppressed after, for example, solid organ transplantation. (Chapter 16)

pre-B-cell receptor   Receptor produced by pre-B cells that includes an immunoglobulin heavy chain, as well as surrogate light-chain proteins, and Igα and Igβ signaling subunits. Signaling through this receptor induces the pre-B cell to enter the cell cycle, to turn off the RAG genes, to degrade the RAG proteins, and to expand by several cell divisions. (Chapter 8)

pre-T cell   The first subset of thymocytes that are fully committed to the T-cell lineage and have lost the ability to develop into B cells, NK cells, or myeloid cells. T-cell receptor β-chain gene rearrangements are completed at this stage. (Chapter 8)

pre-T-cell receptor   Receptor protein produced by developing T lymphocytes at the pre-T-cell stage. It is composed of TCRβ chains that pair with a surrogate α chain called pTα (pre-T-cell α) and is associated with the CD3 signaling chains. Signaling through this receptor induces pre-T-cell proliferation, expression of CD4 and CD8, and cessation of TCR β-chain rearrangement. (Chapter 8)

prednisone A synthetic steroid with potent anti-inflammatory and immunosuppressive activity used in treating acute graft rejection, autoimmune disease, and lymphoid tumors. (Chapter 16)

PrEP (pre-exposure prophylaxis) The daily administration of a combination of two reverse transcriptase inhibitors to uninfected individuals at high risk of HIV infection to lower their risk of contracting HIV infection. (Chapter 13)

PREX1 A guanine nucleotide exchange factor (GEF) activated downstream of small G proteins in response to activation of GPCRs such as the fMLP or C5a receptor. (Chapter 3)

primary focus Site of early antibody production by plasmablasts in medullary cords of lymph nodes that precedes the germinal center reaction and differentiation of plasma cells. (Chapter 10)

primary granules Granules in neutrophils that correspond to lysosomes and contain antimicrobial peptides such as defensins and other antimicrobial agents. (Chapters 2, 3)

primary immune response The adaptive immune response that follows the first exposure to a particular antigen. (Chapters 9, 11)

primary immunization *See* **priming**. (Chapter 1)

primary immunodeficiency A lack of immune function that is caused by a genetic defect. (Chapter 13)

primary lymphoid follicles Aggregates of resting B lymphocytes in peripheral lymphoid organs. Cf. **secondary lymphoid follicle**. (Chapter 10)

primary lymphoid organs *See* **central lymphoid organs**. (Chapters 1, 8)

primary lymphoid tissues *See* **central lymphoid organs**. (Chapters 1, 8)

priming The first encounter with a given antigen, which generates the primary adaptive immune response. (Chapter 9)

pro-B cells A stage in B-lymphocyte development in which cells have displayed B-cell surface marker proteins but have not yet completed heavy-chain gene rearrangement. (Chapter 8)

pro-inflammatory Tending to induce inflammation. (Chapter 3)

profilin An actin-binding protein that sequesters monomeric actin. Protozoan profilins contain sequences recognized by TLR-11 and TLR-12. (Chapter 3)

programmed cell death *See* **apoptosis**. (Chapter 1)

programmed death ligand-1 *See* **PD-L1**. (Chapter 16)

progressive multifocal leukoencephalopathy (PML) Disease in immunocompromised patients caused by opportunistic infection by JC virus, for example as a consequence of immunotherapy. (Chapter 16)

propeptide Inactive precursor form of a polypeptide or peptide, which requires proteolytic processing to produce the active peptide. (Chapter 2)

properdin *See* **factor P**. (Chapter 2)

prostaglandins Lipid products of the metabolism of arachidonic acid that have a variety of effects on tissues, including activities as inflammatory mediators. (Chapters 3, 16)

prostatic acid phosphatase (PAP) Enzyme expressed by prostate cancer cells and used as a tumor-rejection antigen in the vaccine sipuleucel-T (Provenge). (Chapter 16)

pro-T cells In the thymus, ETPs differentiate into pro-T cells. At this stage, the cells begin to lose Kit expression along with their ability to develop into other lineages, such as B cells, NK cells, and myeloid cells. T-cell receptor gene rearrangements begin at this stage. (Chapter 8)

proteasome A large intracellular multi-subunit protease that degrades proteins, producing peptides. (Chapter 6)

protein inhibitors of activated STAT (PIAS) A small family of proteins that inhibit STAT family transcription factors. (Chapter 3)

protein-interaction domains, protein-interaction modules Protein domains, usually with no enzymatic activity themselves, that have binding specificity for particular sites (such as phosphorylated tyrosines, proline-rich regions, or membrane phospholipids) on other proteins or cellular structures. (Chapter 7)

protein kinase C-Θ (PKC-Θ) A serine/threonine kinase that is activated by diacylglycerol as part of the signaling pathways from the antigen receptor in lymphocytes. (Chapter 7)

protein kinases Enzymes that add phosphate groups to proteins at particular amino acid residues: tyrosine, threonine, or serine. (Chapter 7)

protein phosphatases Enzymes that remove phosphate groups from proteins phosphorylated on tyrosine, threonine, or serine residues by protein kinases. (Chapter 7)

proteolytic subunits β1, β2, β5 Constitutive components of the proteasome's catalytic chamber. (Chapter 6)

protein tyrosine kinases Enzymes that specifically phosphorylate tyrosine residues in proteins. They are critical in the signaling pathways that lead to T- and B-cell activation. (Chapter 7)

provirus The DNA form of a retrovirus when it is integrated into the host-cell genome, where it can remain transcriptionally inactive for long periods. (Chapter 13)

P-selectin *See* **selectins**. (Chapter 3)

P-selectin glycoprotein ligand-1 (PSGL-1) Protein expressed by activated effector T cells that is a ligand for P-selectin on endothelial cells and may enable activated T cells to enter all tissues in small numbers. (Chapters 9, 11)

pseudogenes Gene elements that have lost the ability to encode a functional protein but that are retained in the genome and may continue to be transcribed normally. (Chapter 5)

psoriasis Chronic autoimmune disease thought to be driven by T cells manifested in skin, but which can also involve nails and joints (psoriatic arthropathy). (Chapter 16)

psoriatic arthropathy *See* **psoriasis**. (Chapter 16)

pTα *See* **pre-T-cell receptor**. (Chapter 8)

purine nucleotide phosphorylase (PNP) deficiency An enzyme defect that results in severe combined immune deficiency. The deficiency of PNP causes an intracellular accumulation of purine nucleosides, which are toxic to developing T cells. (Chapter 13)

purinergic receptor P2X7 An ATP-activated ion channel that allows potassium efflux from cells when activated, which can trigger inflammasome activation in response to excessive extracellular ATP. (Chapter 3)

pus Thick yellowish-white liquid typically found at sites of infection with some types of extracellular bacteria, which is composed of the remains of dead neutrophils and other cells. (Chapter 3)

pus-forming bacteria Capsulated bacteria that result in pus formation at the site of infection. Also called pyogenic (pus-forming) bacteria. (Chapters 3, 13)

PYHIN A family of four intracellular sensor proteins containing an HIN (hematopoietic expression, interferon-inducible nature, and nuclear localization) domain in place of the LRR domain found in most other NLR proteins. The HIN domain functions in recognition of cytoplasmic dsDNA. Examples are AIM2 and IFI16. (Chapter 3)

pyogenic arthritis, pyoderma gangrenosum, and acne (PAPA) Auto-inflammatory syndrome that is caused by mutations in a protein that interacts with Pyrin. (Chapter 13)

pyogenic bacteria *See* **pus-forming bacteria**. (Chapters 3, 13)

Pyrin An inflammasome sensor protein that becomes dephosphorylated when Rho GTPase is inactivated by toxins produced by certain bacteria such as *Clostridium difficile*, thereby acquiring an active conformation that recruits ASC and leads to caspase 1 activation. (Chapters 3, 13)

pyrin One of several protein-interaction domains, structurally related to but distinct from CARD, TIR, DD, and DED domains. (Chapter 3)

pyroptosis A form of programmed cell death that is associated with abundant pro-inflammatory cytokines such as IL-1β and IL-18 produced through inflammasome activation. (Chapter 3)

Qa-1 determinant modifiers (Qdm) A class of peptides derived from the leader peptides of various HLA class I molecules that can be bound by the human HLA-E and murine Qa-1 proteins, and then are recognized by the inhibitory NKG2A:CD94 receptor. (Chapter 6)

quasi-species The different genetic forms of certain RNA viruses that are formed by mutation during the course of an infection. (Chapter 13)

Rac *See* **Rho family small GTPase proteins**. (Chapter 3)

radiation bone marrow chimera An individual treated with a high dose of radiation to eliminate his or her hematopoietic cells and then transfused with bone marrow or purified hematopoietic stem cells from a different individual, the donor. The donor bone marrow stem cells reconstitute the hematopoietic system in the recipient, who is referred to as a chimera because of the distinct genetic origin of his or her hematopoietic cells compared to all other cells in that individual's body. (Appendix I)

radiation-sensitive SCID (RS-SCID) Severe combined immune deficiency due to a defect in DNA repair pathways, which renders cells unable to perform V(D)J recombination and unable to repair radiation-induced double-strand breaks. (Chapters 5, 13)

radioimmunoassay (RIA) An assay to measure quantities of a specific compound, such as a hormone, in a complex mixture such as serum. The assay uses radioactively labeled antigen and an antibody against that antigen in a competitive binding assay. (Appendix I)

RAE1 (retinoic acid early inducible 1) protein family Several murine MHC class Ib proteins; these are orthologs of human RAET1 family proteins, including H60 and MULT1, and are ligands for murine NKG2D. (Chapter 3)

RAET1 *See* **UL16-binding proteins**. (Chapters 3, 6)

Raf A protein kinase in the Raf–Mek1–Erk signaling cascade that is the first protein kinase in the pathway and is activated by the small GTPase Ras. (Chapter 7)

RAG-1, RAG-2 Proteins encoded by the recombination-activating genes *RAG1* and *RAG2*, which form a dimer that initiates V(D)J recombination. (Chapter 5)

rapamycin An immunosuppressant drug that blocks intracellular signaling pathways involving the serine/threonine kinase mammalian target of rapamycin (mTOR) required for the inhibition of apoptosis and T-cell expansion. Also called sirolimus. (Chapter 16)

Raptor *See* **mTORC1**. (Chapter 16)

Ras A small GTPase with important roles in intracellular signaling pathways, including those from lymphocyte antigen receptors. (Chapter 7)

reactive oxygen species (ROS) Superoxide anion (O_2^-) and hydrogen peroxide (H_2O_2), produced by phagocytic cells such as neutrophils and macrophages after ingestion of microbes, and which help kill the ingested microbes. (Chapter 3)

rearrangement by inversion In V(D)J recombination, the rearrangement of gene segments having RSS elements in an opposing orientation, leading to retention. (Chapter 5)

receptor editing The replacement of a light or heavy chain of a self-reactive antigen receptor on immature B cells with a newly rearranged chain that does not confer autoreactivity. (Chapter 8)

receptor-mediated endocytosis The internalization into endosomes of molecules bound to cell-surface receptors. (Chapter 3)

recessive lethal gene A gene that when inactivated on both alleles of the chromosome encoding the gene results in impaired survival of the homozygous individuals. (Appendix I)

recombination signal sequences (RSSs) DNA sequences at one or both ends of V, D, and J gene segments that are recognized by the RAG-1:RAG-2 recombinase. They consist of a conserved heptamer and nonamer element separated by 12 or 23 base pairs. (Chapter 5)

red pulp The nonlymphoid area of the spleen in which red blood cells are broken down. (Chapters 1, 9)

RegIIIγ An antimicrobial protein of the C-type lectin family, produced by Paneth cells in the gut in mice. (Chapter 2)

regulatory T cells (T$_{reg}$ cells) Effector CD4 T cells that inhibit T-cell responses and are involved in controlling immune reactions and preventing autoimmunity. Several different subsets have been distinguished, notably the natural regulatory T-cell lineage that is produced in the thymus, and the induced regulatory T cells that differentiate from naive CD4 T cells in the periphery in certain cytokine environments. (Chapters 1, 9)

regulatory tolerance Tolerance due to the actions of regulatory T cells. (Chapter 15)

Relish A distinct member of the *Drosophila* NFκB transcription factor family that induces the expression of several antimicrobial peptides in response to Gram-negative bacteria. (Chapter 3)

resistance A general immune strategy aimed at reducing or eliminating pathogens. Cf. **avoidance** and **tolerance**. (Chapter 1)

respiratory burst An oxygen-requiring metabolic change in neutrophils and macrophages that have taken up opsonized particles, such as complement- or antibody-coated bacteria, by phagocytosis. It leads to the production of toxic metabolites that are involved in killing the engulfed microorganisms. (Chapter 3)

restriction factors Host proteins that act in a cell-autonomous manner to inhibit the replication of retroviruses such as HIV. (Chapter 13)

retinoic acid Signaling molecule derived from vitamin A with many roles in the body. It is thought to be involved in the induction of immunological tolerance in the gut. (Chapter 9)

retrotranslocation complex A multi-subunit membrane protein complex in the endoplasmic reticulum that allows the transport of misfolded proteins across the membrane of the endoplasmic reticulum and into the cytosol where ubiquitin-dependent degradation by the proteasome takes place. (Chapter 6)

retrovirus A single-stranded RNA virus that uses the viral enzyme reverse transcriptase to transcribe its genome into a DNA intermediate that integrates into the host-cell genome to undergo viral replication. (Chapter 13)

reverse transcriptase Viral RNA-dependent DNA polymerase that is found in retroviruses and transcribes the viral genomic RNA into DNA during the life cycle of retroviruses (such as HIV). (Chapter 13)

reverse transcriptase–polymerase chain reaction (RT–PCR) A technique for determining the presence and amount of a transcript for a specific gene. mRNA is isolated from cells and converted into cDNA by the enzyme reverse transcriptase (RT). The cDNA is then subjected to a polymerase chain reaction (PCR) in which primers that bind to a specific cDNA sequence are used to amplify a fragment of that gene's sequence. The amplified DNA product can then be visualized on an agarose gel. (Appendix I)

Rheb A small GTPase that activates mTOR when in its GTP-bound form and which is inactivated by a GTPase-activating protein (GAP) complex TSC1/2. (Chapter 16)

rhesus (or Rh) blood-group antigen Individuals in the human population vary in expression of a protein called Rh, expressed on the surface of red blood cells. A subset of individuals lacks expression of the Rh-D protein. When pregnant, an Rh-D–negative mother can make antibodies to the Rh-D protein expressed on her fetus after exposure to fetal blood during delivery. (Appendix I)

rheumatic fever Disease caused by antibodies elicited by infection with some *Streptococcus* species. These antibodies cross-react with kidney, joint, and heart antigens. (Chapter 15)

rheumatoid arthritis (RA) A common inflammatory joint disease that is probably due to an autoimmune response. (Chapter 15)

rheumatoid factor An anti-IgG autoantibody of the IgM class first identified in patients with rheumatoid arthritis, but which is also found in healthy individuals. (Chapter 15)

Rho *See* **Rho family small GTPase proteins**. (Chapter 3)

Rho family small GTPase proteins Several distinct small GTPase family members that regulate the actin cytoskeleton in response to signaling through various receptors. Examples: Rac, Rho, and Cdc42. (Chapter 3)

riboflavin (vitamin B2) A dietary vitamin that is metabolized by intestinal bacteria to generate derivatives that bind to MR1, forming ligands for MAIT cells (Chapter 6)

Rictor *See* **mTORC2**. (Chapter 16)

RIG-I (retinoic acid–inducible gene I) *See* **RIG-I-like receptors (RLRs)**. (Chapter 3)

RIG-I–like receptors (RLRs) A small family of intracellular viral sensors that use a carboxy-terminal RNA helicase–like domain in detection of various forms of viral RNA. These signal through MAVS to activate antiviral immunity. Examples include RIG-I, MDA-5, and LGP2. (Chapter 3)

RIP2 A CARD containing serine/threonine kinase that functions in signaling by NOD proteins to activate the NFκB transcription factor. (Chapter 3)

Riplet An E3 ubiquitin ligase involved in signaling by RIG-I and MDA-5 for the activation of MAVS. (Chapter 3)

rituximab A chimeric antibody to CD20 used to eliminate B cells in treatment of non-Hodgkin's lymphoma. (Chapter 16)

R-loops A structure formed when transcribed RNA displaces the non-template strand of the DNA double helix at switch regions in the immunoglobulin constant-region gene cluster. R-loops are thought to promote class switch recombination. (Chapter 10)

RNA exosome A multi-subunit complex involved in processing and editing of RNA. (Chapter 10)

RORγt RAR-related orphan nuclear receptor γt. One of two isoforms of the liganded transcription factor RORγ, which is a member of the NR1 subfamily of nuclear receptors. RORγt is important for the development of T_H17 cells and ILC3 cells. The ligand bound by RORγt is derived from the cholesterol biosynthesis pathway. (Chapter 9)

ruxolitinib An inhibitor of Jak1 and Jak2 approved for treatment of myelofibrosis. (Chapter 16)

S1P lyase A membrane-bound enzyme that degrades S1P. (Chapter 9)

S1PR1 A G protein–coupled receptor expressed on circulating lymphocytes that binds the chemotactic phospholipid sphingosine 1-phosphate (S1P), which forms a chemotactic gradient that promotes the egress of nonactivated lymphocytes out of peripheral lymphoid tissues into the efferent lymphatics and blood. *See also* **CD69**. (Chapters 8, 9)

SAP (SLAM-associated protein) An intracellular adaptor protein involved in signaling by SLAM (signaling lymphocyte activation molecule). Inactivating mutations in this gene cause X-linked lymphoproliferative (XLP) syndrome. (Chapters 3, 10)

scavenger receptors Receptors on macrophages and other cells that bind to numerous ligands, such as bacterial cell-wall components, and remove them from the blood. The Kupffer cells in the liver are particularly rich in scavenger receptors. Includes SR-A I, SR-A II, and MARCO. (Chapter 3)

scid Mutation in mice that causes severe combined immune deficiency. It was eventually found to be due to mutation of the DNA repair protein DNA-PK. (Chapter 5)

SCID *See* **severe combined immune deficiency**. (Chapter 3)

SDS-PAGE A technique for separating proteins on the basis of their molecular mass. Proteins in a cell lysate are treated with a strong detergent, sodium dodecyl sulfate (SDS), and then subjected to electrophoresis in a polyacrylamide gel (PAGE: polyacrylamide gel electrophoresis). Because the SDS binds relatively uniformly to all proteins, the net charge on the protein reflects the number of SDS molecules bound and, hence, the protein's molecular mass. PAGE then separates the proteins on the basis of this relative charge. (Appendix I)

seasonal allergic rhinoconjunctivitis IgE-mediated allergic rhinitis and conjunctivitis caused by exposure to specific seasonally occurring antigens; for example, grass or weed pollens. Commonly called hay fever. (Chapter 14)

second messengers Small molecules or ions (such as Ca^{2+}) that are produced in response to a signal; they act to amplify the signal and carry it to the next stage within the cell. Second messengers generally act by binding to and modifying the activities of enzymes. (Chapter 7)

secondary granules Type of granule in neutrophils that stores certain antimicrobial peptides. (Chapters 2, 3)

secondary (or recall) immune response The immune response that occurs in response to a second exposure to an antigen. In comparison with the primary response, it starts sooner after exposure, produces greater levels of antibody, and produces class-switched antibodies. It is generated by the reactivation of memory lymphocytes. (Chapters 9, 11)

secondary immunization A second or booster injection of an antigen, given some time after the initial immunization. It stimulates a secondary immune response. (Chapter 1)

secondary immunodeficiency Deficiency in immune function that is a consequence of infection (e.g., HIV infection), other diseases (e.g., leukemia), malnutrition, and so forth. (Chapter 13)

secondary lymphoid follicle A follicle containing a germinal center of proliferating activated B cells during an ongoing adaptive immune response. (Chapter 10)

secondary lymphoid organs *See* **peripheral lymphoid organs**. (Chapters 1, 8)

secondary lymphoid tissues *See* **peripheral lymphoid organs**. (Chapters 1, 8)

secretory component (SC) Fragment of the polymeric immunoglobulin receptor that remains after cleavage and is attached to secreted IgA after transport across epithelial cells. (Chapters 10, 12)

secretory phospholipase A2 Antimicrobial enzyme present in tears and saliva and also secreted by the Paneth cells of the gut. (Chapter 2)

selectins Family of cell-adhesion molecules on leukocytes and endothelial cells that bind to sugar moieties on specific glycoproteins with mucin-like features. (Chapter 3)

self antigens   The potential antigens on the tissues of an individual, against which an immune response is not usually made except in the case of autoimmunity. (Chapter 1)

self-tolerance   The failure to make an immune response against the body's own antigens. (Chapter 15)

sensitization   The acute adaptive immune response made by susceptible individuals on first exposure to an allergen. In some of these individuals, subsequent exposure to the allergen will provoke an allergic reaction. (Chapter 14)

sensitized   In allergy, describes an individual who has made an IgE response on initial encounter with an environmental antigen and who manifests IgE-producing memory B cells. Subsequent allergen exposure can elicit an allergic response. (Chapter 14)

sensor cells   Cells of the innate immune system that detect the presence of pathogens using their innate recognition receptors. In response to triggering of their innate recognition receptors, sensor cells produce inflammatory mediators that promote pathogen clearance and recruit additional cells into the immune response. (Chapter 1)

sentinel goblet cells   Goblet cells present at the entrance of colonic crypts and which sense TLR ligands to activate an NLRP inflammasome to alert adjacent goblet cells deeper in the crypt to secrete MUC2, producing a jet of mucus that expels invading microbes from the crypts. (Chapter 12)

sepsis   Bacterial infection of the bloodstream. This is a very serious and frequently fatal condition. (Chapter 3)

septic shock   Systemic shock reaction that can follow infection of the bloodstream with endotoxin-producing Gram-negative bacteria. It is caused by the systemic release of TNF-α and other cytokines. Also called endotoxic shock. (Chapter 3)

sequence motif   A pattern of nucleotides or amino acids shared by different genes or proteins that often have related functions. (Chapter 6)

serglycin   A proteoglycan found in the secretory granules of many immune cells that serves to protect and store a variety of secreted proteins, such as perforin and granzymes, until they are released by exocytosis. (Chapter 9)

serine protease inhibitor (serpin)   Class of proteins that inhibit various proteases, originally referring to those specific to serine proteases. (Chapter 2)

seroconversion   The phase of an infection when antibodies against the infecting agent are first detectable in the blood. (Chapter 13)

serological assays   Diagnostic tests performed on blood serum, often to detect antibodies. (Appendix I)

serology   The study of components in the serum, often using antibodies to detect specific antigens. (Appendix I)

serotype   Name given to a strain of bacteria or other pathogen that can be distinguished from other strains of the same species by specific antibodies. (Chapter 13)

serum   The fluid phase of clotted blood. Clotting involves fibrinogen and multiple clotting factors. After centrifugation, the clot and cells in the blood are removed, and the fluid phase, or serum, can be recovered. (Appendix I)

serum sickness   A usually self-limiting immunological hypersensitivity reaction originally seen in response to the therapeutic injection of large amounts of foreign serum (now most usually evoked by the injection of drugs such as penicillin). It is caused by the formation of immune complexes of the antigen and the antibodies formed against it, which become deposited in the tissues, especially the kidneys. (Chapters 14, 16)

severe acute respiratory syndrome (SARS)   A coronavirus-caused respiratory illness of zoonotic origin that was responsible for a global disease outbreak in 2003. (Chapter 12)

severe combined immune deficiency (SCID)   Type of immune deficiency (due to various causes) in which both B-cell (antibody) and T-cell responses are lacking; it is fatal if not treated. (Chapters 3, 5, 13)

severe congenital neutropenia (SCN)   An inherited condition in which the neutrophil count is persistently extremely low. This is in contrast to cyclic neutropenia, in which neutrophil numbers fluctuate from near normal to very low or absent, with an approximate cycle time of 21 days. (Chapter 13)

SH2 (Src homology 2) domain   *See* **Src family protein tyrosine kinases**. (Chapters 3, 7)

shear-resistant rolling   The capacity of neutrophils to remain attached to the vascular endothelium under high rates of flow—or shear—enabled by specialized plasma membrane extensions called slings. (Chapter 3)

shingles   Disease caused when varicella-zoster virus (the virus that causes chickenpox) is reactivated later in life in a person who has had chickenpox. (Chapter 13)

SHIP (SH2-containing inositol phosphatase)   An SH2-containing inositol phosphatase that removes the phosphate from PIP₃ to produce PIP₂. (Chapter 7)

shock   The potentially fatal circulatory collapse caused by the systemic actions of cytokines such as TNF-α. (Chapter 3)

short-chain fatty acids (SCFAs)   Fatty acids with fewer than six carbon atoms that are primary metabolic products of bacterial fermentation of dietary fibers and resistant starch in the large intestine. SCFAs can act on intestinal epithelial cells as well as local immune cells to promote intestinal immune homeostasis. (Chapter 12)

SHP (SH2-containing phosphatase)   An SH2-containing protein phosphatase. (Chapter 7)

SHP-1, SHP-2   Intracellular tyrosine phosphatases that are recruited to phosphorylated ITIM domains of various inhibitory receptors and which can remove phosphate residues from other signaling molecules, with effect of reducing signaling. (Chapter 3)

signaling scaffold   A configuration of proteins and modifications, such as phosphorylation or ubiquitination, that facilitates signaling by binding various enzymes and their substrates. (Chapter 3)

signal joint   The noncoding joint formed in DNA by the recombination of RSSs during V(D)J recombination. Cf. **coding joint**. (Chapter 5)

signal peptide   The short N-terminal peptide sequence responsible for directing newly synthesized proteins into the secretory pathway. (Chapter 3)

signal transducers and activators of transcription (STATs)   A family of seven transcription factors activated by many cytokine and growth factor receptors. *See also* **Janus kinase (JAK) family**. (Chapter 3)

single-chain antibody   Referring to the heavy-chain-only IgGs produced by camelids or shark species that lack the light chain present in conventional antibodies. (Chapter 4)

single-nucleotide polymorphisms (SNPs)   Positions in the genome that differ by a single base between individuals. (Chapters 14, 15)

single-positive thymocyte   A mature T cell that expresses either the CD4 or the CD8 co-receptor, but not both. (Chapter 8)

single-stranded RNA (ssRNA)   Usually confined to the nucleus and cytoplasm, this normal molecular form serves as a ligand for TLR-7 and TLR-8 when it is present in endosomes, as during parts of a viral life cycle. (Chapter 3)

sipuleucel-T (Provenge)   Cell-based immunotherapy used to treat prostate cancer that combined prostatic acid phosphatase as a tumor-rejection antigen presented by dendritic cells derived from a patient's monocytes. (Chapter 16)

sirolimus   *See* **rapamycin**. (Chapter 16)

Sjögren's syndrome An autoimmune disease in which exocrine glands, particularly the lacrimal glands of the eyes and salivary glands of the mouth, are damaged by the immune system. This results in dry eyes and mouth. (Chapter 15)

Skint-1 A transmembrane immunoglobulin superfamily member expressed by thymic stromal cells and keratinocytes that is required for the development of dendritic epidermal T cells, which are a type of γδ T cell. (Chapter 6)

SLAM (signaling lymphocyte activation molecule) A family of related cell-surface receptors that mediate adhesion between lymphocytes and which includes SLAM, 2B4, CD84, Ly108, Ly9, and CRACC. (Chapters 3, 10)

slings *See* **shear-resistant rolling**. (Chapter 3)

SLP-65 A scaffold protein in B cells that recruits proteins involved in the intracellular signaling pathway from the antigen receptor. Also called BLNK. (Chapter 7)

SLP-76 A scaffold protein involved in the antigen receptor signaling pathway in lymphocytes. (Chapter 7)

small G proteins, small GTPases Single-subunit G proteins, such as Ras, that act as intracellular signaling molecules downstream of many transmembrane signaling events. (Chapter 7)

small pre-B cell Stage in B-cell development immediately after the large pre-B cell in which cell proliferation ceases and light-chain gene rearrangement commences. (Chapter 8)

somatic diversification theories General hypotheses proposing that the immunoglobulin repertoire was formed from a small number of V genes that diversified in somatic cells. Cf. **germline theory**. (Chapter 5)

somatic DNA recombination DNA recombination that takes place in somatic cells (to distinguish it from the recombination that takes place during meiosis and gamete formation). (Chapter 5)

somatic gene therapy The introduction of functional genes into somatic cells to treat disease. (Chapter 13)

somatic hypermutation Mutations in V-region DNA of rearranged immunoglobulin genes that produce variant immunoglobulins, some of which bind antigen with a higher affinity. These mutations affect only somatic cells and are not inherited through germline transmission. (Chapters 5, 10)

spacer *See* **12/23 rule**. (Chapter 5)

specificity The strength of binding between an antibody and an antigen. When an antibody binds more strongly to some antigens and more weakly to others, it is considered to have greater specificity for the strongly bound antigens. (Appendix I)

sphingolipids A class of membrane lipids containing sphingosine (2-amino-4-octadecene-1,3-diole), an amino alcohol with an unsaturated 18-hydrocarbon chain. (Chapter 6)

sphingosine 1-phosphate (S1P) A phospholipid with chemotactic activity that controls the egress of T cells from lymph nodes. (Chapter 9)

sphingosine 1-phosphate receptor 1 (S1PR1) A G protein–coupled receptor activated by sphingosine 1-phosphate, a lipid mediator in the blood that regulates several physiological processes, including the trafficking of naive lymphocytes from tissues into the blood. (Chapters 10, 12)

spleen An organ in the upper left side of the peritoneal cavity containing a red pulp, involved in removing senescent blood cells, and a white pulp of lymphoid cells that respond to antigens delivered to the spleen by the blood. (Chapter 1)

S-protein (vitronectin) Plasma protein that binds incompletely formed MAC complexes, such as C5b67, preventing bystander complement damage to host membranes. (Chapter 2)

Spt5 A transcription elongation factor required for isotype switching in B cells that functions in association with RNA polymerase to enable recruitment of AID to its targets in the genome. (Chapter 10)

SR-A I, SR-A II *See* **scavenger receptors**. (Chapter 3)

Src family protein tyrosine kinases Receptor-associated protein tyrosine kinases characterized by Src homology protein domains (SH1, SH2, and SH3). The SH1 domain contains the kinase, the SH2 domain can bind phosphotyrosine residues, and the SH3 domain can interact with proline-rich regions in other proteins. In T cells and B cells they are involved in relaying signals from the antigen receptor. (Chapter 3)

staphylococcal complement inhibitor (SCIN) Staphylococcal protein that inhibits the activity of the classical and alternative C3 convertases, promoting the evasion of destruction by complement. (Chapter 2)

staphylococcal enterotoxins (SEs) Secreted toxins produced by some staphylococci, which cause food poisoning and also stimulate many T cells by binding to MHC class II molecules and the V_b domain of certain T-cell receptors, acting as superantigens. (Chapter 6)

staphylococcal protein A (Spa) Staphylococcal protein that blocks the binding of the antibody Fc region with C1, thereby preventing complement activation. (Chapter 2)

staphylokinase (SAK) Staphylococcal protease that cleaves immunoglobulins bound to its surface, thereby preventing complement activation. (Chapter 2)

STAT1 A member of the signal transducer and activator of transcription (STAT) family of transcription factors activated by type I and type II interferon signaling. (Chapters 3, 9)

STAT2 A member of the signal transducer and activator of transcription (STAT) family of transcription factors activated by type II interferon signaling and which heterodimerizes with STAT1 and associates with IRF9 to form a complex called ISGF3. (Chapter 3)

STAT3 *See* **signal transducers and activators of transcription**. (Chapters 9, 10)

STAT3 deficiency A primary immune deficiency with an autosomal pattern of inheritance caused by mutations in the gene *STAT3* that lead to defective STAT3 signaling. *See* also **hyper IgE syndrome**; **Job syndrome**. (Chapter 13)

STAT4 *See* **signal transducers and activators of transcription**. (Chapter 9).

STAT6 *See* **signal transducers and activators of transcription**. (Chapters 9, 10)

statins Drug inhibitors of HMG-CoA reductase used to lower cholesterol. (Chapter 16)

sterile injury Damage to tissues due to trauma, ischemia, metabolic stress, or autoimmunity, bearing many immune features similar to infection. (Chapter 3)

sterilizing immunity An immune response that completely eliminates a pathogen. (Chapter 11)

STIM1 A transmembrane protein that acts as a Ca^{2+} sensor in the endoplasmic reticulum. When Ca^{2+} is depleted from the endoplasmic reticulum, STIM1 is activated and induces opening of plasma membrane CRAC channels. (Chapter 7)

STING (stimulator of interferon genes) A dimeric protein complex in the cytoplasm anchored to the endoplasmic reticulum membrane that functions in intracellular sensing for infection. It is activated by specific cyclic dinucleotides to activate TBK1, which phosphorylates IRF3 to induce transcription of type I interferon genes. (Chapter 3)

stress-induced self *See* **dysregulated self**. (Chapter 3)

stromal cells   The nonlymphoid cells in central and peripheral lymphoid organs that provide soluble and cell-bound signals required for lymphocyte development, survival, and migration. (Chapter 8)

stromal organizer cells   Precursors of fibroblast reticular cells (FRCs) and follicular dendritic cells (FDCs) that develop from mesenchymal cells in response to lymphotoxins produced by lymphoid tissue inducer (LTi) cells. (Chapter 9)

subcapsular sinus (SCS)   The site of lymphatic entry in lymph nodes lined by phagocytes, including subcapsular macrophages, which capture particulate and opsonized antigens draining in from tissues. (Chapters 9, 10)

subcutaneous   Under the epidermal and dermal layers of the skin. (Appendix I)

succinate   A metabolite produced by intestinal parasites that stimulates IL-25 production by tuft cells. (Chapter 11)

sulfated sialyl-Lewis^X   A sulfated tetrasaccharide carbohydrate structure attached to many cell surface proteins, it binds the P-selectin and E-selectin molecules on the surface of cells, such as neutrophils, that mediate interactions with the endothelium. (Chapter 3)

superoxide dismutase (SOD)   An enzyme that converts the superoxide ion produced in the phagolysosome into hydrogen peroxide, a substrate for further reactive antimicrobial metabolites. (Chapter 3)

superoxide radical   A highly reactive form of oxygen having an unpaired electron (making it a radical) and being negatively charged, making it an ion, formed in the phagolysosome by the action of the NADPH oxidase. (Chapter 3)

suppressor of cytokine signaling (SOCS)   Regulatory protein that interacts with Janus kinases (JAKs) to inhibit signaling by activated receptors. (Chapter 3)

supramolecular activation complex (SMAC)   Organized structure that forms at the point of contact between a T cell and its target cell, in which the ligand-bound antigen receptors are co-localized with other cell-surface signaling and adhesion molecules. (Chapter 7)

surface immunoglobulin (sIg)   The membrane-bound immunoglobulin that acts as the antigen receptor on B cells. (Chapter 1)

surface plasmon resonance (SPR)   A technique for measuring the binding kinetics of interaction between two molecules. One molecule is immobilized on the surface of a glass slide, and a solution of the binding partner is streamed over the surface. The instrument measures the binding and then dissociation of the fluid-phase component. (Appendix I)

surfactant proteins A and D (SP-A and SP-D)   Acute-phase proteins that help protect the epithelial surfaces of the lung against infection. (Chapters 2, 3)

surrogate light chain   A protein in pre-B cells, made up of two subunits, VpreB and λ5, that can pair with a full-length immunoglobulin heavy chain and the Igα and Igβ signaling subunits and signals for pre-B-cell differentiation. (Chapter 8)

switch regions   Genomic regions, several kilobases in length each, located between the J_H region and the heavy-chain $C\mu$ genes, or in equivalent positions upstream of other C-region genes (except C_δ), containing hundreds of G-rich repeated sequences that function in class switch recombination. (Chapter 10)

Syk   A cytoplasmic tyrosine kinase found in B cells that acts in the signaling pathway from the B-cell antigen receptor. (Chapter 7)

symbiotic   Relationship between two agents, typically diverse species, that confers benefits to both. (Chapter 1)

sympathetic ophthalmia   Autoimmune response that occurs in the other eye after one eye is damaged. (Chapter 15)

syngeneic graft   A graft between two genetically identical individuals. It is accepted as self. (Chapter 15)

systemic immune system   Name sometimes given to the lymph nodes and spleen to distinguish them from the mucosal immune system. (Chapter 12)

systemic lupus erythematosus (SLE)   An autoimmune disease in which autoantibodies against DNA, RNA, and proteins associated with nucleic acids form immune complexes that damage small blood vessels, especially in the kidney. (Chapters 10, 15)

T10, T22   MHC class Ib molecules expressed by activated lymphocytes and recognized by a subset of γδ T cells. (Chapters 4, 6)

TAB1, TAB2   An adaptor complex that binds K63-linked polyubiquitin chains. TAB1 and TAB2 complex with TAK1, targeting TAK1 to signaling scaffolds where it phosphorylates substrates such as IKKα. (Chapter 3)

TACE (TNF-α–converting enzyme)   A protease responsible for cleavage of the membrane-associated form of the cytokine TNF-α into its soluble form, which can enter the systemic circulation. (Chapter 3)

TACI   A receptor for BAFF expressed on B cells that activates the canonical NFκB pathway. (Chapter 10)

tacrolimus   An immunosuppressant polypeptide drug that binds FK-binding proteins (FKBPs) and inactivates T cells by inhibiting calcineurin, thus blocking activation of the transcription factor NFAT. Also called FK506. (Chapters 7, 16)

TAK1   A serine/threonine kinase that is activated by phosphorylation by the IRAK complex and which activates downstream targets such as IKKβ and MAPKs. (Chapter 3)

talin   An intracellular protein involved in the linkage of activated integrins, such as LFA-1, to the cytoskeleton to allow changes in cellular motility and migration, such as in the diapedesis of neutrophils across the vascular endothelium. (Chapter 3)

TAP-1, TAP-2   Transporters associated with antigen processing-1 and -2. ATP-binding cassette proteins that form a heterodimeric TAP-1:TAP-2 complex in the endoplasmic reticulum membrane, through which short peptides are transported from the cytosol into the lumen of the endoplasmic reticulum, where they associate with MHC class I molecules. (Chapter 6)

tapasin   TAP-associated protein. A key molecule in the assembly of MHC class I molecules; a cell deficient in this protein has only unstable MHC class I molecules on the cell surface. (Chapter 6)

TAPBPR   A quality-control protein in the Golgi apparatus that can recognize improperly folded proteins and cause their re-glucosylation by UDP-glucose:glycoprotein glucosyltransferase 1 (UGT1). It can function to redirect improperly loaded MHC class I back to the endoplasmic reticulum for additional peptide editing by the peptide-loading complex. (Chapter 6)

Tbet   A transcription factor active in many immune cell types but most typically associated with ILC1 and T_H1 function. (Chapters 3, 9, 12)

TBK1 (TANK-binding kinase 1)   A serine/threonine kinase activated during signaling by TLR-3 and MAVS and serving to phosphorylate and activate IRF3 for induction of type I interferon gene expression. (Chapter 3)

T cell, T lymphocyte   One of the two types of antigen-specific lymphocytes responsible for adaptive immune responses, the other being the B cells. T cells are responsible for the cell-mediated adaptive immune reactions. They originate in the bone marrow but undergo most of their development in the thymus. The highly variable antigen receptor on T cells is called the T-cell receptor and recognizes a complex of peptide antigen bound to MHC molecules on cell surfaces. There are two main lineages of T cells: those carrying αβ receptors and those carrying γδ receptors. Effector T cells perform a variety of functions in an immune response, acting always by interacting with another cell in an antigen-specific manner. Some T cells activate macrophages, some help B cells produce antibody, and some kill cells infected with viruses and other intracellular pathogens. (Chapter 1)

T-cell antigen receptor *See* **T-cell receptor**. (Chapter 1)

T-cell areas Regions of peripheral lymphoid organs that are enriched in naive T cells and are distinct from the follicles. They are the sites at which adaptive immune responses are initiated. (Chapters 1, 10)

T-cell clones Expanded populations of cultured T cells in which all cells in a given population derive from a single initial T cell. Each T cell in such a clonal population expresses the same TCR. (Appendix I)

T-cell hybrids Hybridomas of a T cell that was isolated from a T-cell lymphoma cell of an animal fused to a primary antigen-specific T cell to generate an immortalized cell line with a single T-cell receptor specificity. *See also* **hybridoma**. (Appendix I)

T-cell lines Expanded populations of cultured T cells in which all cells in a given population share the same antigen specificity. Each population of T cells in a T-cell line is not necessarily derived from a single initial T cell, and instead is generally composed of a mixture of cells with different TCRs. (Appendix I)

T-cell plasticity Flexibility in the developmental programming of CD4 T cells such that effector T-cell subsets are not irreversibly fixed in their function or the transcriptional networks that underpin those functions. (Chapter 11)

T-cell receptor (TCR) The cell-surface receptor for antigen on T lymphocytes. It consists of a disulfide-linked heterodimer of the highly variable α and β chains in a complex with the invariant CD3 and ζ proteins, which have a signaling function. T cells carrying this type of receptor are often called $\alpha\beta$ T cells. An alternative receptor made up of variable γ and δ chains is expressed with CD3 and ζ on a subset of T cells. (Chapters 1, 4)

T-cell receptor α (TCRα) and β (TCRβ) The two chains of the $\alpha\beta$ T-cell receptor. (Chapter 4)

T-cell receptor excision circles (TRECs) Circular DNA fragments excised from the chromosome during V(D)J recombination in developing thymocytes that are transiently retained in T cells that have recently left the thymus. (Chapter 5)

T-cell zones *See* **T-cell areas**. (Chapter 1)

T-DM1 An antibody–drug conjugate combining trastuzumab (Herceptin) with mertansine used to treat recurrent metastatic breast cancer previously treated with a different trastuzumab drug conjugate. (Chapter 16)

TdT *See* **terminal deoxynucleotidyl transferase**. (Chapter 5)

TEPs *See* **thioester-containing proteins**. (Chapter 2)

terminal deoxynucleotidyl transferase (TdT) Enzyme that inserts non-templated N-nucleotides into the junctions between gene segments in T-cell receptor and immunoglobulin V-region genes during their assembly. (Chapter 5)

tertiary immune response Adaptive immune response provoked by a third injection of the same antigen. It is more rapid in onset and stronger than the primary response. (Chapter 11)

T follicular helper (T$_{FH}$) An effector T cell found in lymphoid follicles that provides help to B cells for antibody production and class switching. (Chapters 1, 9, 12)

TGF-β (transforming growth factor-β) Multifunctional cytokine that is produced in latent form, particularly in the intestinal mucosa. Its activated form is required for the development of T$_{reg}$ and T$_H$17 cells, as well as IgA-producing B cells and plasma cells. (Chapter 9)

T$_H$1 A subset of effector CD4 T cells characterized by the cytokines they produce, notably IFN-γ and TNF-α. They are mainly involved in activating macrophages and promoting inflammation. (Chapters 1, 9, 11)

T$_H$2 A subset of effector CD4 T cells that are characterized by the cytokines they produce, notably IL-4, IL-5, and IL-13. They are involved in recruiting eosinophils and activating mast cells and basophils, and in promoting enhanced barrier protection. (Chapters 1, 9, 11)

T$_H$17 A subset of CD4 T cells that are characterized by production of the cytokine IL-17. They help recruit neutrophils to sites of infection. (Chapters 1, 9, 11)

therapeutic vaccination The use of a vaccine to treat an existing disease, typically in the context of treating a tumor, rather than to prevent the occurrence of a disease. (Chapter 16)

thioester-containing proteins (TEPs) Homologs of complement component 3 (C3) that are found in insects and are thought to have some function in insect innate immunity. (Chapter 2)

thymectomy Surgical removal of the thymus. (Chapter 8)

thymic anlage The tissue from which the thymic stroma develops during embryogenesis. (Chapter 8)

thymic cortex The outer region of each thymic lobule in which thymic progenitor cells (thymocytes) proliferate, rearrange their T-cell receptor genes, and undergo thymic selection, especially positive selection on thymic cortical epithelial cells. (Chapter 8)

thymic stroma The epithelial cells and connective tissue of the thymus that form the essential microenvironment for T-cell development. (Chapter 8)

thymic stromal lymphopoietin (TSLP) Thymic stroma–derived lymphopoietin. A cytokine thought to be involved in promoting B-cell development in the embryonic liver. It is also produced by mucosal epithelial cells in response to helminthic infections and promotes type 2 immune responses through its actions on macrophages, ILC2s, and T$_H$2 cells. (Chapter 3)

thymocytes Developing T cells when they are in the thymus. The majority are not functionally mature and are unable to mount protective T-cell responses. (Chapter 8)

thymoproteasome Specialized form of the proteasome composed of a unique subunit, β5t, that replaces β5i (LMP7) and associates with β1i and β2i in the catalytic chamber. (Chapter 6)

thymus A central lymphoid organ, in which T cells develop, situated in the upper part of the middle of the chest, just behind the breastbone. (Chapters 1, 12)

thymus-dependent (TD) antigens Antigens that elicit responses only in individuals that have T cells. (Chapter 10)

thymus-independent (TI) antigens Antigens that can elicit antibody production without the involvement of T cells. There are two types of TI antigens: the TI-1 antigens, which have intrinsic B-cell activating activity, and the TI-2 antigens, which activate B cells by having multiple identical epitopes that cross-link the B-cell receptor. (Chapter 10)

thymus leukemia antigen (TL) Nonclassical MHC class Ib molecule expressed by intestinal epithelial cells and a ligand for CD8$\alpha\alpha$. (Chapter 12)

TI-1 antigens *See* **thymus-independent antigens**. (Chapter 10)

TI-2 antigens *See* **thymus-independent antigens**. (Chapter 10)

tickover The low-level generation of C3b continually occurring in the blood in the absence of infection. (Chapter 2)

time-lapse video imaging A technique used to capture the movements of cells or molecules over time. A digital camera is combined with two-photon or confocal fluorescent imaging to generate movies of the images. These movies can be sped up for viewing. (Appendix I)

tingible body macrophages Phagocytic cells engulfing apoptotic B cells, which are produced in large numbers in germinal centers at the height of an adaptive immune response. (Chapter 10)

TIR (for Toll–IL-1 receptor) domain   Domain in the cytoplasmic tails of the TLRs and in the IL-1 receptor, which interacts with similar domains in intracellular signaling proteins. (Chapter 3)

tissue-resident memory T (T$_{RM}$) cells   Memory lymphocytes that do not migrate after taking up residence in barrier tissues, where they are retained long-term. They appear to be specialized for rapid effector function after restimulation with antigen or cytokines at sites of pathogen entry. (Chapter 11)

TLR-1   Cell-surface Toll-like receptor that acts in a heterodimer with TLR-2 to recognize lipoteichoic acid and bacterial lipoproteins. (Chapter 3)

TLR-2   Cell-surface Toll-like receptor that acts in a heterodimer with either TLR-1 or TLR-6 to recognize lipoteichoic acid and bacterial lipoproteins. (Chapter 3)

TLR-3   Endosomal Toll-like receptor that recognizes double-strand viral RNA. (Chapters 3, 9)

TLR-4   Cell-surface Toll-like receptor that, in conjunction with the accessory proteins MD-2 and CD14, recognizes bacterial lipopolysaccharide. (Chapter 3)

TLR-5   Cell-surface Toll-like receptor that recognizes the flagellin protein of bacterial flagella. (Chapters 3, 12)

TLR-6   Cell-surface Toll-like receptor that acts in a heterodimer with TLR-2 to recognize lipoteichoic acid and bacterial lipoproteins. (Chapter 3)

TLR-7   Endosomal Toll-like receptor that recognizes single-stranded viral RNA. (Chapter 3)

TLR-8   Endosomal Toll-like receptor that recognizes single-stranded viral RNA. (Chapter 3)

TLR-9   Endosomal Toll-like receptor that recognizes DNA containing unmethylated CpG. (Chapter 3)

TLR-11, TLR-12   Mouse Toll-like receptor that recognizes profilin and profilin-like proteins. (Chapter 3)

TLR-13   A member of the Toll-like receptor (TLR) family expressed in mouse and other rodents, but not in human, that has a specificity for certain bacterial ribosomal RNAs. (Chapter 3)

T lymphocytes (T cells)   *See* **T cell**. (Chapter 1)

TNF family   Cytokine family, the prototype of which is tumor necrosis factor-α (TNF-α, or TNF). It contains both secreted (e.g., TNF-α and lymphotoxin) and membrane-bound (e.g., CD40 ligand) members. (Chapter 3)

TNF receptor–associated periodic syndrome (TRAPS)   An autoinflammatory disease characterized by recurrent, periodic episodes of inflammation and fever caused by mutations in the gene that encodes TNF receptor I. The defective TNFR-I proteins fold abnormally and accumulate in cells in such a way that they spontaneously activate production of TNF-α. *See also* **familial Mediterranean fever**. (Chapter 13)

TNF receptors   Family of cytokine receptors that includes some that lead to apoptosis of the cell on which they are expressed (e.g., Fas and TNFR-I), whereas others lead to activation. (Chapter 3)

tocilizumab   Humanized anti-IL-6 receptor antibody used in treating rheumatoid arthritis. (Chapter 16)

tofacitinib   An inhibitor of Jak3 and Jak1 used to treat rheumatoid arthritis and under investigation in other inflammatory disorders. (Chapter 16)

tolerance   The failure to respond to an antigen. Tolerance to self antigens is an essential feature of the immune system; when tolerance is lost, the immune system can destroy self tissues, as happens in autoimmune disease. (Chapters 1, 8)

tolerant   Describes the state of immunological tolerance, in which the individual does not respond to a particular antigen. (Chapter 1)

tolerogenic   Describes an antigen or type of antigen exposure that induces tolerance. (Chapter 8)

Toll   Receptor protein in *Drosophila* that activates the transcription factor NFκB, leading to the production of antimicrobial peptides. (Chapter 3)

Toll-like receptors (TLRs)   Innate receptors on macrophages, dendritic cells, and some other cells that recognize pathogens and their products, such as bacterial lipopolysaccharide. Recognition stimulates the receptor-bearing cells to produce cytokines that help initiate immune responses. (Chapters 1, 3)

tonsils   *See* **lingual tonsils, palatine tonsils**. (Chapter 1)

toxic shock syndrome   A systemic toxic reaction caused by the massive production of cytokines by CD4 T cells activated by the bacterial superantigen toxic shock syndrome toxin-1 (TSST-1), which is secreted by *Staphylococcus aureus*. (Chapter 6)

toxic shock syndrome toxin-1 (TSST-1)   *See* **toxic shock syndrome**. (Chapter 6)

toxoids   Inactivated toxins that are no longer toxic but retain their immunogenicity so that they can be used for immunization. (Chapters 10, 16)

TRAF3   An E3 ligase that produces a K63 polyubiquitin signaling scaffold in TLR-3 signaling to induce type I interferon gene expression. (Chapters 3, 10)

TRAF6 (tumor necrosis factor receptor–associated factor 6)   An E3 ligase that produces a K63 polyubiquitin signaling scaffold in TLR-4 signaling to activate the NFκB pathway. (Chapter 3)

TRAIL (tumor necrosis factor–related apoptosis-inducing ligand)   A member of the TNF cytokine family expressed on the cell surface of some cells, such as NK cells, that induces cell death in target cells by ligation of the 'death' receptors DR4 and DR5. (Chapter 3)

TRAM   An adaptor protein that pairs with TRIF in signaling by TLR-4. (Chapter 3)

transcytosis   The active transport of molecules, such as secreted IgA, through epithelial cells from one face to the other. (Chapter 12)

transdifferentiation   The transition of one non-stem cell into another cell type. For T cells, this term is often used in the context of the transition of committed T-cell phenotype into another phenotype, such as the transition of T$_H$17 cells into T$_H$1 cells or T$_{reg}$ cells into T$_H$17 cells. (Chapter 11)

transepithelial dendrites (TEDs)   Cellular processes of intestinal macrophages and dendritic cells that extend across the epithelial barrier to sample antigens in the intestinal lumen.   (Chapter 12)

transgenic mice   The process of generating transgenic mice. *See also* **transgenic mice**. (Appendix I)

transgenesis   Mice that are experimentally engineered to carry an extra gene in all of their cells, including germ cells. (Appendix I)

Transib   A superfamily of transposable elements identified computationally and proposed to date back more than 500 million years and to have given rise to transposons in diverse species. (Chapter 5)

transitional B cells   B cells that are newly emerged from the bone marrow into the periphery and are not yet functionally mature. (Chapter 8)

transitional stages   Defined stages in the development of immature B cells into mature B cells in the spleen, after which the B cell expresses B-cell co-receptor component CD21. (Chapter 8)

transporters associated with antigen processing-1 and -2 (*TAP1* and *TAP2*)   *See* **TAP-1, TAP-2**. (Chapter 6)

transposase   An enzyme capable of cutting DNA and allowing integration and excision of transposable genetic elements into or from the genome of a host. (Chapter 5)

trastuzumab   Humanized antibody to HER-2/neu used in treatment of breast cancer. (Chapter 16)

TRECs   *See* **T-cell receptor excision circles**. (Chapter 5)

Trex1   Three-prime repair exonuclease 1 (Trex1) is a DNA exonuclease with 3′-to-5′ activity, which, while playing a proofreading role for DNA polymerase, also has immune activity in degrading cytosolic DNA. The absence of Trex1 can lead to activation of cGAS, causing autoinflammatory disorders resembling lupus erythematosus. (Chapter 3)

TRIF   An adaptor protein that alone is involved in signaling by TLR-3 and which when paired with TRAM functions in signaling by TLR-4. (Chapter 3)

TRIKA1   A complex of the E2 ubiquitin ligase UBC13 and cofactor Uve1A that interacts with TRAF6 in forming the K63 polyubiquitin signaling scaffold in TLR signaling downstream of MyD88. (Chapter 3)

TRIM21 (tripartite motif-containing 21)   A cytosolic Fc receptor and E3 ligase that is activated by IgG and can ubiquitinate viral proteins after an antibody-coated virus enters the cytoplasm. (Chapter 10)

TRIM25   An E3 ubiquitin ligase involved in signaling by RIG-I and MDA-5 for the activation of MAVS. (Chapter 3)

tropism   The characteristic of a pathogen that describes the cell types it will infect. (Chapters 6, 10, 13)

TSC   Tuberous sclerosis complex. Protein complex that acts as a GTPase-activating protein (GAP) for Rheb in its non-phosphorylated state. TSC is inactivated when phosphorylated by AKT. (Chapter 16)

TSLP   Thymic stromal lymphopoietin. A cytokine thought to be involved in promoting B-cell development in the embryonic liver. (Chapter 11)

tuft cells   Chemosensory sentinel cells present in mucosal tissues, such as the intestinal and respiratory tracts, which detect products of helminths and protozoans to activate type 2 immune responses. The ligands recognized by tuft cells share features with tastants/odorants recognized by taste-bud cells and lead to the secretion of IL-25, eicosanoids, and acetylcholine. (Chapters 11, 12)

tumor necrosis factor-α (TNF-α, or TNF)   *See* **TNF family**. (Chapter 3)

tumor-rejection antigens   Antigens on the surface of tumor cells that can be recognized by T cells, leading to attack on the tumor cells. Tumor-rejection antigens are peptides of mutant or overexpressed cellular proteins bound to MHC class I molecules on the tumor-cell surface. (Chapter 16)

tumor-specific antigens   These are newly immunogenic forms of normal proteins that may induce a T-cell response against a tumor. They are expressed by a tumor cell and may arise from mutations in normal genes that alter the expressed amino acid sequence to produce a peptide epitope that can bind to MHC class I molecules and be recognized by T cells. Such peptides may have already been able to bind MHC molecules but become immunogenic by altering a residue recognized by T cells or may become immunogenic by acquiring *de novo* the ability to bind MHC molecules. (Chapter 16)

TUNEL (TdT-dependent dUTP–biotin nick-end labeling) staining   A technique to identify cells undergoing apoptosis on the basis of the DNA fragmentation that occurs in apoptotic cells. The technique labels the 3′ ends of fragmented DNA with biotin. The biotin is detected with enzyme-coupled streptavidin followed by the addition of a substrate that forms a colored precipitate when acted on by the enzyme. (Appendix I)

two-dimensional gel electrophoresis   A solution of proteins is subjected to isoelectric focusing in a narrow tube of polyacrylamide, separating the proteins on the basis of the isoelectric point. This tube is then placed across the top of an SDS-PAGE apparatus and electrophoresed in this second dimension, thereby separating the proteins on the basis of molecular mass. When completed, the proteins are distributed in two dimensions in the rectangular SDS-PAGE gel on the basis of a combination of the protein's isoelectric point and its molecular mass. *See also* **isoelectric focusing**; **SDS-PAGE**. (Appendix I)

two-photon scanning fluorescence microscopy   A fluorescence imaging technique that allows visualization of signals at greater depths in tissues than does standard fluorescent microscopy. Images are captured in thin optical sections from which a three-dimensional image can be built. (Appendix I)

type 1 diabetes mellitus   Disease in which the β cells of the pancreatic islets of Langerhans are destroyed so that no insulin is produced. The disease is believed to result from an autoimmune attack on the β cells. It is also known as insulin-dependent diabetes mellitus (IDDM), because the symptoms can be ameliorated by injections of insulin. (Chapter 15)

type 1 immunity   Class of effector activities aimed at elimination of intracellular pathogens. (Chapters 1, 11)

type 2 immunity   Class of effector activities aimed at elimination of parasites and promoting barrier and mucosal immunity. (Chapters 1, 11)

type 3 immunity   Class of effector activities aimed at elimination of extracellular pathogens such as bacteria and fungi. (Chapters 1, 11)

type 1 LAD (LAD-1)   *See* **leukocyte adhesion deficiency type 1**. (Chapter 13)

type 2 LAD (LAD-2)   *See* **leukocyte adhesion deficiency type 2**. (Chapter 13)

type 3 LAD (LAD-3)   *See* **leukocyte adhesion deficiency type 3**. (Chapter 13)

type 1 NKT cells   A subset of NKT cells restricted by CD1d and having a restricted TCRα chain repertoire. (Chapter 6)

type 2 NKT cells   A subset of NKT cells restricted by CD1d and having a more diverse TCRα chain repertoire. (Chapter 6)

type 1 regulatory (T$_R$1) cells   A poorly characterized population of CD4 T cells that produce immunosuppressive cytokines, such as IL-10, but lack expression of FoxP3. They are thought to regulate inflammatory responses. At steady state, they are most abundant in the small intestine. (Chapter 9)

type I interferons   The antiviral interferons IFN-α and IFN-β. (Chapter 3)

type II interferon   The antiviral interferon IFN-γ. (Chapter 3)

type III secretion system (T3SS)   Specialized appendage of Gram-negative bacteria used to aid infection of eukaryotic cells by direct secretion of effector proteins into their cytoplasm. (Chapter 3)

tyrosinase   Enzyme in melanin synthesis pathway and frequently a tumor-rejection antigen in melanoma. (Chapter 16)

tyrosine phosphatases   Enzymes that remove phosphate groups from phosphorylated tyrosine residues on proteins. *See also* **CD45**. (Chapters 3, 7)

UBC13   *See* **TRIKA1**. (Chapter 3)

ubiquitin   A small protein that can be attached to other proteins and functions as a protein interaction module or to target them for degradation by the proteasome. (Chapter 7)

ubiquitination   The process of attachment of one or many subunits of ubiquitin to a target protein, which can mediate either degradation by the proteasome or formation of scaffolds used for signaling, depending on the nature of the linkages. (Chapter 6)

ubiquitin ligase   Enzyme that attaches ubiquitin covalently to exposed lysine residues on the surfaces of other proteins. (Chapters 3, 7)

ubiquitin–proteasome system (UPS)   A quality-control system in the cell that involves K48-linked ubiquitination of target proteins that are then recognized by the proteasome for degradation. (Chapter 6)

UDP-glucose:glycoprotein glucosyltransferase 1 (UGT1)   An enzyme in the Golgi apparatus that can re-glycosylate proteins detected by TAPBPR as being improperly folded to cause their redirection to the endoplasmic reticulum for additional editing. (Chapter 6)

UL16-binding proteins (ULBPs)   A family of 10 MHC class Ib proteins that are ligands for NKG2D. Also called **RAET1** proteins. (Chapters 3, 6)

ULBP4   *See* **RAET1**. (Chapter 6)

ulcerative colitis (UC)   One of the two major types of inflammatory bowel disease thought to result from an abnormal overresponsiveness to the commensal gut microbiota. *See also* **Crohn's disease**. (Chapters 12, 15)

UNC93B1   A multipass transmembrane protein that is necessary for the normal transport of TLR-3, TLR-7, TLR-8, TLR-9, TLR-11, TLR-12, and TLR-13 from the endoplasmic reticulum, where they are assembled, to the endosome, where they function. (Chapter 3)

unmethylated CpG dinucleotides   While mammalian genomes have heavily methylated the cytosine within CpG sequences, unmethylated CpG is more typically characteristic of bacterial genomes and is recognized by TLR-9 when encountered in the endosomal compartment. (Chapter 3)

uracil-DNA glycosylase (UNG)   Enzyme that removes uracil bases from DNA in a DNA repair pathway that can lead to somatic hypermutation, class switch recombination, or gene conversion. (Chapter 10)

urticaria   The technical term for hives, which are red, itchy skin wheals usually brought on by an allergic reaction. (Chapter 14)

Uve1A   *See* **TRIKA1**. (Chapter 3)

Vα   Variable region from the TCRα chain. (Chapter 5)

V$_\beta$ Variable region from the TCRβ chain. (Chapter 5)

vaccination   The deliberate induction of adaptive immunity to a pathogen by injecting a dead or attenuated (nonpathogenic) live form of the pathogen or its antigens (a vaccine). (Chapters 1, 16)

vacuolar pathway   Relating to the intracellular transport of extracellular materials taken up into endosomes and processed within these and other related membrane compartments such as lysosomes, but excluding entry into the cytosol. (Chapter 6)

variability plot   A measure of the difference between the amino acid sequences of different variants of a given protein. The most variable proteins known are antibodies and T-cell receptors. (Chapter 4)

variable gene segments, V gene segments   Gene segments in immunoglobulin and T-cell receptor loci that encode the first 95 amino acids or so of the protein chain. There are multiple different V gene segments in the germline genome. To produce a complete exon encoding a V domain, one V gene segment must be rearranged to join up with a J or a rearranged DJ gene segment. (Chapter 5)

variable Ig domains (V domains)   The amino-terminal protein domain of the polypeptide chains of immunoglobulins and T-cell receptor, which is the most variable part of the chain. (Chapter 4)

variable lymphocyte receptors (VLRs)   Non-immunoglobulin LRR-containing variable receptors and secreted proteins expressed by the lymphocyte-like cells of the lamprey. They are generated by a process of somatic gene rearrangement. (Chapter 5)

variable region (V region)   The region of an immunoglobulin or T-cell receptor that is formed of the amino-terminal domains of its component polypeptide chains. These are the most variable parts of the molecule and contain the antigen-binding sites. Cf. **constant region**. (Chapters 1, 4, 5)

variolation   The intentional inhalation of or skin infection with material taken from smallpox pustules of an infected person for the purpose of deriving protective immunity. (Chapters 1, 16)

VCAM-1   Vascular cell adhesion molecule-1. An adhesion molecule expressed by vascular endothelium at sites of inflammation; it binds the integrin VLA-4, which allows effector T cells to enter sites of infection. (Chapters 9, 11)

V(D)J recombinase   A multiprotein complex containing RAG-1 and RAG-2, as well as other proteins involved in cellular DNA repair. (Chapter 5)

V(D)J recombination   The process exclusive to developing lymphocytes in vertebrates that recombines different gene segments into sequences encoding complete protein chains of immunoglobulins and T-cell receptors. (Chapter 5)

vesicular compartments   One of several major compartments within cells, composed of the endoplasmic reticulum, Golgi apparatus, endosomes, and lysosomes. (Chapter 6)

viral entry inhibitors   Drugs that inhibit the entry of HIV into its host cells. (Chapter 13)

viral integrase inhibitors   Drugs that inhibit the action of the HIV integrase, so that the virus cannot integrate into the host-cell genome. (Chapter 13)

viral protease   Enzyme encoded by the human immunodeficiency virus that cleaves the long polyprotein products of the viral genes into individual proteins. (Chapter 13)

viral set point   In human immunodeficiency virus infection, the level of HIV virions persisting in the blood after the acute phase of infection has passed. (Chapter 13)

virus   Pathogen composed of a nucleic acid genome enclosed in a protein coat. Viruses can replicate only in a living cell, because they do not possess the metabolic machinery for independent life. (Chapter 1)

virus-neutralizing antibodies   Antibodies that block the ability of a virus to establish infection of cells. (Chapter 10)

vitronectin   *See* **S-protein**. (Chapter 2)

VLA-4   Very late antigen-4. *See* **integrin $\alpha_4\beta_1$**. (Chapter 11)

VLRs   *See* **variable lymphocyte receptors**. (Chapter 5)

VpreB   *See* **surrogate light chain**. (Chapter 8)

V-region gene   The exon encoding the complete variable region sequence of a fully rearranged antigen receptor gene. (Chapter 5)

V-type ATPase   A class of enzymes that use ATP typically to transport H^+ ions across the membrane of organelles to acidify various vacuolar compartments. (Chapter 6)

WAS   *See* **Wiskott–Aldrich syndrome**. (Chapters 10, 13)

WASp (Wiskott–Aldrich syndrome protein)   The protein defective in patients with Wiskott–Aldrich syndrome. When activated, WASp promotes actin polymerization. (Chapter 7)

Weibel–Palade bodies   Granules within endothelial cells that contain P-selectin. (Chapter 3)

western blotting   *See* **immunoblotting**. (Appendix I)

wheal-and-flare reaction   A skin reaction observed in an allergic individual when an allergen to which the individual has been sensitized is injected into the dermis. It consists of a raised area of skin containing edema fluid and a spreading, red, itchy inflammatory reaction around it. (Chapter 14)

white pulp   The discrete areas of lymphoid tissue in the spleen. (Chapters 1, 9)

Wiskott–Aldrich syndrome (WAS)   An immunodeficiency disease characterized by defects in the cytoskeleton of cells due to a mutation in the protein WASp, which is involved in interactions with the actin cytoskeleton. Individuals with this disease are highly susceptible to infections with pyogenic bacteria because of defects in T-follicular helper cell interactions with B cells. (Chapters 10, 13)

XBP1 (X-box binding protein 1)   A transcription factor that induces genes required for optimal protein secretion by plasma cells and is part of the unfolded protein response. XBP1 mRNA is spliced from an inactive to an active form by signals produced by ER stress. (Chapter 10)

XCL1   Chemokine produced by CD8 T cells and NK cells that binds XCR1. (Chapter 9)

XCR1   Chemokine receptor expressed by type 1 conventional dendritic cells (cDC1 cells) that binds XCL1 (lymphotactin). (Chapter 9)

xenografts   Grafted organs taken from a different species than the recipient. (Chapter 15)

xenoimmunity   In the context of immune-mediated disease, refers to immunity directed against foreign antigens of nonhuman species, such as bacteria-derived antigens of the commensal microbiota that are targets in inflammatory bowel disease (IBD). (Chapter 15)

xeroderma pigmentosum   Several autosomal recessive diseases caused by defects in repair of ultraviolet light–induced DNA damage. Defects in Polη cause type V xeroderma pigmentosum. (Chapter 10)

xid   *See* **X-linked immunodeficiency**. (Chapter 8)

X-linked agammaglobulinemia (XLA)   A genetic disorder in which B-cell development is arrested at the pre-B-cell stage and no mature B cells or antibodies are formed. The disease is due to a defect in the gene encoding the protein tyrosine kinase Btk, which is encoded on the X chromosome. (Chapters 7, 8, 13)

X-linked hyper IgM syndrome   *See* **CD40 ligand deficiency**. (Chapter 11)

X-linked hypohidrotic ectodermal dysplasia and immunodeficiency   A syndrome with some features resembling hyper IgM syndrome. It is caused by mutations in the protein NEMO, a component of the NFκB signaling pathway. Also called NEMO deficiency. (Chapters 3, 7)

X-linked immunodeficiency (xid)   An immunodeficiency disease in mice due to defects in the protein tyrosine kinase Btk. Shares the gene defect with X-linked agammaglobulinemia in humans, but leads to a milder B cell defect than that seen in the human disease. (Chapter 8)

X-linked lymphoproliferative (XLP) syndrome   Rare immunodeficiency diseases that result from mutations in the gene *SH2D1A* (XLP1) or *XIAP* (XLP2). Boys with this deficiency typically develop overwhelming Epstein–Barr virus infection during childhood, and sometimes lymphomas. (Chapters 10, 13)

X-linked severe combined immune deficiency (X-linked SCID, or XSCID)   An immune deficiency disease in which T-cell development fails at an early intrathymic stage, and no production of mature T cells or T cell–dependent antibody occurs. It is due to a defect in a gene that encodes the γ_c chain shared by the receptors for several different cytokines. (Chapters 3, 13)

XLP   *See* **X-linked lymphoproliferative syndrome**. (Chapter 13)

XRCC4   A protein that functions in NHEJ DNA repair by interacting with DNA ligase IV and Ku70:Ku80 at double-strand breaks. (Chapter 5)

ζ chain   A subunit of the T-cell receptor:CD3 complex that forms a disulfide-linked dimer. Each monomer of ζ has multiple ITAM signaling motifs in the cytoplasmic tail. (Chapter 7)

ZAP-70 (ζ chain–associated protein)   A cytoplasmic tyrosine kinase found in T cells that binds to the phosphorylated ζ chain of the T-cell receptor and is a key enzyme in signaling T-cell activation. (Chapter 7)

ZFP318   A spliceosome protein expressed in mature and activated B cells, but not immature B cells, that favors splicing from the rearranged VDJ exon of immunoglobulin heavy chain to the C_δ exon, thereby promoting expression of surface IgD. (Chapter 5)

zoonotic   Describes a disease of animals that can be transmitted to humans. (Chapters 2, 12)

zymogen   An inactive form of an enzyme, usually a protease, that must be modified in some way, for example by selective cleavage of the protein chain, before it can become active. (Chapter 2)

Credits

of Immunologists; (center and right panels): Szakal et al. (1989) Ann. Rev. Immunol. 7: 91–109, 1989. Reprinted by permission © Annual Reviews; p. 434: Courtesy of P. Björkman; p. 438 (both): Kenneth H. Roux; p. 443: Photograph courtesy of Anthony Butterworth; p. 445 (both): Photographs courtesy of Dr. Ann M. Dvorak.

Figure 10.29: Courtesy of P. Bjorkman.

Chapter 11

Photos Page 471: Biophoto Associates/Science Source.

Figure 11.23: Reprinted from *Immunity 35*(4), Marion Pepper, Antonio J. Pagán, Botond Z. Igyártó, et al., "Opposing signals from the Bcl6 transcription factor and the interleukin-2 receptor generate T helper 1 central and effector memory cells," 583–595. Copyright © 2011 Elsevier Inc. All rights reserved. With permission from Elsevier. **Figure 11.26**: Reprinted from *Immunity 41*(6), Jason M. Schenkel and David Masopust, "Tissue-resident memory T cells," 886–897. Copyright © 2014 Elsevier Inc. All rights reserved. With permission from Elsevier. **Figure 11.30**: Republished with permission from Annual Reviews, from Ramon I. Klein Geltnik, Ryan L. Kyle, and Erika L. Pearce, "Unraveling the complex interplay between T cell metabolism and function," *Annual Review of Immunology 36*(1): 461–488, 2018; permission conveyed through Copyright Clearance Center, Inc.

Chapter 12

Photos Page 513 (both): Courtesy of Dr. David Lo; p. 521 (all): Bernier-Latmani et al. (2016) Nature Protocols 11:1617–1629. Copyright © 2016, Nature Publishing Group, a division of Macmillan Publishers Limited. All Rights Reserved; p. 526: Johannson et al. (2015) Cell Host Microbe, 18, 582–592. Reprinted with permission © Elsevier; p. 528 (both): Vaishnava et al. (2011) Science 334:255–258. © Reprinted with permission © AAAS; p. 529 (center panel): Brandtzaeg and Pabst. (2004) Trends Immunol. 25, 570–577. Reprinted with permission © Elsevier; (right panel): courtesy of Allan Mowat; p. 545 (both): Casey T. Weaver; p. 572 (center and right panels): Ke et al. (2020) Nature 588, 498–502. Reprinted with permission © Nature.

Figure 12.5a: Adapted by permission from Springer Nature: *Nature*, Les Dethlefsen, Margaret McFall-Ngai, and David A. Relman, "An ecological and evolutionary perspective on human-microbe mutualism and disease." Copyright © 2007, Springer Nature. **Figure 12.5b**: Adapted by permission from Springer Nature: *Nature*, The Human Microbiome Project Consortium, "Structure, function and diversity of the healthy human microbiome." Copyright © 2012 Curtis Huttenhower et al. **Figure 12.15**: Adapted by permission from Springer Nature: Nature, *Nature Reviews Molecular Cell Biology*, Nick Barker, "Adult intestinal stem cells: critical drivers of epithelial homeostasis and regeneration." Copyright © 2013, Nature Publishing Group, a division of Macmillan Publishers Limited. All rights reserved.

Chapter 13

Photos Page 592: Courtesy of Carol Ann Demaret; p. 599 (both): Dr. Raif Geha; p. 619 (both): Whiteley et al. (2001) Nature. 413, 860–864. Reprinted with permission © Nature; p. 623 (both): Photographs courtesy of Gilla Kaplan; p. 634: Figure courtesy of Drs. Beatrice Hahn and Gerald Learn (University of Pennsylvania); p. 636: Photograph courtesy of Dr. Hans Gelderblom; p. 637: NIAID.

Figure 13.32: Courtesy of B. Hahn and G. Learn. **Figure 13.36**: From Haoqing Wang, Christopher O. Barnes, Zhi Yang, et al., "Partially open HIV-1 envelope structures exhibit conformational changes relevant for coreceptor binding and fusion," *Cell Host & Microbe 24*(4): 579–592, 2018. © 2018 The Authors. Published by Elsevier Inc. Available under a Creative Commons Attribution 4.0 International (CC BY 4.0) license. https://doi.org/10.1016/j.chom.2018.09.003 **Figure 13.42**: Adapted by permission from Springer Nature: Nature, *Nature Genetics*, Stephen J. O'Brien and George W. Nelson, "Human genes that limit AIDS." Copyright © 2004, Nature Publishing Group. **Figure 13.44**: From *The New England Journal of Medicine*, Frank J. Palella, Jr., Kathleen M. Delaney, Anne C. Moorman et al., "Declining morbidity and mortality among patients with advanced Human Immunodeficiency Virus infection," 338: 853–860. Copyright © 1998 Massachusetts Medical Society. Reprinted with permission from Massachusetts Medical Society. **Figure 13.47**: Adapted by permission from Springer Nature: *Nature*, Xiping Wei, Sajal K. Ghosh, Maria E. Taylor, et al., "Viral dynamics in human immunodeficiency virus type 1 infection." Copyright © 1995, Nature Publishing Group. **Figure 13.48**: From UNAIDS Data 2018. With permission from UNAIDS.

Chapter 14

Photos Page 667: Sprecher, et al. (2004) Clin. Exp. Dermatol. 29:513–517. Reprinted with permission © Wiley; p. 677: Photograph courtesy of S. R. Durham; p. 681 (both): Photographs courtesy of Thomas Krausz; p. 682 (both): courtesy of Dr Bart Lambrecht and Dr Savvas Savvides; p. 683 (all): Finotto et al. (2002) 295(5553):336–8. Reprinted with permission © AAAS; p. 691: Dr. Raif Geha; p. 692 (both): Photographs courtesy of Allan Mowat.

Chapter 15

Photos Page 716 (both): Casey Weaver; p. 718 (all): Photographs courtesy of H.T. Cook and M. Kashgarian.

Figure 15.29: Courtesy of John Rioux and Ben Weaver. **Figure 15.31**: Adapted by permission from Springer Nature: *Nature*, John D. Rioux and Abul K. Abbas, "Paths to understanding the genetic basis of autoimmune disease." Copyright © 2005, Nature Publishing Group. **Figure 15.35**: Courtesy of Dr. C.J. Thorpe.

Appendix I

Photos Page A-14: Photograph courtesy of M. Solimena and P. De Camilli; p. A-17: Nag et al. (1994) 269(13):10061–70. Journal of Biological Chemistry. CC4.0; p. A-25: Reprinted with permission from Mabtech AB; p. A-27: Courtesy of Dr. Nathan Shaner; p. A-32: Photograph courtesy of R. Budd and J. Russell.

Figure A.50: From Aya Amitai-Lange, Eran Berkowitz, Anna Altshuler, et al., "A method for lineage tracing of corneal cells using multi-color fluorescent reporter mice," *Journal of Visualized Experiments* 106: e53370, 2015. Reprinted with permission from the Journal of Visualized Experiments. **Figure A.51**: Republished with permission of Mary Ann Liebert, Inc. publishers, from Brian Fritz, "High-Definition Immunology: Paired Immune Repertoire Profiling at Single-Cell Resolution with the Chromium V(D)J Solution," *Genetic & Biotechnology News 37*(12), 2017; permission conveyed through Copyright Clearance Center, Inc. **Figure A.52**: From CITE-seq.com. With permission from Peter Smibert and Marlon Stoeckius.

Index

Note: Page numbers in *italics* refer to figures.

2B4 134
4-1BB 292
4-1BBI *375*
4-1BBL A72
5-(2-oxopropylideneamino)-6-d-
    ribitylaminouracil (5-OP-RU) 253
12/23 rule *184,* 185, 189, *189, 198*
19S regulatory caps 220–221, *221*
20S catalytic core 220–221, *221*
777uGads 264, *275,* 275–276

A

Abatacept 787, 790
ABC (ATP-binding cassette) 223, *223*
ABO blood group
    blood typing A8, *A10*
    hyperacute graft rejection 737, *737*
Absent in melanoma 2 (AIM2) *99,* 105–106
Absorptive enterocytes 521, *522,* 523, *523*
Accelerated rejection 733
Accessory effector cells 440
    IgE-mediated activation 445–446
Accessory proteins, Toll-like receptors
    94–95, *95*
ACE2 (angiotensin-converting enzyme 2),
    SARS-CoV-2 *572,* 573–574
Acellular pertussis vaccines 761–762
ACPAs (anti-citrullinated protein antibodies)
    720
Acquired immune deficiency syndrome (AIDS)
    634–656
    decline in spread 635–636, 652–653
    epidemiology 634–636, *635*
    opportunistic infections 471, 649, *649*
    overview 634–636
    progression to 643, 647–648, *648*
    time to development 635
    and zoonotic infections 42, *634,* 634–635
    see also Human immunodeficiency virus
        (HIV)
Acquired immunodeficiency 587, 588,
    615–616, 634–656
Actinobacteria 517, *517,* 518
Actin polymerization *284*
Activating receptors, NK cells 129–130, *130,*
    133, 133–134, *134*
Activation-induced cell death 341
    self-tolerance *700*
Activation-induced cytidine deaminase (AID)
    207–208
    deficiency 421, *590,* 600
    humoral immune response 417, 420–425,
        421, 422, 424, 425
Activator protein 1 (AP-1)
    activation of 280–281, *281*
    costimulatory receptors 290, *291*
    expression of 278–280, *279, 280*

inhibitory receptors 293
pathogen recognition *96,* 96–97
regulatory T cells 387
T-cell activation *371*
Active immunization A35
Acute desensitization 685–686
Acute lymphocytic leukemia (ALL) 774
Acute phase of infection 642–643, *643*
Acute-phase proteins 123, *123*
Acute-phase response 54–55, *122,* 122–124,
    123
Acute rejection 732–733, *736*
ADA (adenosine deaminase)
    deficiency 592–593, *593*
    recombinant 613
Adalimumab 785, *786*
ADAP 283, *283*
Adaptive immune response 5, *6,* 6–7, 37
    agnathans 201, 203–205, *204*
    allergies, autoimmune disease, and organ
        transplant rejection *32,* 32–33
    antigen-receptor gene assembly 14–15
    antigen recognition 13–14, *14*
    cartilaginous fishes 210–211
    cloning of antigen-specific effector cells
        15, *15*
    complement 50–51
    constant and variable regions of antibodies
        and T-cell receptors 13
    course of typical acute infection cleared by
        453, *454*
    defined 2
    different species 207–209, *208, 209*
    effector cell generation 22–24
    evolution 201–211
    gnathostomes 201
    immunoglobulin-like genes in some
        invertebrates *202,* 202–203
    immunological memory 12, 22–24, *23*
    initiation 17–18, *18*
    integration of innate and 453, *454,* 454–462
    interaction of antigens with antigen
        receptors *12,* 12–13
    lymphocyte development 16–17, *17*
    lymphocytes 11–12, *12*
    mucosal surfaces 20–22, *22*
    myeloid cells *7,* 7–8
    principles 11–24
    RAG-dependent 205–207, *206*
    response to antigen 18–20, *19–21*
    role in regulating intestinal immune system
        536–553
    self-reactive receptors *15,* 16
Adaptors 264, *264, 265, 275,* 275–276
ADCC *see* Antibody-dependent cell-mediated
    cytotoxicity (ADCC)
7-ADD (7-amino-actinomycin D) A32–A33
Addison's disease *727*
Adenoid *17,* 20

Adenosine deaminase (ADA)
    deficiency 592–593, *593*
    recombinant 613
Adenosine triphosphatase (ATPase), V-type
    228, *228*
Adenosine triphosphate (ATP)-binding
    cassette (ABC) 223, *223*
Adenovirus 568
    immunoevasins *629,* 630
ADEPT (antibody-directed enzyme/pro-drug
    therapy) 176
ADH(s) (Alcohol dehydrogenases) 544
Adhesins 436, *437*
Adhesion molecules
    effector T cells guided to specific tissues
        and infection sites *463,* 463–467,
        465–467
    T-cell entry into lymphoid tissues
        353–356, *354, 355*
Adjuvants
    adaptive immune response 364
    defined 9
    immunogenicity A3–A4, *A4*
    innate immunity 107
    vaccines 758–759, *759*
Adoptive immunity A36
Adoptive immunization A36
Adoptive T-cell therapy 773–774, *774*
Adoptive transfers
    clonal T-cell populations 485–486, *486*
    lymphocytes A36–A37, *A37*
    protective immunity A36
AEP (asparagine endopeptidase) 228
Aerobic glycolysis, T-cell activation *370,*
    370–372
Afferent lymphatic vessels 19, *20, 512*
Affinity 143, 180, A5
Affinity chromatography A5, *A5*
Affinity hypothesis 339
Affinity maturation 24, 416
Affinity model of T-cell selection *333,* 333–334
Agammaglobulinemia 596
    Bruton's X-linked 309–310, *590,*
        596–597, *598*
    intravenous Ig 613
    X-linked 287
AgDscam 202–203
Age-related macular degeneration (AMD) 72
Agglutinate A8
Agglutination 203
Agglutinin 203
AGM (aorta-gonad-mesonephros) 81
Agnathan(s) 201, 203–205, *204*
Agnathan paired receptors resembling Ag
    receptors (APARs) 207
Agonist selection 531
AHR (aryl hydrocarbon receptor) 534
aHUS (atypical hemolytic uremic syndrome)
    71, 608